McGRAW-HILL
ENCYCLOPEDIA OF
FOOD,
AGRICULTURE &
NUTRITION

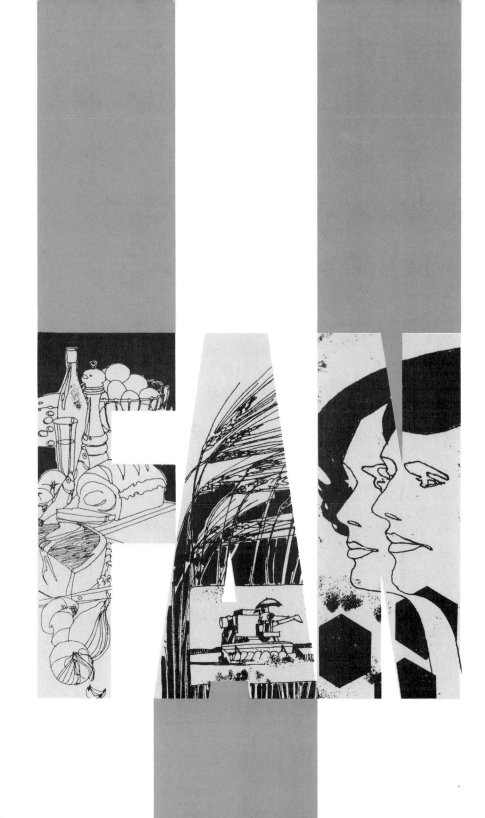

McGRAW-HILL ENCYCLOPEDIA OF
FOOD, AGRICULTURE & NUTRITION

DANIEL N. LAPEDES

Editor in Chief

McGRAW HILL BOOK COMPANY

New York	Auckland	New Delhi
St. Louis	Bogotá	Panama
San Francisco	Düsseldorf	Paris
	Johannesburg	São Paulo
	London	Singapore
	Madrid	Sydney
	Mexico	Tokyo
	Montreal	Toronto

Library of Congress Cataloging in Publication Data

McGraw-Hill encyclopedia of food, agriculture & nutrition.

    Includes index.
    1. Food — Dictionaries.   2. Agriculture — Dictionaries.   3. Nutrition —
Dictionaries.   I. Lapedes, Daniel N.   II. Title: Encyclopedia of food, agri-
culture & nutrition.
TX349.M2   641'.03   77-12181
ISBN 0-07-045263-6

Contents

Editorial Staff

Daniel N. Lapedes, Editor in Chief

Sybil P. Parker, Senior editor

Jonathan Weil, Staff editor

Edward J. Fox, Art director

Joe Faulk, Editing manager

Patricia Albers, Senior editing assistant
Judith Alberts, Editing assistant
Dolores Messina, Editing assistant

Ellen Okin, Editing supervisor

Ann D. Bonardi, Art production supervisor
Richard A. Roth, Art editor
Eda Grilli, Art/traffic

Consulting Editors

Prof. Eric E. Conn. *Department of Biochemistry and Biophysics, University of California, Davis.* BIOCHEMISTRY.

Prof. Harry A. MacDonald. *Professor of Agronomy, Emeritus, Cornell University.* AGRICULTURE.

Dr. Bernard S. Meyer. *Professor of Botany, Emeritus, Ohio State University.* PLANT PHYSIOLOGY.

Dr. N. Karle Mottet. *Professor of Pathology, Department of Pathology, University of Washington.* ANIMAL PATHOLOGY.

Dr. Jerry Olson. *Oak Ridge National Laboratory.* CONSERVATION; PLANT ECOLOGY.

Leonard Trauberman. *Food Engineering Consultant.* FOOD ENGINEERING.

Preface

Food is the source of energy for the maintenance of life. Throughout history, the primary concern of all civilizations has been to produce adequate supplies of food. This has not always been realized, either qualitatively or quantitatively. Today, with 25% of the world population living at or below subsistence food level, a crisis exists.

The problem is complex, having sociological, economic, and technological aspects, and is most acute in the Third and Fourth Worlds. In these regions, population growth outpaces food supply, per capita income is low, and capital investment, particularly in the Third World, has shifted more to industry and away from agriculture, even though these developing countries are agrarian. Where food supplies are limited and poverty prevails, people suffer from chronic malnutrition and starvation, conditions which only serve to reinforce their poverty.

There are several approaches to solving the world food problem. Agriculture plays a key role by providing the means for increasing productivity. Scientific and technological advances in the industrialized world have fostered the development of more efficient farm machinery; more effective chemical fertilizers, insecticides, and herbicides; improved crop varieties and animal breeds; and new farming methods, such as multiple cropping and reduced tillage farming. However, while some of these advances, particularly mechanization and the breeding programs of the Green Revolution, have been successfully applied to large commercial farms, their usefulness must be adapted to subsistence-level farming. Profitable agriculture is thus technologically feasible for the Third and Fourth World countries, but it will require large capital investments from the developed countries and restructuring of the economies within the developing countries.

Another approach in dealing with the problem is to seek new food sources and products, especially those rich in protein. One important source of protein is fish and other seafoods. Another source is vegetables. This type of protein is relatively inexpensive and provides a nutritious substitute for animal protein.

The world population-food crisis is not intractable, but does involve more than increasing food production and decreasing population growth rates. Lack of food also results from crop failures, inefficient food supply systems, maldistribution of food within and between countries, and geographic and climatic restraints. Future success in feeding the world will depend on a coordinated program of action by business and government and on a balanced industrial and agricultural effort.

The *McGraw-Hill Encyclopedia of Food, Agriculture & Nutrition* is designed to inform the student, librarian, scientist, teacher, engineer, and lay person about all aspects of agriculture; the cultivation, harvesting, and processing of food crops; food manufacturing; and health and nutrition—from the economic and political to the technological. The Encyclopedia is arranged in two parts. The first part contains five feature articles which present an overview of the world food problem: Feeding the World, Climate and Crops, Energy in the Food System, Food from the Sea, and The Green Revolution. The second part, with its 400 alphabetically arranged articles written by specialists, contains information on such subjects as food engineering, pesticides, agricultural geography, vitamins, irrigation of crops, breeding of animals and plants, and all important food crops. The articles, some drawn from the *McGraw-Hill Encyclopedia of Science and Technology* (4th ed., 1977) and some written especially for the volume, are included on the recommendation of the Board of Consultants. All articles are signed by the authors, who are listed with their affiliations in the List of Contributors. The articles are cross-referenced to other articles on related subjects. An appendix details the composition of prevalent foods from the standpoint of caloric, protein, carbohydrate, fat, mineral, and vitamin content. There is also an analytical index which provides quick and easy access to the subjects in the volume.

DANIEL N. LAPEDES
EDITOR IN CHIEF

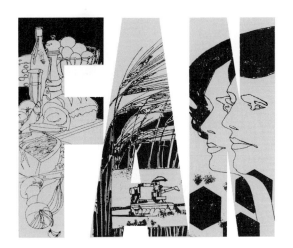

FEEDING THE WORLD

Douglas N. Ross

he population-food crisis in the less-developed regions of the world appears massive and intractable. Despite attention at highest governmental levels in Bucharest at the 1974 World Population Conference and in Rome at the 1974 World Food Conference, serious doubts among groups concerned with both the population and food crises continue to be reported in the public media. Of special concern is the ability and the will of political and economic institutions to respond adequately. The potential for tragedy is great; even if the world succeeds in feeding those presently in need, it may only be deferring the starvation of many more to the future, unless available food supply keeps pace with population growth or population growth is curtailed.

Over 1 billion of the world's 4 billion people live at or below subsistence food levels, mostly in tropical regions which are characterized by high human fertility rates, low per capita income, and low capi-

tal investment in agriculture. These economically marginal regions of South Asia, Central Africa, and South America are grouped into a Third World which has extensive natural resources essential to the industrialized world, and a Fourth World which is deficient in everything but people. The resource-rich Third World has the leverage to force industrial countries' attention to its food and development needs; the Fourth World must rely primarily on humanitarian appeals.

POPULATION AND FOOD

In his 1798 formulation of the population-food dilemma, Thomas Malthus claimed that if the food supply were fixed while the population grew, the only check to the ultimate size of the population would be starvation. While Malthus underestimated the rate of technological change and the effect of human ingenuity, the hypothesis does state the diluting effect on the creation of wealth of changes

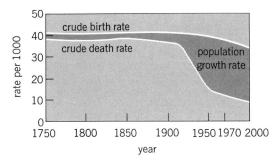

Fig. 1. Antecedents of the population explosion in developing countries. (*From GENERAL ELECTRIC-TEMPO, The Economics of Slowing Population Growth, Center for Advanced Studies, Santa Barbara, CA, 71 TMP-42*)

in population size. and in context, it is not unreasonable. Throughout history, the bane of human existence has been "killer" epidemic disease, such as plague, typhus, cholera, and measles, which usually followed periodic famine. Such natural disasters counterbalanced high birthrates with high death rates, which consequently kept population size in check. In the 17th century something happened: the world's population growth rate (that is, the difference between the birth and death rates — until then about 0.056%, or 560 persons per year for each 1 million population) began to increase. In 18th century Europe, this rate increased first to 0.5% and then to 1.5% (or to 5000 and then to 15,000 per 1 million), due primarily to a decline in death rates (Fig. 1). The population "explosion" has been ascribed to three main factors: (1) public health improvements — largely preventative rather than therapeutic — including means for the detection and containment of infection; (2) the

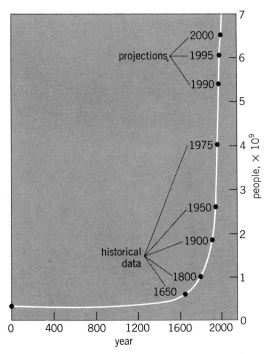

Fig. 2. World population growth. (*From M. Mesarovic and E. Pestel, Mankind at the Turning Point: The Second Report to The Club of Rome. Copyright © 1974 by M. Mesarovic and E. Pestel. Reprinted by permission of the publishers, E. P. Dutton*)

decrease and eventual disappearance in the 19th century of infanticide; and (3) an increase in the food supply. The effect was that instead of taking 1000 years as Malthus predicted, the population doubled within 100 years. By the beginning of the 19th century the Earth's population had reached 1 billion. By 1900 the world's population had reached an estimated 1.7 billion and today is estimated at over 4 billion (Fig. 2). Society has yet to discover and implement socially acceptable means of population control worldwide.

The 20th century has seen the population growth rate of most industrialized countries in the North Temperate Zone fall back to a range of 0.6 to 1.3% (still not a zero population growth rate). Even at this rate the "projective" effect on the United States is still the addition of 25 "Philadelphias" (population 2.3 million) between now and the year 2000.

Current estimates place the world's population growth rate at about 1.8% per year, which means that the world's population may double in about 33 years. Figure 3 illustrates the alternatives. In Fig. 3a, if present population growth rates continue, then by the year 2000 the Population Reference Bureau estimates a world population of 7.2 billion, 75% of whom would be living in less-developed nations. Figure 3b shows that if the world's birthrate could be lowered from present levels to the replacement rate of two children per family, then the world's population could stabilize at about 6 billion by 2020.

Population growth. There is a "development race" between a growing population and an increasing food supply (or capital wealth). The numerical size of a country's population is thus less important to its economic advance than its rate of population growth. It is important to distinguish between them. A "large" or "small" population refers to the total size of the population — or labor force — relative to the availability of natural resources and domestic capital. When a large population also has a high population growth rate, as in India (610 million, with a 2.2% population growth rate) the population-economic situation is at its worst. Rapid population growth means that the population, on average, is younger, and therefore more dependent and less able to work (Fig. 4). Even relatively small-population countries face a tremendous "development race" handicap. Chilean political and economic leaders, for example, face a situation in which less than 25% of Chile's 10.5 million people have sewage facilities and less than 20% have adequate water supplies; 70% of the children are infested by parasites; and the rate of mental retardation approaches 40% in some severely malnourished social groups.

The advantages to a population growth rate below the rate of increase in gross national product (GNP) are that per capita income can increase and, at the same time, a larger percentage of the populace will be of an age to enter the work force (Fig. 5). The danger in a high population growth rate lies in the difficulty of increasing per capita wealth and the benefits of wealth — higher aspirations, greater savings, better education, more food, and more freedom for the mother.

Per capita wealth and population growth rates. In the less-developed nations with annual population increases of 2.5% and GNP increases of 5%, it

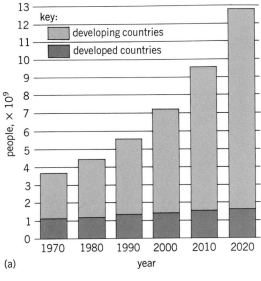

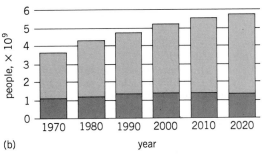

Fig. 3. World population growth, 1970–2020: (a) if number of children per family were to remain at the 1970–1975 level, (b) if an average of two children per family were reached by 1990. (From United Nations, The Population Reference Bureau; and D. N. Ross, Understanding Population: A Short Primer and a Glossary of Terms, Inform. Bull. no. 18, The Conference Board, New York, 1977)

takes about 25 years for per capita GNP to double from $200 to $400. In 1972, according to estimates made by the U.S. Agency for International Development (AID), the world average annual number of births per 1000 people was 32 and the GNP per capita was $904 (Fig. 6).

As Fig. 6 indicates, birthrates in the world's nations show a regular downward trend as GNP per capita increases. More than one-half of the world's people are represented by those countries (in the upper left corner of the figure) where GNP per capita is less than $500 per person per year, and birthrates range from 40 to 50 per 1000 people per year). Recent indications are that less disparity in within-country incomes is also conducive to lower birthrates. While industrialized-country levels of income may not be necessary for lower birthrates, one might conclude from the clustering of countries along the curve in Fig. 6 that a $1000–2000 per capita GNP is the minimum range in which a decline in the birthrate can be expected to occur.

FOOD AVAILABILITY

The problem of feeding people is only one of many interconnected human welfare problems both between and within nations. The solution of any of these problems is critically dependent on the solution of the others. If this approach is not taken, then the food problem either appears unsolvable or proposed solutions are simplistic. As an example, in less-developed countries a significant portion of the population, 62% in 1975, was directly or indirectly involved in agricultural production. Since a main cause of poverty is low agricultural productivity, that is, low yield per worker or per hectare, it is almost astounding that, with respect to nearly two-thirds of the labor force, on the average less than 25% of available investment funds went into agricultural projects. The far greater share, over the past 25 years, has been directed toward urban, industrial development, which has exacerbated population problems by stimulating rural-to-urban migration and which has reduced the food supply by taking capital and credit—one means of production—away from farmers.

Basic food requirements. The most intractable aspect of the food problem is the maldistribution of nutritious foodstuffs between and within countries. Within countries certain vulnerable groups—the poor, particularly women and children—bear the brunt of underconsumption. While climate, physical activity levels, and individual differences affect daily dietary needs, there is still severe undernutrition in terms of dietary energy (protein-calorie) supplies, particularly in Central Africa (Fig. 7). According to the United Nations Protein Advisory Group, the level for the United States—a high-income temperate-zone country—is 2600 cal (10,890 J) and 40 g of protein daily. For tropical-zone developing countries the level is 2300 cal (9630 J) and 38 g of protein per day. Malnutrition places heavy constraints on human potential, whether in a less-developed region of an affluent country or in a poor country. The United Nations World Food Conference Assessment of the World Food Situation estimated that about 25% of the population in developing market-economy countries has an inadequate daily intake of dietary energy as compared with 3% in industrial countries. See MALNUTRITION; NUTRITION; PROTEIN.

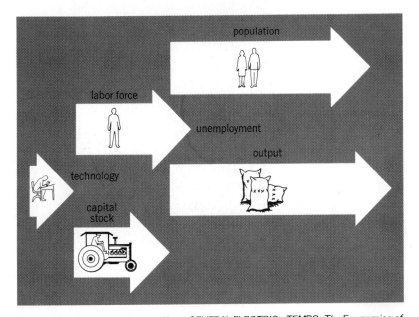

Fig. 4. The development race. (From GENERAL ELECTRIC–TEMPO, The Economics of Slowing Population Growth, Center for Advanced Studies, Santa Barbara, CA, 71 TMP-42)

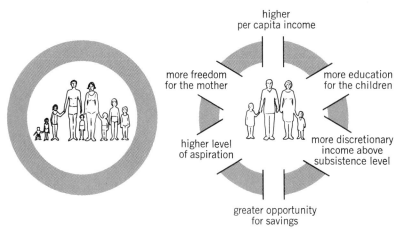

Fig. 5. Qualitative advantages of limiting family size.

decline during the famine of 1966, the situation today still requires constant vigilance and extreme efforts. Food production increases — measured as the food component of crop and livestock production — by FAO estimates have fallen from an average annual increase of 3.1% in the 1950s, through 2.8% in the 1960s, to a 2.2% level in the period 1971–1975. In part, this deteriorating rate of increase reflects the increasing difficulty of producing larger absolute amounts to equal the same percentage increase, and in part, reflects difficulties in extending cultivated areas and in raising yields. By current technological standards, 90% or more of the arable land in the developing regions is already in production (though yields are typically less than half of those obtainable with proper crop selection and fertilizer use). Capital costs which must be incurred to develop land and suitable water supplies depend, of course, upon project size, conditions, and complexity. In Colombia, for example, the average cost for irrigating new lands was $1150/ha in 1967 — a tremendous burden for a country in which yearly per capita income is less than $500 and current capital investment in agrarian areas is not more than $150/ha.

More food — higher energy costs. The quadrupling of oil-energy prices accelerated the arrival of the food crisis. The low-income, high-fertility Fourth World regions do not now generate sufficient foreign exchange earnings to acquire energy resources, chemical fertilizers, and food. In addition, there are more subtle, but profound, difficulties. Scientific agricultural research is carried on primarily in the developed world — 85% of the world's scientists work in developed temperate-zone countries. This has important ramifications. To illustrate, chemical nitrogen fertilizer is a major component of the "green revolution" input package of fertilizer, water, and high-yielding seed vari-

Food versus people. Industrialized and less-developed countries have diverged markedly in per capita food production in recent years due to differences in both population growth rates and agricultural productivity. Of the 96 developing countries for which the Food and Agriculture Organization (FAO, the United Nations agency devoted to promoting efficient production and distribution of food and agricultural products) publishes data, food production kept pace with population increases in 51 and lagged in 45, in the 1961–1974 period. These 45 countries represent 40% of the total population of the developing countries. Figure 8 shows the precarious level of per capita food production in these 96 less-developed countries.

More food — higher capital costs. While the magnitude of the 1972–1973 per capita food production decline which triggered the World Food Conference of 1974 was not nearly so great as the

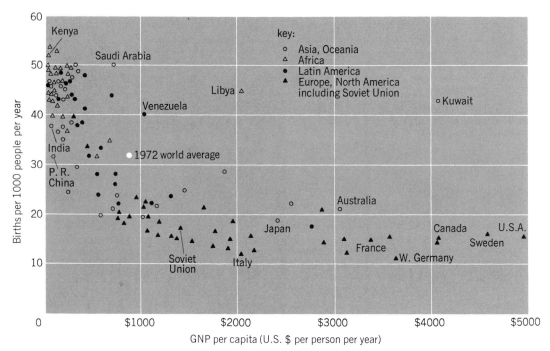

Fig. 6. National birth rates versus per capita GNP. (*From U.S. Agency for International Development, Population Program Assistance Annual Report Fiscal Year 1973, U.S. Government Printing Office, 1974; and The Conference Board, New York*)

eties. The problem with the best commercial method for producing artificial fertilizer is the high energy requirement. Thus, as the price of energy increases, the "appropriateness" of high-energy technology becomes more questionable. *See the feature articles* ENERGY IN THE FOOD SYSTEM; THE GREEN REVOLUTION. *See also* FERTILIZER.

More food—and the weather. In 1972 bad weather was widespread in Europe, the Soviet Union, the Far East, China, and North America, and total world food production declined in absolute terms for the first time in the post–World War II era. Foodstocks, in fact, have declined through 1975, which means that world food supplies have been dependent on current harvests for nearly 4 years. Meteorologists in general are now forecasting a change; some see a trend toward a warmer, others toward a cooler climate. As temperatures drop, the number of people sustainable by arable land also declines. Should the climate return to the level at the "Little Ice Age" of 1600–1850, India could support only three out of four people now living there; the Soviet Union would lose Kazakhstan as a vital grain-producing state; and Canadian grain export capacity would be reduced by 75%. Nevertheless, the world's political and economic leaders are unable to agree upon even emergency food stock reserves. *See the feature article* CLIMATE AND CROPS.

OPTIONS TO PREVENT MALNUTRITION AND STARVATION

This discussion focuses on the less-developed world, particularly the "bottom billion." From the viewpoint of the less-developed countries, there are essentially four interrelated options for improving food availability: (1) decrease the population growth rate; (2) hope for more food aid; (3) import more food; and (4) stimulate the productivity of the food supply system.

Decrease the population growth rate. According to the Population Council, a New York–based research organization, about 30 of 120 developing countries have official policies aimed at reducing population growth rates. Thirty others, which include most Latin America countries, have some family planning policies; the other 60 are "indifferent."

Not everyone agrees on the need to control population growth. Some argue that technology applied to the world's underutilized oceans, deserts, and jungles could provide a base to feed an additional 50 billion people. They suggest that many changes could be made in current practices to enlarge the Earth's carrying capacity. Other political leaders point to the drastic political consequences suffered by Indian Prime Minister Indira Gandhi's Congress Party, at least partly because of government forced-sterilization programs, and see this as an indication for caution in their own population programs.

These views overlook several important considerations: More intensive land use is already threatening ecologically marginal lands. Also, there is evidence that, in the 1974–1975 period of food production decline, the United States activated a "hidden" grain reserve—cereal feeding to livestock decreased 25% due to relative price changes in food and feed grains. In other words, the present food "reserve stock" is slack in the supply system.

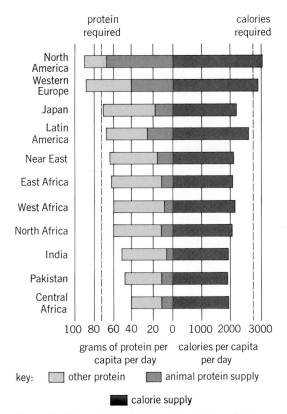

Fig. 7. Protein and caloric intake. Dashed lines indicate estimated North American protein and caloric requirements, based on diets sufficient to enable people to attain full body weight. (*From D. H. Meadows et al., The Limits to Growth: A Report for The Club of Rome's Project on the Predicament of Mankind, A Potomac Associates Book published by Universe Books, New York, 1972. Graphics by Potomac Associates*)

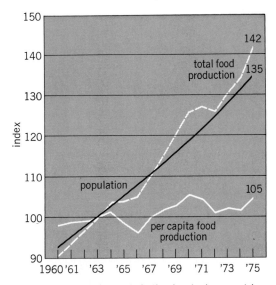

Fig. 8. Food versus people in the developing countries. Index: 1961–1965 = 100. (*USDA*)

Further, there is some evidence that less-developed countries birthrates are declining, due at least in part to the voluntary population programs of the past 15 years in India, Indonesia, Korea, Pakistan, and several Caribbean countries. The

Food shipments under P.L. 480, Title 1, 1960–1974*

Commodity	1960†	1965†	1970	1972	1973	1974‡
Wheat and products	8199	13,705	5765	4615	2517	1005
Milk (dried)	8	42	18	19	2	0
Rice	453	561	884	813	987	620
Corn, sorghum	787	728	1078	1217	1289	454
Vegetable oils	339	364	240	193	107	148

SOURCE: U.S. Department of Agriculture and Lester R. Brown with Erik P. Eckholm, *By Bread Alone*, Praeger Publishing, 1974.
*In thousands of metric tons; all years but 1970 on fiscal-year basis.
†Includes aid under Titles I and IV in previous legislation.
‡Estimate.

United Nations Fund for Population Activities reports increasing requests for population programs assistance.

AID spent $112 million on population programs (of a world total of $200 million spent by United Nations agencies, private groups, and individual countries) in 1974. Both United States and total world expenditures for population programs have increased nearly 50% since then, but the United States still provides the greatest share, and an enthusiastic reception for these programs is hardly found, for cultural and other reasons. United States officials are often frustrated by what they interpret as the developing nations' contradictory position: family planning is guarded as an internal policy matter; at the same time, pleas for more food are made.

More food aid. The United States has been sending more food to developing countries. Under the 1954 Food for Peace Program (P.L. 480), American food surpluses have been sold (under Title 1) and given away as emergency aid (under Title 2). The table summarizes activity under this program for the 1960–1974 period.

Even if requests for more food are a typical reaction of the developing countries, the situation in the United States makes that solution impractical, if not impossible. Because of the energy crisis, the United States agricultural system is facing problems in the very areas responsible for its earlier success.

Fossil fuels—for planting, spraying, fertilizing, and harvesting—are the key to United States food production. Under current circumstances, some see this now as the weakest link in that production system. Many present-day food products require fossil fuels for production. Recently, several oil companies have begun experimental programs to produce single-cell protein directly from fossil fuels, by-passing the fields altogether. Irrigation is another large energy consumer. One comparison indicates that the United States requires eight times as much water as India to produce the daily food for one person.

In any event, more considered forms of assistance are necessary. More-developed country development assistance, for example, in the form of food aid, can have unintended consequences if less-developed country self-help programs are defeated. A study by the U.S. General Accounting Office has found that the food aid program has a large component of farm surplus disposal to it, making it an adjunct to the farm price-support programs rather than an emergency food supply program. This may change, depending upon domestic politics. Aid to less-developed countries must move away from large projects—providing "747" jets and steel mills—toward systematically increasing the productivity of the food supply system, beginning on the farms where most of the world's people still live. If this were to happen, the process of income redistribution would be more likely to occur, as the poorest people would then get an opportunity to become more productive; but this is a joint political decision of the more- and less-developed countries.

Import more food. Population growth in the developing world accounts for 70% of the increase in the demand for the food supply. The remaining 30% is due to higher incomes; that is, as people become more affluent they "upgrade" their food intake. (In the developed countries this population-affluence ratio is 55:45.) In the future the share of the demand for food in less-developed countries due to population pressures is likely to increase. United Nations population projections indicate that 90% of the increase in the world population will occur in the developing countries.

In slightly less than one-half of the less-de-

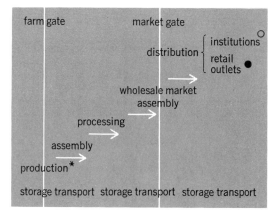

key:

* about 50% retained on typically small (1-10 hectare) farms, where 80% of world's food is grown and 70% of world's people live; only surplus goes beyond the farm gate—of which 20-50% is food loss

○ hospitals, schools, industrial facilities, transportation carriers, facilities for law enforcement, welfare, tourism, national defense, and disaster relief

● 80-85% of total human food consumed

Fig. 9. Simplified representation of food production and food distribution in a developing nation. *(From D. N. Ross, Partners in Agroeconomic Development, The Conference Board, New York, 1977)*

veloped countries the 1961–1974 food supply increase did not meet the estimated domestic demand. As a result, food imports by developing countries in the 1961–1970 period increased 3.3% yearly and, in the 1971–1974 period, 7.1% yearly. Both price of foodstuffs and the quantity demanded are soaring. In 1955 commercial food imports cost developing countries $996 million; in 1967, $3 billion; in 1972–1973, about $4 billion; and in 1973–1974, $10 billion. Coupled with increased oil-energy prices, the non-oil-producing Fourth World countries have accumulated tremendous balance-of-payments deficits in their international current account—merchandise trade, travel expenditures, and income and investment flows. The Fourth World balance-of-payments deficit in 1973 was $9 billion; by 1975 it had reached $35 billion. The capacity of these poorest nations to cover a deficit, from aid and capital inflows, without running down currency reserves or resorting to heavy borrowings from the World Bank or from international markets, is estimated at only $15 billion. The predictable is happening: massive rescheduling of commercial debt and emergency borrowings from the International Monetary Fund.

Food supply system in less-developed countries. People do not simply want food; they want it at particular places at particular times in certain amounts and in accustomed forms. A food supply "system" involves much more than agriculture, although agriculture is still the starting point, and weather and temperature still make the difference between one year's situation and the next. A food system encompasses the entire commodity flow from initial inputs to the final consumer, and all the participants involved in the production, processing, and marketing of a farm product. It includes farm suppliers, farmers, storage operators, processors, wholesalers, and coordinating institutions, as well as agricultural and nutritional research, agricultural extension services, and nutritional education programs.

A simplified system. Increased food production, by itself, does not automatically result in the improved nutritional status of a nation's population. Products must make their way through the entire food system to people who have enough money to buy them. Figures 9–11 illustrate the developmental and technical complexity of the food supply flow.

Figure 9 shows phases of the food supply. All are critical; if one phase such as assembly breaks down, food loss occurs. It is estimated that, depending upon circumstances and countries, post–farm gate food loss varies from 20% to as high as 50% of the food produced.

Figure 10, illustrates the necessary coordination between government programs and business ventures at the initial phase of the food supply system—in the areas of production credit, management, and better seed quality, for example—and links it to other aspects of development.

Figure 11 illustrates the technical aspects of the processing phase, using soybeans as the example. Processing is the first main "value-added" stage in food product manufacture; it is at this level that new domestic employment is created and new products become available domestically and internationally.

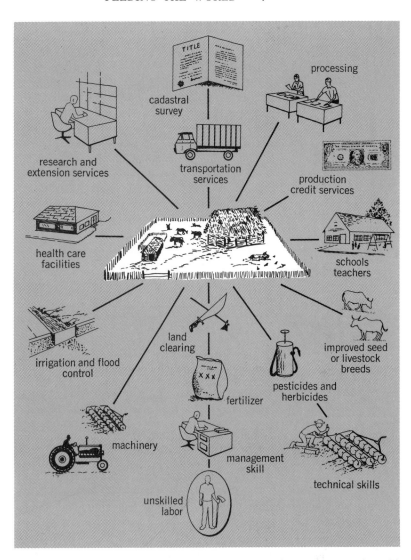

Fig. 10. Production inputs required to create commercial farms to compete in world markets.

Figures 9–11 are intended to illustrate the complexity of the linkage between the food supply flow and the agroeconomic development process. Moreover, most food-related problems are intimately related to, and not distinct from, the development process. Each of the many analyses of the population-food problem may be valid as a part of the whole, yet invalid if, by itself, it purports to explain the problem.

The complex nature of the food problem necessitates the implementation of a coordinated program of action in order to effect a change in the result produced by the food supply system. For example, following the 1965–1966 famine Indian small farmers were pressed by their government to adopt high-yielding varieties of grain and to use fertilizer. The resulting production surplus, however, met with an absence of storage facilities and inadequate marketing channels. Grain prices dropped and many farmers were unable to repay fertilizer loans. The need for complementary institutional roles of government and business is illustrated by this simple yet tragic example.

A government role. Less-developed country policies can affect every aspect of the food supply sys-

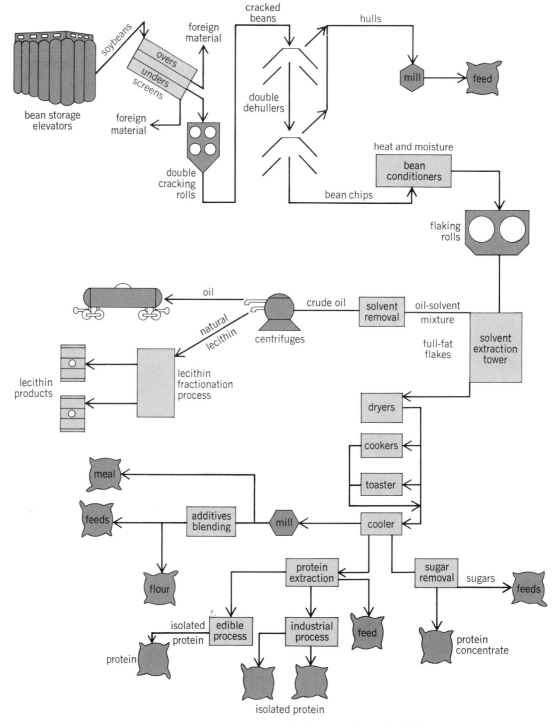

Fig. 11. Technical aspects of modern soybean processing. (From J. D. Long, From farm gate to dining table: A look at central soya, Bus. Horizons, 19(5):12–25, October 1976)

tem. Yet officials at the World Food Council (the United Nations organization charged at the 1974 World Food Conference in Rome with preventing a forecasted 1985 shortfall of 85 million metric tons of grain) claim there is incredible apathy on the part of both more-developed and less-developed country governments. They claim that nations do not want to change their policies, perhaps because policy-makers are not personally affected by the malnutrition problem. Or, it may be a question of priorities, and less-developed country governments may have decided to improve their country's balance of payments by moving products into international trade channels rather than into local utilization. Much of the current debate on nutrition priorities revolves around the efficacy of this choice of priorities.

Less-developed country policies can impede,

rather than promote, the flow of agricultural commodity production. For example, "cheap urban food" programs usually act as anti-incentives by keeping food commodity prices at low levels, thereby encouraging either cash-crop production (such as cotton, coffee, and tea) or the transfer of human efforts and capital resources away from the rural and agricultural sectors toward the urban and industrial sectors. However, in Argentina a reversal of this cheap food policy has resulted in record grain harvests. Farmers, free of export taxes and some price controls, expanded acreage sown to grain by nearly 10%, increased fertilizer use considerably, and produced for the first time since the 1930s a wheat and oilseed (soybean) surplus that in large measure pulled Argentina out of its chronic trade-deficit position.

Possible more-developed country actions in the face of renewed less-developed country competition for world markets pose nagging questions for the future. The United States now relies heavily on receipts from grain sales to cover mounting expenditures for oil. And a new international spirit of sharing is hardly evident in the reactions of United States consumer interest groups to coffee price increases.

A business role. The primary role of business is the development of a viable operation that creates wage-paying jobs and fosters the process of capital formation within a country. While business considers each venture in relation to the entire food supply system, the focus is on specific ventures. Opportunities to increase efficiency, or reduce waste — and thereby make a profit — may occur at any phase of the system. To illustrate, a "food service" company that operates in a less-developed country environment in which the government's number-one priority is feeding the urban masses to avert political unrest concentrates its efforts on institutional markets: hospitals, schools, and the military. The aim is to reduce waste and to provide nutritionally balanced meals from locally grown foods. Product quality specifications, agreed upon by the company and the government, put pressure on all phases of the food supply system — wholesalers, processors, farmers. The result is better meals, less waste, upgraded facilities, and better-quality products available to local markets.

Conclusion. A "doomsayer's" case could be made about the food supply system in less-developed countries, but it would ignore the learning involved in failure and omit the few good examples of systematic, patient and, increasingly, coordinated actions. Some of the gloom may be dispelled by increased sensitivity on the part of developed and less-developed countries, but most of the pessimism will be driven away by a sincere, sustained, environmentally sound, and balanced industrial and agricultural development effort.

CONSEQUENCES OF FAILURE

Achieving a bright long-range future probably will necessitate getting through very troublesome near- and medium-term futures. In the medium term, to 1985, even if less-developed countries' food demands decrease — due to commercial imports, domestic production improvements, and food aid — the number of people suffering from severe protein-calorie malnutrition is projected by the United Nations to increase from about 400 million to nearly 700 million. This is due to the "dilution-effect" that increasing population growth rates have on production increases.

Future-oriented "systems dynamics" groups have become interested in the interrelationships among all the components of the food supply systems. These relationships — usually quantified into numerical variables — are set out in computer-based models. The models are able to project the "results" of various interactions at some long-range future time. In perhaps the best-known prognostication (The Club of Rome's *Limits to Growth*) food production per capita rises to a maximum by about the year 2000 and then drops sharply because of population growth and the rapid depletion of resources (with an attendant population increase), all to the detriment of agriculture. This does not have to happen. The importance of such models is that they enable the cumulative effects of small actions, or inactions, to be seen. In general the studies suggest that real economic growth is essential to the achievement of acceptable and sustainable standards of living for all people. The studies suggest that the nature of economic growth must change and, generally, they underscore the need for political and economic institutions to change as well. In any case, stopping population growth is critical.

The population programs of the 1960s and 1970s appear to be making some headway, but the task of the world's food supply systems in the last quarter of the 20th century is immense. While the specter of Malthus's predictions remains, there is no inexorable process for its materialization. Starvation and malnutrition are not necessary conditions of human existence. What happens depends upon government policies — from population programs to food production incentives — coordinated with business actions, and upon a sustained willingness to address the problem.   [DOUGLAS N. ROSS]

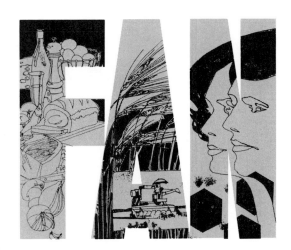

CLIMATE AND CROPS

James D. McQuigg

development of formally organized meteorological networks to provide detailed records of weather events (temperature, wind
speed and direction, atmospheric pressure, cloud type and amount, humidity,
precipitation, and so on) is a very recent occurrence compared with the length of time humans
have cultivated crops or managed herds of livestock. There is ample evidence, however, from
historical writings and folklore and from anthropo-
logical and geological investigations to support the
claim that a number of changes have taken place
in the Earth's climate since humans first appeared.

Five thousand years of records from China include comments about trees and plants flourishing
in certain parts of the country, disappearing for a
time, and then reappearing as the temperature and
precipitation shifted. For example, at one time rice
was grown far north of the present rice region. In
England vineyards flourished in areas that long

since have become unsuitable. Ancient explorers
from Scandinavia established colonies in Green-
land, which had a more hospitable climate at the
time.

The decadal mean annual temperature graph
shown in Fig. 1 was prepared by P. Bergthorsson,
using a series of temperature and historical data.
While one could argue about the precision of temperature data derived from historical accounts,
Bergthorsson's work accurately reflects the magnitude of climatic variability.

While most persons perceive that there have
been shifts in climate over the past thousands of
years, they tend to regard present-day climate as a
"given," to be included in an economic model as a
constant. This tendency exists in part because the
magnitude of meteorologically induced variability
of crop production has been small during a number
of the years following World War II, and in part
because most people are taught a narrow definition

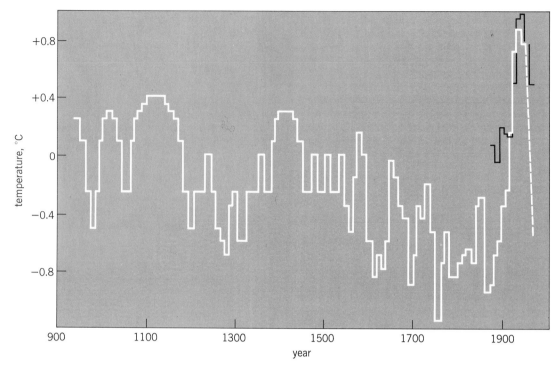

Fig. 1. Decadal mean annual temperature in Iceland over the past millennium. The dashed line indicates the rate of temperature decline in the 1961–1971 period; the black line shows the variation of mean temperature in the Northern Hemisphere plotted to the same relative scale. (*From R. A. Bryson, Environ. Conserv., 2(3):166, Autumn 1975*)

of climate. Traditionally, climate has been defined as "the average weather."

It is becoming increasingly clear that climate should be defined in terms of variability from place to place and from year to year. This type of defini-

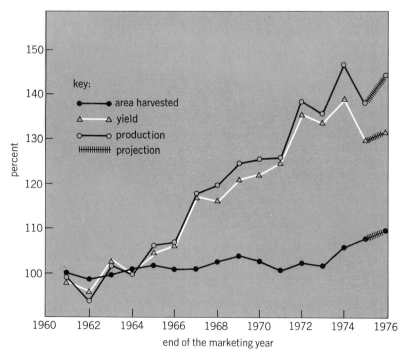

Fig. 2. Total world grain trends. "Percent" is based on a 1961–1965 average of 100%. "End of marketing year" indicates, for example, that 1961 means marketing year 1960–1961. (*USDA*)

tion has been expressed succinctly by the English climatologist H. H. Lamb: Climate is the sum total of weather experienced at a place over the year and over many years; it includes both the sample averages or normals and the range of extremes about the normal.

It is often useful to define climate in terms of some specified range of deviations from the mean. In some instances, this range could include the central third of the frequency distribution of all possible values; if weather events occur within this central third, one could call this normal climate. The problems in using this and other definitions of climate arise because the true mean value or the true range of extremes is not really known; instead a sample of data must be used in most cases. Where this sample is adequate, the statistically defined aspects of climate provide reasonable predictions of future climate.

Climatic variability from region to region within a given year or from year to year can be interpreted in terms of crop production variability, and this approach will be used in the following discussion.

Climatic variability and crop production. Crop production P can be computed as the product of area A and yield Y. In symbolic form, then, $P = AY$. Thus, it is clear that production will vary from year to year as area or yield (or both) varies. The area devoted to a particular crop shifts from year to year because of price, government policy, or weather. For example, as of late winter in early 1977, the price of soybeans in the United States was very high, compared with the price of corn. The commodity news at that time included numerous stories about the amount of acreage that would be shifted from corn to soybeans. Another example would be winter wheat area that had experienced severe cold and inadequate snow cover. This would probably lead to abandonment of winter wheat acreage and possible substitution of another crop. Hail, drought, or prolonged flooding would also lead to shifts in crop area.

The largest contributor to year-to-year crop production variability, however, is weather variability, as illustrated in Fig. 2. Here three data series on world grain are shown: area, yield, and production. Values are plotted on a common scale, where the average of the period 1961–1965 is set at 100. The change in area has been small compared with changes in yield and production values.

The values in Fig. 3 are a series of corn yield data for the United States Corn Belt. Two patterns are apparent in this illustration: First, there is a flat trend in yields during the years prior to World War II, followed by a definite trend toward higher yields since that time. Second, there is a significant amount of variability around the trend. Similar patterns appear when the yields of other crops, such as wheat, rice, and other grains, are presented graphically.

The trend toward higher yields began after World War II for grains grown in most developed regions of the world. This increase can be explained in terms of several factors, among which are genetic improvements, increased use of chemical fertilizers, better management, and improved machinery. These factors are often grouped together under the term "technology." A significant portion of the year-to-year yield variability about the technology trend can be "explained" as the impact of year-to-year crop weather variability.

Two basic approaches have been used to model the impact of meteorological variability on crop yields: the physiological approach and the correlative approach. The physiological approach is an attempt to describe the detailed impact of weather events on the biological and physical processes that occur within a typical plant or within a plant canopy. Ideally, this description is based on precise knowledge of the interactions between the plant and its immediate soil-atmospheric environment. Models of this type are very useful for a variety of purposes, serving as scientific tools for studying the potential impact of climatic change, studying the effects of deliberate genetic engineering, estimating crop yields, or estimating the progress of a crop, given knowledge of weather conditions.

There are two major disadvantages to this modeling approach. (1) Knowledge of detailed causal relationships between weather events and biological and physical processes within the plant is incomplete. (2) The detailed measurements needed to estimate the coefficients in this kind of model are expensive. The problem of extending results obtained from small-plot experiments over a short period of time to aggregated estimates for large crop areas over a very long period of time has not been solved.

The correlative, or statistical, approach is based on long series of climatological data and a concurrent series of yield data. Coefficients are estimated by using a statistical technique such as multiple regression. At its worst, such an approach is a "cut-and-try" effort. At its best, the specification

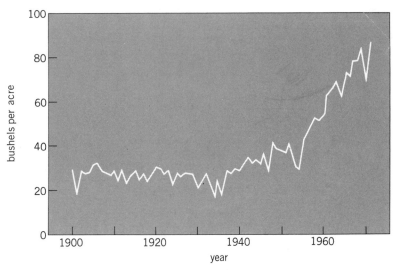

Fig. 3. Average corn yields by year for the United States Corn Belt (Iowa, Illinois, Indiana, Ohio, and Missouri); 20 bu/acre = 12.52 quintals/ha.

of the model is based on sound agronomic knowledge.

Future trends in crop area. There are still some land areas in the world which have not been fully developed for agricultural production, and it is reasonable to assume that continuing attempts will be made to put these areas into production. But it is also true that most of the highly productive land is already under cultivation.

Much land that is not currently used for crop production lies in climatic zones that present serious problems to development, including a high risk of drought or flood, or temperature-humidity patterns that are conducive to frequent outbreaks of plant disease or insect infestation.

A large portion of the land area of the world that is not currently used for crop production lies in tropical latitudes in countries such as Brazil, in the tropical areas of Africa, or in the Malaysian area. Another example of land that has only recently been put into production is the "new lands" regions of the Soviet Union where temperature and rainfall are at the outer fringe of the range of values for which crop production is possible.

Examples of existing productive farmland that has been put to urban or nonagricultural use can be found near any of the major cities in the midlatitude regions of the world. The construction of superhighways, urban housing, airports, shopping centers, and so forth has used up about 1,000,000 acres (400,000 hectares) of productive land in the United States in each of the most recent years.

Future trends in yields. Projections of future yields have to take into account the future trend of agricultural technology as well as future climate. There is little doubt that future genetic, chemical, and engineering developments will result in higher yields per unit area for many crops. Researchers working in the early 1940s with United States corn yield data series for the period 1900–1930 might have projected a "flat" technology into the period 1945–1965, but such a projection would have been wrong. Hybrid seed, chemical fertilizer, and better management all contributed to a spectacular increase in yields without precedent in agricultural

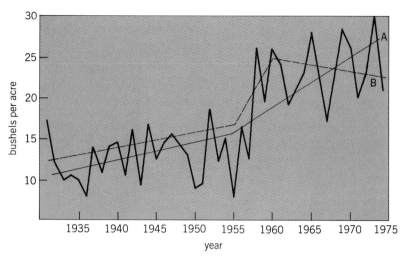

Fig. 4. Oklahoma wheat yields and technology trends; 5 bu/acre = 3.36 quintals/ha. Curve A represents estimate of the technology trend resulting from regressing yields on year. Curve B represents the impact of technological improvement.

history. Likewise, the problem of projecting future agricultural technology for the period 1980–2000 is not simply a matter of projecting a continuation of the trend which occurred in the preceding 2 or 3 decades.

Consider the series of wheat yield data for Oklahoma as an example. In Fig. 4 these data are shown for the period 1931–1974. It is relatively easy to recognize the impact of technological improvements in this series by observing the comparatively flat trend in yields from 1931 to 1955. This is followed by a sharp trend toward higher yields beginning about 1956. The mid-1950s saw the introduction of several improved wheat varieties, together with an increase in application of chemical fertilizer, and the use of herbicides and improved machinery.

The same series of Oklahoma wheat yield data were used to fit a piece-wise trend line by regressing yields on year. This regression resulted in an estimate of the technology trend shown in Fig. 4 (curve A). The difficulty with this analysis is that this trend line is influenced by shifts in weather from the drought years of the 1930s to more favor-

able wheat weather in the 1960s. In other words, in this form the trend line does not represent the impact of technology alone.

The impact of year-to-year weather and the impact of changes in technology were estimated concurrently, and the "best" statistical fit of the sample data to the model is shown in Fig. 4 (curve B). Here, the impact of technological improvement that started in the mid-1950s was realized in about 5 years, followed by a trend toward somewhat lower yields in the last 10 or 15 years of the data series.

A similar slowdown of the technological trend has been revealed through statistical analysis of corn yields in the central United States, and of wheat yields in the Soviet Union and Canada. In these analyses the leveling-off period of the technological trend apparently began in the late 1960s or early 1970s.

It is a very difficult statistical problem to produce strong evidence for the hypothesis that there has been a shift toward a flatter technological trend in recent years, but there is enough evidence to cause an investigator to suspect that the trend toward higher yields that began in the mid-1950s will not continue unbroken into the mid-1980s and beyond.

Future climate impact on grain production. J. M. Mitchell has studied large-scale change in annual temperatures over the Northern Hemisphere. There is still much uncertainty (and some controversy) about how to sketch in future annual temperatures in a graphical presentation such as the one in Fig. 5. Even if the annual average temperature for the coming decade or two could be plotted on such a graph without any forecast error, interpreting the impact on grain production would be difficult for two reasons.

First, year-to-year variability of grain yields in a large region, such as the United States Corn Belt or the Soviet spring wheat area, is related to year-to-year weather variability in a complex, nonlinear manner. When viewed in more detail month by month, and allowing for regional variability as well, the climate change patterns are much more complex. In Fig. 6 an example of the change in average precipitation from the 1931–1960 to the 1941–1970 "normals" is shown. In Fig. 7 the differences in monthly temperature average between these same two sample periods are shown for Unionville, in northern Missouri.

A useful statement about future climate can be made by taking a sample of past climate and using it as a model for climate during some future period. Traditionally, economists and agronomists have reduced the sample of past climate to an average and then have used this an estimate of future value. However, it is very difficult to find even one year of past climate where all the temperature and precipitation values, month by month, are even close to the expected value. If, instead of just projecting future climate, one is trying to project the future impact of climate on grain yields, choosing an adequate sample of past years becomes more important.

As an example, most of the advances in agricultural technology have taken place during 1953–1973. For this reason, a sample of tempera-

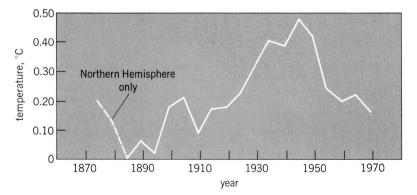

Fig. 5. The variation of global mean surface air temperature, expressed as deviation from the mean, in successive 5-year averages from 1880–1884 to 1965–1969. (After computations by J. M. Mitchell updated at the National Center for Atmospheric Research, Boulder, CO)

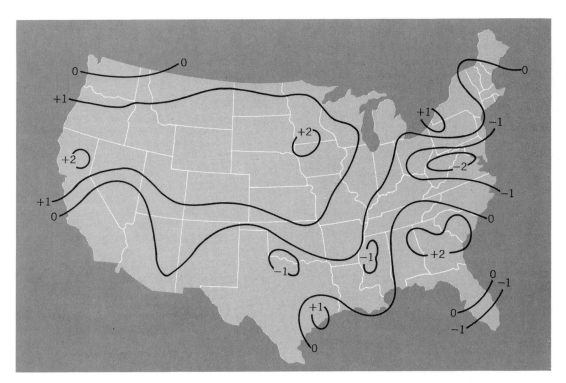

Fig. 6. Graph showing the difference between the average of 1931–1960 and the average of 1941–1970 annual precipitation levels, as expressed in inches (1 in. = 2.5 cm).

ture and precipitation data could be selected from that period, and that sample average and variance could be projected into the coming 20 years. If this were done for the United States Corn Belt, it would be hard to find a less representative sample. Consider the result of a simulation model experiment conducted by J. D. McQuigg and L. M. Thompson. In this simulation, agricultural technology was assumed to be fixed at the 1973 level. A long series of weather data, for the period 1894–1973, was then used as input to a weather–corn yield model. Results are shown as Fig. 8. The vertical scale is expressed in bushels per acre, but it could just as well have been labeled "corn-weather index." The important point is that the 20-year period ending with 1973 exhibits a higher sample mean and a much smaller variance about the mean than any 20-year sample drawn from the period prior to 1953.

In a presentation on Dec. 10, 1974, to the National Outlook Conference sponsored by the U.S. Department of Agriculture, McQuigg approached the problem with the following explanation.

There are several primary agricultural production regions that did have a very favorable crop weather from about the mid-1950s to the early 1970s. The exact length of the period varies from place to place. A particular example of this is the Corn Belt of the United States, which had unusually favorable weather from the mid-1950s to early 1970. Not only were yields higher on average, but the variability around the average yields was much smaller than one would expect from the sample of years prior to the mid-1950s.

Many projections of yields or grain production into the coming decades are based on agricultural data collected from the most recent decade or two

because this is the period within which most of the important developments in agriculture have taken place. These important developments include improved seed; increased use of chemical fertilizer, insecticides, and herbicides; and a trend toward more effective machinery and more effective management of farms. It may be a coincidence that these decades were also a period of highly favorable weather, but when the agricultural yield and production data are projected into the future, on the basis of this small sample, a highly favorable climate is implicit in the projections. The results of such projections would be quite different if the one or two most recent decades had been more like the period prior to 1955. In many areas of the

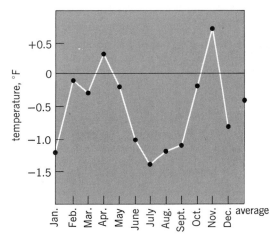

Fig. 7. Differences between the 1931–1960 and the 1941–1970 monthly mean temperatures; 0.5°F = 0.9°C.

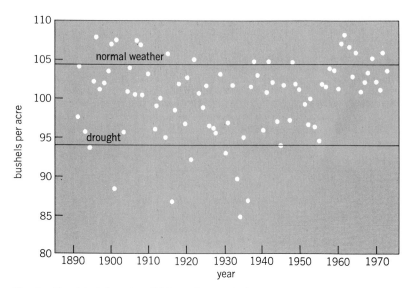

Fig. 8. Simulated five-state (Ohio, Indiana, Illinois, Iowa, and Missouri) weighted corn yields using 1973 technology and harvested acreage; 5 bu/acre = 3.14 quintal/ha.

world, this earlier sample included a much larger range of variability from year to year of crop season weather. It also included less favorable weather in a larger proportion of years than had been the case in the most recent decade or two.

The two years that have followed the 1974 Outlook Conference have included: (1) a massive shortfall of food grain production in the Soviet Union in 1975; (2) the most serious drought in the European region in many years in 1975–1976; (3) an abundant wheat crop on a worldwide basis in 1976, with favorable weather in the Soviet Union, India, and North America; (4) a serious 2-year drought in California and surrounding states in 1975–1976; and (5) prolonged drought in the United States Corn and Wheat belts in the winter of 1976–1977, coupled with severe cold in January over the east half of the United States. Rather than perceive these most recent events as some anomaly, researchers would be well advised to consider them as a sample of the kind of climatic variability that can be expected in the future.

[JAMES D. MC QUIGG]

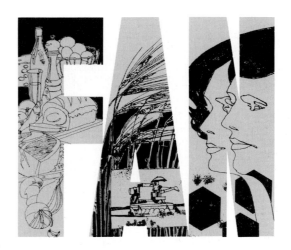

ENERGY IN THE FOOD SYSTEM

Ivan L. Kinne; Thomas A. McClure

food production is essentially a process of energy transformation. Whether of animal or vegetable origin, food basically is derived from a crop or plant source. Crop production, of course, uses solar energy in a number of ways to transform carbon dioxide, soil nutrients, and water into plant tissues, sugars, and other materials that are used either directly or indirectly for food. *See* PHOTOSYNTHESIS.

In primitive agricultural systems these processes are carried out in virtually their natural state, that is, the principal energy source is solar, augmented only slightly by human or animal energy inputs. In "modern" agricultural systems, however, in order to achieve greater levels of output, other energy inputs are used to enhance solar energy transformations. It is these added energy inputs, ultimately derived mainly from fossil fuel reserves, that are the subject of much controversy today.

Because energy historically has been inexpensive relative to labor or land inputs in the developed world, and relative to the value of food and other agricultural outputs, energy use has increased steadily. Figure 1 shows the approximate increases in energy use by agriculture in the United States from 1940 through 1970.

With the dramatic rise in fossil fuel prices since the Organization of Petroleum Exporting Countries (OPEC) boycotts of 1973, much attention has been focused on measuring energy inputs in the food system, devising more efficient and effective means for energy utilization, and seeking alternative energy sources. This is, indeed, a complex process that is difficult to understand completely and to measure accurately. Estimates in this article, while taken from sources currently considered as authoritative, should be viewed principally as indicators of relative energy use rather than as absolute measures.

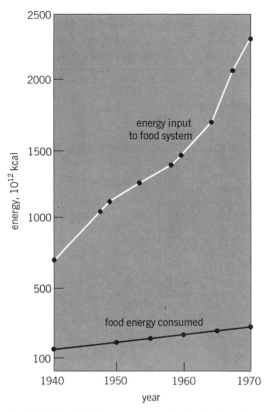

Fig. 1. United States energy use in the food system (1940–1970) compared with the caloric content of food consumed; 10^{12} kcal = 4.19×10^{15} J. *(From J. S. Steinhart and C. E Steinhart, Energy use in the U.S. food systems, Science, 184:308, 1974)*

ENERGY USES

A food system, whether primitive or quite advanced, can be analyzed in terms of sets of principal activities or components: (1) agricultural services and "off-farm" inputs; (2) agricultural production itself; (3) processing and manufacturing agricultural products; (4) marketing, distribution, and storage; and (5) consumption itself. Obviously, in primitive systems these functions are very simplified and, in the case of purely subsistence systems, may even be carried out mostly by a family on an individual plot of land. However, in modern society this is a highly complex, interactive system, with individual functions carried out by a large number of independent yet interlocking organizations.

Agricultural inputs. Inputs to agriculture include such items as machinery and equipment, fuels, fertilizers, pesticides, seeds, and animal feedstuffs, and such services as veterinary, farm management, credit, insurance, and irrigation. Energy is utilized in a number of ways, including that required for manufacture of these items, as well as for transportation from the point of manufacture through marketing and distribution systems to the farm or place of utilization. Some input items are a direct transformation of energy sources. For example, present-day manufacture of ammonia, which is used directly as a nitrogenous fertilizer in crop production or as a feedstock in the manufacture of other fertilizers, utilizes natu-

ral gas as a direct input. A number of petroleum by-products are also used in the production of other inputs such as pesticides. Plastics, which are used in many ways in the agricultural production process, are derived from a petroleum base.

Farm production. Energy use in the production sector of agriculture is divided into two parts: direct use in the production function itself, and use for farm family living. The requirements for family living are similar to those in other sectors of society. On the production side, energy is required for land preparation and seeding, irrigation, fertilizer and pesticide application, weed control and cultivation, harvesting, materials handling, crop drying, transportation, and product storage, and in some cases for greenhouse operation, heating and lighting, maintenance and repair, and equipment use. Specific applications of energy, of course, vary tremendously among the different types of agriculture and among the different locations in which agricultural activity takes place throughout the United States.

Food processing and manufacturing. Just as energy is critical to food production, it also is vital to food processing and manufacturing. In this sector, energy is used for heat, power, materials handling, and transportation, as well as for refrigeration and storage of perishable products. Heat for processing is extremely important because most current food preservation techniques require cooking, water removal, and other similar activities. Again, because there are a large number of different types of manufacturing and processing industries, the specifics of energy use vary considerably from industry to industry and from plant to plant. *See* FOOD ENGINEERING; FOOD MANUFACTURING.

Marketing and distribution. Energy is required to move fresh and processed foods through the various marketing channels. Transportation, maintaining frozen or refrigerated storage space, moving materials within storage, and the controlled-environment requirements of warehouses, supermarkets, and grocery stores require energy, as do packaging and further processing activities.

Consumption. Food consumption in modern society takes place either at home or away from home. In this sector, energy is required for basic food preparation (cooking), for storing, and for the operation of auxiliary activities involved in the food process. In those establishments that are directed mainly toward food consumption, one must also consider energy required for heating and air conditioning, lighting, and general operation.

Uses and sources in the United States. As indicated previously, the process of measuring energy use in the very complicated United States food system is difficult. Problems include data availability and coverage, identification of direct uses, and identification and apportionment of indirect uses.

One of the most comprehensive attempts at compiling information in this area is a 1976 report of the Federal Energy Administration (FEA). This report draws on a large body of literature, reconciling estimates and converting them to a 1971 base (Fig. 2 and Table 1). The energy data are inflated or deflated to 1971 by Eqs. (1) and (2), where e = energy consumption in sector, E = total United States energy consumption, t = year for which data were

Table 1. Relative energy consumption in the United States food system in 1971*

Sector	Total use, 10^{12} Btu†	Percent of total
Food production	1,993	18
Food manufacturing	3,290	30
Wholesale trade	348	3
Retail trade	572	5
Food consumption	4,885	44
Total system	11,088	100

*From Federal Energy Administration, Office of Industrial Programs, *Energy Use in the Food System*, May 1976.
†10^{12} Btu = 1.055×10^{15} J.

given, and $P =$ fraction of total United States energy consumption. The FEA compilation indicates that over 1.1×10^{16} Btu (1 Btu = 1055 J) of energy

$$e_t/E_t = P \qquad (1)$$

$$P \times E_{1971} = e_{1971} \qquad (2)$$

were consumed in the United States food system in 1971. This total is probably understated because of significant data gaps. A number of boxes in Fig. 2 have been left blank, indicating no available data source.

Food consumption is the system component utilizing the largest amount of energy, about 44% of the total. Of this figure, 2.93×10^{15} Btu, or about 60%, is consumed in in-home preparation and the remainder in away-from-home food preparation and consumption. In in-home preparation 2.285×10^{15} Btu, or approximately 78%, of energy is consumed directly in the food preparation process. Of this direct energy use, some 34% (7.77×10^{14} Btu) is used in the cooking process itself. The indirect uses of energy include that required to produce the capital equipment needed for in-home food preparation (about 1.79×10^4 Btu, or 6% of the subsector total), or for transportation including transportation from supermarket to home (about 4.66×10^{14} Btu, or 17% of the subsector total).

The next most important energy consumption sector in the food system is manufacturing and processing, amounting to some 30% of the total. Within this sector 1.246×10^{15} Btu, or slightly less than 40%, of the energy is directly consumed in the processing function itself. Over 50% of the energy (1.746×10^{15} Btu) is consumed by inputs to the production process (packages, other ingredients, and so on), with the remainder being made up by the energy used to provide capital inputs to manufacturing and for transportation. Energy consumption tends to be relatively evenly divided over the various subsectors of the manufacturing portion of the system. Those that consume the most are those that require power in the production process, such as grain milling; or that require either heat or refrigeration, such as canning and freezing of fruits and vegetables and processing of meat products; or that must separate relatively large amounts of water, such as in sugar refining.

The food production sector uses only about 18% of the total amount of energy consumed in the food system. Approximately 35% (6.87×10^{14} Btu) of this is direct energy consumed in the production process, about 38% (7.56×10^{14} Btu) is energy consumed in the manufacture and provision of pro-

duction inputs, and the remainder is made up of that required for capital inputs and for transportation. Within the production sector the largest consumer of energy is the production of cash grains such as wheat, corn, and soybeans. The next largest is the production of other field crops, followed by livestock production and commercial fishing. Other agricultural activities such as vegetables and melons, fruits, and poultry are relatively minor consumers of energy.

Examining this energy consumption in a different way (Table 2) indicates that direct consumption of fuels and other energy in the food system amounts to some 58% of total consumption. Inputs from outside the system amount to approximately 24% of energy consumption. Energy requirements for provision of capital equipment are 5% of the total, while requirements for transportation, other than transportation in the marketing and distribution sectors, are some 13%.

The above estimates indicate that approximately 17% of all United States energy requirements are consumed by the food system. This estimate may be understated in several ways. There are gaps in data availability, and some factors in the food system may have become more energy-intensive since these estimates were made. Also, it should be noted that almost all of the studies referenced utilized data from the pre−petroleum embargo era. Therefore, any upward or downward shifts within the various sectors that have resulted from price changes brought about by the embargo have not been taken into account. However, this is also true for other energy-consuming sectors of the United States economy.

The FEA study concludes that research to date on energy in the food system is inadequate, particularly relative to capital inputs and transportation. Its recommendations are to improve estimates for these portions of the food system energy use pattern, and to measure the shifts in energy use due to price changes, conservation measures, and so on, that have occurred since 1973.

In reference to the future, a U.S. Department of Agriculture (USDA) study conducted in 1974 indicated that in the decade 1970−1980 farm production use of energy would increase slightly but food processing and manufacturing, marketing and distribution, and production input manufacturing all would increase from 15 to 20%, making for a total increase in energy use of over 11%. However, again, these estimates were made utilizing pre-embargo era data and therefore do not truly reflect changes brought about by price increases and conservation measures.

Table 2. Percent of energy used for selected purposes in the United States food system in 1971*

Purpose	Percent
Direct consumption	58†
Production inputs	24
Transportation	13
Capital inputs	5
Total	100

*From Federal Energy Administration, Office of Industrial Programs, *Energy Use in the Food System*, May 1976.
†Assumes that energy consumed in wholesale and retail trade is all direct.

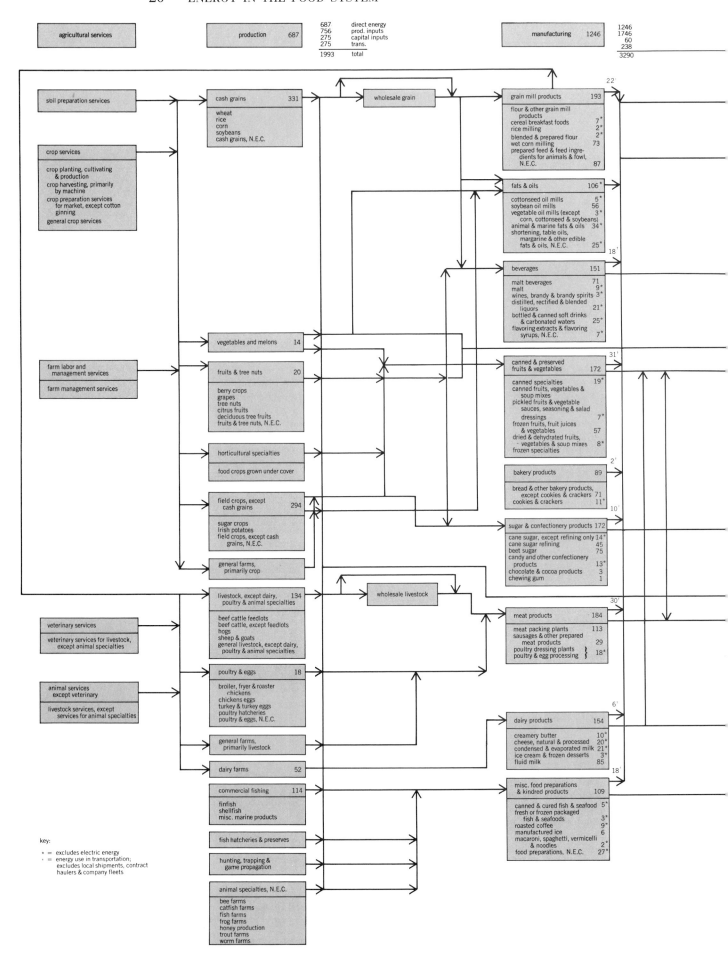

agricultural services

production   687

687	direct energy
756	prod. inputs
275	capital inputs
275	trans.
1993	total

manufacturing   1246

1246	
1746	
60	
238	
3290	

soil preparation services

cash grains   331
wheat
rice
corn
soybeans
cash grains, N.E.C.

wholesale grain

grain mill products   193
flour & other grain mill
  products   22'
cereal breakfast foods   7*
rice milling   2*
blended & prepared flour   2*
wet corn milling   73
prepared feed & feed ingredients for animals & fowl,
  N.E.C.   87

crop services
crop planting, cultivating
  & production
crop harvesting, primarily
  by machine
crop preparation services
  for market, except cotton
  ginning
general crop services

fats & oils   106*
cottonseed oil mills   5*
soybean oil mills   56
vegetable oil mills (except
  corn, cottonseed & soybeans) 3*
animal & marine fats & oils 34*
shortening, table oils,
  margarine & other edible
  fats & oils, N.E.C.   25*

beverages   151
malt beverages   71
malt   9*
wines, brandy & brandy spirits 3*
distilled, rectified & blended
  liquors   21*
bottled & canned soft drinks
  & carbonated waters   25*
flavoring extracts & flavoring
  syrups, N.E.C.   7*

vegetables and melons   14

farm labor and
  management services

farm management services

fruits & tree nuts   20
berry crops
grapes
tree nuts
citrus fruits
deciduous tree fruits
fruits & tree nuts, N.E.C.

canned & preserved
fruits & vegetables   172   31'
canned specialties   19*
canned fruits, vegetables &
  soup mixes
pickled fruits & vegetable
  sauces, seasoning & salad
  dressings   7*
frozen fruits, fruit juices
  & vegetables   57
dried & dehydrated fruits,
  vegetables & soup mixes   8*
frozen specialties

horticultural specialties
food crops grown under cover

bakery products   89   2'
bread & other bakery products,
  except cookies & crackers   71
cookies & crackers   11*

field crops, except
  cash grains   294
sugar crops
Irish potatoes
field crops, except cash
  grains, N.E.C.

sugar & confectionery products 172   10'
cane sugar, except refining only 14*
cane sugar refining   45
beet sugar   75
candy and other confectionery
  products   13*
chocolate & cocoa products   3
chewing gum   1

general farms,
  primarily crop

livestock, except dairy,   134
  poultry & animal specialties
beef cattle feedlots
beef cattle, except feedlots
hogs
sheep & goats
general livestock, except dairy,
  poultry & animal specialties

wholesale livestock

meat products   184   30'
meat packing plants   113
sausages & other prepared
  meat products   29
poultry dressing plants
poultry & egg processing   } 18*

veterinary services
veterinary services for livestock,
  except animal specialties

poultry & eggs   18
broiler, fryer & roaster
  chickens
chickens eggs
turkey & turkey eggs
poultry hatcheries
poultry & eggs, N.E.C.

animal services
  except veterinary
livestock services, except
  services for animal specialties

general farms,
  primarily livestock

dairy products   154   6'
creamery butter   10*
cheese, natural & processed   20*
condensed & evaporated milk   21*
ice cream & frozen desserts   3*
fluid milk   85

dairy farms   52

commercial fishing   114
finfish
shellfish
misc. marine products

misc. food preparations   109   18'
& kindred products
canned & cured fish & seafood   5*
fresh or frozen packaged
  fish & seafoods   3*
roasted coffee   9*
manufactured ice   6
macaroni, spaghetti, vermicelli
  & noodles   2*
food preparations, N.E.C.   27*

fish hatcheries & preserves

key:
* = excludes electric energy
' = energy use in transportation;
  excludes local shipments, contract
  haulers & company fleets

hunting, trapping &
  game propagation

animal specialties, N.E.C.
bee farms
catfish farms
fish farms
frog farms
honey production
trout farms
worm farms

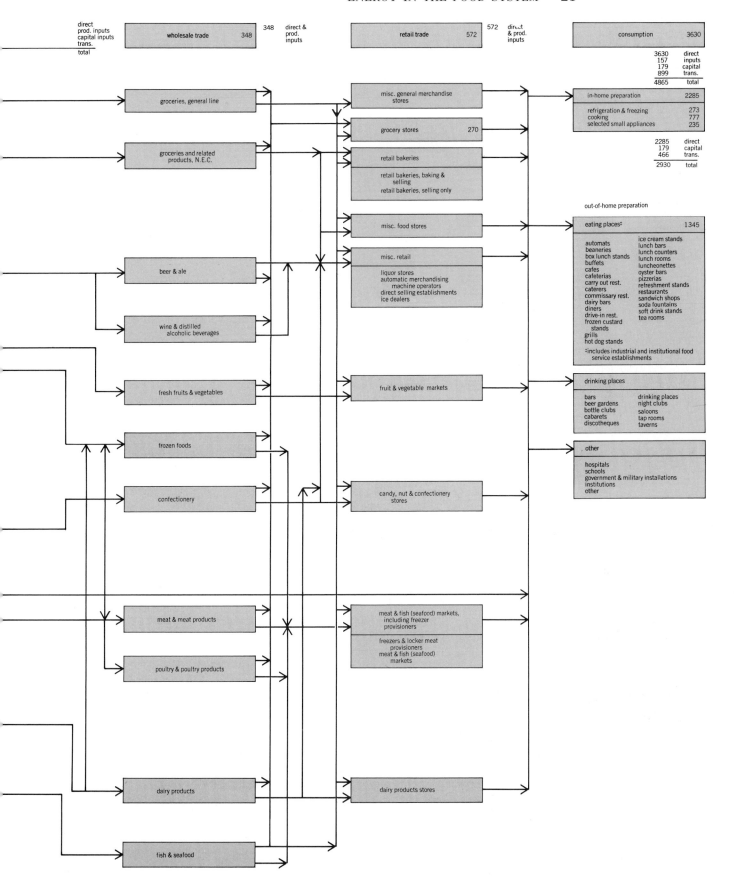

Fig. 2. Energy consumption in the food system, in 10¹²
Btu = 1.055 × 10¹⁵ J. (*From Federal Energy Administration,
Office of Industrial Programs, Energy Use in the Food Sys-
tem, May 1976*)

Table 3. Btu used in United States food and fiber sector by major types of industries and energies in 1970 or later and 1980 (USDA estimates)*

Item	1970† 10¹² Btu‡	Percent	1980 10¹² Btu‡	Percent	Change in percent
Type of industry or use					
Farm production	1,051.4	22.5	1,095.3	21.1	+4.2
Farm family living	554.6	11.9	499.2	9.6	−10.0
Food and kindred product processing	1,302.9	27.9	1,548.3	29.8	+19.8
Marketing and distribution	832.7	17.9	988.9	19.0	+18.8
Input manufacturing§	925.3	19.8	1,063.8	20.5	+15.0
Total	4,666.9	100.0	5,195.5	100.0	+11.3
Type of energy					
Liquid fuels and LPG	2,334.5	50.0	2,502.3	48.2	+7.2
Residual fuel oil	97.5	2.1	115.0	2.2	+17.9
Natural gas	1,414.4	30.3	1,652.7	31.8	+16.8
Electricity	643.0	13.8	738.6	14.2	+14.9
Coal and coke	165.8	3.6	173.6	3.3	+4.7
Other	11.6	0.2	13.3	0.3	+14.7
Total	4,666.9	100.0	5,195.5	100.0	+11.3

*From *The U.S. Food and Fiber Sector: Energy Use and Outlook,* Economic Research Service, U.S. Department of Agriculture for Subcommittee on Agricultural Credit and Rural Electrification of the Committee on Agriculture and Forestry, U.S. Senate, Sept. 20, 1974.
†For some industries data are for 1971, 1972, or 1973.
‡10^{12} Btu $= 1.055 \times 10^{15}$ J.   §Includes estimates for six selected industries.

Sources of energy. It is evident from available estimates that the United States food system relies heavily upon fossil fuels as a primary energy source. According to the previously quoted USDA estimate, 50% of all energy used in the food system in 1970 was represented by liquid fuels and liquefied petroleum gas (LPG), and an additional 30% was represented by natural gas. Electricity is a major source, amounting to some 14%; all other energy sources identified in this study amounted to less than 6% of total consumption (Table 3).

A breakdown of energy sources by function is found in Table 4, with projections to 1980 indicating that energy consumption will increase but will shift somewhat away from liquid fuels and LPG to residual fuel oils, natural gas, electricity, and other energy sources. Again, however, these estimates were made in consideration of the prevailing situation prior to 1973. With the current problems with natural gas, and with the increased prices of other petroleum products, these patterns may change considerably. For example, the food processing and manufacturing industries are major consumers of natural gas. With the current curtailments of natural gas deliveries, many of these industries, especially new processing plants, will likely be shifting to other energy sources and to processes that are more energy-conserving. Similarly in the fertilizer industry a great deal of attention is being given to alternative sources of hydrogen for the production of nitrogenous fertilizers.

United States versus world food system. Comparison of energy consumption in the United States food system with that of the rest of the world is difficult. Data are even less available and coverage even more inadequate in most other parts of the world. G. Leach has attempted to make some comparisons of energy outputs of various types of food systems. His study centers primarily on the United Kingdom, but also attempts to put its agriculture into perspective with the rest of the world. Leach classifies agriculture into four types of systems; preindustrial crops, semi-industrial crops, full industrial crops, and full industrial crops plus animal agriculture combined.

Systems. In preindustrial systems the primary inputs are land and labor or animal power, with very little fossil fuel utilization. Energy use is mainly in the form of human food or animal feeds. These preindustrial systems include hunter-gatherers and subsistence crop production, and are found largely in the tropical zone. The semi-industrial systems are those in which some machinery and fertilizers are used, this being a transition sys-

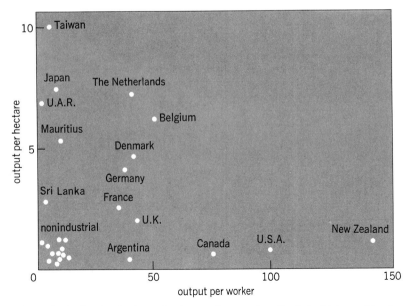

Fig. 3. Agricultural outputs per hectare and per worker. Nonindustrial countries include Brazil, Sri Lanka, Chile, Colombia, Greece, India (which has the lowest output per worker), Mexico, Paraguay, Peru, Spain, Syria, Turkey, and Venezuela (which has the lowest output per hectare). (From G. Leach, *Energy and Food Production, IPC Science and Technology Press Ltd., 1976*)

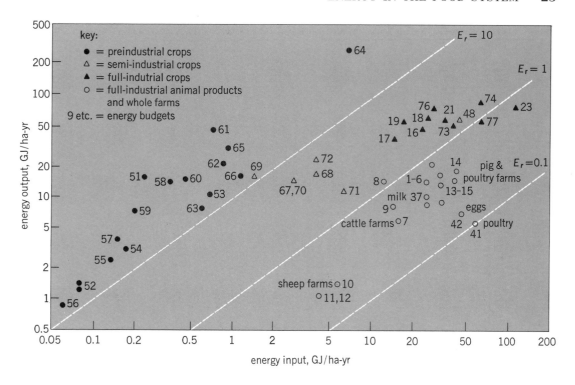

Fig. 4. Comparison of different types of food systems in terms of energy inputs and outputs per unit of land area in world food production. (*From G. Leach, Energy and Food Production, IPC Science and Technology Press Ltd., 1976*)

key:
1-16 whole farms (England and Wales, 1970-1971)
1- 6 dairy farms
7- 9 cattle and sheep farms
10-12 sheep farms
13-15 swine and poultry farms
16 cereal
17 barley (U.K.)
18 maize grain (U.K.)
19 wheat (U.K.)
21 average potatoes (U.K.)
23 sugar (from beet) (U.K.)
37 milk (U.K.)
41 poultry: broiler meat (U.K.)
42 poultry: battery eggs (U.K.)

48 allotment garden (U.K.)
51 shifting cultivators (Congo)
52 Tsembaga (shifting cultivators) (New Guinea)
53 subsistence (India)
54-63 subsistence + shifting, various
54 rice (Dayak)
55 rice (Dayak)
56 rice (Iban)
57 rice (Tanzania)
58 maize (Africa)
59 millet (Africa)
60 sweet potato (Africa)
61 cassava (Africa)
62 yams (Africa)

63 groundnut (Africa)
64 peasant farming (China, 1935-1937)
65 corn (Mexico)
66 corn (Guatemala)
67 corn (Mexico)
68 corn (Guatemala)
69 corn (Nigeria)
70 corn (Philippines)
71 wheat (Uttar Pradesh, India)
72 rice (Philippines)
73 intensive rice (Surinam)
74 intensive rice (U.S.A.)
76 corn (U.S.A., 1970)
77 rice + vegetables (Hong Kong, 1971)

tem between subsistence and commercial production. Some of the crop is marketed, but a large proportion of the agricultural activity is also devoted to providing foodstuffs for the extended farm family. Fully industrial cropping systems are found in the United States, the United Kingdom, Japan, and other countries. In these systems there is a very high degree of substitution of machinery, pesticides, and fertilizer for labor and comparatively high energy use either per unit of land or per farm worker. In combined crop-animal systems most of the output of the cropping systems is fed to animals, and animal products are the final stage.

Energy outputs and inputs. Focusing first on overall productivity of these types of agricultural systems, Fig. 3 indicates that as one moves away from the nonindustrial systems, output increases and the resource base of the individual country determines whether or not the emphasis is on increasing output per unit of land or per unit of la-

bor. In the United States the emphasis is on increasing output per unit of labor, whereas in Japan and Taiwan the reverse is true. Europe falls midway between these extremes.

Table 5 indicates the energy outputs per hour of farm labor for various types of agricultural systems. As one would expect, as more energy-related inputs are substituted for labor, the output per unit of farm labor increases dramatically; as one moves into less output-efficient systems, such as animal production systems, the output per unit of labor decreases in terms of food energy.

Figure 4 compares the different types of food production systems in terms of energy inputs and outputs per unit of land in food production. The preindustrial systems rank very low in terms of output and input, but the ratio of output to input (energy ratio, E_r) is very high—greater than 10 in most cases. But, again, total production is small. As one moves up the scale to more intensive crop

Table 4. Summary of Btu used in United States food and fiber sector, by functions, in 1970 and 1980 (USDA estimates), in 10⁹ Btu (1.055 × 10¹² J)[a]

Function	Gasoline		Diesel		Distillate fuel oil		LPG	
	1970[b]	1980	1970[b]	1980	1970[b]	1980	1970[b]	1980
Farm production								
Crops	377,372	375,215	280,451	300,668	. . . .	. . . .	93,113	100,275
Livestock	125,791	125,071	93,483	100,222	. . . .	. . . .	31,037	33,425
Total farm production	503,163	500,286	373,934	400,890	(c)	(c)	124,150	133,700
Family living								
Transportation	179,603	179,603	968	968	. . . .	. . . .	. . . .	. . . .
Home uses	. . . .	. . . .	. . . .	. . . .	118,442	68,374	104,381	114,504
Total family living	179,603	179,603	968	968	118,442	68,374	104,381	114,504
Food and kindred products[d]								
Processing—14 selected industries:								
Meat packing	. . . .				3,966	. . . .	2,523	. . . .
Sausage; other prepared meat	23				1,848	. . . .	274	. . . .
Dairy products[e]	4,838				19,594	. . . .	4,354	. . . .
Canned fruits and vegetables	. . . .				529	. . . .	1,704	. . . .
Frozen fruits and vegetables[f]	. . . .				242	. . . .	483	. . . .
Wet corn milling	. . . .				3,378	. . . .	225	. . . .
Cane sugar refining	. . . .				142	. . . .	. . . .	
Beet sugar refining	. . . .				75	. . . .	. . . .	
Malt beverages	. . . .				3,641	. . . .	412	. . . .
Total, 14 selected industries	4,861	5,403			33,415	39,624	9,975	11,707
Total, 28 other industries	2,956	3,887			23,912	28,501	6,962	8,421
Total, 42 industries	7,817	9,290			57,327	68,125	16,937	20,128
Marketing and distribution								
Transporting farm products to cities of final consumption	47,027	53,781	470,009	561,108	. . . .	. . . .	. . . .	. . . .
Transporting farm inputs from plants and warehouses to firms	28,766	32,518	286,845	341,449	. . . .	. . . .	. . . .	. . . .
Total marketing and distribution	75,793	86,299	756,854	902,557	. . . .	. . . .	. . . .	. . . .
Input manufacturing[b]								
Prepared feeds and ingredients	1,073	1,183			3,415	3,765	2,927	3,227
Animal and marine fats and oils	238	299			2,274	2,861	272	341
Fertilizer	. . . .				2,286	3,037	. . . .	. . . .
Farm machinery	. . . .				1,136	1,200	. . . .	. . . .
Pesticides	. . . .				309	324	. . . .	. . . .
Petroleum	. . . .				1,200	1,268	. . . .	. . . .
Total input manufacturing	1,311	1,482			10,620	12,455	3,199	3,568
Grand total	767,687	776,960	1,131,756	1,304,415	186,389	148,954	248,667	271,900

[a]From *The U.S. Food and Fiber Sector: Energy Use and Outlook*, Economic Research Service, U.S. Department of Agriculture for Subcommittee on Agricultural Credit and Rural Electrification of the Committee on Agriculture and Forestry, U.S. Senate, Sept. 20, 1974.
[b]Data vary by subsectors from 1970 to 1973.
[c]Included with diesel fuel.
[d]The distribution of total Btu for 1980 by fuel type was assumed to be the same as 1971. No distribution was made for individual industries.
[e]Includes five industries.
[f]Includes frozen specialties.

cultivation, but still in relatively primitive systems, both inputs and outputs per hectare tend to increase but the ratio tends to remain the same. Some of these systems, such as corn production in Mexico or cassava production in Africa, achieve energy outputs per hectare that are equivalent to some of the most advanced farming systems. In fact, the greatest energy output per hectare is found (at least in Leach's budgets) in Chinese peasant agriculture in the pre–World War II era.

Again, moving to the more industrialized systems, outputs increase somewhat but inputs increase more rapidly, and the ratio of output to input tends to decline on a per hectare basis. In animal production systems the energy output/input ratios decline even further; and in Leach's budgets the lowest ratios are found in poultry production in the United Kingdom.

These analyses led Leach to the conclusion that there are diminishing returns in the utilization of energy as agriculture moves from primitive to fully industrialized systems. Therefore, society should examine means of energy conservation, alternative energy sources, and the merits of systems having energy ratios greater than 1 with high productivity.

PETROLEUM PRICES AND AGRICULTURAL PRODUCTION

United States agricultural production has become increasingly energy-intensive over the past 2 decades. One important reason behind this trend was the relatively stable energy prices prevailing until 1973 (Fig. 5). A second reason is that the effects of agricultural commodity programs have been capitalized into land prices and have imposed constraints on land input that make it profitable to substitute fertilizer, pesticides, and machinery inputs. Also, the social costs of waste and residue disposal and farm labor displacement have been undervalued and not fully internalized into agricultural costs.

Table 4. Summary of Btu used in United States food and fiber sector, by functions, in 1970 and 1980 (USDA estimates), in 10⁹ Btu (1.055 × 10¹² J)ᵃ (cont.)

Function	Residual fuel oil 1970 or later	1980	Natural gas 1970 or later	1980	Electricity 1970 or later	1980	Coal 1970 or later	1980	Other 1970 or later	1980	Total 1970 or later	1980
Farm production												
Crops					12,539	15,098					763,475	791,256
Livestock					37,617	45,294					287,928	304,012
Total farm production					50,156	60,392					1,051,403	1,095,268
Family living												
Transportation											180,571	180,571
Home uses			37,260	44,505	87,006	81,438	26,936	9,828			374,025	318,649
Total family living			37,260	44,505	87,006	81,438	26,936	9,828			554,596	499,220
Food and kindred products												
Processing — 14 selected industries:												
Meat packing	6,249		58,643		36,652		12,137				120,170	137,923
Sausage; other prepared meat	844		11,045		8,581		205				22,820	25,864
Dairy products	9,918		84,425		110,792		7,983				241,904	248,041
Canned fruits and vegetables	3,995		40,888		9,634		1,997				58,747	72,880
Frozen fruits and vegetables	1,353		20,341		24,157		1,739				48,315	83,658
Wet corn milling	976		33,183		10,586		26,727				75,075	96,061
Cane sugar refining	14,341		32,718		285						47,486	48,624
Beet sugar refining	1,790		49,458		1,044		19,246		2,984		74,597	89,749
Malt beverages	7,901		26,312		25,625		4,809				68,700	97,750
Total, 14 selected industries	47,367	56,735	357,013	424,159	227,356	270,165	74,843	89,155	2,984	3,602	757,814	900,550
Total, 28 other industries	34,715	40,808	256,644	305,087	163,509	194,323	54,142	64,126	2,228	2,591	545,068	647,744
Total, 42 industries	82,082	97,543	613,657	729,246	390,865	464,488	128,985	153,281	5,212	6,193	1,302,882	1,548,294
Marketing and distribution												
Transporting farm products to cities of final consumption											517,036	614,889
Transporting farm inputs from plants and warehouses to firms											315,611	373,967
Total marketing and distribution											832,647	988,856
Input manufacturing												
Prepared feeds and ingredients	2,341	2,582	51,999	57,334	35,511	39,155	293	323			97,559	107,569
Animal and marine fats and oils	3,123	3,928	22,372	28,136	5,398	6,789	272	341			33,949	42,695
Fertilizer	930	1,215	491,044	581,477	58,743	70,086	1,150	1,518	1,554	2,025	555,707	659,358
Farm machinery	660	700	18,009	18,400	4,436	4,500	5,345	5,400	1,798	1,800	31,384	32,000
Pesticides	390	409	6,417	6,747	921	967	1,593	1,672	696	731	10,326	10,850
Petroleum	8,000	8,665	173,700	186,834	10,000	10,779	1,200	1,268	2,300	2,536	196,400	211,350
Total input manufacturing	15,444	17,499	763,541	878,928	115,009	132,276	9,853	10,522	6,348	7,092	925,325	1,063,822
Grand total	97,526	115,042	1,414,458	1,652,679	643,036	738,594	165,774	173,631	11,560	13,285	4,666,853	5,195,460

While United States farm output from 1960 through 1976 increased by 22%, the use of farm labor declined by 44% and the use of farm real estate by 6%. On the other hand, mechanical power and machinery inputs increased by 6%, and the use of agricultural chemicals by a staggering 172% (Fig. 6). However, during the first half of the 1970s there has been no growth in crop and livestock production. Crop production per acre has also remained static during the 1971–1976 period (Fig. 7).

Since the initial impacts of the energy crisis during the early 1970s, numerous suggestions have been made for energy-conserving practices in agriculture. However, in all cases the trade-off between energy conversion, yields, and other input requirements and costs must be considered. Therefore, it does not follow that United States farmers have been economically irrational in their use of energy. The migration of people away from farming as a way of life served to stimulate a trend toward larger farm units and, consequently, a higher degree of mechanization to maintain productivity levels. New technologies in pesticides and fertilizers offered another avenue for greatly

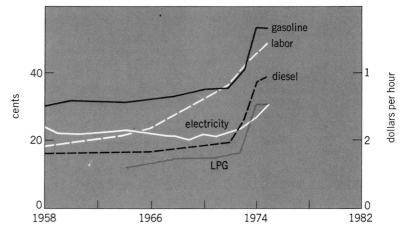

Fig. 5. Energy prices paid by farmers. Electricity in cents per 10 kWh (10 kWh = 3.6 × 10⁷ J), and gasoline, diesel, LPG in cents per gallon (1 gal = 3.8 liters). (From U.S. Department of Agriculture, Handbook of Agricultural Charts, Agr. Handb. no. 504, 1976)

increasing crop productivity during the past 25 years. The low energy prices prevailing during the 1950s and 1960s greatly stimulated the adoption of

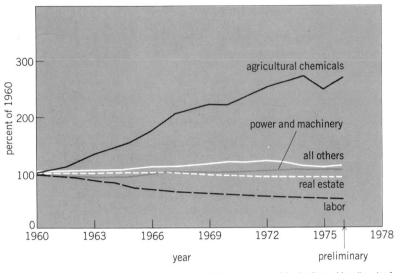

Fig. 6.   Use of selected farm inputs. *(From U.S. Department of Agriculture, Handbook of Agricultural Charts, Agr. Handb. no. 504, 1976)*

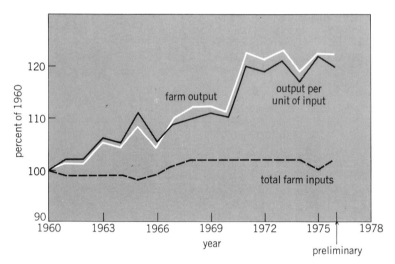

Fig. 7.   Farm productivity. *(From U.S. Department of Agriculture, Handbook of Agricultural Charts, Agr. Handb. no. 504, 1976)*

Table 5. Food energy outputs per worker-hour of farm labor*

Agricultural system	Output, megajoules per worker-hour
Preindustrial crops	
Ikung Bushmen, hunter-gatherers	4.5
Subsistence rice, tropics	11 – 19
Subsistence maize, millet, sweet potato, tropics	25 – 30
Peasant farmers, China	40
Semi-industrial crops	
Rice, tropics	40
Maize, tropics	23 – 48
Full-industrial crops	
Rice, U.S.A.	2800
Cereals, U.K.	3040
Maize, U.S.A.	3800
Full-industrial crops plus animal	
Sheep, cattle, pig and poultry, dairy farms, U.K.	50 – 170
Cereal farms, U.K. (small animal output)	800
U.K. allotment garden, approx.	4.3
U.K. food system, approx.	30 – 35

*From G. Leach, *Energy and Food Production*, IPC Science and Technology Press Ltd., 1976.

these technologies. The pattern of land ownership that has developed over this period is not adaptable to labor-intensive production, except for limited acreages of high-value specialty crops.

Impacts on agricultural chemicals. Increased usage of agricultural chemicals, including fertilizers, has been a primary factor behind higher crop productivity per acre. For example, the application of fertilizers and pesticides to corn has resulted in increasing average United States corn yields from 55 bu/acre (4.8 m³/ha) in 1960 to 87 bu/acre (7.6 m³/ha) in 1976—an increase of almost 60%. The stimulus behind increased fertilizer usage has been its price relative to other farm inputs (Fig. 8). Thus, fertilizer offered an economically effective means of increasing crop yields. Beginning in 1974, fertilizer prices began to increase sharply. However, in 1976 a decline in average fertilizer prices and an increase in corn production acreage again stimulated fertilizer consumption to record highs.

Fertilizers account for about one-third of cultural energy requirements for food, feed, and fiber production (Fig. 9). Nitrogen fertilizers are most widely used and require 85% of the total energy used to produce all fertilizers. Although 90% of the energy used to produce nitrogen fertilizer, especially anhydrous ammonia, comes from natural gas, this represents only 2% of total United States natural gas consumption. Manufacture of all fertilizers requires about 1% of total United States energy requirements.

Approximately 35,000 ft³ (990 m³) of natural gas is necessary to produce 1 ton (0.9 metric ton) of anhydrous ammonia (NH_3). If the price of natural gas were assumed to double from $1 to $2 per 1000 ft³ (28.3 m³), the cost of producing 1 ton of ammonia would rise by approximately $35 per ton. Furthermore, if the initial price of ammonia were $200 per ton at the farm level, the price after the doubling of natural gas costs would be about $235 per ton, assuming that marketing and distribution margins remained unchanged. Since fertilizers represent approximately one-half of total cultural energy requirements to produce corn, a farmer applying 200 lb per acre (224 kg/ha) of NH_3 on corn would have a cost increase of $3.50 per acre ($8.65/ha) as a direct result of the doubling of natural gas prices. However, total production costs for corn grain in the Midwest are approximately $275–300 per acre ($680–740/ha), including fixed costs of land and machinery ownership. Therefore, the $3.50-per-acre increase attributable to a doubling in natural gas prices represents an increase in total corn production costs of only slightly over 1.2%

The above example indicates that (1) higher fertilizer prices are not entirely attributable to higher energy prices, and (2) sharp increases in energy prices exert a significantly smaller impact on final crop production costs. However, a simultaneous increase in natural gas, gasoline, diesel fuel, and propane gas prices (these fuels are used in drying corn grain) will naturally exert a greater impact than price increases for just one fuel source.

Impact on food costs. One recent study estimated the energy inputs for food commodities produced in the state of Washington (Fig. 10). This study indicated that a 100% increase in petroleum prices would result in a 2% increase in the cost of transporting food to the consumer; a 100% change in electricity prices would increase food costs by 2.3%; a 100% increase in natural gas prices would increase food costs about 0.7%; and a 100% rise in all energy prices would increase food costs by 5%.

It should be noted that retail food prices might increase more than the actual change in total costs affected by energy price increases due to changes in absolute marketing margins. However, it is apparent that energy still contributes a relatively small share of total food costs. It is possible that the income effect of an energy price increase on the demand for food may be more significant than the direct cost effect. That is, a doubling of energy prices could significantly affect the disposable income of consumers in other non-food-related ways. This reduction in disposable income theoretically would cause reductions in the demand for food, particularly in the demand for luxury-type food items as compared with basic staples.

ALTERNATE SOURCES OF ENERGY

Because agricultural production depends heavily upon the type of energy in shortest supply, there is considerable interest in broadening the energy base so that restricted availability of petroleum-based fuels will not inhibit United States capabilities as a world food supplier. A number of alternative energy sources are under development.

Solar radiation. The temperatures that can be obtained by using flat-plate collector technology appear to make solar energy most applicable to uses where low-grade heat is required, such as in heating livestock shelters, greenhouses, and rural residences, and in artificial crop drying. However, it is conceivable that advanced concentrator-collector technology might be developed that would permit use of solar energy for high-temperature applications, such as steam generation and high-speed drying.

Solar energy is currently used for grain drying; however, existing systems can be cumbersome and costly. The use of solar heat appears more feasible than natural air drying east of the Mississippi River because of more humid natural air conditions.

Another potential use of solar energy is in powering irrigation pumps. The commercial application of solar energy to irrigation could be especially important in the southwestern region of the United States, where many crops must be irrigated and a relatively large number of cloud-free sunny days occur. The potential for energy savings is significant. For example, nearly three times more fuel is used in growing irrigated than nonirrigated sorghum. More than twice as much fuel is used on irrigated alfalfa, soybeans, and wheat, and about 50% more fuel is used to grow irrigated corn, cotton, and fruit. Research is also underway on utilizing a complete solar system to heat farm homes and adjacent buildings.

Wind. Although wind is a potential alternative power source, currently available wind-driven generating systems are not sufficiently efficient to make such systems practical under present conditions. However, as fuel costs increase, the wind turbine system may become competitive with other power generation systems. The potential for development of wind power varies among regions

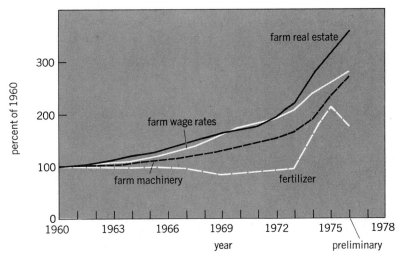

Fig. 8. Prices of selected farm inputs. (*From U.S. Department of Agriculture, Handbook of Agricultural Charts, Agr. Handb. no. 504, 1976*)

in the United States. The High Plains, the New England coast, and the Pacific Northwest offer the greatest potential for wind power, while the Southeast has the lowest potential.

Biomass. There are several categories of plants possessing inherent capabilities for capturing and storing large quantities of solar energy. For example, sugarcane can produce 35–90 metric tons of dry matter per hectare per year. Energy systems utilizing this biomass as sources of liquid fuels (such as ethanol and methanol) and of gaseous fuels (such as substitute natural gas and ammonia) are under investigation (Fig. 11). Biomass can also be used for direct combustion to generate electric power. In fact, this practice has been followed in Hawaiian sugarcane mills for years to dispose of the bagasse residues remaining after raw sugar has been extracted from the cane.

In addition to sugar crops, several potential sources of plant biomass are available and conceivably could be useful as energy feedstocks.

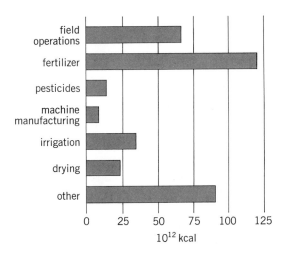

Fig. 9. Energy for food, feed, and fiber production; 10^{12} kcal = 4.19×10^{15} J. (*From L. F. Nelson et al., Recognizing Productive, Energy-Efficient Agriculture in the Complex U.S. Food System, Amer. Soc. Agr. Eng. Pap. no. 75–7505, December 1975*)

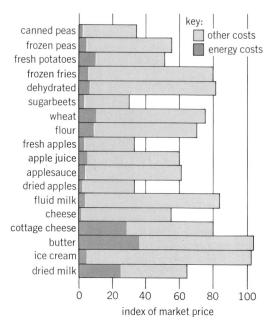

Fig. 10. Relative proportions of total energy cost, other costs, and gross marketing margins. (From N. K. Whittlesey and C. Lee, Impacts of Energy Price Changes on Food Costs, Coll. Agr. Res. Center Bull. no. 822, Washington State University, April 1976)

These include trees, various grains and grasses, and various forms of marine vegetation. Formal plantations for the cultivation of selected high-yield plant species for the sole purpose of biomass production offer the greatest potential in terms of yield per unit area or time. The state of the art of technology is much more advanced in terrestrial plantations; hence, biomass production costs are currently much lower than on marine plantations. However, the concept of marine plantations is intriguing in that they are essentially free of two important restrictions imposed on terrestrial plantations—namely, limited availability of land and adequate moisture.

The cost of biomass material for energy feedstocks varies according to the crop species and its productivity per unit area. The estimated costs of biomass derived from sugarcane, delivered to a processing plant, are approximately $50–60 per metric ton. One metric ton (dry weight) of sugarcane will yield an estimated 0.21 metric ton of ethanol, 0.13 metric ton of ethylene, and 0.23 metric ton of ammonia or methanol.

The conversion of biomass into ammonia could directly benefit farmers since ammonia is an important source of nitrogen fertilizer. This use of biomass could free natural gas for other uses. However, in order to produce ammonia the biomass would have to be dried, which would entail an energy input.

Agricultural wastes and residues. The estimated annual production of agricultural wastes and residues in the United States has been estimated to range between 6 and 8×10^8 dry metric tons. Primarily these include residues from crops left in the field following harvest, livestock and poultry manures, and forestry residues. The theoretical energy potential from animal wastes alone is indicated in Table 6. It should be noted that not all of the waste is readily collectable and that inefficiencies of conversion reduce the total potential considerably. Research investigation of the application of known anaerobic digester technologies may eventually result in part of this potential being realized.

The use of agricultural residues has several apparent advantages: (1) Residue production is not restricted by geography and occurs wherever crops are grown. (2) Costs of residue production are partially defrayed by the sales value of the commodity being produced. (3) Residue sales could provide additional income to farmers. (4) Often residue use would eliminate costly and environmentally sensitive disposal problems. (5) No new land or water development would be required for residue production.

Disadvantages of agricultural residues for energy purposes are also readily apparent: (1) Uses have already been found for many residues, including livestock feeds, field mulches, erosion control, fertilizer, and manufacture of various wood products. (2) Residue production, especially crop residues, is highly seasonal, resulting in discontinuity of supplies. (3) Annual production in localized areas depends on market conditions and normal crop rotation practices, thus resulting in fluctuating supplies. (4) Most residues have high moisture contents which inhibit burning efficiency and prohibit storage unless dried artificially, which requires large quantities of energy. (5) The widespread distribution of residues results in high collection and transportation costs in many cases. These costs, combined with the value of the residues in alternative end uses, may exceed the economic value of the residues as an energy feedstock.

FERTILIZER ALTERNATIVES

Since fertilizer accounts for such a large amount of energy used in agricultural production, various methods for reducing fertilizer requirements are under investigation.

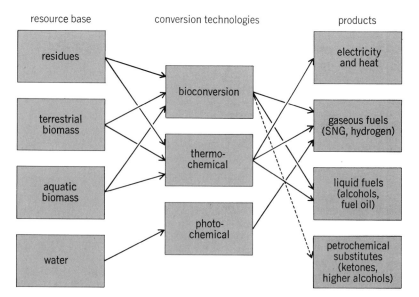

Fig. 11. Fuels from biomass. (From R. Ward, Energy Research and Development Administration, Fuels from Biomass Program, a speech delivered at the "Biomass—A Cash Crop for the Future?" Conference, Kansas City, MO, Mar. 2–3, 1977)

Table 6. Energy potential from animal wastes in the United States*

Production	Beef, 1000 lb weight	Dairy, 1000 lb weight	Poultry, 5 lb weight	Swine, 100 lb weight
Waste, lb/animal/day	10	6	0.70	0.70
Methane gas†, ft³/animal/day	27	18	0.18	3.6
Number of animals to produce the equivalent of 1 gal of gasoline/day	8	12	1250	60
Total United States potential, 10⁶ gal of gasoline/day	8.6	0.975	2.5	1.4

*1 lb = 0.454 kg; 1 ft³ = 0.0283 m³; 1 gal = 3.8 liters; 1 Btu = 1055 J.
†The heat value of anaerobic digester gas is approximately 600 Btu/ft³.
SOURCE: W. J. Jewell, *Energy from Agricultural Wastes — Methane Generation*, Cornell Univ. Agr. Eng. Ext. Bull. 397, 1974.

Methods of fertilizing. Increasing use is being made of soil tests and tissue analysis to determine the optimum rates of fertilization. Although the implementation of these techniques is not likely to decrease total chemical fertilizer usage, they serve as guides to maximization of net economic returns.

Attention also is being given to timing and method of application of fertilizers. The objective of timing is to provide nutrients to plants when needed with a minimum nutrient loss from the soil or with a minimum loss of availability to the plant due to nutrient interactions with the soil. This is particularly true with nitrogen, which may be lost in drainage water and by change to gaseous forms escaping into the atmosphere. However, there is a certain trade-off between efficiency of nitrogen fertilization and time needed to accomplish other essential farming operations.

Localized placement of fertilizer, such as in a band close to the crop row, can increase the efficiency of absorption of phosphorus and, to a lesser extent, potassium. The greatest benefit from localized application is derived in soils that interact strongly with these elements to reduce their availability; only small amounts of fertilizer are applied to these soils. Under current economic conditions, the quantity of fertilizers that yield such differences in efficiency are below those that yield the maximum net return. The comparative advantage of localized application over broadcast application will increase with an increase in the ratio of fertilizer cost to crop price. See FERTILIZING.

Crop interplanting. Interplanting of crops, such as corn with a legume that fixes atmospheric nitrogen, presents an alternative way to meet some or all of the nitrogen needs without use of nitrogen fertilizer. One experimental system uses crown vetch, a long-lived perennial legume, which is planted and allowed to grow in a solid stand for a year. The stand is then weakened by spraying with a herbicide in the spring of the second year, and corn is planted by minimum tillage methods. The corn outgrows the crown vetch, and by early fall, when the corn is maturing, the crown vetch has recovered from the herbicide treatment and again is growing. Corn is grown each year, and the crown vetch is allowed to remain on the land without being plowed. Experimental corn yields with this system, where 50 lb of nitrogen fertilizer are used per acre (57 kg/ha) with the corn, have been similar to those with about 150 lb (161 kg/ha) of nitrogen fertilizer without the crown vetch. Once the crown vetch is established, therefore, the potential saving of nitrogen fertilizer appears to be about 100 lb per acre (114 kg/ha).

Plant genetics. A longer-term development for reducing fertilizer use is genetic manipulation of plants. Leguminous crops, such as soybeans, do not require nitrogen fertilizer and ultimately require less energy for production than nonleguminous crops. For example, soybeans have the ability to extract nitrogen from the air and make it available for plant growth. The development of corn, sorghum, wheat, and rice capable of biological nitrogen fixation would reduce the requirement for fertilizer nitrogen and thus release fuel for other purposes. Similarly, genetic incorporation of insecticide resistance into crop plants would reduce insecticide requirements and the energy used in their production. *See the feature article* THE GREEN REVOLUTION.

Animal manure and sewage sludge. The application of animal manures and urban sewage sludge are other possibilities for reducing fertilizer use. Animal manures and sewage sludge have the disadvantage that they cannot be formulated and tailored to specific nutrient requirements, such as chemical fertilizers. Thus, use of these materials to correct a single nutrient deficiency may cause excesses and imbalances in nutrients not deficient. Concentration of nutrients in these materials are generally much lower than in chemical fertilizers, and this increases transportation costs. Nitrogen is the major plant nutrient contained in manure. Volatilization of ammonia from animal manure is a large flow of nitrogen that decreases manure's value as a fertilizer replacement.

Sewage sludge application has been practiced in various parts of the United States on a limited basis. The greatest limitation to land application of sewage sludge is the difficulty of distribution on the land because of either wet conditions or a growing crop. Soil compaction is another limitation, and balloon tires, irrigation equipment, or other means must be used to distribute the load to minimize soil compaction. The biggest advantage of sewage sludge application appears to be the addition of humus material to the soil.

IMPROVING ENERGY EFFICIENCY

Obviously, over the long term, there will be an increasing pressure on the United States system to increase its total agricultural production, although demand will fluctuate from year to year depending upon production conditions in the rest of the world. With changing supply and price conditions for energy, it is evident that attention must be given to increasing the energy efficiency of agricultural production processes while maintaining their overall productivity and economic efficiency. Conceptually, one can approach this either by increasing production with the same energy input or by decreasing energy input for the same production. In recommending changes in the agricultural system, however, one must be sure that the changes recommended will have the desired effect.

Alternative energy sources. At the moment, the principal concern is over the availability and prices of fossil fuels, particularly those based on petroleum or natural gas. The increased use of alternative sources is also being debated. Increased use of solar and other nonexhaustible energy sources would alleviate the energy availability problem. However, none of these alternative sources will be available at zero cost, and it is likely that the cost of all energy sources will increase. Therefore, alternative energy sources may only be a temporary solution. At the same time, attention must be given to energy efficiency.

Minimum tillage methods. Changing the conventional system for field crop production to minimize the number of steps, especially those that have relatively high energy demands such as plowing and cultivating, is being researched and increasingly applied. There are a number of so-called minimum tillage systems. Most involve substituting a disking operation for plowing and substituting herbicide applications for weed-control cultivation. Others minimize the land-filling operation by utilizing techniques which seed directly into a sod or relatively undisturbed field. By making these changes it is possible under certain conditions to reduce the fuel requirements for this stage of the crop production process by 60 to 75%. However, this is only one phase in the total cropping system, and minimum tillage does not exert any impact on the other stages.

There are several drawbacks to the application of minimum tillage methods. The increased use of herbicides requires petroleum and other energy sources for herbicide manufacture. This is almost an even trade-off with the energy required for conventional weed-control cultivation. In many circumstances, minimum tillage results in yield reductions of 5 to 15%. Furthermore, these methods are not suitable to all soil conditions—for example, some of the heavier soil types, such as those found in the central part of the United States Corn Belt. In addition, the producer runs a greater risk of problems with certain insects and diseases, and thus experiences a greater need for pesticides or a further reduction yield—both of which reduce the energy efficiency of this method.

If properly applied, these methods can reduce labor requirements in the field crop production process and, therefore, can improve labor efficiency. But they also require a higher degree of control and greater sophistication of management practices.

While, on balance, it is difficult to accurately pinpoint the potential for energy saving by reduced tillage, it appears that a significant portion of United States cropping areas are suitable for some reduced tillage. Application of these methods would result in fuel savings, particularly in the spring and early summer months. Because of these savings, minimum tillage methods are being increasingly applied, particularly in the Great Plains wheat areas. If these methods were extended to corn and soybean cultivation, further savings

could result. For example, if farmers could eliminate an average of one field operation on 25% of the 1.325×10^8 acres (5.364×10^7 ha) that were planted to corn and soybeans in 1975, there would be a savings of some 1.65×10^7 gal (6.25×10^7 liters) of diesel fuel equivalent per year. *See* RE-DUCED TILLAGE AGRICULTURE.

Irrigation improvements. Changes in the efficiency and management of irrigation practices could result in energy savings in two directions—the fuels and other energies required for pumping and distributing water, and reduction of nitrogen and other fertilizer losses as a result of excessive water use. Possible changes include improvements in the pumping efficiencies and pumping mechanisms themselves and application of improved distribution systems, such as trickle and subsurface irrigation. Such systems, while costly to install, will reduce the amount of water required and will apply the water to proper locations in plant root zones for maximum plant utilization. This reduces leaching of soil nutrients while saving water. Further, there are improvements possible in irrigation management practices to avoid untimely irrigation or overwatering.

Research in Nebraska on the field performance of irrigation systems indicates that relatively simple adjustments (tuning) of pumping plants under field operations could reduce the energy required by 13% in the state of Nebraska alone. Further, replacing older, less efficient plants with newer ones would permit an even greater efficiency, providing for approximately a 24% reduction in energy. Other studies have shown that better irrigation management and scheduling practices can save from 15 to 35% of the water presently being pumped in Nebraska, thus effecting substantial energy savings up to 35%. Lowering the pressures of sprinkling systems is another way to save energy in irrigation. Other Nebraska work indicates that pressure reduction in that state is possible and could save up to 50% of the energy requirement in those systems where pressure reduction is feasible. *See* IRRIGATION OF CROPS.

Alternative crop-drying technologies. In the past several decades, there has been a shift away from field drying of farm crops to heated-air drying, particularly for tobacco, soybeans, corn, and to some extent, other grains. These systems have been adopted because of their increased overall productivity and the improved flexibility that is afforded the crop production process. They are another factor in helping the farmer combat variable weather conditions. Substantial amounts of energy are used in this process as in any water removal process (Table 7). Systems could be developed to minimize the requirement for crop drying; however, these will take time to evolve and may have adverse impacts on the overall productivity of the cropping system.

Considerable attention is being paid to increasing the energy efficiency of various drying techniques. In Table 8 several of these techniques are identified and their relative energy efficiency is indicated.

Another approach is to increase the utilization of higher-moisture-content grains, particularly corn and other feed grains. The problem is that wet grains deteriorate more rapidly than grains with moisture content below 10–14%, unless they are

Table 7. Fuel requirements for crop drying in 1973[a]

Commodity	Total production, 10^6	Total dried, 10^6	Fuel used (LPG equivalents)[b], 10^6 gal
Corn	5661 bu	3963 bu	609[c]
Tobacco (flue-cured)	0.575 acre	0.575 acre	348[d]
Soybeans	1539 bu	277 bu	20.2[e]
Rice	220 bu	220 bu	10.9[f]
Peanuts	131 bu	131 bu	10.4[g]
Sorghum	936 bu	94 bu	7.3[h]

[a]1 bu = 0.0352 m^3, 1 gal = 3.8 liters, 1 acre = 4047 m^2, 1 Btu = 1055 J.
[b]Natural gas = 1050 Btu/ft^3, LPG = 92,000 Btu/gal, gasoline = 128,000 Btu/gal.
[c]10 points removal of water, 6.5 bu/gal of fuel.
[d]Assumes 443 gal of gasoline equivalent per acre (South Carolina unpublished data).
[e]Assumes 18% of total production was dried 4 points, 13.7 bu/gal of fuel.
[f]Assumes 6 points removal, low temperature, 50% dried on farm, balance dried continuous-flow, 2 pass, 150°F (66°C) temperature, 20.2 bu/gal of fuel.
[g]Assumes all production dried (South Carolina unpublished data), 12.6 bu/gal of fuel.
[h]Assumes 10% of production was dried, 12.0 bu/gal of fuel.
SOURCE: Council for Agricultural Science and Technology, *Potential for Energy Conservation in Agricultural Production*, Rep. no. 40, Ames, IA, February 1975.

Table 8. Energy efficiencies of various drying techniques[a]

Drying technique	Drying efficiency[b], bu/gal of LPG	Comments
1. Batch or continuous flow with cooling in dryer (180–220°F; 82–104°C)	6.5	High-capacity, flexible, high kernel stress from fast drying and cooling, incomplete air saturation
2. Batch or continuous flow with dryeration[c] (180–220°F; 82–104°C)	8.1	Increased capital investment, two handlings to storage, 50 to 60% increase in throughput, improved product quality
3. Bin drying without stirring device (10°F, or 5°C, rise with 55% RH humidistat control)	9.2	Overdrying in bottom layers, difficult to manage for optimum performance
4. Bin drying with stirring device (110–140°F; 43–60°C)	9.2	Mechanical reliability may be a problem, flexible in grain depth, fast batch procedures
5. Bin batch drying with cooling in bin (120–140°F; 49–60°C)	9.2	Modest price, medium capacity, additional manual labor for daily leveling and unloading
6. Electric bin drying[d] (2–7°F, or 1–3.5°C, rise)	7.7	Slow drying rate, mold increase, dependent on weather, good grain quality, limits on grain moisture content
7. Combination system, 5% with batch or continuous flow drying, 2% with dryeration, 3% with aeration[e]	12.6	Same as technique 1 or 5 except final drying (without heat) and cooling done in another bin, increase in potential for mold during final drying
8. Drying with ambient air (2°F, or 1°C, rise)	—	Slow drying, grain must be below 20% in moisture content, vulnerable to mold, weather conditions critical
9. Solar heat drying	—	Technology is still in the developmental stage and potential use is not yet known, potential for use as a supplemental source of heat may be practical with development of technology

[a]1 bu = 0.0352 m^3, 1 gal = 3.8 liters.
[b]Based on drying 10 points (25 to 15% wet basis), 2100 Btu/lb of water for high-temperature dryer, and 1500 Btu/lb of water for bin-drying systems.
[c]Dryeration response is a constant 2 points of drying, assuming a kernel temperature of 120 to 140°F (49 to 60°C).
[d]Electric drying based on 0.35 kWh per bushel per point of moisture removed.
[e]Based on dryeration air flow of 1 ft^3 per bushel per minute for 20 hr plus aeration air flow of 0.5 ft^3 per bushel per minute for 30 days.
SOURCE: Council for Agricultural Science and Technology, *Potential for Energy Conservation in Agricultural Production*, Rep. no. 40, Ames, IA, February 1975.

stored under special conditions. Many of these storage techniques require utilization of increased amounts of energy; therefore, the trade-offs have to be carefully evaluated. Furthermore, the potential for introducing increased amounts of wet grains into the livestock feeding pictures is limited, although wet grain feeding can be increased over present amounts.

Increasing energy conversion efficiency in plants. The total productive efficiency of a plant can be increased in a number of ways. For exam-

ple, most of the dry weight of plants comes from the assimilation of carbon dioxide through photosynthetic processes. The efficiency of this process varies among the plant species and among varieties within species. On a short-term basis, productivity can be increased by selecting varieties that are the most efficient under the conditions of planting and cultivation. Furthermore, respiration of plants occurs both in light and in darkness. "Dark respiration" tends to waste energy, CO_2, water, and nutrients because photosynthesis cannot take place at this time. Photorespiration (which occurs in light) may outrun the ability of the photosynthetic processes to deal with CO_2 in the plant system, especially under warm light conditions. This then results in inefficient CO_2 assimilation. Some plants, such as corn, have built-in regulatory mechanisms to reduce these inefficiencies. There may be both genetic and chemical means to achieve a greater balance between the respiration processes and the photosynthetic process, thus achieving greater carbon and energy efficiency in a wider range of plants.

Other mechanisms, such as improved plant geometry, to increase access to sunlight and therefore improve ability to capture more solar energy for the photosynthetic processes, will aid in increasing efficiency. Also, new crops might be introduced that will aid in the overall energy conservation effort in agriculture and perhaps add to the energy resource base. In sum, greater attention to energy-related perimeters in plant breeding, plant selection, and genetic improvement programs can result in greater plant energy efficiencies and, therefore, increases in both productivity and energy conservation. Many of these changes will require relatively long time periods, but some can be brought about in a few years. *See* BREEDING (PLANT).

Animal systems. A high proportion of United States crop production, especially the so-called feed grains, is converted by animals into products that are more desirable to consumers. One way, recommended by many, to increase the energy efficiency in the total agricultural system in the United States would be to change this pattern and utilize more crop products directly as food products. However, this would require a major change in eating habits not only of Americans but also of most other Western populations.

Another alternative may be to increase the feed efficiency of the animal by improving the conversion of plant to animal tissues. Means of effecting this include development of improved criteria and knowledge in breeding and animal improvement systems, more effective disease control, increased reproductive efficiency, and improved knowledge of nutrition. *See* BREEDING (ANIMAL).

Reduction of waste. There are a number of ways in which agricultural production systems could be "tightened up" and wasteful practices eliminated. These include more effective utilization of the total plant (the so-called biomass concept), improved utilization of animal waste, improved disease and pest control, and reduction of postharvest losses. Virtually all agricultural enterprises in the United States could reduce waste and increase waste utilization, given proper incentives.

Management practices. Management practices in agriculture can also be "fine-tuned" to adjust for increased energy cost and decreased energy availability. More effective control throughout the food system undoubtedly would result in greater energy efficiency. This would involve taking energy parameters into greater account in decision-making and management control process. To do this may require the application of more sophisticated management practices in all sectors of the food system.

Conclusion. These are but a few indicative ways to increase energy efficiency in the food system. They are mainly relevant to the production and inputs sectors of the system. The listing is not exhaustive, and further study will undoubtedly uncover even more ways than are known today. A similar enumeration can be developed for other sectors of the system. Therefore, there is substantial scope for increasing energy efficiency, even though in comparison with other sectors of the United States economy the amount of energy used in agriculture and the total food system is relatively small. However, it is likely that as final demand pressures on the United States food system increase, the total amount of energy used will grow despite efficiency improvements.

[IVAN L. KINNE; THOMAS A. MC CLURE]

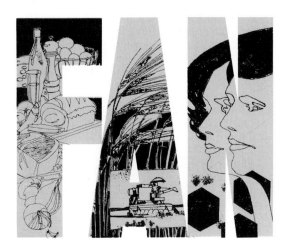

FOOD FROM THE SEA

Frederick J. King

nutritionists estimate that food production is becoming less adequate to meet the demand for good-quality protein at moderate prices. Most seafoods are excellent resources for meeting this demand. However, there is a growing awareness that the ocean's resources for traditional forms of seafood may be nearing maximum harvest.

The purpose of this article is to describe the capacity of the oceans to feed the world, and to discuss the concern regarding overfishing of certain popular species, the technological developments to increase utilization of the food harvest, and ocean ranching or farming.

CAPACITY OF THE OCEANS

Harvests of ocean fish have been increasing at a rate of about 7% per year since 1950 (doubling every 10 years; Fig. 1). For some resources of traditional species, harvests have already approached a maximum sustainable yield. Several examples of

near-depleted resources can be found in the often used fishing grounds of the Northwest and Northeast Atlantic. The relation between catches and potential sustainable yield is less certain for other, less frequently used areas or the oceans as a whole. Various estimates of potential sustained yield range from 5.5×10^7 tons up to 2×10^9 tons (5×10^7 to 1.8×10^9 metric tons). Much of this variability is due to different opinions on what species to include. For example, one may include all plants and animals except the smaller zooplankton, all fish, or only those fish harvestable with present techniques.

To predict future harvests or the potential for future harvest, three general methods are recognized: (1) extrapolate present trends in total harvests; (2) extrapolate resource estimates from a known area to other, less well-known areas (Woods Hole method); and (3) estimate primary production and production at each successive stage in the food chain.

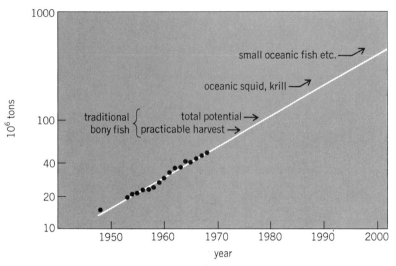

Fig. 1. Trends in world marine fish catch, in relation to the potential of various groups; 10⁶ tons = 9 × 10⁵ metric tons. *(From J. A. Gulland, ed., The Fish Resources of the Ocean, Fishing News (Books) Ltd., Food and Agriculture Organization, 1971)*

Extrapolate present trends. Extrapolation of present trends in total harvest (Table 1) gives the most accurate estimate for the short-range future. For individual species or stocks, the pattern is much less reliable. Harvests from several species do not change appreciably from year to year. Those from many other species have oscillated due to year-class fluctuations or other environmental effects. Still other stocks have shown extremely rapid increases when fishing efforts turned to them to supplement traditional sources which were becoming overexploited. The Peruvian anchovy fishery is an example from the 1960s, and other examples are likely in the near future.

Extrapolate known resources. Extrapolation from known resource areas depends on obtaining a reliable figure for maximum potential yield or yield per unit area in one fishing region and applying this figure to the world's oceans, or more specifically, to the world's continental shelves (Fig. 2). Researchers at Woods Hole derived a figure of 20

lb/acre (22 kg/ha) from the relatively well-known areas of the Northwest Atlantic. They estimated that the total potentially productive area of the world's oceans is 6×10^9 acres (2.4×10^7 km²) and derived a figure of 1.2×10^{11} lb, or 5.5×10^7 tons, for the total world potential.

Events since this estimate of 22 kg/ha was made suggest that this figure is less than the maximum sustainable yield even for the Northwest Atlantic. In the last 20 years, catches of traditional species have increased due to larger and better-equipped fishing vessels (Fig. 3), and more attention has been given to exploiting abundant resources of species which were scarcely considered in the 1950s, such as squid, capelin herring, sand launce, and whiting.

Estimate primary production. Estimates from primary production show clearly how estimates are derived. Thus, they can be revised more easily if one changes the assumptions on which they are based. Such estimates start with phytoplankton which convert the Sun's energy to carbohydrates and with minerals dissolved in the ocean which support their growth. Extrapolating from this basic trophic level to the zooplankton trophic level, and beyond to the several levels of fishes feeding on plankton and fishes feeding on fishes, creates two basic problems. The first is to define the trophic level or levels which are of interest in harvesting for food. The second problem is to quantify the ecological efficiency factor or conversion of food eaten to body weight.

Defining trophic levels. Difficulties in quantitating trophic levels of interest are based on the fact that the potential harvest should be less than the total production at that level. The harvest may be considered part of the assumption otherwise needed by the next higher trophic level, but attempts to increase the proportion taken run the risk of imperiling the future viability of the next trophic level.

Although the potential for production of human food is greater in the early stages of the ocean's food chain, harvesting at these stages is considerably less feasible; innovations in catching, processing, and marketing are usually needed for such lower-trophic-level species. An example is krill, a very small animal which is food for baleen whales in Antarctic waters. The large size of the krill resource has already attracted the interest of fishing enterprises in several nations. Exploratory fishing efforts have thus far demonstrated that humans are less efficient than the baleen whale in catching krill. There are additional problems in processing or preserving krill to transport it from the Antarctic to nations in the Northern Hemisphere, as well as in marketing this unfamiliar source of food.

Ecological efficiency factor. The ecological efficiency factor is subject to more guesswork than the trophic level of interest. This factor may be defined as the ratio of total annual production between successive trophic levels (Table 2). It is less than the efficiency of food utilization, or ratio of growth increment or maintenance to food consumed, since part of each trophic level is destroyed by disease or other natural causes, and may never appear in a form usable by humans. This factor is probably higher at the beginning lev-

Table 1. World fish catch, 1975*

Country	Catch, metric tons
Japan	10,058,451
Soviet Union	9,876,173
China	6,880,800
Peru	3,447,485
United States	2,798,703
Norway	2,550,438
India	2,328,000
South Korea	2,133,371
Denmark	1,767,039
Spain	1,532,878
South Africa	1,401,383
Indonesia	1,389,861
Thailand	1,369,900
Philippines	1,341,636
Canada	1,023,750
Vietnam	1,013,000
Iceland	994,791
United Kingdom	981,280
France	805,787
Poland	800,737

*From *Fishing News*, Feb. 11, 1977.

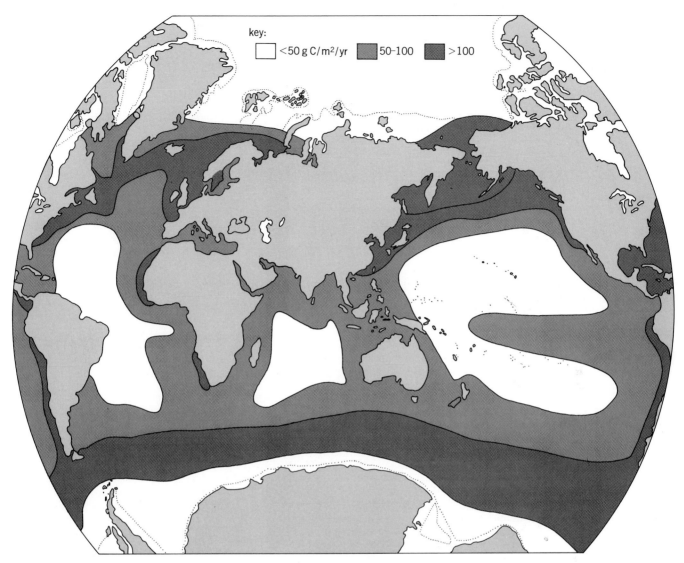

Fig. 2. Generalized chart showing the world net primary production of marine fish. (*From H. W. Graham and R. L. Edwards, World Biomass of Marine Fishes, National Marine Fisheries Service, Woods Hole, MA, 1962*)

els (phytoplankton to zooplankton, for example) that have smaller organisms and shorter life cycles and thus use a greater proportion of food intake for growth rather than maintenance. Fishing itself may affect this factor by increasing the mortality of adults, thereby leaving a greater proportion of younger fish with faster growth and smaller maintenance requirements. The ecological efficiency factor may also vary in a systematic way from region to region. It is probably higher in reproductive regions which have upswelling to increase production of phytoplankton compared with areas such as the open ocean which have a low primary production. It may also be affected by changes in species present, their nutritional status, and their ease of assimilation as food by the next higher trophic level. Thus, a single value of the ecological efficiency factor is most useful in suggesting an order of magnitude to the potential harvest.

Summary. Published estimates of potential harvest based on trophic levels and ecological efficiency factors vary between 2×10^8 and 2×10^9 tons (1.8×10^8 to 1.8×10^9 metric tons) of fish at the first carnivore level. These results are more useful in describing an order of magnitude than in obtaining a specific figure. Principal sources of uncertainty concern assigning values to the ecological efficiency factor, locating the precise position of fish species being considered in the food chain, and determining what proportion of the total production at any trophic level might be economically harvestable or might become desired for human use.

Table 2. Estimated annual production (live weight, 10^6 tons*) at various trophic levels†

Level	Ecological efficiency factor		
	10%	15%	20%
Phytoplankton (net carbon fixation)	1.9×10^4	1.9×10^4	1.9×10^4
Herbivores	19,000	28,000	38,000
First-stage carnivores	1,900	4,200	7,600
Second-stage carnivores	190	640	1,520
Third-stage carnivores	19	96	304

*10^6 tons $= 9 \times 10^5$ metric tons.

†From J. A. Gulland (ed.), *The Fish Resources of the Ocean*, Fishing News (Books) Ltd., Food and Agriculture Organization, 1971.

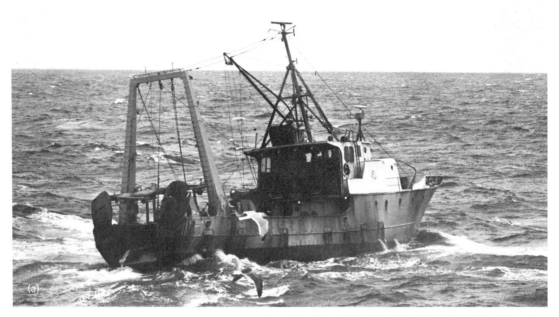

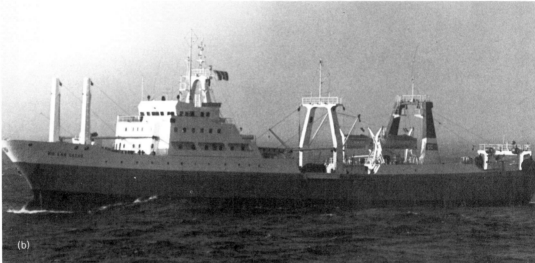

Fig. 3.   Modern stern trawlers. (*a*) United States trawler. (*b*) Cuban trawler. (*National Marine Fisheries Service*)

NATIONAL ECONOMIC ZONES

The year 1977 marks the change from the freedom of unlimited offshore fishing to the restriction of a recognized area, usually up to 200 mi (320 km) offshore, under the economic jurisdiction of a coastal state. Chile, Peru, and Ecuador were the original claimants to 200-mi zones, some 25 years previously. Their claims were greeted at first with derision and were later contested by other countries. As countries such as Peru began to exploit their coastal stocks to the limit, other coastal countries began to realize that rich fishing areas off their own shores might become depleted by others. During the 1960s, several voluntary international commissions were created for some of the world's richest fishing grounds, but these mutual fishing efforts were overwhelmed by increasingly larger and more efficient leviathan harvests.

In the early 1970s, the United Nation began a series of conferences on a Law of the Sea to find some consensus on fair sharing of the oceans' re-

sources by member countries. By the mid-1970s, the failure of these conferences to find an acceptable solution prompted several countries with major coastal interests on the richest fishing grounds to declare unilateral 200-mi economic or exclusive zones. With the Soviet Union, United States, Canada, Norway, European Economic Community (EEC) countries, Iceland, Mexico, India, and other coastal nations making claims or preparing to do so, the concept of economic zones has become a recognized reality, regardless of its legality in international law. The international commissions have been reduced to scientific advisory groups without authority to set quotas. The United Nations Law of the Sea conferences may continue, but these unilateral actions of 1977 by major coastal nations will certainly change the nature of these conferences.

Overlapping claims. Setting boundaries for economic zones has its problems. It is comparatively easy for a coastal nation to draw a line 200 mi out from its coastline into the open ocean, but when its neighbors draw their 200-mi lines some overlap is almost certain to occur. Bilateral negotiations between Canada and the United States, the United States and Mexico, and India and Sri Lanka are examples of nations attempting to solve overlapping claims. A more extreme case of overlapping claims concerns the islands of St. Pierre and Miquelon, which are part of France but are located well within Canada's 200-mi zone. France participates in the EEC's economic zone of the Northeast Atlantic as a member of the EEC. If Canada were to consent to France or the EEC's control of fishing within 200 mi of St. Pierre and Miquelon, many original claims of Canada in the Northwest Atlantic would be lost. At the present time, not surprisingly, Canada and France have agreed to a status quo arrangement.

EEC "fishing pond." A different set of boundary problems has occurred within the EEC. Although Iceland, the Faroe Islands, and Norway are accommodating themselves to the EEC's "fishing pond," those member countries of the EEC who depend on commercial fishing for part of their national wealth, such as Great Britain, France, the Federal Republic of Germany, Denmark, and Iceland, have been engaged in sometimes heated discussions among themselves and with other member nations of the EEC concerning exclusive fishing areas within the EEC's "pond." For example, Great Britain has favored a 50-mi (80 km) exclusive zone off its shores to compensate for harvests lost when Iceland, Canada, and the United States made their 200-mi claims, but is has gained little sympathy for its views from most other member nations.

Allocating resources. Other recent discussions among member nations of the EEC illustrate the problems of allocating the stocks of available resources. A fishery for industrial applications (fish meal and oil) may take species which are needed or are potentially useful for human consumption. This fishing effort may damage the breeding grounds of more valuable species and may deprive these species of the food they need for growth or maintenance. Thus, Denmark's recent large harvests of sand launce in the eastern part of the North Sea for reduction to fish meal was protested by other EEC member nations since the area fished is a well-known spawning and nursery ground for more valuable species such as cod, sole, and herring.

Joint ventures. As countries adjust to the spread of economic fishing zones, new patterns are emerging. Some overseas countries are setting up joint ventures with the United States and Canada to harvest fish within these economic zones, land them in the two countries, and "export" these "naturalized" fish overseas. Another example of mutual cooperation concerns Japan and Australia. Japan wants to restrict imports of Australian beef due to high cost. On the other hand, it realizes that any restrictions on beef imports may prompt Australia to reduce Japan's fishing effort in the emerging Australian economic zone.

It is a bit early to estimate the degree of success of these national economic zones in preventing overfishing. Fishing nations are beginning to appreciate the costs of the surveillance necessary to enforce regulations. Efforts of international cooperation may be the only alternative to depletion or exhaustion of valuable traditional resources.

BETTER UTILIZATION OF OCEAN RESOURCES

The preceding sections have focused on the world's food needs in the sense of traditional resources. However, the oceans' potential capacity to produce food is much greater. Less conventional alternatives include the use of more of the edible parts of fish already harvested and landed; of fish which are harvested but thrown back into the ocean; and of other species of fish which for one reason or another are not sought by fishing vessels. Any uncertainty in implementing these alternatives to increase the oceans' potential rests in finding consumer acceptance of less traditional food products.

More edible parts. More of the edible parts of fish already landed and harvested can be used. For many traditional species, the most popular edible portion is the fillet, which is a piece of muscle cut from the backbone. The skin may be removed or left on. Present-day filleting operations (by hand or machine) remove about 30 to 40% of these fish for food use, depending on the size and shape of the species. There is about 20 to 30% more edible muscle left over after filleting. Most of it is between segments of the backbone and an attached fleshy area (nape) that was originally located between the outer skin and the visceral cavity of the fish. Another potential source of additional edible flesh is created when the fillets themselves are given a V-shaped cut to remove pin-shaped bones.

Minced fish. The meat industry has already demonstrated the profitability of increasing the yield of edible flesh from each animal that has been harvested. In the seafood industry, some products have already emerged that are based on minced fish which has been removed from filleting leftovers by means of a meat-bone separator (Fig. 4). These products are generally patterned after fish sticks or fish portions, which have become increasingly popular since their introduction in the 1950s. The typical appearance, taste, and texture of sticks and portions made from fillet (regular) blocks have become well established. The resemblance of products made from minced fish to these "regular" sticks and portions depends mainly on the type of raw material used.

Some European countries are making fish blocks containing mixtures of fillets and minced fish. In most of these blocks, the amount of minced fish represents a natural proportion to the headed and gutted fish from which it and the fillets were obtained. When the minced fish is spread evenly on the surface of the fillet, it is difficult to distinguish fish sticks made from these blocks from those made from 100% fillet blocks. These blocks, sometimes called laminated blocks, represent a more efficient use of fish as food.

Minced fish obtained from V-cuts (fillet trimmings) is the most suitable material to prepare a minced fish product which resembles a regular fish stick. Headed and gutted fish are sometimes used to make stick- or portionlike products. In comparison, fish frames (filleting leftovers) represent a potentially good source of minced fish if problems of color and texture can be solved. The color problem is due to the concentration of blood tissues near the spinal column, while the texture problem results from using a strainer to improve its appearance.

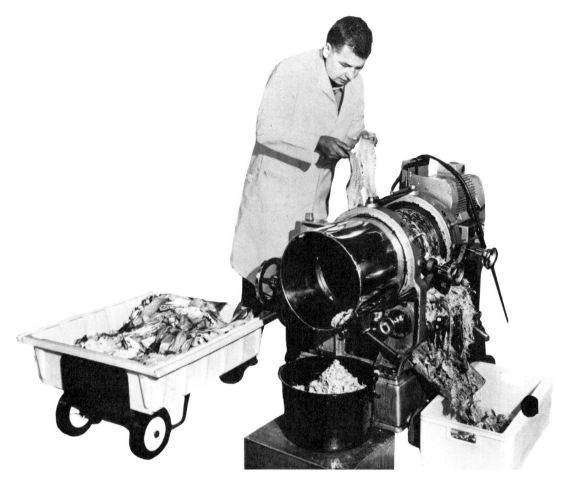

Fig. 4. Making minced fish with a meat-bone separator. (*National Marine Fisheries Service*)

Thus a series of grades (and prices) can be visualized for minced blocks from different sources of machine-separable flesh based on the suitability for making fish sticks and related items. On the basis of appearance (whiteness) and texture, at least, it can be assumed that minced blocks made from V-cuts would be near the top and blocks from frames would be near the bottom of this series. Techniques for improving the suitability of minced fish blocks from pigmented sources have merit. However, they are vulnerable to criticism for reasons of increasing cost or reducing yield to unacceptable levels compared with the present sources of supply for the fish stick trade.

New products. Instead of altering minced fish derived from frames or headed and gutted fish to suit requirements for fish sticks, food products which take advantage of this material's natural characteristics can be developed. For example, its color (due to blood pigments) suggests a resemblance to red meats, especially beef. Economic considerations definitely favor the mixing of beef and blood-colored fish. Nutritionally, there are several positive advantages in mixing ground fish with ground beef: The protein value of fish is comparable to beef both in quantity and in quality as well as being more easily digestible. The fat content of fish is typically lower than beef and contains less cholesterol. Fish fats also contain a greater proportion of unsaturated fatty acids in comparison with the "hard" saturated fatty acids of beef.

Despite the importance of nutritional and economic considerations, consumer acceptance is the major factor in development of any new product. The presence of several main dish items based on ground beef in American diets attests to the popularity of these dishes. Soy protein has already gained a degree of acceptance in American diets when mixed with ground beef. Preliminary new product development work suggests that many main dish items can be made from mixtures of ground beef and minced fish ("beefish"). In some countries, such as Japan, Poland, Uruguay, and Argentina, the mixtures are being seriously considered either to supplement expensive imported beef or to increase the supply of beef available for export in exchange for foreign trade credits.

Minced fish from blood-colored sources of material can be made into salted fish by a quick process because the muscle fibers have already been broken into chunks. The salted product is used to make food items such as fish cakes. In such items, it is a satisfactory replacement for the traditional salted fish fillets, which have to be broken into chunks when mixed with the other ingredients.

Using "discards." Fish that are usually thrown back into the ocean can also be used. A typical catch of fish contains a mixture of species and sizes. Up to 20–30% of such catches are often discarded at sea because the fish are too small or are not marketable under present conditions. A few fishing vessels convert these discards into fish meal (which becomes an ingredient in feeds used to raise poultry and other animals). However, on too many vessels all but the larger or more valuable species are thrown away—a significant waste of fishing effort.

Methods for preserving these "discards" at sea and landing them as food-quality fish are being developed. Since there usually is no time to sort all of the catch between tows, these discards are stored in bulk and sorted after they are landed ashore. The most successful storing method is to immerse them in a mixture of sea water and ice. Advantages of this method are that a minimum of mechanical equipment is needed and that the fish can be quickly unloaded by a dockside pump. Mechanically refrigerated sea water has been used but involves costly equipment and runs the risk of mechanical failure. Ice alone is impractical because too much time is needed to unload the vessel by traditional basket methods and to separate the fish from the ice.

After separating these bulk loads ashore by species and size, they can be headed and gutted and either used in this form or put through a meat-bone separator to recover edible flesh as minced fish.

Other species. Many other species of ocean fish are not presently sought by fishing vessels. The potential of this resource for food use is undoubtedly large, but its magnitude can only be estimated. As mentioned previously, most knowledge about the oceans' resources is based on past fishing efforts along certain parts of the continental shelves. Less is known about resources along other parts of the shelves and in deeper waters. With the obvious exception of the tuna fishery, very little is known about mid-water depths and near-surface dwellers especially in mid-ocean areas. The developing blue whiting fishery in the United Kingdom shows that harvesting is feasible when a resource congregates by itself or if a means is found to induce it to congregate sufficiently for practical catch rates.

Proccesing. Recent exploratory fishing efforts suggest that a significant part of these resources, when found, should be converted into minced fish for food use. Some species, such as flying fishes, have been satisfactorily preserved by drying or salting. For other species such as grenadier and cutlass fish, food additives may be required to improve the textural quality of minced flesh. These and many other, "newer" species have a greater proportion of dark muscle and lipids in their edible flesh than the well-known, white-muscle, lean gadoid fishes. It may be necessary to add antioxidants to prevent lipid oxidation and development of rancid flavors during preservation of the minced flesh. In some cases, it may be feasible to mix fillets with minced fish from the same species or from different species as long as they have similar or complementary edibility characteristics.

Mixing species. The concept of mixing species is gaining acceptance, especially for these underutilized recources. Many of the physical characteristics which distinguish one species of fish from another disappear as a consequence of meat-bone separation. The flesh itself is more readily identified as minced than as coming from a particular species. However, there are practical limits in mixing certain species together for food applications.

A chemical aspect of these limits concerns the mixing flesh of species whose quality deteriorates rapidly during frozen storage as a result of enzymic activity with flesh of another species which when stored by itself retains its initial quality for a long period. On the other hand, arrow tooth flounder or soft Dover sole can be blended with firmer-textured species such as rockfish to take advantage of the desirable taste of the flounder or sole while eliminating the problems associated with these soft-textured species.

End products. It is important to recognize that products made from minced fish blocks are more recognizable as an end product than as the species of fish from which they were taken. By analogy to the meat industry, an average consumer recognizes hamburger or ground beef more readily than whether it came from Angus, Hereford, or some other breed of cattle. Similarly, a fish stick or a seafood pattie is readily identified as such, but few consumers can tell whether it was made from cod, haddock, or some other gadoid species.

Such identification of end product rather than the species from which it was taken may help solve the complicated problem of finding suitable, attractive names for those species which are now, for the first time, being considered for food uses. Some of these species have unattractive names, based on their external anatomy (for example, ratfish, flathead, cutlass fish) instead of their edibility characteristics, while others have only taxonomic names.

Group names. The National Marine Fisheries Service has started a Plan for Market Names of Fishery Products, which calls for a fishery product to be identified by an appropriate group name. Each group would have a descriptive one-word name, and the total of food groups would not exceed 30. These group names would be based on edibility characteristics instead of biological or taxonomic ones. Thus, each group would include several species—as many as appropriate—as long as they were based on similar characteristics of appearance, taste, and texture of their edible flesh.

Efficient utilization of resources. All of the foregoing considerations lead to the concept of total oceanic production of seafood which advocates the use of all species harvested. Traditional or conventional species and market forms of seafood are included, as well as unconventional sources. Obviously, these unconventional sources should be tailored to present consumer tastes, rather than trying to educate consumers to accept a particular species whose future availability is questionable. Successful applications also would increase efficiency of the harvesting effort and thereby maintain the oceans' food resources in a more healthy condition for future human needs.

The Japanese seafood industry has already demonstrated ways to increase the efficiency of utilizing marine food resources for food. To meet their increasing demands for good-quality protein foods, a family of machines and appropriate technology were developed. The machines remove edible flesh from bones and skin and convert the minced flesh into a "universal" food material that can be preserved by freezing. This food material is called "surimi." It is a basic ingredient in manufacturing food items such as fish cake or paste ("kamaboko"), several kinds of sausages ("chikuwa"), and several kinds of deep-fat-fried products.

Products made in Japan from surimi are relatively unknown in the United States, but the relevant technology and equipment have spread throughout the world. Other countries are adapting this technology, especially meat-bone separators, to their own conditions. Outside of the Orient, the nearest to a "universal" basic ingredient in manufacturing seafood products is the minced fish block. It has potential for many applications other than the fish sticks, fish portions, fish cakes, and seafood patties in which it is presently used.

AQUACULTURE

Thus far this article has discussed the oceans' resources for food in terms of humans as hunters. For land-based food resources, humans have long since turned to ranching and farming to increase productivity. The oceans have a greater theoretical potential than the land since the buoyancy of water allows for ranching or farming in three dimensions as opposed to the two dimensions of land. This potential has hardly been tapped because the long-standing tradition of freedom of the seas is antithetical to the concept of property ownership on which ranching and farming are based.

Ocean aquaculture. Present-day ocean aquaculture or mariculture enterprises are limited to estuarine or other near-shore areas in which national sovereignty is universally recognized. Many of these enterprises are devoted to raising shellfish instead of fish because they are relatively immobile animals and can be sold for high prices. An example is raising oysters, mussels, and clams in North America, Europe, and Asia. For some species, methods for raising an animal through a complete life cycle are not known. Natural or "wild" stocks have to be gathered to start raising species such as shrimp in the United States and Japan, eels in Japan, plaice in Scotland, and salmon in the United States. Ocean aquaculture is not limited to animals; several species of plants (algae, seaweeds, or kelp) are harvested for food or industrial uses.

Fresh-water aquaculture. Present knowledge of raising species of fish or shellfish has been gained mainly from ranching or farming in fresh-water areas rather than the oceans. In the United States, fresh-water aquaculture is in its infancy, but it is an ancient and well-established practice in the Orient and Southeast Asia. It comprises a significant portion of the total fisheries harvest in China (40%), India (38%), Indonesia (22%), the Philippines (10%), and Japan (6%).

Ranching versus farming. Most fresh-water production relies on ranching, or "extensive," methods in which there is little or no control over the environment. This contrasts with farming, or "intensive," methods which use full environmental control.

In ranching, fish or invertebrates are trapped in special enclosures such as pens or tidal ponds, and held to marketable size. The animals depend on natural food sources. Labor input is restricted to the initial collection and final harvest. Survival rates tend to be low (20–50%) but can be improved by influencing the environment during the growing period. Advantages of this method are lower environmental and labor costs as well as a lower product cost for food uses.

Differences between farming and ranching fish or invertebrates are similar to those between farming and ranching animals on land. In fresh-water farming, culture techniques are used to increase a dependable supply of larvae or juveniles. A higher yield per unit area and a faster growth rate are possible, but these advantages weigh against problems such as water purity feeding costs, disease control, and higher labor costs. Examples of fresh-water fish farming in the United States include trout, channel catfish, crayfish, and macrobrachium (a fresh-water prawn).

High seas. If humans are to ranch or farm on the high seas, some sort of property rights will have to be established to protect investments made to start and raise animals for harvest. Recent national declarations of 200-mi economic zones suggest that, in the future, the traditional concept of freedom of the seas will not include poaching. On land, fences are a traditional symbol of ownership, but in the oceans building fences may not be necessary. For example, species accustomed to living on the continental shelf are not likely to migrate to the deeper areas of mid-ocean, and major ocean currents (such as the Gulf Stream) help to control population distribution.

It seems probable that humans will start ranching the high seas before they start farming them. As on land, finding ways to increase food supply should increase harvest productivity. Present rich fishing areas are characterized by natural mixing of warm upper layers of water, in which phytoplankton use the Sun's energy for growth, with lower layers of water which contain those dissolved minerals needed by phytoplankton to support their growth. Some other areas of the oceans, such as the Caribbean Sea, could be made more productive if the warm upper layer of water which lacks dissolved minerals could be mixed with the lower, nutrient-laden layers of water. This would increase the availability of phytoplankton to support the well-known food chain of the ocean's animals. This concept of "upwelling" has already been tested in the Caribbean by pumping the lower layers of water up to the surface through a vertical pipe. The costs of operating these pumps are surprisingly low. Controlling predators is another problem of ranching but, in the absence of artificial fences, the only visible solution appears to be to capture the predators for food or industrial use.

OUTLOOK

The capacity of the oceans' resources for food uses is highly speculative if ranching or farming were universally substituted for hunting. It is obvious that a high degree of international effort and cooperation would be required for these efforts In any case, the world's population growth suggests that future generations will need to focus more attention on increasing the oceans' harvests.

[FREDERICK J. KING]

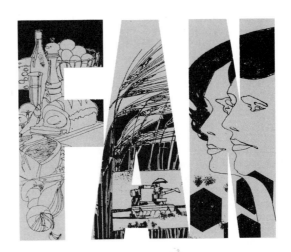

THE GREEN REVOLU- TION

H. Garrison Wilkes

The Green Revolution is the most recent of a long series of environmental rearrangements to increase the food-producing systems of the human population. The term "Green Revolution" was first used by William S. Gaud, former Director of United States Aid for International Development (USAID), in a speech given to the Society of International Development in 1968. The expression gained extensive publicity in 1970 when the Nobel Peace Prize was awarded to Norman E. Borlaug, "who, through his work in the laboratory and in the wheat fields, has helped to create a new food situation in the world, and who has turned pessimism into optimism in our dramatic race between the population explosion and the production of food."

Specifically, the Green Revolution consists of the introduction of yield-responsive wheat and rice varieties to the underdeveloped countries of the world. There are two classical methods to increase agricultural yield: increase the area under cultiva-tion or the yield per unit area. Since most of the favorable crop land in the world (with a few exceptions) has already been cleared of its natural vegetation cover and is under cultivation, the best approach to feeding the world's growing population is to increase the yields in specific crops.

DOMESTICATION AND FOOD PLANTS

Food production is the most time-consuming activity of humans worldwide, and agriculture has the greatest environmental impact. Present control over food production is a comparatively recent event, dating back only 10 millennia with the Neolithic or Agricultural Revolution. Prior to that time humans, like all other animals, secured food from wild plants and animals by gathering and hunting. Then about 10,000 years ago humans began to cultivate, independently in different parts of the world, a diversity of crop plants—maize, beans, and squash in Mexico; wheat, barley, and peas in the Near East; and rice, millets, and soybeans in the Far East. The earliest domestic crops were probably not much more productive than their wild progenitors, but the act of cultivation was a radical break with the past. The human species was restructuring its food supply.

Selection of food plants. Through thousands of years of experience various civilizations have selected for cultivation and subsequent domestication a relatively small number of plants upon which the world's food production is now based. Today the entire world is fed by domesticated plants which did not exist except as wild progenitors 400 human generations ago. Most of the present food plants are the product of a very long selection process by which they have become completely dependent on human care for their survival. This change is called domestication, and in the course of this process food plants have crossed a threshold. Their survival is now keyed to human preparation of the ground, provision of required nutrients or fertilizer, diminished competition with other plants, sowing of the seed in the right season, protection of the plants during growth, and finally the collection of their seed or other useful parts. Domestication has made these plants human captives, but the human population has increased so dramatically that it is now impossible to meet food needs with such plants alone. So, ironically, humans are held captive by the food plants that have been domesticated, and have become dependent on their high yields.

Key crops. The actual number of plants that feed the human population is amazingly small. A list of as few as 15 plants accounts for three-quarters of all plant calories consumed. They include 5 grasses: rice, wheat, corn, barley, and sorghum; 3 legumes: soybeans, common beans, and peanuts; 2 sugar sources: sugarcane and sugar beet; 2 tropical tree crops: coconuts and bananas; and also 3 starchy root crops: potatoes, yams, and cassava. Although the above list does not include many vegetables (which are high in vitamins and minerals but relatively low in calories), these 15 food plants literally stand between subsistence and starvation for the human population. Not only is the number of plants that feed the world becoming smaller, so are the diversity and genetic variation which are the basis of breeding new varieties. These trends are coming at a time when the human population is expanding rapidly, and all available options will be needed to meet world food demand. *See* articles on each plant named.

High yield and genetic uniformity. The reasons for this decrease in genetic variation are complex, but they have to do in part with an ever-increasing population, rising expectations of rural peoples, and intensive efforts to increase production on all the world's arable land. The result has been a push to develop plants that respond to fertilizers, require less water to develop, and are uniform so that they can be easily machine-harvested. For the most part, the emphasis has been on breeding new, improved, and usually genetically uniform varieties. In terms of yield, the benefits of this process are obvious. But the price has been the genetic limitation—and consequent increased vulnerability—of major food crops. *See the feature article* FEEDING THE WORLD.

Throughout the world there exists an unstable "truce" between basic food plants and their patho-gens. Genetic changes, whether mutations or recombinations, are constantly taking place in individual pathogens, and if one grows successfully on a previously resistant plant host, it will be able to spread across the entire population of genetically similar plants. However, in many parts of the world entire plant population diversity may exist in a single field, the fields of one village, or a district. As a result, the pathogen can make only small inroads in the crop. But in advanced agricultures, such as in the United States and with the high-yielding varieties (HYVs) of the Green Revolution, the genetic uniformity and high-density planting of crops creates ideal conditions for insects, nematodes, bacteria, viruses, fungi, and rodents to flourish. In the present agricultural system, the plant's genetic uniformity and vulnerability extend nationwide or worldwide. The price for maintaining high yields is a whole arsenal of insecticides, fungicides, and herbicides, and a constant commitment to change genetic material and breeding to achieve resistance to new races of a pathogen, a new biotype of an insect pest, or common environmental stress. There is nothing biologically unsound about breeding for high yields, and using a narrow genetic base is a plant breeding expediency necessary to obtain the most uniform high-yielding crop in the shortest period of time. But this type of plant breeding demands a constant commitment to crop improvement to maintain equilibrium.

Indigenous agriculture with primitive varieties or land races is the largest depository of genes for food crops. Generally these land races perform poorly under large doses of fertilizers, water, and intensive cultivation because they are the product of a long evolutionary history lacking these factors. However, they have a wide range of ability to withstand cold temperatures, drought, disease, insect damage, and other variables. These are the raw materials with which the plant breeder works.

PLANT BREEDING

Plant breeding has been one of the most distinctive elements in the Green Revolution's strategy of high-yielding crops for developing nations. Traditional land races of wheat and rice do not make effective use of fertilizer since it causes them to lodge (grow too tall and topple over). The high-yielding varieties incorporate dwarfing genes which give the plant short, stiff straw and enable it to respond to fertilizer without lodging to produce higher grain yields. Other genetic improvements include resistance to certain pests (but chemical pesticides must be applied and are part of the agricultural improvement package), insensitivity to day length, and rapid maturation so that a second crop or double cropping can be practiced. Besides fertilizers, herbicides, and pesticides, most HYVs yield best under a controlled supply of water, which requires the land to be irrigated, often necessitating the digging of tube wells so that the dependence on unpredictable rainfall is eliminated. *See* BREEDING (PLANT).

Criticism of the technologies. These technologies are relatively simple, but their impact has been dramatic on the developing countries. Food supply has increased, but there has also been an increase in population, so the Green Revolution has not been a solution to the world population problem, but only a means to alleviate the crisis for a few years. In addition, the Green Revolution technologies have been criticized because they more frequently benefit rich farmers, who can get credit for fertilizer and pesticides and can consolidate large tracts of land and mechanize more readily than the poor. A second major criticism, which has not been clearly substantiated, is that the Green Revolution displaces labor and increases rural unemployment. However, probably the most serious criticism is the increased crop vulnerability created by genetic uniformity and its energy-intensive technology. The Green Revolution is essentially a Western technology to increase food yields, and as such is dependent on high energy inputs in the form of fertilizers, pesticides, and fossil fuels used in cultivation practices and in transport and lifting of water for irrigation. This technology, in turn, is dependent on abundant and low-cost oil—a resource that suddenly no longer exists. Taken as a whole, the new agricultural technologies of the Green Revolution have certainly helped the poor countries of the world to feed their expanding populations. But it has not solved their social and economic problems, and it is not the ultimate solution to feeding a hungry world where one out of four people is still undernourished. *See the feature article* ENERGY IN THE FOOD SYSTEM.

Wheat program in Mexico. The beginnings of the Green Revolution date back to 1943 when the Rockefeller Foundation, in collaboration with the Mexican Ministry of Agriculture, began a research program designed to increase the production of Mexico's basic crops: corn, beans, potatoes, and wheat. A broad-based breeding program was initiated with each of these crops. Borlaug headed the wheat program at the International Maize and Wheat Improvement Center (Centro Internacional de Mejoramiento de Maiz y Trigo, or CIMMYT), and since most wheat grown in Mexico was highly susceptible to stem rust the initial breeding focused on increasing stem rust resistance in existing Mexican varieties. The development of new wheats possessing rust resistance and improved cultural practices such as the use of fertilizers and pesticides had made a substantial impact on wheat yields by 1957, the year Mexico achieved self-sufficiency in wheat. Over a 10-year period the average yield rose from 740 kg/ha in 1945–1946 to 1440 kg/ha in 1957–1958. Then the yield response began to level off because the most productive fields at 4 metric tons/ha lodged when nitrogen fertilizer was applied at 80 kg/ha or more. To increase the yields further, more fertilizer-responsive wheat varieties would have to be bred.

GREEN REVOLUTION WHEAT

The first extensive breeding program to develop semidwarf spring wheats was started by Borlaug in 1954 when a wheat Norin 10 × Brevor was crossed with indigenous Mexican varieties. The dwarf wheat Norin × Brevor came from the United States, and the dwarfing trait in Norin 10 from Japan. Following World War II, an agricultural adviser to the United States Occupation Army in Japan observed the Japanese farmers growing short, stiff-strawed wheat varieties that remained erect under heavy fertilizer application. This wheat variety, Norin 10, has an international ancestry. The dwarfing short-stature gene came from

a Japanese wheat which in 1917 was crossed with Glassy Fultz, a selection of the American soft red winter variety Fultz, at the Central Agriculture Experiment Station (Nishigahara, Tokyo) to produce Fultz-Daruma. This variety in turn was crossed with the American hard red winter variety Turkey-Red, which Mennonite immigrants (1873–1875) to the plains of Kansas had brought from their homeland in the Crimea, at the Ehime Perfectural Agricultural Experiment Station in 1925, in an effort to produce rust-resistant, short-stemmed, early-maturing varieties. Following seven cycles of selection by plant breeders, Norin 10 was registered and released in 1935 for Japanese farmers. (The Japanese word "norin" means "agriculture and forestry," and varieties officially released are so named and given a number.) The Norin 10 brought to the United States in 1946 was not adapted for direct planting in American fields, but was introduced into breeding nurseries.

The first American semidwarf variety developed at Pullman, WA, was a soft winter wheat from the cross [(Norin 10 × Brevor) × (Orfed × hybrid 50) −3] × Baart. The final selection was made in 1956, and in 1961 the variety named Gaines was released. (Orville Vogel, who was the breeder of Gaines, had supplied the Norin 10 × Brevor cross to Borlaug.)

An extensive breeding program to develop semidwarf spring wheats was started using already developed disease-resistant Mexican varieties. The result was a new type of wheat with higher yield potential. The selected progenies not only received semidwarf stature from Norin 10 × Brevor lines, but also inherited genes that increased the number of fertile florets per spikelet and the number of tillers per plant (Fig. 1).

The introduction of Norin 10 genes into the Mexican program led to the development of the first short-statured and lodging-resistant spring wheat varieties, Pitic 62 and Penjamo 62, which began to be grown by Mexican farmers in 1962. They were followed by the release of Sonora 63, Tobari 66, Jaral 66, Siete Cerros, Inia 66, Noreste 66, and Norteño 67. Mexican wheat yields which leveled

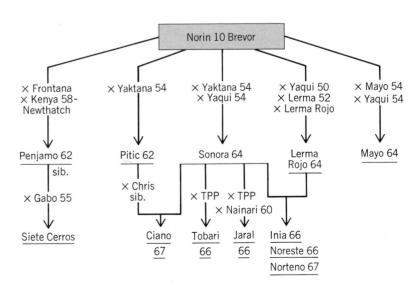

Fig. 1. Genealogy of early semidwarf CIMMYT wheat varieties. *(From D. G. Dalrymple, Development and Spread of High-Yielding Varieties of Wheat and Rice in the Less Developed Nations, 5th ed., Foreign Agr. Econ. Rep. no. 95, August 1976)*

off after 1958 because of lodging started rising again. These varieties broke the yield barrier, and yields as high as 8 metric tons/ha were not uncommon.

International diffusion of these varieties began almost immediately at the experimental level. India and Pakistan were involved in the program from an early date. New Mexican wheats were first grown in India in 1962. In 1963, 100-kg samples of Sonora 63, Sonora 64, Lerma Rojo, and Mayo were grown in experimental planting. By 1964 India had purchased 250 metric tons of Mexican wheat seed for planting, and Pakistan 350 metric tons. By 1965 India had an order for 18,000 metric tons of Mexican wheat, and Pakistan for 42,000 metric tons. This successful rapid transfer of technology halfway around the world was the break in static yield potentials which marked the Green Revolution.

The Mexican varieties proved remarkably well adapted to India and Pakistan because in accelerating the Mexican wheat program two generations of the breeding material were grown each year at very different climatic and day-length regimes. A valuable side effect of this system was to establish a relatively photoperiod-insensitive plant. The normal winter crop was grown on the northeast coast in Sonora essentially at sea level. The summer crop was grown at high elevations (2600 m) in central Mexico near Toluca. The Toluca site has heavy rainfall and severe epidemics of both stem and stipe rust. Selection for broad disease resistance and the use of widely adapted varieties that were not bred to pure-line standards meant that these semidwarf Mexican lines possessed a reservoir of genetic diversity that could be incorporated into national breeding programs. The adaptation and use of these wheats now occurring in developing nations is a continual process of crossing with indigenous varieties and of selection for local growing conditions, disease resistance, and grain quality tailored to national needs.

GREEN REVOLUTION RICE

The break with the static yield potentials for rice in developing countries has also been based on

plant breeding. The HYVs of rice have a history of origin very similar to that of wheat. In Taiwan in 1949 at the Taichung District Agricultural Improvement Station a cross between semidwarf Dee-geo-woo-gen, a Chinese variety, and a tall native indica variety of rice was made. An outstanding selection from this cross, Taichung Native 1, (TN-1), was the first semidwarf fertilizer-responsive indica variety developed through breeding, and was released in 1956. Prior to this time only dwarf fertilizer-responsive japonica-type varieties with short sturdy straw and dark-green, thick, narrow, and somewhat erect leaves were known, primarily in Japan, Korea, and Taiwan. However, these varieties were not adapted to the tropics. By 1961 TN-1 was recording yields in excess of 8 metric tons/ha, and by 1964 about one-third of Taiwan was planted to this variety.

In 1962 the International Rice Research Institute (IRRI), founded by the Ford Foundation and the Rockefeller Foundation in cooperation with the government of the Philippines, began research on rice production in the tropics. From the start there was a recognition that one of the most important single reasons for the low yields of tropical rice was the lack of lodging-resistant varieties. The traditional tropical varieties are tall and leafy and lodge under heavy nitrogen application.

The IRRI's geneticist T. T. Chang, who came from Taiwan, was familiar with the breeding work then in progress in his homeland, and the rice varieties Dee-geo-woo-gen, I-geo-tse, and TN-1 were used in the earliest crosses. The most successful crosses that first year (1962) were between Peta, a tall Indonesian Indica type which had disease resistance and heavy tillering, and the Chinese Dee-geo-woo-gen (Fig. 2). Less than 3 years after the first cross IR-8 was released. IR-8 responded favorably to fertilizer and produced its maximum yield of 9477 kg/ha at 120-kg/ha nitrogen application. By 1966 developing rice-eating nations had a new plant type, Indica rice, which has short height, stiff straw, short erect leaves, and a grain/straw ratio of about 1 compared with a ratio of about 0.5 for Peta. After the new plant type demonstrated a radical improvement in rice yields for the tropics, the major rice-breeding emphasis shifted to improving grain quality and disease, insect, and cold resistance, and new releases such as IR-20, IR-22, and IR-28 were made.

SUCCESS OF THE GREEN REVOLUTION

The key element in the Green Revolution has been the HYV's of wheat and rice. The impact of these improved varieties and optimal agricultural practices has been to increase production dramatically, two- to five-, sometimes tenfold, over broad areas of India, Pakistan, and Iraq for wheat; and Indonesia, Philippines, Sri Lanka, and Bangladesh for rice (Tables 1 and 2). Prior to the Green Revolution these countries had been part of a general pattern of yield stagnation in the developing countries. In fact, per capita grain production had actually decreased over the last 25 years. Prior to World War II these countries had been net exporters of grain. By the close of the war they had become net importers. This trend continued, and in 1948–1952 average imports for the developing world were 4×10^6 tons of food grains, in 1957–1959 1.3×10^7 tons, and in 1961 2×10^7 tons. HYVs

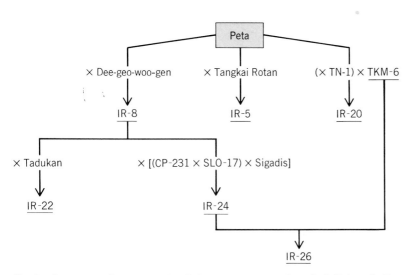

Fig. 2. Genealogy of early semidwarf IRRI rice varieties. (*From D. G. Dalrymple, Development and Spread of High-Yielding Varieties of Wheat and Rice in the Less Developed Nations, 5th ed., Foreign Agr. Econ. Rep. no. 95, August 1976*)

Table 1. Percentage of total wheat area planted to high-yielding varieties in Asia and the Near East

Country	Crop year									
	1965–1966	1966–1967	1967–1968	1968–1969	1969–1970	1970–1971	1971–1972	1972–1973	1973–1974	1974–1975*
Asia										
Bangladesh	–	–	–	7.2	7.6	11.3	11.8	17.7	23.1	23.4
India	negl.	4.2	19.6	30.0	30.1	35.9	41.1	51.4	57.4	61.7
Nepal	1.2	5.2	12.9	25.9	33.5	43.0	52.3	65.6	75.5	84.9
Pakistan	0.1	1.9	16.0	38.0	43.0	52.3	56.7	56.5	59.0	62.5†
Near East										
Afghanistan	–	negl.	0.8	4.3	5.1	9.2	10.1	15.0	16.1	17.4
Algeria	–	–	–	–	2.2	6.7	14.5	27.9	not avail.	not avail.
Egypt	–	–	–	–	–	negl.	0.3	3.5	39.8	14.3
Iran	–	–	–	0.2	0.9	1.6	2.9	3.2	6.1†	6.7†
Iraq	–	–	0.3	2.0	9.6	9.0	45.2	49.6	42.9	50.0
Lebanon	–	–	negl.	0.7	4.1	11.7	18.8	31.3	not avail.	not avail.
Morocco	–	–	negl.	0.3	2.5	4.8	10.0	14.4	19.6	16.7
Saudi Arabia	–	–	–	–	–	–	–	negl.	2.0	10.0
Syria	–	–	–	–	–	4.3	6.8	10.1	14.9	17.0
Tunisia	–	–	0.1	1.8	7.1	10.7	6.0	9.4	5.5	5.5
Turkey	–	negl.	2.1	7.0	7.6	7.8	8.0	not avail.	not avail.	not avail.

*Preliminary   †Based on unofficial estimates of HYV area.
SOURCE: D. G. Dalrymple, *Development and Spread of High-Yielding Varieties of Wheat and Rice in the Less Developed Nations*, 5th ed., Foreign Agr. Econ. Rep. no 95, August 1976.

Table 2. Percentage of total rice area planted to high-yielding varieties in Asia and the Near East

Country	Crop year									
	1965–1966	1966–1967	1967–1968	1968–1969	1969–1970	1970–1971	1971–1972	1972–1973	1973–1974	1974–1975*
Asia										
Bangladesh	–	negl.	0.7	1.6	2.6	4.6	6.7	11.1	15.6	14.9
Burma	–	–	negl.	3.3	2.9	2.6	3.6	4.2	5.1	6.4
India	negl.	2.5	4.9	7.3	11.3	14.6	19.3	23.2	25.6	29.9
Indonesia	–	–	–	2.4	10.4	11.0	15.8	22.8	36.6	40.3
South Korea	–	–	–	–	–	–	0.2	15.6	11.7	25.5
Laos	–	negl.	0.2	0.3	0.2	6.0	3.3	5.5	not avail.	not avail.
Malaysia	10.0	14.7	20.6	20.1	26.4	30.9	35.8	37.1	36.7	not avail.
Nepal	–	–	–	3.7	4.4	5.8	6.3	14.8	17.1	18.6
Pakistan	–	negl.	0.3	19.8	29.9	36.6	50.0	43.7	42.1	40.3
Philippines	–	2.7	21.2	30.4†	43.5	50.3	56.3	54.0	63.4	64.0
Sri Lanka	–	–	–	1.0	3.9	4.6	10.6	33.2	64.5	52.8
Thailand†	–	–	–	–	negl.	0.4	1.3	4.2	5.0	5.5
South Vietnam	–	–	negl.	1.6	8.3	19.9	25.9	32.1	31.1	29.9†
Near East										
Egypt	–	–	–	–	–	–	–	–	negl.	0.1
Iraq	–	–	–	–	–	–	–	5.0	12.6	15.8

*Preliminary   †Based on unofficial estimates of HYV area.
SOURCE: D. G. Dalrymple, *Development and Spread of High-Yielding Varieties of Wheat and Rice in the Less Developed Nations*, 5th ed., Foreign Agr. Econ. Rep. no 95, August 1976.

of wheat and rice arrested and in some cases dramatically reversed food import dependency in the developing nations.

The use of HYVs of wheat developed at CIMMYT in Mexico under Borlaug and rice developed in the Philippines at IRRI under Chang has expanded rapidly in the developing nations since 1965–1966 when these varieties first came into wide use (Table 3). As of 1974–1975 the HYV wheat and rice area in non-Communist nations (for which there is no reliable data) in Asia and the Near East (including North Africa) totaled about 4.09×10^7 ha (1.01×10^8 acres). Of this about 1.93×10^7 ha (4.77×10^7 acres) were wheat and 2.16×10^7 ha (5.33×10^7 acres) were rice. In addition, several million hectares of HYV wheat and about 770,000 ha (1.9×10^6 acres) of rice were planted in Latin America (exclusive of Cuba). HYV area in Africa was relatively minor.

A measure of the success of the HYVs in the Green Revolution is to map their adoption by native cultivators. Altogether, HYVs in the 1974–1975 crop year accounted for about 38.4% of the total wheat area and 26% of the total rice area in Asia and the Near East. Over half of the HYV area for both wheat and rice was in India, followed by Pakistan for wheat and by Indonesia and the Philippines for rice. In the Western Hemisphere virtually all of Mexico's wheat acreage was in HYVs, and thoughout Latin America use of HYVs of rice was expanding.

INTERNATIONAL AGRICULTURAL RESEARCH

The improvement of major crops by deliberate breeding programs, along with experiments in improving agricultural practices at research institutions, started in the late 18th century in Europe and parallels in time the Industrial Revolution. By the first decades of the 20th century most of the arable land of industrialized Europe and North

Table 3. Estimated high-yielding wheat and rice area, in Asia and Near East from 1965–1966 to 1974–1975[a]

Crop year	Area		
	Wheat	Rice	Total
	Hectares		
1965–1966	9,300	49,400	58,700
1966–1967	651,100	1,034,300	1,685,400
1967–1968	4,123,400	2,653,500	6,776,900
1968–1969	8,012,600	4,707,500	12,720,100
1969–1970	8,879,300	7,764,300	16,643,600
1970–1971	11,219,700	9,972,100	21,191,800
1971–1972	13,930,000	13,052,900	26,982,900
1972–1973	16,561,300[c]	15,624,900	32,186,200
1973–1974	18,194,100[c,d]	19,715,100[e]	37,909,200
1974–1975[b]	19,288,300[c,d]	21,587,300[e,f]	40,875,600
	Acres		
1965–1966	22,900	122,100	145,000
1966–1967	1,608,800	2,555,900	4,164,700
1967–1968	10,188,800	6,557,000	16,745,800
1968–1969	19,799,500	11,631,800	31,431,300
1969–1970	21,941,000	19,185,900	41,126,900
1970–1971	27,723,900	24,640,900	52,364,800
1971–1972	34,421,100	32,254,000	66,675,100
1972–1973	40,922,600[c]	38,609,000	79,531,600
1973–1974	44,957,700[c,d]	48,716,200[e]	93,673,900
1974–1975[b]	47,661,200[c,d]	53,342,300[e,f]	101,003,500

[a]Excludes Communist countries (except South Vietnam), developed nations, and Taiwan.
[b]Preliminary.
[c]Includes Turkey at 1971 and 1972 levels.
[d]Includes Algeria and Lebanon at 1972–1973 level.
[e]Includes Laos at 1972–1973 level.
[f]Includes Malaysia at 1973–1974 level.
SOURCE: D. G. Dalrymple, *Development and Spread of High-Yielding Varieties of Wheat and Rice in the Less Developed Nations*, 5th ed., Foreign Agr. Econ. Rep. no. 95, August 1976.

America was planted to varieties which had been bred or selected by plant breeders. Yet even by the middle of the 20th century the people of the developing nations were little affected by the improvements that had been made in the temperate regions. The introduction of HYVs of wheat from CIMMYT and rice from IRRI in the 1960s was a revolution in the historically static yields of the developing nations.

CGIAR. In 1971 international aid to agricultural research and development was strenghtened by the formation of the Consultative Group on International Agricultural Research (CGIAR). CGIAR is cosponsored by the World Bank, Food and Agriculture Organization (FAO), and the United Nations Development Program. Among its 34 members are, in addition to the sponsors, 14 donor governments, 3 regional development banks, the European Economic Community, the Ford, Rockefeller, and Kellogg foundations, the International Development Research Centre (Ottawa), and 2 representatives from each of 5 major developing regions. At present CGIAR mobilizes funds from its members to finance nine institutions, eight of which are crop research centers. The cost of these institutions exceeded $70,000,000 in 1976.

International institutes. The concept underlying these international agricultural institutes is to have a core staff of plant breeders, geneticists, physiologists, chemists, pathologists, agronomists, entomologists, engineers, and economists in a central location with excellent facilities all focused on a specific crop or group of related agricultural problems. The goals of the institutes are to produce improved crop varieties with general agronomic recommendations and technologies suitable to farming conditions of low-income countries, to train personnel for national institutions, and to facilitate international cooperation in agricultural production. The experimental varieties developed at the institutes are tested at many locations around the world, along with materials developed in cooperating national programs, to permit selection of specific varieties best suited for release to specific environmental and national needs. The international institutes are a means to hasten the development of new technologies. A listing of the

Table 4. International agricultural institutes for the development of improved crop varieties*

International institute	Year founded	Location	Research area	Region of the world served
International Rice Research Institute (IRRI)	1960	Philippines	Rice, multiple cropping	Rain-fed and irrigated subtropics/tropics
International Maize and Wheat Improvement Center (CIMMYT)	1967	Mexico	Wheat, barley, maize	Rain-fed and irrigated temperate/tropics
International Center of Tropical Agriculture (IITA)	1968	Nigeria	Maize, rice, root and tuber crops, cowpeas, soybeans, lima beans, farming systems	Rain-fed and irrigated lowland tropics
International Center of Tropical Agriculture (CIAT)	1969	Colombia	Beans, corn, rice, cassava, beef and forages, pigs	Rain-fed and irrigated tropics (sea level to 1000 m)
International Potato Center (CIP)	1972	Peru	Potatoes	Rain-fed and irrigated temperate to tropic
International Crops Research Institute for the Semi-Arid Tropics (ICRISAT)	1972	India	Sorghum, millets, peanuts, chickpeas, pigeon peas	Semiarid tropics
International Laboratory for Research on Animal Diseases (ILRAD)	1974	Kenya	Blood diseases of cattle	Mainly semiarid tropics
International Livestock Centre for Africa (ILCA)	1974	Africa	Cattle production	Humid to dry tropics
International Center for Agricultural Research in Dry Areas (ICARDA)	Planning stage	Lebanon	Wheat, barley, broad beans, lentils, oilseeds, cotton, sheep production	Mediterranean

*Compiled from working papers of the Rockefeller Foundation.

eight institutes, and a ninth in the planning stage, their locations, and research areas is summarized in Table 4.

Outlook. The present world food crisis has provoked doubt about the capability of present and expanding populations to feed themselves. This challenge will be met by increases in yield potentials of specific crops and not by acreage expansion. In many cases the failure to achieve higher yields is due to the inadequacy of institutional arrangements (land policies, credit structure, techni-cal assistance to farmers, and so on); in other instances the technology is not transferable from the temperate regions to the tropics, or is simply not worked out and available. HYVs of wheat and rice which started the Green Revolution are not a final solution to the world's food problem. Yet it is hoped that research at the nine international institutions will focus on continued agricultural yield improvement, so that the Green Revolution will not be an isolated event but a continuous process.   [H. GARRISON WILKES]

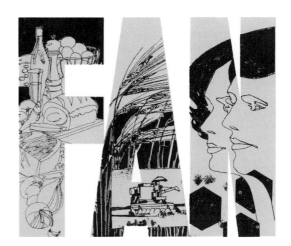

A-Z

Abscisic acid

One of the five major plant hormones. It has a number of important functions in plant growth and development. The name abscisic acid (ABA) is derived from the ability of the substance to promote abscission. It is also a potent inhibitor of growth. In this capacity it helps to induce and prolong dormancy of buds. It is a powerful inhibitor of seed germination and has an important role in the closure of stomata. *See* ABSCISSION.

Abscisic acid is distributed throughout the plant body but is found in highest concentrations in leafy tissues, fruits, and seeds. The principal site of ABA synthesis is the chloroplast (which is also the site of synthesis of related chemicals such as the gibberellins and carotenoids). Synthesis of ABA increases markedly when the plant is under stress.

The chemical structure of ABA is shown in the illustration. ABA is a member of the terpenoid family of chemicals, which includes a number of essential oils, insect hormones, steroids, gibberellins, carotenoids, and natural rubber. It is a weak organic acid, as are two other plant hormones, auxin and gibberellin. Natural ABA is dextrorotatory, hence the "+" in front of the name. *See* AUXIN; GIBBERELLIN.

Hormonal activity. Early experiments demonstrated that ABA is a plant hormone; that is, it is a naturally occurring organic compound that functions at very low concentrations and coordinates important plant functions. It was first shown to be a hormone of young fruit of cotton and lupin; it serves as a natural thinning agent to promote the abscission of excessive numbers of young fruit. In preventing seed germination, ABA also functions as a hormone, usually being produced by seed coats or nearby tissues. Another striking hormonal function is the closure of stomata, induced by ABA

ABSCISIC ACID

Structural formula for
+-abscisic acid, which is
the naturally occurring
form.

synthesized in leaves in response to water stress. Other experiments indicate that ABA may also have a hormonal role in some aspects of senescence, dehiscence, and permeability, and in the geotropic response of roots.

Abscission. ABA is a strong promoter of abscission. Its action has been studied extensively with explants (excised abscission zones) of leaves. There have also been many experiments that demonstrate the ability of ABA to promote the abscission of young fruit. With mature fruit and with vigorously growing leaves, experimental applications of ABA sometimes have little effect. Such organs possess considerable intrinsic ability to prevent their abscission. This ability appears due largely to high levels of nutrients and growth-promoting hormones (such as auxin, gibberellin, and cytokinin) that are normally present in vigorous leaves and fruit, making them unresponsive to applied ABA. However, if the leaves and fruit are weakened through competition, disease, or aging, ABA accelerates the processes of abscission. *See* CYTOKININS.

Stress. When placed under stress, the plant synthesizes increased amounts of ABA. A variety of stress conditions can induce this response; ABA responses to water stress have been studied in greatest detail. Within a few minutes of the onset of water stress, levels of ABA rise rapidly and can increase to more than 40 times the original level within 2 hr. The almost immediate response to the increased ABA is the closure of stomata. Thus, ABA has a key function in the plant mechanism that protects the plant from excessive water loss. A mutant tomato (*flaca*) has been discovered whose leaves remain wilted almost continuously; it cannot synthesize ABA and hence is unable to close its stomata when subjected to even mild water stress. The action of ABA appears to increase the permeability of the guard cells, with the result that turgor drops and the stomata close.

Growth. ABA can strongly inhibit the growth of plants, organs, and tissues being grown in culture. However, when ABA is applied to vigorously growing intact plants, its inhibition may be only transitory. In such plants, ABA can be rapidly inactivated, and often there are high levels of auxin and other hormones that can counteract ABA.

Dormancy and flowering. If sufficient ABA is applied to growing shoots, growth is arrested and a kind of dormancy is induced, with the dormant shoots resembling somewhat the dormant shoots and buds that are normally formed in the autumn. The results suggest that ABA could be one of the factors that combine to induce the development of dormant buds in the autumn. Applications of ABA have influenced the flowering behavior of a number of plants. For example, in some species, flowering can be promoted by ABA and by other factors which retard vegetative growth and thereby encourage earlier flowering. In other species, where flowering is more closely correlated with vegetative growth, ABA tends to retard flowering. Such results appear due to general effects of ABA on the growth of the experimental plants rather than to specific effects on the induction of flowering.

Germination. Well over 100 chemicals occurring in plants have inhibitory effects on seed germination. Among these chemicals, ABA is one of the most widespread. It occurs naturally in the seeds, seed coats, and other tissues close to the seed, and has now been implicated as a seed germination inhibitor of a number of species. In laboratory experiments, ABA completely inhibits germination as long as it is present in the water about the seeds. However, as soon as the ABA solutions are rinsed away, germination proceeds normally. There are no deleterious effects from even prolonged exposure to ABA solutions, indicating that ABA has little toxicity to plant tissues. Its physiological action in inhibiting germination appears primarily to be that of preventing the synthesis of the digestive enzymes required to solubilize the reserve foods of the seed. *See* SEED (BOTANY).

Senescence. ABA is able to accelerate a number of changes associated with the senescence of plants and plant organs. Increases in ABA often precede the abortion of young fruit, the senescence of plants and plant organs, and the senescence and the dehiscence of fruit. Applications of ABA hasten the chemical and biochemical changes of senescence, including chlorophyll degradation, and increase the activity of enzymes such as ribonuclease and acid phosphatase. The promotion of senescence by ABA can sometimes be reduced or prevented by the growth hormones, auxin, gibberellin, and cytokinin.

Mode of action. Clearly ABA has profound effects on the physiology and biochemical activities of plant tissues. The precise manner in which ABA acts has not been discovered, although there has been much research on the problem. However, there are significant indications of the ways in which physiological activities are controlled by ABA. It is a powerful inhibitor of the growth-promoting and other functions of auxin, gibberellin, and cytokinin. In many situations, ABA is able to completely block responses to those hormones. One of its major effects is to counteract biochemical reactions promoted by the growth hormones; and further, ABA itself promotes other biochemical reactions. In particular, it promotes the synthesis of hydrolases associated with senescence and abscission. Some of the effects of ABA are similar to those of ethylene, but ABA appears to function via pathways different from those of ethylene.

There appear to be two basic kinds of responses to ABA. One is a direct, rapid response that leads to changes in the permeability of cell membranes, often in the course of a very few minutes. One such change is the rapid loss of turgor from guard cells. The other kind of response to ABA is slower and may develop over a period of hours or days. This involves ABA's inhibition of the synthesis of some groups of enzymes and promotion of the synthesis of other groups of enzymes. Such enzymatic changes can have far-reaching effects on the physiology and metabolism of the plant. *See* PLANT GROWTH; PLANT HORMONES.

[FREDRICK T. ADDICOTT]

Bibliography: F. T. Addicott, Biochemical aspects of the action of abscisic acid, in D. J. Carr (ed.), *Plant Growth Substances*, pp. 272–280, 1972; F. T. Addicott et al., On the physiology of abscisins, *Colloq. Int. Centre Nat. Rech. Sci. Paris*, no. 123, pp. 678–703, 1964; B. V. Milborrow, The chemistry and physiology of abscisic acid, *Annu. Rev. Plant Physiol.*, 25:259–307,

1974; S. T. C. Wright, Physiological and biochemical responses to wilting and other stresses, in Rees et al., (eds.), *Crop Processes in Controlled Environments*, pp. 349–359, 1972.

Abscission

The process whereby a plant sheds one of its parts. Leaves, flowers, seeds, and fruits are parts commonly abscised. Almost any plant part, from very small buds and bracts to branches several inches in diameter, may be abscised by some species. However, other species, including many annual plants, may show little abscission, especially of leaves.

Abscission may be of value to the plant in several ways. It can be a process of self-pruning, removing injured, diseased, or senescent parts. It permits the dispersal of seeds and other reproductive structures. It may also serve an excretory function by the removal of parts in which waste or toxic substances have accumulated.

In most plants the process of abscission is restricted to an abscission zone at the base of an organ (see illustration); here separation is brought about by the disintegration of the walls of a special layer of cells, the separation layer. Less than an hour may be required to complete the entire process for some flower petals, but for most plant parts several days are required for completion of abscission. The portion of the abscission zone which remains on the plant commonly develops into a corky protective layer that becomes continuous with the cork of the stem.

In general, a healthy organ inhibits its own abscission. Only after it is injured, diseased, or senescent is an organ abscised. In many instances abscission is also a correlation phenomenon, its occurrence being correlated with events elsewhere in the plant. For example, the abscission of flower petals usually follows closely after pollination and fertilization; and in some broad-leaved evergreen trees, such as live oaks, the camphor tree, and *Magnolia grandiflora*, the major flush of leaf abscission follows closely after the appearance of new buds and leaves in the spring.

Abscission is a typical physiological process requiring favorable temperatures, oxygen, and energy-yielding respiration. The energy is required for the synthesis of hydrolytic enzymes. These enzymes function to soften the pectins and other constituents of the cell wall. When the cell walls of the separation layer are sufficiently weakened, the leaf (or other organ) falls from the plant by its own weight.

Agricultural regulation. Regulation of abscission by means of chemicals is an important practice. Chemical growth regulators such as naphthaleneacetic acid are used to delay abscission of leaves, fruits, and other plant parts. Most notable among these applications are the spraying of apple orchards to prevent the premature drop of fruit, and the dipping of cut holly to prevent abscission of berries and leaves during shipment. Chemicals are used also to accelerate abscission. Chemical defoliation of cotton plants is widely practiced in the United States, as it facilitates mechanical harvest. In some regions defoliation of young nursery plants is used to facilitate earlier digging and shipping. Similar chemicals are used to thin fruit from some varieties of apples and peaches and to remove undesired young fruits from ornamentals such as horse chestnut, catalpa, and honey locust.

Factors affecting abscission. Abscission is affected by a number of environmental and internal factors. It can be initiated or accelerated by extremes of temperature, such as frost; by extremes of moisture, such as drought or flooding; by deficiency of mineral elements in the soil, particularly nitrogen, calcium, magnesium, potassium, and zinc; by the shortening photoperiod in the fall; by oxygen concentrations above 20%: by volatile chemicals, such as ethylene and air pollutants; and by moderately toxic chemicals. Abscission can be retarded or inhibited by excessive nitrogen from the soil; by high carbohydrate levels in the plant; by oxygen concentrations below 20%; and by application of growth-regulator chemicals, such as naphthaleneacetic acid. *See* PLANT, MINERAL NUTRITION OF; PLANT PHYSIOLOGY.

Hormones. Although a number of internal chemical changes regularly precede the abscission of an organ, at most only a few of the changes appear to be directly related to the process of abscission. Of the changes, a decrease in the level of the growth hormone auxin appears to be the most important. Auxin applied experimentally to the distal (organ) side of an abscission zone retards abscission, while auxin applied to the proximal (stem) side accelerates abscission. From this and related evidence it is considered that the gradient of auxin across the abscission zone is the major internal factor controlling abscission. Further, many other factors affecting abscission appear to act through effects on the auxin gradient. *See* AUXIN.

The gibberellins are growth hormones which influence a number of plant processes, including abscission. When applied to young fruits or to leaves, they tend to promote growth, delay maturation, and thereby indirectly prevent or delay abscission. *See* GIBBERELLIN.

Abscisic acid is a different type of hormone and has the ability to promote abscission and senescence and to retard growth. Like auxin, it is synthesized in fruits and leaves; however, it tends to counteract the effects of the growth-promoting hormones, auxin, gibberellin, and cytokinin. *See* ABSCISIC ACID; CYTOKININS.

Another hormonal chemical is the gas ethylene. Small amounts of ethylene have profound effects on the growth of plants and can distort and reduce growth and promote senescence and abscission.

Thus the process of abscission is strongly influenced by interaction of several plant hormones. Frequently the hormones that tend to retard or delay abscission (auxin, gibberellin) are counteracted by the hormones that tend to promote and accelerate abscission (abscisic acid, ethylene). These interactions are further influenced by many environmental and external factors, as mentioned above. Depending on circumstances, any one of several factors may at times be the key factor controlling the entire process of abscission. *See* PLANT HORMONES.

In agricultural practice, retardation of abscission is obtained by applying growth regulators or

ABSCISSION

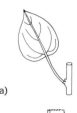

(a)

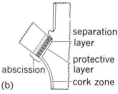

abscission

(b)

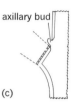

separation layer

protective layer

cork zone

axillary bud

(c)

Diagrams of the abscission zone of a leaf. (*a*) A leaf with the abscission zone indicated at the base of the petiole. (*b*) The abscission zone layers shortly before abscission and (*c*) the layers after abscission.

by heavy fertilization with nitrogen, which leads to high levels of auxin. Acceleration of abscission is obtained by applying toxic chemicals, by employing cultural methods which lower the levels of auxin, or by applying ethylene.

[FREDRICK T. ADDICOTT]

Bibliography: F. T. Addicott, Plant hormones in the control of abscission, *Biol. Rev.*, 45:485–524, 1970; T. T. Kozlowski (ed.), *Shedding of Plant Parts*, 1973; R. J. Weaver, *Plant Growth Substances in Agriculture*, 1972.

Agricultural chemistry

The science of chemical compositions and changes involved in the production, protection, and use of crops and livestock. As a basic science, it embraces in addition to test-tube chemistry all the life processes through which man obtains food and fiber for himself and feed for his animals. As an applied science or technology, it is directed toward control of those processes to increase yields, improve quality, and reduce costs. One important branch of it, chemurgy, is concerned chiefly with utilization of agricultural products as chemical raw materials.

Scope of field. The goals of agricultural chemistry are to expand man's understanding of the causes and effects of biochemical reactions related to plant and animal growth, to reveal opportunities for controlling those reactions, and to develop chemical products that will provide the desired assistance or control. So rapid has progress been that chemicalization of agriculture has come to be regarded as a 20th-century revolution. Augmenting the benefits of mechanization (a revolution begun in the mid-19th century and still under way), the chemical revolution has advanced farming much further in its transition from art to science.

Every scientific discipline that contributes to agricultural progress depends in some way on chemistry. Hence agricultural chemistry is not a distinct discipline, but a common thread that ties together genetics, physiology, microbiology, entomology, and numerous other sciences that impinge on agriculture. Chemical techniques help the geneticist to evolve hardier and more productive plant and animal strains; they enable the plant physiologist and animal nutritionist to determine the kinds and amounts of nutrients needed for optimum growth; they permit the soil scientist to determine a soil's ability to provide essential nutrients for the support of crops or livestock, and to prescribe chemical amendments where deficiencies exist. *See* FERTILIZER; SOIL.

Chemical materials developed to assist in the production of food, feed, and fiber include scores of herbicides, insecticides, fungicides, and other pesticides, plant growth regulators, fertilizers, and animal feed supplements. Chief among these groups from the commercial point of view are manufactured fertilizers, synthetic pesticides (including herbicides), and supplements for feeds. The latter include both nutritional supplements (for example, minerals) and medicinal compounds for the prevention or control of disease. *See* HERBICIDE; PESTICIDE.

Important chemicals. Chemical supplements for animal feeds may be added in amounts as small as a few grams or less per ton of feed, but the tremendous tonnage of processed feeds sold, coupled with the high unit value of some of the chemical supplements, makes this a large market. *See* ANIMAL-FEED COMPOSITION.

Of increasing importance since their commercial introduction have been chemical regulators of plant growth. Besides herbicides (some of which kill plants through overstimulation rather than direct chemical necrosis), the plant growth regulators include chemicals used to thin fruit blossoms, to assist in fruit set, to defoliate plants as an aid to mechanical harvesting, to speed root development on plant cuttings, and to prevent unwanted growth, such as sprouting of potatoes in storage. *See* DEFOLIANT AND DESICCANT.

Striking effects on growth have been observed in plants treated with gibberellins. These compounds, virtually ignored for two decades after they were first isolated from diseased rice in Japan, attracted widespread research attention in the United States in 1956; first significant commercial use began in 1958. The gibberellins are produced commercially by fermentation in a process similar to that used to manufacture penicillin. *See* GIBBERELLIN.

In the perennial battle with insect pests, chemicals that attract or repel insects are increasingly important weapons. Attractants (usually associated with the insect's sexual drive) may be used along with insecticides, attracting pests to poisoned bait to improve pesticidal effectiveness. Often highly specific, they are also useful in insect surveys; they attract specimens to strategically located traps, permitting reliable estimates of the extent and intensity of insect infestations.

Repellents have proved valuable, especially in the dairy industry. Milk production is increased when cows are protected from the annoyance of biting flies. Repellents also show promise as aids to weight gain in meat animals and as deterrents to the spread of insect-borne disease. If sufficiently selective, they may protect desirable insect species (bees, for instance) by repelling them from insecticide-treated orchards or fields.

Agricultural chemistry as a whole is constantly changing. It becomes more effective as the total store of knowledge is expanded. Synthetic chemicals alone, however, are not likely to solve all the problems man faces in satisfying his food and fiber needs. Indeed, many experts are coming to the view that the greatest hope for achieving maximum production and protection of crops and livestock lies in combining the best features of chemical, biological, and cultural approaches to farming. *See* AGRICULTURAL SCIENCE (ANIMAL); AGRICULTURAL SCIENCE (PLANT); AGRICULTURE.

[RODNEY N. HADER]

Agricultural engineering

The principal engineering discipline which serves the agricultural industry. Agricultural engineering is directly concerned with developing means for providing food and fiber for mankind's needs. With the world population explosion and the desire for higher standards of living, the efficiency of food and fiber production must be continually increased. *See* AGRICULTURE.

The agricultural industry is the oldest and largest industry in the world. It encompasses much more than just farming in the United States. Agriculture and related businesses that serve agriculture account for approximately 40% of the gross national product, one-third of the labor force, and involve about one-half of the total agricultural and industrial financial investment. The segment of the agricultural industry which provides the machines, chemicals, buildings, and materials-handling equipment, and the many products and services that farm producers demand, requires a great number of agricultural engineers.

History and training. The agricultural engineering profession had its origin in 1907, when the American Society of Agricultural Engineers was founded at Madison, Wis. In 1906 Iowa Agricultural College offered a program leading to the bachelor's degree in agricultural engineering. Approximately 52 colleges and universities in the United States and Canada offer undergraduate curricula, and an increasing number of institutions in foreign countries are initiating similar programs. A majority of the curricula in the United States are accredited by the Engineers Council for Professional Development, the nationally recognized accrediting agency for engineering degree programs. Many of these institutions also offer programs on the graduate level in agricultural engineering.

Applications. Nearly all problems that agricultural engineers deal with involve biological materials, systems, and processes. Application of physical and engineering sciences to the solution of such problems is the distinguishing feature of agricultural engineering.

Mechanization of agricultural production has been responsible in large measure for the productivity record of agriculture. The product output per man-hour of an agricultural worker is nearly twice that of most manufacturing industries. *See* AGRICULTURE, MACHINERY IN.

While great progress has been made in the application of mechanical power to the production and harvesting of field crops, there is constant demand for new machines and techniques to produce additional saving of labor, human energy, and increased efficiency. The production of many crops, such as fruits and vegetables, still requires expensive and increasingly scarce hand labor, especially in harvesting operations. To develop complete mechanized systems for all agricultural crops is a challenging goal for agricultural engineers.

Environmental control. One of the areas of great importance for the future is modification and control of the soil, water, and air environment of plants. As greater production is demanded from an ever-decreasing available land area, more and more attention is being given to modifying the natural environment to produce conditions which are more nearly ideal for plant growth. Many agricultural engineers are actively working to accomplish this goal in environmentally controlled chambers and greenhouses and by use of special tillage methods, plastic and petroleum-derivative mulches, irrigation, drainage, and other means for controlling soil and air temperature and moisture conditions to increase plant growth. *See* AGRICULTURAL SCIENCE (PLANT); AGRICULTURE, SOIL AND CROP PRACTICES IN; LAND DRAINAGE (AGRICULTURE).

Controlled environment for animal production

within confined housing systems is another area of activity of major concern to agricultural engineers. Providing optimum animal environment offers much promise for increasing the efficiency of production at reduced cost per unit of animal product. Many research studies are being conducted to determine the best conditions of temperature, humidity, and light, as well as systems to provide these conditions economically. *See* AGRICULTURAL SCIENCE (ANIMAL).

Livestock farming. The modern livestock farm can be likened to a factory with various imputs for poultry and dairy and meat animals. All of the problems of a factory, including buildings, materials handling, storages, and disposal of waste products are encountered. Add to this the fact that many operations in these enterprises are intermittent, such as feeding and milking, and thus they present a multitude of engineering problems. Mechanization of the modern farmstead has become a reality and agricultural engineers have been largely responsible. Automation is now the goal that challenges agricultural engineers. *See* CATTLE PRODUCTION, BEEF; CATTLE PRODUCTION, DAIRY; DAIRY MACHINERY; POULTRY PRODUCTION; SWINE PRODUCTION.

Resource management. An important phase of agricultural engineering involves the management and beneficial use of soil and water resources. Food and water are basic to mankind. It is recognized that these resources are limited and must be managed wisely. Agricultural engineers are involved in research to develop new techniques and design systems to control soil erosion, to control soil moisture for crop production, to prevent floods, to prevent water pollution, and to provide pure water supplies for human use. *See* SOIL CONSERVATION.

Produce processing. Although much agricultural engineering work is involved with the development and design of power machinery for crop production, many engineering problems are encountered after the crops are harvested. Postharvest processing, such as drying of grains and forages; washing, grading, and storage of fruits and vegetables, including controlled atmosphere systems; and ginning of cotton are typical of on-the-farm applications of agricultural engineering. *See* AGRICULTURE, STRUCTURES IN.

An increasingly large volume of food products are being processed prior to purchase by the consumer. This is resulting in rapid growth of the food processing industry, which has found that agricultural engineers are especially well qualified for many of the required engineering, technical, and management positions. *See* FOOD ENGINEERING.

Forest products. Another relatively new field of activity within the agricultural engineering profession is concerned with the design and development of equipment for the production, harvesting, and handling of forest products prior to their processing.

Fields of work. A great variety of employers hire agricultural engineers to work on problems such as outlined above. Some typical employers are farm equipment manufacturers and distributors, electrical power suppliers, electrical equipment manufacturers, the farm buildings industry, processors of agricultural products, processors and distributors of agricultural supplies, universities, and branches of the state and Federal governments. With these employers, agricultural engineers may engage in design, development, testing, sales and service, teaching, research, or other activities. Many foreign countries need agricultural engineers to assist in the development of an efficient agriculture to provide food for their rapidly increasing populations.

[ORVAL C. FRENCH]

Bibliography: American Society of Agricultural Engineers, *Agr. Eng. Yearb.*, 1968; O. C. French, *Automot. Ind.*, 136:12, 1967; H. F. McColly and J. W. Martin, *Introduction to Agricultural Engineering*, 1955; C. B. Richey, *Agricultural Engineering Handbook*, 1961.

Agricultural geography

Farming systems are an amalgam of climatic, geographical, historical, and cultural features. The evolution of these systems has led to the characterization of distinct types of agricultural activity, each with its own developmental trends that sometimes diminish or even erase differences between systems.

Agricultural systems involve one-third of the Earth's land area—one-third of which is tilled land $(1.47 \times 10^9$ ha) and two-thirds of which is pasture $(2.9 \times 10^9$ ha). Rarely, however, are more than $8.5-9 \times 10^8$ ha actually harvested in any year, due to floods, droughts, pests, and diseases. In addition, it is anticipated that 3×10^8 ha of tilled land will become unsuitable prior to the year 2000 due to ongoing soil erosion, salination, spread of waterborne diseases, and the mounting force of urbanization. Another loss involves rangeland and pasture, more than half of which are currently overgrazed and are evolving into steppe or desert.

Every society, however, is dependent directly or indirectly on agriculture for survival. On a global scale more people (half the working population) are engaged in agriculture than in any other economic activity. Without agriculture the type of culture with which most of the world's inhabitants are familiar could not exist.

ORIGIN OF AGRICULTURAL SYSTEMS

Most present-day agricultural systems can be traced back 10,000 years to the beginnings of agriculture: the first domestication of plants and animals. While today most cultivated crops and domesticated animals are distributed worldwide, they were internationalized fairly late in human history, mostly within the last 4 or 5 centuries. The Indians of the Western Hemisphere contributed several major crops to the world: corn, potato, manioc, beans, groundnut, and tomato. Wheat, barley, and rye originated in the Near East, rice and bananas in southern Asia, sugarcane in India, and sorghum in Africa.

A distinction should be made at this point between "seed agriculture" and "vegeculture." Seed agriculture refers to plant reproduction from seed. In seed agriculture, cereals dominate as staple food crops in all but a few parts of the world. Such crops are predominantly annuals and are harvested in one short period, necessitating storage between crops. Seed agriculture formed the basis of the major agricultural civilizations of history. There were three major centers of cereal domestication in the Old World: southwestern Asia, north-

ern China, and southeastern Asia; and possibly two in the New World: southern Mexico and Peru. *See* CEREAL.

Vegeculture refers to plant reproduction by vegetative propagation. The principal crops of vegeculture are tropical roots such as taro, manioc, yams, sweet potatoes, and arrowroot. In vegeculture, rhizomes are cut from the growing plant and individually planted. There are two distinct advantages of this system: First, there is less need to completely clear the natural vegetation, because if a mixture of roots is grown, crops may be harvested when needed; and second, storage is less imperative.

Vegeculture developed in the tropics, on the boundary between forest and grassland, in the Americas, Africa, and southeastern Asia. Over the years, it has contracted as seed agriculture expanded from the heartlands of these regions. The best-known tropical vegeculture is that of southeastern Asia and includes not only the mainland, but also the Malaysian archipelago, Assam (India), and southern China. Root and tree crops indigenous to this region include taro, the greater yam, breadfruit, sago palm, bamboo, coconuts, and bananas. *See* ROOT AND TUBER FOOD CROPS.

The Middle East was the origin of all domesticated food-producing animals except the water buffalo and the llama. In the 1530s European pioneers brought cattle to the Western Hemisphere, initially close to present-day Buenos Aires. This early trial failed, but a renewed effort was made in 1569 when horses were also introduced. Cattle reached the North American continent with the early European settlers in 1610, and sheep in 1633. Australia, today's leading sheep-producing nation, received its first sheep as late as 1797 (possibly 1788).

CLIMATIC FEATURES

Climate, as defined by temperature and precipitation patterns, is the major factor in the selection of specific crops to satisfy human needs. Agricultural geography tries to define these physical limits for crop cultivation. The limits of cultivation have persistently been extended by developing crop strains which are resistant to cold, drought, or excessive moisture. Where economic forces or incentives are sufficiently strong, adverse climatic conditions may be overcome by irrigation, pest control, and other means. Production is basically determined by the vegetation period, mostly the frost-free period. In warmer latitudes this period is extended, allowing for multicropping. *See the feature article* THE GREEN REVOLUTION; *see also* MULIPLE CROPPING.

The environment as shaped through climate is the basis for each kind of agriculture as it has evolved in various regions of the world. Soils have been shaped by topography and the composition of parent materials in an intricate interplay with climate. Soils have also been affected by the vegetation cover. This pattern has been the operational basis for agricultural pursuits. With time, agricultural systems evolved which were profoundly modified by plants and soils to increase production, originally with the double aim of feeding humans and livestock; more recently these systems have become increasingly specialized for the production of crops or the raising of livestock. Specialization itself has evolved into monocultures, as well as into mass raising of a single category of livestock. *See* AGRICULTURAL METEOROLOGY.

SYSTEM CLASSIFICATION

The most widely accepted classification of agricultural systems dates back to the 1930s when D. Whittlesey recognized two main factors as basic: environmental conditions (such as climate, soil, and slope) and human and social factors (such as population density, technological advances, and traditional practices). These factors interact to create circumstances that provide the functional basis for every type of agriculture.

There are several areas of the world in which the land is totally unsuitable for agricultural use. Such environments, termed restrictive or negative, include high mountains, with rugged surfaces, shallow stony soils, restricted flat land, and inhospitable climates; deserts, where water for irrigation is nonexistent; icecaps; and tundras, with permafrost and poor drainage.

Thirteen distinct types of agricultural activity were originally identified. Later developments somewhat modified this early classification, and also reduced the validity of distinctive features. This review identifies 11 major types: (1) subsistence tillage—shifting cultivation, transition forms, and intensive variants; (2) subsistence crop and livestock farming; (3) wet rice cultivation; (4) pastoral nomadism; (5) Mediterranean agriculture; (6) mixed farming (crop and livestock farming); (7) dairying; (8) plantation agriculture; (9) specialized horticulture and truck farming; (10) large-scale grain production; and (11) livestock ranching.

Subsistence tillage: shifting cultivation. Shifting cultivation is mostly practiced in isolated areas in the tropics. Three major subtypes may be identified.

The least advanced type usually consists of hunting-gathering tribes that supplement their major sources of livelihood with primitive agricultural pursuits. Few if any tools are employed, and the ground is not plowed. Wherever there is a natural clearing in the forest, seeds are placed in holes dug by hand or stick. The growers do not till or care for their crops and return only for harvesting. Due to pests and diseases, crop yields are low.

In a slightly more advanced type of shifting cultivation, the tribes occupy semipermanent dwellings for about 3 to 4 years, and agricultural activities occur in the immediate vicinity of the settlement.

In the third and most common type of shifting agriculture, the tribe stays in the same area for periods of up to 20 to 30 years. The forest is cleared in patches with one clearing used at a time. Within a year or two, however, weeds and pests become serious or fertility declines, at which time the land is abandoned and a new clearing is made. After several clearings are made and their soil resources depleted, the dwellings and fields are abandoned and a new area is sought. This category of subsistence growers numbers approximately 54×10^6, with the approximate number (in millions of tillers) per region as follows: Africa, 30; Indonesia, 10; Southeast Asia, 5.5; India, 5; South America, 1.1; Madagascar, 1; New Guinea, 0.5; Central America, 0.25; and the Philippines, 0.2.

As a rule only one or two vegetable crops are planted per family in the wet tropics, although a wide variety of tree crops (coconuts, breadfruit, oil palm, mangos, avocados, bananas, plantains, cacao, and guavas) and vegetable crops (yams, sweet potatoes, pumpkins, beans, and peanuts) are encountered. Some rice and corn are grown in a few places when introduced from outside. Here and there sugarcane and millet are raised. Bread is made from cassava or manioc, which frequently is a staple in the diet. Bananas, yams, and sweet potatoes provide abundant starch; coconuts and oil palms supply needed fats.

Transitional forms. Throughout areas inhabited by hunter-gatherers practicing shifting cultivation, some changes have gradually taken place, evolving into rudimentary and sedentary tillage systems. The main driving forces for change are a lowered standard of living resulting in a switch to other forms of resources; migration to other areas; and changes in socioeconomic activities.

Production of foodstuffs and other plants solely for local use takes many forms in terms of products (rice, tubers, fruits), techniques (hand tools, irrigation, use of work animals), intensity (settled agriculture, minor gardening), organization (ownership of land, financing, work methods), and other variables. Native communities often supplement their subsistence cropping to some extent with marketable products. For example, growing rubber or pepper or making copra from coconuts provides communities with money to help fill minimum needs for imported goods.

Much of the sedentary subsistence farming in Latin America is still characterized by extensive employment of human labor, little use of machinery, forest destruction, and soil depletion or erosion. Three or four crops, such as corn, beans, rice, manioc, and even cotton, are planted and harvested with a hoe or stick. After the soil is depleted, grasses are planted to be grazed until scrubby trees choke them out, or the land is simply abandoned for a newly cleared plot.

In African sedentary subsistence farming, the cultivated crops of the wet-dry savanna lands are mainly shrubs such as the cotton bush, small plants such as tobacco and peanut, or domesticated grasses such as maize and millet. Other primary crops include corn, wheat, barley, rice, sorghum, sweet potatoes, and various types of beans which are diet staples. Secondary crops commonly grown in the savanna lands are manioc, sesame, artichokes, peppers, tomatoes, and pumpkins.

Intensive variants. India and China are classic examples of intensively cultivated, densely populated lands with the bulk of their labor force engaged in subsistence agriculture. Although cultivated intensively, much of interior India, dry inland portions of southeastern Asia, and regions of China north of the Yangtze River differ in the nature and methods of crop production. Rice is dominant where water is supplied either through irrigation systems or by natural rainfall and flooding. Other grains become the staples of diet where precipitation is inadequate or undependable and irrigation is too costly.

In India, most cultivators remain involved in subsistence agriculture. The land tenure system provides little incentive to the cultivator. However, recent land reform, agricultural extension services, better seed, and the rapidly expanding use of fertilizer have resulted in an increase in food production which is slightly ahead of the increase in population. However, there are still extensive problems and the population pressure on the land is getting worse. There are an estimated 45×10^6 landless agricultural laborers in India; crop failures in various sections have been a recurrent feature; and approximately four-fifths of the cultivatable land area is dependent on the rainy seasons or monsoons.

The major subsistence grains cultivated in the drier parts of India are sorghum, millet, and wheat. Sorghum is widely distributed over the Deccan Plateau but is most heavily concentrated on the black soils in the central part of the Indian peninsula. Millet is the major grain in the extreme northwest and Rajasthan portions of India bordering Pakistan. Wheat is grown mainly in northwestern and central India. Secondary crops include gram or chickpea, grown from the Punjab plains eastward to the delta region; peanuts, which are highly concentrated in the southern half of the peninsula; and cotton, produced mostly in the northwestern and central parts of the Deccan Plateau.

A clear-cut separation exists in China between the areas north and south of the Yangtze Valley. Rice predominates to the south in a climate which has a more dependable rainfall and is moist and warm throughout most of the year. To the north is a region of fertile but often barren plains and bare mountains, except for a short-lived green revival where the Hwang River approaches the sea. Like the southern region, there is much rich soil, but rainfall is infrequent. Prolonged droughts may parch the soil and burn crops out before harvest. Sudden outbursts of rain produce devastating floods.

Despite this climate, northern China is a highly productive region. The area near the coast, the famous North China Plain, is one of the most densely populated and most intensively cultivated parts of the world. This is the winter wheat–kaoliang region and it comprises most of the provinces of Hopei, Shantung, and Honan. Due to a high percentage of usable land (60% or more under cultivation), this region produces a wide variety of crops without irrigation. Fortunately, the maximum rainfall of 24 in. (61 cm) occurs during the hot summer. Winter wheat is the principal crop and occupies almost half the cultivated land, while barley and peas are grown in a few districts. Kaoliang, a type of millet, is the chief summer crop, with soybeans, cotton, corn, and sweet potatoes also covering a considerable acreage. Persimmons and hard pears are key fruits; peanuts are cultivated in several districts, especially in Shantung and Honan; and tobacco is grown in a few localities.

To the west of this region are the Loess Highlands, an area of windblown silt deposits 300 or more feet (90 meters) thick in places, with fertile soils, steep slopes, and marginal rainfall. More than one-third of the cropland is terraced to check erosion of the steep hillsides. The best agricultural districts are situated along the Hwang River in southern Shansi and northern Honan, extending west into Shensi. Winter wheat, the major crop, is confined to the plains and valleys; other winter

crops are rapeseed, peas, and barley. Millet is the most widely grown summer crop, followed by corn, soybeans, sesame, and buckwheat; cotton is important in some of the more productive agricultural districts.

The spring wheat region forms a fringe along the Mongolian frontier, lying on either side of the Great Wall. The percentage of cultivable land is small, owing to the cold climate and limited rainfall. Spring wheat is the principal crop, interspersed with millet, oats, peas, flax, and buckwheat.

Subsistence crop and livestock farming. Subsistence crop and livestock farming occupies large tracts of semidesert, hill, or mountainous lands in the Anatolian and Iranian plateaus in southwestern Asia, portions of Soviet Siberia bordering the Mongolian People's Republic, and small segments in Soviet Europe north of the 55th parallel. The Carpathian and Rhodope mountain areas of east-central and southeastern Europe also have small tracts of land that are still classified as subsistence crop and livestock farming areas. The only area of corresponding size outside the Eurasian realm is the Mexican plateau.

Few people are engaged in this type of agriculture. In the past, most of them followed a nomadic way of life, but inroads are constantly being made on the occupied lands through government intervention, improvement in agricultural techniques, and resettlement programs. The Kurds of eastern Turkey and Armenia, the Buryats of southeastern Siberia, and the Yakuts north and west of Lake Baikal in the Soviet Union are former nomadic herders who have become sedentary yet still dependent on livestock farming.

For the most part, agriculture and animal husbandry tend to split into separate occupations. The mixed type of farming characteristic of many parts of the world is practiced only on a minor scale, and many villages maintain one or more shepherds to look after a common herd, while the great majority of owners devote themselves entirely to crop cultivation. All tillable land is devoted to growing cereals, and vegetables and fruits are cultivated wherever possible.

Herding tends to be restricted to less favorable regions. People who still engage in this endeavor have become seminomadic villagers who move their flocks in summer to hillsides or mountain slopes where the animals graze until cold weather threatens.

Wet rice cultivation. Rice is the predominant crop in the dry and cool monsoon regions. The staple food of well over half the world's people, rice is so prevalent that an agricultural system has been developed around it.

The task of clearing and maintaining rice fields, which are small (often averaging less than 2 acres or 0.8 ha per farm), is relatively easy. The young trees and dry grass are burned near the close of the dry season and the ground is hoed. Prior to monsoon rains, the fields are tilled and flooded with water. The rice is then planted and the fields remain flooded until a few days before harvest.

The soils are generally alluvial in nature and mainly hold key drainage basins, such as those of the Irrawaddy, Salween, Menam, Mekong, Red, Yangtze, and Si river basins. These soils are naturally fertile, but owing to intensive tillage they require large amounts of fertilizing from animal manure and night soil (human excrement). The latter is by far the most widely used fertilizer in southeastern Asia, where the population is so dense that animals are relatively few.

Rice cultivation of this kind covers much of Sri Lanka, southern India, Bangladesh, the delta of mainland southeastern Asia, Java, Sumatra, the Philippines, and southern China and Japan. The total area under wet rice cultivation exceeds 10^8 ha.

As rice exists in so many varieties, it can be grown under widely varying conditions, from brackish or even saline soils to deeply flooded deltas like those of Thailand and southern Vietnam. In many places, given enough water, rice can supply two crops from the same land each year. It can give worthwhile yields on the same land year after year for generations without fertilizer, although yields may be greatly increased by the judicious use of manure. Dry crops under similar conditions in the tropics tend to give declining yields that often stabilize at an uneconomic level. *See* RICE.

Pastoral nomadism. The principal regions of pastoral nomadism are in the arid lands of the Old World, extending from northern Africa through Saudi Arabia to inner Asia. This type of highly specialized livelihood involves frequent movement of livestock in response to the need for grazing lands and water. Settlement is generally characterized by small clusters of homesteads temporarily established near a common watering point and pasture. Subsistence is maintained almost entirely by domestic stock, such as cattle, camels, goats, and sheep.

In many areas, nomadism is a product of cultural associations that may be as dominant a factor in the activity as the physical landscape. Many Moslem Arabs prefer nomadism to a sedentary way of life because of long tradition. In other areas, without the benefits of modern technology and capital investment, nomadism is the only economic system that can survive.

There has been a conscious effort on the part of some governments to make nomads sedentary. Egypt has attempted this with moderate success. Iran and Iraq have taken measures to permanently settle more than 3,000,000 nomads. Somali, Israel, Tanzania, and the Soviet Union also have experimented with settling nomads.

Mediterranean agriculture. This refers to a diverse crop-livestock economic system that is practiced most extensively around the Mediterranean Sea and in four other non-Mediterranean areas with similar climatic patterns: southern California, central Chile, southwest of Capetown in South Africa, and southern parts of South Australia and the area around Spencer Gulf. From a geographic standpoint, this system is the most clearly defined. The climate is characterized by mild, wet winters and hot, dry summers. Unless crops are irrigated, they must either be sown in the autumn and harvested by early summer or be drought-resistant.

Mediterranean agriculture has many distinctive features. Winter grains, such as wheat and barley, and all-year crops, such as olives, grapes, and carob, are grown without irrigation. All-year or summer crops that are generally irrigated include oranges, lemons, deciduous fruits, corn, rice, and vegetables. Livestock, mainly sheep, goats, and some cattle, are brought to the highlands for grazing in summer and kept on the lowland plains in winter. This transhumance is less significant today but still is practiced in parts of Greece, Italy, Yugoslavia, Spain, and North Africa.

Both subsistence and cash crops are important in the economy of every region of Mediterranean agriculture, although not on every farm. The relative emphasis on the several products varies with the amount of rainfall. Thus, northern Africa produces more barley and goatskins, and southern Europe more wheat and sheepskins. Citrus and vine crops have long been important in world trade (Table 1). Southern France, Italy, California, and Chile are important wine producers; California and Spain stress oranges.

Despite the importance of agriculture, only about one-fifth of the land in the Mediterranean climatic regions is intensively cultivated. Due to the restricted rainfall, no less than 40% of the grainlands are kept in fallow each year. Much land is too steep, dry, or rocky. Due to these constraints, a definite pattern of land use has evolved over the centuries: small fruits and vegetables occupy the lowlands; wheat and barley are grown in the more arid portions of the lower slopes; and tree and vine crops dominate the upper slopes. Frequently, interculture is practiced to make the most of the usable land.

Livestock grazing is based primarily on natural vegetation. Generally, cattle tend to predominate in the wetter areas; sheep, which far outnumber other domestic animals, dominate vast areas of the arid zone; and goats predominate in the driest, more rocky areas. During the wet winter season,

Table 1. Global production of grapes and citrus fruits in top producers, in 10^6 metric tons*

Producer	1961–1965	1973–1974	Percent change
Grapes			
France	9.6	13.1	+ 36.5
Italy	9.8	11.3	+ 15.2
Spain	4.2	6.2	+ 47.5
Soviet Union	2.8	4.7	+ 67.5
Turkey	3.1	3.2	+ 3.2
United States	3.3	3.8	+ 15.1
Argentina	2.4	3.1	+ 29.5
World total	50.6	63.2	+ 25.0
Oranges			
United States	4.5	8.9	+ 19.8
Brazil	2.0	3.2	+ 60.0
Spain	1.6	2.0	+ 25.0
Mexico	1.2	2.0	+ 66.5
Italy	0.9	1.5	+ 66.8
Israel	0.6	1.2	+100.0
World total	17.5	28.5	+ 63.2
Lemons and limes			
Italy	0.55	0.84	+ 52.5
United States	0.55	0.72	+ 31.0
India	0.44	0.45	+ 2.3
Argentina	0.08	0.28	+250.0
Mexico	0.17	0.23	+ 35.3
Spain	0.11	0.24	+118.0
World total	2.8	4.1	+ 46.5

*From *FAO Production Yearbook*, 1974.

the lush green lowlands with mild temperatures are ideal for grazing livestock. In summer, when the lowland pastures are dry and dormant, the cool grassy upper slopes are utilized.

Livestock farming in Mediterranean agriculture is based on irrigated meadows planted in alfalfa, hay, clover, sown grasses, or other forage crops. The animals are stall-fed. Meat, milk, and cheese are produced both for local consumption and export in northern Algeria, northern Italy, southern France, and southern and eastern Spain. Dairying is especially important near the larger cities. In other areas of the Mediterranean Basin, such as southern Italy, central Spain, northern Greece, Yugoslavia, Turkey, and Syria, subsistence livestock farming prevails. Large-scale commercial livestock farming is important in California. Irrigated pastures and imported grain support huge dairies and meat-packing plants near Los Angeles and San Francisco. The San Joaquin Valley is a major milk-producing center.

Crop and livestock farming. This mode of agriculture, also called mixed farming, is based on a combination of crop cultivation and animal husbandry. It is extensive and occupies the humid middle latitudes of all continents. The monetary return is generally less than that for commercial dairy farming or specialized agriculture. Periodic rather than daily shipment to market is the rule. Farm population density is high, and large urban centers are dispersed within the mixed farming belts. Smaller cities, towns, and villages dot the landscape, providing market outlets and services.

China and India are top-ranking in total number of livestock, but the Soviet Union and the United States lead in commercial production. The two largest commercial livestock and crop farming regions are in the United States and Eurasia. In the United States, this activity is prevalent in the Midwest (Ohio, Indiana, Illinois, Iowa, and Nebraska), the South (Virginia, Tennessee, and Georgia), and Southwest (Oklahoma and much of Texas). In Eurasia, this system is encountered in much of northern Portugal and Spain, the Po River plain of Italy, a large portion of the Danube basin countries of Hungary, Yugoslavia, and western Romania, and the Amur Valley in the Soviet Union. Minor regions are found in Argentina, southeastern Brazil, south-central Chile, and South Africa.

The commercial crop and livestock farming system concentrates on breeding and plant selection and a well-established crop rotation in which legumes and hay play an important part in proper soil management. Some farmers produce grains such as wheat, corn, or soybeans for sale as a cash crop; others produce only corn as feed for livestock. Farm animals use roughage, which may be produced in any mixed farming system. On a typical midwestern farm with a rotation of corn, oats, and clover, approximately 1.75 tons of roughage are produced for every ton of grain (1.95 metric tons for every metric ton). In Eurasia, root crops planted in rotation with grain crops in order to maintain soil fertility are fed to farm animals. Hay is a substitute for corn in most of Eurasia; corn is an important feed crop only in the Danube Valley. Elsewhere potatoes, turnips, sugarbeets, and oats are the major feed crops.

Farms in Eurasia are smaller and less mechanized than their United States couterparts, with higher production per acre but lower output per worker. Average livestock-grain operations in the United States range from 120 to 200 acres (50 to 80 ha); in South America and South Africa, they are about the same size; and in Eurasia, about half as large.

Livestock and crop production are complementary activities. They make possible a more even seasonal distribution of labor. Cattle raising plays an important role in the intensive agriculture of northwestern Europe and the American Midwest.

Dairying. Commercial dairy farming is profitable only where the products can be sold to an urban market, and is generally located near densely populated industrial areas. Fresh milk cannot be shipped distances farther than 12 hr away and requires refrigerated tank cars; some milk is presently flown into major cities, such as New York. Refrigerated butter can be shipped great distances. Cheese will keep for up to 3 or 4 years, depending on the type.

Dairying is an intensive form of agriculture. It is elaborately mechanized, and the capital investment in buildings and equipment on high-grade dairy farms exceeds that in any other type of agriculture. The labor requirement for dairying is exceeded only in few other agricultural activities. Every step in feeding, milking, and processing is critical since dairy cattle must be milked twice a day to produce their maximum capacity.

The Soviet Union has become the world's leader in producing milk, followed by the United States (Table 2). The major European producers of dairy products are France, West Germany, Poland, the United Kingdom, Italy, the Netherlands, East Germany, Czechoslovakia, and Denmark. The chief dairy regions of the Soviet Union are in the Baltic countries. In North America, the north-central United States and adjacent parts of Canada, in particular the state of Quebec, contribute most of the milk. Production in Australia and New Zealand is about equally divided. *See* CATTLE PRODUCTION, DAIRY.

Plantation agriculture. Plantation agriculture is usually a corporate enterprise that organizes the production of valuable commercial crops, such as

Table 2. Global production of cow milk in top producers, in 10⁶ metric tons*

Producer	1961–1965	1973–1974	Percent change
Soviet Union	63.8	89.8	+40.1
United States	57.0	52.3	− 8.2
France	25.1	29.1	+11.6
India (includes buffalo)	19.6	24.1	+12.3
West Germany	20.6	21.4	+ 3.5
Poland	12.9	16.6	+28.8
United Kingdom	12.0	14.3	+19.1
Canada	8.4	7.6	− 9.5
Brazil	5.9	7.3	+23.7
World total	324.4	382.2	+11.8
Europe	135.7	158.9	+11.7
North America	65.4	60.0	− 8.3
	%		%
Satisfied world	282.6	87	329.8	86
Hungry world	41.8	13	52.4	14

*From *FAO Production Yearbook*, 1974.

cotton, rubber, rice, sugarcane, sugarbeets, pineapple, bananas, coconut, tea, cacao, and citrus fruits. This system is not characterized by a predominant crop, but by the manner in which crops are produced and the land is managed. Plantation agriculture is not strictly a phenomenon of the tropics or subtropics; the system is employed in a wide range of extratropical regions. The type of plantation ranges from those producing bananas or rubber in the wet tropics to state and collective enterprises in the Soviet Union, China, and Cuba.

The tropical plantation system initially evolved to meet the world demand for certain staple crops. As part of the colonial era, it rested on European acquisition of land areas that would make economically attractive units. Manual labor was held cheap, so that the product could be sold at a price that would ensure large and growing volumes. These conditions no longer prevail. Some plantation crops are grown and even harvested by small individually owned farms, but the output is channeled into major marketing enterprises; examples are cacao and peanuts in Nigeria and Senegal, rubber in Amazonas and Malaysia, bananas in Central America, and tea in Ceylon. Monoculture no longer prevails. Crop diversification has taken place in order to minimize crop failures, hurricane destruction, or attacks by pests and diseases. For example, rubber and bananas are produced in tandem on plantations in British Honduras; cacao and oil palms in other parts of Central America; and sugarcane, citrus fruits, and cattle in Florida.

The three most important commercial tropical plantation crops are bananas, sugarcane, and rubber. Brazil leads the world in production of bananas, but Ecuador is the major exporter. While India is the largest producer of sugarcane, the bulk of it is consumed domestically. Cuba, once the major producer of sugarcane, has reduced its acreage because of economic pressures and loss of the United States market. Malaysia continues to dominate the production of natural rubber.

Specialized crop production on a much smaller scale is encountered in some dry regions where irrigation is employed. Cotton is grown in this manner in parts of Central Asia, southern Kazakhstan and Transcaucasus (Soviet Union), the coastal oases of Peru, sections of the lower Colorado Basin, and the Argentine Chaco. In the same manner sugarbeets are produced in the Platte River and Salt Lake oases of the western United States, and sugarcane in coastal Peru and northern Argentina.

Specialized horticulture and truck farming. Early types of commercial fruit and vegetable production hinged on either closeness to city markets or a rapid transportation system in order to meet the demand for perishables. Until about 1900, such gardening was mainly restricted to an area lying within 10–15 mi (16–24 km) of a city, but since then production has been extended to distances of several hundred miles. The increased use of trucks—mostly refrigerated—and the development of improved roads have been important factors in this widened range. The development of such specialized horticulture is most clearly evident in parts of the Po Valley (northern Italy), the Rhone Valley of southern France, Sicily, and the Campania—often a result of railroads and highways linking production areas and large commerce centers.

Market gardening, a very intensive form of cultivation, is carried out on land adjacent to cities. Such production close to the market benefits from lower transportation costs and less packing, compared with production at greater distances. The market gardener supplies principally in-season vegetables; out-of-season vegetables may be raised in hothouses. Most major cities have outlying market garden areas. For example, Long Island and northern New Jersey serve the New York City region. London receives a large portion of its vegetables from the nearby counties of Middlesex and Bedfordshire and from the Isle of Ely. All of England receives early potatoes from the Channel Islands. East and West Ridings of Yorkshire are important sources of vegetables for the northern sections of Great Britain. In the Netherlands vegetables are grown over such wide areas that it would be difficult to define those supplying each city.

Truck farming is characterized by high specialization, mostly a single crop, applies less intensive methods, and as a rule is located further from the markets. Each producer concentrates on a crop particularly adapted to the soil conditions and seasonal climate of the region. In each trucking region, crops are grown at a time of year when there is little competition with crops grown in other sections. For instance, vegetables from Mexico and the West Indies reach the eastern cities of the United States first, and then crops are successively received from Florida, Georgia, South and North Carolina, and as far north as Canada.

The most important trucking sections of the United States are the Atlantic Coastal Plain from southern New Jersey to Florida; the Gulf Coastal Plain from Alabama to Texas; California; and certain north-central states. Important trucking areas are also found in Algeria, Tunisia, Egypt, and the French Riviera. Other such areas are located near the major cities of South Africa and southwest of Australia.

Large-scale grain production. Commercial grain farms lie on the border between humid and semiarid climates, where summers are short and winters cold. Most of these regions are deep in the interior of continental land masses. Wheat is the dominant grain crop, being well adapted to the conditions of scarce labor and extensive cultivation on vast tracts of land, distant from markets. These factors explain the importance of wheat in the North American Great Plains region (United States and Canada), Argentina, Australia, the Ukraine, and Kazakhstan.

Three technological developments which made possible the cultivation of the vast grasslands of the world's chief wheat-growing regions are transportation facilities (such as railroads, highway trucks, and barges) for handling the wheat; agricultural machinery for cultivating large tracts of land; and well-drilling machinery to make water available in semiarid regions.

The major regions of commercial grain farming are concentrated in the middle latitudes of the Northern and Southern hemispheres, between 30 and 55°. Eurasia's commercial grain area stretches from west to east for some 2000 mi (3200 km) and

Table 3. Average 1973–1974 production of main grain producers, in 10^6 metric tons

Producer	Amount
Cereals	
World total	1,345.9
China	227.1
United States	220.9
Soviet Union	200.3
India	113.3
France	41.4
Asia	515.3
North America	255.2
Europe	229.7
Latin America	75.4
Africa	61.5
Australia and New Zealand	17.8
Wheat	
World total	368.8
Soviet Union	96.8
United States	47.6
China	36.5
India	23.4
France	18.4
Canada	15.3
Asia	89.5
Europe	86.4
North America	63.0
Rice	
World total	323.9
China	113.6
India	63.6
Indonesia	22.3
Bangladesh	18.3
Japan	15.8
Thailand	14.0
United States	4.7
Asia	296.0
Latin America	11.8
Corn	
World total	301.7
United States	130.8
China	30.7
Brazil	15.1
Soviet Union	12.7
Argentina	9.8
France	9.8
North America	133.5
Asia	49.9
Europe	44.9
Latin America	38.2
Africa	22.3
Barley	
World total	170.1
Soviet Union	54.6
China	20.3
France	10.4
Canada	9.4
Great Britain	9.0
West Germany	6.8
Denmark	5.7
Europe	58.7
Asia	30.8
North America	17.4

north to south for 700 mi (1120 km). It includes all of the Ukraine except its extreme southeastern corner, the Crimea; much of the northern Caucasus Mountains and the irrigated regions of Central Asia and Transcaucasia; the middle and lower Volga Basin; the southern Ural Mountains; western Siberia; and Kazakhstan.

The Soviet Union is by far the world's leading wheat producer—surpassing the United States in most years by 60–100%. Canada's wheat production declined drastically from 1963 to 1972, while India showed the greatest percentage of gain (Table 3). *See* WHEAT.

Livestock ranching. In general, livestock ranching involves extensive grazing by cattle or sheep. Ranching is practiced in the humid margins of steppelands in the middle latitudes and the savanna areas of the tropics, tending to occupy regions where land values are low and population is sparse. This type of economic activity is characterized by the use of relatively large land areas, as opposed to smaller areas for field agriculture and livestock farming. Economic factors play a more immediate role in the magnitude of operation than in other systems.

Major ranching areas are the semiarid parts of the Great Plains, stretching from Texas through the prairie provinces of Canada, and throughout the intermontane basins and plateaus between the Rocky Mountains and the Sierra Nevada—Cascades from Canada to central Mexico: the llanos of Venezuela and Colombia, the sertão of Brazil, the pampa of Uruguay, the southeastern Argentine pampa, the Chaco, and Patagonia; the Karoo of South Africa; the big arid interior of Australia; and the high parts of the South Island of New Zealand. Livestock ranching is largely absent from the Eurasian realm, and has largely been the mode of occupying expanding frontiers.

Carrying capacity varies considerably. In deserts, 40 ha or more is required for forage to support one steer. Steppes and mountain meadows vary from 10 to 30 ha, depending on availability of moisture. In the subhumid part of the Great Plains, each steer averages 4 to 6 ha. When carrying capacity is low, large acreages are required. In western Texas many ranches have 8000 ha, and in southern Texas even more land is required. In Arizona and New Mexico many ranches have from 12,000 to 16,000 ha. The world's largest ranches are found in Australia.

The United States is the chief producer of beef in the world, followed by the Soviet Union (Table 4). The considerable percentage of increase in beef production in the Soviet Union, Australia, and Brazil from 1961–1965 to 1973–1974 should be noted. *See* CATTLE PRODUCTION, BEEF.

WORLD HUNGER AND AGRICULTURE

No issue confronting modern society is more complex than that of ensuring an adequate global food supply in the decades which lie immediately ahead. More than 500,000,000 people live under near-famine conditions in various parts of the world. Double that number of people live on a critically low standard which becomes still more precarious in poor crop years or between growing seasons.

The risk of expanded starvation will become greater toward the end of the century with another

Table 4. Total production of beef and veal in top producers, in 10⁶ metric tons*

Producer	1961–1965	1973–1974	Percent change
United States	8.1	10.2	+25.9
Soviet Union	3.5	6.1	+73.5
Argentina	2.2	2.2	–
Brazil	1.4	2.2	+37.5
France	1.4	1.6	+ 7.3
China	1.4	1.5	+ 7.3
Australia	0.88	1.37	+56.0
World	31.0	40.8	+31.5

*From *FAO Production Yearbook*, 1974.

3,000,000,000 expected to be added to a current world population of 4,000,000,000. It is generally agreed that the food crisis is global in nature and requires a comprehensive well-coordinated program of urgent, cooperative worldwide action. Food has become a central element of the international economy. A world characterized by energy shortages, rampant inflation, and a weakening trade and monetary system will be plagued by food scarcities as well.

During the 1950s and 1960s global food production consistently increased. Per capita output expanded even in the food-deficit nations, and the world's total output increased by more than half. But at the precise moment when growing populations and rising expectations made a continuation of this trend essential, a dramatic change occurred. Since 1974 world cereal production has fallen, and reserves have dropped to the point where major crop failures will be disastrous. In 1976 some recovery was noticeable.

The long-term picture remains grim. Since increases in food production are not evenly distributed, the absolute number of malnourished people is in fact probably greater today than ever before.

The world faces a challenge unprecedented in severity, pervasiveness, and global dimension. The minimum objective of the next quarter century must be to more than double world food production and to improve its quality; yet even this would not remove the "hunger gap" unless drastic measures are taken to change current distribution patterns and to channel less grain into the excessive animal production of the affluent world, which now utilizes three times more tilled land to feed each person than the developing world. *See the feature article* FEEDING THE WORLD; *see also* AGRICULTURE. [GEORG BORGSTROM]

Bibliography: J. R. Borchert, The Dust Bowl in the 1970's, *Ann. Ass. Amer. Geogr.*, 61:1–22, 1971; E. Boscrup, *The Conditions of Agricultural Growth*, 1965; C. Clark and M. R. Hascell, *The Economics of Subsistence Agriculture*, 1964; J. C. Dickinson, Alternatives to monoculture in the humid tropics of Latin America, *Prof. Geogr.*, 24:217–222, 1973; A. N. Duckham and G. B. Masefield, *Farming Systems of the World*, 1971; D. B. Grigg, *The Agricultural Systems of the World: An Evolutionary Approach*, 1974; F. Hart, The Middle West, *Ann. Ass. Amer. Geogr.*, 62:258–282, 1972; M. U. Igbozurike, Ecological balance in tropical agriculture, *Geogr. Rev.*, 61:519–529, 1971; E. Mather, The American Great Plains, *Ann. Ass. Amer. Geogr.*, 62:237–257, 1972; C. O. Sauer, The agency of man on Earth, in W. L. Thomas, Jr. (ed.), *Man's Role in Changing the Face of the Earth*, pp. 56–64, 1956; J. E. Spencer and N. R. Stewart, The nature of agricultural systems, *Ann. Ass. Amer. Geogr.*, 63:529–544, 1973; H. L. Trueman, The hungry seventies, *Can. Geogr. J.*, 83:114–129, 1971; D. Whittlesey, Major agricultural regions of the Earth, *Ann. Ass. Amer. Geogr.*, 26:199–240, 1936; G. C. Wilken, Microclimate management by traditional farmers, *Geogr. Rev.*, 62:544–560, 1972.

Agricultural meteorology

The study and application of relationships between meteorology and agriculture. It involves simple concepts such as timing the planting of crops to avoid damage from freezing temperatures, and more complicated problems such as the combined effects of temperature and humidity in producing an outbreak of a disease such as potato blight. *See* GROWING SEASON.

Here, meteorology is used in its broadest sense to include observing, reporting, and forecasting day-to-day variations in weather, as well as the study and use of past climatological data. Agriculture includes all farming, ranching, orchard, nursery, and forestry operations concerned with the production, harvesting, processing, and shipping of foods, fibers, flowers, leather, and lumber. Protection from and control of plant and animal diseases and insect pests are also included.

Major participating agencies. The U.S. Department of Agriculture and the state agricultural colleges and experiment stations are active in research in this field. The U.S. Weather Bureau assists in many of these projects, operates various service programs, and conducts research through cooperative agreements.

International cooperation and exchange of information are carried out through the Commission for Agricultural Meteorology (CAgM) of the World Meteorological Organization (WMO). This commission promotes meteorological development and standardizes methods, procedures, and techniques in the application of meteorology to problems in agriculture.

Microfocus of investigation. Microclimatology is of major importance in the study of agricultural meteorology. The interrelationships of climate and soil and the many important phenomena involved in the interchange of heat and moisture at the air-soil interface are of critical importance to vegetation and animal life in the biosphere.

Water and moisture problems. Water is often the most critical limiting factor in food production. More than 25,000,000 acres of land is irrigated in the United States. Much of this is in arid regions of the West and Southwest but a surprisingly large and increasing amount of irrigation is in the more humid East.

Moisture is withdrawn from the soil by direct evaporation from the soil surface and by transpiration through the plants. The first process is capable of quickly drying a shallow surface layer of soil, and in hot summer weather the water from brief showers can be removed by evaporation before it can enter the root zone. Transpiration removes moisture from the soil layers penetrated by roots. *See* EVAPOTRANSPIRATION.

The rate of loss by both processes (evapotranspiration) is closely related to the energy available for evaporation. Sunshine and temperature are used as indicators. Wind and humidity are also critical. Evapotranspiration rates of 0.25–0.30 in./day are not uncommon during warm summer seasons. Several methods have been suggested for computation of these rates from meteorological parameters. None has been completely accepted but several give approximations useful in determining irrigation requirements.

Precipitation data for agricultural planning include more information than simple monthly and annual average amounts. The range and the frequency distribution of various amounts about the mean are necessary in planning land use and crop risks. The duration and frequency of drought periods are needed in planning potential irrigation requirements.

Temperature factors. Temperature, both of the air and the soil, is an important factor in agricultural meteorology. The length of growing season and the average temperature during the season often determine the choice of crop species or variety. Sugarcane requires temperatures high enough to permit rapid growth for at least 8 months. Rice requires a warm moist environment with mean temperatures of 70°F or higher for 4–6 months. Cotton requires warm summer months (75–80°F), a long (180–200 days) growing season, and warm sunny days during harvest. Corn is considered to be of tropical origin but varieties have been developed for widely differing climates. However, the principal corn belt lies in a region having warm summer months (70–80°F) and a growing season of 140–160 days. Wheat production is divided into winter-wheat and spring-wheat areas largely on the basis of the severity of the winter.

The frequency and duration of freezing temperatures at certain seasons are of critical importance in many areas. The U.S. Weather Bureau operates localized frost-warning services in winter citrus- and truck-producing areas of Florida and California, in apple and other fruit regions of Washington and Oregon, and in summer in cranberry areas of Wisconsin and Massachusetts.

The temperature range of 60–80°F is optimum for milk production in dairy cattle. At 85°F production is reduced by as much as 25%, and at 95°F it is reduced 50%. Hogs gain little or no weight at 90°F. At 95°F or higher, fattened animals lose weight. When high temperatures are expected, hog shipments are postponed or arrangements are made for artificial cooling en route.

Diverse responses to weather. It is difficult to generalize in agricultural meteorology. Species and varieties of crops and breeds of animals all have their own peculiar responses to weather factors. Effects are often cumulative. For these reasons, many special problems are isolated and studied separately.

Maleic hydrazide (MH-30) acts as a growth regulator on some plants. Used as a spray, it controls the growth and development of suckers on tobacco, runners on strawberries, branches and shoots on trees, and new growth in grasses. Turgidity of plants and the weather (moisture, temperature, sunshine) during a period following application are important in determining final effectiveness. Much experimentation is being concentrated on this and similar problems to determine optimum spraying weather conditions.

Rapid increases in the use of aircraft for agricultural purposes have brought new meteorological problems. Weather reports and forecasts are needed to determine optimum times of application for control of diseases, insects, and weeds and also to determine conditions of wind, visibility, and temperature for the safe and effective operation of aircraft.

Potato blight, a fungus disease caused by *Phytophthora infestans*, occurs in serious to epidemic outbreaks in many areas. It can be controlled by spraying above-ground plant parts with a fungicide, but economical and effective protection depends upon application at the right time. If too early, it wastes the spray and permits new unprotected growth to be exposed to later infections. If too late, the crop may be lost. Timing is based on certain critical combinations of temperatures and moisture which favor spore germination. Special warning services are developed to assist farmers in timing their spraying programs.

In the forests there are many special problems. Forecast services are established to warn of low humidity, high temperatures, and winds which favor the outbreak and rapid spread of fires. Forest insect pests are favored by certain weather conditions. For example, the spruce budworm emerges in largest numbers after a snowy cold winter which is followed by a warming period with rain in the spring. The tent caterpillar is favored by a warm sunny spring followed by warm humid weather.

Principal technical literature. The sources of literature references and reports on recent work in agricultural meteorology in the United States are varied and numerous. Examples are publications of the American Meteorological Society and the U.S. Weather Bureau, *Agronomy Journal, Soil Science Society of America Proceedings, Agricultural Engineering, American Geophysical Union Transactions, Journal of Agricultural Research,* and *Agricultural Meteorology.*

[MILTON L. BLANC; WOODROW C. JACOBS]

Bibliography: *Agricultural Meteorology*, WMO no. 310, 1972; R. Geiger, *The Climate near the Ground*, 4th ed., 1965; J. W. Smith, *Agricultural Meteorology: The Effect of Weather on Crops*, 1920; Soil Science Society of America, American Agronomy Society, *Plant Environment and Efficient Water Use*, 1967; A. C. True, *A History of Agricultural Experimentation and Research in the United States 1607–1925*, USDA Misc. Publ. no. 251, 1937; R. O. White, *Crop Production and Environment*, 1960; Jen-Yu Wang, *Agricultural Meteorology*, San Jose, Calif., Agricultural Weather Information Service, 1967; Jen-Yu Wang and G. L. Barger, *Bibliography on Agricultural Meteorology*, 1962.

Agricultural science (animal)

The science which deals with the selection, breeding, nutrition, and management of domestic animals for economical production of meat, milk, eggs, wool, hides, and other animal products. Horses for draft and pleasure, dogs and cats and rabbits for meat production, and bees for honey production may also be included in this group. *See* BEEKEEPING; CATTLE PRODUCTION, BEEF; CATTLE PRODUCTION, DAIRY; FOOD ENGINEERING; POULTRY PRODUCTION; SHEEP; SWINE PRODUCTION.

When primitive man first domesticated animals, they were kept as means of meeting his immediate needs for food, transportation, and clothing. Sheep probably were the first and most useful animals to be domesticated, furnishing milk and meat for food, and hides and wool for clothing.

As chemistry, physiology, anatomy, genetics, nutrition, parasitology, pathology, and other sciences developed, their principles were applied to the field of animal science. Since the beginning of the 20th century, great strides have been made in livestock production. Today, farm animals fill a highly important place in the life of man. They convert raw materials, such as pasture herbage, which are of little use to man as food, into animal products having nutritional values not directly available in plant products.

Ruminant animals (those with four compartments or stomachs in the fore portion of their digestive tract, such as cattle and sheep) have the ability to consume large quantities of roughages because of their particular type of digestive system. They also consume large tonnages of grains, as well as mill feeds, oil seed meals, industrial and agricultural by-products, and other materials not suitable for human food. Estimates indicated that in the United States on July 1, 1975, there were 140,000,000 cattle and calves, of which 16,000,000 were dairy cattle; there were also 15,000,000 sheep and lambs, 42,000,000 hogs, and 1,000,000 goats and kids. On Jan. 1, 1971, there were 443,000,000 chickens and 7,500,000 turkeys. These figures do not include over 2,000,000,000 broiler chickens and 100,000,000 turkeys raised for the fresh and frozen turkey market. The total value of all cattle, hogs, sheep, chickens, and turkeys on farms was estimated to be $23,800,000,000 as of Jan. 1, 1971. Estimates of total numbers of pleasure horses were difficult to obtain in the 1970s, but between 6,000,000 and 7,000,000 were available in 1968. Between 2,000,000 and 3,000,000 tons of grains, mill feeds, and high protein feeds were consumed per year by these livestock.

Products of the animal industry furnish raw materials for many important processing industries, such as meat packing, dairy manufacturing, poultry processing, textile production, and tanning. Many services are based on the needs of the animal industry, including livestock marketing, milk deliveries, poultry and egg marketing, poultry hatcheries, artificial insemination services, feed manufacturing, pharmeutical industry, and veterinary services. Thus, animal science involves the application of scientific principles to all phases of animal production, furnishing animal products efficiently and abundantly to consumers. Products from animals are often used for consumer products other than food, for example, hides for leather, and organ meats for preparation of drugs and hormones.

Livestock breeding. The breeding of animals began thousands of years ago. During the last half of the 19th century, livestock breeders made increasing progress in producing animals better suited to the needs of man by simply mating the best to the best. However, in the 20th century animal breeders began to apply the scientific principles of genetics and reproductive physiology. Some progress made in the improvement of farm animals resulted from selected matings based on knowledge of body type or conformation. This method of selection became confusing due to the use of subjective standards which were not always related to economic traits. This error was corrected, however, and many breeders of dairy cattle, poultry, beef cattle, sheep, and swine in the mid-1970s made use of production records or records of performance. Some of their breeding plans were based on milk fat production or egg production, as well as on body type or conformation. The keeping of poultry and dairy cow production records began in a very limited way late in the 19th century. The first Cow-Testing Association in the United States was organized in Michigan in 1906. Now over 1,500,000 cows are tested regularly in the United States. *See* BREEDING (ANIMAL).

Many states now have production testing for beef cattle, sheep, and swine, in which records of rate of gain, efficiency of feed utilization, incidence of twinning, yield of economically important carcass cuts, and other characteristics of production are maintained on part or all of the herd or flock. These records serve as valuable information in the selection of animals for breeding or sale.

Breeding terminology. A breed is a group of animals that has a common origin and possesses characteristics that are not common to other individuals of the same species.

A purebred breed is a group that possesses certain fixed characteristics, such as color or markings, which are transmitted to the offspring. A record, or pedigree, is kept which describes their ancestry for five generations. Associations have been formed by breeders primarily to keep records, or registry books, of individual animals of the various breeds. Purebred associations have taken a more active role in promoting and improving the breeds.

A purebred is one that has a pedigree recorded in a breed association or is eligible for registry by such an association. A crossbred is an individual produced by utilizing two or more purebred lines in a breeding program. A grade is an individual having one parent, usually the sire, a purebred and the other parent a grade or scrub. A scrub is an inferior animal of nondescript breeding. A hybrid is one produced by crossing parents that are genetically pure for different specific characteristics. The mule is an example of a hybrid animal produced by crossing two different species, the American jack, *Equus asinus*, with a mare, *E. caballus*.

Systems of breeding. The modern animal breeder has genetic tools which he may apply, such as selection and breeding, and inbreeding and outbreeding. Selection involves directly the retaining or rejecting of a particular animal for breeding purposes, being based largely on qualitative characteristics. Inbreeding is a system of breeding related animals. Outbreeding is a system of breeding unrelated animals. When these unrelated animals are of different breeds, the term crossbreeding is usually applied. Crossbreeding is in common use by commercial swine producers. About 80–90% of the hogs produced in the Corn Belt states are now crossbred. Crossbreeding is also used extensively by commercial beef and sheep producers.

Grading-up is the process of breeding purebred sires of a given breed to grade females and their female offspring for generation after generation. Grading-up offers the possibility of transforming a nondescript population into one resembling the purebred sires used in the process. It is an expedient and economical way of improving large numbers of animals.

Formation of new breeds. New breeds of farm animals have been developed from crossbred foundation animals. Montadale, Columbia, and Targhee are examples of sheep breeds so developed. The Santa Gertrudis breed of beef cattle was produced by crossing Brahman and Shorthorn breeds on the King Ranch in Texas. In poultry, advantage has been taken of superior genetic ability through the development of hybrid lines.

Artificial insemination. In this process spermatozoa are collected from the male and deposited in the female genitalia by instruments rather than by natural service. In the United States this practice was first used for breeding horses. Artificial insemination in dairy cattle was first begun on a large scale in New Jersey in 1938. In 1958 over 6,000,000 cows were bred artificially in the United States. Freezing techniques for preserving and storing spermatozoa have been applied with great success to bull semen, and it is now possible for outstanding bulls to sire calves years after the bulls have died. The use of artificial insemination for beef cattle and poultry (turkeys) has become more common since 1965. Drugs are being developed which stimulate beef cow herds to come into heat (ovulate) at approximately the same time. This will permit the insemination of large cow herds without the individual handling and inspection which is used with dairy cattle. Although some horses are bred by artificial insemination, many horse breed associations allow only natural breeding.

Livestock feeding. Scientific livestock feeding involves the systematic application of the principles of animal nutrition to the feeding of farm animals. The science of animal nutrition has advanced rapidly since 1930, and the discoveries are being utilized by most of those concerned with the feeding of livestock. The nutritional needs and responses of the different farm animals vary according to the functions they perform and to differences in the anatomy and physiology of their digestive systems. Likewise, feedstuffs vary in usefulness depending upon the time and method of harvesting the crop, the methods employed in drying, preserving, or processing them, and the forms in which they are offered to the animals.

Chemical composition of feedstuffs. The various chemical compounds that are contained in animal feeds have been divided into groups called nutrients. These include proteins, fats, carbohydrates, vitamins, and mineral matter. Proteins are made up of amino acids. Twelve amino acids are essential for all nonruminant animals and must be supplied in their diets. Fats and carbohydrates provide mainly energy. In most cases they are interchangeable as energy sources for farm animals. Fats furnish 2.25 times as much energy per pound as do carbohydrates because of their higher proportion of carbon and hydrogen to oxygen. Thus the energy concentration in poultry and swine diets can be increased by inclusion of considerable portions of fat. Ruminants cannot tolerate large quantities of fat in their diets, however.

Vitamins essential for health and growth include fat-soluble A, D, E, and K, and water-soluble vitamins thiamine, riboflavin, niacin, pyrodoxine, pantothenic acid, and cobalamin. *See* VITAMIN.

Mineral salts that supply calcium, phosphorus, sodium, chlorine, and iron are often needed as supplements, and those containing iodine and cobalt may be required in certain deficient areas. Zinc may also be needed in some swine rations. Many conditions of mineral deficiency have been noted in recent years by using rations that were not necessarily deficient in a particular mineral but in which the mineral was unavailable to the animal because of other factors in the ration or imbalances with other minerals. For example, copper deficiency can be caused by excess molybdenum in the diet.

By a system known as the "proximate analysis," developed prior to 1895 in Germany, feeds have long been divided into six fractions including moisture, ether extract, crude fiber, crude protein, ash, and nitrogen-free extract. The first five fractions are determined in the laboratory. The nitrogen-free extract is what remains after the percentage sum of these five has been subtracted from 100%. Although proximate analysis serves as a guide in the classification, evaluation, and use of feeds, it gives very little specific information about particular chemical compounds in the feed.

The ether extract fraction includes true fats and certain plant pigments, many of which are of little nutritional value. *See* FAT AND OIL, EDIBLE.

The crude fiber fraction is made up of celluloses and lignin. This fraction, together with the nitrogen-free extract, makes up the total carbohydrate content of a feed. *See* CARBOHYDRATE.

The crude protein is estimated by multiplying the total Kjeldahl nitrogen content of the feed by the factor 6.25. This nitrogen includes many forms of nonprotein as well as protein nitrogen. *See* PROTEIN.

The ash, or mineral matter fraction, is determined by burning a sample and weighing the residue. In addition to calcium and other essential mineral elements, it includes silicon and other nonessential elements.

The nitrogen-free extract (NFE) includes the more soluble and the more digestible carbohydrates, such as sugars, starches, and hemicelluloses. Unfortunately, most of the lignin, which is not digestible, is included in this fraction.

A much better system of analysis has been developed for the crude fiber fraction of feedstuffs. This system separates more specifically the highly digestible cell-soluble portion and the less digestible fibrous portion of plant cell walls. This system of nonnutritive residue analysis was developed at the U.S. Department of Agriculture laboratories in Maryland.

Digestibility of feeds. In addition to their chemical composition or nutrient content, the nutritionist and livestock feeder should know the availability or digestibility of the different nutrients in feeds. The digestibility of a feed is measured by determining the quantities of nutrients eaten by an animal over a period of time and those recoverable in the fecal matter. By assigning appropriate energy values to the nutrients, total digestible nutrients

(TDN) may be calculated. These values have been determined and recorded for many feeds.

Formulation of animal feeds. The nutritionist and livestock feeder finds TDN values of great use in the formulation of animal feeds. The TDN requirements for various classes of livestock have been calculated for maintenance and for various productive capacities. However, systems have been developed for expressing energy requirements of animals or energy values of feeds in units which are more closely related to the body process being supported (such as maintenance, growth, and milk or egg production). New tables of feeding standards are being published using the units of metabolizable energy and net energy, which are measurements of energy available for essential body processes. Recommended allowances of nutrients for all species of livestock and some small animals (rabbit, dogs, and mink) are published by the National Academy of Sciences – National Research Council. These are assembled by experts in the field of animal science and are available for distribution through the Superintendent of Documents, Washington, D.C.

Nutritional needs of different animals. The nutritional requirements of different classes of animals are partially dependent on the anatomy and physiology of their digestive systems. Ruminants can digest large amounts of roughages, whereas hogs and poultry, with simple stomachs, can digest only limited amounts and require more concentrated feeds, such as cereal grains. In simple-stomached animals the complex carbohydrate starch is broken down to simple sugars which are absorbed into the blood and utilized by the body for energy.

Microorganisms found in the rumen of ruminant animals break down not only starch but the fibrous carbohydrates of roughages, namely, cellulose and hemicellulose, to organic acids which are absorbed into the blood and utilized as energy. Animals with simple stomachs require high-quality proteins in their diets to meet their requirements for essential amino acids. On the other hand, the microorganisms in ruminants can utilize considerable amounts of simple forms of nitrogen to synthesize high-quality microbial protein which is, in turn, utilized to meet the ruminant's requirement for amino acids. Thus, many ruminant feeds now contain varying portions of urea, an economical simple form of nitrogen, which is synthesized commercially from nonfeed sources. Simple-stomached animals require most of the vitamins in the diet. The microorganisms in the rumen synthesize adequate quantities of the water-soluble vitamins to supply the requirement for the ruminant animal. The fat-soluble vitamins A, D, and E must be supplied as needed to all farm animals. Horses and mules have simple stomachs but they also have an enlargement of the cecum (part of the large intestine), in which bacterial action takes place similar to that in the rumen of ruminants. The requirements for most nutrients do not remain the same throughout the life of an animal but relate to the productive function being performed. Therefore, the requirements are much higher for growth and lactation than they are for pregnancy or maintenance. *See* ANIMAL-FEED COMPOSITIONS.

Livestock judging. The evaluation, or judging, of livestock is important to both the purebred and the commercial producer.

Show-ring judging. The purebred producer usually is much more interested in show-ring judging, or placings, than is the commercial producer. Because of the short time they are in the show-ring, the animals must be placed on the basis of type or appearance by the judge who evaluates them. The show-ring has been an important influence in the improvement of livestock by keeping the breeders aware of what judges consider to be desirable types. The shows have also brought breeders together for exchange of ideas and breeding stock and have helped to advertise breeds of livestock and the livestock industry. The demand for better meat-animal carcasses has brought about more shows in which beef cattle and swine are judged, both on foot and in the carcass. This trend helps to promote development of meat animals of greater carcass value and has a desirable influence upon show-ring standards for meat animals. The standards used in show rings have shifted toward traits in live animals which are highly related to both desirable carcass traits and high production efficiency.

Selection of animals for breeding. The evaluation or selection of animals for breeding purposes is of importance to the commercial as well as to the purebred breeder. In selecting animals for breeding, desirable conformation or body type is given careful attention. The animals are also examined carefully for visible physical defects, such as blindness, crooked legs, jaw distortions, and abnormal udders. Animals known to be carriers of genes for heritable defects, such as dwarfism in cattle, should be discriminated against.

When they are available, records of performance or production should be considered in the selection of breeding animals. Some purebred livestock record associations now record production performance of individual animals on their pedigrees.

Grading of market animals. The grading on foot of hogs or cattle for market purposes requires special skill. In many modern livestock markets, hogs are graded as no. 1, 2, 3, or 4 according to the estimated values of the carcasses. Those hogs grading no. 3 are used to establish the base price, and sellers are paid a premium for better animals. In some cases the grade is used also to place a value of the finished market product. For example, the primal cuts from beef cattle are labeled prime, choice, or good on the basis of the grade which the rail carcass received. A trend is underway toward pricing market animals on the basis of grade and yield, which also takes into account factors associated with yield of lean cuts.

Livestock pest and disease control. The innumerable diseases of farm livestock require expert diagnosis and treatment by qualified veterinarians. The emphasis on intensive animal production has increased stresses on animals and generally increased the need for close surveillance of herds or flocks for disease outbreaks. Both external and internal parasites are common afflictions of livestock but can be controlled by proper management of the animals. Sanitation is of utmost importance in the control of these pests, but under most circumstances sanitation must be supplemented with effective insecticides, ascaricides, and fungicides. See FUNGISTAT AND FUNGICIDE; INSECTICIDE; PESTICIDE.

Internal parasites. Internal parasites, such as stomach and intestinal worms in sheep, cannot be controlled by sanitation alone under most farm conditions. They are a more critical problem under intensive management systems and in warm, humid climates. For many years the classic treatment for sheep was drenching with phenothiazine and continuous free choice feeding of one part phenothiazine mixed with nine parts of salt. New drugs have been developed which more effectively break the life cycle of the worm and have a broader spectrum against different classes of parasites.

Control of gastrointestinal parasites in cattle can be accomplished in many areas by sanitation and the rotational use of pastures. In areas of intensive grazing, animals, especially the young ones, may become infected. Regular and timely administration of antiparasite drugs is the best means of controlling the pests. Otherwise their effects will seriously decrease productivity of animals.

The use of drugs to control gastrointestinal parasites and also certain enteric bacteria in hogs is commonplace. Control is also dependent on good sanitation and rotational use of nonsurfaced lots and pastures. Similarly, because of intensive housing systems, the opportunities for infection and spread of both parasitism and disease in poultry flocks are enhanced by poor management conditions. The producer has a large number of materials to choose from in preventing or treating these conditions, including sodium fluoride, piperazine salts, nitrofurans, and arsenicals and antibiotics such as penicillin, tetracyclines, hygromycin, and tylosin.

External parasites. Control of horn flies, horseflies, stable flies, lice, mange mites, ticks, and fleas on farm animals has been in the process of rapid change with the introduction of many new insecticides. Such compounds as DDT, methoxychlor, toxaphene, lindane, and malathion were very effective materials for the control of external parasites. The use of these materials was wisely restricted to certain conditions and classes of animals by the provisions of Public Law 518, which is the Miller Amendment to the Federal Food, Drug, and Cosmetic Act. For example, use of DDT was not permitted on dairy animals. Reliable information should be obtained before using these materials for the control of external parasites. Pressure from various nonscientific lobby groups has prompted legislative prohibition of an increasing number of these chemicals.

Control of cattle grubs, or the larvae of the heel fly, may be accomplished by dusting the backs of the animals with powders or by spraying them under high pressure. Systemic insecticides for grub control have been given approval if used according to the manufacturer's recommendation.

Fungus infections. Actinomycosis is a fungus disease commonly affecting cattle, swine, and horses. In cattle this infection is commonly known as lumpy jaw. The lumpy jaw lesion may be treated with tincture of iodine or by local injection of streptomycin in persistent cases. Most fungus infections, or mycoses, develop slowly and follow a prolonged course. A veterinarian should be consulted for diagnosis and treatment.

General animal health care. Numerous other disease organisms pose a constant threat to livestock. Although many of these organisms can be treated therapeutically, it is much more advisable economically to establish good preventive medicine and health care programs under the guidance of a veterinarian.

Management. Economic changes have continued to narrow the profit margins for economic livestock producers. This has increased the necessity for attention to good management practices in all aspects of production.   [RONALD R. JOHNSON]

Bibliography: J. R. Campbell and J. F. Lasley, *The Science of Animals That Serve Mankind*, 1969; J. R. Campbell and R. T. Marshall, *The Science of Providing Milk for Man*, 1975; H. H. Cole, *Introduction to Livestock Production*, 2d ed., 1966; E. W. Crampton and L. E. Harris, *Applied Animal Nutrition*, 2d ed., 1969; M. E. Ensminger, *Beef Cattle Science*, 4th ed., 1968; M. E. Ensminger, *Horses and Horsemanship*, 1969; M. E. Ensminger, *Sheep and Wool Science*, 1964; J. L. Krider and W. E. Carroll, *Swine Production*, 4th ed., 1971; L. A. Maynard and J. K. Loosli, *Animal Nutrition*, 6th ed., 1969; Merck and Co., Inc., *The Merck Veterinary Manual*, 4th ed., 1973; F. B. Morrison, *Feeds and Feeding*, 22d ed., 1961; M. O. North, *Commercial Chicken Production Manual*, 1972; R. R. Snapp and A. L. Newmann, *Beef Cattle*, 5th ed., 1965.

Agricultural science (plant)

The pure and applied science that is concerned with botany and management of crop and ornamental plants for utilization by humankind. Crop plants include those grown and used directly for food, feed, or fiber, such as cereal grains, soybeans, citrus, and cotton; those converted biologically to products of utility, such as forage plants, hops, and mulberry; and those used for medicinal or special products, such as digitalis, opium poppy, coffee, and cinnamon. In addition, many plant products such as crambe oil and rubber are used in industry where synthetic products have not been satisfactory. Ornamental plants are cultured for their esthetic value.

The ultimate objective of plant agriculture is to recognize the genetic potential of groups of plants and then to manipulate and utilize the environment to maximize that genetic expression for return of a desirable product. Great advancements in crop culture have occurred by applying knowledge of biochemistry, physiology, ecology, morphology, anatomy, taxonomy, pathology, and genetics of plants. Contributions of improved plant types by breeding, and the understanding and application of principles of atmospheric science, soil science, and animal and human nutrition, have increased the efficiency and decreased the risks of crop production.

Domestication of crop plants. All crops are believed to have been derived from wild species. However, cultivated plants as they are known today have undergone extensive modification from their wild prototypes as a result of the continual efforts to improve them. These wild types were apparently recognized as helpful to humans long before recorded history. Desirable plants were continually selected and replanted in order to improve their growth habit, fruiting characteristics, and growing season. Selection has progressed so far in cases such as cabbage and corn (maize) that wild ancestors have become obscure.

Centers of origins of most crop plants have been determined to be in Eurasia, but many exceptions exist. This area of early civilization apparently abounded with several diverse plant types that led to domestication of the crops known today as wheat, barley, oats, millet, sugarbeets, and most of the cultivated forage grasses and legumes. Soybeans, lettuce, onions, and peas originated in China and were domesticated as Chinese civilization developed. Similarly, many citrus fruits, banana, rice, and sugarcane originated in southern Asia. Sorghum and cowpeas are believed to have originated in Africa. Crops which were indigenous to Central and South America, but which migrated to North America with Indian civilization, include corn, potato, sweet potato, pumpkin, sunflower, tobacco, and peanut. Thus, prior to 1492 there was little, if any, mixing of crop plants and cultural practices between the Old and the New Worlds. Most of the major agricultural crops of today in the United States awaited introduction by early settlers, and later by plant explorers.

During domestication of crop plants the ancient cultivators in their geographically separated civilizations must have had goals similar to present-day plant breeders. Once valuable attributes of a plant were recognized, efforts were made to select the best types for that purpose. Desirable characters most likely included improved yield, increased quality, extended range of adaptation, insect and disease resistance, and easier cultural and harvesting operations. About 350,000 species of plants exist in the world, yet only about 10,000 species can be classified as crops using the broadest of definitions. Of these, about 150 are of major importance in world trade, and only 15 make up the majority of the world's food crops. On a world basis, wheat is grown on the most acreage, followed by rice, but rice has a higher yield per area than wheat so their total production is about equal. Other major crops are corn, sorghum, millet, barley; sugarcane and sugarbeet; potato, sweet potato, and cassava; bean, soybean, and peanut; and coconut and banana.

Redistribution of crop plants. Crop distribution is largely dictated by growth characters of the crop, climate of the region, soil resources, and social habits of the people. As plants were domesticated by civilizations in separate parts of the world, they were discovered by early travelers. This age of exploration led to the entrance of new food crops into European agriculture. The potato, introduced into Spain from the New World before 1570, was to become one of the most important crops of Europe. When introduced into Ireland, it became virtually the backbone of the food source for that entire population. Corn was introduced to southern Europe and has become an important crop. Rice has been cultivated in Italy since the 16th century. Tobacco was also introduced to European culture, but continued to provide a major source of export of the early colonial settlements in America.

European agriculture reciprocated by introducing wheat, barley, oats, and several other food and feed crops into the New World. In the new environment, plants were further adapted by selection to meet the local requirements. Cultural technology regarding seeding, harvesting, and storing was transferred along with the crops. This exchange of information oftentimes helped allow successful culture of these crops outside of their center of origin and domestication. Today the center of production of a crop such as wheat in the United States and potato in Europe is often markedly different from its center of origin.

The United States recognized early the need for plant exploration to find desirable types that could be introduced. Thomas Jefferson wrote in 1790, "The greatest service which can be rendered to any country is to add a useful plant to its culture." Even today the U.S. Department of Agriculture conducts many plant explorations and maintains plant introduction centers to evaluate newly found plants. Explorations are also serving a critical need for preservation of germplasm for plant breeders, as many of the centers of origin are becoming agriculturally intensive, and wild types necessary to increase genetic diversity will soon be extinct.

Adaptation of crop plants. Crop plants of some sort exist under almost all environments, but the major crops on a world basis tend to have rather specific environmental requirements. Furthermore, as crop plants are moved to new locations the new environment must be understood, and cultural or management changes often must be made to allow best performance. More recently, varieties and strains of crops have been specifically developed that can better cope with cold weather, low rainfall, diseases, and insects to extend even further the natural zone of adaptation.

Temperature. Temperature has a dominant influence on crop adaptation. The reason is that enzyme activity is very temperature-dependent and almost all physiological processes associated with growth are enzymatically controlled. Crops differ widely in their adapted temperature range, but most crops grow best at temperatures of 15 to 32°C. Optimum day temperature for wheat, however, is 20 to 25°C, while for corn it is about 30°C and for cotton about 35°C.

The frost-free period also influences crop adaptation by giving an indication of the duration of the growing season. Thus a growing season for corn or soybeans might be described as one with mean daily temperatures between 18 and 25°C, and with an average minimum temperature exceeding 10°C for at least 3 months. Small grains such as wheat, barley, and oats tolerate a cooler climate with a period of only 2 months when minimum temperatures exceed 10°C. Because of optimum growth temperatures and frost-free periods, it is easily recognized why the spring wheat belt includes North Dakota and Montana, the corn belt Iowa and Illinois, and the cotton belt Mississippi and Alabama. Farmers use planting dates and a range in maturity of varieties to match the crop to the growing season. *See* PLANT GROWTH.

In many winter annual (the plants are sown in fall, overwinter, and mature in early summer), biennial, and perennial crops, cold temperatures also influence distribution. The inherent ability of the crop to survive winter limits distribution of crops. As a generalized example, winter oats are less able to survive cold winters than winter barley, followed by winter wheat and then winter rye. Thus oats in the southern United States are mostly winter annual type, while from central Arkansas northward they are spring type. The dividing line for barley is about central Missouri and for wheat about central South Dakota. Winter rye can survive well into Canada.

A cold period may be required for flowering of winter annual and perennial crops. This cold requirement, termed vernalization, occurs naturally in cold environments where the dormant bud temperature is near 0°C for 4 to 6 weeks during winter. Without this physiological response to change the hormonal composition of the terminal bud, flowering of winter wheat would not occur the following spring. Bud dormancy is also low-temperature-induced and keeps buds from beginning spring growth until a critical cold period has passed. The flower buds of many trees such as peach, cherry, and apple require less chilling than do vegetative buds, and therefore flower before the leaves emerge. The intensity and duration of cold treatment necessary to break dormancy differs with species and even within a species. For example, some peaches selected for southern areas require only 350 hr below 8°C to break dormancy, while some selected for northern areas may require as much as 1200 hr. This cold requirement prevents production of temperate fruit crops in subtropical regions, but in temperate climates its survival value is clear. A physiological mechanism that prevents spring growth from occurring too early helps decrease the possibility of cold temperature damage to the new succulent growth.

Temperature of the crop environment can be altered by date of planting of summer annuals, by proper site selection, and by artificial means. In the Northern Hemisphere the south- and west-facing slopes are usually warmer than east- or north-facing slopes. Horticulturists have long used mulches for controlling soil temperature, and also mists and smoke for short-term low-temperature protection.

Water. Water is essential for crop production, and natural rainfall often is supplemented by irrigation. Wheat is grown in the Central Plains states of the United States because it matures early enough to avoid the water shortage of summer. In contrast, corn matures too late to avoid that drought condition and must be irrigated to make it productive. In the eastern United States where rainfall is higher, irrigation is usually not needed to produce good yields. *See* IRRIGATION OF CROPS.

Crops transpire large amounts of water through their stomata. For example, corn transpires about 350 kg of water for each kilogram of dry weight produced. Wheat, oats, and barley transpire about 600 kg, and alfalfa about 1000 kg for each kilogram of dry weight produced. Fallowing (allowing land to be idle) every other season to store water in the soil for the succeeding crop has been used to overcome water limitations and extend crops further into dryland areas. *See* PLANT, WATER RELATIONS OF.

Light. Light intensity and duration also play dominant roles. Light is essential for photosynthesis. The yield of a crop plant is related to its efficiency in intercepting solar radiation by its leaf tissue, the efficiency of leaves in converting light energy into chemical energy, and the transfer and utilization of that chemical energy (usually sugars) for growth of an economic product. Crops differ markedly in the efficiency of their leaves. Photosynthetic rate of corn or sorghum leaves may be as high as 60 mg CO_2/dm^2 of leaf area/hr with full sunlight. Photosynthesis of wheat, soybeans, or rice is about $25-35$ mg/dm²/hr, while that of pineapple or tree nut crops is about $8-15$ mg/dm²/hr. *See* PHOTOSYNTHESIS.

Crops also differ markedly in leaf area and leaf arrangement. Humans greatly influence the photosynthetic area by altering number of plants per area and by cutting and pruning. Corn producers have gradually increased plant population per area about 50% since about 1950 as improved varieties and cultural methods were developed. This has increased the leaf area of the crop canopy and the amount of solar energy captured. Defoliation and pruning practices also influence solar energy capture and growth rate. Continued defoliation of pastures by grazing may reduce the photosynthetic area to the point that yield is diminished. In these perennial plants, carbohydrates are stored in underground organs such as roots, rhizomes, and stem bases to furnish food for new shoots in spring and following cutting. Availability of water and nitrogen fertilizer also influences the amount of leaf area developed.

Photoperiodism, the response of plants to day length, also has a dramatic effect on plant distribution. Such important adaptive mechanisms as development of winter hardiness, initiation and maintenance of bud dormancy, and floral initiation are influenced by photoperiod. Plants have been classified as long-day, those that flower when day lengths exceed a critical level; short-day, which is opposite to long-day; and day-neutral, those that are not affected by day length. Photoperiod also has a controlling influence on formation of potato tubers, onion bulbs, strawberry runners, and tillers of many cereal grains and grasses. Farmers select varieties bred for specific areas of the country to ensure that they flower properly for their growing season. Horticulturists, in a more intensive effort, provide artificial lighting in greenhouses to lengthen the photoperiod, or shorten it by shading, to induce flowering and fruit production at will; for example, to ready poinsettias for the Christmas holiday trade or asters for Easter. Natural photoperiods are important in plant breeding when varieties of day-length-sensitive crops must be developed for specific localities. Soybeans are day-length-sensitive and have been classified into several maturity groups from north to south in latitude. *See* PHOTOPERIODISM IN PLANTS.

Pathogens. Pathogens of plants that cause diseases include fungi, bacteria, viruses, and nematodes. These organisms are transmitted from plant to plant by wind, water, and insects and infect the plant tissue. Organisms infect the plant and interfere with the physiological functions to decrease yield. Further, they infect the economic product and decrease its quality. Pathogens are most economically controlled by breeding resistant varieties or by using selective pesticides. Insects decrease plant productivity and quality largely by mechanical damage to tissue and secretion of toxins. They are also usually controlled by resistant varieties or specific insecticides. *See* PLANT DISEASE; PLANT DISEASE CONTROL.

Soil. The soil constitutes an important facet of the plant environment. Soil physical properties such as particle size and pore space determine the water-holding capacity and influence the exchange of atmospheric gases with the root system. Soil chemical properties such as pH and the ability to supply nutrients have a direct influence on crop productivity. Farmers alter the chemical environment by addition of lime or sulfur to correct acidic or basic conditions, or by addition of manures and chemical fertilizers to alter nutrient supply status. Soil also is composed of an important microbiological component that assists in the cycling of organic matter and mineral nutrients. *See* SOIL.

Management. During and following domestication of crop plants, humankind has learned many cultural or management practices that enhance production or quality of the crop. This dynamic process is in operation today as the quest continues to improve the plant environment to take advantage of the genetic potential of the crop. These practices have made plant agriculture in the United States one of the most efficient in the world. Some major changes in technology are discussed in the following sections.

Mechanization. In 1860 an average United States farm worker produced enough food and fiber for fewer than 5 other persons. In 1950 it was enough for 25, and today exceeds 50 other persons. Mechanization, which allowed each farm worker to increase the area managed, is largely responsible for this dramatic change.

A model of a grain reaper in 1852 demonstrated that nine men with the reaper could do the work of 14 with cradles. By 1930 one man with a large combine had a daily capacity of 20–25 acres (1 acre = 4047 m²), and not only harvested but threshed the grain to give about a 75-fold gain over the cradle-and-flail methods of a century earlier. In 1975 one man with a faster-moving combine could harvest 50–75 acres per day. The mechanical cotton picker harvests a 500-lb (1 lb = 0.45 kg) bale in 75 min, 40–50 times the rate of a hand picker. The peanut harvester turns out about 300 lb of shelled peanuts per hour, a 300-hr job if done by hand labor. Hand setting 7500 celery plants is a day's hard labor for one person. However, a modern transplanting machine with two people readily sets 40,000, reducing labor costs by 67%. Today crops such as cherries and tomatoes are machine-harvested. When machines have been difficult to adapt to crops such as tomatoes, special plant varieties that flower more uniformly and have tougher skins on the fruit have been developed. *See* AGRICULTURE, MACHINERY IN.

Fertilizers and plant nutrition. No one knows when or where the practice originated of burying a fish beneath the spot where a few seeds of corn were to be planted, but it was common among North American Indians when Columbus discovered America and is evidence that the value of fertilizers was known to primitive peoples. Farm manures were in common use by the Romans and have been utilized almost from the time animals were first domesticated and crops grown. It was not until centuries later, however, that animal fertilizers were supplemented by mineral forms of lime, phosphate, potassium, and nitrogen. Rational use of these substances began about 1850 as an outgrowth of soil and plant analyses.

Justus von Liebig published *Chemistry and Its Application to Agriculture and Physiology* in 1840, which led to concepts on modifying the soil by fertilizers and other amendments. These substances soon became the center of crop research. In 1842 John Bennet Lawes, who founded the famous Rothamsted Experiment Station in England, obtained a patent for manufacture of superphosphates and introduced chemical fertilizers to agriculture. As research progressed, crop responses to levels of phosphate, lime, and potassium were worked out, but nitrogen nutrition remained puzzling. The nitrogen problem was clarified in 1886, when H. Hellriegel and H. Wilfarth, two German chemists, reported that root nodules and their associated bacteria were responsible for the peculiar ability of legume plants to use atmospheric nitrogen. These findings collectively allowed rational decision-making regarding nutrition of crop plants and were understandably very significant in increasing crop productivity.

By the early 20th century 10 elements had been identified as essential for proper nutrition. These were carbon, hydrogen, and oxygen, which are supplied by the atmosphere; and nitrogen, potassium, phosphorus, sulfur, magnesium, calcium, and iron, supplied by the soil. The first 40 years of the 20th century witnessed the addition of manganese, boron, copper, zinc, molybdenum, and chlorine to the list of essential mineral nutrients. These 6 are required only in very small amounts as compared with the first 10 and have been classified as micronutrients. From a quantitative view they are truly minor, but in reality they are just as critical as the others for plant survival and productivity. Many early and puzzling plant disorders are now known to be due to insufficient supplies of micronutrients in the soil, or to their presence in forms unavailable to plants.

An important result of discoveries relating to absorption and utilization of micronutrients is that they have served to emphasize the complexity of soil fertility and fertilizer problems. In sharp contrast to early thoughts that fertilizer practices should be largely a replacement in the soil of what was removed by the plant, it is now recognized that interaction and balance of mineral elements within both the soil and plant must be considered for efficient crop growth. Usage of chemical fertilizers has become more widespread with time. In 1967, 37,000,000 tons (1 short ton = 0.9 metric ton), and in 1974, 47,000,000 tons of mineral fertilizer were applied to crop and pasture lands in the United States. Major crops usually receive the most fertilizer: 94% of the corn acreage was fertilized in 1974, 79% of the cotton, 66% of the wheat, and 30% of the soybeans. *See* FERTILIZER; FERTILIZING; PLANT, MINERAL NUTRITION OF; PLANT, MINERALS ESSENTIAL TO.

Pesticides. Total destruction of crops by swarms of locusts and subsequent starvation of many people and livestock have occurred throughout the world. Pioneers in the Plains states suffered disastrous crop losses from hordes of grasshoppers and marching army worms. An epidemic of potato blight brought hunger to much of western Europe and famine to Ireland in 1846–1847. The use of new insecticides and fungicides has done much to prevent such calamities. Various mixtures, really nothing more than nostrums (unscientific concoctions), were in use centuries ago, but the first really trustworthy insect control measure appeared in the United States in the mid-1860s, when paris green was used to halt the eastern spread of the Colorado potato beetle. This was followed by other arsenical compounds, culminating in lead arsenate in the 1890s.

A major development occurred during World War II, when the value of DDT (dichlorodiphenyltrichloroethane) for control of many insects was discovered. Although this compound was known to the chemist decades earlier, it was not until 1942 that its value as an insecticide was definitely established and a new chapter written in the continual contest between humankind and insects. Three or four applications of DDT gave better season control of many pests at lower cost than was afforded by a dozen materials used earlier. Furthermore, DDT afforded control of some kinds of pests that were practically immune to former materials. In the meantime other chemicals have been developed that are even more effective for specific pests, and safer to use from a human health and ecological viewpoint. See PESTICIDE.

Dusts and solutions containing sulfur have long been used to control mildew on foliage, but the first highly effective fungicide was discovered accidentally in the early 1880s. To discourage theft, a combination of copper sulfate and lime was used near Bordeaux, France, to give grape vines a poisoned appearance. Bordeaux mixture remained the standard remedy for fungus diseases until relatively recently when other materials with fewer harmful side effects were released.

Today new pesticides are being rapidly developed by private industry and are carefully monitored by several agencies of the Federal government. Besides evaluation for its ability to repel or destroy a certain pest, influence of the pesticide on physiological processes in plants, and especially long-range implications for the environment and human health, are carefully documented before Federal approval for use is granted.

Herbicides. Because they are readily visible, weeds were recognized as crop competitors long before microscopic bacteria, fungi, and viruses. The time-honored methods of controlling weeds have been to use competitive crops or mulches to smother them, or to pull, dig, hoe, or cultivate them out. These methods are still effective and most practical in many instances. However, under many conditions weeds can be controlled chemically much more economically. A century ago regrowth of thistles and other large weeds was prevented by pouring salt on their cut stubs. Salt and ashes were placed along areas such as courtyards, roadsides, and fence rows where all vegetation needed to be controlled. However, until the 1940s selective weed control, where the crop is left unharmed, was used on a very limited scale. The first of these new selective herbicides was 2,4-D (2,4-dichlorophenoxyacetic acid), followed shortly by 2,4,5-T (2,4,5-trichlorophenoxyacetic acid) and other related compounds. This class of herbicides is usually sprayed directly on the crop and weeds and kills susceptible plants by upsetting normal physiological processes, causing abnormal increases in size, and distortions that eventually lead to death of the plant. As a group, these herbicides are much less toxic to grasses than to broad-leaved species, and each one has its own character of specificity. For instance, 2,4-D is more efficient for use against herbaceous weeds, whereas 2,4,5-T is best for woody and brushy species.

Today's herbicides have been developed by commercial companies to control a vast array of weeds in most crop management systems. Some herbicides such as atrazine are preemergence types that are sprayed on the soil at time of corn planting. This herbicide kills germinating weed seeds by interfering with their photosynthetic system so they starve to death. Meanwhile metabolism of the resistant corn seedlings alters the chemical slightly to cause it to lose its herbicidal activity. Such is the complexity that allows specificity of herbicides. The place that herbicides have come to occupy in agriculture is indicated by the fact that farmlands treated in the United States increased from a few thousand acres in 1940 to over 150,000,000 acres in 1974, not including large areas of swamp and overflow lands treated for aquatic plant control and thousands of miles of treated highways, railroad tracks, and drainage and irrigation ditches. See HERBICIDE.

Growth regulators. Many of the planters' practices in the past hundred years may be classified as methods of regulating growth. Use of specific substances to influence particular plant functions, however, has been a more recent development, though these modern uses, and even some of the substances applied, had their antecedents in century-old practices in certain parts of the world.

Since about 1930 many uses have been discovered for a considerable number of organic compounds having growth-regulating influences. For instance, several of them applied as sprays a few days to several weeks before normal harvest will prevent or markedly delay dropping of such fruits as apples and oranges. Runner development in strawberries and sucker (tiller) development in tobacco can be inhibited by sprays of maleic hydrazide. Another compound called CCC (2-chloroethyl trimethyl ammonium chloride) is used to shorten wheat plants in Europe to allow higher levels of fertilizer. Many greenhouse-grown flowers are kept short in stature by CCC and other growth regulators. Striking effects from gibberellins and fumaric acid have also been reported. The first greatly increase vegetative growth and the latter causes dwarfing. In practice, growth-inhibiting or growth-retarding agents are finding wider use than growth-stimulating ones. In higher concentration many growth-retarding agents become inhibiting agents.

There are marked differences between plant species and even varieties in their response to most plant growth regulators. Many, if not most, growth regulators are highly selective; a concentration of even 100 times that effective for one species or variety is necessary to produce the same response in another. Furthermore, the specific formulation of the substances, for example, the kind or amount of wetting agent used with them, is important in determining their effectiveness. In brief, growth regulators are essentially new products, though there are century-old instances of the empirical use of a few of them. Some influence growth rate, others direction of growth, others plant structure, anatomy, or morphology. With the discovery of new ones, indications are that it is only a matter of time before many features of plant growth and development may be directly or indirectly controlled by them to a marked degree. Applications of these substances in intensive agriculture are unfolding rapidly, and their use is one of the many factors making farming more of a science and less of an art. *See* GIBBERELLIN; PLANT HORMONES.

Plant improvement. From earliest times humans have tried to improve plants by selection, but it was the discovery of hybridization (cross-mating of two genetically different plants) that eventually led to dramatic increases in genetic potential of the plants. Hybridization was recognized in the early 1800s, well before Mendel's classic genetic discoveries, and allowed the combination of desirable plants in a complementary manner to produce an improved progeny. Plant breeding had a dramatic flourish in the early 20th century following the rediscovery of Mendel's research and its implications, and has had much to do with the increased productivity per area of present-day agriculture.

Corn provides the most vivid example of how improvement through genetic manipulation can occur. Following the commercial development of corn hybrids about 1930, only a few acres were planted, but by 1945 over 90% of the acreage was planted to hybrids, and today nearly 100% is planted. It has been conservatively estimated that hybrids of corn have 25% more yield potential than old-style varieties. Subsequently, plant breeders have utilized hybridization for development of modern varieties of most major crop species.

While very significant changes through crop breeding have occurred in pest resistance and product quality, perhaps the character of most consequence was an increase in the lodging (falling over) resistance of major grain crops. Corn, wheat, and rice have all been bred to be shorter in stature and to have increased stem resistance to breaking. These changes have in turn allowed heavier fertilization of crops to increase photosynthetic area and yield. The impact of this was recognized when Norman Borlaug was awarded the Nobel Peace Prize in 1970 for his breeding contribution to the "green revolution." His higher-yielding wheats were shorter and stiff-strawed so they could utilize increased amounts of nitrogen fertilizer. They were also day-length-insensitive and thus had a wide adaptation. New varieties of rice such as IR-8 developed at the International Rice Research Institute in the Philippines are shorter, are more responsive to nitrogen fertilizer, and have much higher potential yield than conventional varieties. With those new wheat and rice varieties many countries gained time in their battle between population and food supply. *See* BREEDING (PLANT).

Often in tree crops and high-value crops it is not feasible to make improvements genetically, and other means are utilized. Grafting, or physically combining two or more separate plants, is used as a method of obtaining growth control in many fruit trees, and also has been used to provide disease resistance and better fruiting characteristics. This technique is largely limited to woody species of relatively high value. Usually tops are grafted to different rootstocks to obtain restricted vegetative growth, as in dwarf apple and pear trees which still bear normal-sized fruit. Alternatively, junipers and grapes are grafted to new rootstocks to provide a better root system. In both cases the desirability of the esthetic or economic portion warrants the cost and effort of making the plant better adapted to environmental or management conditions. *See* GRAFTING OF PLANTS.   [CURTIS J. NELSON]

Bibliography: R. J. Delorit, L. J. Greub, and H. L. Ahlgren, *Crop Production*, 1974; J. R. Harlan, *Crops and Man*, 1975; J. Janick et al., *Plant Science: An Introduction to World Crops*, 1969; J. H. Martin and W. H. Leonard, *Principles of Field Crop Production*, 2d ed., 1967; U.S. Department of Agriculture, *Yearbook of Agriculture: After a Hundred Years*, 1962.

Agriculture

The production of plants and animals useful to human beings, including the cultivation of soil, management of crops, and the feeding, breeding, and managing of livestock. To a variable extent, agriculture also includes the preparation of plant and animal products for use by humans, and the disposal of these products by marketing.

Many different environmental factors influence the kind of agriculture practiced in a particular community. Among these factors are climate, soil, topography, nearness to markets, transporta-

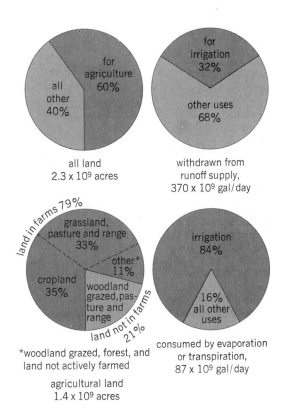

Fig. 1. Use of land and water resources in the United States. (*USDA*)

tion facilities, and cost of the land.

Climate, soil, and topography vary widely throughout the world. In turn, this variation brings about a wide range in agricultural production enterprises. Certain areas tend toward a specialized agriculture, whereas other areas engage in a more diversified agriculture. As new technology is introduced and adopted, environmental factors are less important in influencing agricultural production patterns.

Rapid growth in the world's population, coupled with medical progress promising further success in reducing death rates, makes critically important the continuing ability of agriculture to provide needed food and fiber.

AGRICULTURE IN THE UNITED STATES

Agriculture is the means by which the resources of land and water are converted into those things needed by people for food, fiber, shelter, and recreation. These land resources must be carefully managed to maintain and enhance the productivity of areas suitable for crops and for pasture and grazing, as well as to ensure effective use of the rain that falls on these lands so that the water needs of the nation will be met (Fig. 1).

The United States has developed the most efficient agricultural system in the world, but this system continues to change through scientific discoveries and new technology.

The chronology of American agriculture is highlighted in Table 1. The nation has evolved from a predominantly agricultural society in 1790 to a highly industrialized one in 1970. The farm population grew in actual numbers up to 1940, but the percentage of the total population engaged in agricultural production steadily decreased as American farmers became more productive. The number of people on the farm in 1970 does not include the large and growing population that is engaged in supporting agriculture by providing tractors and trucks, machinery and equipment, petroleum products, fertilizers, lime, pesticides and other agricultural chemicals, seeds, and other essential materials. A still larger group of people is engaged in agricultural industries that store, process, distribute, and sell farm products to the consumer. The number of people employed by these supporting industries is much greater than the number working on farms. Nowadays, the United States has an even greater dependence on its lands and waters for the well-being of its people than in earlier eras. In addition, the United States has

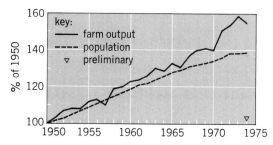

Fig. 2. United States farm output and population. (*USDA*)

become the world's greatest producer of foodstuffs both for export to other nations and to relieve food shortages in less fortunate countries.

Farm output has more than kept pace with the population growth of the nation, as shown by Fig. 2. The output per man-hour of farm workers has continued to increase (Fig. 3) because of the greater use of power and machinery, more effective use of fertilizers and lime to enhance soil fertility, use of higher-yielding crop strains, more efficient feeding and management of livestock, and similar advances.

It is significant that the output of farm products has increased more rapidly than the inputs have, owing to the application of new knowledge and skills in farm operations. The major inputs are shown in Fig. 4. Labor costs have been reduced by the use of power and machinery; there have been great improvements in the use of fertilizers and lime and other items such as chemical compounds to control insect pests, diseases, and weeds, and in the use of livestock feed supplements. Figure 5 shows that the total farm output and the output per unit of the various products that constitute inputs are closely related. This means that the inputs were effective in increasing the efficiency of production, which is a measure of the skill of the farmer in applying modern science and technology.

American agriculture has provided a great diversity of foodstuffs, as well as industrial products, of good quality at lower costs than are enjoyed by other nations. Figure 6 indicates the major categories of crop products and the per capita trends in their use. Figure 7 shows the changes in the use of selected livestock products. There has never been a shortage of essential animal protein in the United States.

Table 1. A chronology of American agriculture

| Year | Total population, 10^6 | Farm population | |
		Numbers, 10^6	Percent of total
1790	3.9	3.5	over 90
1820	9.6	6.9	72
1850	23.2	11.7	50
1880	50.1	24.5	49
1910	92.0	28.5	31
1940	131.8	30.8	23.4
1950	151.0	25.0	16.5
1960	180.0	15.6	8.7
1970	205.0	9.7	4.7

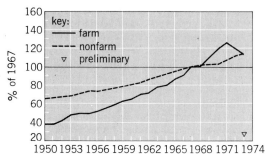

Fig. 3. United States farm and nonfarm output per man-hour. (*USDA*)

Characteristics and trends. To the people on the land, farming is still a way of life. However, the skills and knowledge of the successful farmer have changed drastically with the advent of tractors and trucks to replace horses, the development of more effective machines to replace much of the previous hand labor, the breeding of more productive crops and livestock, the development of chemical fertilizers to supplement native soil fertility, and the advent of chemical compounds to control insect pests, diseases, and weeds. The progressive development of processing of all agricultural products not only saved these products from spoilage and losses but also converted them into goods more readily utilized in meeting human needs. These agricultural industries have been removed from the farm and now constitute a large segment of the agricultural industries located in factories and processing plants in urban areas. They are a vital part of the entire national system for channeling agricultural products to the consuming population of the nation. *See* AGRICULTURAL SCIENCE (ANIMAL); AGRICULTURAL SCIENCE (PLANT); AGRICULTURE, MACHINERY IN; FERTILIZER; FOOD MANUFACTURING; PESTICIDE.

Nature of agricultural products. Agricultural products basically include crop plants, livestock products, and feedstuffs for livestock. The crop plants are divided into 10 categories: grain crops (wheat, for flour to make bread, many bakery products, and breakfast cereals; rice, for food; corn, for livestock feed, syrup, meal, and oil; sorghum grain, for livestock feed; and oats, barley, and rye, for food and livestock feed); food grain legumes (beans, peas, lima beans, and cowpeas, for food; and peanuts, for food and oil); oil seed crops (soybeans, for oil and high-protein meal; and linseed, for oil and high-protein meal); root and tuber crops (principally potatoes and sweet potatoes); sugar crops (sugar beets and sugar cane); fiber crops (principally cotton, for fiber to make textiles and for seed to produce oil and high-protein meal); tree fruits (apples, peaches, oranges, lemons, prunes, plums, cherries); nut crops (walnuts, almonds, pecans); vegetables (melons, sweet corn, cabbage, cauliflower, lettuce, celery, tomatoes, eggplant, peppers, onions, and many others); and forages (for support of livestock pastures and range grazing lands and for hay and silage crops). The forages are dominated by a wide range of grasses and legumes, suited to different conditons of soil and climate.

Livestock products include cattle, for beef, tallow, and hides; dairy cattle, for milk, butter, cheese, ice cream, and other dairy products; sheep, for mutton (lamb) and wool; pigs, for pork and lard; chickens, for broilers and eggs; other poultry (turkeys, ducks), principally for meat; and horses, primarily for recreation.

Livestock are raised principally on crops and pastures. They consume feedstuffs unsuited for humans, and produce highly nutritious products (meat, milk, eggs, and so on). Humans require that about one-fourth of their dietary protein be obtained from animal sources to supply amino acids not found in proper balance in crop products.

In the United States, 65–90% of all feed units for cattle, sheep, and goats is provided by forage

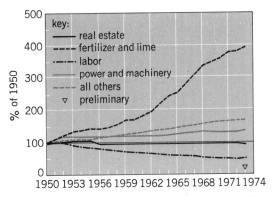

Fig. 4. Quantities of selected farm inputs in the United States. (*USDA*)

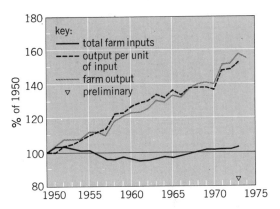

Fig. 5. United States farm productivity. (*USDA*)

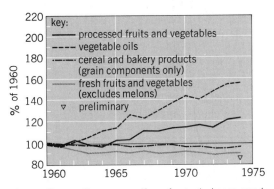

Fig. 6. Per capita consumption of selected crop products in the United States; items combined in terms of 1957–1959 retail prices. (*USDA*)

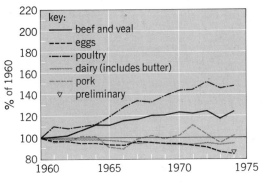

Fig. 7. Per capita consumption of selected livestock products in the United States; items combined in terms of 1957–1959 retail prices. (*USDA*)

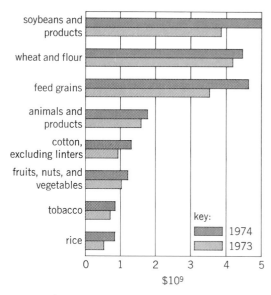

Fig. 8. United States agricultural exports, by commodity group. (*USDA*)

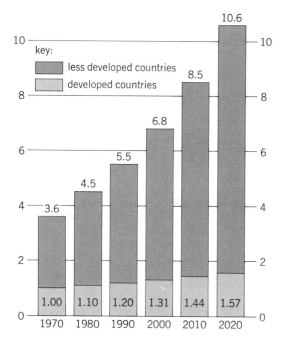

Fig. 10. World population (billions of people). Less-developed countries' growth projected at the current annual rate of 2.5%, developed countries at 0.9%. (*From U.S. Agency for International Development,* War on Hunger, *December 1974*)

crops (grazing lands, hay, and silage), and the remainder from feed grains and other concentrated feeds. In most of the less-developed countries, such livestock subsist solely on forages.

Livestock play a vital role in using lands not suited for crops, to produce animal products that are indispensable to humans. However, commercially produced pigs and poultry are dependent on supplies of grains and concentrates. *See* ANIMAL-FEED COMPOSITION.

Exports. The United States is the world's largest exporter of agricultural products. The value of agricultural exports for the year ending June 30, 1975, totaled $21,000,000,000, which provided the necessary foreign exchange for imports of minerals and petroleum from other countries (see Fig. 8).

Food Relief Program. In addition to commercial sales of agricultural products, the United States has had a major role in providing foods and other supplies for relief and rehabilitation in develop-

ing countries wherever the need arises. Such supplies are sent as outright grants or as long-term loans with no interest and a long grace period. Wherever food shortages or famines occur, or wherever there is devastation from storms, floods, earthquakes, or civil disruption, the United States has been responsive. In 1975 a world program for meeting food shortages was organized, with strong participation by the United States, but in cooperation with other countries that can supply food. Western European countries, Canada, and Australia are other contributors.

For the period covering fiscal years 1974, 1975, and 1976, the United States contributed between $750,000,000 and $950,000,000 yearly to assistance programs. This food, medical assistance, shelter, and other essential services are provided largely from United States reserves. They were channeled to about 26 nations that were in greatest need of assistance. Special assistance beyond these budgets is provided in other areas where disaster strikes. The United States works in cooperation with other countries in mitigating the impact of distressful conditions. Since food plays an important role in such relief and rehabilitation, it is essential that the agriculture of the United States continue to produce food surpluses.

WORLD AGRICULTURAL CONDITIONS

Since 1960 a very large number of countries that were once colonies became self-governing. These countries, together with others that have been independent for longer periods but are relatively undeveloped, have been increasing their total food production (Fig. 9). However, a tremendous increase in population growth has resulted in food production per capita barely keeping pace. In

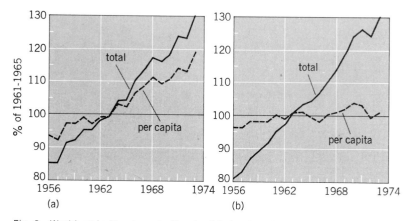

Fig. 9. World agricultural production in: (*a*) developed countries, North America, Europe, the Soviet Union, Japan, Republic of South Africa, Australia, and New Zealand; and (*b*) less-developed countries, Latin America, Asia (except Japan and Communist Asia), and Africa (except South Africa). (*USDA*)

Table 2. Indexes of world population and food production*

Year	World			Developed countries			Developing countries		
	Popula-tion	Food production		Popula-tion	Food production		Popula-tion	Food production	
		Total	Per capita		Total	Per capita		Total	Per capita
1955	85.7	80	93	90.3	81	90	82.5	78	95
1960	94.2	94	100	96.3	96	100	92.8	92	99
1965	103.9	104	100	102.3	104	102	105.0	104	99
1970	114.2	121	106	107.3	119	111	119.0	126	106
1973	120.9	133	110	110.2	133	121	128.5	132	103

SOURCE: U.S. Department of Agriculture, Economic Research Service, *The World Food Situation and Prospects to 1985,* Foreign Agricultural Economic Report no. 98, December 1974.
*1961–1965 = 100.

contrast, the developed countries in North America and Western Europe, and Australia have had food surpluses since 1964 (Table 2). This imbalance between agricultural production and population growth is a matter of worldwide concern. The application of science and technology to agriculture in the less-developed countries has great potential, but it will have a greater effect if companion programs of population control can become effective. World population growth is shown in Fig. 10.

Effects of science and technology. A worldwide program to adapt agricultural, biological, and physical sciences to the needs of less-developed countries is continually expanding. The United States has been a major contributor of funds, trained manpower, and physical supplies and facilities, and doubtless will continue to be a strong partner with other world agencies. In addition to the United Nations Development Program and the UN Food and Agricultural Organization, there were six international agricultural research institutes operating in 1975, and two in early stages of development. They are all dedicated to solving the urgent agricultural problems in the tropics and subtropics. In addition, agricultural development programs are being supported by the World Bank and by the regional banks in Latin America, Africa, and Asia. The bilateral assistance program of the U.S. Agency for International Development of less-developed countries is also being supplemented by bilateral programs of Western European countries and by Canada.

These programs deal not only with agricultural production and marketing but also with the health, education, and general development of less-developed countries. See AGRICULTURAL ENGINEERING. [HOWARD B. SPRAGUE]

Bibliography: Food and Agriculture Organization of the United Nations, Rome, *The State of Food and Agriculture,* 1974; H. B. Sprague (ed.), *The Grasslands of the United States,* 1974; U.S. Agency for International Development, *War on Hunger,* June 1975; U.S. Department of Agriculture, *Agricultural Handbook,* no. 477, 1974; U.S. Department of Agriculture, *This Land of Ours,* The Farm Index, March 1975; U.S. Department of Agriculture, Economic Research Service, *The World Food Situation and Prospects to 1985,* Foreign Agr. Econ. Rep. no. 98, December 1974; U.S. Department of Commerce, *Agriculture and Population: World Perspective and Problems,* 1975.

Agriculture, machinery in

Machines that are utilized for agricultural crop production involving tillage of the soil, planting of the crops, cultural practices during the growing season, and harvesting of the crops. Many of the machines are independently powered by tractors; however, an increasing number are self-propelled with their own specially designed power units, such as grain combined harvesters (Fig. 1), threshers, cotton harvesters, forage harvesters (Fig. 2), and numerous other special machines. *See* AGRICULTURE, SOIL AND CROP PRACTICES IN.

Implements such as plows, cultivators, and seeders may be mounted integrally on a tractor, and some of the functions of the tool are controlled by hydraulic systems with fingertip control by the tractor operator. Implements are also available that are pulled by a tractor. The tractor may also supply power through a power takeoff shaft that provides rotating force to drive rotating elements of the implement, such as hay balers, mowing machines, hay rakes, and others.

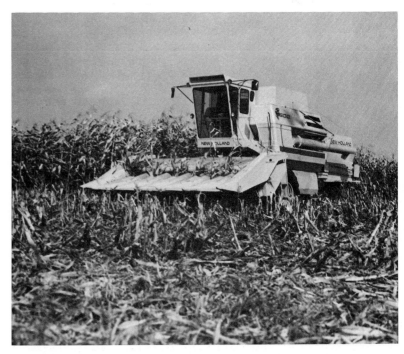

Fig. 1. Self-propelled combine (*Sperry New Holland, Div. of Sperry Rand Corp.*)

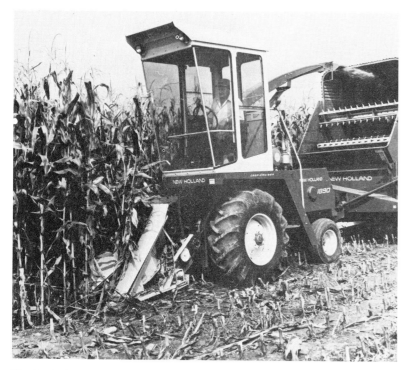

Fig. 2. Self-propelled forage harvester gathering corn for silage. (*Sperry New Holland, Div. of Sperry Rand Corp.*)

Farmstead machinery and equipment. Operations around and within production buildings on farms are nearly all or partially mechanized. Machines for these functions are usually classified as materials-handling equipment. Some may be powered by tractors, such as portable feed grinders (Fig. 3), manure spreaders, silage blowers, and numerous others (Fig. 4). Machines that do not require mobility are usually powered with electric motors. Such machines include silo unloaders, livestock feeding equipment, and milking machines. *See* DAIRY MACHINERY.

Machinery development. Economic and sociological forces have been the principal factors that have accelerated the demand for, and hence the development of, agricultural machinery. The availability of farm labor has been constantly decreasing, and costs continue to rise. An obvious solution has been to rely on power-operated machines to reduce the dependence on labor to increase individual productivity and to accomplish timely field operations during periods when climatic conditions permit.

Sizes of agricultural machines have been increasing because farm operations are becoming larger. With power-operated machines one operator can manage a large machine as easily as a small one; hence his productivity increases. To further increase the efficiency of field operations, several machine units may be combined to perform multiple functions simultaneously. For example, one such unit may include a rotary tiller to prepare a seedbed, planter units to seed the crop, units to place fertilizer in the soil near the seed, and an applicator to apply preemergence herbicide to control weeds. All of these are combined in one unit, pulled by one tractor. Such a unit size may cover a width of 20–24 ft.

Fruit and vegetable harvesting. Extensive research and development has been underway since 1950 to provide mechanical systems for harvesting and handling fruit and vegetable crops to eliminate dependence on hand labor. A considerable number of tree and vine fruits are now being harvested mechanically by means of devices which shake the tree or vine, and the fruit is collected on special collecting frames and then transferred to bulk bins or tanks (Figs. 5 and 6). This system is known as the mass removal method.

Generally, most harvesting machines are nonselective; that is, the entire crop is harvested in one operation. Exceptions to this include a selective lettuce harvester that electronically selects heads of lettuce that are mature and leaves immature heads for later harvesting. Another selective-

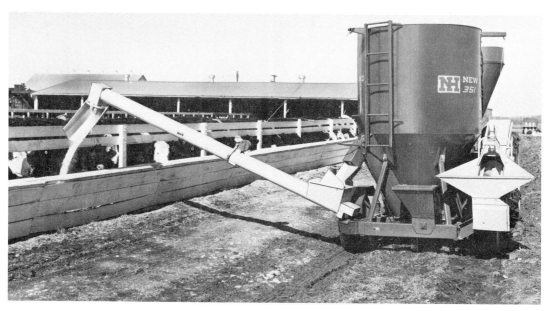

Fig. 3. Portable feed grinder-mixer delivering processed feed. (*Sperry New Holland, Div. of Sperry Rand Corp.*)

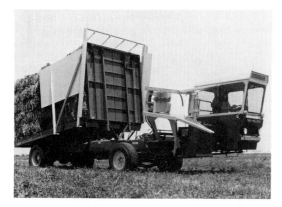

Fig. 4.   Machine to automatically pick up, load, and stack hay bales. (*Sperry New Holland, Div. of Sperry Rand Corp.*)

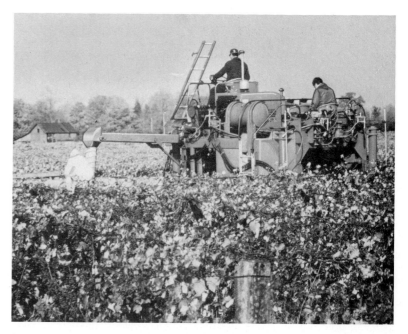

Fig. 6.   Juice grapes being harvested mechanically at the rate of an acre or more per hour.

type machine is a cucumber harvester that removes only the larger cucumbers, leaving small ones for later harvest. Tomato harvesters pick up the entire tomato plant and remove the fruit on the machine. Some hand labor is required on the machine for sorting ripe and green fruits, since not all are of equal maturity. This same principle is employed on potato harvesters for sorting out imperfect tubers, clods, and stones.

Some fruit and vegetable crops still have to be harvested by hand, such as citrus fruits, cauliflower, broccoli, and watermelons. Experimental and development work is being done on most of these, and in the near future they too will be mechanized.

Cost and productivity. Investment in agricultural machinery, including tractors and motor trucks, has been increasing at a rate of about $1,500,000,000 per year during the recent past and now approaches about $30,000,000,000. If a depreciation of 15% is assumed, this means that United States farmers invest about $5,000,000,000 annually in machinery and equipment. Farmers have nearly twice as much invested in machinery per worker as compared to most manufacturing industries. This is a major reason that the productivity per farm worker is greater than that in any other major industry. The adoption and use of modern agricultural machinery is also a major factor re-

sponsible for reducing the unit cost of food production. The American food consumer could purchase his food in 1968 with less than 18% of his disposable income—the lowest percentage in the world and in the nation's history.

[ORVAL C. FRENCH]

Bibliography: R. Bainer et al., *Principles of Farm Machinery*, 1955; C. B. Richey, P. Jacobson, and C. W. Hall, *Agricultural Engineers' Handbook*, 1961.

Agriculture, soil and crop practices in

The techniques and methods used in plowing, harrowing, planting, tilling, harvesting, drying, storing, and processing of agricultural crops.

PLOWING

Cutting and turning a furrow with a plow is usually the first and most effective operation of tillage. There are two types of plow, the moldboard (Fig. 1) and the disk.

Moldboard plow. The working part of the moldboard plow is the plow bottom. The plow furrow is cut or broken loose on the land side by the shin of the plow or by a coulter or jointer attached to the plow beam, and on the bottom by the point and edge of the plow share. The advancing plow moldboard exerts pressure on the furrow slice, pulverizing it and causing it to move upward and to the side in a spiraling path so that it is partially or completely inverted. The shape of the moldboard may be described as a section cut from a warped cylinder, on the inside of which the soil spirals. The selection of design of the moldboard depends upon the physical reaction of the kind of soil and sod cover on which it is to be used. Because precise information of soil physical reaction is inadequate and the amount of pulverization and placement, or throw, of the furrow slice depends upon the speed of plowing, plows have been designed largely by the cut-and-try method. This has result-

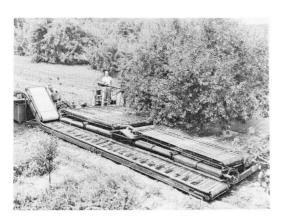

Fig. 5.   Mechanical harvester for tree fruits, shown harvesting tart cherries. (*Cornell University*)

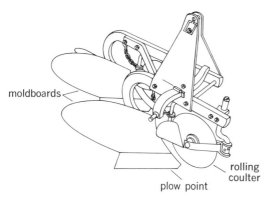

Fig. 1.   One type of moldboard plow. (*Tractor and Implement Division, Ford Motor Co.*)

ed in a great variety of shapes. Moldboard plows have largely been adapted to power farming by the selection of bottoms suitable for certain soils and combination of these bottoms into gangs sufficiently large to use the power of the tractor at the approximate speed for which the bottoms were designed. The power required at normal speed of 4 mph varies from 2–3 psi of cross section of furrow slice for sand, to 20 psi for tough clay. Modifications of shape have permitted a speed of 5–6 mph.

Moldboard plow bottoms are designated as right-hand or left-hand bottoms, depending upon the direction of throw. Both may be combined on one frame so that the plow can be pulled back and forth, always throwing the furrow downhill, or in one direction. Sizes range from 8 to 20 in. in width of cut; the 10–12 in. size is suitable for use with animal power, and the 14–16 in. size is largely used with power equipment. Although a plow may be used to plow at different depths, most have been designed to work at a depth of approximately one-half the width of the furrow.

The effectiveness of plowing may be materially increased by attachments. A jointer, or a jointer

and coulter combination, which cuts a small furrow in front of the plow shin, permits complete coverage of sod. Where there are large amounts of rubbish or crop residue, a weed chain or wire can be used to drag the debris into the furrow and hold it there until covered. A furrow wheel may reduce land-side friction, and a depth gage on the beam helps secure uniform depth. A modified form of plow bottom, called a lister, is in effect a right and a left moldboard joined at the shin so as to throw soil both to the right and to the left. This produces a furrow or trough, called a list, in which seed is planted. Because it concentrates rainfall in the furrow, this method is used largely in areas of light rainfall.

Disk plow. The disk plow consists of a number of disk blades attached to one axle or gang bolt. This plow is used for rapid, shallow plowing. In fields where numerous rocks and roots are present, the disk plow, which rolls over obstacles, is substituted for the moldboard. The disk is also used for sticky soils that will not scour on a moldboard. The disk plow is manufactured in widths of from 2-1/2 to 20 ft. The disks are commonly spaced 8–10 in. apart. The angle between the gang bolt and the direction of travel is usually adjustable from 35 to 55°.

HARROWING

Soil preparation for planting usually involves the pulling of an implement called a harrow over the plowed soil to break clods, level the surface, and destroy weeds. A wide variety of implements are classified as harrows; the most common kinds are the disk harrow, the spike-tooth harrow, the spring-tooth harrow, and the knife harrow. Previously the function of seedbed preparation was performed almost entirely by the implements classified as harrows. With the introduction of power, farming is now performed in large part by field cultivators, rod weeders, rotary hoes, or treaders, subsurface packers, and various designs of rollers. Power-driven rotary tillers perform the function of both plowing and harrowing.

Kinds of harrows. The spike-tooth is the oldest form of commercial harrow and consists of spikes or teeth (usually adjustable) extending downward from a frame. The teeth extend into the soil, and when the harrow is pulled forward, they cut through clods and break them. The teeth also stir and level the soil surface and kill weeds. This type of harrow has light draft and is built in sections, many of which may be joined together so that large areas can be covered quickly. This implement is most effective if used before clods dry; it is frequently attached behind the plow.

The spring-tooth harrow is similar to the spike-tooth type but has long curved teeth of spring steel. The spring action renders it suitable for rough or stony ground. It is particularly useful in bringing clods to the surface, where they can be pulverized. It is also used to bring the roots of weeds and obnoxious grasses to the surface for destruction, and to renovate and cultivate alfalfa fields. The knife harrow consists of a frame holding a number of knives which scrape and partly invert the surface to smooth it and destroy small weeds.

The disk harrow is probably the most universally used type (Fig. 2). It cuts clods and trash

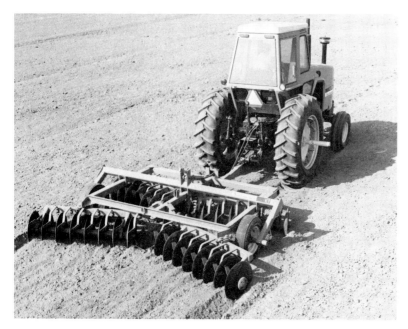

Fig. 2.   One type of disk harrow. (*Allis-Chalmers*)

effectively, destroys weeds, cuts in cover crops, and smoothes and prepares the surface for other farming operations. The penetration of the disk harrow depends largely upon weight. The disk blades are commonly 16–24 in. in diameter and are spaced 6–10 in. apart in gangs of 3–12 disks. Disk harrows can be obtained in widths up to 20 ft. A single-acting disk harrow has two opposed gangs throwing soil outward from the center; a tandem or double-acting disk has two additional gangs which throw the soil back toward the center. An important advancement in the design of the disk harrow is the offset disk. A right-hand offset disk harrow has a gang in front which throws to the right and a rear gang which throws to the left. It may be adjusted to pull to one side and to the rear of the tractor so as to harrow beneath the low limbs of orchard trees.

Other soil-preparation equipment. The field cultivator is used to perform many of the jobs of harrows before planting. It usually consists of a number of adjustable standards with sweeps or scrapes attached to tool bars in such a fashion that the soil is stirred from underneath, killing the weeds and creating a surface mulch for moisture conservation. The rod weeder is a power-driven rod, usually square in cross section, which also operates beneath the surface of loose soil, killing weeds and maintaining the soil in a loose mulched condition. It is adapted to large operations and is used in dry areas of the Northwest. A variety of rollers and packing wheels and clod crushers have been designed.

PLANTING

The practice of placing seed or vegetative propagating material in soil for multiplication through growth and reproduction is usually a seasonal operation. Its success depends upon soil preparation and placing of the seed in an environment favorable to growth. The seed, which is an embryonic plant enclosed in a protective membrane, usually contains enough nutritional material to start growth. It must have suitable temperature, adequate air, and sufficient moisture to overcome its dormant condition and induce vigorous growth. In general, the seeding process consists of opening a furrow in properly prepared soil to the correct depth, metering and distributing the seed or planting material, depositing the seed in the furrow, and covering and compacting the soil around the seed to a degree suitable to the crop. Fertilizer is usually placed in the soil sufficiently near the seed that it will be available to the young plants after germination.

Kinds of planters. There are five general methods of planting based on five special types of machinery: (1) broadcasters; (2) seed drills used for small seed and grains; (3) planters for cultivated row crops such as corn or cotton; (4) special planters for parts of plants used for propagation, such as potato planters; and (5) transplanters used to set out small plants that have been grown in beds from small seed. The last is commonly used for tobacco, sweet potatoes, cabbage, trees, and many horticultural crops.

Broadcasters. Small grains, grasses, and clovers are planted by broadcasting or drilling. The broadcaster is usually a rotating fanlike distributor which throws the seed over a wide area by

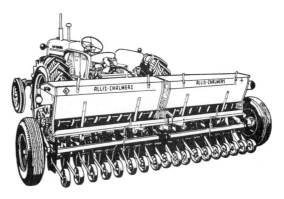

Fig. 3.   All-crop drill with rubber press wheels to push seeds into soil. (*Allis-Chalmers*)

centrifugal force. Like hand seeding, this method requires the absence of gusty wind for most effective distribution. Under proper conditions, broadcasting can be done from airplanes. Broadcasting is especially suited to sowing seed in another crop without unduly disturbing the soil, such as sowing clover seed in wheat.

Drills. The grain drill opens a furrow and places the seed in it. Attachments, such as covering chains and wheels to press seed into the soil, are commonly used (Fig. 3). The seed is metered by a special apparatus into rows 6–14 in. apart. Several types of furrow openers adapted to different soil and crop conditions are available. Grain drills are also commonly equipped for fertilizer distribution and grass seeding.

Row-crop planters. Such crops as corn and cotton are planted with special planters in rows to simplify cultivation. Because yield may be greatly affected by the stand's being too thick or too thin, precision planting is important to avoid the cost of thinning or interplanting. Delinting of cotton-seed and sizing of seed corn and other seeds are important to precision planting. Planters usually are equipped for dropping in hills or drilling in rows. The hills may be check-rowed, that is, spaced equally apart on the corners of squares so that the crop can be cultivated in two directions, thus avoiding hoeing. The precision necessary for this type of planting is secured by opening valves in the planter shank at measured intervals by means of buttons on a check wire.

Transplanters. Special kinds of equipment designed for the planting of cuttings or small plants are known as transplanters. Such machines usually transport one or more men who assist the action of the machine in placing the plants in a furrow and properly covering them. Transplanters commonly supply a small quantity of water to each plant.

TILLAGE

The mechanical manipulation of the soil to improve its physical condition as a habitat for plants is called tillage. It includes plowing, inversion, loosening, harrowing, pulverization, packing, and rolling the soil, all to improve aeration and temperature conditions and to produce a firm seedbed (Fig. 4). Subsurface tillage is the loosening of soil by sweeps or blades pulled beneath the surface without inversion of the soil. This practice, especially adapted to dry areas, fragments the soil and

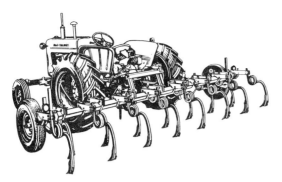

Fig. 4. Coil-shank field cultivator. (*Allis-Chalmers*)

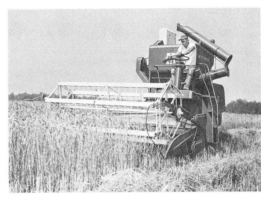

Fig. 8. Combine-harvester. (*International Harvester Co.*)

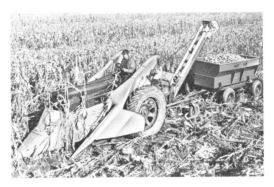

Fig. 5. Corn picker. (*New Idea Farm Equipment Co.*)

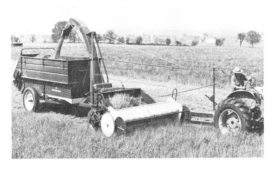

Fig. 6. Forage harvester equipped with a sickle-bar attachment. (*Sperry New Holland, Div. of Sperry Rand Corp.*)

HARVESTING

The practice of severing and reaping the plant or any of its parts is called harvesting.

Crops harvested for grain. The process of gathering such crops as corn, sorghums, wheat, oats, barley, rye, buckwheat, and rice is called grain harvesting.

Ear corn is harvested by means of a corn picker (Fig. 5). The ears are snapped off by specially designed rollers which pass around the standing stalks. The husks are removed by a husking bed consisting of rolls of various types, over which the ears are passed.

Shelled corn is harvested by a picker-sheller or by the combine harvester. The picker-sheller snaps the ears from the stalks in the same manner as the picker, but the husking bed is replaced by a shelling unit. A trailing shelling unit attached to the picker can also be used.

Corn is also harvested by a self-propelled combine harvester. The header can be removed and replaced with a snapping unit, or the header can remain in place with the whole plant passing through the machine. Grain sorghums and cereals are harvested largely with the combine harvester, a machine that severs the standing crop, shells the grain, separates grain from straw, and removes chaff and trash in one operation. Sometimes these crops are severed and windrowed, allowed to dry, and threshed later.

Grain crops harvested for ensilage. This operation is used for corn, sweet sorghums, and cereals such as oats, wheat, barley, and rye.

Row crops, such as corn and some sorghums, are harvested with a forage harvester equipped

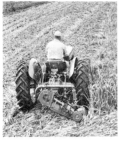

Fig. 7. Mowing machine. (*Massey Ferguson Co.*)

leaves a mulch of stubble or other plant residues on the soil surface to conserve water and help control erosion.

Effective tillage eliminates competitive vegetation, such as weeds, and stimulates favorable soil microbiological activities. Natural forces of heating and cooling, swelling and shrinkage, wetting and drying, and freezing and thawing account for the major pulverization of soil and assist in the production of a favorable crumb structure. Wise practice dictates the avoidance of tillage when soil is so wet and plastic that its crumb structure is easily destroyed, as well as the use of those operations which put the soil in the most favorable condition for natural forces to act. This results in the minimum amount of time and power for soil preparation. Manipulation of the soil by machinery is an essential part of soil management, which includes such soil-building practices as grass and legume rotations, fertilization, and liming.

[MARK L. NICHOLS]

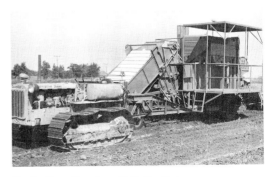

Fig. 9. Bean thresher. (*C. B. Hay Co.*)

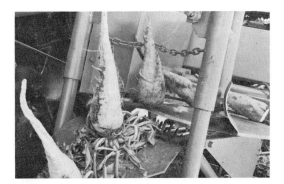

Fig. 10. Detail of spiked-wheel harvester gathering sugar beets. (*Blackwelder Manufacturing Co.*)

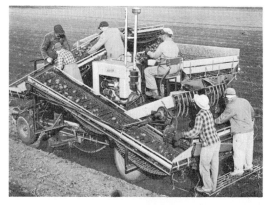

Fig. 11.   Potato harvester. (*USDA Agricultural Research Service, Red River Valley Potato Research Center*)

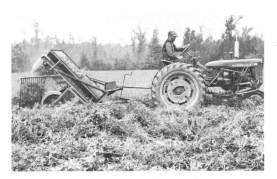

Fig. 12.   Peanut digger-shaker-windrower. (*Department of Agricultural Engineering, North Carolina State College*)

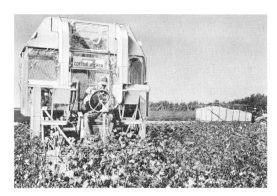

Fig. 13.   Cotton stripper. (*Allis-Chalmers*)

with a row-crop attachment. High-moisture corn may be shelled by a picker-sheller and stored as ensilage.

Drilled crops and some row crops are harvested with the forage harvester equipped with a sickle-bar attachment (Fig. 6). Rotary-type harvesters are also used. The plants are severed at or near the soil surface and cut or shredded into short lengths.

Crops for silage, soilage, and hay. This type of harvesting is used for legumes (other than edible-podded legumes) and grasses (excluding corn, sorghums, and cereals). The sickle-bar or rotary-type forage harvester is used. It severs the crop near the ground surface and chops it into desired lengths for silage or soilage. It also chops hay from the windrow. The crop may be wilted slightly in the windrow to reduce moisture for silage preservation. The conventional mower, or the mower-crusher designed to speed up drying, is used to harvest crops for hay (Fig. 7).

Legumes and grasses for seed. Legumes and grasses are harvested largely by the combine harvester, either by direct or windrow methods (Fig. 8). Windrowing becomes necessary when the crop fails to ripen evenly. Because some seeds are lighter than cereal grains, machine adjustments differ widely. To increase overall efficiency, two combines may be hooked together in tandem. All straw and chaff from the lead combine passes through the rear one.

Podded legumes which are harvested include soybeans, dry edible beans, and peas. Soybeans are harvested exclusively by the combine-harvester direct method. Peas and beans may be harvested by the combine harvester or by bean threshers with multiple shelling cylinders (Fig. 9). In many cases, beans or peas may be removed or severed from the soil and windrowed prior to threshing. To prevent the cracking of seeds, cylinder speeds are reduced and concave clearance increased. Rubber-covered rolls, placed ahead of the cylinder, may be used to squeeze beans from pods.

Harvested root crops include sugar beets, potatoes, and peanuts. Sugar beets are gathered by special harvesters. One type tops the beets in place, after which the beets are lifted by specially designed blades or fingers. Another type lifts the beets by gripping the tops or by impaling the beets on a revolving spiked wheel (Fig. 10). The beets are then topped in the machine. An elevator conveys the beets to trucks for bulk handling.

Potatoes are harvested by several methods. They may be (1) dug with a one- or two-row digger and picked up by hand; (2) dug, sorted, and placed into containers by machine (vines, trash, and clods are removed mechanically and by men riding the machine); (3) harvested by a fully mechanized procedure which includes digging, sorting, removal of vines, trash, and clods, and loading into bulk trucks (Fig. 11); and (4) dug with a standard digger, windrowed for drying, and picked up later by an indirect harvester. Sweet potatoes are harvested largely by the first method.

Peanuts are harvested by the following methods: (1) pole-stack method, in which the peanuts are dug and hand-shaken, stacked around poles, and later picked; (2) a method in which they are dug with a one- or two-row digger, windrowed, and harvested later with a peanut picker (Fig. 12); and (3) the once-over method, in which all operations are accomplished with the same machine.

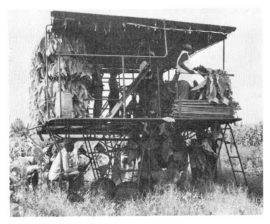

Fig. 14. Tobacco harvester. (*Department of Agricultural Engineering, North Carolina State College*)

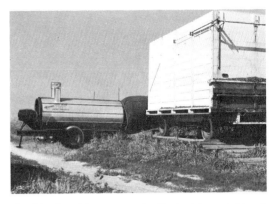

Fig. 16. Special wagon rack attached to portable oil-burning crop drier for finish-drying chopped forage.

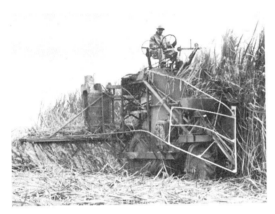

Fig. 15. Sugarcane harvester. (*Agricultural Engineering Department, Louisiana State University*)

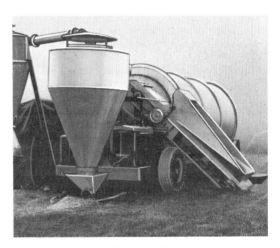

Fig. 17. Portable alfalfa-dehydrating equipment.

Crops harvested for fiber. Cotton is harvested by two methods: (1) pulling lint from the bolls by means of the cotton picker, a method which requires several pickings and is accomplished by broached spindles revolving rearward on which the lint is wound; and (2) pulling the entire boll from plants by a cotton stripper (Fig. 13), a onceover method accomplished by rolls of various types (steel, rubber paddle, or brush) which strip the bolls from the plants.

Special crops. There are several crops requiring special methods to be harvested. These include tobacco, castor beans, and sugarcane. Tobacco is harvested by two general methods. (1) Leaves may be primed from the stalks as they mature, in several primings starting with the lower, more mature, leaves; or (2) the stalks may be severed near the base (Fig. 14), upended, and speared, after which laths are inserted to handle the plants and support them in the curing barn. Machines have been developed to speed up the priming process; workers ride rather than walk.

Castor beans are harvested by special machines that straddle the rows, with revolving beaters that strip the beans from the standing stalks.

Sugarcane is harvested by self-propelled harvesters which sever the cane at or slightly below the soil surface (Fig. 15). Additional knives top the cane. Tops and trash are removed by fans and dis-

tributed over the soil. Conveyors move the cane into heap rows or directly into trucks or wagons. Some machines cut the cane into short lengths for easier handling and processing.

[EDWARD A. SILVER; R. B. MUSGRAVE]

DRYING AND STORAGE

Farm crops may be harvested at the most desirable stage of maturity and stored for weeks or months if properly dried or preserved. Field drying is an inexpensive procedure. However, in cool, humid areas a fine crop may deteriorate to a low-value feedstuff if it is damaged by rain during field drying; loss of quality may also occur as a result of mold or spontaneous heating in storage. To reduce such losses in forage crops, many farmers partially cure grasses or legumes in the field and then finish drying them in hay mows, bins, special wagons, or drying buildings by passing heated or unheated air through the forage with a power-driven fan unit attached to an air-duct system (Fig. 16).

Forage. Forage containing 70–80% moisture at harvest time is field-dried to 30–40% and finish-dried to 22–25% for safe storage as chopped or long hay, or to 20% as baled hay. Hay processed in this manner is superior to field-dried material in color, carotene content, and leafiness.

Because hay quality is to some extent a function

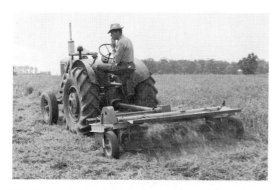

Fig. 18. Forage crusher for cracking or shredding stems to accelerate field drying rate of forage crops.

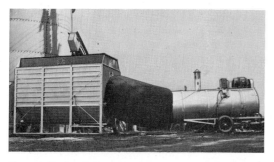

Fig. 19. Perforated metal bin for drying small grain and shelled corn with heated air from portable crop drier.

of the rapidity of drying, heated air usually produces the best product. Very rapid drying can be accomplished with dehydrating equipment which can dry material from 75 to 10% moisture in 20 min or less. The quality of a dehydrated product is high; however, costs of labor and fuel are also high. Alfalfa to be used in mixed feed is the most frequently dehydrated crop (Fig. 17).

Field drying can be accelerated by the use of crushing machines which crack or shred the freshly cut forage as it passes through one or more pairs of crushing rollers (Fig. 18). Overall drying time is shortened because the stems, if crushed, will dry almost as fast as the leaves which, if the hay was improperly dried, often shatter and drop off.

Small grains and shelled corn. Small grains and shelled corn are dried to 12% moisture or less in either continuous or batch driers and stored in bins. Ear corn stored in an open crib must be dried to 16% moisture if mold growth in storage is to be prevented. Generally, temperatures of drying should not exceed 100°F for seed and malting grains, 130°F for milling corn, and 200°F for feedstuffs (Fig. 19). Frequently rice drying is carried on in two stages to prevent cracking.

Ensiling. The anaerobic fermentation process of ensiling is used to preserve immature green corn, legumes, grasses, and grain plants. The crop is chopped and packed while at about 70–80% moisture and put into cylindrical tower-type silos, horizontal trenchlike structures, or other containers to exclude the air. This tightly packed, juicy material is preserved by proper bacterial fermentation. Desirable microorganisms in grass and legume silage can be encouraged by field-wilting the crop to 70% moisture, or by adding chemical preservatives, sugar, and starch materials, such as ground corn or small grain. Shelled or chopped ear corn is occasionally stored under similar anaerobic conditions.   [HJALMAR D. BRUHN]

PROCESSING CROPS

Crop processing involves such operations as shelling, cleaning, separating, sorting, washing, treating, scarifying, testing, grinding, and ginning.

Shelling. The separation of corn kernels from the cob or the removal of the shell from nuts such as peanuts, walnuts, and hickory nuts is called shelling. This can be done with two types of machines, the spring type in which the kernels are rubbed from the ears by a notched metal bar called a rag iron, and the power-driven cylinder-type machine into which the ears are fed between a revolving shelling cylinder and stationary bars called concaves (Fig. 20). The kernels are rubbed off and separated before the cobs are removed. Proper shelling is obtained by control of the rate of feeding, tension of the shelling bar, choice of shelling concave, cleaning-air control, and cob-outlet control. The practice of picking high-moisture corn in the field and shelling it with a picker-sheller or combine-sheller is increasing.

Cleaning and separation. These procedures include the removal of foreign material, such as weed seeds, chaff, dead insects, and broken stems. The fanning mill, consisting of two vibrating screens and an air blast, is used on the farm for cleaning (Fig. 21). The most common methods of cleaning are by size, using a screen; by length,

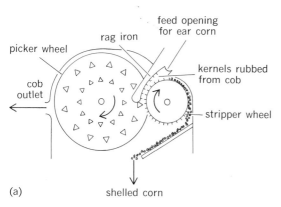

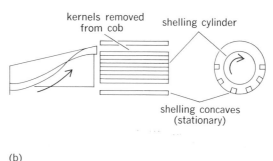

(a) shelled corn   (b)

Fig. 20. Operation of two types of corn shellers. (a) Spring. (b) Cylinder.

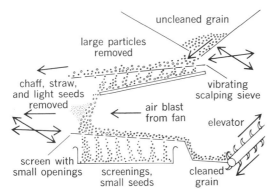

Fig. 21. Fanning mill operation.

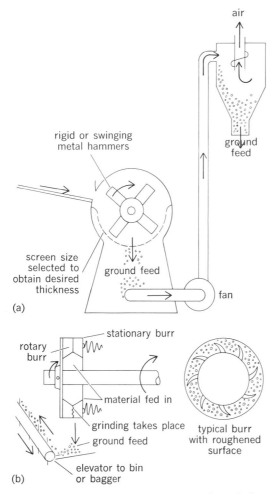

Fig. 22. Operation of two machines for grinding. (a) Hammer mill. (b) Burr mill.

using a cylinder or disk with indented pockets to accept only short, small grain; by specific gravity, using a vibrating screen or inclined deck through which air is blown to remove the light material from the top; and by brine solutions of such density as to float light material and permit heavy material to settle. Seeds which become sticky when wet are separated from other seeds (for example, buckhorn seed from cloverseed) by moistening of the seed surfaces with wet iron filings or sawdust. The wetted seeds and iron filings or sawdust stick together, forming large clumps which are then removed by screening. Buckhorn seeds are removed in this manner from clover seeds. Seed shape can also be used as a means of separation because the round seeds roll and the flat seeds slide. Smooth and rough materials may be separated by using velvet- or velveteen-fabric-covered rolls, or by air in which the materials with irregular and rough surfaces are removed from those with smooth surfaces. Fruits may be cleaned by brushing, wet or dry, and by flailing.

Sorting. The separation of products into prescribed standards is called sorting. Grading is sorting to meet state and Federal agency regulations. Grading, particularly of fruits and vegetables, is done by machinery to obtain the proper size or weight. Size grading is practiced to obtain desired diameter by using a belt with holes, a link chain, a diversion belt, diversion rollers, or spool units. Apples, peaches, potatoes, onions, lemons, and oranges are commonly sized. The weight method is sometimes used to place products in appropriate grades. For beans, coffee, and lemons, color sorting is accomplished by scanning with an electric-eye device which rejects the materials possessing undesirable light-reflecting properties.

Washing. Foreign materials are removed from fruits, seeds, nuts, and vegetables by washing, often with a detergent and chlorine solution. Washing is done by soaking in tanks, spraying with high-pressure nozzles, or moving the materials through a washing solution in a rotary cylinder.

Treating. Seeds are treated for disease or growth control. Treating was formerly performed by heating the seeds in water, but now it is usually done with a chemical. The treating material may be applied as a chemical slurry, dust, liquid, or vapor. Mercury compounds are often used, but seed treated with mercury cannot be used for animal or human feed. Legume seeds are often inoculated with bacteria which convert the nitrogen of the soil air into a form which is suitable for use by the plant.

Scarifying. This process, usually preceded by hulling, is an operation in which hard seed, such as that of legumes, is scratched or scarred to facilitate water absorption and to speed germination.

Testing. Usually testing is performed on batches of seeds to determine the purity, moisture content, weight, and germination potential. The major problem in testing is to obtain a representative sample. The moisture content of grains and seeds indicates the keeping quality in storage and is a basis for estimating their commercial value. Weight per bushel is an important commercial criterion used for grain and is known as the test weight.

Grinding. Reduction in size of the material to improve utilization by animals and to make handling easier is called grinding. Measurement of the fineness of the ground material is designated by fineness modulus numbers from 1 (fine) to 7 (coarse). Units for size reduction include the hammer mill, a rotating high-strength beater which crushes the material until it will pass through a screen mounted above, below, or around the rotating hammer; the burr or attrition mill, in which two ribbed plates or disks rub or crush the material between them; and the roller mill, in which grain passes between pairs of smooth or corrugated rolls (Fig. 22). The last is used extensively for flour manufacture. The crimper-roller is used on farms to crush grains. The roller-crusher is also used to reduce the size of ear corn before it is fed into the hammer mill or burr mill.

Ginning. Separation of lint from cottonseed is called ginning. The cotton gin cleans the cotton and seed in addition to separating them. The saw gin, which consists of about 100 saws per gin stand mounted about 5/8 in. apart on a shaft, is the most commonly used. The 12-in. diameter saws are made up of spikes on wheels which pull the cotton through huller ribs, but the seed cotton (cotton containing seed) is not pulled through. The lint is removed from the saw blades with air or with a high-speed brush. *See* AGRICULTURAL ENGINEERING; AGRICULTURAL SCIENCE (PLANT); AGRICULTURE, MACHINERY IN. [CARL W. HALL]

Agriculture, structures in

All buildings used on the farm for human habitation and agricultural enterprises. Extremes of climate make buildings necessary. Climatic building zones have been established by the American Society of Agricultural Engineers to aid in the planning of farm buildings in the United States (Fig. 1). These zones are based on the average temperature for the month of January, zone 1 being the coldest. Superimposed on the zones are the symbols A, B, C, D, and E, which indicate the number of hours per year when the temperature is 85°F or higher, zone A representing the greatest.

Kinds of housing. Variations in management and in size and age of animals require different degrees of environmental control. Three principal kinds of housing take care of these variations.

First, open housing, provided with open-front sheds facing south or east and protected yards, is used in the warmer zones (Fig. 2). Such housing partially protects animals from winter wind, snow, and rain and furnishes some heat from the manure pack maintained during the winter season. The yards are protected by the building and by windproof fences. In zones A, B, and C sheds are open on both the north and south sides in summer to allow free circulation of air. These sheds are covered with highly reflective material to reduce absorption of solar heat.

Second, a variation of open housing with warming of a small area in each pen is used for young animals. Both types of open housing require acclimated animals, that is, animals housed in open sheds or yards during the fall season to prepare them for winter. Animals that are not acclimated cannot adjust readily to changes in the weather, and are dependent on the barn for protection.

Third is the type called closed housing which is used principally in the colder zones, and is designed to provide protection for animals in extremes of temperature.

Barns are used in animal husbandry and for the storage of agricultural products and equipment (Fig. 3). The lower boundary of the optimum environment for closed dairy barns and milking rooms is 35°F, 60% relative humidity, and 1/2 mph air movement. This is based primarily on the needs of the operator, the machines for operating the enter-

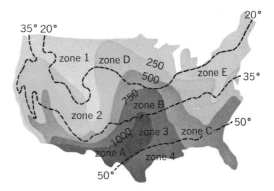

Fig. 1. Climatic building zones. (Broken lines mark divisions between low-temperature zones; shading marks divisions between high-temperature zones.) Low-temperature zones based on average January temperature: 1, 5–20°F; 2, 20–35°F; 3, 35–50°F; 4, over 50°F. High-temperature zones based on number of hours per year with 85°F or higher temperature: A, over 1000; B, 750–1000; C, 500–750; D, 250–500; E, less than 250.

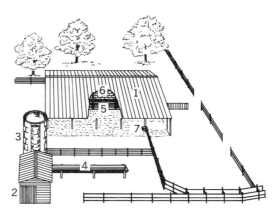

Fig. 2. Housing for a cow- and calf-raising project: 1, open-front shed facing south; 2, feed-storage and -processing building; 3, silo; 4, feed bunk; 5, hay-feeding manger; 6, baled hay or straw; 7, watering place.

prise, and the maintenance of sanitation, rather than the needs of the cows. Acclimated cows will produce satisfactorily at a temperature of 5°F or even colder. Maintenance of optimum environment in closed barns requires building insulation to reduce heat loss and automatic ventilation to control humidity.

Enterprises involving adult poultry, swine, or sheep require much the same environment in closed-type buildings as that for the dairy enterprise. However, the animals in these enterprises, being smaller, may require somewhat more protection from cold than do the larger dairy animals.

Barns of the closed type for housing young stock must provide a higher temperature than that needed for producing cows. At birth the body temperature-regulating mechanisms of young animals are not developed, and the animals are dependent on the barn for assistance in maintaining the needed body temperature. With slight changes, the barn for young stock also meets the needs for young poultry, swine, and sheep.

Grain-storage and -processing buildings. Each grain contains a living embryo enclosed by food tissues. Storage of grain requires the maintenance

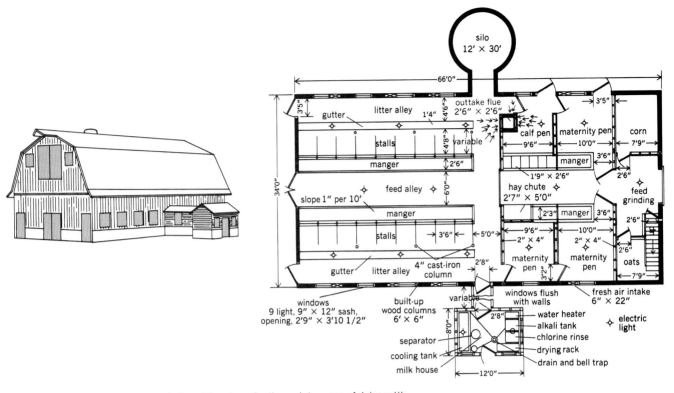

Fig. 3. A closed-type barn for the maintenance of dairy cattle.

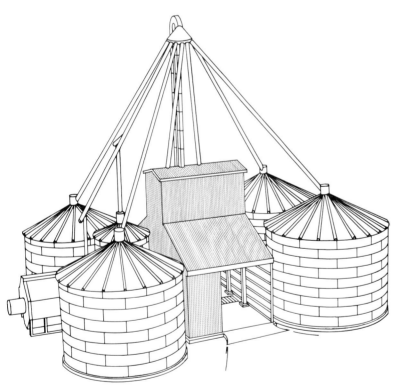

Fig. 4. A grain-handling, -conditioning, and -processing center.

of an environment sufficiently dry and low in temperature that it will not cause the embryo to begin active growth (or germinate). Such an environment is also needed to reduce the development of mold on the grain. Bins must be constructed so as to permit fumigation of the grain to destroy fungi and prevent insect infestation in addition to providing adequate circulation of air for drying.

Grain is placed in storage at harvest time by use of mechanical power. It is dried if necessary, handled, ground and mixed in the proportions desired, and often delivered by mechanical power to buildings where it is needed.

The group of storage units shown in Fig. 4 is made up of standard-size bins and can be assembled to suit the needs of any farm. Such equipment enables the farmer to balance his ability at the farmstead with that in the fieldwork.

Processing of feed may require facilities for promoting chemical change, such as the making of silage. A silo is a semiairtight container which is used to provide conditions for lactic and acetic acid fermentation and for preventing oxidation or decay of the ensiled material until it is needed for feed. The walls of the silo must be made air- and watertight. In the past the silos were open at the top, with or without a roof. The air seal was secured by covering the silage with straw or other materials which would rot and form a seal, thus keeping the silage until needed for feed, at which time the seal was removed. From then on, enough silage was removed from the surface each day to prevent spoilage.

The gastight silos were then developed and are completely closed. A door is provided in the top cover for use when the silo is filled. The silage is removed from the bottom of the silo and distributed along a feed trough, making this chore a semi-automatic process (Fig. 5).

Silos of the horizontal type are either a trench in the ground or a bunker built above ground. The silage may be covered with earth or straw, which rots and forms a seal, or with a plastic material to

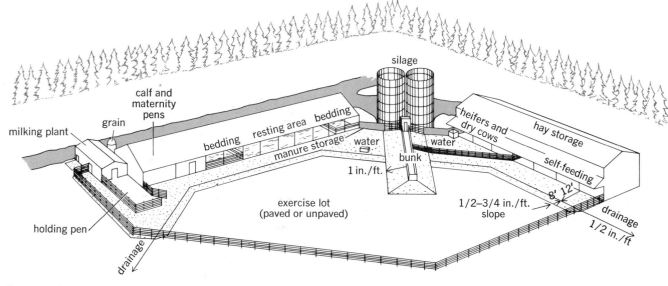

Fig. 5. Vertical silos with feeding equipment for dairy cattle, arranged for most efficient use of space.

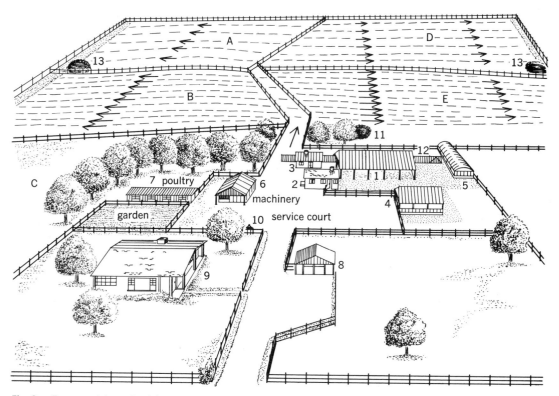

Fig. 6. Farm and farmstead layout where dairy and poultry are the principal enterprises: 1, resting barn for dairy cows; 2, combined milking and milk room; 3, feed-storage and -processing building; 4, combined hay-storage, -curing, and self-feeding barn; 5, bunker silo equipped for self-feeding; 6, farm machinery storage and repair building; 7, laying house; 8, double garage; 9, farmhouse; 10, hydrant to connect pump for fire protection; 11, pond to supply farmstead; 12, watering place; 13, ponds with watering places in fields (A, B, D, and E); C, pasture.

provide the seal; a movable manger may be used to self-feed the silage if desired.

The initial cost of the horizontal type is much less than the modern vertical silo; however, the waste is greater, the quality of the silage is lower, and the amount of labor in feeding is greater.

Machinery storage. Large machines which are used for seeding and harvesting require a building with an unobstructed floor space, high clearance, and extra height and width in the doors.

Since the tractor is used frequently and in all seasons, it should have a place in a separate building or section of the machinery building, on or near to the central service court of the farmstead. If kept in the machinery storage building, it should have a partitioned space, equipped with concrete floor, workbenches, and storage places for tools and materials required for maintenance. This building can then be the farm shop for general repair and maintenance of all farm equipment.

Service buildings. Individually or as a group, these structures must meet the need for efficiency in the use of the farmer's time and energy. New machines have increased efficiency in the field from 100 to 500% in some enterprises. For full advantage to be taken of these improvements, a like increase in efficiency of facilities for converting field crops into meat, milk, and eggs must be available to the farmer.

Buildings, yards, lanes, and fields should be laid out so that crops can be stored easily in buildings provided with self-feeding equipment, so that animals can be routed to the feed, whether it be in the field or at the farmstead, and so that they can be moved to a central holding or handling area for operations such as milking, testing, or treating (Fig. 6). Buildings, yards, and gates must also be arranged so that barns and yards can be cleaned with machine power. *See* AGRICULTURAL ENGINEERING; AGRICULTURE, MACHINERY IN.

Farm homes. Since 1935 the number of farms in the United States has decreased from 6,800,000 to 3,700,000 in 1960. In all probability the number of farm homes in 1968 was less than one-half the number in 1935. The type of building has changed from a two-and-one-half-story house, with full basement, to a one-story ranch type.

The Housing and Home Financing Agency reported in 1953 that a majority of these one-story homes were built with a concrete floor slab and a crawl space, plank and beam construction, prefabricated roof trusses, fitted window and door units including frames, and complete kitchen and workroom cabinets. Dry wall construction with veneer-finished plywood was used in practically all cases.

[JOHN C. WOOLEY]

Bibliography: J. S. Boyd, *Practical Farm Buildings: A Text and Handbook*, 1973; H. E. Gray, *Farm Service Buildings*, 1955; R. J. Lytle et al., *Farm Builders Handbook*, 2d rev. ed., 1973.

Agronomy

The principles and procedures of field crop improvement, management, and production. This includes production and care of such field-crop plants as wheat, potatoes, corn, alfalfa, timothy, sorghum, and cotton, as well as many others. Agronomy is also concerned with the improvement and management of special-purpose plants, such as turf grasses for home lawns, recreational areas, highway embankments, drainage ditches, and waterways. Soil characteristics, properties, uses, and conservation are part of agronomy, and management of soils for efficient production of specific crops is a major interest. *See* AGRICULTURE, SOIL AND CROP PRACTICES IN.

Regarding crops, primary consideration is given to relationship among crop plants as conditioned by their heredity, physiology, and ecology. Soil genesis, classification, and morphology; soil physical, chemical, and biological properties; and water relationships are of prime importance with respect to soils.

The following are only a few of the many problems in agronomy to which science and technology

are being applied: the molecular structure of soil minerals and their relations to the availability of soil nutrients to plants; the development of hybrid wheats with higher yield potential than present self-pollinated varieties; improvements in calibration of chemical soil tests in terms of fertilizer needs of crops; the development of new corn hybrids containing more amino acids, lysine and tryptophan, which are needed by man in areas where corn is a major food crop but are deficient in present corns; the movement, retention, and availability to plants of water in soils; improved varieties of all crop species with greater resistance to diseases and pests and greater yield ability; the differences in the abilities of different varieties of the same crop plant to absorb or exclude nutrients from the soil, including radioactive materials which may be harmful to animals or man; the domestication of wild plants not heretofore used by man. *See* BREEDING (PLANT); FERTILIZER; PLANT, WATER RELATIONS OF; PLANT DISEASE CONTROL; SOIL.

[WALTER I. THOMAS]

Bibliography: R. W. Pearson, *Soil Acidity and Liming*, Agron. Monogr. no. 12, 1966; W. H. Pierre, S. R. Aldrich, and W. P. Martin (eds.), *Advances in Corn Production*, 1966; L. P. Reitz (ed.), *Wheat and Wheat Improvement*, Agron. Monogr. no. 13, 1967.

Alanine

An amino acid. The amino acids are characterized physically by the following: (1) the ˙pK$_1$, or the dissociation constant of the various titratable groups; (2) the isoelectric point, or pH at which a dipolar ion does not migrate in an electric field; (3) the optical rotation, or the rotation imparted to a beam of plane-polarized light (frequently the D line of the sodium spectrum) passing through 1 dm of a solution of 100 in 100 ml; (4) solubility.

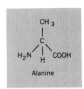

Physical constants of the L isomer at 25°C:

pK$_1$(COOH): 2.34; pK$_2$(NH$_3^+$): 9.69

Isoelectric point: 6.00

Optical rotation: $[\alpha]_D(H_2O)$: +1.8; $[\alpha]_D$(5 N HCl) +14.6

Solubility (g/100 ml H$_2$O): 16.51

The biosynthesis of alanine starts with pyruvic acid, by transamination or reductive amination. During metabolic degradation, alanine is deaminated to pyruvic acid. For pathways of pyruvic acid breakdown *see* CARBOHYDRATE METABOLISM. *See also* AMINO ACIDS.

[EDWARD A. ADELBERG]

Albumin

A type of globular protein that is characterized by its solubility in water and in 50% saturated aqueous ammonium sulfate. Albumins are present in mammalian tissues, bacteria, molds, and plants, and in some foods. Serum albumin, which contains 584 amino acid residues, is the most abundant protein in human serum, and it performs two very important physiological functions. This protein is responsible for about 80% of the total osmotic regulation in blood, and it transports fatty acids between adipose tissues. When excessive amounts of albumin are found in the urine upon clinical examination, some form of kidney disease is usually indicated.

Another important albumin, ovalbumin, is found in egg white. This protein is about two-thirds the size of serum albumin, and it contains sugar residues in addition to amino acid residues (that is, it is a glycoprotein). *See* PROTEIN.

[JAMES M. MANNING]

Alcoholism

The continuous or excessive use of alcohol with associated pathologic results. In the past decade the emphasis of the research in alcoholism has shifted to biological aspects. Although alcoholism has been classically considered a problem of the soul with implications in the soma, both soul and soma are known to be reflections of cellular properties of the biological system and therefore separate distinctions can no longer be drawn. Thus the type of interaction of alcohol with the biological system and the frequency of interaction combine to project the image commonly referred to as alcoholism, and will be thus analyzed.

Absorption of alcohol. Alcohol, contained in different beverages, is absorbed most rapidly from solutions in the order of 15–30% (30–60 proof) and less rapidly from beverages containing below 10% and over 30%. At the lower concentrations this is to be expected since the rate of absorption depends on the concentration gradient across the mucosal surface. At the higher concentrations ethanol abolishes the rhythmic opening of the pylorus, thus preventing the passage to the intestine, where absorption is faster. The presence of foods in the stomach is also known to delay gastric emptying and thus to slow absorption. Once in the bloodstream, alcohol is distributed evenly in all tissues, according to their water content.

Effects of alcohol on nervous system. The exact mechanisms of the pharmacological actions of alcohol are not known. Alcohol can act as a stimulant at lower doses and as a depressant at higher doses. Even at very low doses alcohol can impair the sensitivity to odors and taste. Also, low doses are known to alter motor coordination and time and space perception, important aspects of car driving. Pain sensitivity is diminished with moderate doses. Doses in the order of 0.6 g/kg (about 35 oz of 100-proof per person of 150 lb) are normally lethal by depression of respiratory activity. Alcohol is known to release feelings of self-criticism and to inhibit fear and anxiety, effects which are probably related to an alcohol-induced sociability. These desirable effects act, no doubt, as psychological reinforcers for the increasing use of alcoholic beverages.

Studies in isolated nerve tissue have shown that ethanol can inhibit the sodium permeability in the action potential and inhibit the active extrusion of Na^+ and the recovery of K^+ (sodium-potassium pump) that follows the electrical activity. The carrier of Na^+ and K^+, an adenosinetriphosphatase activated by Na^+ and K^+, is inhibited by moderate concentrations of alcohol. Low concentrations of alcohol enhance the spontaneous and elicited release of acetylcholine in motoneurones at the presynaptic level of the neuromuscular junction and also activate the Renshaw cells, a known spinal inhibitory neurone innervated by a side branch of the motoneurones. The activation of these structures may conceivably add to the central effects of ethanol to produce motor incoordination.

Studies in the laboratory show that alcohol depresses, rather than increases, acetylcholine liberation in brain cortex. Alcohol has been shown to release norepinephrine and epinephrine from their peripheral storage sites, increasing the urinary excretion of these substances. It has been proposed that this peripheral effect is mediated by acetaldehyde, an intermediate in the metabolism of alcohol. Alcohol also changes the excretion pattern of the metabolites of norepinephrine and serotonin. Due to changes in the liver to a more reduced state and to the production of acetaldehyde, the aldehyde products of the monoamine oxidase reaction tend to undergo a reduction rather than an oxidation, as in the normal state. Acetaldehyde can condense with catecholamines to form compounds that act as false neurotransmitters and to form other pharmacologically active compounds. However, the relative importance of these in the overall picture of alcohol intoxication or in alcoholism remains to be determined. In the living brain an alcohol-induced reduction in norepinephrine can be seen only when the synthesis of the neurotransmitter is blocked. This reduction may reflect an increased release or a depressed active uptake of the neuroamine. Studies in the laboratory have shown that alcohol does not depress the spontaneous or the electrically stimulated release but inhibits the active uptake.

In humans and animals, continuation of alcohol ingestion produces adaptive changes which act by opposing the effects of alcohol in the brain. This leads to nervous-tissue tolerance. In this new state larger doses of alcohol are required to produce effects similar to those obtained in the initial phases of drinking. Discontinuation of alcohol use leaves an unbalanced biological state which appears to be responsible for the withdrawal syndrome. Characteristic of this state are a marked hyperexcitability, hallucinations, insomnia, sleep fragmentation, and moderate to extreme tremor as seen in delirium tremens. The person is now physically dependent on alcohol. It has been postulated that the mechanism of physical dependence is an increased enzyme synthesis (enzyme induction) or receptor synthesis (receptor expansion) that occurs to compensate for the inhibitory effects of alcohol but that does not rapidly reverse to normal when the alcohol is discontinued.

Nutritional complications. Since alcohol has a large caloric value, a person drinking 25 oz of a 100-proof beverage per day ingests about 2000 cal, or 70–80% of his total caloric intake as alcohol. However, since alcoholic beverages are normally devoid of essential food factors such as proteins, vitamins, and trace metals, malnutrition is very common in alcoholics. Further, it has been shown that heavy alcohol consumption reduces, both directly and indirectly, the capacity of the intestine to absorb various nutrients such as the vitamins B_1 and B_{12} and some essential amino acids, thus accentuating the malnutrition state. Encephalopathies, beriberi, pellagra, anemia, scurvy, and other hypovitaminoses are very often observed in alcoholics. The encephalopathies are among the most

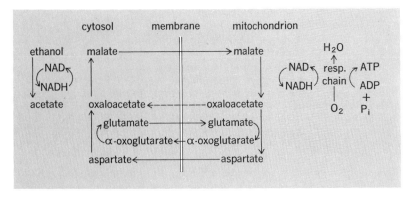

Fig. 1. Metabolic routes for the oxidation of hydrogen equivalents of alcohol in the mitochondria.

serious complications associated with alcoholism. Among them Wernicke-Korsakoff's encephalopathy is most common. It is characterized by mental disorientation, failure of memory, ataxia of gait, and paralysis of the eye nerves. This complication can be effectively treated with thiamine. Other nutritional complications can also be treated in their early stages. *See* NUTRITION.

Alcohol metabolism. Of the alcohol ingested, 80–90% is metabolized in the liver. Ethanol is first oxidized to acetaldehyde in a reaction catalyzed by alcohol dehydrogenase, an enzyme located in the cell cytosol. Nicotinamide adenine dinucleotide (NAD), the cofactor in this reaction, is reduced to the NADH form. Acetaldehyde reacts with another molecule of NAD, and by a reaction catalyzed by acetaldehyde dehydrogenase, it yields acetate plus a second molecule of NADH. Since the second reaction is faster than the first one, little acetaldehyde accumulates. A minor

proportion of the acetate is oxidized to carbon dioxide and water, or it is incorporated into fats in the liver; the rest is mostly oxidized in the peripheral tissues (skeletal muscle, heart, brain, and so on). Indirect measurements show that in the presence of alcohol the relative proportion of NADH/NAD in the liver cell cytosol increases. NADH molecules in the cytosol are oxidized by mitochondria to NAD plus water. However, since mitochondria are not permeable to NADH, the hydrogen equivalents are transferred to molecules (which are then reduced) that can cross the mitochondrial membranes. Once inside the mitochondria, the hydrogen equivalents are incorporated into NADH and the transporting molecules leave the mitochondria in the oxidized form. These transporting systems are called shuttle mechanisms, of which one of the most important is the malate-aspartate shuttle (Fig. 1).

The mitochondrial oxidation of NADH seems to be the rate-limiting step of ethanol removal. Increasing the mitochondrial oxidative capacity by means of uncouplers of oxidative phosphorylation or by increasing the availability of adenosinediphosphate increases the oxidation of NADH and thus more NAD is available to start a new cycle at the alcohol dehydrogenase step.

The rate at which alcohol is metabolized in the body increases, in some cases doubles, after chronic consumption of alcohol. This explains in part the fact that alcoholics can ingest substantially larger amounts of alcoholic beverages for prolonged periods than nonalcoholics (metabolic tolerance). Animal experiments have shown that the increased rate of ethanol metabolism after chronic treatment with ethanol can be explained by the finding that mitochondria in the liver of these animals consume oxygen (and thus oxidize NADH and alcohol) at

Apparent consumption, in 20 countries, of each major beverage class, and of absolute alcohol from each class, in U.S. gallons per person in the drinking-age population (listed in descending order of total)*

Country	Year	Distilled spirits	Absolute alcohol	Wine	Absolute alcohol	Beer	Absolute alcohol	Total absolute alcohol
France	1966	2.35	1.18	43.03	4.52	20.10†	0.83	6.53
Italy	1968	[1.11]	0.55	41.29	3.30	3.54	0.16	4.01
Switzerland	1966	1.53	0.61	13.61	1.43	29.73†	1.35	3.39
West Germany	1968	[2.35]	0.89	4.04	0.40	44.65	1.97	3.26
Australia	1966	0.54	0.31	2.58	0.44	42.86	2.14	2.89
Belgium	1967	0.67	0.33	3.14	0.44	42.07†	2.10	2.87
United States	1970	2.56	1.15	1.84	0.29	25.95	1.17	2.61
New Zealand	1964	0.79	0.45	0.98	0.17	39.28	1.96	2.58
Czechoslovakia	1968	[0.83]	[0.42]	[3.51]	[0.49]	[30.91]	[1.54]	2.45
Canada	1967	[1.86]	0.75	[1.12]	0.18	[25.47]	1.27	2.20
Denmark	1968	0.78	0.34	1.53	0.22	29.03	1.38	1.94
United Kingdom	1966	0.51	0.29	1.08	0.18	31.77	1.43	1.90
Sweden	1968	2.13	0.85	1.77	0.24	15.57	0.65	1.74
Japan	1968	[1.10]	0.35	[5.10]‡	0.81	8.22	0.37	1.53
Netherlands	1968	[1.38]	[0.69]	[0.86]	[0.15]	[15.38]	[0.69]	1.53
Ireland	1966	0.70	0.40	0.56	0.09	22.26	1.00	1.49
Norway	1968	1.20	0.52	0.70	0.10	10.82	0.51	1.13
Finland	1968	1.33	0.52	1.06	0.17	6.85	0.34	1.03
Iceland	1966	2.11	0.73	0.62	0.08	4.26	0.15	0.96
Israel	1968	0.89	0.44	1.66	0.20	3.58	0.18	0.82

*Bracketed data converted from source terms.

†Includes cider.

‡Includes sake.

SOURCE: *Alcohol and Health*, U.S. Department of Health, Education, and Welfare, 1971.

higher rates than those from nontreated animals.

The increase in NADH and decrease in NAD caused by ethanol in the liver produce marked alterations in several reactions that require these cofactors. Mitochondria oxidize preferentially NADH produced by ethanol rather than from glucose or fatty acids. This may explain in part the accumulation of fat that occurs in the liver after consumption of large amounts of alcohol.

Liver pathology. It was formerly believed that only about 1 out of 10 alcoholics developed cirrhosis. However, it has been shown that the production of cirrhosis is correlated with the amount of ethanol ingested multiplied by the period (years) of ingestion. Thus, an alcoholic that has consumed 200 g of ethanol (18 oz of 100-proof beverage) daily for 20 years has a 50% chance of developing cirrhosis. Deaths due to cirrhosis in different geographic areas are directly correlated with the consumption of (absolute) alcohol per person regardless of the type of alcoholic beverage consumed. The table lists the types of beverages consumed in different countries.

Cirrhosis is characterized by a diffuse deposition of collagen (scar tissue) in the liver. The tissue gradually hardens and the blood flow is restricted, giving rise to a variety of metabolic and circulatory disturbances which are ultimately fatal. The initial stage that sets the conditions for collagen deposition is alcoholic hepatitis. This condition is characterized by cell death, cell ballooning, and polymorphonuclear leukocytic infiltration. In some, but not all, cases of alcoholic hepatitis, a microfilament mesh with a treelike structure called an alcoholic hyaline or Mallory body also appears in the liver. All these changes occur in the centrilobular area (periphery of the acinus), which is the area farthest from the site of entrance of oxygenated blood into the microcirculatory unit. It has been proposed that cell death and other changes are produced by lack of proper oxygenation in this area. In fact, experiments in rats have shown that hepatitis can be triggered in this zone in alcohol-treated but not in control animals by a variety of conditions that reduce the availability of oxygen to the liver. The hepatitis found in these animals could be prevented or cured by administration of propylthiouracil, an antithyroid drug that reduces the rate of oxygen consumption by the cells. If this animal model proves to be similar to human alcoholic hepatitis, it should be possible to halt this disease and its further progression to cirrhosis.

For a long time it was believed that the production of alcoholic cirrhosis was the result of the severe malnutrition often found in alcoholics. However, experiments with monkeys receiving 50% of their caloric intake as pure alcohol, along with a well-balanced diet, have shown that these animals develop alcoholic hepatitis and cirrhosis with characteristics that are identical to those found in humans. Therefore, these experiments show that dietary malnutrition is not responsible for the development of these lesions and that alcohol itself has hepatotoxic effects. The possibility of an alcohol-induced "internal" malnutrition cannot, however, be discarded.

Statistics. In the United States about 21% of adult men and 5% of adult women are considered heavy drinkers, and about 6% of the combined to-

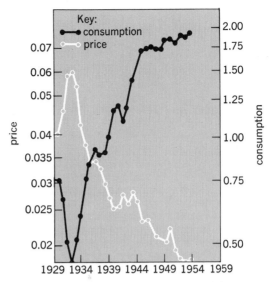

Fig. 2. Alcohol price and consumption in Ontario, Canada, during 1929–1954. Price is that of an average gallon of absolute alcohol expressed as a fraction of average disposable income. Consumption is expressed in gallons of absolute alcohol per person 20 years and older. *(From J. de Lint and W. Schmidt, in Y. Israel and J. Mardones (eds.), Biological Basis of Alcoholism, Wiley-Interscience, 1971)*

tal number of drinkers are alcoholics, as defined by a loss of control over drinking. Since the percentage of alcoholics correlates well with the per person consumption of the population, approximate values can be calculated for other countries using the table. Another interesting correlation is the one showing that alcohol consumption varies inversely with the price of alcoholic beverages (Fig. 2). Theoretically the rates of alcoholism and cirrhosis should be reduced in a population by a simple increase in price.

[YEDY ISRAEL]

Bibliography: Alcohol and Health, U.S. Department of Health, Education and Welfare, 1974; Y. Israel et al., *Proc. Nat. Acad. Sci. U.S.,* 72: 1137–1141; Y. Israel and J. Mardones (eds.), *Biological Basis of Alcoholism,* 1971; J. M. Khanna, Y. Israel, and H. Kalant (eds.), *Alcoholic Liver Pathology,* 1975; F. A. Seixas, F. A. Williams, and S. Eggleston (eds.), *Medical Consequences of Alcoholism,* Ann. N.Y. Acad. Sci., 252:1–399, 1975.

Alfalfa

The world's most valuable forage legume, *Medicago sativa* L., known also as lucerne. In the United States alone it is grown for hay, pasture, and silage on about 27,000,000 acres annually (Fig. 1), where it produces the equivalent of 75,000,000 tons of hay. Valued highly as livestock feed, alfalfa hay cut at a late bud or early bloom stage (and cured properly) contains 17–24% protein and is a good source of certain vitamins and minerals.

World cultivation of alfalfa is estimated at approximately 80,000,000 acres; in each of 27 countries more than 90,000 acres are grown annually (see table).

History. Alfalfa originated in the Near East, in the area extending from Turkey to Iran and north

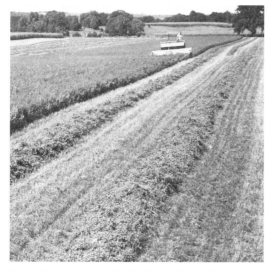

Fig. 1. Harvesting alfalfa. (*Northrup, King and Co.*)

into the Caucasus. From the great diversity of forms within the genus *Medicago*, two species, *M. sativa* and *M. falcata*, have become important forage plants. These species are mainly tetraploid, with 32 chromosomes, although diploid forms are known. Alfalfa species are composed of ecotypes,

Estimated acreage (and hectarage) in countries growing 90,000 acres or more annually*

Continent and country	Acreage	Hectarage
Europe		
Austria	111,000	45,000
Bulgaria	494,000	200,000
Czechoslovakia	694,000	281,000
East Germany	180,000	73,000
France	3,551,000	1,437,000
Greece	445,000	180,000
Hungary	806,000	326,000
Italy	4,935,000	1,997,000
Poland	603,000	244,000
Romania	1,100,000	445,000
Soviet Union (European)	8,340,000	3,375,000
Spain	494,000	200,000
Switzerland	91,000	37,000
West Germany	250,000	101,000
Yugoslavia	887,000	359,000
North America		
Canada	4,915,000	1,989,000
Mexico	395,000	160,000
United States	27,171,000	10,993,000
South America		
Argentina	18,533,000	7,500,000
Chile	208,000	84,000
Peru	304,000	123,000
Asia		
Iran	247,000	100,000
Soviet Union (Siberian)	2,780,000	1,125,000
Turkey	183,000	74,000
Africa		
South Africa, Republic of	425,000	172,000
Oceania		
Australia	2,807,000	1,133,000
New Zealand	198,000	80,000

*Adapted from J. L. Bolton, B. P. Goplin, and H. Baenziger, World distribution and historical developments, in C. H. Hanson (ed.), *Alfalfa Science and Technology*, American Society of Agronomy, Madison, 1972.

population complexes adapted to the environment of a given climatic region or to definite habitats within a region. There is a great diversity of forms, in both wild and cultivated alfalfas in the Near East, which offer a potential source of germplasm highly valuable to plant breeders seeking to develop improved varieties.

Earliest cultivation of alfalfa (2000–1000 B.C.) probably began in ancient Armenia and a little later in Anatolia, Mesopotamia, and Yemen. Alfalfa was introduced into Greece by 490 B.C. and into Italy, northern Africa, and Spain shortly thereafter. From Italy and Spain alfalfa spread to Switzerland, France, Great Britain, and much of northern and central Europe. The Spanish explorers took alfalfa to Mexico, where it spread to Peru, Chile, Uruguay, and Argentina.

Alfalfa was introduced to United States by two routes: It was carried by gold prospectors from Chile and Peru to California, where it spread eastward, and it was introduced directly into the midwestern and eastern states from Europe. The Chilean type from South America became source material for natural selection of many regional strains, such as Arizona Common, Kansas Common, and Dakota Common, which differed mainly in degree of winterhardiness. An introduction from Germany into Minnesota in 1857 resulted in the development of Grimm alfalfa, the first of the truly winter-hardy alfalfas.

Description. Alfalfa is a herbaceous perennial legume characterized by a deep taproot, which shows a varying degree of branching (Fig. 2). Erect

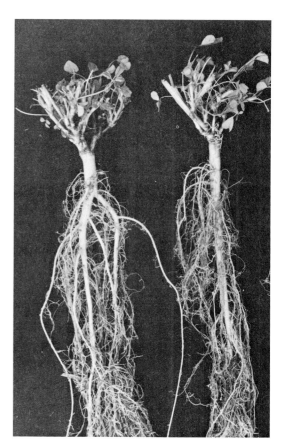

Fig. 2. Buffalo alfalfa, showing crown and root in 8-month-old plants. (*Iowa State University Photo Service*)

or semierect stems, bearing an abundance of leaves, grow to a height of 2–3 ft (Fig. 3). The number of stems arising from a single woody crown may vary from just a few to 50 or more. New stems develop when older ones are mature or have been cut or grazed.

Flowers are borne on axillary racemes which vary greatly in size and number of flowers. Flower color is predominantly purple, or bluish-purple, but white, cream, yellow, green, lavender, and reddish-purple occur. Crossing of *M. sativa* (purple flowers) and *M. falcata* (yellow flowers) results in an array of flower colors, including many that are truly variegated.

The fruit is a legume, or pod, usually spirally coiled in *M. sativa*, but crescent-shaped or straight in *M. falcata*. Seeds are small, with about 220,000/lb, and the color varies from yellow to brown.

Reproduction in alfalfa is mainly by cross-fertilization. Pollination is effected largely by bees, including species of bumblebee (*Bombus*), alkali bee (*Nomia*), leaf-cutter bee (*Megachile*), and honeybee (*Apis*). Seed production is favored by bright sunny days, cool nights, an abundance of bees, and dry weather for harvesting. Such conditions are found in certain irrigated valleys of the Pacific Coast and intermountain regions of the United States and Canada.

Adaptation. Alfalfa is widely adapted to temperate and subtropical climates and soils. It is grown from 40°S in Argentina and New Zealand to 60°N in Canada, Sweden, and the Soviet Union. It is not well adapted to humid tropical conditions.

Deep fertile loams are best and good drainage is essential. The water requirement for sustained high yields is great, and moisture deficiency often is a serious limiting factor in areas dependent on natural rainfall.

Alfalfa requires considerable plant nutrients for high yields of forage. A crop of 5 or 6 tons (dry matter) per acre removes approximately 200 lb of nitrogen, 150 lb of calcium, 40 lb of phosphorus, and 200 lb of potassuim. Nitrogen usually is not limiting because alfalfa roots and certain strains of *Rhizobium* have an effective symbiotic relationship, which results in fixation of atmospheric nitrogen needed by the plant. Acid soils should be limed to bring the pH up to about 7; the necessary phosphorus and potassium should be supplied by fertilizer. *See* NITROGEN FIXATION (BIOLOGY).

Management and harvesting. Alfalfa is grown from seed, usually planted at the rate of 10–15 lb/ acre. Often it is grown with grasses, especially bromegrass (*Bromus inermis*) or orchard grass (*Dactylis glomerata*), and the seeding rate of alfalfa reduced to 7 or 8 lb/acre. The bulk of the alfalfa crop in the United States is harvested for hay, although much is used for pasture and silage. About 1,540,000 tons of artificially dehydrated alfalfa, commonly known as "dehy," are also produced annually in the United States. At one time all dehy was fed in the form of meal, but now more than 90% is pelleted. Much of this high-quality product is used in mixed feeds for poultry and other livestock.

Alfalfa is cut in early bloom and may be recut at intervals of 30–40 days. The number of cuttings per season varies from one or two in central

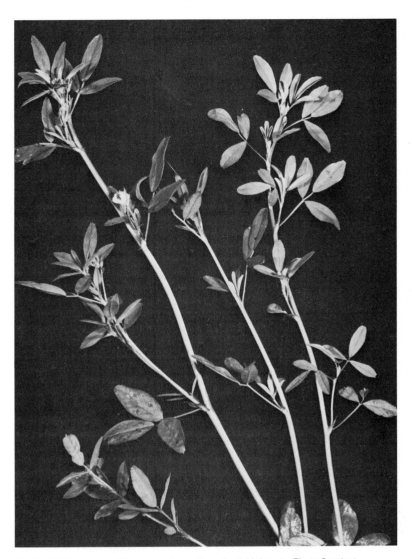

Fig. 3. Alfalfa stems at flowering stage. (*Iowa State University Photo Service*)

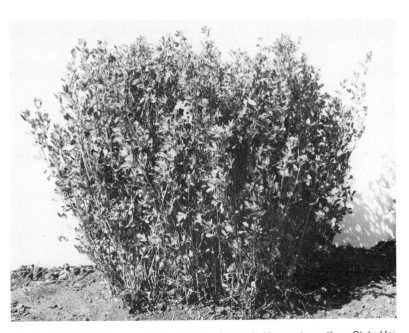

Fig. 4. Alfalfa of wide crown type at late bud or early bloom stage. (*Iowa State University Photo Service*)

insect pests of alfalfa. Cultivars or breeding lines are now available with resistance to diseases such as bacterial wilt, common leaf spot, anthracnose, phytophthora root rot, rust, and downy mildew, and to insects such as the spotted alfalfa aphid and the pea aphid. Resistance to bacterial wilt alone contributes more than $100,000,000 annually to agricultural production in the United States. Urgently needed is greater resistance to other insect pests, especially the alfalfa weevil and leafhopper. Other breeding objectives are high yield of improved quality forage, resistance to important diseases, and a creeping root character for dry regions. *See* BREEDING (PLANT).

Geographic specificity. Three general regions of adaptation of alfalfa, based largely on requirements of winterhardiness, have been designated in the United States. The northern region demands a high level of winterhardiness. Moderately hardy cultivars are grown in the central region. In the southern region (especially in the Southwest) little winter hardiness is necessary, and nonhardy cultivars are highly productive. Different combinations of disease and insect resistance are required in each region.

Seed standards. Since alfalfa varieties cannot be distinguished by seed characters, an effective system of seed certification offers a safeguard for obtaining seed that is true to variety name. Certified seed is grown from authentic planting stock. Specific standards are established by the International Crop Improvement Association and its state member organizations. These standards provide for the number of generations of seed increase, volunteer plants, isolation from other alfalfa, viability, and mechanical purity, and assure the alfalfa grower that he is getting a specific variety of good seed quality.

Diseases of alfalfa. Alfalfa is susceptible to at least 75 diseases incited by fungi, bacteria, viruses, and nematodes. Some of these occur sporadically and are rarely destructive; however, several are responsible for appreciable losses.

Root and crown diseases. Bacterial wilt is one of the best-known and most damaging diseases (Fig. 5). The bacteria enter plants principally through

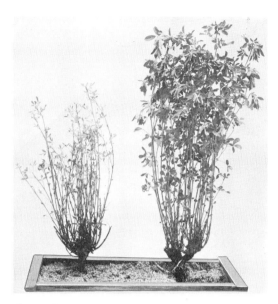

Fig. 5. Damaging effect of bacterial wilt of alfalfa, contrasted with healthy plant on the right.

Canada to eight or more in Imperial Valley, Calif. Research results suggest the optimum stage for harvesting is the 10% bloom stage (Fig. 4) based on percentage protein, total digestible nutrients, yield of forage, persistence of stand, and gains of livestock fed on the forage.

Cultivars. More than 80 improved cultivars of alfalfa are recognized as eligible for seed certification in the United States. These trace to three basic stocks: *M. sativa,* purple-flowered, narrow-crowned, and erect; *M. falcata,* yellow-flowered, somewhat prostrate, with deep-set crown and branching roots; and an intermediate form, often called variegated, derived from crossing *M. sativa* and *M. falcata.*

Breeding. Plant breeders have used these three sources of germplasm to develop superior varieties for the changing needs of the farmer. Breeding for resistance is the most practical and economical means of controlling most diseases and

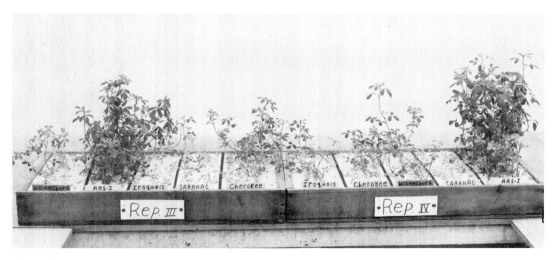

Fig. 6. Resistance to anthracnose made the difference in this test. ARS-I had been bred for resistance. Other cultivars demonstrated varying degrees of susceptibility. (*USDA*)

wounds in the roots. They cause stunting and reduce yield and longevity of stands. Wilt-resistant varieties have been developed for the northern, central, and southwestern alfalfa-growing regions of the United States.

Root and crown rot fungi occur in all areas in which alfalfa is grown. They are among the most destructive pathogens and may cause injury at all stages of plant growth. Some, such as *Sclerotinia*, are active during cool, moist weather; in contrast, *Fusarium* and *Rhizoctonia* flourish during warm weather. Plants are frequently attacked by these fungi following injury from cold, insects, or harvesting machinery. Because these fungi occur in most soils, the diseases they incite are among the most difficult to control, and no highly resistant varieties of alfalfa have been developed.

Stem and foliage diseases. Many organisms attack the stem and foliage of alfalfa. Some, such as the fungi causing anthracnose and blackstem, attack the stems, but sometimes they spread into the crown and upper part of the taproot, weakening or killing the plant. Anthracnose, favored by warm, humid weather, occurs principally in the southern and eastern states. The disease is associated with summer weakening and death of plants. Resistance to anthracnose has been incorporated into improved varieties for the eastern United States (Fig. 6). Blackstem occurs in most alfalfa-growing areas and is particularly damaging in the cooler, humid regions. The causal fungus can attack any part of the plant, but the shiny black streaks or spots characteristic of the disease are most conspicuous on stems and petioles.

Several leaf diseases occur widely and they frequently damage alfalfa. Common leafspot, yellow leaf blotch, and pseudoplea leafspot may develop so abundantly that they cause serious loss of leaves. Most varieties of alfalfa contain some resistant plants. Early harvest sometimes reduces spread of leaf and stem diseases.

Some less prevalent but occasionally locally important foliar diseases are downy mildew, summer blackstem, and leaf rust.

Virus diseases. Alfalfa mosaic virus occurs generally in the United States. Diseased plants become weakened and are unable to withstand the rigors of repeated harvests, drought, and winter injury. The leaves of some diseased plants exhibit yellow blotching, while other infected plants are stunted but may show no visible symptoms.

Mycoplasma and Rickettsia diseases. Some diseases formerly thought to be caused by viruses are now known to be due to *Mycoplasma* or *Rickettsia*. Witches' broom is caused by a *Mycoplasma* and is important in the western states. Alfalfa dwarf has the same cause, a *Rickettsia*, as Pierce's disease of grapevine.

Sporadic outbreaks of witches'-broom have occurred in seed fields of the western states since 1925. Destroying diseased plants, which have many spindly stems, prevents the further spread of the disease.

Nematode diseases. Nematodes are widely distributed but are destructive to alfalfa only in certain areas. The stem nematode (*Ditylenchus dipsaci*) thrives best under the cool moist conditions of spring and fall and is destructive to irrigated alfalfa in the West. However, some areas of infestation also occur in Virginia and North Carolina. Nematodes can infect plants of any age. In older plants infected crown buds become thickened and deformed and ultimately rot off. Several alfalfa cultivars highly resistant to the stem nematode disease are available.

The root knot nematodes (*Meloidogyne* sp.) frequently attack alfalfa in regions where these parasites are abundant. They are most prevalent in mild climates; hence they are of greatest concern in the South and Southwest. Gall-like enlargements on roots are a characteristic symptom. *See* LEGUME FORAGES; PLANT VIRUS.

[CLARENCE H. HANSON]

Bibliography: J. L. Bolton, *Alfalfa Botany, Cultivation and Utilization*, 1962; C. H. Hanson (ed.), *Alfalfa Science and Technology*, American Society of Agronomy, Madison, 1972 (this monograph of 35 chapters contains basic and applied information available on alfalfa and is authored by specialists in various fields); C. H. Hanson and D. K. Barnes, Alfalfa, in M. E. Heath, D. S. Metcalfe, and R. E. Barnes (eds.), *Forages*, 1973.

Allspice

The dried, unripe fruits of a small, tropical, evergreen tree, *Pimenta officinalis*, of the myrtle family (Myrtaceae). This species (see illustration) is a native of the West Indies and parts of Central and South America. The spice, alone or in mixtures, is much used in sausages, pickles, sauces, and soups. The extracted oil is used for flavoring and in

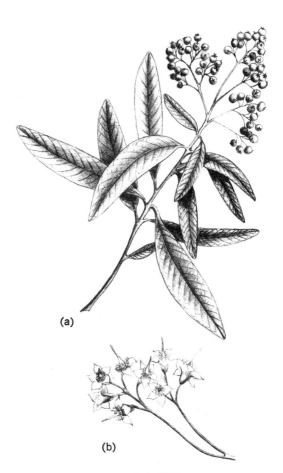

(a)

(b)

Allspice. (*a*) Branch with fruit. (*b*) Flowers.

perfumery. Allspice is so named because its flavor resembles that of a combination of cloves, cinnamon, and nutmeg. *See* SPICE AND FLAVORING.

[PERRY D. STRAUSBAUGH/EARL L. CORE]

Almond

A small deciduous tree, *Prunus amygdalus*, closely related to the peach and other stone fruits and grown widely for its edible seeds. The fruit, classified botanically as a drupe, is like that of the peach except that the outer fleshy layer becomes dry at maturity and splits, releasing the seed or nut (see illustration).

Probably native to central Asia, the almond spread very early throughout the milder, drier parts of the Old World temperate zone. It is now grown commercially in Mediterranean Europe, particularly Spain and Italy, and in the United States. In the United States commerical production is limited to California.

Because of the trees' early spring flowering habit, commercial culture of the almond is limited to areas with mild winters and few late spring frosts. The trees thrive under high summer temperatures and withstand considerable drought, though better crops are secured with adequate rainfall or irrigation. All varieties of almonds need cross-pollination, and in grafted orchards it is essential to plant combinations of varieties that will bloom at the same time and pollinate each other. *See* BREEDING (PLANT).

In the Mediterranean region culture and harvest of the almond are for the most part still primitive, using hand labor. But there has been a rapid shift to mechanical shelling and better handling of the crops for export. In California there are machines to cover nearly all phases of the industry. The older method of knocking the nuts off the trees onto ground cloths has been largely superceded by mechanically sweeping nuts shaken from the trees into windrows on a smooth soil surface and then picking them up with another machine. The mixture of hulls and nuts is run through a machine which hulls and cleans the nuts. These are taken to the cooperative, where they are shelled and the kernels electronically sorted for defects, graded for size, and packaged. The California Almond Grower's Exchange establishes grades, controls quality, and markets the crop.

Almonds are of two general types: bitter, which is a source of prussic acid and flavoring extracts;

and sweet, which is used in a variety of products in confectionery, particularly chocolate bars, and bakery goods and other cookery. Only about 7% of the crop is used in whole nut mixtures. Sweet almonds may be either soft-shell or hard-shell, the former furnishing the bulk of the California crop. For diseases of almond *see* APRICOT. *See also* NUT CROP CULTURE.

[L. H. MAC DANIELS]

Amino acids

Organic compounds possessing one or more basic amino groups and one or more acidic carboxyl groups. Of the more than 80 amino acids which have been found in living organisms, about 20 serve as the building blocks for the proteins.

All the amino acids of proteins, and most of the others which occur naturally, are α-amino acids, meaning that an amino group (—NH_2) and a carboxyl group (—COOH) are attached to the same carbon atom. This carbon (the α carbon, being adjacent to the carboxyl group) also carries a hydrogen atom; its fourth valence is satisfied by any of a wide variety of substituent groups, represented by the letter R in Fig. 1.

In the simplest amino acid, glycine, R is a hydrogen atom. In all other amino acids, R is an organic radical; for example, in alanine it is a methyl group (—CH_3), while in glutamic acid it is an aliphatic chain terminating in a second carboxyl group (—CH_2—CH—COOH). Chemically, the amino acids can be considered as falling roughly into nine categories based on the nature of R (see table).

Occurrence of conjugated amino acids. Amino acids occur in living tissues principally in the con-

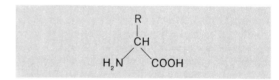

Fig. 1. Structural formula for an amino acid.

Amino acids of proteins, grouped according to the nature of R

Amino acids*	R
Glycine	Hydrogen
Alanine, valine, leucine, isoleucine	Unsubstituted aliphatic chain
Serine, threonine	Aliphatic chain bearing a hydroxyl group
Aspartic acid, glutamic acid	Aliphatic chain terminating in an acidic carboxyl group
Asparagine, glutamine	Aliphatic chain terminating in an amide group
Arginine, lysine	Aliphatic chain terminating in a basic amino group
Cysteine, cystine, methionine	Sulfur-containing aliphatic chain
Phenylalanine, tyrosine	Terminates in an aromatic ring
Tryptophan, proline, histidine	Terminates in a heterocyclic ring

*See articles on the individual amino acids listed in the table; the articles give the structure, biosynthetic origin, special properties, special functions, and pathways of metabolic degradation.

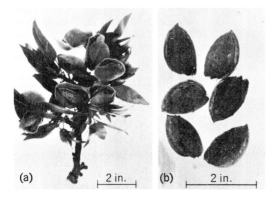

Almond. (*a*) Twig with leaves and fruit. (*b*) Hulled nuts.

jugated form. Most conjugated amino acids are peptides, in which the amino group of one amino acid is linked to the carboxyl group of another. This type of linkage is known as a peptide bond; a molecule of water is split out when a peptide bond is formed, and a molecule of water must be added when a peptide bond is broken, as shown in the reaction below.

$$
\begin{array}{c}
\text{R}_1 \qquad \text{(water)} \\
| \qquad\qquad\qquad \text{H} \quad \text{O} \\
\text{CH} \qquad\qquad\qquad | \quad || \\
\text{HN}\!-\!\text{C}\!-\!\overline{[\text{OH} + \text{H}]}\text{N}\!-\!\text{C}\!-\!\text{OH} \\
| \quad || \qquad\qquad\qquad | \\
\text{H} \quad \text{O} \qquad\qquad\qquad \text{CH} \\
\qquad\qquad\qquad\qquad | \\
\qquad\qquad\qquad\qquad \text{R}_2
\end{array}
$$

$$
\begin{array}{c}
\text{R}_1 \\
| \qquad\quad \text{H} \quad \text{O} \\
\text{CH} \qquad | \quad || \\
\text{HN}\!-\!\text{C}\!\overrightarrow{}\!\text{N}\!-\!\text{C}\!-\!\text{OH} + \text{H}_2\text{O} \\
| \quad || \quad | \\
\text{H} \quad \text{O} \quad \text{CH} \\
\qquad\qquad\quad | \\
\qquad\qquad\quad \text{R}_2
\end{array}
$$

(peptide bond)

Since each amino acid possesses both an amino group and a carboxyl group, the acids are capable of linking together to form chains of various lengths, called polypeptides. Proteins are polypeptides ranging in size from about 50 to many thousand amino acid residues. The process by which peptides are formed from free amino acids actually cannot be as simple as pictured in the equation, for a considerable amount of energy is required. This process is discussed later in this article.

Although most of the conjugated amino acids in nature are proteins, numerous smaller conjugates occur naturally, many with important biological activity. The line between large peptides and small proteins is difficult to draw, with insulin (molecular weight = 7000; 50 amino acids) usually being considered a small protein and adrenocorticotropic hormone (molecular weight = 5000; 39 amino acids) being considered a large peptide. In addition to their role as hormones, peptides often occur in coenzymes (such as folic acid and glutathione), bacterial capsules (the polyglutamic acid capsule which contributes to the pathogenicity of *Bacillus anthracis*), fungal toxins (the tomato wilt toxin of *Fusarium* and the toxins of the poisonous mushroom *Amanita phalloides*), and antibiotics (chloramphenicol, penicillin, bacitracin, and polymixins). Elucidation of the structure of bacterial cell walls has shown that they are composed in part of a series of cross-linked peptides, the cross-linking providing the wall with a large part of its rigidity. The action of penicillin in inhibiting this cross-linking reaction accounts for its antibiotic activity. Finally, a considerable part of the phospholipid fraction of any organism contains serine linked by phosphoester bond to glycerol phosphate.

Occurrence of free amino acids. Free amino acids are found in living cells, as well as in the body fluids of higher animals, in amounts which vary according to the tissue and to the amino acid. The amino acids which play key roles in the incor-

poration and transfer of ammonia, such as glutamic acid, aspartic acid, and their amides, are often present in relatively high amounts, but the concentrations of the other amino acids of proteins are extremely low, ranging from a fraction of a milligram to several milligrams per 100 g wet weight of tissue. In view of the fact that amino acid and protein synthesis go on constantly in most of these tissues, the presence of free amino acids in only trace amounts points to the existence of extraordinarily efficient regulation mechanisms. Each amino acid is ordinarily synthesized at precisely the rate needed for protein synthesis. The regulation mechanism has been found most often to be one of feedback control; each amino acid acts as an inhibitor of its own biosynthesis. If any amino acid is formed in excess of that required for protein synthesis, the biosynthesis of that amino acid is slowed down until the excess has been used.

In addition to the amino acids of protein, a variety of other free amino acids occurs naturally. Some of these are metabolic products of the amino acids of proteins; for example, γ-aminobutyric acid occurs as the decarboxylation product of glutamic acid. Others, such as homoserine and ornithine, are biosynthetic precursors of the amino acids of protein. However, the origin and role of many unusual free amino acids is not yet known.

General properties. At ordinary temperatures, the amino acids are white crystalline solids; when heated to high temperatures, they decompose rather than melt. They are stable in aqueous solution, and with few exceptions can be heated as high as 120°C for short periods without decomposition, even in acid or alkaline solution. Thus, the hydrolysis of proteins can be carried out under such conditions with the complete recovery of most of the constituent free amino acids. The exceptions are as follows: Acid hydrolysis of protein destroys most of the tryptophan and some of the serine and threonine, oxidizes cysteine to cystine, and deamidates glutamine and asparagine; alkaline hydrolysis destroys serine, threonine, cystine, cysteine, and arginine, and also causes deamidations.

Enantiomorphs. Since all of the amino acids except glycine possess a center of asymmetry at the α carbon atom, they can exist in either of two optically active, mirror-image forms or enantiomorphs. All of the common amino acids of proteins appear to have the same configuration about the α carbon; this configuration is symbolized by the prefix L-. The opposite, generally unnatural, form is given the prefix D-. Some amino acids, such as isoleucine, threonine, and hydroxyproline, have a second center of asymmetry and can exist in four stereoisomeric forms. The prefix allo- is used to indicate one of the two alternative configurations at the second asymmetric center; thus, isoleucine, for example, can exist in the L, L-allo, D and D-allo forms.

Unlike chemical syntheses, which lead to mixtures of D and L forms, biosynthetic processes invariably produce optically active amino acids. For most amino acids, only the L isomer occurs naturally; but in a few cases, the D isomer is found also. For example, the cell walls of certain bacteria contain D-alanine and D-glutamic acid, and the D isomers of phenylalanine, leucine, serine, and valine occur in some antibiotic peptides.

Ionic state. Another important general property of all amino acids is their ionic state (Fig. 2). The basic amino group can bind a proton from solution

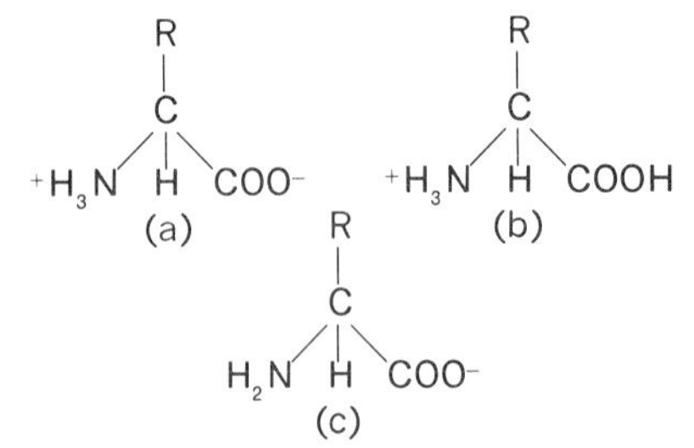

Fig. 2. The ionic states of an amino acid. (*a*) Zwitterion. (*b*) Cation. (*c*) Anion.

and become a cation; the acidic carboxyl group can release a proton into solution and become an anion. At the isoelectric point (the pH at which the molecule has no net charge), amino acids exist as dipolar ions or zwitterions, while in strong acid solution, the carboxyl group exists in the undissociated form, and the molecule becomes a cation. If such an acidic solution is titrated with strong alkali, two dissociations of protons are observed. The carboxyl group, having the weakest affinity for its proton, dissociates at a fairly low pH; its pK (the pH at which half of the molecules are dissociated) in most cases is close to 2.0. As more alkali is added, the proton on the amino group begins to dissociate; pK values for this dissociation are generally found close to 9.5. When sufficient alkali has been added to pull off all the dissociable protons, the amino acid exists as an anion.

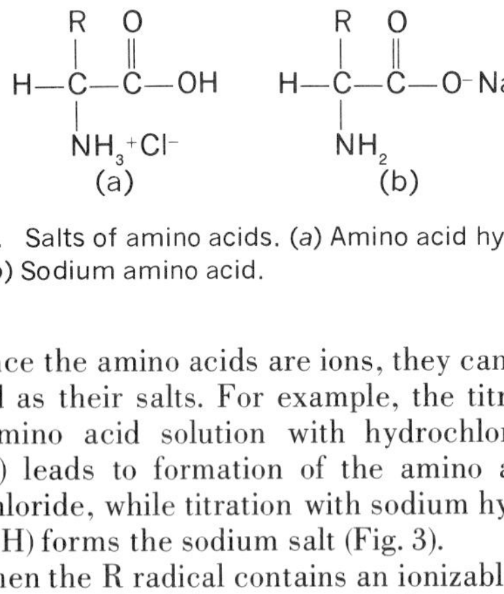

Fig. 3. Salts of amino acids. (*a*) Amino acid hydrochloride. (*b*) Sodium amino acid.

Since the amino acids are ions, they can be prepared as their salts. For example, the titration of an amino acid solution with hydrochloric acid (HCl) leads to formation of the amino acid hydrochloride, while titration with sodium hydroxide (NaOH) forms the sodium salt (Fig. 3).

When the R radical contains an ionizable group, the amino acid will have correspondingly more ionic forms. Those amino acids whose radicals contain carboxyl groups (aspartic and glutamic acids) are known as the acidic amino acids, since a solution of the zwitterion will be strongly acidic. Similarly, histidine, lysine, and arginine are known as the basic amino acids, and the rest as the neutral amino acids. (It is important to note that a solution of the zwitterion of a neutral amino acid will in fact be slightly acidic.)

The salts are, in general, more soluble in water or alcohol than the corresponding zwitterions.

Isolation and determination. Since most amino acids occur in conjugated form, their isolation usually requires their prior release in free form by acid or alkaline hydrolysis. Hydrolysates of proteins or other polypeptides, or crude extracts of plant, animal, or microbial materials, serve as the starting point for the isolation in pure form of single amino acids. Prior to the application of chromatography in the early 1940s, the isolation of an amino acid depended on slight differences in the solubilities of amino acid salts in various solvents and at different pH values. For example, the isolation of aspartic acid was accomplished by adding an excess of calcium hydroxide to an aqueous solution of amino acids and then precipitating the calcium aspartate with alcohol.

Such methods, although used successfully to isolate each of the common amino acids of protein, are difficult as well as tedious, and require relatively large amounts of starting material. Chromatography, on the other hand, is simple, rapid, and capable of isolating amino acids even when they are present in microgram quantities. Thus chromatography has been the method of choice for amino acid isolation ever since its first application by A. J. P. Martin and R. L. M. Synge in 1941.

Chromatography is carried out by using either cylindrical glass tubes (columns) packed with a porous solid or by using sheets of filter paper. In the former method, the column is packed with any of a variety of substances, such as starch, powdered cellulose, or cation-exchange resin, and is saturated with the chosen solvent. A solution of amino acids is allowed to percolate into the top of the column, and then solvent is forced through the column at a controlled rate. The solvent is allowed to flow out through an opening at the bottom of the column, and the eluate is caught in a series of test tubes.

A given amino acid will have been eluted from the column at a time depending on its own characteristic rate of movement, and will have been caught in one or a few tubes; a different amino acid will have been eluted into a separate set of tubes. To detect their presence, as well as to determine their exact quantity, a substance which reacts with amino acids to give a visible color is then added to each tube. The best such reagent is ninhydrin, which reacts with amino acids to produce carbon dioxide, ammonia, and aldehyde, and forms a purple compound with the liberated ammonia. The amount of color which develops under standard conditions can then be measured in a photoelectric colorimeter, and the precise amount of amino acid determined by comparison with a standard curve based on reactions with known quantities. Figure 4 shows a typical separation achieved by passing water adjusted to different pH values and temperatures through a column of cation-exchange resin, collecting fractions and determining the amount of amino acid in each with ninhydrin.

The column method described above is capable of giving the most precise quantitative data, and can handle relatively large quantities of amino acids. For the analysis of mixtures containing only a few micrograms of each amino acid, however, paper chromatography is the simplest and rapidest procedure, and can also be made quantitative. In this procedure, the mixture of amino acids is applied as a drop of solution to a spot close to one

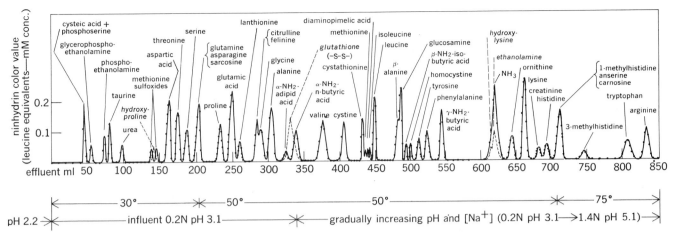

Fig. 4. A typical protein fractionation into amino acids shown in a cation-exchange resin column chromato-gram. (*From S. Moore and W. H. Stein, J. Biol. Chem., 211: 893–906, 1954*)

corner of a sheet of paper. The sheet is then placed in a vapor-tight chamber with one edge of the paper dipping into a chosen, water-saturated organic solvent. The solvent flows through the paper by capillarity, water becoming bound to the paper and the organic solvent flowing past it. The amino acids travel through the paper as discrete spots, exactly as described above for their travel through a column. When the solvent has traveled to the opposite edge of the paper, the sheet is removed, dried, and sprayed with a reagent such as ninhydrin. The position of each amino acid is then revealed by a colored spot which appears when the sheet is heated.

If the solvent used brings two or more amino acids to the same position, two-dimensional chromatography is employed. The dried sheet is not sprayed, but is rotated 90° and is placed with the edge along which the amino acids are located in a second solvent. This solvent flows through the paper at right angles to the direction taken by the first solvent, and if correctly chosen, will separate those amino acids which stayed together in the first solvent. The sheet is then dried and sprayed to locate the amino acids, and then the spots can be cut out with scissors and eluted with water in separate tubes for colorimetric determination. A two-dimensional chromatogram of the amino acids of a protein is shown in Fig. 5.

The determination of total α-amino acids in extracts of natural materials can be carried out by using the ninhydrin method, described above, or the Van Slyke method, which measures the amount of nitrogen gas given off on treatment with nitrous acid. Specific determinations of a given amino acid were previously carried by means of sensitive microbiological assays which measured the growth of a microorganism dependent on the amino acid as a function of the concentration of the unknown material. Nowadays this rather difficult and cumbersome method has been largely replaced by ion-exchange chromatography.

There are relatively specific color reactions for many amino acids; while still used to some extent as quantitative assays, these now find most widespread use as qualitative tests for the presence of the amino acids.

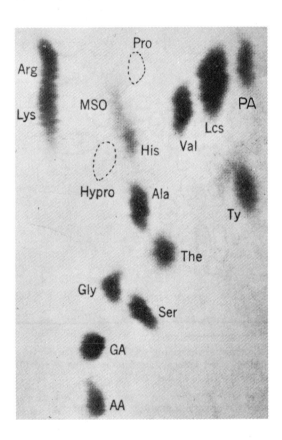

KEY:

Arg = arginine	His = histidine
Lys = lysine	Ala = alanine
MSO = methionine	The = threonine
sulfoxide	Se = serine
Hypro = hydroxyproline	Val = valine
Gly = glycine	Lcs = leucines
GA = glutamic acid	Ty = tyrosine
AA = aspartic acid	PA = phenylalanine
Pro = proline	

Fig. 5. Two-dimensional chromatogram of a protein; solvents: phenol and lutidine. (*From R. J. Block, E. L. Durrum, and G. Zweig, A Manual of Paper Chromatography and Paper Electrophoresis, 2d ed., Academic, 1958*)

AMINO ACID METABOLISM

Although amino acids and some other charged molecules can enter a cell passively by means of simple diffusion, there are present in all cells so far examined special systems for concentrating such small molecules inside the cell. These systems, called permeases, are localized in the cell membrane. They are protein complexes, probably containing at least two parts, which utilize metabolic energy to transport small molecules against the concentration gradient. Bacterial amino acid permeases are capable of achieving a concentration inside a cell 1000 times greater than that outside the cell.

The criteria for a permease, or active transport system, are (1) it must require energy, (2) it must be relatively specific, and (3) it must concentrate the transported substance against a gradient. Most permeases obey the classical Michaelis-Henry enzyme kinetics. Portions of the system which concentrates valine, isoleucine, and leucine in *Escherichia coli* have been purified; thus the mechanism of action of this permease may soon be clear.

Biosynthesis. Since amino acids, as precursors of proteins, are essential to all organisms, all cells must be able to synthesize those they cannot obtain from their environment. The selective advantage of being able rapidly to shift from endogenous to exogenous sources of these compounds has led to the evolution in bacteria and many other organisms of very complex and precise methods of adjusting the rate of synthesis to the available level of the compound. These regulatory mechanisms can be divided according to whether they require a short or a long time to take effect.

The immediately effective control is that of feedback inhibition. As Figs. 9–14 show, the biosynthesis of amino acids is relatively complicated and usually requires at least three enzymatic steps. In most cases so far examined, the amino acid end product of the biosynthetic pathway inhibits the first enzyme to catalyze a reaction specific to the biosynthesis of that amino acid. This inhibition is extremely specific; the enzymes involved have special sites for binding the inhibitor. This inhibition functions to shut off the pathway in the presence of transient high levels of the product, thus saving both carbon and energy for other biosynthetic reactions. When the level of the product decreases, the pathway begins to function once more.

If a microorganism is grown for several generations in the presence of an amino acid, the levels of the enzymes of the biosynthetic pathway decrease considerably. This phenomenon is called enzyme repression, and it comes about because the synthesis of the enzymes is decreased in the presence of the end product. However, the enzyme already present in the cell is stable; therefore several generations are required before it is diluted to its lowest level by being apportioned among daughter cells at each division. (The level of such enzymes never reaches zero.) If at any time during this process the amino acid ceases to be available to the microorganism, synthesis of the enzyme immediately begins and continues until the proper intracellular concentration of the amino acid is reached. At this point the biosynthesis of the enzyme slows down and an equilibrium is reached such that the level of the enzyme remains constant until there is another alteration in the exogenous level of the amino acid. In contrast to feedback inhibition, which requires only milliseconds to act, repression and derepression require from one-half to several generations to reach a new equilibrium.

The actual metabolic pathways by which amino acids are synthesized are presented in diagrammatic form in Figs. 9–14. These pathways generally are found to be the same in all living cells investigated, whether microbial or animal. Biosynthetic mechanisms thus appear to have developed soon after the origin of life and to have remained unchanged throughout the divergent evolution of modern organisms. The major exception is lysine, which is formed from aspartic acid via diaminopimelic acid in bacteria, but from α-ketoglutaric acid in the fungi. Indeed, the occurrence of diaminopimelic acid as a precursor of lysine, or as a constituent of proteins, or both, is a major taxonomic property of the bacteria and the related blue-green algae.

Formation and transfer of amino groups. The biosynthetic pathway diagrams reveal only one quantitatively important reaction by which organic nitrogen enters the amino groups of amino acids: the reductive amination of α-ketoglutaric acid to glutamic acid by the enzyme glutamic acid dehydrogenase. All other amino acids are formed either by transamination (transfer of an amino group, ultimately from glutamic acid) or by a modification of an existing amino acid. An example of the former is the formation of valine by transfer of the amino group from glutamic acid to α-ketoisovaleric acid; an example of the latter is the reduction and cyclization of glutamic acid to form proline.

Two other direct conversions of inorganic nitrogen to amino acid nitrogen are known: the reductive amination of pyruvic acid to alanine and the addition of ammonia to fumaric acid to form aspartic acid. However, there is no evidence that either of these reactions is quantitatively important in amino nitrogen formation. In any case, ammonia is the only form of inorganic nitrogen which has been clearly shown to enter organic compounds directly; nitrate (NO_3^-), nitrite (NO_2^-), and nitrogen gas (N_2) are probably reduced to free intracellular ammonia before being converted to organic form in those plants and microorganisms which can use them as nutritional sources of nitrogen.

The principal mechanism of amino group transfer, transamination, is extremely important in

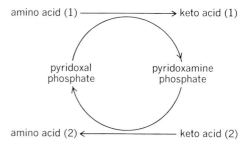

Fig. 6. Graphic representation of transamination mechanism by true transaminase.

many phases of nitrogen metabolism. Although a great many transamination reactions are known (all or most naturally occurring amino compounds probably participate in transamination in one tissue or another), the actual number of transaminases involved is uncertain. The few transaminases which have been highly purified all catalyze amino group exhange between more than just one pair of amino acids.

A true transaminase uses pyridoxal phosphate or pyridoxamine phosphate as coenzyme; the amino group is transferred to the former, which then gives it up to the keto acid acceptor (Fig. 6). A different mechanism of amino group transfer occurs in the biosyntheses of arginine and of adenylic acid; here, aspartic acid is added to a keto group to form a stable intermediate; a second enzyme then cleaves the intermediate to fumaric acid plus the new amino compound (see Fig. 10, showing the pathway of arginine biosynthesis).

One other important route by which ammonia enters organic compounds is by way of the amide group of glutamine. This group is formed by the direct addition of ammonia to glutamic acid, the necessary energy coming from the breakdown of adenosinetriphosphate (ATP), first to adenosinediphosphate (ADP), then to inorganic phosphate. Once formed, amide nitrogen can be transferred to suitable acceptors to form precursors of the purine and histidine rings, as well as to hexose 6-phosphate to form glucosamine 6-phosphate.

Asparagine is another important amide, but the mechanism of asparagine formation is still in some doubt, and the only known product of the asparagine amide group is free ammonia. Glutamine is also readily deamidated to ammonia; both glutamine and asparagine serve as important storage forms of ammonia in higher plants and animals, as well as being constituent amino acids of proteins.

Degradation. Most organisms are capable of degrading some amino acids, and metabolic pathways leading to degradation to CO_2 and H_2O are known for each of the common amino acids. These pathways are detailed in the articles on the individual amino acids. There are, however, general features (Fig. 7) characteristic of degradative pathways which are discussed below.

The first step in the degradation of all amino acids, with the exception of tyrosine and phenylalanine, is the labilization of one of the four groups

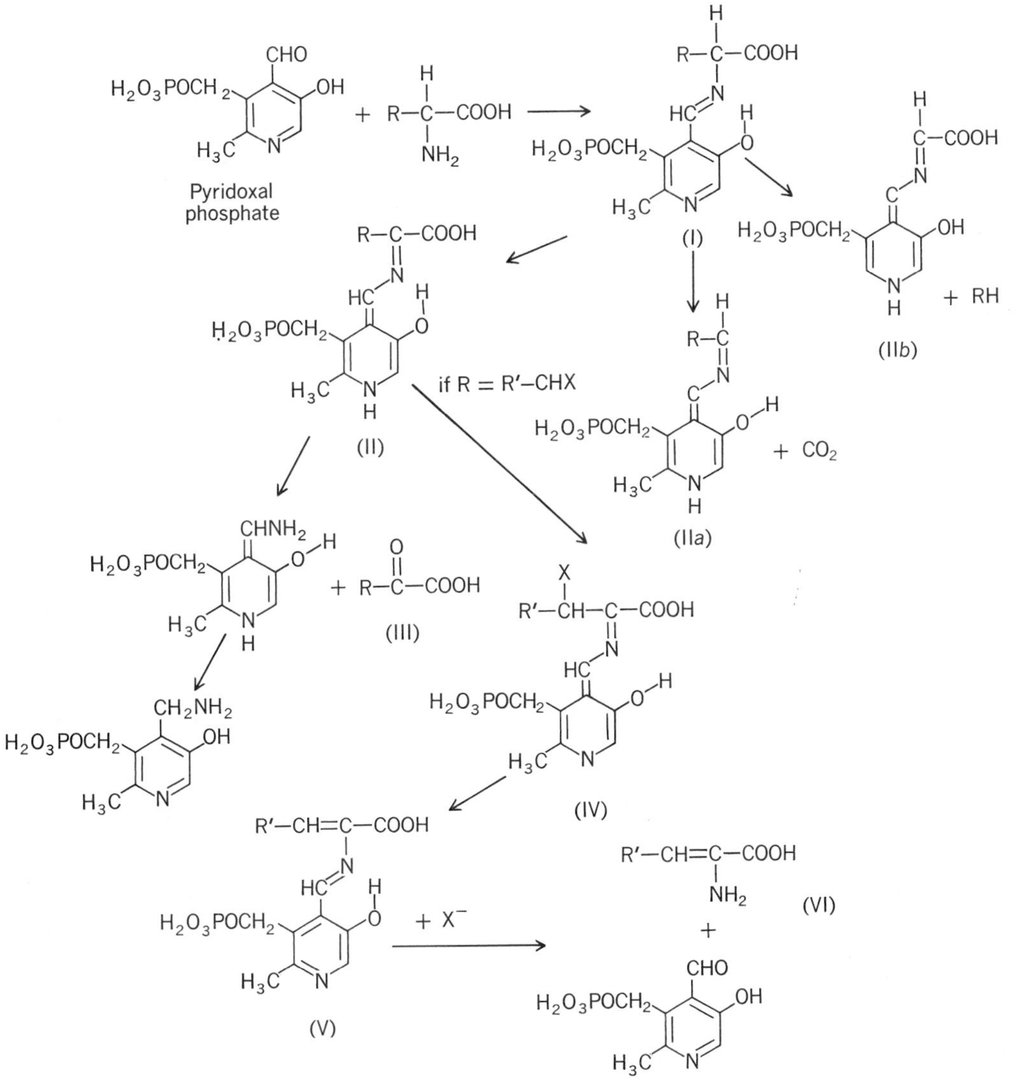

Fig. 7. General features of degradative pathways for amino acids.

on the α carbon atom. The labilization always involves an enzyme containing pyridoxal phosphate as a cofactor, except in the case of oxidative deamination where a flavoprotein is involved. Pyridoxal phosphate acts by forming a Schiff's base (shown as I in Fig. 7) with the amino acid, as shown in Fig. 7. By a rearrangement of electrons and protons (a tautomerization) the double bond moves to the position shown in II, with a concomitant alteration in the electron distribution in the pyridine ring of pyridoxal phosphate and the loss of the hydrogen on the α carbon to the solvent. Intermediate II may now be hydrolyzed to yield the α-keto acid (III) corresponding to the amino acid, or it may return to intermediate I. In the latter case there is often a racemization, since II is a symmetric compound and the reversal of the tautomerization is not always carried out in an asymmetric manner.

If, instead of the hydrogen atom, the carboxyl group is labilized by donating its electrons to form the new double bond, intermediate IIa is formed. A reversal of the tautomerization cannot regenerate an amino acid in this case; the reaction is a decarboxylation and the product is an amine. Similarly, the organic radical R may be lost (IIb) whereupon the reversal of the tautomerization yields glycine. The last reaction is possible only when the radical is substituted with a hydroxyl group on the β carbon (adjacent to the α carbon). A final variation on the basic reactions of pyridoxal phosphate takes place when the R group contains an electronegative substituent on the β carbon (IV). In this case it is possible to expel the substituent, leading to an allyl amino acid, intermediate V, analogous to I. Intermediate V is now hydrolyzed to yield the extremely unstable intermediate VI which rearranges to give the keto acid, ammonia, and X^- from the amino acid.

Transamination. Transamination is accomplished by hydrolysis of intermediate II to yield the keto acid and pyridoxamine phosphate. The latter compound reacts with another keto acid, yielding pyridoxal phosphate and the new amino acid. Transaminase enzymes are relatively nonspecific, reacting with groups of amino acids with similar R groups (for example, the aromatic amino acids or the branched-chain amino acids). The equilibrium constant of a transaminase reaction is usually very close to 1, reflecting the similarity in the free energies of formation of keto acids from amino acids. Transamination is much commoner than deamination in nature, since a deamination without a subsequent transfer of the amino group to another keto acid renders the coenzyme inactive. Most transaminase reactions involve aspartate or glutamate as one partner, with alanine also being rather common.

Decarboxylation. Decarboxylations are carried out by rather specific enzymes and their products are often biologically active substances. Histamine, tryptamine (serotonin), and dopamine are all examples of decarboxylation products which are very active in animal tissues.

β-Elimination. These reactions result in the loss of an electronegative group, such as OH^- or SH^-, from the carbon adjacent to the α carbon. Usually the net result is a deamination as well, since α,β-unsaturated amino acids rapidly tautomerize to α,β-saturated imino acids, which hydrolyze to yield the corresponding keto acid. Sometimes, however, there is addition to the α,β double bond of the pyridoxal phosphate – amino acid complex, so that the net result is a β-substitution. This type of reaction is important in the synthesis of tryptophan.

β-Cleavage. Instead of the α hydrogen or the carboxyl group, the β carbon can be eliminated, giving rise to glycine. These reactions only occur when the β substituent is electronegative, as in serine or threonine.

Conjugation. Until 1956 the mechanism of protein synthesis was totally unknown. Since then most of the details have been elucidated. A brief outline of the steps involved follows. The brevity of the outline precludes mention of many of the details.

The structure of a protein is determined by the arrangement of bases in the portion of the deoxyribonucleic acid (DNA) making up the gene for that protein. This sequence of DNA is transcribed into a complementary molecule of ribonucleic acid (RNA). The specific RNA, called messenger RNA (m-RNA), binds to ribosomes, which are complex subcellular particles composed of a different sort of RNA, ribosomal RNA (r-RNA), and protein. The ribosomes serve as the sites where conjugation of the amino acids takes place.

The amino acids are activated by reaction with a molecule of ATP to form an amino-acyl adenylate (Fig. 8) that remains temporarily bound to the enzyme which catalyzes the activation, an amino-acyl-t-RNA synthetase (t-RNA indicates transfer RNA). The amino-acyl moiety is then transferred to a specific molecule of RNA, that is, to t-RNA. The linkage of the amino acid to the t-RNA takes place by esterification to the 2'-hydroxyl of the ribose moiety of the 3'-terminal end. The t-RNA molecule has a complex secondary structure which exposes a sequence of three bases in the interior of the molecule. These three bases are called the anticodon. The nature and order of these bases are specific for the amino acid involved. The amino-acyl-t-RNA synthetase contributes the specificity which ensures, with a very high degree of certainty, that the amino acid is attached to a t-RNA with the proper anticodon.

The amino-acyl-t-RNA interacts with the ribosome messenger complex when there is a sequence of three bases (the codon) on the messenger complementary, in the Watson-Crick sense, to the anticodon. The t-RNA is aligned on the ribosome in such a way that the nascent protein chain, held by a C-terminal amino acid still linked to its t-

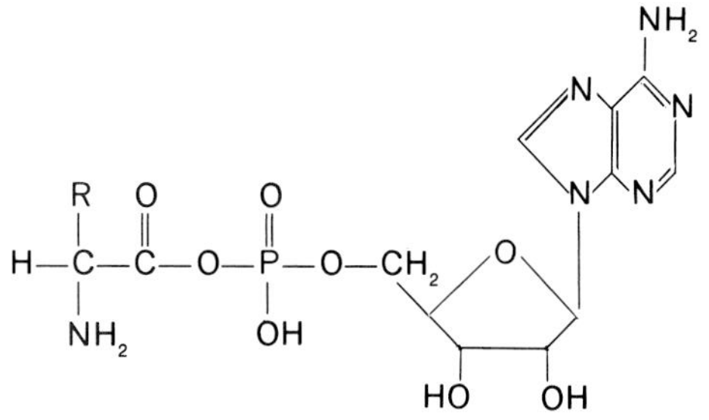

Fig. 8. Structural formula for amino-acyl adenylate.

RNA, is brought into proximity with the free α-amino group of the amino acid. A series of enzymes effects formation of the peptide bond, and the nascent protein chain has been elongated by one amino acid. The chain is now held to the ribosome by the t-RNA of the latest residue added, and it is ready to accept the amino acid specified by the next codon. Thus the ribosome progresses along the m-RNA, "reading" it, until all the amino acids specified by the original DNA gene have been added. It then reaches a codon which signifies termination of the chain, and a soluble protein is released.

The nascent protein chain begins in bacteria with a special methionyl-t-RNA complex, in which the amino group of methionine is blocked with a formyl group. This is the first amino-acyl-t-RNA to bind to the ribosome, and apparently all genes begin with the codon specific for this t-RNA. In the first peptide bond formed, the N-formyl-methionyl-t-RNA plays the part of the nascent protein chain.

For smaller peptides, such as glutathione and the mucopeptide of bacterial cell walls, the conjugation process is catalyzed by specific enzymes and involves different intermediates. Necessarily this means separate enzymes for each such peptide, in contrast to protein synthesis where the same machinery (except for the m-RNA) serves for all chains of whatever sequence.

AMINO ACIDS IN NUTRITION

The nutritional requirement for the amino acids of protein can vary from zero, in the case of an organism which synthesizes them all, to the complete list, in the case of an organism in which all the biosynthetic pathways are blocked. There are 8 or 10 amino acids required by certain mammals; most plants synthesize all of their amino acids, while microorganisms vary from types which synthesize all, to others (such as certain lactic acid bacteria) which require as many as 18 different amino acids. *See* NUTRITION; PROTEIN METABOLISM.

It seems likely that, when life first originated, amino acids were taken from the rich organic medium which the oceans then offered, and biosynthetic abilities evolved only slowly as the supply of exogenous materials became depleted. A stage must have eventually been reached, however, at which all the amino acids were being synthesized metabolically, and none was required nutritionally. As evolution progressed, food chains developed, and some forms of life became adapted to obtain many of their organic nutrients at the expense of other living forms, either directly or indirectly. In these dependent types, mutations had occurred, causing the loss of specific biosynthetic enzymes and hence the gain of nutritional requirements. It is easy to duplicate this process in the laboratory: A microorganism with full biosynthetic ability can be induced to undergo random mutations, and selective methods can then be used to isolate mutants requiring amino acids, vitamins, or other normal metabolites. In every case, it is found that a given mutation deprives the cell of a single biosynthetic enzyme, blocking the reaction which that enzyme catalyzes and thus the entire pathway of which that reaction is a part.

In summary, the nutrition of many organisms must include the provision of growth factors, which are defined as organic compounds which the organism requires for its growth but which it cannot synthesize. Growth factor requirements reflect the heritable loss of biosynthetic enzymes, as the result of gene mutations. Amino acids are typical growth factors for many organisms.

The one exception to this general rule is the growth factor requirement which results from the presence in the environment of a metabolic inhibitor. For example, a certain strain of bacterium is very sensitive to inhibition by valine, and this inhibition can be overcome by isoleucine. In the presence of valine, then, this strain requires isoleucine for growth. There are many such antagonisms between amino acids, with the result that organisms which require several amino acids must receive them in balanced amounts; any one in excess may prove inhibitory.

GRAPHIC PRESENTATION OF BIOSYNTHESIS OF AMINO ACIDS

The amino acids are grouped into families on the basis of their common biosynthetic origins. Lysine is shown in two families, because its biosynthesis in bacteria differs from that in fungi.

Intermediates which are hypothetical are shown in brackets. The notation $-2H$ or $+2H$ refers to the removal or addition of two electrons and two hydrogen ions with the aid of either diphosphopyridine nucleotide (DPN) or triphosphopyridine nucleotide (TPN), both of which are coenzymes of hydrogen transfer.

Symbols used are $\sim$Ac, coenzyme A–bound acetate; PRPP, phosphoribosyl pyrophosphate; CAP, carbamyl phosphate; and ATP, adenosinetriphosphate.

An arrow between two compounds in the diagrams does not necessarily imply a single enzymatic reaction. In many cases, the arrow represents a sequence of reactions for which the intermediates are unknown.

[EDWARD A. ADELBERG; PAUL T. MAGEE]

Aromatic family. This family is composed of phenylalanine, tyrosine, tryptophan, and two other important metabolites, p-aminobenzoic acid and p-hydroxybenzoic acid. The initial precursors for the biosynthesis of these amino acids, phosphoenol pyruvate and D-erythrose 4-phosphate, are metabolites of glucose catabolism.

Although the intermediates shown in Fig. 9 have all been isolated and identified, not all of the enzymes (particularly those involved in chorismic acid metabolism) have been studied. It is probable that p-hydroxybenzoic acid and prephenic acid are synthesized directly from chorismic acid by a single enzymatic reaction, and p-aminobenzoic acid may also be a direct metabolite. It is certain that other as yet unidentified intermediates exist in the pathway between chorismic acid and anthranilic acid.

Two different enzymes for the conversion of chorismic acid to prephenic acid have been demonstrated in microorganisms. One of these enzymes is controlled by the pool size of tyrosine, while the other is controlled by phenylalanine.

The glycerol phosphate side chain of indoleglycerol phosphate derived from phosphoribosyl pyrophosphate can be exchanged directly for serine

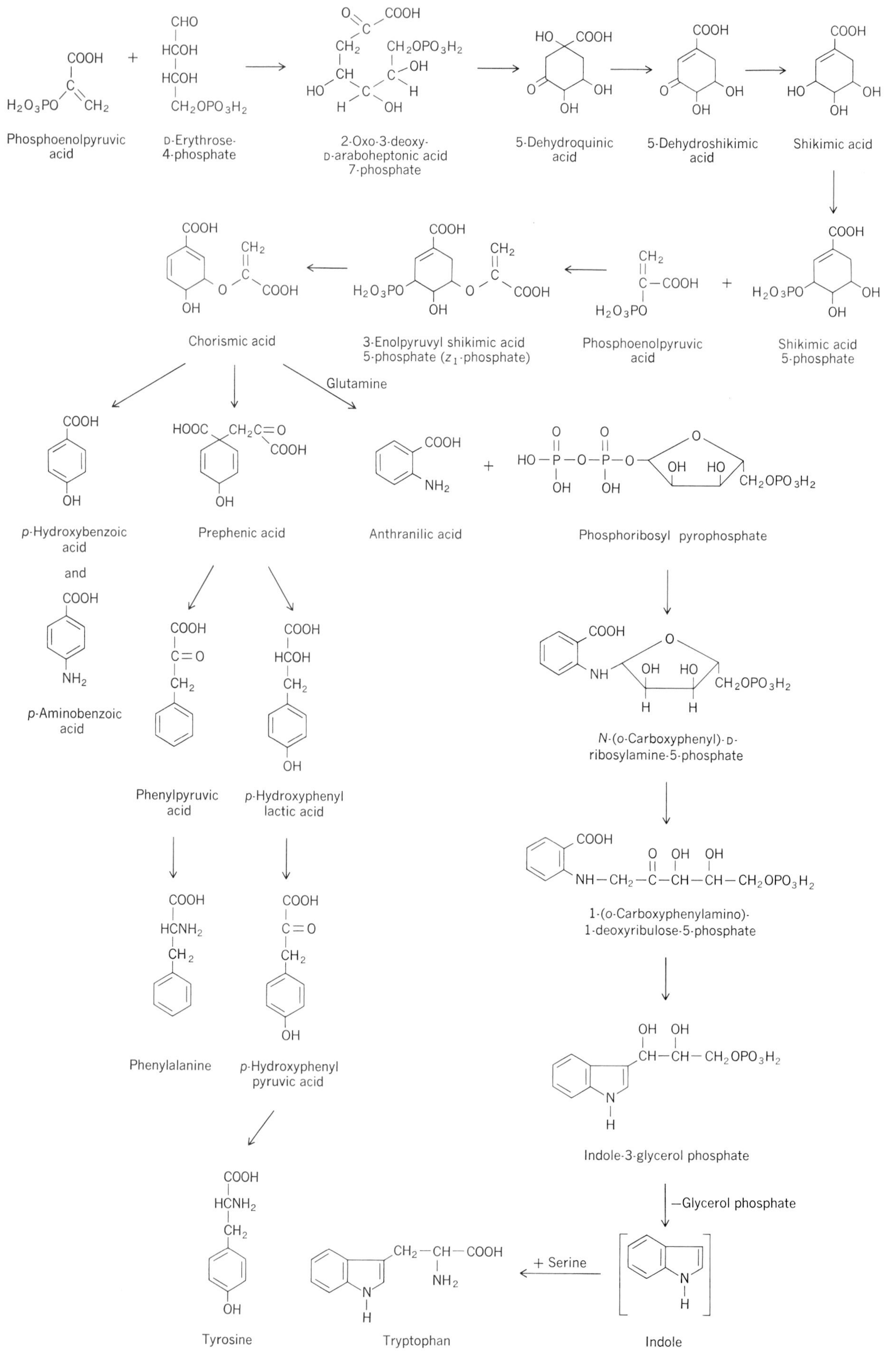

Fig. 9. Metabolic pathways for the aromatic family of amino acids.

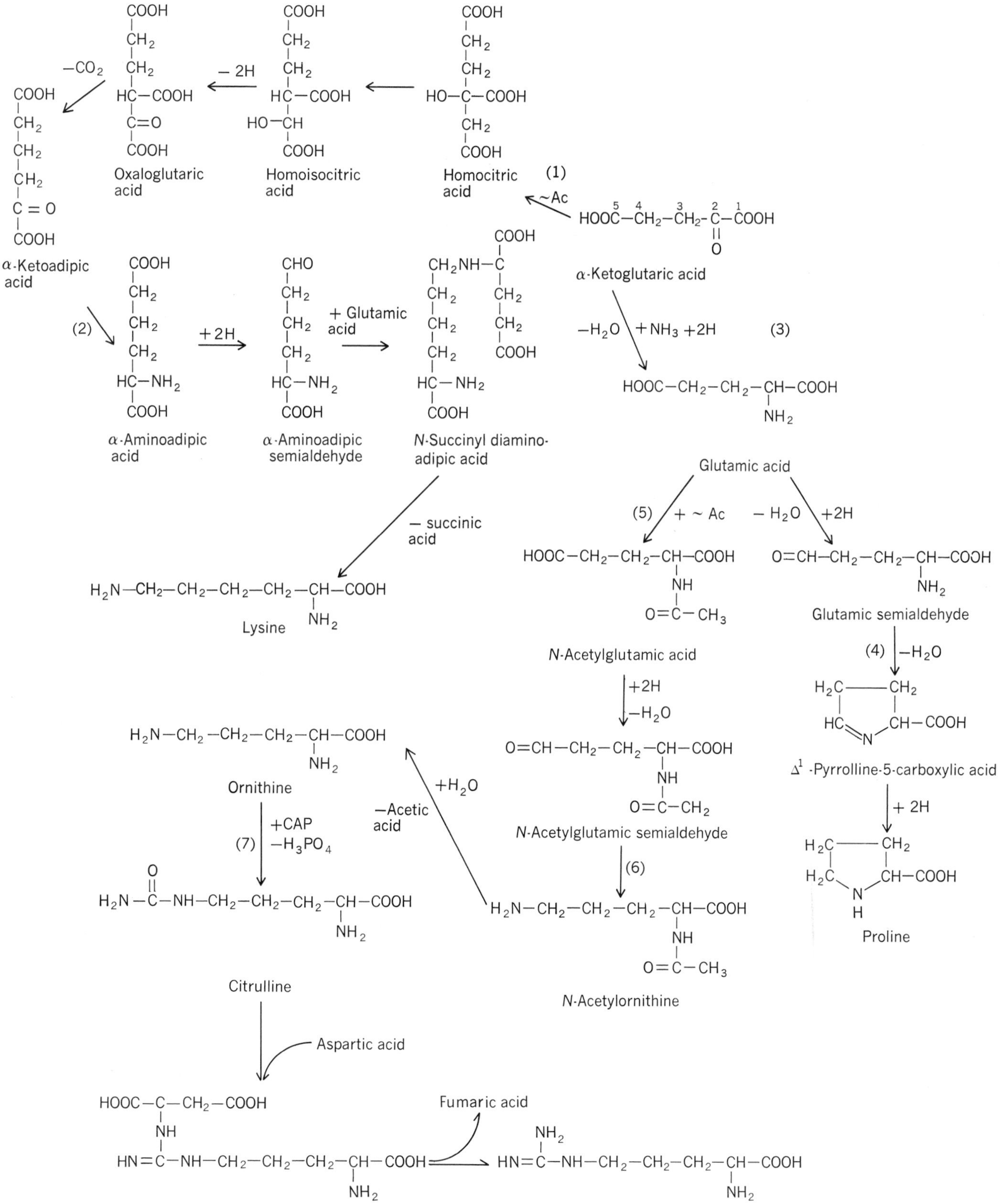

COOH
CH$_2$
CH$_2$
HC—COOH
C=O
COOH
Oxaloglutaric acid

$-$ 2H

COOH
CH$_2$
CH$_2$
HC—COOH
HO—CH
COOH
Homoisocitric acid

COOH
CH$_2$
CH$_2$
HO—C—COOH
CH$_2$
COOH
Homocitric acid   (1)

$-$CO$_2$

COOH
CH$_2$
CH$_2$
CH$_2$
C = O
COOH
α-Ketoadipic acid

$\sim$Ac

HOOC$-$CH$_2$$-CH_2$$-C-$COOH
‖
O
5 4 3 2 1
α-Ketoglutaric acid

(2)

COOH
CH$_2$
CH$_2$
CH$_2$
HC—NH$_2$
COOH
α-Aminoadipic acid

$+$2H

CHO
CH$_2$
CH$_2$
CH$_2$
HC—NH$_2$
COOH
α-Aminoadipic semialdehyde

$+$ Glutamic acid

COOH
CH$_2$NH—C
CH$_2$ CH$_2$
CH$_2$ CH$_2$
CH$_2$ COOH
HC—NH$_2$
COOH
N-Succinyl diamino-adipic acid

$-$H$_2$O $+$NH$_3$ $+$2H   (3)

HOOC$-$CH$_2$$-CH_2$$-CH-$COOH
NH$_2$
Glutamic acid

$-$ succinic acid

H$_2$N$-$CH$_2$$-CH_2$$-CH_2$$-CH_2$$-CH-$COOH
NH$_2$
Lysine

(5) $+$ $\sim$ Ac

HOOC$-$CH$_2$$-CH_2$$-CH-$COOH
NH
O=C$-$CH$_3$
N-Acetylglutamic acid

$+$2H
$-$H$_2$O

O=CH$-$CH$_2$$-CH_2$$-CH-$COOH
NH
O=C$-$CH$_3$
N-Acetylglutamic semialdehyde

(6)

H$_2$N$-$CH$_2$$-CH_2$$-CH_2$$-CH-$COOH
NH
O=C$-$CH$_3$
N-Acetylornithine

$-$ H$_2$O $+$2H

O=CH$-$CH$_2$$-CH_2$$-CH-$COOH
NH$_2$
Glutamic semialdehyde

(4) $-$H$_2$O

H$_2$C——CH$_2$
HC=N   CH—COOH
Δ^1-Pyrroline-5-carboxylic acid

$+$ 2H

H$_2$C——CH$_2$
H$_2$C   CH—COOH
N
H
Proline

H$_2$N$-$CH$_2$$-CH_2$$-CH_2$$-CH-$COOH
NH$_2$
Ornithine

$+$H$_2$O

$-$Acetic acid

(7) $+$CAP $-$H$_3$PO$_4$

O
‖
H$_2$N$-$C$-$NH$-$CH$_2$$-CH_2$$-CH_2$$-CH-$COOH
NH$_2$
Citrulline

Aspartic acid

HOOC$-$C$-$CH$_2$$-$COOH
NH
HN=C$-$NH$-$CH$_2$$-CH_2$$-CH_2$$-CH-$COOH
NH$_2$

Fumaric acid

NH$_2$
HN=C$-$NH$-$CH$_2$$-CH_2$$-CH_2$$-CH-$COOH
NH$_2$

Fig. 10.   Metabolic pathways for the α-ketoglutaric family of amino acids.

without the formation of free indole as an intermediate. In the absence of serine, the enzyme liberates free indole from indoleglycerol phosphate, and the same enzyme will condense indole with serine to form tryptophan.

There is some evidence for the existence of an anthranilic acid–tryptophan cycle in microorganisms. Formylkynurenine produced by the action of tryptophan pyrrolase on tryptophan can regenerate anthranilic acid by the combined action of kynureninase and kynurenine formamidase.

[R. G. MARTIN]

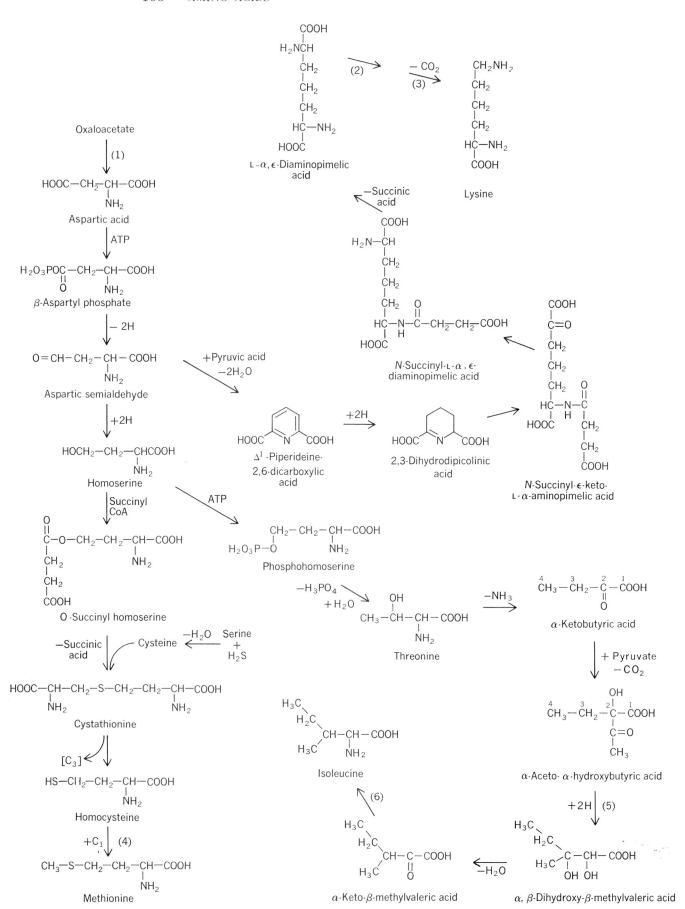

Fig. 11.   Metabolic pathways for the aspartic acid family of amino acids.

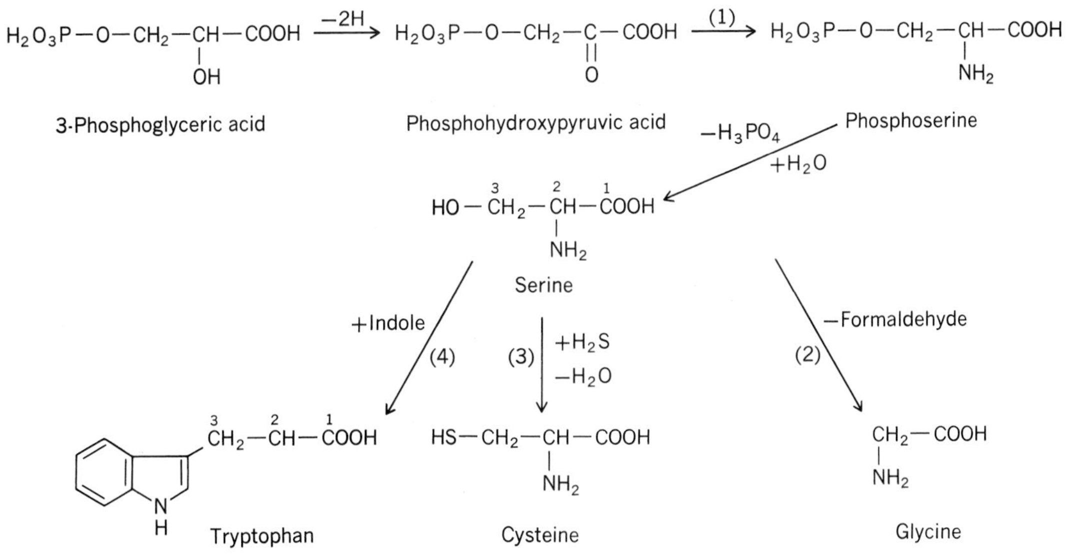

$$\text{H}_2\text{O}_3\text{P}-\text{O}-\text{CH}_2-\underset{\overset{|}{\text{OH}}}{\text{CH}}-\text{COOH} \xrightarrow{-2\text{H}} \text{H}_2\text{O}_3\text{P}-\text{O}-\text{CH}_2-\underset{\overset{||}{\text{O}}}{\text{C}}-\text{COOH} \xrightarrow{(1)} \text{H}_2\text{O}_3\text{P}-\text{O}-\text{CH}_2-\underset{\overset{|}{\text{NH}_2}}{\text{CH}}-\text{COOH}$$

3-Phosphoglyceric acid   Phosphohydroxypyruvic acid   Phosphoserine

$-\text{H}_3\text{PO}_4$ / $+\text{H}_2\text{O}$

$$\text{HO}-\overset{3}{\text{CH}_2}-\underset{\overset{|}{\text{NH}_2}}{\overset{2}{\text{CH}}}-\overset{1}{\text{COOH}}$$

Serine

+Indole (4)   (3) $+\text{H}_2\text{S}$ / $-\text{H}_2\text{O}$ −Formaldehyde (2)

$$\overset{3}{\text{CH}_2}-\overset{2}{\text{CH}}-\overset{1}{\text{COOH}}$$ (indole ring)

Tryptophan

$$\text{HS}-\text{CH}_2-\underset{\overset{|}{\text{NH}_2}}{\text{CH}}-\text{COOH}$$

Cysteine

$$\text{CH}_2-\text{COOH} \atop \underset{\text{NH}_2}{|}$$

Glycine

Fig. 12. Metabolic pathways for the serine family of amino acids.

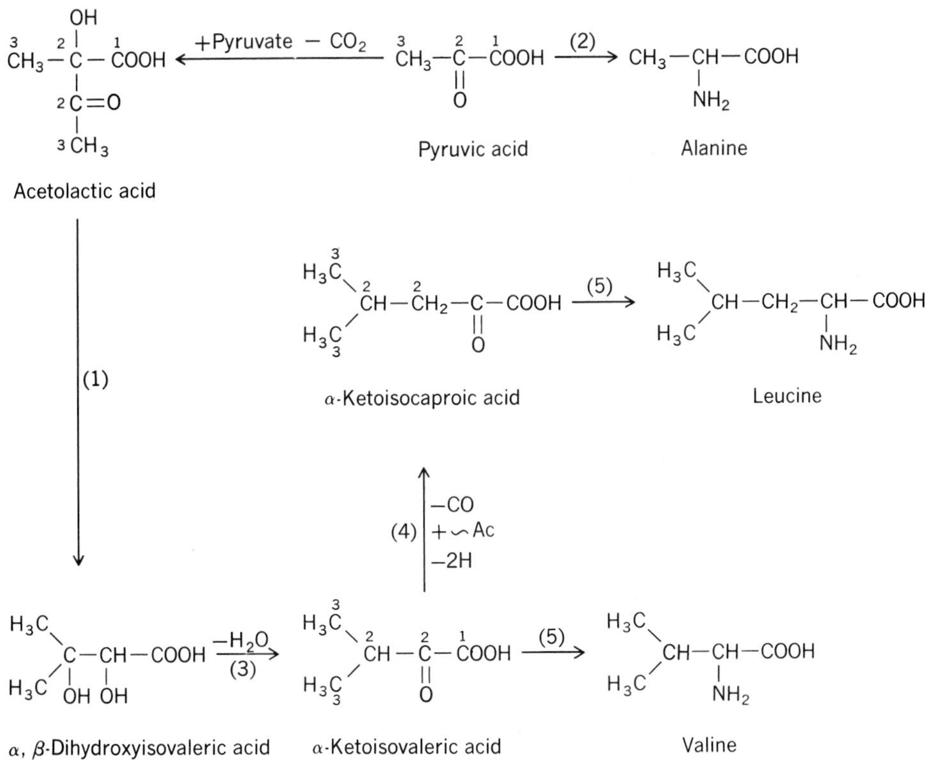

$$\underset{\overset{|}{\text{2C}=\text{O}}\,\overset{}{\underset{\text{3CH}_3}{|}}}{\overset{3}{\text{CH}_3}-\overset{\overset{\text{OH}}{|}}{\text{C}}-\overset{1}{\text{COOH}}} \xleftarrow{+\text{Pyruvate}\,-\text{CO}_2} \overset{3}{\text{CH}_3}-\underset{\overset{||}{\text{O}}}{\overset{2}{\text{C}}}-\overset{1}{\text{COOH}} \xrightarrow{(2)} \text{CH}_3-\underset{\overset{|}{\text{NH}_2}}{\text{CH}}-\text{COOH}$$

Acetolactic acid   Pyruvic acid   Alanine

$$\underset{\text{H}_3\text{C}}{\overset{\text{H}_3\text{C}}{}}\text{CH}-\text{CH}_2-\underset{\overset{||}{\text{O}}}{\text{C}}-\text{COOH} \xrightarrow{(5)} \underset{\text{H}_3\text{C}}{\overset{\text{H}_3\text{C}}{}}\text{CH}-\text{CH}_2-\underset{\overset{|}{\text{NH}_2}}{\text{CH}}-\text{COOH}$$

α-Ketoisocaproic acid   Leucine

(4) $-\text{CO}$ $+\sim\text{Ac}$ -2H

(1)

$$\underset{\text{H}_3\text{C}}{\overset{\text{H}_3\text{C}}{}}\underset{\overset{|}{\text{OH}}\,\overset{|}{\text{OH}}}{\text{C}}-\text{CH}-\text{COOH} \xrightarrow[(3)]{-\text{H}_2\text{O}} \underset{\text{H}_3\text{C}}{\overset{\text{H}_3\text{C}}{}}\text{CH}-\underset{\overset{||}{\text{O}}}{\text{C}}-\text{COOH} \xrightarrow{(5)} \underset{\text{H}_3\text{C}}{\overset{\text{H}_3\text{C}}{}}\text{CH}-\underset{\overset{|}{\text{NH}_2}}{\text{CH}}-\text{COOH}$$

α, β-Dihydroxyisovaleric acid   α-Ketoisovaleric acid   Valine

Fig. 13. Metabolic pathways for the pyruvic acid family of amino acids.

α-Ketoglutaric acid family. This family is composed of glutamic acid, proline, lysine, and arginine. The numbered items refer to Fig. 10.

(1) In yeast and other fungi, lysine is formed from α-ketoglutaric acid plus a C_2 fragment derivable from acetate. It is formed by a different pathway in bacteria (see section on aspartic acid).

(2) Presumably by transamination.

(3) This reductive amination is the main source of organic nitrogen for most microorganisms.

(4) The cyclization takes place spontaneously.

(5) The acetylation of glutamic acid prevents cyclization at the next step and permits the eventual formation of ornithine. This mechanism has been demonstrated in *Escherichia coli*, but does not take place in the fungus *Neurospora*; the fungus appears able to form ornithine via the nonacetylated intermediates.

(6) Transamination.

(7) Carbamyl phosphate (CAP).

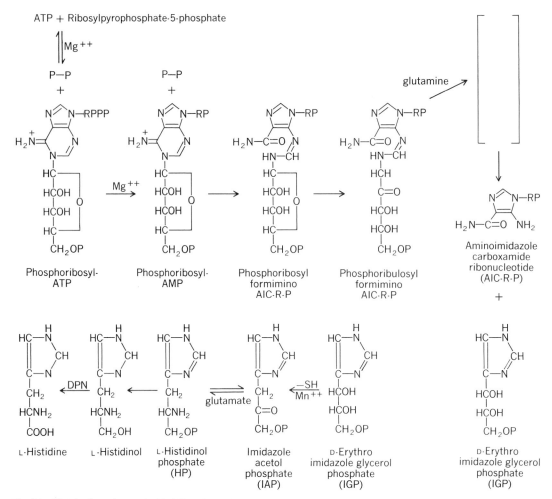

Fig. 14.   Metabolic pathways in histidine biosynthesis.

Aspartic acid family. This family is composed of aspartic acid, lysine, threonine, methionine, and isoleucine. The numbered items refer to Fig. 11.

(1) Aspartate arises principally by the transamination of oxaloacetate. In plants and in some microorganisms, it is formed by the direct amination of fumaric acid.

(2) The compound formed by the transamination at carbon 6 and subsequent desuccinylation is L,L-diaminopimelic acid. For the decarboxylase to function, the compound must be racemized to form *meso*-diaminopimelic acid.

(3) In bacteria, and presumably in blue-green algae, lysine is formed by decarboxylation of diaminopimelic acid. In fungi and in higher animals, lysine is formed by a different route as seen in the α-ketoglutaric acid family (Fig. 10).

(4) A series of reactions probably involves transfer of an active formaldehyde group from serine, followed by reduction.

(5) Intramolecular rearrangement and reduction in α-aceto-α-hydroxybutyric acid take place in one step. The same enzyme catalyzes the analogous step in valine biosynthesis (Fig. 13).

(6) Transamination from glutamic acid. The same transaminase functions for the keto acids of both isoleucine and valine.

Serine family. The serine family is composed of serine, glycine, cysteine, and tryptophan. The numbered items refer to Fig. 12.

(1) Transamination from alanine. There is equal evidence for a second pathway in which dephosphorylation precedes transamination.

(2) The terminal group of serine is transferred to tetrahydrofolic acid (THFA) to form *N*(10)-hydroxymethyl-THFA. In this form, it can be transferred at various levels of oxidation for biosynthesis of compounds methionine, purine, and thymine.

(3) This reaction, inferred to occur in microorganisms, is yet to be directly demonstrated. In animal tissues, serine receives the sulfhydryl group by transsulfuration from homocysteine, which is formed in animal tissues from dietary methionine.

(4) See the aromatic family for considerations of this reaction.

Pyruvic acid family. This family is composed of valine, leucine, and alanine. The numbered items refer to Fig. 13.

(1) Intramolecular rearrangement and reduction take place in one step.

(2) Generally by transamination from glutamate, although cases of direct reductive amination with ammonia have been cited.

(3) A single enzyme, dihydroxy acid dehydrase, catalyzes the dehydration of both the isoleucine and valine dihydroxy acid precursors.

(4) The complex series of reactions involved in the formation of α-ketoisocaproic acid is exactly analogous to the steps in the citric acid cycle leading to formation of α-ketoglutarate, with the keto acid taking the place of oxaloacetate.

(5) Transamination from glutamate. The valine transaminase also functions in isoleucine biosynthesis.

[EDWARD A. ADELBERG; PAUL T. MAGEE]

Histidine biosynthesis. The pathway of histidine biosynthesis shown in Fig. 14 is known to occur in the mold *Neurospora* and in coliform bacteria. It should be noted that the imidazole ring of histidine is formed by the pathway and is not derived from the five-membered ring of adenosinetriphosphate (ATP).   [DAVID W. E. SMITH]

Bibliography: B. N. Ames and P. E. Hartman, *Cold Spring Harbor Symp. Quant. Biol.*, 28:349, 1963; A. Meister, *The Biochemistry of Amino Acids*, 2d ed., 1965; D. W. E. Smith and B. N. Ames, *J. Biol. Chem.*, 239:1848, 1964.

Amylase

An enzyme which breaks down (hydrolyzes) starch, the reserve carbohydrate in plants, and glycogen, the reserve carbohydrate in animals, into reducing fermentable sugars, mainly maltose, and reducing nonfermentable or slowly fermentable dextrins. Amylases are classified as saccharifying (β-amylase) and as dextrinizing (α-amylases). The α- and β-amylases are specific for the α- and β-glucosidic bonds which connect the monosaccharide units into large aggregates, the polysaccharides. The α-amylases are found in all types of organs and tissues, whereas β-amylase is found almost exclusively in higher plants. *See* CARBOHYDRATE; GLYCOGEN.

Animals. In animals the highest concentrations of amylase are found in the saliva and in the pancreas. Salivary amylase is also known as ptyalin and is found in man, the ape, pig, guinea pig, squirrel, mouse, and rat. Pig pancreas is rich in amylase, whereas cattle, sheep, and dog pancreases have lower concentrations.

Starch is one of the most important constituents of human food. The food prepared by the mouth for swallowing (the bolus) is converted by the gastric juices into chyme (a semiliquid paste). Chyme is passed through the pylorus into the duodenum, where intestinal digestion occurs. Part of this digestion is caused by pancreatic amylase, which, like ptyalin, hydrolyzes starch to maltose. A maltase also found in pancreatic juice hydrolyzes maltose to glucose. Glucose is picked up by the bloodstream for use in the tissues for respiration and for conversion to glycogen in the liver for storage.

Plants. Starch is broken down during the germination of seeds (rich in starch) by associated plant enzymes into sugars. These constitute the chief energy source in the early development of the plant. β-Amylase occurs abundantly in seeds and cereals such as malt. It also is found in yeasts, molds, and bacteria.

Industry. Amylase is also used as a diastase in industry. It is used (1) in brewing and fermentation industries for the conversion of starch to fermentable sugars, (2) in the textile industry for designing textiles, (3) in the laundry industry in a mixture with protease and lipase to launder clothes, (4) in the paper industry for sizing, and (5) in the food industry for preparation of sweet syrups, to increase diastase content of flour, for modification of food for infants, and for the removal of starch in jelly production. The amylase enzyme used in industry comes from many sources: fungi, malt, bacteria, and the pancreas gland of cattle.

[DANIEL N. LAPEDES]

Animal-feed composition

The chemical composition of animal feeds can be considered as falling into three categories: water content (moisture), certain groups of natural organic compounds, and inorganic or mineral elements.

The principal organic groups are proteins, carbohydrates, and fats. A further group of essential but unrelated organic compounds, occurring in smaller concentration, consists of vitamins. In addition, a large number of organic compounds for which no essential nutritive function has been discovered have been isolated from animal feeds; acids, waxes, gums, lignins, hemicelluloses, and sterols. Small quantities of volatile oils contribute to the flavor of many feedstuffs.

Mineral elements. Although exacting chemical and spectrographic analysis of animal feeds reveals the presence of a long list of elements other than carbon, hydrogen, nitrogen, and oxygen, only those elements which are known to be essential in the nutrition of animals are usually included in tables of chemical composition of foods.

When feeds are carefully heated to destroy all organic matter, there is left an ash containing varying amounts of the essential elements, calcium, magnesium, potassium, sodium, sulfur, phosphorus, and chlorine (called major constituents), and smaller concentrations of iron, manganese, zinc, copper, cobalt, and iodine (called minor elements, micro elements, or trace elements).

A small group of elements is constantly present in low but highly variable concentration in the tissues and fluids of higher animals and plants. Several of these, namely, molybdenum, fluorine, selenium, and chromium, have had physiological significance ascribed to them. In certain lower forms of animal life, vanadium must be added to the list of essential elements. The physiological level of these elements is very low and excesses are known to be toxic.

Although the ashing process is carried out at moderate temperatures, a portion of some of the elements may be lost. Special techniques must be employed to determine their true content in the feeds analyzed.

The water content of feeds may vary from a low of 10% in many dry roughages to as high as 96% in stock melons.

Organic constituents. These include carbohydrates, proteins, fats, and oils.

Carbohydrates. In most animal feeds about three-fourths of the dry matter is made up of carbohydrates. They furnish the bulk of the energy for livestock. The simplest carbohydrates—sugars and starches—are highly digestible, but the more complex ones, such as the celluloses forming the woody parts of plants, must be digested by action of bacteria such as inhabit the paunch of ruminants and to a lesser degree the large intestine and cecum of herbivorous animals like the horse.

Proteins. Most of the nitrogenous compounds of animal feeds are proteins, which are among the most complex of all the known natural organic compounds. When completely digested, the proteins are broken down into 20 or more simpler compounds called amino acids.

Some commercial feeds for livestock contain synthetic urea, $CO(NH_2)_2$, which can be used by some rumen microorganisms as a source of nitrogen, and can be eventually converted to protein in their growth. Protein, thus synthesized, becomes food for the host. Urea is useful in this way only to ruminants such as cattle and sheep.

Examples of high-protein feeds are oil-cake meals (cottonseed meal, peanut meal, and soybean meal) and packing-house by-products such as meat meal.

Fats and oils. These are esters of glycerol and a number of fatty acids. They are called fats if they are solids at room temperature and oils if they are liquid at room temperature. The fats and oils have the highest energy value per unit weight of any of the three groups of food constituents. Much of the flavor of foods is found in the fat, which may be expressed from the feed at higher temperatures by mechanical means or extracted with a fat solvent, such as ethyl ether. The fat-soluble vitamins, if present in the foods, will also be found in this extract.

Feed analyses. A typical chemical analysis of animal feeds, such as is used for regulatory purposes or in nutrition studies for rough comparisons of food composition, includes the following constituents as percentages: moisture, ash, crude protein, crude fat, crude fiber, and nitrogen-free extract.

The methods used in determining these constituents vary, but for regulatory purposes in food control work, official methods are used which have been established by the Association of Official Agricultural Chemists.

Moisture represents loss of weight on drying. Ash is the residue remaining on combustion. Crude protein signifies the amount of total nitrogen multiplied by the factor 6.25. This does not represent the true protein content, but is based upon the average content of nitrogen found in a number of proteins which have been isolated in pure form. The term crude fat is the sum of all ether-soluble material and includes a number of substances other than true fats or oils. Crude fiber is a rough measure of the cellulose and cellulose-like woody part of the plant cells. It is the organic part of the ether-extracted feed which is not digested by first boiling with dilute sulfuric acid solution followed by boiling with dilute sodium hydroxide solution. The term nitrogen-free extract is a name with no particular significance. It has been used for many years to represent the sum of all the remaining undetermined constituents of the feedstuff.

Feed supplements. The manufacture of commercial mixed feeds has become a very important industry in the United States. Prior to 1949 the principal feed additives used in these mixed feeds were minerals and protein concentrates. Since that date, there has been enormous expansion in large-scale manufacture of vitamins, antibiotics, hormones, and essential amino acids. These substances have been added to mixed feeds as supplements having either direct action on metabolism and growth or indirect action through control of bacterial growth and infection. Although hundreds of compounds have been studied in experiments, relatively few have been cleared by the Federal Food and Drug Administration for general use in commercial feeds.

Antibiotic feed supplements. Antibiotics are substances which have a distinctive action against pathogenic or saprophytic bacteria, yeast, and molds. Among those most commonly used in animal feeds are chlortetracycline, oxytetracycline, a stabilized form of penicillin, and bacitracin. A suitable antibiotic supplement will generally, but not always, increase the rate of gain of pigs, chicks, and young calves less than 3 months old. The cause of growth stimulation is not fully known. It is generally believed that the antibiotic causes a reduction in undesirable bacteria in the digestive tract, especially under unsanitary conditions of poor management. Direct growth effects have also been ascribed to these antibiotics. Some synthetic compounds are claimed to have effects similar to those of the antibiotics. An example is the insoluble, nontoxic tetraalkylammonium stearate derived from animal fat.

Because of the possibility that uncontrolled use of antibiotics in animal feeds may contribute to the evolution of resistant strains of bacteria, the Food and Drug Administration regulations have been under review. For this reason only the latest regulations should be consulted on the use of antibiotic supplements in feedstuffs. Withdrawal of antibiotics from the ration several days before slaughter seems to allow clearance from the tissues. Cooking destroys antibiotic residues.

Vitamin supplements. Although it has been shown that an ample supply of all vitamin requirements of livestock usually can be made up through the use of common feeds, vitamins are becoming more general as feed additives in commercial feeds. The principal water-soluble vitamins manufactured for this purpose are nicotinic acid, riboflavin, thiamine, pantothenic acid, pyridoxine, choline chloride, and folic acid concentrates. These vitamins are added to some commercially mixed feeds for poultry, swine, and to a limited extent, for calves; but since adult ruminants are furnished with an adequate supply through synthesis by microorganisms in the rumen, no advantage has been shown for addition of synthetic water-soluble vitamins to their ration. Vitamin B_{12} (cobalamine) is present in some antibiotic supplements. Organisms in the rumen of cattle and sheep can synthesize vitamin B_{12}, provided sufficient cobalt is present in the ration. Increasing amounts of fat-soluble vitamin A are being produced for all types of livestock. This vitamin, which formerly was supplied as a fish liver oil to be fed separately because of the rapid destruction of the vitamin on oxidation, is now available in a stabilized form in which small particles of the concentrated vitamin are coated by a protective covering of a synthetic wax, gelatin, or other material. The antirachitic vitamin (vitamin D) in the form of irradiated ergosterol is also included as an additive in some mixed feeds for poultry, swine, and young calves.

Vitamin E (or α-tocopherol) is less common as

an added vitamin. Certain feeds may also contain menadione, the synthetic antihemorrhagic vitamin.

Amino acids. Methionine (α-aminomethylthiobutyric acid) is the only pure amino acid now being manufactured at a price low enough to permit its use as an additive in commercial rations. This amino acid has been added to some mixed feeds for poultry and swine. It has little or no application in ruminants' feed since rumen microorganisms can synthesize methionine from other amino compounds and sulfur compounds.

Fat. With a growing surplus of by-product animal fats in the United States, prices of tallows and greases have fallen to levels which make it practical to add limited quantities to livestock feeds. From 2 to 5% of the fat, stabilized by addition of an approved antioxidant, is added to some formula feeds. The added fat, in addition to its nutritional value, reduces dustiness of the feed, helps to reduce abrasion of machinery, and reduces the cost of pelleted feeds. The addition of fat to swine rations is less popular since it tends to increase the proportion of carcass fat, which is undesirable. Addition of greases also produces soft, undesirable pork carcasses.

Mineral additives. The addition of calcium and phosphorus in various mineral mixtures has been common practice for many years. Ground limestone or oyster shells have been the principal sources of calcium, while various forms of calcium phosphate, such as bone meal and defluorinated rock phosphate, furnish phosphorus as well as calcium. Iodinated salt is widely used in mixed feeds and salt blocks. Unless the iodine is present in some stable form, such as iodate or as an iodide protected from oxidation by a covering material, its presence in a mixed feed is temporal. Claims have been made for some types of organic iodine compounds as superior sources of nutritional iodine. Following the discoveries that certain mineral elements in trace amounts were essential for the animals' nutrition, there has been widespread addition, at low cost, of small quantities of salts of all trace elements (iron, copper, manganese, zinc, and cobalt) to formula feeds for all types of livestock.

Hormonelike substances. Hormones are specific chemical substances produced by living cells in limited areas of the organism. They are generally liberated into the bloodstream and carried to other parts of the body, where they produce specific effects. A number of synthetic chemical substances not produced in nature have hormonelike effects. Some of these synthetic substances added to rations of livestock in very small amounts have appeared to stimulate gains. One such substance is diethylstilbestrol, an estrogen. Another group of hormonelike substances affects the thyroid gland and its production of thyroxine. Iodinated casein may produce a slight hyperthyroidism, whereas a goitrogen such as thiouracil produces a hypothyroidism.

Tranquilizers. This term applies to a series of drugs which produce a sedative or calming action without enforcement of sleep. Certain of these compounds have been fed orally in experimental rations of livestock because the claim has been made that their tranquilizing effect causes greater weight gains. The two substances most generally used are reserpine (trimethoxybenzoylmethyl reserpate) and hydroxyzine. *See* NUTRITION.

[HAROLD GOSS]

Bibliography: E. W. Crampton and L. E. Harris, *Applied Animal Nutrition: The Use of Feedstuffs in the Formulation of Livestock Rations*, 2d ed., 1969; E. W. Crampton and L. E. Lloyd, *Fundamentals of Nutrition*, 1960; R. Ewing, *Poultry Nutrition*, 1963; L. A. Maynard and J. K. Loosli, *Animal Nutrition*, 6th ed., 1969; E. J. Underwood, *Trace Elements in Human and Animal Nutrition*, 3d ed., 1971.

Anthrax

An acute infectious disease, primarily of animals from which man may be secondarily infected. It is caused by *Bacillus anthracis*, a spore-forming bacterium. In animals the disease, known as splenic fever, occurs when spores of *B. anthracis* are eaten with forage. Man contracts the disease by contact with infected animals or animal products, such as bone meal, meat, hide, and fur.

Cause. *B. anthracis* is gram-positive, rod-shaped, $3-8\ \mu$ in length by $1-1.2\ \mu$ in diameter, and belongs to the family Bacillaceae. In infected animals, the microorganism occurs as chains of $2-8$ bacilli surrounded by a large capsule (see illustration). When grown on artificial media, the chains contain more bacilli, and the capsule is lost. Under conditions unfavorable for growth, the bacilli form small, ellipsoidal spores which are very resistant to temperature extremes and to dehydration. The spores, which remain capable of growth for about 12 years, are ingested by animals grazing on pastureland contaminated with the droppings of sick animals. The spore capsule contains polyglutamic acid. This, plus an extracellular toxin which produces edema, combats the host defense mechanism. The toxin may later kill the host by producing secondary shock.

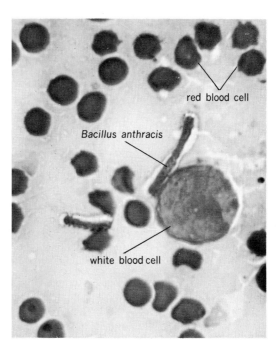

Photomicrograph of blood from a sheep that died of anthrax (splenic fever). (*USDA*)

In animals (splenic fever). The most susceptible animals are herbivora, especially cattle, sheep, pigs, horses, and goats. Usually septicemia, or blood poisoning, occurs. The effects vary from a sudden apoplectic attack (with death occurring a few minutes after the appearance of the first symptoms) to a subacute but eventually fatal illness manifesting fever, an enlarged spleen, and frequently intestinal disturbances. Sometimes local manifestations, which are less often fatal, occur. For example, in cattle and horses circumscribed cutaneous carbuncles may appear, and in swine similar lesions are commonly found in the throat.

In man. The disease in man occurs almost exclusively from contact with animals or animal products. It takes three main forms: malignant pustule, pulmonary anthrax, and intestinal anthrax.

Malignant pustule (cutaneous anthrax), the commonest form, results from contamination of the skin. An area of inflammation forms and necroses in the center which becomes brown, purplish, or black, and is surrounded by an area of edema and by vesicles containing yellow fluid. There is no true pus and little pain. Fatality is low and occurs only if generalized septicemia ensues.

Pulmonary anthrax (wool-sorter's disease) is caused by the inhalation of dust containing spores. Patchy areas form in the lungs. These areas hemorrhage and become solid, the hilar lymph nodes are enlarged, septicemia develops, and, if diagnosis is not made early, death follows.

Intestinal anthrax may follow the eating of infected food. Carbunclelike lesions in the ileum and cecum have been noted; the intestine also shows local areas of hemorrhage. A septicemia develops and death follows if an early diagnosis is not made.

The two latter types of anthrax are rare but almost invariably fatal. Treatment is difficult because of the short period of time between onset of symptoms and death.

Immunization, diagnosis, and therapy. Live spores of attenuated virulence form an effective vaccine for cattle and other animals. A cell-free protective vaccine has been produced for use in man. This vaccine is a sterile filtrate from a culture of *B. anthracis* grown in a chemically known medium with controlled incubation time and temperature.

The disease is diagnosed by microscopic identification of bacteria in the blood and by the Ascoli thermoprecipitin test. In the Ascoli test, a precipitate forms when a boiled saline extract of infected tissue is added to a suitable immune serum.

If used early, penicillin and streptomycin cure anthrax.

[HARRY SMITH]

Antioxidant

An inhibitor which is effective in preventing oxidation by molecular oxygen (autoxidation). Such inhibitors have great commercial significance in the preservation of food and food products and in the prevention of deterioration of petroleum products, rubber, and plastics.

Autoxidations are free-radical chain reactions characterized by the interaction of the radicals with oxygen to yield peroxy radicals, organic peroxides, and a broad spectrum of stable oxygenated products. The latter, in the case of foods, are usually of unpleasant taste and odor and render the food unpalatable. It is of interest that antioxidants for foods were known and used long before their function was appreciated. Spices from the Orient served not only to mask unpleasant tastes and odors, but also to prevent the reactions which led to their formation. Modern studies have shown that sage, cloves, oregano, rosemary, and thyme, to name but a few, prevent peroxide development and increase the stability of fats toward oxidation. The active constituents in these spices are phenolic compounds. The autoxidation of gasoline yields gums which foul internal combustion engine fuel systems and which increase combustion chamber deposits. These results increase the octane requirement for the engine. The autoxidation of lubricating oils yields acidic products which accelerate corrosion and engine wear. Oxidation of rubber and plastic products causes chain fission with resultant loss of strength. Discoloration often accompanies this degradation. Hydrocarbon polymers such as polyethylene and polypropylene are particularly subject to such attack and require the addition of appropriate antioxidants to give satisfactory performance. *See* SPICE AND FLAVORING.

Mechanism of autoxidation. The reaction of hydrocarbons and their oxidized derivatives with oxygen at low temperatures can be summarized by the reactions shown in Eqs. (1), (2), and (3).

$$RH + O_2 \rightarrow R\bullet + HO_2 \qquad (1)$$
$$R\bullet + O_2 \rightarrow ROO\bullet \qquad (2)$$
$$ROO\bullet + RH \rightarrow ROOH + R\bullet \qquad (3)$$

The initiation reaction (1) is uncertain, but it is definite that some such process must intervene to produce alkyl radicals ($R\cdot$). Attack is directed at the most labile C—H linkage. In order of reactivity these linkages are allyl > benzyl > tertiary alkyl > secondary alkyl > primary alkyl > aryl. Ample proof exists for the succeeding steps (2) and (3). The free radical $R\cdot$ is regenerated by reaction (3) and repeats the cycle (2) and (3) indefinitely, giving rise to a chain reaction. It is stopped when $R\cdot$ is consumed in some competing reaction. Both the peroxy radical ($ROO\cdot$) and the hydroperoxide ($ROOH$) may undergo further reaction to yield more stable oxidized products. These may be alcohols, aldehydes, ketones, acids, and esters. The peroxides themselves, though often used as catalysts for autoxidations and other free-radical chain reactions, can be inert reaction products at relatively low temperatures. Under these conditions, hydroperoxides may function as nonchain oxidants by reaction with aldehydes and olefins present to yield acids and epoxides.

Autoxidation chains are often long, so that a single initiating event may produce many stable product molecules. Thus only a very small amount of an effective antioxidant need be employed for the protection of a large quantity of a substrate. The role of the antioxidant is to provide an alternate path for oxidation which does not involve the substrate. The antioxidant is destroyed in the process and thus does not function indefinitely.

Interruption of the autoxidation chain by an antioxidant takes place at the peroxy radical stage of the chain. Proof of this mechanism was the demonstration that inhibitor (In) efficiency is independent of oxygen partial pressure. The inhibited oxidation process then becomes the reactions shown in Eqs. (1) and (2), followed by that of Eq. (4) in place of

ROO• + In→
stabilized radical or stable product   (4)

Eq. (3). In this way, the chain-carrying radical (R·) is not regenerated as long as antioxidant remains.

The critical features of oxidation inhibition are the relative reactivity of the antioxidant and the substrate toward the peroxy radical, the stability of the initial product of the radical antioxidant reaction, and the number of radicals with which a given quantity of inhibitor will interact. The first two features determine the efficiency of the inhibition; the third feature determines how long a given quantity of antioxidant will be effective.

Many naturally occurring substances contain antioxidants in their crude states. These inhibitors produce an induction period in autoxidations. During this induction period, absorption of oxygen by the substrate may be so slow as to escape observation. Upon exhaustion of the inhibitor, however, the rate of oxidation quickly increases to a steady level. This level is the same as that for steady-state oxidation of the purified substrate. The length of the induction period observed when an antioxidant is added to a purified substrate has been used extensively as a criterion of antioxidant effectiveness. A quantitative comparison of the relative efficiencies of a series of inhibitors involves a determination of the rate of oxygen absorption during the initial stages of the inhibition period. The efficiency, when measured by this technique, varies considerably with the nature of the antioxidant, as shown in the table.

Types and action of antioxidants. The study of the kinetics of inhibitor action, together with isolation and identification of the products of oxidation of antioxidants has led to the scheme for inhibition shown in Eqs. (5) and (6).

$$ROO• + InH \rightleftarrows ROOH + In \quad (5)$$
$$In• + ROO• \rightarrow InOOR \quad (6)$$

Products of the oxidation of some typical antioxidants are shown in Fig. 1.

The major types of antioxidants now in use are the phenols, the aromatic amines, sulfur compounds, and a variety of naturally occurring materials. The latter find particular use in the protection of foods and cosmetics from oxidation. The structural formulas of some phenolic antioxidants

Inhibition of the oxidation of cumene at 62.5°C and 1 atm O$_2$ pressure*

Inhibitor	Relative efficiency
Phenol	1.00
2,6-Di-*tert*-butyl-*p*-cresol	3.3
Diphenylpicrylhydrazyl	1.6
4-*tert*-Butylcatechol	14.
N-Methylaniline	1.2
p-Methoxydiphenylamine	6.1
Diphenylamine	2.1
N,N'-Diphenyl-*p*-phenylenediamine	16.
p-Hydroxydiphenylamine	5.6

*G. S. Hammond et al., *J. Amer. Chem. Soc.*, 77:3238, 1955.

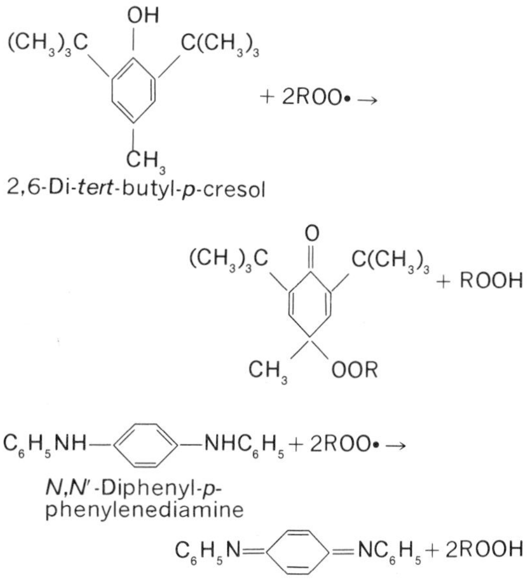

Fig. 1. Oxidation products of typical antioxidants.

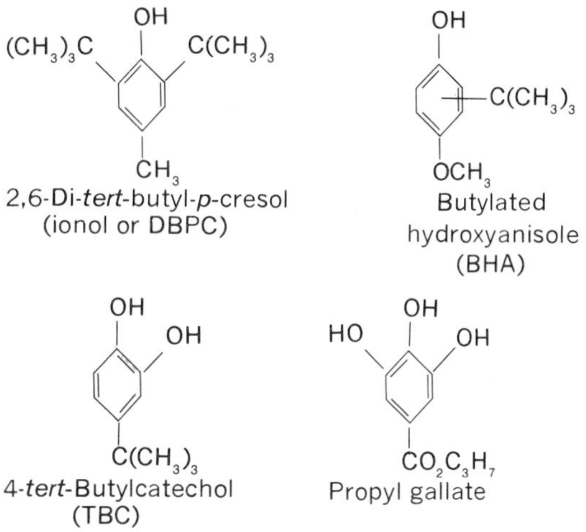

Fig. 2. Phenolic antioxidants.

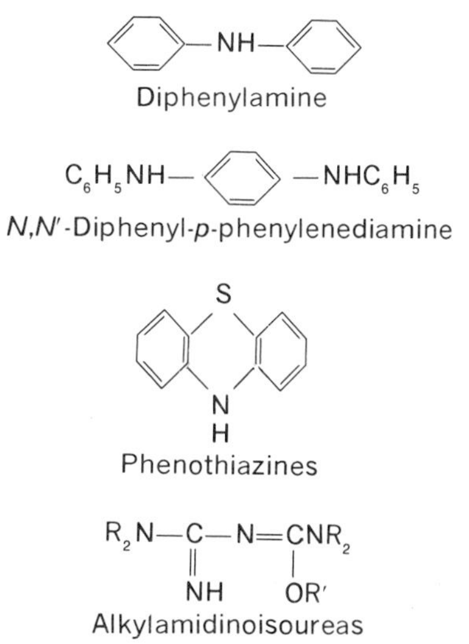

Fig. 3 Nitrogen- and sulfur-containing antioxidants.

are shown in Fig. 2, and of some nitrogen- and sulfur-containing antioxidants in Fig. 3.

Naturally occurring antioxidants include raw seed oils, wheat germ oil, tocopherols, and gums. The activity of the last-named category may often be increased by the use of synergists. These are substances which have little or no activity alone but which enhance the activity of stronger antioxidants. Some effective synergists are phosphoric, citric, and ascorbic acids.

The wide variety of antioxidants now available is necessitated by the extreme range of conditions under which protection from oxidation is required. An antioxidant which can delay the development of rancidity in stored butter will seldom prove to be suitable for the protection of hot lubricating oil in the crankcase of an automobile. The design of antioxidants for specific uses, however, is still more of an art than a science. Even the qualitative behavior of certain classes of compounds is not always predictable in this connection.

[LEE R. MAHONEY]

Bibliography: W. O. Lundberg, *Autooxidation and Antioxidants*, 2 vols., 1961–1962.

Apple

A fruit *(Malus domestica*, also designated *M. malus, M. sylvestris, M. pumila,* and *Pyrus malus)* which is native to western Asia or eastern Europe. Apples were grown by the Greeks as early as the 4th century B.C.

By the time America was discovered, apples were central and northern Europe's most important cultivated fruit. Early explorers and settlers from Europe brought the apple to North America, where it was further spread by explorers, Indians, and pioneer settlers.

Distribution in North America. Apples are produced commercially in 35 states, as well as in Mexico and Canada, but the apple does not grow well in regions having either long, hot summers or temperatures below −20°F (−29°C).

Principal apple-growing areas in the United States are the Okanogan, Wenatchee, and Yakima valleys in Washington; Sebastapol and Watsonville areas of California; Champlain and Hudson valleys of eastern New York; western New York; western Michigan; Appalachian regions of Pennsylvania, Maryland, West Virginia, Virginia, and North Carolina; and important but lesser production in New England, New Jersey, Ohio, Indiana, Illinois, Oregon, Idaho, and Colorado. The major production areas in Canada are Nova Scotia, the Niagara Peninsula of Ontario, and the Okanagan Valley of British Columbia.

Varieties. Most early apple trees developed from seed, but grafted varieties were known by the middle of the 17th century. Superior types were selected from thousands of seedlings. Nearly all the major varieties grown today originated as chance seedlings before 1900. Delicious (see illustration), Golden Delicious, McIntosh, Rome Beauty, Jonathan, York Imperial, Stayman Winesap, Winesap, Cortland, and Rhode Island Greening account for over 85% of United States apple production, more than half of which is contributed by Delicious and Golden Delicious.

Propagation and rootstocks. Since apple varieties do not come true from seed, scions of desired varieties are budded or grafted onto seedling rootstocks or onto clonal (standardized) rootstocks. The seedling rootstocks are grown from seed of native apples of Europe (such as French Crab) or from the standard varieties (such as Golden Delicious). The clonal rootstocks are often dwarfing types, usually Malling (M) or Malling-Merton (MM) rootstocks from East Malling, England.

Most varieties propagated on seedling rootstocks become large trees, whereas the "dwarfing" stocks of East Malling may result in a small garden tree about 6 ft (1.8 m) tall or an intermediate-sized tree similar in size to a peach tree.

Culture. The apple may be grown in a wide range of conditions but it does best in deep, well-aerated loam soils which have abundant supplies of irrigation water or rainfall during the growing season. Apples are highly subject to spring frost injury and therefore should be planted on frost-free sites or in areas with minimum susceptibility to late spring freezes.

Year-old nursery trees on seedling rootstocks are planted with the bud (graft) union 1–2 in. (2.5–5.0 cm) below ground level. The bud union for dwarf trees must be placed above the soil level or the scion may root and the dwarf character of the tree may be lost. The newly planted trees should be pruned to a whip about 30 in. (76 cm) above the ground. In subsequent years, it is best to train the tree to a modified central leader, leaving four to five well-spaced laterals to form the permanent scaffold branches.

Tree spacings in commercial orchards range from 6 to 12 ft (1.8 to 3.6 m) for dwarfed trees to 20 to 30 ft (6 to 9 m) for standard-sized trees. Present trends are toward semidwarf trees planted at in-row spacings of 8 to 12 ft (2.4 to 3.6 m) and between-row spacings of 16 to 20 ft (4.8 to 6 m), which

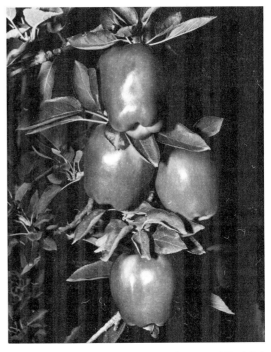

Red Delicious apple which accounts for 35% of the total United States apple production.

provides for 180 to 425 trees per acre (445 to 1050 trees per hectare).

Most commercial apple orchards are grown in grass-sod, without any cultivation. In younger orchards, grass and weed competition is removed by chemical weed control. Grass centers are mowed two or three times each season. Commercial nitrogen fertilizers are applied in nearly all apple orchards at the rate of approximately 50 lb of nitrogen per acre (57 kg per hectare), depending on the individual orchard need. In some areas apple trees need applications of other nutrients such as potassium, calcium, magnesium, boron, zinc, and sulfur. *See* FERTILIZER.

Since the first apple tree was cultivated, diseases and insects have been a constant plague. Over 80 separate diseases or insect pests cause problems in American apple orchards. Their control requires a sophisticated program of chemical sprays combined with biological protection of certain insect predators. Modern research and improved chemicals have made it possible to produce the world's highest-quality apples without injury from diseases such as apple scab or insects such as the ubiquitous apple worm (codling moth).

Sprays of hormone-type chemicals are used to thin apples in the spring, prevent preharvest drop in the fall, promote earlier flowering and fruiting, control excessive growth of young trees, enhance fruit color, and prolong fruit storage life.

Handling, storage, and marketing. Nearly all apples are picked by hand, after which they are moved in large 20-bu (0.7 m²) bins into warehouses for grading, packaging, and storage. Apples may be stored in regular refrigerated storage (31 to 34°F; −1 to 1°C) for approximately six months or in controlled-atmosphere storage for nearly a year. Controlled atmosphere storages are airtight, refrigerated rooms where carbon dioxide and oxygen can be controlled to ensure maximum extension of an apple's life and quality. Prior to controlled atmosphere storage the bulk of the United States fresh apple crop had to be marketed in the fall and winter. Now, about 40% of fresh market apples can be held in controlled atmosphere, thus providing a year-round quality apple.

Production and utilization. During 1972–1976, 61% of the United States apple crop was marketed fresh, 19% canned, 4% frozen or dried, and 16% for juice or cider. The average commercial production for the same period was 3,239,000 short tons (2,912,000 metric tons), of which Washington produced 29%, New York 13%, and Michigan 10%. *See* FRUIT, TREE. [R. PAUL LARSEN]

Bibliography: N. F. Childers, *Modern Fruit Science*, 5th ed., 1973; R. P. Larsen, The quiet revolution in the apple orchard, *U.S. Department of Agriculture Yearbook of Agriculture*, 1975.

Apricot

Prunus armeniaca, a stone fruit, or drupe, related to peaches, plums, and cherries (see illustration). It is orange or yellow, about 1¼ to 2 in. (3 to 5 cm) in diameter, and has a characteristic sweet rich flavor. It originated in China and spread across Asia to Europe, the Americas, and Australia. There are other, closely related species in Asia, but the important cultivars have come from *P. armeniaca*.

Production. Although apricots are grown commercially on every continent, Europe is first in production and North America is second. Statistics are not available for the Soviet Union and China, but production in these countries is believed to be considerable. In 1972, 116,000 metric tons were produced in the United States, compared with 159,000 tons in Spain and 101,000 tons in France. Total world production in countries from which data were available was 741,000 tons.

Cultivation. The climatic requirements of apricots are rather narrow. They will withstand slightly lower temperatures in the winter than peaches, but they also must be exposed to a longer period of low temperatures than many peach varieties before they will start to grow normally in the spring. They are usually not grown where winter temperatures are lower than −10 to −15°F (−23 to −26°C), or where there are fewer than approximately 700 hr of temperature below 45°F (7°C). Apricots are the earliest of the tree fruits to bloom in the spring and are thus frequently injured by late spring frosts. In areas where such frosts occur regularly, apricots should not be grown. They require warm weather to properly mature, but exhibit a form of injury called pit burn when the fruit matures in hot weather. The apricot will withstand drought better than many fruits, but it requires a steady supply of moisture for good production. When grown in humid climates, brown rot, a fungus disease very difficult to control, may develop. For this reason, most apricots are grown in dry climates but under irrigation.

Use and varieties. Apricots are used as fresh fruit or are canned, dried, or frozen. Of the total 1976 crop, 8% was used fresh, 75% canned, 14% dried, and 3% frozen. The chief cultivars grown in

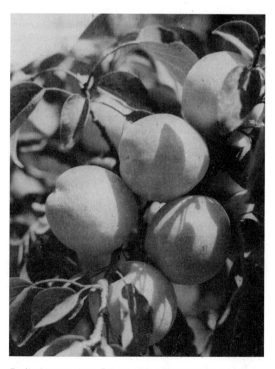

Fruit of the apricot, *Prunus armeniaca*, showing the manner in which the fruit is borne and the leaves. (*New York State Agricultural Experiment Station, Geneva*)

California, the largest-producing state, are Tilton, Royal, and Blenheim. Some apricots have sweet kernels that can be eaten like almonds; other varieties have bitter-tasting kernels. The bitter taste is amygdalin which is poisonous, and these kernels should not be eaten. Most of the varieties grown in the United States have bitter pits.

Research at several agricultural experiment stations in the United States and Canada is being carried on with a view to producing varieties which are better adapted to colder areas. Blenril, Earliril, Rival, and Goldgiant from Washington, Goldcot from Michigan, Veecot and Viceroy from Ontario, Skaha and Sundrop from British Columbia, and Alfred and Farmingdale from New York are some of these newer varieties. They have not been tested sufficiently to determine their economic importance.   [ROBERT C. LAMB]

Apricot and almond diseases. These two closely related fruits are affected by many of the same diseases. The almond (*P. amygdalus*) is a stone fruit in which the seed is eaten instead of the flesh. *See* ALMOND.

Even under relatively arid conditions, brown rot caused by the fungus *Monilinia laxa* is a major problem. Losses result from blighting of the blossoms and twigs in the spring. Before the buds open, a solution containing monocalcium arsenite is sprayed on the apricot trees, and sodium pentachlorophenate is sprayed on the almonds to control this disease. For additional protection sprays containing copper compounds are used after the buds open. *See* FUNGISTAT AND FUNGICIDE.

The fungus *Coryneum beijerinckii*, causing pustular spot or coryneum blight, defoliates the trees and spots the fruit. This serious disease is controlled by spraying with copper fungicides during the dormant period. *See* FUNGI.

Bacterial canker, caused by *Pseudomonas syringae*, and the fungus root rots, caused by *Armillaria mellea* and *Dematophora necatrix*, are other destructive diseases. No effective, economical control measures are available for the root rots. *See* BACTERIA.

The virus diseases, ring pox, almond calico, and drake bud failure, affect commercial production by reducing the size and quality of the crop. Removal of affected trees and use of bud wood from virus-free trees retard the spread of these virus diseases. *See* FRUIT, TREE; FRUIT (TREE) DISEASES; PLANT DISEASE CONTROL; PLANT VIRUS.

[JOHN C. DUNEGAN]

Arginine

An amino acid. The amino acids are characterized physically by the following: (1) the pK_1, or the dissociation constant of the various titratable groups; (2) the isoelectric point, or pH at which a dipolar ion does not migrate in an electric field; (3) the optical rotation, or the rotation imparted to a beam of plane-polarized light (frequently the D line of the sodium spectrum) passing through 1 dm of a solution of 100 g in 100 ml; and (4) solubility.

Arginine forms a red color when treated with sodium hypochlorite and α-naphthol (Sakaguchi reaction). The amino acid's special functions are: (1) Arginine is an intermediate in the process of urea formation from ammonia and carbon dioxide, by virtue of its position in the urea cycle. Arginine is cleaved to ornithine and urea: The former ac-

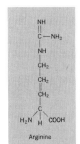

Physical constants of the L isomer at 25°C:
pK_1 (COOH): 2.17; pK_2 (NH₃⁺): 9.04; pK_3 (NH₃⁺): 12.48
Isoelectric point: 10.76
Optical rotation: [α]$_D$(H₂O): +12.5; [α]$_D$(5 N HCl): +27.6
Solubility (g/100 ml H₂O): 15.0 (21°C)

cepts ammonia and carbon dioxide to form arginine again. The net result of the cycle is the formation of urea from two molecules of ammonia plus one of carbon dioxide. (2) Arginine is probably the source of the guanidine groups of streptomycin.

The biosynthesis of arginine starts with glutamic acid and proceeds by way of ornithine and citrulline. The metabolic degradation begins with the hydrolysis of arginine to ornithine and urea. Ornithine can be deaminated to glutamic acid semialdehyde. This compound is oxidized to glutamic acid, which is catabolized via α-ketoglutaric acid and the Krebs cycle. *See* AMINO ACIDS.

[EDWARD A. ADELBERG]

Arrowroot starch

A product derived from different plant species. Rhizomes (underground stems) of *Maranta arundinacea* in the arrowroot family (Marantaceae) of tropical America supply the West Indian arrowroot. Florida arrowroot is the flour made from the rhizomes of the cycad, *Zamia floridana* (Cycadaceae), the Seminole bread plant. Queensland arrowroot is obtained from the edible rhizomes of *Canna edulis* (Cannaceae). The tubers of *Curcuma angustifolia* in the ginger family (Zingiberaceae) yield the East Indian arrowroot. Arrowroot starch is of no importance in the industries, but because it is very easily digested, it is valued highly as a food for infants and invalids.

[PERRY D. STRAUSBAUGH/EARL L. CORE]

Artichoke

Cynara scolymus, a herbaceous perennial plant, in the family Compositae; also called globe artichoke. Its origin is in the Mediterranean region. Artichoke requires a mild winter and cool summer with fog and little bright sunshine. It is a delicacy in Europe, Africa, and North and South America. Artichoke is also a medicinal plant; it is rich in the cynarin and ortho phinols constituents. There are 273,626 acres (110,718 ha) planted worldwide, of which 56%, 14%, and 12% are planted in Italy, France, and Spain, respectively.

The marketable portion of the plant, the so-called bud, is actually the immature flower head, made up of numerous closely overlaid bracts or scales (see illustration). The edible portion consists of the tender bases of the bracts, the young flowers, and the receptacle or fleshy base upon which the flowers are borne. The bud can be various shapes, from round to oblong to flat, and the color can be light green to dark green, often with purple or red.

Artichoke is grown readily from seed, but the seedlings are highly variable and plants tend to throw back to the wild; hence, vegetative propaga-

ARTICHOKE

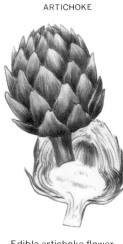

Edible artichoke flower heads. The bottom one is shown in cross section.

tion by means of stumps (rootstocks), offshoots, or ovoli is recommended. The latter two are believed to produce earlier crops. The plant grows to a height of 3 or 4 ft (0.9 or 1.2 m), and sends up seasonal shoots from a permanent crown—as many as 12 or more in plants that are 4 or 5 years old. Each shoot forms a cluster of large basal or rosette leaves, from the center of which the stem grows. Buds are produced terminally on this elongated stem and on the lateral branches. If the buds are not removed, they develop into purple-centered thistlelike flowers and viable seeds are produced.

In the United States, artichokes are grown in the Pacific Coast area between south San Francisco and Los Angeles, mainly Monterey County, where there are about 10,000 acres (4050 ha), with total annual value of $12,000,000. The production per acre fluctuates according to weather conditions. The average production is 200 to 400 boxes, 22.5 lb (10 kg) each, averaging 6750 lb per acre (7500 kg/ha).   [ALY M. IBRAHIM]

Ascorbic acid

A vitamin also known as vitamin C. It is a white crystalline compound, highly soluble in water, which is a stronger reducing agent than the hexose sugars, which it resembles chemically. Vitamin C deficiency in man has been known for centuries as scurvy. The compound has the structural formula shown in the illustration.

The stability of ascorbic acid decreases with increases in temperature and pH. This destruction by oxidation is a serious problem in that a considerable quantity of the vitamin C content of foods is lost during processing, storage, and preparation. Biological methods for estimating ascorbic acid are rarely used. The vitamin is determined chemically by making use of its reducing properties.

While vitamin C is widespread in plant materials, it is found sparingly in animal tissues. Of all the animals studied, only the guinea pig, the red vented bulbul bird, the fruit-eating bat, and the primates, including humans, require a dietary source of vitamin C. The other species studied are capable of synthesizing the vitamin in such tissues as liver and kidneys. Some drugs, particularly the terpenelike cyclic ketones, stimulate the production of ascorbic acid by rat tissues.

Vitamin C–deficient animals suffer from defects in their mesenchymal tissues. Their ability to manufacture collagen, dentine, and osteoid, the intercellular cement substances, is impaired. This may be related to a role of ascorbic acid in the formation of hydroxyproline, an amino acid found in structural proteins, particularly collagen. People with scurvy lose weight and are easily fatigued. Their bones are fragile, and their joints sore and swollen. Their gums are swollen and bloody, and in advanced stages, their teeth fall out. They also develop internal and subcutaneous hemorrhages. See SCURVY.

The biochemical role of ascorbic acid is obscure. It seems reasonable to expect that it functions metabolically in oxidation-reduction systems, since it has been shown that ascorbic acid and dehydroascorbic acid are readily interconverted in plant and animal tissues. It may also act as an antioxidant, protecting hydrogen carriers from destructive oxidation. Ascorbic acid has a role in tyrosine metabolism. It also appears to function in

the conversion of folic to folinic acid. See FOLIC ACID; TYROSINE.

There has been great difficulty in establishing the human requirements for vitamin C. Usually, vitamin requirements are based on data obtained from dietary surveys accompanied by blood or urine analyses and often by saturation tests. There is evidence that vitamin C may play roles in stress reactions, infectious disease, or in wound healing. Therefore, many nutritionists believe that the human intake of ascorbic acid should be many times more than that intake level which produces deficiency symptoms.

The recommended dietary allowances of the Food and Nutrition Board of the National Research Council are 30 mg per day for 1- to 3-month infants, 80 mg per day for growing boys and girls, and 100 mg per day for pregnant and lactating women. These values represent an intake which tends to maintain tissue and plasma concentrations in a range similar to that of other well-nourished species of animals. The Accessory Food Factors Subcommittee of the British Medical Research Council does not believe that a dietary intake of more than 30 mg per day has beneficial effects. See VITAMIN.   [STANLEY N. GERSHOFF]

Industrial production. Most processes for the large-scale synthesis of ascorbic acid follow the method proposed by T. Reichstein. Technical dextrose is hydrogenated to sorbital. Biological oxidation converts sorbitol to sorbose. The next step is diacetone sorbose, which is oxidized to diacetone gulosonic acid. Diacetone gulosonic acid is hydrolyzed to gulosonic acid. The methyl ester of the latter is reacted with sodium methylate to form the sodium salt of ascorbic acid.

[WERNER A. LINDENMAIER]

Asparagine

An amino acid. The amino acids are characterized physically by the following: (1) the pK_1, or the dissociation constant of the various titratable groups; (2) the isoelectric point, or pH at which a dipolar ion does not migrate in an electric field; (3) the opt-

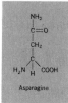

Physical constants of the L isomer at 25°C:
pK_1 (COOH): 2.02; pK_2 (NH_3^+): 8.80
Isoelectric point: 5.41
Optical rotation: $[\alpha]_D(H_2O)$: −5.3; $[\alpha]_D$(3 N HCl): +33.2
Solubility (g/100 ml H_2O): 3.11 (28°C)

ical rotation, or the rotation imparted to a beam of plane-polarized light (frequently the D line of the sodium spectrum) passing through 1 dm of a solution of 100 g in 100 ml; and (4) solubility.

Asparagine forms a brown color with ninhydrin. The amide group of asparagine presumably serves as a storage site for nitrogen, especially in plants. Although it is known that asparagine is formed biosynthetically from aspartic acid, it is not certain whether the mechanism involves amide transfer from glutamine, transamination, or ammonia incorporation. Asparagine is deamidated to aspartic acid, which is further catabolized by way of oxaloacetic acid and the Krebs cycle. See AMINO ACIDS.

[EDWARD A. ADELBERG]

ASCORBIC ACID

The structural formula of ascorbic acid.

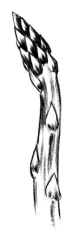

The top of a spear of asparagus.

Asparagus

A dioecious perennial monocot (*Asparagus officinalis*) of Mediterranean origin belonging to the plant order Liliales. Asparagus is grown for its young shoots or spears, which are canned, frozen, or cooked fresh as a vegetable (see illustration). These aerial stems arise from rhizomes (underground stems). The rhizomes and the fleshy and fibrous roots constitute the massive underground part of the plant.

Propagation. Asparagus is propagated by seed with 1-year-old crowns transplanted to the field and spaced 8–18 in. apart in 4–8-ft rows. Although male plants outyield female plants, separating crowns on the basis of sex has not been economical. Mary Washington is the principal variety cultivated; several new varieties developed by the University of California are widely planted. Blanched or white asparagus is grown by ridging soil over the rows and cutting the spears beneath the soil surface. Chemical weed control is commonly used.

Harvesting. The length of the annual harvest season varies with age of the crowns and with climatic conditions. Generally, spears are cut for 8–10 weeks each spring after the crowns are 3–4 years old. In areas with longer growing seasons, such as California, harvesting begins earlier and continues 10–12 weeks. Commercial plantings are often harvested for 12–16 years. In most areas special knives are used for harvesting; however, spears for canning and freezing are sometimes snapped off by hand above the ground level. Several types of mechanical harvesters are now in commercial use.

Commercial production is limited to areas where crowns will have a dormant period of 3–5 months each year. Dormancy in the northern states is induced by low temperatures and in California by withholding irrigation. California, New Jersey, and Washington are important asparagus-producing states. The total annual farm value in the United States from approximately 140,000 acres is approximately $50,000,000. *See* VEGETABLE GROWING.

[H. JOHN CAREW]

Aspartic acid

An amino acid. The amino acids are characterized physically by the following: (1) the pK_1, or the dissociation constant of the various titratable groups; (2) the isoelectric point, or pH at which a dipolar ion does not migrate in an electric field; (3) the opt-

COOH
CH₂
|
C
H₂N   H   COOH

Aspartic acid

Physical constants of the L isomer at 25°C:
pK_1 (COOH): 1.88; pK_2 (COOH): 3.65; pK_3 (NH_3^+): 9.60
Isoelectric point: 2.77
Optical rotation: $[\alpha]_D(H_2O)$: +5.0; $[\alpha]_D(5\ N\ HCl)$: +25.4
Solubility (g/100 ml H_2O): 0.50

ical rotation, or the rotation imparted to a beam of plane-polarized light (frequently the D line of the sodium spectrum) passing through 1 dm of a solution of 100 g in 100 ml; and (4) solubility.

Aspartic acid forms an alcohol-insoluble calcium salt. The amino acid functions are as follows: (1) It

Carbamyl phosphate   Aspartic acid

Carbamyl aspartate

Dihydroorotic acid

Chemical reaction to form pyrimidines.

is a key intermediate in many transamination reactions and is a product of ammonia incorporation in plants and some microorganisms (the aspartase-catalyzed reaction: fumaric acid + ammonia → aspartic acid). (2) It functions as a source (from the amino group) of one of the ring nitrogens of purines and of the amino group of adenylic acid.

Aspartic acid also undergoes reaction with carbamyl phosphate to form carbamyl aspartate, a precursor of pyrimidines (see illustration). (3) Aspartic acid can be amidated to form asparagine; it is also the biosynthetic precursor of methionine, threonine, isoleucine, and, in bacteria, of lysine. *See* AMINO ACIDS; ISOLEUCINE; LYSINE; METHIONINE; THREONINE.

Aspartic acid is formed, biosynthetically, by transamination of oxaloacetate or by the addition of ammonia to fumaric acid.

The metabolic degradation pathway is by deamination to oxaloacetate, or by decarboxylation. Two different decarboxylases are known, one forming α-alanine, the other β-alanine.

[EDWARD A. ADELBERG]

Atmospheric pollution

Air pollutants of various types adversely affect living organisms, both animals and plants, and also cause deterioration of inanimate materials such as stone, metal, rubber, paint, and fabric. Pollutants within an atmospheric system must exist in sufficient concentrations and remain long enough to have an adverse effect on biological organisms or on other materials. Thus, particular pollution problems frequently occur within regions or areas where severity and incidence depend upon a number of factors.

NATURE OF POLLUTION

Air pollutants can be in the form of particulates, aerosols, or gases in varying concentrations and combinations mixed in the air.

Origin of pollutants. There are many natural sources of air pollutants. Biological decay and metabolic respiration release H_2S, N_2O, NH_3, and CO_2; forest fires and reactions involving terpene which is formed from plant vegetation release appreciable amounts of CO; oceans serve as relatively large sources of CO_2 and CO, with ocean spray releasing particulate sulfur; bacterial activity in soil releases NO and NO_2; air turbulence transfers ozone from higher altitudes to the Earth's surface; and volcanoes emit H_2S and considerable amounts of SO_2, although amounts of SO_2 from volcanic activity are negligible compared with those released by human technology. Many of these natural pollution sources far overshadow human activity in amounts of pollutants released into the atmosphere. However, because natural sources are widely dispersed and usually are not released near human population centers, their effects may not be readily apparent.

Pollutants resulting primarily from human activity and causing greatest concern include oxides of sulfur and nitrogen, photochemical oxidants, and fluorides. Many other pollutants of less importance may under given conditions cause considerable damage.

These human-caused air pollutants result primarily from the transfer of energy from fossil fuels for transportation, heat, light, and so on, and from the conversion of raw products into usable materials such as in smelting, electrolysis, and ceramic and glass manufacture. Air pollution is becoming a burden to the economy of nations, and costs must be assessed not only by evaluating direct detrimental effects on agricultural production, animal and plant health, and deterioration of materials, but also by considering expenses for various pollution abatement control practices and the high cost of fuels of relatively low pollution potential.

Pollutants may originate at a point source such as a power plant or a smelter. Other pollutants such as those emitted by internal combustion engines originate from many sources, with the result that high concentrations may be distributed over wide areas. Pollutants may in their original state be relatively innocuous, but become much more toxic after chemical transformation in the atmosphere. This is particularly true of the photochemical oxidants, in which sunlight transforms precursor compounds through complex chemical reactions into ozone, peroxyacetyl nitrate (PAN), and related compounds.

Distribution of pollutants. Atmospheric conditions and land configuration affect the distribution and accumulation of air pollutants within limited to relatively large geographical areas. They also influence long-distance transport. Atmospheric drainage patterns associated with valleys, fiords, deep canyons, or land basins tend to confine pollutants to such areas. Accumulation of toxicants within these locations may damage agricultural crops and impair human health.

Normal convection currents associated with daily warming and cooling of land masses as well as winds usually disperse and dilute pollutants to nontoxic levels. Winds may also cause long-distance transport of pollutants so that they are present in toxic concentrations many kilometers from their source. Prevailing winds may move pollu-

tants so that injury becomes progressively less severe away from the point source. Many pollutants are emitted from tall smokestacks. Thus, they may not be returned to the land surface until they have been transported considerable distances.

Inversions are of at least two types: ground inversions with warm layers of air above a cool land surface; and subsidence inversions associated with relatively large, high-atmospheric-pressure areas. Inversions inhibit vertical air currents and can also impair horizontal air movement. These conditions entrap pollutants and provide stagnant air in which toxicants accumulate to damaging concentrations. Because of this, "episodes" of air pollution (periods of a few days, usually less than a week, characterized by high concentrations of pollutants) may be present only once or twice during the growing season, or they may be separated by years. Damage to plants, animals, or humans may be slight or severe depending upon a number of factors, including concentration of pollutants, environmental conditions, duration of exposure, and stage of growth during the episode.

The term "sink" refers to mechanisms which remove pollutants from the atmosphere or transform them into less toxic materials. Sinks include physical mechanisms such as solubility in rain, lake, or sea water; dilution in the larger air masses; and absorption or adsorption to surfaces of soil, plants, and solids; as well as microbiological action in soils and chemical reactions in which the pollutant is modified. Because of these factors, the "residence time," or length of time pollutants survive in the atmosphere, ranges from a few days for many pollutants to years for others.

Diagnosis of damage. Considerably more information is available concerning air pollution damage to plants than to animals because plant damage is more readily observed and better documented. Accurate diagnosis of air-pollution injury to plants is difficult because of differences in plant response to dosage intensity, duration, frequency, stage of plant growth at time of exposure, environmental stress, varietal and species differences in sensitivity or tolerance, and similarities of symptoms between the several pollutants. Another complicating factor is symptom similarity with disorders caused by factors other than pollution.

Diagnosis of air pollution damage solely on the basis of symptoms is subject to many possible errors, and assessment of the extent of damage is difficult. Also, it has not yet been possible to find natural pollution-free environments to serve as controls for direct comparison with naturally polluted air under natural field conditions.

EFFECTS ON PLANTS

The following discussion describes several of the important air pollutants and their most obvious effects on plants as they are presently understood. Air pollutants enter plant leaves primarily through small openings in the leaf surface (stomata). These are usually much more numerous on the lower surface than on the upper. The mesophyll cells within the leaf are usually the first to show injury (Fig. 1).

Sulfur oxides. Damage to plant foliage by sulfur oxides has been recognized for many years. Sulfur pollution largely originates from combustion of fos-

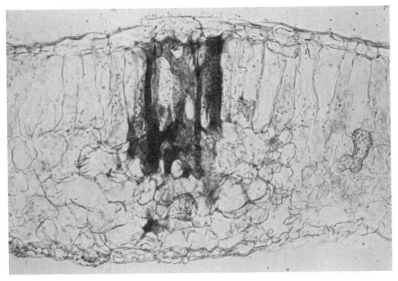

Fig. 1. Cross section of potato leaf from the field. Some of the palisade mesophyll cells have been killed by photochemical oxidants. *(From W. J. Hooker, T. C. Yang, and H. S. Potter, Air Pollution Effects on Potato and Bean in Southern Michigan, Mich. State Univ. Agr. Exp. Sta. Res. Rep. 167, 1972)*

sil fuels or smelting at point sources. Plant injury is usually most severe near and downwind from the source.

Chemical reactions involving SO_2 give rise to a number of compounds, including SO_3, H_2SO_3, and H_2SO_4, with the last existing largely as aerosol. A number of chemical pathways, including photochemical reactions, are apparently involved.

Losses to sulfur pollution of cultivated agricultural crops, home gardens, forests, and ornamental plants may be severe. Lichens and bryophytes are

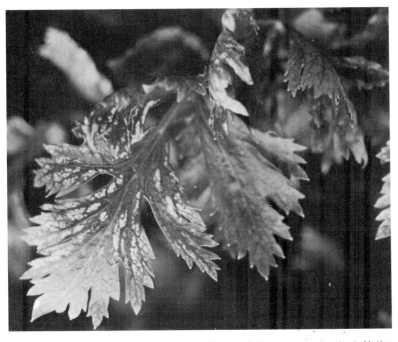

Fig. 2. Sulfur oxide injury of celery leaves from a field near a power plant. Notice characteristic interveinal bleaching and yellowing. Although the edible celery was not injured, damage to leaves reduced market value of the crop.

extremely sensitive to sulfur oxides and usually do not survive in even slightly polluted air. Differences in species tolerance are known. The presence of lichens or bryophytes on trees gives a fairly reliable indication of relatively pollutant-free air. Most higher plants are considerably more tolerant and may not show injury under conditions where lichens and bryophytes cannot survive. Damage to sensitive higher plants can result from exposures of 0.5 parts per million (ppm) SO_2 or less for 8 hr, whereas more tolerant plants require longer exposures at higher concentrations.

Chronic plant injury results from exposure to low concentrations and is evident as a mild general chlorosis and a silvering or bronzing of the lower leaf surface. The injury may somewhat resemble senescence. Leaf tissue of herbaceous plants develops acute injury between the larger veins. Tissue becomes white, appears bleached, and may become necrotic (Fig 2). In some species affected tissue becomes dark-colored. Grasses and needles of conifers typically respond by tip dieback with some cross banding of the leaf. Young conifer needles may escape injury and old needles drop prematurely. Grasses and conifers are relatively nonspecific in symptom responses, and symptoms closely resemble other types of injury not necessarily related to air pollution.

When plants are grown for the leaf crop—for example, ornamentals or leafy vegetables—losses may be severe with injury on only a few leaves. However, a similar amount of leaf injury may have little influence on the yield potential of root or fiber crops. Continual partial defoliation of forest trees results in reduced growth rates and even eventual death.

Photochemical oxidants. This heterogeneous group of chemicals is formed by the action of sunlight, particularly in the ultraviolet wavelengths, on precursors such as oxides of nitrogen or hydrocarbon radicals. These precursors are transformed by complex chemical reactions into ozone (O_3), PAN, and related compounds, all of which are highly reactive with biological materials (Figs. 3 and 4). PAN and related compounds normally are present in much lower concentrations than is ozone. However, on the basis of molecular activity they are much more injurious. Photochemical oxidants in air form smog, often seen as a heavy, cloudy haze which is irritating to the eyes. When nitrogen oxides are present in high concentration, especially in the morning before smog has become severe, a brownish-orange cast may be seen hovering over the affected area.

Nitrogen oxides are formed in high-temperature combustion processes and are chiefly produced in automobile exhausts. Compared with the several photochemical oxidants, nitrogen dioxide is relatively low in toxicity to plants, requiring for injury approximately 1000 ppm over a 1-hr exposure. However, nitrogen oxides are important because they serve as precursors for the more toxic photochemical oxidants.

Ozone injury is first evident on the upper leaf surface as small water-soaked (and later necrotic) spots, with cells of the palisade mesophyll the first to be affected. Later necrosis extends through the spongy mesophyll, and spots appear on the lower leaf surface. These spots are at first water-soaked but soon turn gray or brown. Frequently leaves become bronze-colored, later turn chlorotic, dry out, and fall from the plant. Additional symptoms of affected plants include premature senescence accompanied by losses in yield. Chronic, nonacute injury causes reduced growth rates and yield, sometimes in the absence of well-defined symptoms. For example, needles of conifers become necrotic and drop from the tree, causing dwarfing, reduced growth, and lowered productivity.

Ozone concentrations necessary to cause plant injury vary and depend on a number of factors. Levels above 80 parts per billion (ppb) for 6 hr or more are usually sufficient to cause injury in sensitive varieties of bean and tobacco. If levels recur for several days, the amount of air pollution injury is greatly increased. If ozone and sulfur dioxide are both present, they act synergistically to cause greater injury than either pollutant could produce alone. Symptoms under these circumstances usually resemble those caused by ozone.

Typical PAN injury is evident as a glazing or bleaching and, later, bronzing of the leaf undersurface associated with the collapse of spongy mesophyll cells. Usually the young leaves are most sensitive. Severely injured areas may extend as a transverse band across the leaf because sensitivity is closely related to tissue maturity at time of exposure.

Fluorides. Compounds containing fluorine are released into the atmosphere from numerous industrial processes, including production of fertilizers, ceramics, aluminum, and phosphorus-containing chemicals. Fluorides may be emitted either as gases or as particulates containing fluorine in various chemical combinations; the particulates may release water-soluble fluorine, causing injury when leaves become wet. Fluoride usually enters the leaf as a gas and may gradually accumulate until toxic levels are reached. Fluoride concentrations of 2 ppb for extended periods of time are sufficient to cause damage to leaves of many plants.

Tip burn is a common response of leaves exposed to toxic levels of fluorine, with certain varieties of gladiolus being highly sensitive. Broad-leaved plants develop dull, gray-green discoloration; at first the leaf margins are water-soaked but later turn brown. A narrow, dark brown zone less than 1 mm wide, particularly evident in apricot leaves, may develop between necrotic and healthy tissue. Sometimes the necrotic tissue may drop from the leaf, but leaf abscission is not as common as with many other pollutants. Citrus leaves frequently become chlorotic. Peach fruit develops soft suture, but factors other than fluorides can cause somewhat similar injury. Fluoride accumulation on leaf surfaces of forage crops becomes a problem because of toxicity of the forage to livestock.

Plants exposed to fluorides frequently have higher fluorine content than unexposed plants. Although this may be useful in diagnosis, high levels of fluorine do not necessarily confirm fluoride toxicity to plants. Plant responses to fluorine are variable and are determined by exposure intensity and duration; species; variety; stage of plant

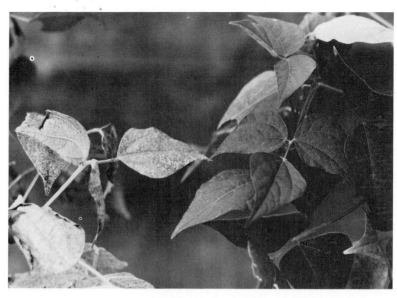

Fig. 3. Leaves of bean plants (left) grown in ambient, naturally polluted field air have been injured by photochemical oxidants. Plants (right) grown in air freed from photochemical oxidants by filtering through charcoal are unaffected. (*From W. J. Hooker, T. C. Yang, and H. S. Potter, Air Pollution Effects on Potato and Bean in Southern Michigan, Mich. State Univ. Agr. Exp. Stat. Res. Rep. 167, 1972*)

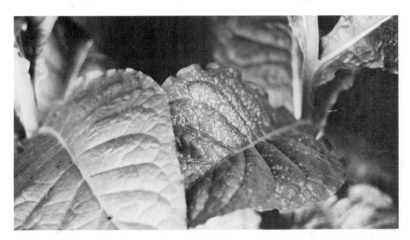

Fig. 4. Weather fleck in tobacco is caused by photochemical oxidants. The plant at left was grown in charcoal-filtered air, and the one at right showing weather fleck was grown in naturally polluted field air. (*From W. J. Hooker, T. C. Yang, and H. S. Potter, Air Pollution Effects on Potato and Bean in Southern Michigan, Mich. State Univ. Agr. Exp. Sta. Res. Rep. 167, 1972*)

growth at time of exposure; and environmental conditions, particularly water stress.

[WILLIAM J. HOOKER]

Bibliography: R. J. Bibbero and I. G. Young, *Systems Approach to Air Pollution Control*, 1974; J. S. Jacobson and A. C. Hill (eds.), *Recognition of Air Pollution Injury to Vegetation: A Pictorial Atlas*, 1970; J. B. Mudd and T. T. Kozlowski (eds.), *Responses of Plants to Air Pollution*, 1975; J. H. Seinfeld, *Air Pollution, Physical and Chemical Fundamentals*, 1975.

Auxin

The generic term originally suggested by F. Kögl and A. J. Haagen-Smit in 1931 to refer to substances which were capable of promoting plant growth in a manner similar to that of the native growth hormone. The currently accepted definition is that of an organic compound which promotes growth along the longitudinal plant axis when applied in low concentrations to shoots freed as far as practical from indigenous growth-promoting substances. Auxins may, and generally do, influence other plant systems, but the effect on plant growth is critical to characterizing an organic compound, synthetic or natural, as an auxin. *See* PLANT GROWTH.

Occurrence in plants. Demonstrations that growth-promoting substances could be extracted from plants formed the basis in the early 1940s for research on chemical characterizations of auxins. Because of the minute amounts of auxin present in plants, chemical identifications of auxins have been few and far between. It was not until 1946 that indole-3-acetic acid (IAA), now considered the most widely occurring auxin, was proven by good chemical characterization techniques to occur in higher plants. However, the presence was suspected long before this from comparative analysis between the active fractions from higher plants and IAA isolated and identified from urine and lower plants.

The advancement in knowledge of the natural occurrence of IAA and other compounds with growth-promoting activity has depended a great deal on the development of chromatography. This technique has allowed physiologists to compare the mobilities of solutes in minute quantities in several solvent systems without chemical alteration of the compounds so that subsequent biological and chemical assays are possible. By comparisons of physical characteristics during chromatography, and of microchemical and biological characteristics between growth-promoting fractions from plants and known chemicals, it has often been

possible to establish the identity of the active compound. At the present time several compounds active in the *Avena* straight-growth bioassay have been identified, including indole-3-acetic acid, indole-3-acetamide, indole-3-pyruvic acid, ethyl indole-3-acetate, 1-(indole-3-acetyl)-β-D glucose, indole-3-acetylaspartic acid, and indole-3-acetonitrile. Formulas for these compounds are reproduced in Fig. 1; the *Avena* bioassay is outlined in Fig. 2, along with a dose-response curve for IAA.

There are other bioassays for auxin activity other than just the coleoptile explant from *Avena*, such as the pea stem test, or the *Avena* curvature test. Taking these biological tests into account, several other indolic compounds can be named that have been isolated from plants and identified. A few of the others are glycosides of IAA in addition to glucose, peptides of IAA in addition to aspartate, ascorbigen, and glucobrassicin. On a chemical basis many of these compounds may have activity because they are easily converted to IAA. Whether any of the indolic compounds, other

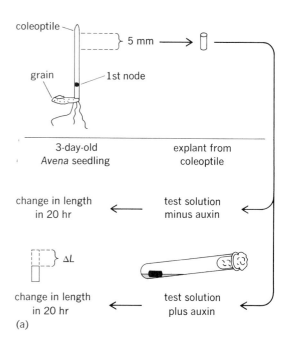

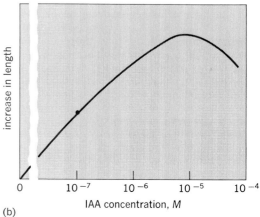

Fig. 1. Indolic compounds which have been isolated and identified from higher plants that have auxin activity in the *Avena* straight-growth bioassay.

Fig. 2. (*a*) Diagrammatic outline of the *Avena* straight-growth bioassay. (*b*) A dose-response curve for the effect of IAA on the growth of *Avena* coleoptile sections.

than IAA, have auxin activity per se is a moot question, and the final answer may depend on an understanding of the biochemical mechanism of auxin action. In addition to the indolic compounds, chromatographic studies indicate that there are other natural auxins occurring that do not possess an indolic ring structure, but these have not been identified.

The most widely isolated and identified auxin is IAA. It has been isolated from fruits, seeds, pollen, root tips, young leaves, and buds. In general, plant organs, just prior and during cellular expansion, are good sources of auxin, particularly actively growing buds. This has been one of the facts which supports the idea that IAA is a growth hormone for many of the higher plants, especially for cellular systems undergoing primarily unidirectional expansion.

Synthetic auxins. Many synthetic auxins have been produced and a great deal of information has been gleaned from studies with them, both from the standpoint of basic and applied physiology. Several examples of synthetic auxins are shown in Fig. 3. The relation of structure to activity of the auxins has received much attention in hopes of unraveling the mystery of the nature of auxin action. Three general features of the molecule are ordinarily needed for auxin activity: an unsaturated ring structure, an acidic side chain, and some spatial relationship between the two. Although there are exceptions to each of these parameters and studies of the action of auxins as related to structure have not revealed the biochemical basis for activity, much has been learned of uptake, translocation, and metabolism of auxins and of the effects of auxin on cellular metabolism. From comparative analyses of IAA and synthetic auxins, it is apparent that IAA is polarly transported in plant tissues in much greater quantities than any of the synthetic auxins studied, that IAA is not very stable in tissues, especially the highly differentiated systems, and that the action of synthetic auxins resembles that of IAA to varying extents. These and other observations have given rise to the concept that correlative growth and development of plants are very intimately involved with auxin genesis; destruction; binding to other chemicals which may take them out of the system permanently or temporarily; movement, especially polar translocation; cellular sensitivity to auxins themselves; and interaction with other chemical regulators.

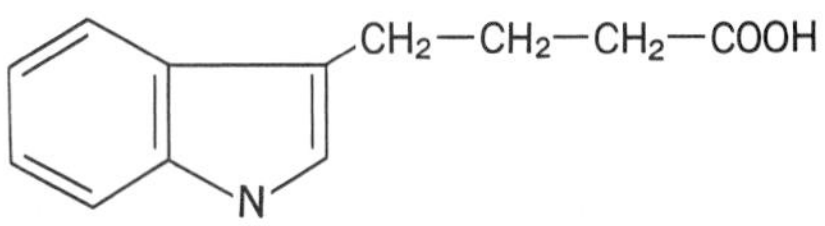

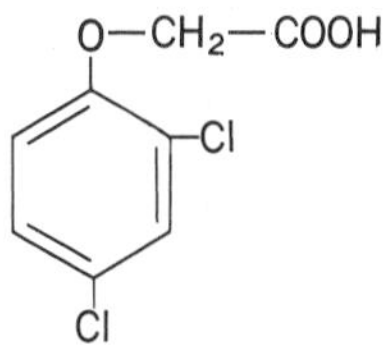

Action of auxin. Many theories have been proposed for the mechanism of action of auxin on plant tissues, but at the present time no one theory reconciles the many known facts concerning the effects of auxin on plant systems. In the case of the effects of auxin on growth, the concept of the primary site of auxin action is cloudy; but research has demonstrated some of the basic physical changes and chemical reactions at the cellular and subcellular level that occur very early in the chain of events leading to growth. Some of these are localized changes in the plasticity and elasticity of the cell wall, protoplasmic streaming, increased respiration, and alteration in the patterns of synthesis of certain macromolecules within the cell, particularly ribonucleic acids and proteins. In the case of the changes in the cell wall, there are ap-

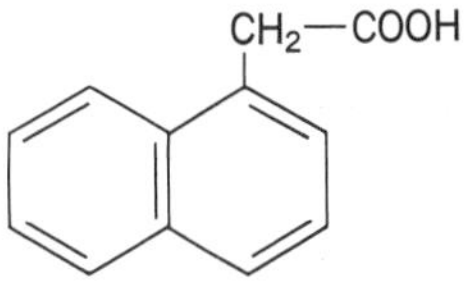

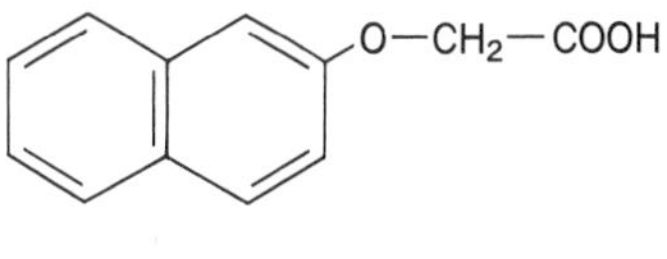

Fig. 3. Examples of synthetic auxin.

parently alterations in both the pectic and the cellulosic substances, the basic structural materials of the cell wall at the expansion stage. These changes are catalyzed by enzymes, and an unanswered question is whether the enzymes are influenced directly by auxins or indirectly through effects on the genetic material, on catalytic protein synthesis, or other intermediates. In either case a knowledge of the nature of the enzymic system could help with the answers.

Although the primary reaction, or reactions, for auxin is unknown, it is known that it plays major roles in controlling tissue differentiation and correlative growth and development of plants, in addition to its control of growth. Examples of the effects of auxin on organ and tissue differentiation are the stimulation of root formation and of xylem development.

In the area of the regulatory actions exerted by one plant part on another, numerous investigations have been made, probably because of the striking effects auxin has on correlative growth and development. Apical dominance, that is, alterations of the growth of lateral buds caused by the terminal bud of a shoot, is a good example of the correlative influence of one organ on another. Other examples are regulation of rooting on the basal end of shoots; control of abscission by subtended organs, (buds, flowers, fruits, and leaves); and plant tropisms, such as roots growing downward (geotropism) and shoots curving toward light (phototropism). These correlative effects have been shown to be intimately involved with patterns of auxin production, destruction, translocation, and accumulation.

The observations by Darwin in 1881 of a correlative effect, the alteration by light of the direction of growth by a grass shoot, gave rise to the first glimmering of the existence of a growth hormone in plants. With lateral illumination the intact grass shoot (coleoptile) curved toward the light. If the shoot apex was severed and removed from the plant, there was no curvature toward the light. This classical experiment demonstrated that, when seedlings are exposed to a lateral light, some influence is transmitted from the upper to the lower part, causing the latter to bend. This bending is now known to be caused by an accumulation of auxin on the shaded sides of the shoot which results in more growth of that side, leading to curvature. For the occurrence of this correlation effect, as well as many others, translocation of auxin is involved. This transport of auxin has several remarkable qualities, such as being polar in movement from apex to base, moving auxin considerably faster than diffusion (1 cm/hr), and being highly selective (many synthetic auxins are not transported polarly). Movement in the opposite direction does take place, but by diffusion or through the xylem of conductive tissues. The latter is the principal route of applied synthetic auxins.

Uses. Starting with the first practical use of plant-regulating substances, the stimulation of rooting, the importance of auxins for plant production has steadily increased. In the United States alone over 35 growth-regulating chemicals have been approved for over 100 different agricultural uses. A large portion of the 35 chemicals are either auxins, chemicals that are converted to auxins by certain plants, auxin antagonists, or chemicals that interact with auxins in modifying growth.

Herbicides. The largest use of auxins has been as herbicides. Here the chlorinated phenoxyacetic acids, particularly 2,4-D (2,4-dichlorophenoxyacetic acid) and 2,4,5-T (2,4,5-trichlorophenoxyacetic acid), have been used in the greatest quantity during the past decade. These chemicals cause death of plants at very low concentrations, but they are more lethal against broadleaf plants (dicots) than against grasses (monocots). Thus by proper application, it is possible to kill broadleaf weeds in fields of such crops as corn, oats, wheat, and other grains. The auxins used initially as herbicides are thus used to a lesser extent today, even though the overall use of herbicides has increased steadily. In general, this has resulted from the advent of more selective herbicides, many of which have auxin activity, for use with broadleaf row and tree crops. The chlorinated phenoxyacetic and benzoic acids are still used extensively with the grain crops. *See* HERBICIDE.

Crop improvement. A few other uses for auxins are enumerated to give an idea of the scope of development in this area. Many of the applications are based on the correlative action of auxin on tissue differentiation: rooting of cuttings; organ abscission, both promotion and inhibition; fruit development; induction of flowering; and alteration of fruiting patterns. Commercially, auxins, particularly naphthaleneacetic acid (NAA) and indolebutyric acid (IBA), have been used to stimulate rooting of asexually propagated materials, including

many woody species that are difficult to root. Premature fruit drop is prevented by preharvest application of low concentrations of 2,4,5-trichlorophenoxypropionic acid to apples and of 2,4-D to "pineapple" oranges. Beta-naphthoxyacetic acid has been used to increase the number of fruits set and developed by the first cluster of field-grown tomatoes. Fruit thinning of peaches is feasible by application of 3-chlorophenoxypropionic acid and its amide salt in low concentrations to peach fruits when the ovules are in the process of cytogenesis. This results in embryo abortion which subsequently leads to fruit drop. Correct thinning depends on timing the application so that some fruits are undergoing cytogenesis—number to approximate the degree of thinning required—and others are in the prior-to or post stage of cytogenesis, preferably post stage. The yield of Anjou and Bartlett pear trees can be increased through the use of 2,4,5-trichlorophenoxypropionic acid. This acid increases the number of flowers that develop fruit (fruit set) as a result of spray application during the bloom period. As an inducer of flowering, NAA has been used commercially on pineapples. In this case flowering action may be through auxin stimulation of ethylene production, another growth regulator, by the plant. A pronounced change in growth pattern of fruits from auxin application is exemplified by figs. Application of 2,4,5-T to unpollinated Calimyrna figs at the beginning of a period of depressed growth rate completely eliminates that period, resulting in mature fruit in only 15 days—60 days before untreated fruits. When minute amounts of 2,4,5-T are sprayed on soybean plants in full bloom, the regulator indirectly brings about an increased yield by causing the early-formed flowers to absciss. The plants subsequently produce new flowers in greater numbers which set and produce a much larger crop. A compound that interferes with auxin transport, 2,3,5-triiodobenzoic acid, has been registered by the U.S. Department of Agriculture for use on apples to promote flower formation and to increase the branch angle of nonflowering trees.

Future. It has become increasingly evident that complex interactions between various growth regulatory substances are involved in the growth and development of plant organs. With the realization that interactions of auxins, cytokinins, gibberellins, growth inhibitors, and other regulatory substances may be involved in a given physiological system, the correct alteration in any one, or several simultaneously, may elicit the desired response. Thus the usefulness of auxins and compounds that interact with auxin for the practical production of crops is being realized, and new ways of advantageously controlling plant growth and development with auxins and other plant regulators are sure to be discovered. *See* ABSCISSION; CYTOKININS; GIBBERELLIN; PLANT HORMONES; PLANT PHYSIOLOGY.   [ROBERT H. BIGGS]

Bibliography: L. J. Audus, *Plant Growth Substances*, vol. 1: *Chemistry and Physiology*, 3d ed., 1962; W. M. Laetsch and R. E. Cleland, *Papers on Plant Growth and Development*, 1967; A. C. Leopold, *Auxins and Plant Growth*, 1955; A. C. Leopold, *Plant Growth and Development*, 1964; M. B. Wilkins (ed.), *Physiology of Plant Growth and Development*, 1969.

Avocado

A tender evergreen subtropical tree, *Persea americana*, native to Central America and southern Mexico. It bears oval or round, green or black fruits 1–9 in. or more in diameter, containing a single large seed (see illustration). Three horticultural races are recognized by the type of skin: thin (Mexican), thick (Guatemalan), or leathery (West Indian). The Mexican race is hardiest to frost, the West Indian most tender, and the Guatemalan intermediate. The fruit, which does not soften until picked, is utilized fresh, usually in salads, and contains 5–30% oil. Commercial production is limited to the milder sections of California and Florida, which produce an annual crop valued at approximately $8,490,000. *See* FRUIT, TREE.

[CHARLES A. SCHROEDER]

Baking powder

A yeast substitute made of baking soda (sodium bicarbonate) plus cream of tartar (potassium acid tartrate), tartaric acid, and alum (in modern baking powders, usually anhydrous sodium aluminum sulfate), or monocalcium phosphate, or any combination of these acids so formulated as to release carbon dioxide from the baking soda when moistened. Baking powder causes breadstuffs to rise without the fermentation effects of yeast. Commercial baking powders contain some inert materials, such as starch or flour, to slow down the chemical reactions between the active ingredients. *See* FOOD MANUFACTURING. [FRANK H. ROCKETT]

Bamboo

The common name of various perennial, ornamental grasses (Gramineae). There are five genera with approximately 280 species. They have a wide distribution, but occur mainly in tropical and subtropical parts of Asia, Africa, and America, extending from sea level to an elevation of 15,000 ft. Their greatest development occurs in the monsoon regions of Asia. The plants grow very rapidly. From the jointed rhizome, numerous straight, usually erect, stems arise, which at their full height produce dense masses of horizontal branches. The giant bamboo (*Dendrocalamus giganteus*), the largest known grass, attains a height of 120 ft and a diameter of 8–12 in. Most are woody; a few are herbaceous or climbing. The economic uses of bamboo are numerous and varied. The seeds and young shoots are used as food and the leaves make excellent fodder for cattle. In varying sizes, the stems are used for pipes, timber, masts, bows, furniture, bridges, cooking vessels, buckets, wickerwork, paper pulp, cordage, and weaving. Entire houses are made of bamboo stems. Certain bamboos have been naturalized in California, Louisiana, and Florida.

[PERRY D. STRAUSBAUGH/EARL L. CORE]

Banana

A large tropical plant; also its edible fruit, which occurs in hanging clusters, is usually yellow when ripe, and is about 6–8 in. long. The banana belongs to the family Musaceae. The banana of commerce (*Musa sapientum*) believed to have originated in the Asian tropics, was one of the earliest fruits cultivated by man. For commercial production the plant requires a tropical climate within the temperature range 50–105°F and a constant supply of moisture by rainfall or irrigation. Bananas are subject to mechanical injury by strong winds which tear the leaves or blow down the plants. *See* IRRIGATION OF CROPS.

The plant portion above the ground is a false stem (pseudostem) consisting of several concentrically formed leaves, from the center of which develops the inflorescence stalk (Fig. 1). The rhizome or true stem is underground. Near the tip of the flower stalk are several groups of sterile male flowers subtended by brilliant purple bracts. The lower female flower clusters on the same stalk give rise to the fruit and contain aborted stamens (male organs). The single fruits are called fingers, a single group of 8–12 fingers is termed a hand, and the several (6–18) hands of the whole inflorescence make up a stem.

After the single fruiting stalk has produced the fruit bunch, the whole pseudostem is cut off at the ground, allowing one of several new buds or suckers from the underground stem to develop into a new plant. The fruit bunch requires 75–150 days to mature and must be removed from the plant to ripen properly. Chilled banana fruits do not soften normally; hence for best edibility the fruit is kept well ventilated at room temperature.

Kinds and distribution. Banana fruits of commerce set without pollination, by parthenocarpy, and hence are seedless. When mature, most varieties are yellow, although fine red-skinned types are well known. There are several hundred varieties grown throughout the world. The Cavendish banana (*M. nana*, variety Valery) is becoming important in the American tropics. The more starchy bananas, known as plantains, must be cooked before they can be eaten.

Yearly world production averages nearly 100,000,000 bunches, over 60% of which is consumed in the United States. Three-fourths of the world's bananas is grown in the Western Hemisphere. The greatest production occurs in Ecuador, Guatemala, Honduras, and other tropical Central and South American countries. Commercial production of bananas has been attempted in Florida, but climatic conditions there do not allow continuous economical cultivation of the fruit. *See* FRUIT, TREE.

[CHARLES A. SCHROEDER]

Diseases. Some of the most devastating plant disease epidemics recorded in the history of plant pathology have affected the banana industry at various times. Some diseases, like Panama disease, have attained epidemic proportions wherever susceptible varieties, such as Gros Michel, have been planted. In Central America, before resistant varieties such as Valery became available, the average productive life of a banana farm was only 5 years because of the inroads of Panama disease. Other diseases, like Sigatoka disease, became epidemic only during certain years, since the development of the pathogen is intimately associated with favorable moisture conditions. In recent years Moko disease has reached epidemic proportions in many parts of Central and South America because of the appearance of an insect-transmitted strain of the pathogen. Together, these

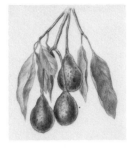

Avocado foliage and fruit.

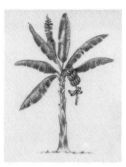

Fig. 1. Pseudostem of commercial banana plant (*Musa sapientum*), showing characteristic foliage and single stem of bananas. Plant grows to height of 30 ft or more.

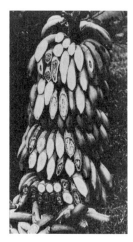

Fig. 2. Moko disease, with internal browning of banana fruit (Gros Michel variety).

diseases have caused losses estimated in many millions of dollars, and demand a continuous, costly program of control. The industry has survived because of the availability of wide tracts of virgin soils and because of the methods of control developed by both private and governmental agencies.

Etiology. Diseases of the banana plant and of the banana fruit are caused mainly by fungi, bacteria, viruses, and nematodes. The more important plantation diseases are Panama disease or fusarial wilt (*Fusarium oxysporum* f. *cubense*), Moko disease or bacterial wilt (*Pseudomonas solanacearum*) (Fig. 2), Sigatoka disease or leaf spot (*Mycosphaerella musicola*) (Fig. 3), bunchy top (bunchy top virus), infectious chlorosis (cucumber mosaic virus), and root and rhizome necrosis (*Radopholus similis*). The banana fruit is subject to spotting and rotting by numerous fungi before and after harvest. Of particular importance are the stem end rot and crown rot problems associated with fungi that attack the fruit after it is boxed for transport and storage.

Microbial strains. Most of these pathogens occur in the form of distinct strains or races, each with different characteristics, including pathogenic potential. For example, the bacterial wilt organism occurs as two well-defined strains: one being transmitted mainly by mechanical means, such as agricultural tools; the other mainly by insects that are attracted to inflorescences, where they become contaminated by the bacteria oozing out of wounds left by shedding bracts and flowers.

Soil pathogens. Both bacterial and fusarial wilt diseases are induced by soil-inhabiting microorganisms which are extremely persistent; thus, once an area becomes infested, it is extremely difficult to rid the soil of these root pathogens. For many years intentional flooding of large areas was practiced to reduce populations of *Fusarium* in the soil, but the procedure proved uneconomical. *See* SOIL MICROBIOLOGY.

Control measures. Although varieties of banana resistant to fusarial wilt had been known for many years, they did not come into extensive use until the late 1950s. These bananas, of the Cavendish-Lacatan group, have many undesirable features,

such as poor carrying qualities and short shelf life. Research provided methods for transportation and ripening which allowed the use of these resistant varieties. They are now well established throughout the world and have given excellent control of the disease. However, all commercial banana varieties are susceptible to Sigatoka, and to control this disease it is necessary to spray the foliage with fungicides on a regular basis. Eighteen to twenty spray cycles per year may be required in the more humid localities. Banana companies have pioneered in the development of high-volume or low-volume procedures to apply fungicides to banana foliage. Mixtures of orchard oil and dithiocarbamate fungicides, applied at low-volume by helicopter or fixed-wing aircraft, have proven the most effective. Commercial banana varieties are also susceptible to bacterial wilt, but effective control procedures have been devised. These consist mainly of sanitation procedures to prevent contamination of tools, the use of clean seed pieces, and the removal of the male inflorescences to reduce the possibilities of attracting insects which may carry the bacteria. Virus diseases are most effectively controlled by the complete eradication of infected plants. Fungi causing storage problems are controlled by dipping the fruit in fungicide solutions or by applying fungicide paste to cut surfaces at the stem ends.   [LUIS SEQUEIRA]

Bibliography: N. W. Simmonds, *Bananas*, 2d ed., 1966; R. H. Stover, *Fusarial Wilt (Panama disease) of Bananas and other Musa Species*, Commonwealth Mycological Institute, Kew, England, 1962; C. W. Wardlaw, *Banana Diseases, Including Plantains and Abaca*, 2d rev. ed., 1972.

Barley

A cereal grass plant whose seeds are useful to humans. It is grown in nearly all cultivated areas of the temperate parts of the world, and is an important crop in Europe, North and South America, North Africa, much of Asia, and Australia. Barley is the most dependable cereal crop where drought, summer frost, and alkali soils are encountered. In the United States, barley is grown to some extent in 49 states, with the most important production areas in North Dakota, Montana, and California. The average annual production in the United States for 1966–1975 was over 4.03×10^8 bu (8.9×10^6 metric tons), grown on about 9.5×10^6 acres (3.85×10^6 ha) with a yield of 42 bu/acre (1.1 metric tons/ha). Worldwide production in 1975 was estimated at 1.44×10^8 metric tons on more than 8.4×10^7 ha. Principal uses of barley grain are as livestock feed, for the production of barley malt, and as human food. It is also used in some areas for hay and silage.

Origin and description. Barley is probably one of the most ancient cultivated cereal grains. Its origin is still debated. Archeological evidence in the form of heads, carbonized grains, and impressions of grains on pottery have been found in several areas of the world. Some in Egypt are dated over 5,000 years ago. Barley was probably grown by the Swiss Lake Dwellers between 2000 and 3000 B.C., in China about 200 B.C., and in Greek and Roman areas about 300 B.C.

Taxonomically barley belongs to the family Gramineae, subfamily Festucoideae, tribe Hor-

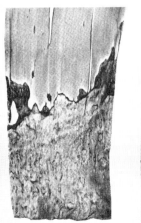
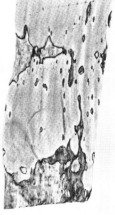

Fig. 3. Sigatoka disease, banana with spotting and necrosis of marginal areas on leaves of Gros Michel variety. (*Division of Tropical Research, United Brands Co.*)

deae, and genus *Hordeum*. Most of the modern cultivated barleys are *H. vulgare* (six-rowed) or *H. distichum* (two-rowed; Fig. 1). All cultivated barleys are annuals, are naturally self-pollinated, and have seven pairs of chromosomes. Figure 2 shows a typical barley plant. Cultivated barleys can be readily crossed by emasculating before pollen is shed or through genetic male sterility. There are also two wild species having chromosomes homologous with the cultivated species which are crossable with each other and with the cultivated species. Both of these, *H. spontaneum* (two-rowed) and *H. agriocrithon* (six-rowed), have brittle rachis and readily reseed themselves in the wild state. There are also a number of wild grasslike species which belong to the genus *Hordeum*. The basic chromosome number of these species is 7, and 2n numbers of 14, 28, and 42 have been observed. These species do not cross readily with the cultivated species, although in recent years there has been marked advancement in artificial crosses with the use of colchicine techniques and in growing excised embryos on artificial media. Among this group of wild barleys are annuals including *H. murinum*, *H. gussoneanum*, *H. glaucum*, *H. leproinum*, *H. depressum*, and *H. geniculatum*. Perennial types are *H. jubatum*, *H. bulbosum*, and *H. montanese*.

Varieties. In the cultivated varieties, a wide diversity of morphological, physiological, and anatomical types are known. There are spring, facultative, and winter growth habits; hulled and naked grain; awned, awnless, and hooded lemmas; black,

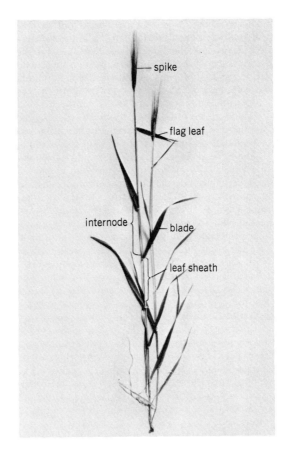

Fig. 2. Typical barley plant. (*USDA*)

purple, and white kernels; and also a wide range of plant heights, spike densities, and resistances to a wide range of diseases and insects. There are in excess of 150 cultivars presently commercially grown in the United States and Canada alone, and many additional cultivars are grown in other parts of the world. New and improved varieties produced by barley breeders are constantly replacing older varieties. Several barley collections are being maintained in different countries as germplasm sources for breeding and research. These include both collections made by direct exploration in many barley-growing areas of the world and lines from barley breeding programs. Among the largest of these collections is one maintained by the U.S. Department of Agriculture which presently includes more than 17,000 individual strains.

Cultural practices. The best soils for growing barley are well-drained fertile loams and clay loams. This grain is the most tolerant of the cereal grains to alkaline soils (pH 6.0 to 8.0), and the least tolerant to acid soils (below pH 5.0), especially if there is soluble aluminum in the soil solution. Liming may be necessary to correct acidity and to precipitate aluminum, and lime should be applied at the time of seedbed preparation. Soil tests will determine if phosphorus or potash is needed. Nitrogen will generally be needed for good production, depending on the previous crop and climatic conditions. Time and rate of seeding, seedbed preparation, and rotations vary widely with geographical area. In the United States, spring varieties are grown in the Midwest, northern Great Plains, and Pacific Northwest. Seeding should be

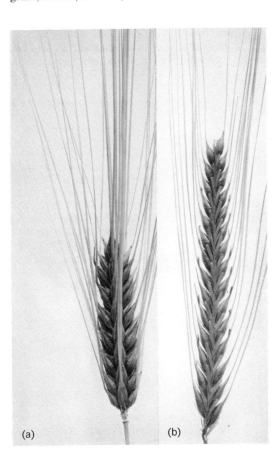

Fig. 1. Barley spikes: (*a*) six-rowed *Hordeum vulgare*; (*b*) two-rowed *H. distichum*. (*USDA*)

done as early as the seedbed can be prepared. This will vary from about March 1 to 15 in the Kansas-Nebraska area, the Great Basin, and the Pacific Northwest to late April or early May in the northern Great Plains. Spring varieties are commonly sown in the late fall or winter in the southwestern states, the Atlantic seaboard, the southern Great Plains, and in the milder areas of the Pacific Northwest. Generally the planting date will be 1 to 2 weeks ahead of the earliest fall frost-free date. Common seeding rates are 4 to 8 pecks per acre (0.087 to 0.174 m³/ha), depending on expected moisture conditions. Barley can be grown in a variety of rotations with other crops common to a particular region. In areas with long growing seasons, it is possible to double-crop (growing two crops in 12 consecutive months on the same land) with summer crops such as soybeans or cotton. Barley is ideally suited to this purpose because it is usually the earliest maturing of the small grains. The variety of the alternate crop should also be early-maturing. *See* GRAIN CROPS.   [DAVID A. REID]

Diseases. Barley is one of the cereals most subject to diseases, especially in the humid areas. For this reason the varieties grown in the humid areas have been less consistent in yields than other grains. Because of diseases, barley production has shifted westerly from the Corn Belt to northwestern Minnesota, through North Dakota, Montana, northern Idaho, and California, where humidity is lower.

The annual loss from diseases in the United States is estimated at 5%, or almost 20,000,000 bu, with a monetary loss to growers of about $18,000,000. Destructive epidemics are not uncommon. In 1945 barley production in Minnesota decreased from an annual average of about 50,000,000 bu to less than 13,000,000, and the yield dropped more than 30% because of two successive epidemics of root rot and foliage diseases.

Seed-borne disease. In the 1930s seed-borne diseases such as covered smut (*Ustilago hordei*), loose smut (*U. nuda*), and barley stripe (*Helminthosporium gramineum*) (Fig. 3) were of great economic importance. Today these diseases are controlled to a large extent by treating the seed with chemical fungicides and growing varieties with some degree of resistance. A seed-treatment chemical has been developed that gives virtually 100% control of both smuts.

Foliage disease. The foliage diseases such as spot blotch (*H. sativum*; Fig. 4), net blotch (*H. teres*), leaf blight (*Septoria passerinii*), and scald (*Rhynchosporium secalis*) have become very prevalent and are more difficult to control. However, real progress has been made since the late 1950s in developing varieties with some resistance to foliage diseases. *See* FUNGISTAT AND FUNGICIDE.

Root disease. Root rots, including basal stem rot, are among the most destructive diseases of barley, particularly in the United States. Their importance varies tremendously with the season, locality, and variety. The plants are exposed to attack from the time the seeds are sown until the barley matures. The pathogens are of many types and attack all underground parts of the plant, inducing seedling blight, root decay, stem rot, and premature death.

Grain disease. In the more humid regions of the United States kernel blight occurs in most years. This is another reason for the shift of barley production to the less humid areas of the West. Kernel blight, caused chiefly by *Gibberella zeae*, *H. sativum*, and *Alternaria* sp., shrivels and discolors the grain, thus reducing storage, marketing, and particularly malting qualities (Fig. 5). Storage molds, caused by many fungi, often cause rapid

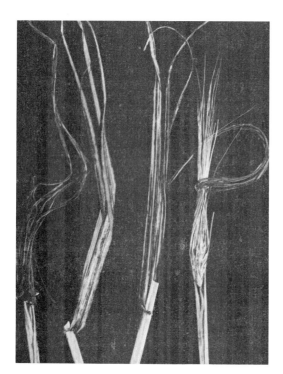

Fig. 3.   Barley stripe, caused by *Helminthosporium gramineum*. (*Minnesota Agricultural Experiment Station*)

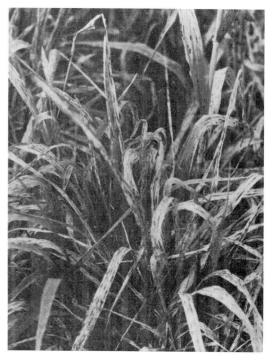

Fig. 4.   Barley spot blotch, caused by *Helminthosporium sativum*. (*Minnesota Agricultural Experiment Station*)

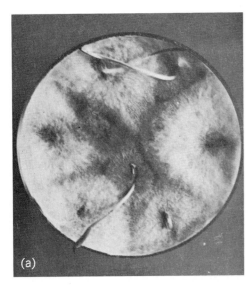
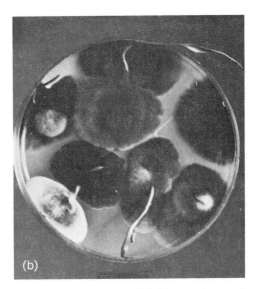

Fig. 5. Infected barley seed planted out on nutrient agar. (a) Gibberella zeae. (b) Helminthosporium sp. and Alternaria sp. These kernel blights occur in more humid regions. (Minnesota Agricultural Experiment Station)

deterioration of barley seeds in storage.

Other types. Although both stem rust (*Puccinia graminis*) and leaf rust (*P. hordei*) are common diseases of barley, they seldom cause severe epidemics. Powdery mildew (*Erysiphe graminis*) is widespread and sometimes causes heavy losses in certain regions. Yellow dwarf is caused by a virus and has become widespread and destructive. It has also been discovered that the aster yellow virus infects barley, and this disease can be quite destructive, especially if it occurs in combination with yellow dwarf. Nematodes are widely distributed, but their economic importance on barley is not known. *See* PLANT VIRUS.

Changing problem. Disease problems in barley are continually changing, primarily because new, disease-producing organisms are introduced or new, virulent strains or races of established pathogens are developed or introduced into new regions. Sometimes disease problems change because minor diseases become major diseases with the introduction of new varieties or changes in farming practices, cropping systems, or mechanization. Seed storage problems, for instance, have become more intensified since farmers do not dry and cure the grain in shocks and stacks, but harvest by windrowing and combining either from the windrow or directly.

Disease control. Although losses from many diseases can be reduced by planting sound, disease-free seed, by treating seed with fungicides, and by using appropriate crop sequences and cultural practices, including proper fertilizers, the most feasible practical method of disease control of barley is growing disease-resistant varieties. As no variety is resistant to all diseases, a control program involves the development of varieties resistant to the major diseases. Much progress has been made since the late 1950s in getting barley varieties resistant to spot blotch, net blotch, and Septoria leaf blight. *See* PLANT DISEASE; PLANT DISEASE CONTROL. [MILTON F. KERNKAMP]

Pot and pearl barley. The term pot barley is applied to the food product which results after the husk has been removed by coarse grinding. Pearled barley is obtained by a more involved, dry-milling process.

Barley is pearled in a machine consisting of a perforated cylinder, with indentations smaller than the kernels, and a cylindrical revolving millstone, rotating in the opposite direction at faster speed. The perforations cause the grain to turn rapidly, while the revolving millstone grinds off the hull. From the pearler the barley passes through reels which separate the hulls. Dust and fine particles are removed by aspiration, and the pearled barley is then transferred to cooling bins. Pearled barley is small, round, and white. It is classified according to size by passage through a grading reel. Normally, 100 lb of barley will yield about 65 lb of pot barley or 35 lb of pearled barley. In the manufacture of pearled barley, some flour is produced as a by-product.

Malting. For malting purposes the brewing industries in the United States use different types of barley from those desired throughout the remainder of the world. Outside the United States the demand is for large-kerneled barley of the two-row type which is high in starch and low in nitrogen content. In North America the demand is for the six-row, small-kernel type with higher nitrogen and enzyme content.

There are two systems of malting: flour malting and pneumatic or drum malting. The malting process involves the germination of the barley in a controlled state, followed by drying under conditions that retain enzymatic activity. The basic steps taken during malting are as follows: The barley is cleaned, graded for uniformity of size, and steeped in cold water until the moisture content reaches about 45%. The steeped grain is germinated in compartments or drums under suitable moisture, temperature, and aeration conditions to modify the kernels. Germination usually is stopped when the acrospire has grown to the length of the kernel, which requires several days. During this period enzyme development takes place.

The next step is drying the germinated grain

under conditions which will stop germination and any further chemical change. Drying temperatures vary from 120 to 180°F with the final moisture content reduced to about 6%. The rootlets are then removed by cleaning, and the malt is ready for industrial use.

During malting there are certain losses of dry substances from barley. Steep loss is usually 1.5–2.0%, respiration loss equals 3–5%, and removing the rootlets contributes another 3–5% loss. At the start of the malting process, barley moisture is likely to be from 10–18%, whereas the moisture of the finished malt is low.

Industrial value of malt depends on its starch-splitting and protein-degrading enzymes. Brewers' malts are used to produce beer and ale and, to a lesser extent, for malt syrups and evaporated malt extracts. Distillers' malts are employed for starch conversion in the production of distilled beverages and industrial alcohol and for converting starch for the sizing of paper and textiles.

[JOHN A. SHELLENBERGER]

Bibliography: A. H. Cook, *Barley and Malt: Biology, Biochemistry, Technology*, 1962; J. G. Dickson, *Diseases of Field Crops*, 2d ed., 1956; W. H. Leonard and J. H. Martin, *Cereal Crops*, 1963; S. A. Matz, *Cereal Science*, 1969; S. A. Matz, *Cereal Technology*, 1970; U.S. Department of Agriculture, *Barley*, Agri. Handb. 338, 1968.

Bean

Any of several leguminous plants, or their seeds, long utilized as food by humans or livestock. Some 14 genera of the legume family contain species producing seeds termed "beans" and useful to humans. Twenty-eight species in 7 genera produce beans of commercial importance, which implies that the bean can be found in trade at the village level or up to and including transoceanic commerce.

Varieties. The principal Asiatic beans include the edible soybeans, *Glycine* sp., and several species of the genus *Vigna*, such as the cowpea *(V. unguiculata)* and mung, grams, rice, and adzuki beans. The broad bean *(Vicia faba)* is found in Europe, the Middle East, and Mediterranean region, including the North African fringe. Farther south in Africa occur *Phaseolus* beans, of the *vulgaris* (common bean) and *coccineus* (scarlet runner) species. Some *Phaseolus* beans occur in Europe also. The cowpea, used as a dry bean, is also found abundantly in Nigeria. *See* COWPEA; SOYBEAN.

In the Americas, the *Phaseolus* beans, *P. vulgaris* and *P. lunatus* (lima bean), are the principal edible beans, although the blackeye cowpea, mung bean, and chick pea or garbanzo *(Cicer arietinum)* are grown to some extent. *P. coccineus* is often grown in higher elevations in Central and South America, as is *Vicia faba*. The tepary bean *(P. acutifolius)* is found in the drier southwestern United States and northern Mexico.

Characteristics. Bean plants may be either bush or vining types, early or late in maturity, with white, yellow, red, or purple flowers. The seed itself is the most differentiating characteristic of bean plants. It may be white, yellow, black, red,

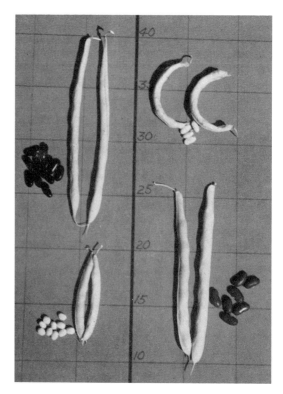

Fig. 1. Pod and seed types in dry beans.

tan, cream-colored, or mottled, and range in weight from 125 to over 700 mg per seed. Seeds are grown in straight or curved pods (fruit), with 2–3 seeds per pod in *Glycine* to 18–20 in some *Vigna* (Fig. 1). Pods vary in fiber content; the immature pods of low-fiber types are often used as a green vegetable. Beans are normally self-pollinated, although a small amount of natural crossing may occur. Scarlet runner bean is normally highly cross-pollinated.

Production statistics. The United States dry bean crop in 1976 amounted to 17,246,000 hundredweight (cwt; 783,000,000 kg) produced on 1,485,300 acres (601,546 ha), primarily in 13 northern and western states (see table). In 1975 some 354,000 acres (143,370 ha) were devoted to snap

Production of commercial classes of dry edible beans in the United States in 1976

Class	Production, 100-lb bags (45.4 kg), cleaned
Navy (pea)	4,315,000
Great Northern	1,771,000
Small white	329,000
Flat small white	6,000
Pinto	5,716,000
Red kidney	1,433,000
Pink	990,000
Small red	437,000
Cranberry	280,000
Black turtle	118,000
Large lima	552,000
Baby lima	378,000
Blackeye	607,000
Garbanzo	46,000
Other	268,000
Total	17,246,000

beans. (These figures do not include mung beans or soybeans.)

Most navy beans in the United States are produced in Michigan; Great Northern beans in Nebraska, Wyoming, and Idaho; pinto beans in Colorado, North Dakota, and Idaho; red kidneys in New York, Michigan, and California; and large and baby limas in California. Such regional distribution of bean classes is partly historical and partly due to climatic and disease factors.

Culture. Most beans are a temperate-season crop, with major producing areas in the United States having a mean August temperature of 70°F (21°C) or less and a mean July temperature of between 72° (22°C) and 74°F (23°C), except for the central valley of California. With higher temperatures there is extensive flower and pod abscission, except for those species such as *P. acutifolius* and *Vigna* sp. that require the higher temperature for seed development. Flower initiation in beans may be affected by the length of day, there being long-day-, day-neutral-, and short-day-requiring types. Many types suffer a delay in flowering with lower mean temperature.

Beans are grown on a wide variety of soil types, the most productive being the well-drained loams, silt loams, and clay loams abundantly supplied with organic matter. It is important that the soils not be compacted. Sandy soils are satisfactory where rainfall is sufficient and well-distributed throughout the season. Beans grow best in soils of pH 6.5–7.2 that are also high in phosphorus and potassium. Zinc and manganese are minor elements that may be the first to become limiting in the lake bed or outwash soils of the United States.

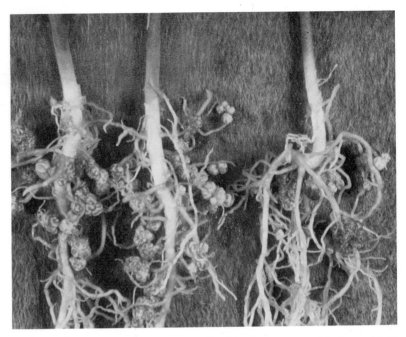

Fig. 2. Bacterially induced nodules on roots of beans are responsible for symbiotic nitrogen fixation. (*Courtesy of Joe Burton, The NITRAGIN Company, Milwaukee*)

Except where a special nutrient deficiency exists, beans do not respond well to added fertilizer.

Beans are normally planted after danger of frost is past and when soil temperature has reached 65°F (18°C). Inoculation with nitrogen-fixing bacteria (*Rhizobium* sp.) is generally unnecessary since most bean soils are naturally supplied with nodu-

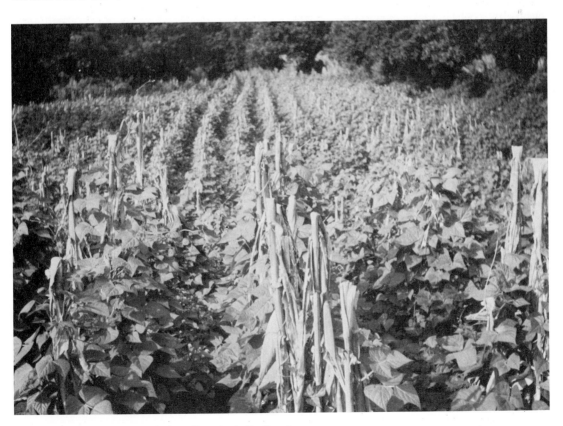

Fig. 3. Beans growing in association with maize in Guatemala.

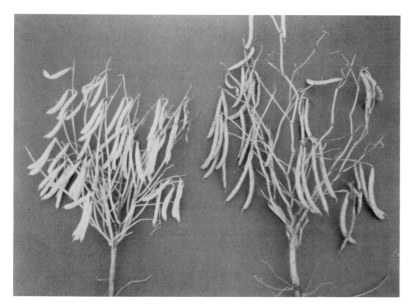

Fig. 4. Some typical plant types of *Phaseolus* beans at maturity.

pulled plants are formed into windrows and cured for a few hours in bright clear weather before threshing with a grain combine or special bean harvester. In some countries all the harvesting operations are carried out by hand, and winnowing of the seed is still practiced. A product of high physical quality usually results from this process. In the United States field-run beans require screening, and, for highest quality, "picking," that is, the removal of seed-sized foreign matter and off-colored, stained or damaged seeds. This was formerly done by hand but presently is accomplished by electric-eye machines in the cleaning plants or elevators. *See* AGRICULTURE, MACHINERY IN.

Utilization. Beans are consumed as food in several forms. Lima beans and snap beans are used as fresh vegetables, or they may be processed by canning or freezing. Limas are also used as a dry bean. Mung beans are utilized as sprouts.

Usage of dry beans *(P. vulgaris)* for food is highly dependent upon seed size, shape, color, and flavor characteristics, and is often associated with particular social or ethnic groups. Popular usage includes soups, mixed-bean salads, pork and beans, beans boiled with meat or other vegetables or cereals, baked beans, precooked beans, and powder, and, in the Peruvian Andes, parched or roasted beans. Per capita consumption of dry beans in the United States is 6.7 lb/yr (3 kg/yr).

Dry beans range in protein content from 17 to

lating bacteria (Fig. 2). Beans under irrigated or humid conditions are usually grown in rows 50 to 70 cm apart, with plants from 5–10 cm apart in the row. Under dryland conditions the spacing is greater. In much of the tropics a considerable portion of the production is from beans grown in association with another crop, such as maize (Fig. 3).

Weed control. One of the main cultural requirements for successful bean growing is weed control. Cultivation by hand or by mechanical means is the time-honored method, but selective chemical herbicides are available which, under favorable temperature and soil moisture conditions, are capable of giving almost 100% control of most annual grasses and broadleaved weeds. Widely used preplant herbicides are EPTC (S-ethyl dipropylthiocarbamate) and Trifluralin (α,α,α-trifluoro-2,6-dinitro-N,N dipropyl-P-toluidine) for many broadleaved weeds and annual grasses. Combinations of a preplant herbicide with a preemergence herbicide such as Chloramben (3-amino-2,5-dichlorobenzoic acid) or CDAA (N,N-diallyl-2-chloroacetamide) are currently proving capable of excellent long season weed control with a high safety factor for the bean plant. However, perennial weeds are still a serious problem in bean fields. Plant diseases continue to be a major hazard in production, although progress toward disease control by developing resistant varieties is being made. *See* HERBICIDE; PLANT DISEASE CONTROL.

Harvesting. Most bean crops will mature in from 80 to 120 days; in higher elevations or cooler seasons they may take up to 150 days. Beans are ready for harvest when the pods and upper portion of the plants have changed color from green to tan or brown and seeds have dried to under 20% moisture (Fig. 4). Bean seeds split or break easily when threshed mechanically at under 14% seed moisture. The ripened plants are pulled from the soil by hand or by a machine called a puller which has two sets of heavy steel knives set at an angle to the row and positioned to intercept the roots about 2 in. (5 cm) below the soil surface. The

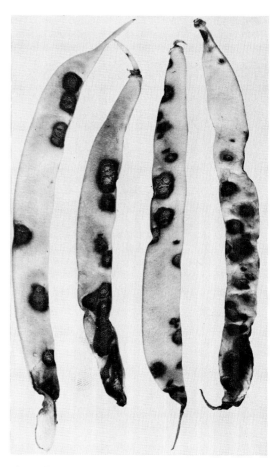

Fig. 5. Anthracnose on bean pods (fruits).

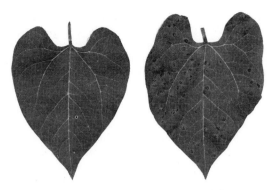

Fig. 6. Bean leaves. (a) Healthy. (b) Rust-infected.

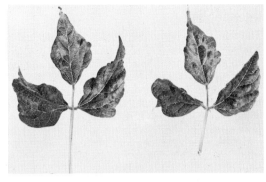

Fig. 7. Virus infection of bean leaves.

32%. Commercial types average around 23–25%. The sulfur-containing amino acids methionine and cystine are the first limiting factors in bean protein, from a nutritional standpoint. The dry beans have less than 2% oil (except soybeans) and some 61–63% carbohydrate, and are rich sources of fiber, calcium, and phosphorus. Because of the presence of heat-labile growth retardants, beans must be thoroughly cooked before being used as food. Newer developments are in the areas of cooking time, the manufacture of precooked dry powders that can be readily rehydrated to make a palatable soup, and new research impetus to identify the flatulence factors in dry beans. *See* Food Engineering.

Developments. Since the food grain legumes are an important protein source in human diets, intensive efforts are being made in research and development, both on a national and international level. Broadly based production research is presently being conducted on the *Phaseolus* beans at CIAT (Centro Internacional de Agricultura Tropical, Cali, Colombia); on ground nuts, chick pea, pigeon pea, grams, and mung beans at ICRISAT (International Center for Research in Semi-Arid Tropics, Hyderabad, India); and on edible soybeans, peas, and Asiatic beans at AVRDC (Asian Vegetable Research and Development Center, Tainan, Taiwan). National research programs in Latin American, African, and United States institutions are often linked in these research efforts with the international centers. *See* Breeding (Plant); Legume; Vegetable growing.

[M. W. Adams]

Bean diseases. There are two types of bean diseases, the parasitic and nonparasitic. Parasitic diseases are caused by fungi, bacteria, and viruses, and nonparasitic by unfavorable environment, mineral deficiencies, and related conditions. Of some 40 parasitic field diseases of beans, only 18 are of major importance. About 20 nonparasitic diseases are recognized, few of which regularly cause serious losses. These diseases cost the American farmer an estimated $35,000,000 annually. Some common diseases kill young seedlings, others cause injury or death of older plants, and some produce spots on pods and seeds that make the product unsalable.

Fungus diseases. The most important worldwide fungus diseases of beans are anthracnose, root rots, and rust. Anthracnose (*Colletotrichum linde-*

muthianum) causes dark sunken cankers on pods and angular dead spots on leaves (Fig. 5). The causal fungus is spread by such means as infected seed, wind, rain, and insects. Root rots are caused by several organisms which produce black or reddish-brown lesions on the roots and some root decay. Infected plants are often stunted and their leaves turn yellow, or they may suddenly wilt and die. Rust (*Uromyces phaseoli* var. *typica*) is chiefly a disease of leaves (Fig. 6). It appears as small rust-colored lesions that may be so numerous that they cause the leaves to shrivel and drop. Each lesion contains thousands of reddish-brown spores which are carried by the wind and spread the disease.

Bacterial diseases. Blights and wilts, caused by bacteria, are important wherever rain falls frequently during the growing season. The blights, caused principally by *Xanthomonas phaseoli* and *Pseudomonas phaseolicola*, show up most strikingly on leaves as small, water-soaked spots which later merge and form extensive brown, dead areas. The pods also show very small water-soaked spots that later form dry and sunken lesions with reddish-brown or brick-red margins. The bacteria may infect the hinge, or upper suture, of the pod and cause discoloration and water-soaking of tissue. Through the hinge they may attack the seed. Bacterial wilt (*Corynebacterium flaccumfaciens*) causes shriveling of plants. Seedlings produced by infected seeds may be stunted or may not emerge from the soil.

Virus diseases. These diseases, including the important common bean mosaic and curly top, are characterized by leaf mottling and malformation, stunting of the plants, and sometimes death (Fig. 7). Viruses are spread from plant to plant chiefly by aphids and other insects. Some are carried in seeds.

Disease control. Use of disease-free seed is one important method of control. Some seed-borne diseases, such as anthracnose, and bacterial blights and wilt do not develop where rainfall is low and temperatures are high during the growing season; therefore, seeds produced in the mountain and Pacific states are freer of these diseases than seeds grown east of the Rocky Mountains. Other control measures include use of resistant varieties, crop rotation, field sanitation, spraying plants, or treating seeds with chemicals. *See* Plant disease; Plant virus.

[William J. Zaumeyer]

Beekeeping

The management and maintenance of colonies of honeybees. Beekeeping is an ancient art. Although the commonly known honeybee species is native to Europe and Africa only, humans have transported them to other continents, and in most places they have flourished. The natural home for a honeybee colony is a hollow tree (Fig. 1), log, or cave. European strains of the honeybee build a nest only in locations which are dry and protected from the wind and sunlight (Fig. 2). African bees are less

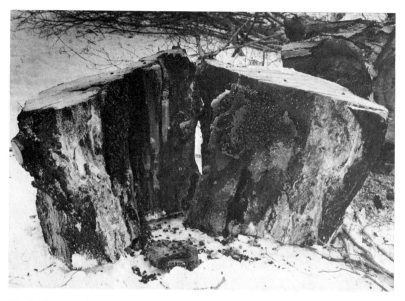

Fig. 1. A hollow tree, the original, natural home for honeybees; this tree trunk has been split apart to expose the nest. The bees used today are not domesticated and can easily revert to their old ways. Beekeeping is possible because of present-day understanding of bee biology. *(New York State College of Agriculture, Cornell University, Ithaca, NY)*

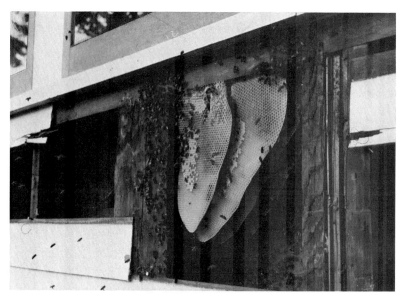

Fig. 2. A swarm which escaped from a beekeeper's hive and took up residence in the side of a house. The house boards have been removed to photograph the swarm. A swarm can live successfully in the side of a house, though the bees may be a nuisance.

selective and may nest in hollowed-out termite mounds, rock piles, and locations which are less well protected. It is not known when humans first started to husband bees. However, there is much archeological and historical evidence that there were beekeepers among all of the ancient European and African civilizations.

Bees are important plant pollinators, but early beekeepers were not concerned with pollination and cross pollination of agricultural crops since their fields were small and they conducted diversified farming. For them, the importance and value of honeybees lay in the various hive products, especially honey, which was used as a sweetener, in making a fermented beverage, in medicine, and in conducting rituals. Beeswax was civilization's first plastic, and was used as a polish, in the preparation of molds for metal casting, for waterproofing, and in many other ways. Some ancient peoples ate honeybee brood, the developing larvae and pupae in the hive. Brood eating has never been widely practiced, but even today the habit is found among some African and Asian peoples.

Honey. Honey was a precious commodity in early Roman, Greek, and Egyptian civilizations. For people 2000 to 4000 years ago, it was the main source of sugar. Thus, in the ancient Mediterranean world, honey and beekeepers were held in extremely high esteem. Today, honey is still valued as a sweetener and is used to some extent in medicine.

Production. The honey which beekeepers harvest is made from nectar, a sweet sap or sugar syrup produced by special glands in flowers, collected from both wild and cultivated plants. Nectar, the honeybees' source of sugar or carbohydrate, and pollen, their source of protein and fat, make up their entire diet.

Nectar contains 50–90% water, 10–50% sugar (predominantly sucrose), and 1–4% aromatic substances, coloring material, and minerals. To transform nectar into honey, bees reduce its moisture content, so that the final honey produced contains between 14 and 19% water, and also add two enzymes which they produce in their bodies. One enzyme inverts the sucrose, a sugar with 12 carbon atoms, into two 6-carbon sugars, levulose and dextrose. The second enzyme added by bees is glucose oxidase, which is inactive when honey has a normal moisture content (14–19%). However, when the honey is diluted, as when it is fed to honeybee larvae, the enzyme becomes active, resulting in the breakdown of dextrose into hydrogen peroxide and gluconic acid. Hydrogen peroxide prevents or slows the growth of bacteria and thus protects the diluted honey from attack by microbes. Glucose oxidase is also active while the bees are in the process of reducing the nectar's moisture content, a process which may take 24 hr or more. The gluconic acid produced during this time, along with other acids present in honey, gives honey a pH of 3.5 to 4.0 which, among food products, is quite acid and makes honey an inhospitable medium for bacterial growth. Also, since it is a supersaturated sugar solution, honey has a high osmotic pressure. Therefore, any microorganisms present in honey are plasmolyzed and die.

Use in medicine. Honey has been used in medicines for thousands of years. Since honey is about half levulose, the sweetest of the common sugars, it is sweeter than cane sugar or corn syrup. Even today, honey is used in certain medicinal compounds because the sweet levulose covers up harsh, bitter flavors better than other sugars. The most popular honey for use by drug manufacturers is tupelo honey, which is produced only along the banks of the Apalachicola River in west Florida. Tupelo honey is the sweetest of the commercially produced honeys in the United States. Honeys high in levulose granulate much more slowly than do honeys high in dextrose; this is an added advantage for the drug manufacturer, who does not want the produce to granulate or contain sugar crystals.

Before the discovery of modern salves and creams, honey was widely used as a wound dressing. It was an ingredient in over half of the medicinal compounds and cures made by Egyptian physicians 2000 to 5000 years ago. Honey is an effective dressing, not only because bacteria cannot live in it, but also because honey on a wound creates a physical barrier through which bacteria cannot pass. Some of the ancient Egyptian salves called for a mixture of honey and grease. Lint was sometimes added to help bind the mixture. If the honey was diluted with water, the glucose oxidase became active, producing hydrogen peroxide and again giving the wound some protection. Honey also prevented dried blood from adhering to a bandage and kept the bandage soft. Thus, dressings could be removed from a wound periodically, and the wound treated with more salve and rebandaged.

Use in baking. About half the honey produced in the world is sold as table honey and is used as a sweetener on bread, cereal, or desserts. The remaining half is used in the baking trade. Honey is hygroscopic, that is, it absorbs moisture. When honey is added to a baked product some of this property is retained, helping to keep the bread or cake moist. Bakers are also concerned with the browning qualities of their product, and the sugar levulose in honey has the desired browning qualities. Because the price of honey is many times that of sugar, it is too expensive to use in all baked products. Thus, honey is added only in specialty products.

Biology of the honeybee. Honeybees are social animals. A minimum of about 200 worker bees and a queen must live together for social order to exist; however, such a small number of bees could not survive for long without human assistance.

A colony of bees in an artificial hive, or living wild, contains about 10,000 worker bees, all females, in midwinter. The same colony would have a peak population of 30,000 to 60,000 workers in early summer. In addition to the workers, a normal colony has a single queen and 0 to 3000 drones (males). The sole function of the drones is to mate, and their presence in the hive is not tolerated by the workers during nonmating seasons. In the fall, the drones are deprived of food by the workers and are driven from the hive. The rearing of new drones in the spring starts well after bees have initiated the rearing of workers.

It is generally accepted that, in most situations, all the bees in a colony develop from eggs laid by the single queen. The size and composition of the colony population is regulated by how many eggs are reared during each season. In the Northern Hemisphere, bees rear the least number of young, called brood, in October and November. The least number of adult bees is found in the hive about 3 to 4 months later. Pollen first becomes available in the spring, February in the southern states and April in the northern states. The availability of pollen controls brood rearing, for without large quantities only a small number of young are reared. The natural seasonal population fluctuation which takes place in a colony is referred to as the cycle of the year.

Honeybees separate their young and their food, which is one of the factors which makes beekeeping possible. Honey and pollen are usually stored above the brood-rearing area, which is called the brood nest. The brood nest, which contains the eggs, larvae and pupae, is a compact area more or less the shape of a ball. Brood is reared in many combs at the same time, but always in combs which are side by side. Honeybees maintain a constant brood-rearing temperature of about 92–95°F (24–36°C). This allows them to rear their young in a set period of time (see table) regardless of seasonal and climatic temperature variations. A few other species of social insects exercise some control over brood-rearing temperature, but none so precisely as the honeybee.

When cool weather prevails, the bees form an insulating shell of live bees around the outside of the brood nest. Bees in the center of the brood-rearing area make physical movements to generate heat. If the temperature drops, more bees generate heat and the shell of bees around the area becomes more compact. In this manner the heat is retained within the cluster; bees do not heat the inside of the whole hive. Bees can survive severe winters, even in Alaska, if they have sufficient honey. However, because so much honey is required for energy, usually in excess of 100 lb (45 kg) per colony in Alaska, it is considered uneconomical to keep bees there. In the summer when the temperature is high, bees collect water, deposit it in droplets around the hive, and fan their wings, causing masses of air to pass through the hive, evaporating the water and preventing excessive temperatures in the brood nest. Colonies of bees have survived in the Arizona desert, where temperatures may reach 120°F (49°C). In such cases, a colony may need to collect and evaporate as much as 1 or 2 gal (3.8 or 7.6 liters) of water per day.

Remarkably, the largest, most important individual in the colony, the queen, is reared in the shortest period of time. Evolution has favored this fast development. If a queen dies, a replacement must be produced rapidly or the colony will perish. Queens and workers develop from identical eggs. In fact, a queen can be made from a larva that is from 24 to about 48 hr old. Larvae destined to be-

Development time for honeybee castes, in days

Stage	Queen	Worker	Drone
Egg	3	3	3
Larva	5½	6	6½
Pupa	7½	12	14½
Total	16	21	24

come queens are fed a special food, royal jelly, which is produced by glands in the heads of worker bees; larvae destined to become worker bees receive less of this glandular secretion and more honey and pollen in late larval life. Thus, in a colony that loses its queen but has young larvae present, a queen may be produced in 11 or 12 days.

Pollination. Pollination is the process by which pollen, comprising the male germ cells, is transferred from the male part of a flower (anthers) to the female part (stigma) on the same plant. The process of transferring the pollen from the flower of one plant to that of another is called cross pollination. Pollen may be carried by wind, water, or animals. While only a small number of plants are water-pollinated, wind pollination is fairly common.

Many plants, however, require animals agents for cross pollination. Certain birds, especially hummingbirds, are especially adapted for this purpose, but insects, especially bees, are the most efficient pollinators. Most bees are solitary insects, living and making their nests in hollow twigs, under bark, in stone crevices, or in tunnels in the ground. These insects pollinate many of the flowers which produce seeds, nuts, and fruit. Some species of social bees, however, including bumblebees and honeybees, are important pollinators. In many areas in the United States the solitary twig- and ground-nesting bees and the bumblebees outnumber honeybees.

The honeybee is especially well adapted to gathering large quantities of pollen and nectar and, in the process, bringing about efficient cross pollination. A honeybee is a very hairy creature, the hairs on its body being plumose, or branched, so that pollen grains are easily caught. When a honeybee collects pollen, it actually wallows in the flower parts, dusting itself thoroughly with pollen. It then hovers above the flower and used its legs to clean its body of pollen; the pollen is raked into areas of longer hairs, called pollen baskets, one on each of its hindlegs. Bees pack pollen into the baskets until they become large, round balls; bright colored pollen balls may be seen with the naked eye on foraging bees, both as they collect more pollen in the field and as they later enter their hive.

When the pollen balls on the two hindlegs are large enough, the bee carries the pollen back to the hive, where it is deposited in cells and becomes food for adult bees and larvae. A bee never cleans its body so thoroughly that all the pollen grains are removed, and does not clean itself after visiting every flower. Thus, in the process of moving from one flower to another, large numbers of pollen grains are transferred.

Modern beekeeping. Scientific beekeeping started in 1851 when an American, L. L. Langstroth, discovered bee space and the movable frame hive. Bee space is the open space which is about 1 cm wide and maintained around and between the

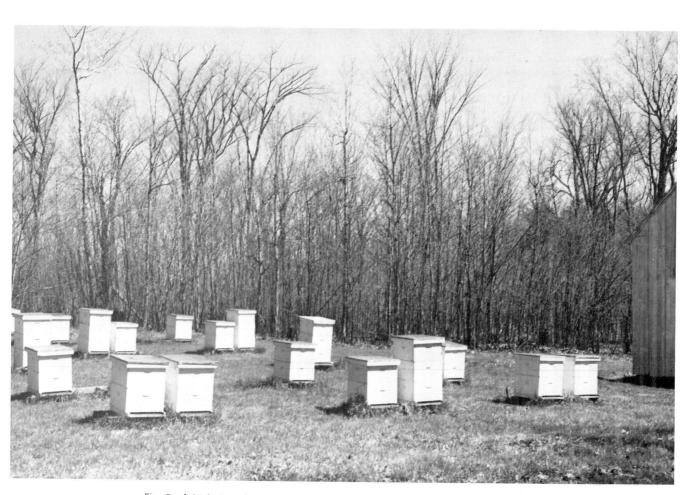

Fig. 3. A typical modern-day commercial apiary. Beekeepers often select apiary sites surrounded by woods so as to protect bees from damage by wind; hidden apiaries are also less likely to be vandalized.

combs in any hive or natural nest and in which the bees walk. If this space is smaller or larger than 1 cm, the bees will join the combs. When the combs are stuck together, the hive is not movable, and it is not possible for beekeepers to manipulate a colony or to examine a brood nest. Prior to 1851, beekeeping methods were crude and the quantity of honey harvested per hive was probably one-quarter of that obtained by modern beekeepers.

It was found, in 1857, that bees could be forced to build a straight comb in a wooden frame by giving them a piece of wax, called foundation, on which the bases of the cells were aready embossed. Bees use these bases to build honeycomb, the cells of which are used for both rearing brood and for storing honey. When a hive of bees is given a frame of foundation, they are forced to build the comb where the beekeeper wants it and not where they might otherwise be inclined to build it.

Another discovery, made in 1865, was that honey can be removed from the comb by placing a comb full of honey in a centrifugal force machine, called an extractor. Approximately 16 lb (7 kg) of honey must be consumed by the bees in order for them to make 1 lb (0.45 kg) of wax comb. If the beekeeper can return an intact comb to a hive after removing the honey from it, the bees are saved the time and trouble of building a new comb, and the honey harvest is increased.

The next discovery, in 1873, was the modern smoker. When bees are smoked, they engorge with honey and become gentle. Without smoke to calm a hive, normal manipulation of the frames would not be possible. While smoke has been used to calm bees for centuries, the modern smoker has a bellows and a nozzle which allows a beekeeper to use smoke more effectively by directing the smoke where it is needed.

Within the short span of 22 years, these four discoveries laid the basis for the modern beekeeping industry. Prior to 1851, only a few individuals in the United States owned a hundred or more colonies of bees. By 1880, several people owned a thousand or more colonies each, and honey, which had once been a scarce commodity, became abundant.

Hives for bees. All beehives used in the industry today are made of wooden boxes (Fig. 3) with removable frames of comb, and 90% of these are 10-frame Langstroth hives. Beekeepers have standardized their equipment so that parts will be interchangeable within an apiary and from one commercial operation to another. The dimensions of the modern-day hive (Fig. 4) were determined in 1851 by Langstroth, who made a box based on the size of lumber available to him and on what he thought was an easy unit to lift and handle. The honeybee is remarkably adaptable. While it may show a preference for a nest of about 40 liters in volume, it will live almost anywhere it can keep its combs dry and protected.

Commercial practice. To be successful in commercial beekeeping, beekeepers must move to those areas where nectar-producing plants abound. The best-known honey in the United States is clover honey. Clovers grow in almost every state and, where abundant, they may produce large quantities of nectar. Alfalfa is also a good nectar-producing plant and it too is a major

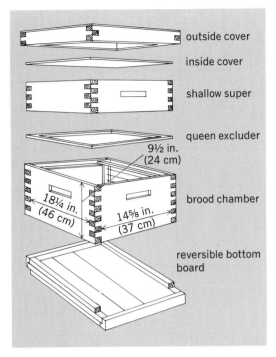

Fig. 4. Construction and dimensions of a 10-frame beehive. (*Apiculture Research Branch, Plant Industry Station, Agricultural Research Service, U. S. Department of Agriculture, Beltsville, MD*)

source of honey. Oranges grown in Florida, Arizona, and California are also known for the high quantity and quality of nectar which they produce. Just as each flower is different in its color, shape, and design, so each flower produces a unique nectar. Thus, orange honey does not taste like clover honey, and clover honey is different from that produced by buckwheat, sage, gallberry, and so on. Bees collect nectar from hundreds of kinds of flowers, and thus there are a great variety of honey flavors.

In agricultural regions where land use is intense, large areas of land are cleared, removing hedgerows and woodlots in which many insects nest and grow. Large acreages of such monocrops as apples, oranges, alfalfa, almonds, cantaloupes, and watermelons are planted, decreasing the diversity of the vegetation and eliminating many indigenous insect pollinators. In these areas there are few solitary bees.

Thousands of colonies of honeybees are rented each year by growers of crops needing cross pollination. When the plants are coming into bloom the beekeeper moves the bees, usually at night when all the bees are in the hive, and places them in groups in groves, orchards, and fields. While beekeepers make most of their living producing honey, the real importance of their bees in the agricultural economy is as cross pollinators. Without cross pollination the abundance and variety of food and flowers would not exist.

It is estimated that there are about 2000 commercial, full-time beekeepers and 200,000 persons for whom beekeeping is a part-time job or hobby in the United States. As mentioned, to be successful in beekeeping one must move to areas where nectar-producing plants are numerous. One may plant some flowering trees, bushes, and ground plants on which bees may forage, but a colony needs so much foraging area during the course of a year that a beekeeper cannot plant all that is needed. Most commercial beekeepers agree they need to harvest an average of 60 to 100 lb (27 to 45 kg) of honey per colony per year to be successful. In addition 30 to 60 colonies are needed in an apiary to be economically efficient. Not all locations have sufficient nectar forage to support that number of colonies. Commercial beekeepers feel they need to own 500 to 2000 colonies to make a living, depending on how they market their honey. Some beekeepers sell their honey on the wholesale market only, while others pack their honey themselves and devote a great deal of time to sales.

[ROGER A. MORSE]

Beet

The red or garden beet (*Beta vulgaris*), a cool-season biennial of Mediterranean origin belonging to the plant order Caryophyllales (Centrospermales). This beet is grown primarily for its fleshy root, but also for its leaves, both of which are cooked fresh or canned as a vegetable. The so-called seed is a fruit containing 2–6 true seeds. Detroit Dark Red strains predominate. Beets are only slightly tolerant of acid soils and have a high boron requirement. Cool weather favors high yields of dark red roots. Exposure to temperatures of 40–50°F for 2 weeks or more encourages undesirable seed-stalk development. Roots are harvested when they are 1–3 in. in diameter, generally 60–80 days after planting. Wisconsin, New York, and Texas are important beet producing states. The total annual farm value in the United States from about 20,000 acres is approximately $5,000,000. *See* SUGAR-BEET; VEGETABLE GROWING.

[H. JOHN CAREW]

Belladonna

The drug and also the plant known as the deadly nightshade, *Atropa belladonna* (see illustration), which belongs to the nightshade family (Solanaceae). This is a coarse, perennial herb na-

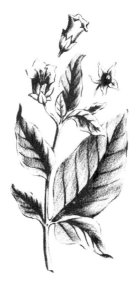

Belladonna (*Atropa belladonna*), flowering branch and isolated flowers (two views).

tive to the Mediterranean regions of Europe and Asia Minor, but now grown extensively in the United States, Europe, and India. During the blooming period, the leaves, flowering tops, and roots are collected and dried for use. The plant contains several important medicinal alkaloids, the chief one being atropine, which is much used to dilate the pupils of the eye.

[PERRY D. STRAUSBAUGH/EARL L. CORE]

Beriberi

A disorder resulting from a deficiency of vitamin B₁ (thiamine), due usually to idiosyncrasies of diet or excessive cooking or processing of food. Vitamin B₁ is a coenzyme involved in decarboxylation of alpha-keto acids (pyruvic and alpha-ketoglutaric acid) and is important in normal carbohydrate metabolism. It also acts as a factor in maintaining the integrity of the normal conductivity of the nerve fiber for transmission of neural impulses. *See* CARBOHYDRATE: CARBOHYDRATE METABOLISM: THIAMINE.

Beriberi is characterized by neurologic symptoms, such as tingling of the extremities and muscular weaknesses. Actual inflammation of the nerve fibers occurs and this neuritis, in turn, leads to other alterations in reflexes, in coordination, and in sensory perception, as well as the appearance of occasional psychic states.

When beriberi occurs suddenly, the symptomatology frequently centers about the heart. Derangement of rhythm, decreased blood pressure, the appearance of valvular murmurs, and electrocardiogram changes are typical. These may lead, somtimes precipitously, to cardiac failure and death. In many of these cardiac cases resulting from beriberi, there is associated digestive upset and irregularity and sometimes a paralysis of the diaphragm.

A progressive edema of the legs which finally involves the entire body is a common occurrence in severe cases. Such edema may also involve body cavities, producing pleural, pericardial, or peritoneal fluid formation.

The prognosis depends upon the severity and duration of the deficiency and is unfavorably affected by a tendency for sudden, often fatal, cardiac involvement to occur.   [N. KARLE MOTTET]

Bermuda grass

A long-lived perennial, *Cynodon dactylon*, native to the Old World. Bermuda grass is now common in all tropical and subtropical regions and was introduced to southern United States in colonial days.

Bermuda grass is propagated by surface runners, underground rootstocks, and seed (see illustration). Common Bermuda grass grows 6–8 in. tall; it has short, flat leaves and somewhat wiry stems, and flowers are borne on slender spikes, three to six in a cluster. The grass grows on any soil that is fertile and not too wet, but does best on heavier soils. It requires warm weather for growth, and therefore is adapted to the southern half of the United States. It endures hot dry periods well and thrives under irrigation.

Although formerly regarded as a pest in row crops, Bermuda grass is now grown as a valuable forage plant. It responds strongly to such soil im-

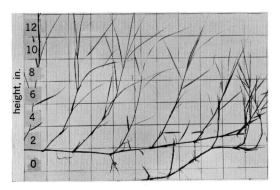

Common Bermuda grass, showing its surface runners, characteristic seedheads, and short leaves. (*From G. W. Burton, Coastal Bermuda Grass, Ga. Agr. Exp. Sta. Bull. N.S. 2, 1954*)

provements as lime and complete fertilizers, particularly those that are high in nitrogen. Improved strains of Bermuda grass have been developed at Tifton, Ga., of which Coastal, Suwanee, and Tift have been most widely used. These strains are much superior to common Bermuda for both hay and pasture. Under adequate fertilization and management, the forage is highly nutritious and supports high production by both dairy and beef cattle. *See* GRASS CROPS.

[HOWARD B. SPRAGUE]

Betel nut

The dried, ripe seed of the palm tree *Areca catechu* (Palmae), a native of Ceylon and Malaya, which attains a height of 30–50 ft. The nuts, slightly larger than a chestnut, when broken open have a faint odor and a somewhat acrid taste. Betel nuts are chewed by the natives together with the leaves of the betel pepper, *Piper betle* (Piperaceae), and lime. The mixture discolors and eventually destroys the teeth. Frequently, habitual chewers of the nut are toothless by the age of 25. The seeds contain a narcotic that produces some stimulation and a sense of well-being.

[PERRY D. STRAUSBAUGH/EARL L. CORE]

Bioclimatology

A study of the effects of the natural environment on living organisms. These effects may be direct, such as the influence of ambient temperature on body heat, or indirect, such as the influences on composition of food. Only direct effects are discussed in this article. Natural and artificial elements cannot be sharply distinguished. For example, smoke from a lightning-induced forest fire is natural, but smoke from a chimney is artificial.

Bioclimatology encompasses biometeorology, climatophysiology, climatopathology, air pollution, and other fields. The interplay between disciplines, such as meteorology and physiology, is emphasized. Concerning the time scale, the study of events enduring for hours to days is called biometeorology; for years to centuries, bioclimatology; for millennia and more, paleobioclimatology. For intrinsic reasons bioclimatology should serve as an overall term. Bioclimatology falls naturally into the two areas of plants and of animals and man.

In plant bioclimatology solution of any problem involves study of the natural climatic values, such as air temperature, precipitation, and wind speed and its variations; the transfer mechanism, such as the eddy diffusivity; and the effect of these agents on the plant. The most important mechanisms are (1) photochemical effects, such as photosynthesis and (blue) phototaxis: photosynthesis needs blue and red light, water from the roots (and possibly from the air), and CO_2 from the air; all these components vary with weather and climate; (2) evapotranspiration through integument and stomata of plants, a process depending highly on availability of water, transfer of liquids from root to leaf, temperature of the leaf, water vapor of the air, and ventilation; (3) picking up compounds of N, K, P, Ca, and others from the ground; and (4) avoidance of destructive conditions, such as freezing, drying out of leaves (if water supply is smaller than evaporative demand), and overheating. *See* AGRICULTURAL METEOROLOGY.

Although considerable work has been done on bioclimatology of domestic animals, the following discussion focuses on humans.

Photochemical bioclimatology. Essentially this is the investigation of the effects of light from the Sun and sky. Sunburn of the skin and cornea of the eye is initiated by denaturization of nucleic acid and skin proteins, causing a local histaminelike action. In nature the effect is restricted and is induced by ultraviolet radiation with wavelengths around $0.3-0.31\ \mu$. Sunburn is delayed or prevented by three screeening agents in the skin: pigment, horny layer, and urocanic acid. The pigment of permanently brown or black races, as well as the radiation-induced pigment in variably colored races (the so-called white race), acts as a protective filter. The horny layer of the skin reportedly grows in thickness by ultraviolet exposure. It is still debated how much protection is offered this way. The third screen is urocanic acid, a substance derived by enzymatic action from the amino acid L-histidine in the sweat. A 1-mm sweat layer absorbs 50% of the natural ultraviolet at 300 mm and nearly 100% of the mercury lamp ultraviolet at 250 mm. Artificial ultraviolet sources, such as the cold mercury lamp, act very differently from these sources. Solar erythema can be seen within minutes of exposure. A simple rule to avoid solar overexposure is this: As soon as the dividing line between exposed and shielded (clothed) areas can be discerned, stop sun bathing.

There are two kinds of solar pigmentation, late and direct. The late seems more prevalent in fair races; it occurs in conjunction with sunburns days later. The direct type is found more in southern Europeans and Japanese. It occurs, without sunburn, during a 30-min exposure, and is caused by long-ultraviolet ($0.32-0.4\ \mu$) and possibly visible light.

Frequent exposure over years leads to skin elastosis (sailor's skin) and finally skin cancer. Skin carcinomas occur more frequently on facial skin exposed to sun. Proof that exposure to sun is carcinogenic comes from statistical evidence and from the results of animal experiments, in which rodents were exposed to very strong artificial ultraviolet radiation.

Although bacteria are easily killed with artificial ultraviolet radiation of short wavelength, natural sunlight probably has very little bactericidal action because it does not contain these short wave-lengths.

Vitamin D is produced from natural sterols in plant and animal foodstuffs and in human skin by short-wavelength solar ultraviolet radiation (0.3 μ). *See* VITAMIN D.

It has been claimed that solar ultraviolet radiation favorably affects blood circulation and general health, but sunbather faddism has not been conductive to serious research. It is difficult to separate the effects of ultraviolet radiation, thermohygric exposure, and mental stimuli on a sunbather.

Most sunlight and sky light received by the eye is that reflected by clouds and surfaces. The intensity of the incoming light, its angle of incidence, and the amount and kind (specular or diffuse) of albedo control the amount of light received by the eye. The specular reflections of water, ice, metals, snow, clouds, and white sand are bright enough to irritate the eye. Most sunglasses dampen the whole visible spectrum uniformly and eliminate ultraviolet and infrared rays.

All the important ultraviolet effects mentioned above occur at about 0.3 μ, near the end of the solar spectrum. This ultraviolet radiation is controlled by absorption in stratospheric ozone and scattering by air molecules, clouds, and smog. Dependence of ultraviolet radiation on solar and geometric altitude is pronounced. Usually, the scattered sky ultraviolet radiation exceeds that of the Sun. Snow reflects both ultraviolet rays and visible light to cause snow blindness and sunburn below the chin. No other natural substance reflects more than a few percent of natural ultraviolet; however, metals reflect highly.

Natural penetrating ionizing radiation is composed of β- and γ-rays from radioactive minerals, including their emanations and secondary rays from cosmic radiation, mainly mesons and neutrons. Ionization by both effects at altitudes below 18 km is less than 40 milliroentgens per day, probably an insignificant figure.

Air bioclimatology. Gaseous air constitutents, such as oxygen and water vapor, influence body chemistry and heat balance. The oxygen partial pressure (pO$_2$) of inhaled air is vital for blood oxygenation and depends mainly on altitude. At or above an altitude of about 3000 m, the pO$_2$ is low enough to cause air sickness, or mountain sickness. Residence at an altitude of 1–2 km is supposed to benefit circulation, but may be harmful for some heart patients.

Low water vapor pressure may cause drying of the skin and of the mucous membranes of upper respiratory organs. Water vapor pressure, even indoors, is especially low when outdoor air temperatures are low. Many skin and respiratory complaints in winter are caused more by dryness than by cold. Water vapor influence on heat balance is discussed below.

Carbon dioxide, CO_2, water, H_2O, and organic vapors emitted by man contribute to the unpleasantness of crowded and ill-ventilated rooms, which may also be overheated.

Man's industries, volcanoes, fires, dust storms, and other more or less violent events spew large amounts of matter into the air known as fallout, smog, air pollution, and so forth. No bioclimatic problem in this field can be reported as solved un-less source, transfer mode, change in transfer concentration near the sink, the mode of intake by the sink, and the biological and chemical action of the sink are clear.

Ozone, O_3, may serve as an example. It is produced by solar ultraviolet radiation in the higher stratosphere, by lightning, and by sunlight falling on smog (Los Angeles). Stratospheric ozone is brought down by turbulence, and might reach toxic levels for crews of airplanes at about 15-km altitude. Ozone is blamed for some smog-induced injuries, for example, ocular pain in Los Angeles. A very important sink action is the inhalation into the respiratory organs, where especially the lung's surface is changed by oxidation. This causes coughing at first and tiredness later. Amounts of O_3 less than 0.5 part per million are toxic.

Carbon monoxide, unburned hydrocarbons, NO, NO$_2$, SO$_2$, and other by-products are prevalent where there is incomplete combustion. Many by-products are also highly hygroscopic, and serve as nuclei of condensation to cause the low-humidity type of smog, such as that occurring in Los Angeles. This smog condition is further complicated by the occurrence of light-induced reactions between hydrocarbons and NO$_2$ and other pollutants. The high-moisture type of smog seems typical for London.

Very few gases, in fact very little of any gas, pass the skin, with the exception of more easily permeated areas such as chapped lips, scrotum, and labia.

Aerosol bioclimatology. Solid or liquid suspensions in the air affect breathing organs or skin. Widely discussed elements of the atmospheric aerosols are the ions, which are particles containing one or more electrical charges. For a long time beneficial or dangerous effects of an abundance of particles of one charge type have been claimed. These electrical space charges reportedly have influenced results of physiological tests, growing of living cells, and severity of hay fever attacks. As a rule, negative space charge of the order of 1000–10,000 ions/cm³ is reportedly beneficial. These results are expected to explain some observations of statistical bioclimatology. *See* ATMOSPHERIC POLLUTION.

Thermal bioclimatology. This subdiscipline concerns the heat balance of man as controlled by his environment. The basic relation is shown by Eq. (1), where M is metabolic heat production; C is

$$M - Cd\theta_b/dt + H_h = H_r + H_a + H_e + R \quad (1)$$

body heat capacity; H is heat exchanged through skin; R is respiratory heat exchange; θ is temperature (°C); b refers to total body; h refers to solar radiation; r refers to infrared radiation; s refers to skin; a refers to air (convection); e refers to evaporation; and t is time. The H terms are defined in Eq. (2), where S is visible and near-infrared radiant

$$\begin{aligned} H_h &= S \cdot \epsilon_h \cdot A_h & H_r &= h_r \cdot A_r(\theta_s - \theta_r) \\ H_a &= h_a A_a(\theta_s - \theta_a) & H_e &= h_e \cdot A_e(e_s - e_a) \end{aligned} \quad (2)$$

heat flow from the Sun, sky, and environment; and ϵ_h is absorptivity of skin (0.6 for white and 0.9 for black skin). The A factors, that is, the respective surface areas, depend on body posture and on the process involved, such as radiation or convection; these areas are always smaller than the geometric surface. The terms e_s and e_a are the vapor pressures of skin and air, respectively.

The h factors are heat conductances at absolute temperature T, as shown by Eq. (3), where ϵ_r is

$$h_r = \epsilon_r \sigma (T_s^4 - T_r^4)/(\theta_s - \theta_r) \qquad (3)$$

0.98 (infrared absorptivity of skin), and σ is Stefan's constant, 4.9 kcal-m²/(hr)(deg⁴). From experiments with men, and using kilocalorie units (kcal), $h_a = 6.3\sqrt{v}$ kcal/(m²)(hr)(deg) for wind velocity v m/sec; further, $h_a = 3.3$ in calm. Equation (4)

$$h_e = 1.63 h_a \text{ kcal}/(\text{m}^2)(\text{hr})(\text{mb})(\text{deg}) \qquad (4)$$

follows from h_a. These data are valid for supine adults at sea level, and refer to the heat- or vapor-exchanging area.

Equation (5) applies for the clothed body, if h_e is

$$\theta_s - \theta_a = M/A_a h_c + (M + H_h)/A_a(h_a + h_r) \qquad (5)$$

conductance of clothes, and if $\theta_r = \theta_a$, $A_r = A_a$, $H_c = 0$, and $d\theta_b/dt = 0$. The absorptivity of the clothing is inserted for ϵ_h. If $h_a \gg h_e$ (strong wind, thick clothes), solar heating H_h becomes unimportant.

H_e can be measured directly with a good balance. The relative skin humidity $r_s = e_s/e_s^*$, where e_s^* is saturation vapor pressure at skin temperature, can be measured with a hair hygrometer or can be derived from H_e, h_e, e_a, and e_s. During sweating r_s is 100%; otherwise, it is usually below 60%. If skin relative humidity is below 10%, the skin may crack.

Skin water transfer is accomplished by sweating and diffusion. The latter corresponds usually to 1 kcal/(m²)(hr); it may reverse, so that water or vapor is transferred into the skin. Sweat is a powerful emergency measure capable of producing $H_e = 600$ kcal/(m²)(hr) or more. Bioclimatic sweat control works two ways, via body temperatures and via water coverage. The prime control for the amount secreted seems to be the temperature of a section of the hypothalamus, skin temperature acting as a moderator. These temperatures are of course bioclimatologically controlled. Skin totally covered with sweat or bath water lowers its sweat water loss strongly, about 4:1. The effect is absent in saline or with sweat highly concentrated by evaporation.

The respiratory heat and vapor loss is small except during hyperventilation at reduced pressure. Ordinarily, this loss varies little because the exhaled temperature drops as θ_a and e_a fall.

Of the climatic elements, S, h_a (wind), and precipitation are easiest to control. High values of θ_a, θ_r, and e_a are much harder to influence than low values. To ensure a constant θ_b, the body alters the peripheral blood flow and thus alters θ_s. In low temperatures M is raised by shivering or work; in a hot environment H_e is raised by sweat. These emergency regulations are effective only for certain periods. Short-time limits are set by variations of θ_b and finally θ_s (skin burn or freezing). All body controls vary with age, sex, health, exercise, and adaptation. Reportedly, frequent limited exposures to adverse thermal conditions, particularly cold, invigorate many body functions, especially if exposure is combined with exercise.

The most important climatic element is local air temperature; in the cold, wind increases the rate of body cooling. For a well-insulated man or house, Eq. (5), air temperaute alone is the deciding factor. The house heating bill is proportional to the number of degree days, that is, time multiplied by $(\alpha - \theta_a)$, where α is the preferred room temperature, about 22°C. No usable formula for the cooling effect of open air on average individuals can be derived because clothing styles change.

At temperatures greater than 25°C sweating starts. Its evaporation is restricted by high values of e_a. Hence, the combination of θ_a and e_a describes livability in the heat. Tests on sensation experienced by young men exposed to different pairs of θ_a and e_a led to the effective temperature (ET), which approximately equals $(\theta_a + \text{dew-point temperature})/2$. The area of high ET or extreme summer discomfort in the United States is the Gulf Coast, especially the lower Rio Grande Valley (average ET, 26–27°C). In the Indus Valley ET is 28.5°C; and the world maximum is in Zeila, Somali Coast, where ET is 29.7°C. Figure 1 shows a United States map of the sum of heating and cooling degrees days. Since cooling also involves drying, the cooling degree days are multiplied by two. Large numbers of the sum mean climatic hardship for the outdoors man and high bills for heating fuel and cooling wattage.

The microclimate can enhance discomfort. The values of θ_a and θ_r are much below normal on calm clear nights, especially when the terrain is concave. The Sun can raise the surface temperatures of such features as sand, walls, and vehicles to as much as 40° above the air temperature.

Extreme climates and microclimates. Certain climatic conditions can be tolerated only for a limited time, since they either overrun the physiological defense mechanism or injure and destroy body parts directly. The first mechanism usually leads to a breakdown of temperature regulation and of the body circulation, and the latter usually involves skin injuries.

The safe survival time depends primarily on air and wall temperature, if there is no artificial ventilation and no radiation other than the walls. Other conditions may suitably be converted into equivalent temperature data. Figure 2 contains such data, listing safe times between seconds (in a fire) to life-span. Some case studies are listed below.

1. The hot desert: Temperatures are in the fifties, vapor pressure is 10–15 mb, and there is sunshine and wind. Over a period of a few hours no equilibrium of body data is reached, and especially heart rate and core temperatures rise. The skin is dry and salt covered. The skin water loss is much below the level needed to compensate by evaporation for the large heat input by solar and infrared radiation and convection.

2. The jungle: Normal jungle is the habitat of a large segment of people. However, extreme jungle conditions are around 35°C and 40 mb vapor pressure. The skin is totally wet, but evaporation becomes insufficient due to external moisture. The effective temperature is a good measure for this danger signal. Worst in this respect are locally wet areas surrounded by a hot desert.

3. Fire: A forest or house fire has flame and glowing fuel temperatures of 600–900°C. Injury comes from skin burns via contact, convection, or radiation. The latter can be warded off by

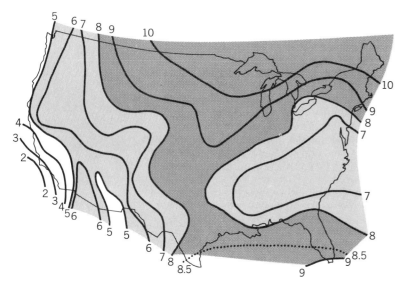

Fig. 1. Sum of heating degree days plus two times cooling degree days. The larger the sum, the larger is the integrated year-round outdoors discomfort, and also total fuel and power bill for heating and air conditioning. Units 1000°F times days. (*From K. J. K. Buettner, Human aspects of bioclimatological classification, in S. W. Tromp, ed., Biometeorology, Pergamon Press, 1962*)

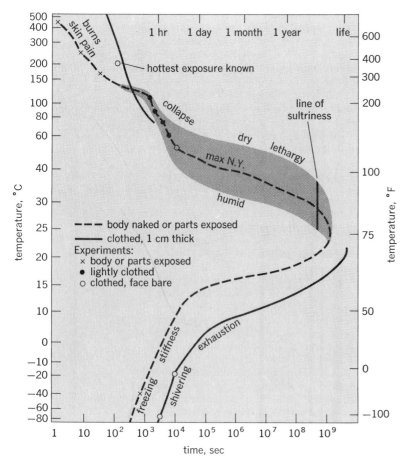

Fig. 2. Safe heat and cold exposure times in seconds for healthy, normal men at rest, with body wholly or partly exposed. Room is free from artificial ventilation and radiation; air and walls have identical temperature. Humidity influence is shown by shading. Max N.Y. = highest data of temperature and humidity in New York City. (*From K. J. K. Buettner, Space medicine of the next decade as viewed by an environmental physicist, U.S. Armed Forces Med. J., 10:416, 1959*)

aluminum-covered suits. Near a large fire radiant heat of 40,000 kcal m^{-2} hr^{-1} may cause skin pain in 1 sec and burns in a few seconds. This heat transfer is superior to flame contact. Inhaling of hot air and lack of O_2 are frequently minor problems compared to poisoning by CO.

4. Frostbite and freezing fast: Strong convective cooling by wind and low temperatures may overrun the local defenses, causing defective circulation in the skin and breakdown of small vessels and blood particles. Developing of ice crystals may puncture cells. Skin touching metals below $-30°C$ freezes on contact, causing mechanical loss of skin layers upon removal.

5. Weather accident and disaster: Yearly average of fatalities by weather catastrophes for the United States during 1901–1960 are as follows: hurricanes, 100; tornadoes, 150; lightning, 175; floods, 80; and snowstorms, blizzards, and ice storms, 200. There are probably deaths of similar numbers from heat waves and smog periods. Weather-caused farming disasters have produced many mass-killing famines. These figures fortunately have declined, as have death figures from hurricanes and tornadoes and, probably, lightnings. All others mentioned here have risen.

Statistical bioclimatology. This aspect of bioclimatology investigates correlation between weather and climate phenomena and their effects on man. The most important work concerns clinical data correlated with daily weather. Two weather types seem to be involved: Fronts, central low, and ascending air coincide with frequent attacks of angina pectoris and embolism; incidence of foehn and cyclogenesis to the west are found to correlate with increasing circulatory disorders, mental troubles, increase of accidents, and kidney colic. It has been claimed that there is a correlation between increased solar activity and all deaths in big cities, especially deaths from mental diseases.

Climatotherapy. This health treatment is more venerated than exact. Going to a resort is intimately connected with nonclimatic changes of housing, mode of living, food, exercise or rest, and psychological stimuli.

A health climate location should avoid extremes of temperature, especially high effective temperature felt as sultriness. Air should be free of smoke, smog, allergens, ozone, car exhausts, and industrial and volcanic effluents.

Solar ultraviolet and natural radioactive substances and rays are generally harmful. Beneficial outdoor living usually involves exposure of parts of the skin to solar ultraviolet, and the ensuing pigment is then taken as proof of health, a rather doubtful conclusion. A certain moderate thermal stimulation by wind, waves, and temperature changes may be helpful to most people. Adaptation to the new time zone may severely interfere with adaptation of intercontinental East-West travelers.

If a physician prescribes a very balmy climate for a weak elderly patient, the patient should be aware of the difference between the dry summer heat of for example, El Paso, Texas, and the moist heat of the Lower Rio Grande.

Paleobioclimatology. This deals with possible environmental influences on the development of species, especially of man. The local microclimate has to be considered. A cave, for example, has a very constant temperature and humidity and no sunlight. Fire, as an adjunct, was introduced in China and Hungary more than 500,000 years ago. In a tropical jungle one is not exposed to solar rays. The reduction of fur in man seems correlated with the perfection of eccrine sweating as part of a well-developed cranial temperature control. It might also permit man to utilize his skin temperature sensors to function as infrared "eyes" in the dark of a cave.

In most animals skin and fur color seem to promote camouflage or its opposite. Should this be true for man, one would find dark skin in the tropical jungle; while in a temperate maritime clime white in winter and brown in summer seems adequate. Thermally, a black skin is less suited for sunny hot climate than is a lighter one. Fair-skinned but unprotected man at a latitude of 40–50° may seasonally adapt himself to the varying solar ultraviolet. Sunburn is unlikely if daily exposure is routine. During the ultraviolet-rich summer season a sufficient deposit of vitamin D can be produced in the body to last for the darker seasons. There might have been sufficient vitamin D in the food of Stone Age man. So neither sunburn nor vitamin D seems to have affected evolution.

Ideal bioclimate. There is no ideal climate for all men. One's physiological and psychological preference seems to be set in childhood. History starts, long before effective room heating, in such subtropical climates as Egypt, Mesopotamia, and southern China, or in tropical lowlands, for example, Yucatan, or in tropical highlands, as Peru. It moves in the Old World to higher latitudes, where Romans developed heating. Later, civilized power centers around the 45° latitude, where the house microclimate was adequate the year around, even before air cooling.

Statements that culture best develops in a particular climate are of little value.

In the United States people entirely free to settle where they like the climate seem to prefer the Mediterranean climate of Southern California and the desert of Arizona. A large immigration proves this preference.

[KONRAD J. K. BUETTNER/H. E. LANDSBERG]

Bibliography: F. Becker et al., *A Survey of Human Biometeorology*, World Meteorol. Organ. Tech. Note no. 65, 1964; K. Buettner et al., Biometeorology today and tomorrow, *Bull. Amer. Meteorol. Soc.*, 48:378–393, 1967; G. E. Folk, *Textbook of Environmental Physiology*, 2d ed., 1974; H. E. Landsberg, *Weather and Health*, 1969; S. Licht (ed.), *Medical Climatology*, 1964; S. W. Tromp, *Medical Biometeorology*, Elsevier, Amsterdam, 1963; S. W. Tromp and J. J. Bouma (eds.), *Progress in Biometeorology 1963–1970*, Div. A, vol. 1, Swets and Zeitlinger, Amsterdam.

Biotin

A vitamin, widespread in nature, whose deficiency causes dermatitis and other disturbances in animals and man. It is only sparingly soluble in water (0.03 g/100 ml H_2O at 25°C). It is stable in boiling water solutions, but can be destroyed by oxidizing agents, acids, and alkalies. Under some condi-

tions, it can be destroyed by oxidation in the presence of rancid fats. Its structural formula is shown in the illustration.

Occurrence. Biotin's occurrence in nature is so widespread that it is difficult to prepare a natural deficient diet. Studies of egg-white injury resulted in the discovery of biotin deficiencies in animals. Raw egg white contains a protein, avidin, which combines with biotin to form an indigestible complex. The feeding of large amounts of raw egg white has been used in producing experimental biotin deficiencies. Heating of egg white denatures avidin, destroying its biotin complexing ability. Although the avidin biotin complex is stable to intestinal enzymes, it is hydrolyzed when administered parenterally.

Bioassay. Chemical and physical methods for biotin analyses are not available. Rat and chick assays are not very good and are seldom used. Microbiological assays using yeast or *Lactobacillus arabinosus* are commonly used.

Nutritional value. Biotin deficiency in animals is associated with dermatitis, loss of hair, muscle incoordination and paralysis, and reproductive disturbances. Biotin deficiency produced in human volunteers by feeding large amounts of egg white resulted in dermatitis, nausea, depression, muscle pains, anemia, and a large increase in serum cholesterol.

Biochemistry. Biotin occurs in nature mainly in bound forms. One of these isolated from yeast, biocytin, is ε-*N*-biotinyl-L-lysine. Biocytin can replace biotin as a growth factor for many organisms. Although the metabolic role of biocytin is unknown, its structure and concentration in some materials suggest that it is more than an oddity. Biotin functions as a coenzyme in carbon dioxide fixation and decarboxylation enzymes, as illustrated by the reversible reaction: pyruvic acid + $CO_2 \rightleftharpoons$ oxaloacetic acid. The amino acid aspartic acid can replace biotin for some microorganisms because the bacteria require aspartic acid for growth, and the oxaloacetic acid produced by biotin-containing enzymes can be converted by transamination to aspartic acid. Biotin is also involved in deamination of some amino acids: aspartic acid $\rightleftharpoons NH_3$ + fumaric acid. Some microorganisms require oleic acid if biotin is not supplied. Biotin may be important for oleic acid synthesis or vice versa. Under normal conditions, biotin is synthesized to such a degree by intestinal bacteria that a dietary source is probably not necessary. Most diets contain 25–50 μg per day, but 2–5 times as much is excreted in the urine and feces. *See* VITAMIN B$_6$.

[STANLEY N. GERSHOFF]

Structural formula for biotin.

Industrial synthesis. The structure of biotin was established and the vitamin synthesized by V. du Vigneaud and coworkers in a masterpiece of technical management of a highly complicated synthesis. *meso*-Dibenzylaminosuccinic acid is reacted with phosgene to close the imidazolidone ring. The two carbocyclic groups enable closing the adjacent thiophanone ring by reduction and sulfonation. A three-carbon chain is then introduced by reaction with ethoxypropylmagnesium bromide. Upon closing a third (thiophanium) ring, resolution of the optical antipodes is possible. A malonic ester condensation providing the necessary side chain is followed by dibenzylation, saponification and decarboxylation, giving the naturally occurring dextrorotatory biotin. *See* VITAMIN.

[ROGER A. MERCANTON]

Blackberry

Those species of the genus *Rubus*, plant order Rosales, having fruits that persist on the receptacles (see illustration). The plants are upright or trailing shrubs, usually thorny, with perennial roots and biennial canes (stems). Horticulturally, these fruits, derived from species native to or introduced into the United States, are classified as upright and trailing blackberries and black-fruited and red-fruited dewberries, the latter being closely related to the raspberry, with which there are a few hybrids. Propagation of the upright types is by suckers and root cuttings; for the dewberries and trailing blackberries, propagation is by tip layers.

Blackberries are grown in home gardens over most of the United States, except for the coldest parts of the Great Plains area and the hottest part of the South. Commercial production is extensive in many states; the annual value of the crop usually exceeds $3,000,000. The upright types are grown in the North, whereas the more tender dewberries and trailing blackberries are grown in the South and along the Pacific Coast. States usually leading in blackberry production are Oregon, Tex-

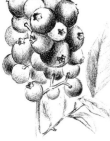

A cluster of blueberries.

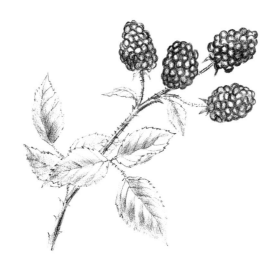

Blackberry shrub with thorny, biennial stems.

as, California, Washington, Michigan, Arkansas, Oklahoma, Alabama, and North Carolina. Although the fruit is sold fresh or canned for dessert purposes and is made into jelly or jam, quick-freezing is the largest outlet for the crop.

For diseases of blackberry *see* RASPBERRY. *See also* FRUIT GROWING, SMALL.

[J. H. CLARKE]

Blackleg

An acute, usually fatal, disease of cattle and occasionally of sheep, goats, and swine, but not man. The infection is caused by *Clostridium chauvoei* (*C. feseri*), a strictly anaerobic, spore-forming bacillus of the soil. The disease is also called symptomatic anthrax or quarter-evil. The characteristic

lesions in the natural infection consist of crepitant swellings in involved muscles, which at necropsy are dark red, dark brown, or blue black. Artificial immunization is possible by use of blackleg aggressin or whole-culture bacterin. Animals surviving an attack of blackleg are permanently immune to recurrence of the disease.

[LELAND S. MC CLUNG]

Bibliography: W. A. Hagan and D. W. Bruner, *Infectious Diseases of Domestic Animals*, 4th ed., 1961; I. A. Merchant and R. A. Packer, *Veterinary Bacteriology and Virology*, 7th ed., 1967.

Blueberry

Several species of the genus *Vaccinium*, plant order Ericales, ranging from low-growing, almost prostrate plants to vigorous shrubs reaching a height of 12–15 ft. The fruit, a berry, is usually black and covered with bluish bloom, generally occurring in clusters (see illustration), and has numerous small seeds, a characteristic that distinguishes the blueberry from the huckleberry, which has 10 rather large, gritty seeds. Although there are blueberry species on other continents, all cultivated varieties in the United States are American in origin.

Types. The dryland blueberry (*V. ashei*) is adapted to relatively dry soils and has been brought under cultivation in Florida and Georgia.

In the Northeast the lowbush blueberry (*V. lamarckii*) grows wild over thousands of acres of dry hillsides, where it is harvested commercially, especially in Maine, but also in other New England states, Michigan, Minnesota, and a few others. Some berries are sold fresh, but most are canned or frozen to be used for pies. In some areas the plants are burned over every 3 years to kill certain weeds and to remove the old wood, thus stimulating vigorous new growth. Lowbush blueberries are harvested with a small scoop, resembling a cranberry scoop, which combs the berries from the plants, whereas most of the highbush and dryland berries are picked by hand.

In the Northwest fruit of the evergreen blueberry (*V. ovatum*) is harvested in the wild, and large tonnages of the leafy twigs are shipped for use as florists' greens.

The highbush blueberry, represented by *V. australe* and *V. corymbosum*, provides most of the cultivated plants. These are bushes reaching 6–8 ft in height, and normally propagated by hardwood or softwood cuttings. The highbush blueberry is found in swampy land, usually on hummocks, so that its roots are not actually submerged. It does best in an acid soil, preferably sand and peat, and must have an ample water supply and good drainage. It can be grown on ordinary mineral soils if the water is properly regulated and the soil acidity is kept in the range pH 4–6. Nitrogen is utilized as ammonium rather than nitrate. The highbush blueberry has been under cultivation since 1910, when the first experiments on its culture were reported. Production in the United States is greatest in New Jersey, followed by Michigan, North Carolina, and Washington. The fruit is sold fresh, canned, and frozen. The blueberry is becoming increasingly popular in home gardens, although its cultural requirements are rather exacting. For garden culture, mulching with sawdust or other organic matter is desirable because the roots are shallow.

Value of crop. The annual crop value of cultivated blueberries is close to $15,000,000, and the value of blueberries harvested in the wild is about $5,000,000. *See* FRUIT GROWING, SMALL.

[J. HAROLD CLARKE]

Bluegrass

A common name applied to several species but particularly to Kentucky bluegrass (*Poa pratensis*) and to Canada bluegrass (*P. compressa*). Kentucky bluegrass is widely grown in temperate humid regions, doing best on fertile soils that are loamy or heavy in texture. Canada bluegrass is more abundant on less fertile soils in cooler regions. Both species are perennial, form sod by underground creeping stems, and have extensive root systems which are finely branched and comparatively shallow (see illustration). Top growth is 1–2 ft tall and leafy, except for seed stalks. These grasses are utilized primarily for pasture and lawns. Bluegrasses respond to fertilizers, especially those supplying nitrogen, and the herbage generally is high in the mineral elements, particularly phosphorus. Growth occurs from early spring to late fall, except for near-dormancy during the hot, dry summer period.

Kentucky bluegrass is the most important species in permanent pastures, recreation areas, and lawns in the northern half of the United States, where moisture is adequate from rainfall or irrigation. However, in pastures grown in rotation with crops in humid regions, it has been largely replaced by orchard grass and bromegrass. Several varieties have been developed specifically for turf use with special emphasis on disease resistance. *See* BROMEGRASS; GRASS CROPS.

[HOWARD B. SPRAGUE]

Bluestem grass

The most important forage grasses in those parts of the Great Plains which have 15–30 in. annual rainfall from mid-Canada to Mexico. The two major species of the bluestem group are big bluestem (*Andropogon furcatus*) and little bluestem (*A. scoparius*). Big bluestem is a large perennial, 3–5 ft tall, with somewhat coarse stems. It thrives on the more fertile soils and produces nutritious forage. Little bluestem is a tufted perennial (bunchgrass), 1–2 ft tall, with wiry stems. It tolerates moderately poor soils and droughty sites, but makes nutritious feed on the better soils. Although both species may be injured by heavy continuous grazing, under controlled management they are important range grasses for summer grazing, and also for winter range where grasses are cured on the stem. *See* GRASS CROPS.

[HOWARD B. SPRAGUE]

Botulism

A type of food poisoning due to intoxication by the extremely potent exotoxin produced by the anaerobic bacteria *Clostridium botulinum* and *C. parabotulinum*. These species, differentiated on the basis of the ability to hydrolyze protein, both produce an exotoxin of similar pharmacologic and immunologic properties. Six antigenic types of the toxin exist, most of which have been chemically purified, and toxoid or antitoxin immunization is type-specific. Immunization against botulism is generally not considered necessary since the disease is comparatively rare. The disease in humans most commonly follows ingestion of unheated, improperly processed food, with pH above 4.5, in which growth and toxin production has occurred. It is characterized by respiratory failure. The disease may occur spontaneously in a variety of animals, including chickens, ducks, minks, cattle, and horses.

The causal organism is isolated from suspected food, and the toxin type is determined by neutralization tests with antitoxin of known types. Cell-free filtrates of incriminated food may also be used for toxin typing. In humans, an acute gastroenteritis may or may not precede the principal symptoms of extreme weakness, dry mucosa, loss of accommodation, ocular muscle paralysis, and difficulty in swallowing. These symptoms commonly occur within 48 hr after the ingestion of the toxic food.

Prevention of botulism is best accomplished by safe procedures of food preservation. In established cases, serum therapy is useful only in massive doses and is effective only if toxin is not bound to motor nerve terminals.

[LELAND S. MC CLUNG]

Brassin

A lipid complex from rape pollen that is biologically active on a wide range of crop plants. Plants produce hormones which control their growth and behavior. Synthetically prepared growth-regulating substances have been used for many years to supplement endogenous hormones, and they change to some extent the behavior of crop plants to suit the needs of humans. But hormones produced by crop plants themselves so far have not been used in place of synthetic substances for this purpose, mainly because they occur in extremely small amounts and are difficult to extract. Tons of plant material are required to produce a few milligrams of hormones. However, some hormones made by plants eventually may be useful in plant control because sources have been discovered from which relatively large amounts of endogenous regulators can be obtained. Brassins, for example, are hormones that may eventually be useful; they have been discovered in pollen of rape (*Brassica napus*), a widely grown crop plant. Furthermore, endogenous hormones induce some responses that cannot be obtained with synthetic growth-regulating substances. Also of importance for food crops is the fact that these hormones, which are present in plants consumed by humans and animals, are relatively nontoxic substances.

Detection. A bioassay, devised to aid in the search for hormones in crop plants, is based on the following principles: The entire plant, rather than an explant, is used, thus making possible the expression of a variety of responses by the test plant. The test compound is applied to an undeveloped portion of a stem (internode) just as the portion is beginning to grow rapidly, thus taking advantage of the extreme sensitivity of immature plant parts to the effects of hormones. An oily carrier is used. This carrier is suitable for all known hormones and also for any lipoidal compounds that may have growth-regulating properties. Brassins

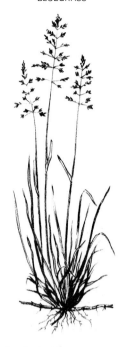

Kentucky bluegrass (*Poa pratensis*).

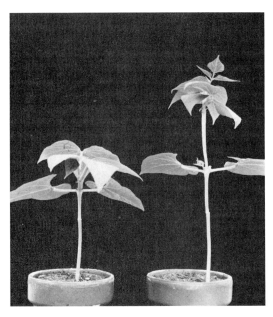

Accelerated stem growth induced in bean plant (right) with 10 μg of a fatty hormone complex (brassins) obtained from rape pollen, compared with that of an untreated bean plant (left).

and similar hormones have been detected in rape and other crop plants with this bioassay.

Isolation. Cotton fibers contain some hormones, but yields from this source are insufficient. Corn pollen contains relatively large amounts of growth-accelerating substances, but obtaining the pollen of this wind-pollinated plant is difficult. Bees have been used to facilitate the collection of pollen for most of these hormone studies.

Pollen from 39 kinds of plants were tested; 18 of these plants contained substances that accelerated plant growth in the assay used. Of these, pollen from the rape plant proved to be most promising both in terms of biological activity and availability. Since rape plants are grown extensively for the oil obtained from them, it is possible to collect large amounts (hundreds of pounds if needed) of pollen from them.

Marked acceleration of stem growth resulted when crude extracts of rape pollen, made by soaking rape pollen in ether, were tested. Chromatographic purification of the hormones obtained resulted in an oily product, 10 μg of which accelerated stem elongation three- to fivefold, sometimes as much as tenfold (see illustration). Methods have been developed whereby brassins can be purified using column and plate chromatography; 6–10 mg of the brassin complex is obtained from 60 g of rape pollen. *See* RAPE.

Pollen from other plants may contain hormones similar to brassins. For example, pollen from alder (*Alnus glutinosa*) contains hormones that behave like brassins chromatographically and induce plant responses typical of those caused by brassins.

Chemistry. The brassins contain a complex mixture of lipids. The constituent fatty acids have varying chain lengths and are presumably present in the ester form, as determined by spectroscopic

and chromatographic methods. Separation of brassins by Florisil column chromatography gives five fractions, each with hormonal activity. Saponification of brassins yields fatty acids, some of which are linked to polyhydroxyl-containing compounds such as sugars. These acids are converted into corresponding methyl esters, which are then analyzed by gas-liquid chromatography. There are five major peaks on the chromatogram. Comparison of these peaks with those of standard methyl esters shows that the major methyl esters in brassins have chain lengths of C_{16} to C_{20}. These results suggest that the brassin complex contains several compounds which seem to be fatty acids in the form of esters. At present it is not known how many of these compounds are active in producing biological activity.

Growth responses. Knowledge about the way plants respond to brassins is very limited because only small amounts of these hormones are available. Both leaves and stems of bean plants respond to treatment with brassins. An internode treated with 10 μg of brassin complex usually begins to show an increase in growth rate, compared with that of an untreated plant, in about 24 hr. About 4 days after treatment, this internode will be both longer and in most cases, larger in diameter at the top than comparable parts of untreated plants (see illustration). Histological studies show that brassins induce both cell elongation and cell division within the same internode. This dual effect (elongation plus division) is unique among the natural plant hormones. Stimulation of cell division is unusual, since, in untreated plants, growth of the internodes mainly involves cell enlargement rather than cell division. Cell division in the stem usually involves parenchyma cells of the cortex, phloem, xylem, and pith. *See* PLANT GROWTH.

When applied to the stem, brassins also stimulate cell division in the pulvinus, petiole, and veins of bean leaves. When relatively large amounts of brassins are used (10 μg), leaves assume a distorted shape, and tissue arrangement, particularly that of the vascular tissues, is greatly modified when viewed histologically.

Responses to brassins have occurred over a hundredfold concentration range (1–100 μg), and the hormone complex is not toxic to bean plants even when applied directly and undiluted with the lanolin carrier. *See* PLANT HORMONES.

[J. F. WORLEY; N. MANDAVA]

Bibliography: N. Mandava et al., *I & EC Prod. Res. Develop.*, 12:138–139, 1973; N. Mandava and J. W. Mitchell, *Chem. Ind.*, 23:930–931, Dec. 2, 1972; J. W. Mitchell et al., *Nature*, 225:1065–1066, 1970; J. W. Mitchell and L. E. Gregory, *Nature New Biol.*, 239:253–254, 1972; J. F. Worley and D. T. Krizek, *Hortscience*, 7:480–481, 1972; J. F. Worley and J. W. Mitchell, *Amer. Soc. Hort. Sci.*, 96:270–273, 1971.

Brazil nut

A large broad-leafed evergreen tree, *Bertholettia excelsa*, that grows wild in the forests of the Amazon valley of Brazil and Bolivia. The fruit is a spherical capsule, 3–6 in. in diameter and weighing 2–4 lb which, when mature, consists of an outer hard indehiscent husk about 1/2 in. thick enclosing an inner hard-shelled container or pod filled with about 20 rather triangular seeds or nuts.

Although there are a few plantations in Brazil, almost the entire production is gathered from wild trees. The quantity that gets into commercial channels varies with the price paid on the world market. The nuts are gathered either by local people who live in the forest or migrants who come into the area for the harvest season. The ripened capsules fall to the ground, and because of their weight and the height of the trees are a hazard to the harvesters. The fruits are carried to the stream bank and transported in small boats to local huts, where the capsules are split open to free the nuts. These are sold to traders who ship them downstream to brokers. Total average yearly production is reported to be 43,000 short tons of nuts in shell. They are mostly exported to Europe, Canada, and the United States. About one-fourth of the crop is shelled in Brazil before export.

Brazil nuts have a high oil and protein content and require careful handling and refrigeration to prevent spoilage. The nuts are used in confectionery, baked goods, and nut mixtures. See NUT CROP CULTURE.

[LAURENCE H. MAC DANIELS]

Breadfruit

The multiple fruit of an Indo-Malaysian tree, *Artocarpus altilis*, of the mulberry family (Moraceae), now cultivated in tropical lowlands around the

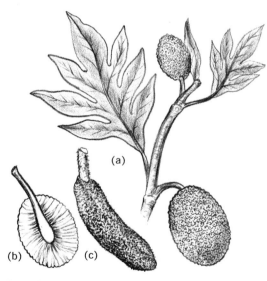

Breadfruit (*Artocarpus altilis*). (*a*) End of branch with multiple fruits. (*b*) Longitudinal section of multiple fruit. (*c*) Staminate flower cluster.

world (see illustration). Captain William Bligh was bringing plants from Tahiti to America when the mutiny on the *Bounty* occurred. The perianth, pericarp, and receptacle are all joined in a multiple fruit having a high carbohydrate content. The fruits vary considerably in size and are often borne in small clusters. Breadfruit is a wholesome food for both man and beast. It is eaten fresh or baked, boiled, roasted, fried, or ground up and made into bread. There are many varieties, both with and without seeds.

[EARL L. CORE]

Breeding (animal)

The theory and application of quantitative and Mendelian genetics to the genetic and economic improvement of farm animals for such traits as growth rate and meat quality in beef cattle, sheep, and swine; egg yield and quality in chickens; and milk yield and composition in dairy cattle. Although farm animals have been domesticated and improved for thousands of years, the theory for genetic improvement was not developed until after Gregor Mendel's laws were rediscovered in 1901. Before then, however, Robert Bakewell (1726–1795), in England, is credited with development of several improved breeds of livestock by application of his still true axioms, "Like begets like" and "Breed the best to the best." The ideas of Charles Darwin on natural selection in the middle 1800s also anticipated the effects of selection controlled by humans on the genetic improvement of farm animals.

History. The first applications of Mendel's genetic laws involved the qualitative effects of only a pair of genes, but most economic traits are controlled by many genes, each with relatively small effects. This form of inheritance, while following Mendel's principles, is called polygenic or quantitative inheritance. Although Bakewell is sometimes called the father of animal breeding, the honor in the modern era more fittingly belongs to Jay L. Lush, who in the 1920s and 1930s developed most of the theory of modern animal breeding. The mathematical basis of these principles can be credited to Sewell Wright, certainly the grandfather of modern animal breeding. The theory for more complicated statistical situations has been developed by C. R. Henderson and Alan Robertson, both of whom studied with Lush.

Principles of selection. Selection of superior parents can be very effective in improving a single trait or combination of traits weighted by the economic values of the traits. The principles are the same in either case, although the application is more complicated for a combination of traits. Animals must show differences (variation) or selection is impossible. A fraction of the variation (heritability) must also be due to genetic differences. Gain from selection per year can be predicted as the product of accuracy of selection, a factor related to the fraction of animals selected (the selection intensity factor), and the standard deviation of the trait (a standard measure of variation) which is divided by the interval measured in years between when an animal is born and when its replacement is born. The accuracy of evaluation, which may range between 0 and 100%, increases as more records on the animal and close relatives are used for evaluation, and is higher for traits with high heritability.

Selection. Generally, mass selection (selection on the animal's own record) is efficient for traits with heritability above 25%. Progeny testing is more effective for traits with low heritability and those that are limited to only one sex such as milk production.

For most traits, male selection will contribute 90% or more to total genetic gain because fewer and thus more highly selected males are needed as compared with females. The most striking gains

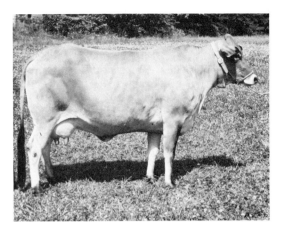

The result of a cross between a Red Sindhi bull (a Zebu breed, *Bos indicus*) and a Jersey cow (a European breed, *B. taurus*). *(From G. H. Schmidt and L. D. Van Vleck, Principles of Dairy Science, W. H. Freeman and Company; copyright © 1974)*

from selection have been made in dairy cattle because of the primary importance of a single trait, the accuracy of selection made possible by an excellent records system for progeny testing, and the use of artificial insemination which makes intense selection of males practical since up to 50,000 matings per year are possible to each accurately evaluated bull. *See* CATTLE PRODUCTION, DAIRY.

Rapid genetic change from intense selection is also possible in swine breeding because of the rapid rate of reproduction — two litters of 8 to 10 pigs per year. Progress has been limited, however, by the necessity of selecting simultaneously for several traits and because of changing goals of selection. *See* SWINE PRODUCTION.

Progress in beef cattle has been slow because different parts of the industry consider different traits to have primary importance. In addition, reproductive rate is low, and the potential of artificial insemination has not been exploited due to management difficulties. *See* CATTLE PRODUCTION, BEEF.

Most economic traits of farm animals fall into three groups: production traits such as milk yield or growth rate; quality of product traits such as carcass quality or milk composition; and reproductive traits such as calving interval or services per conception. The quality traits generally have high heritability and exhibit little heterosis; production traits usually have moderate heritability and heterosis; and reproductive traits have low heritability and relatively high heterosis. Heterosis is defined as the difference of crossbred offspring from the average of purebred offspring of the same breeds of parents.

Crossbreeding. Crosses between breeds can be used to improve traits which exhibit positive heterosis. Crossbreeding is also used when the optimum for a trait is intermediate between the average for the two breeds (see illustration). Problems with crossbreeding involve the maintaining of pure breeds, the lack of selection possible in the pure breeds, and the difficulty of finding enough breeds with desirable characteristics to use as males on crossbred females. Thus, after three to four crosses or less of different breeds of males on succeed-

ing generations of crossbred females, the breeds of sires are usually repeated in rotation. Most commercial swine and sheep are produced by crossbreeding because of heterosis for reproductive rate and also for growth rate. Beef cattle production has recently increased the use of crossbreeding, especially for terminal crosses where a large breed of sire is used to produce offspring, all of which are marketed, and also because of heterosis for reproductive rate and for improved mothering ability of crossbred cows.

Crossbreeding is also used to upgrade native breeds. An imported or exotic breed with more desirable production characteristics is mated to native breeds of low productivity but high adaptability to the local conditions. These crossbred offspring can then be mated to sires of the same imported breed — a process that can be continued until the genes of the population are nearly all from the imported breed. Since the imported breed is often not adapted to the local conditions, management often must be improved to allow for increased productivity of the upgraded animals. If the management is increased only slightly, the first cross, in many cases, will be more productive than crosses with three-fourths or more of imported genes; in such situations, a rotational system maintaining three-eighths to five-eighths imported genes may be optimum. Matings and selection among the crossbred animals also can be used to form a synthetic breed with the desirable characteristics of the parent breeds — productivity of the imported breed and adaptability of the native breed. *See* AGRICULTURAL SCIENCE (ANIMAL).

[DALE VAN VLECK]

Bibliography: D. S. Falconer, *Introduction to Quantitative Genetics*, 1960; J. F. Lasley, *Genetics of Livestock Improvement*, 1972; G. H. Schmidt and L. D. Van Vleck, *Principles of Dairy Science*, 1974.

Breeding (plant)

The application of genetic principles to the improvement of cultivated plants, with heavy dependence upon the related sciences of statistics, pathology, physiology, and biochemistry. The aim of plant breeding is to produce new and improved types of farm crops or decorative plants, to better serve the needs of the farmer, the processor, and the ultimate consumer. New varieties of cultivated plants can result only from genetic reorganization that gives rise to improvements over the existing varieties in particular characteristics or in combinations of characteristics. In consequence, plant breeding can be regarded as a branch of applied genetics, but it also makes use of the knowledge and techniques of many aspects of plant science, especially physiology and pathology. Related disciplines, like biochemistry and entomology, are also important, and the application of mathematical statistics in the design and analysis of experiments is essential.

Plant breeding has made major contributions to increasing the yields of crops and to diminishing their susceptibility to hazards that limit their productivity. It has been estimated that the annual production of corn in the United States has been increased by 750,000,000 bu by plant breeding methods, especially by the exploitation of hybrid corn. In western Europe the yields of wheat and barley have been increased by approximately 1% per annum since the late 1940s. Perhaps the most dramatic impact of plant breeding occurred during the 1960s in Mexico where, as the result of the stimulus from a Rockefeller Foundation program, a wheat-importing country was changed into a wheat-exporting country because of a surplus of wheat.

Scientific method. The cornerstone of all plant breeding is selection. By selection the plant breeder means the picking out of plants with the best combinations of agricultural and quality characteristics from populations of plants with a variety of genetic constitutions. Seeds from the selected plants are used to produce the next generation, from which a further cycle of selection may be carried out if there are still differences. Much of the early development of the oldest crop plants from their wild relatives resulted from unconscious selection by the first farmers. Subsequent conscious acts of selection slowly molded crops into the forms of today. Finally, since the early years of the 20th century, plant breeders have been able to rationalize their activities in the light of a rapidly expanding understanding of genetics and of the detailed biology of the species studied.

Plant breeding can be divided into three main categories on the basis of ways in which the species are propagated. Species that reproduce sexually and that are normally propagated by seeds occupy two of these categories. First come the species that set seeds by self-pollination, that is, fertilization usually follows the germination of pollen on the stigmas of the same plant on which it was produced. The second category of species sets seeds by cross-pollination, that is, fertilization usually follows the germination of pollen on the stigmas of different plants from those on which it was produced. The third category comprises the species that are asexually propagated, that is, the commercial crop results from planting vegetative parts or by grafting. Consequently, vast areas can be occupied by genetically identical plants of a single clone that have, so to speak, been budded off from one superior individual. The procedures used in breeding differ according to the pattern of propagation of the species.

Self-pollinating species. The essential attribute of self-pollinating crop species, such as wheat, barley, oats, and many edible legumes, is that, once they are genetically pure, varieties can be maintained without change for many generations. When improvement of an existing variety is desired, it is necessary to produce genetic variation among which selection can be practiced. This is achieved by artificially hybridizing between parental varieties that may contrast with each other in possessing different desirable attributes. All members of the first hybrid (F_1) generation will be genetically identical, but plants in the second (F_2) generation and in subsequent generations will differ from each other because of the rearrangement and reassortment of the different genetic attributes of the parents. During this segregation period the breeder can exercise selection, favoring for further propagation those plants that most nearly match the ideal he has set himself and discarding the remainder. In this way the genetic structure is remolded so that some generations

later, given skill and good fortune, when genetic segregation ceases and the products of the cross are again true-breeding, a new and superior variety of the crop will have been produced.

This system is known as pedigree breeding, and while it is the method most commonly employed, it can be varied in several ways. For example, instead of selecting from the F_2 generation onward, a bulk population of derivatives of the F_2 may be maintained for several generations. Subsequently, when all the derivatives are essentially true-breeding, the population will consist of a mixture of forms. Selection can then be practiced, and it is assumed, given a large scale of operation, that no useful segregant will have been overlooked. By whatever method they are selected, the new potential varieties must be subjected to replicated field trials at a number of locations and over several years before they can be accepted as suitable for commercial use.

Another form of breeding that is often employed with self-pollinating species involves a procedure known as backcrossing. This is used when an existing variety is broadly satisfactory but lacks one useful and simply inherited trait that is to be found in some other variety. Hybrids are made between the two varieties, and the F_1 is crossed, or backcrossed, with the broadly satisfactory variety which is known as the recurrent parent. Among the members of the resulting first backcross (B_1) generation, selection is practiced in favor of those showing the useful trait of the nonrecurrent parent and these are again crossed with the recurrent parent. A series of six or more backcrosses will be necessary to restore the structure of the recurrent parent, which ideally should be modified only by the incorporation of the single useful attribute sought from the nonrecurrent parent. Backcrossing has been exceedingly useful in practice and has been extensively employed in adding resistance to diseases, such as rust, smut, or mildew, to established and acceptable varieties of oats, wheat, and barley. *See* PLANT DISEASE.

Cross-pollinating species. Natural populations of cross-pollinating species are characterized by extreme genetic diversity. No seed parent is true-breeding, first because it was itself derived from a fertilization in which genetically different parents participated, and second because of the genetic diversity of the pollen it will have received. In dealing with cultivated plants with this breeding structure, the essential concern in seed production is to employ systems in which hybrid vigor is exploited, the range of variation in the crop is diminished, and only parents likely to give rise to superior offspring are retained.

Inbred lines. Here plant breeders have made use either of inbreeding followed by hybridization (see illustration) or of some form of recurrent selection. During inbreeding programs normally cross-pollinated species, such as corn, are compelled to self-pollinate by artificial means. Inbreeding is continued for a number of generations until genetically pure, true-breeding, and uniform inbred lines are produced. During the production of the inbred lines rigorous selection is practiced for general vigor and yield and disease resistance, as well as for other important characteristics. In this way desirable attributes can be maintained in the

first year

pollen
from A

detasseled

second year

detasseled

pollen from
(C × D)

first year

pollen
from D

detasseled

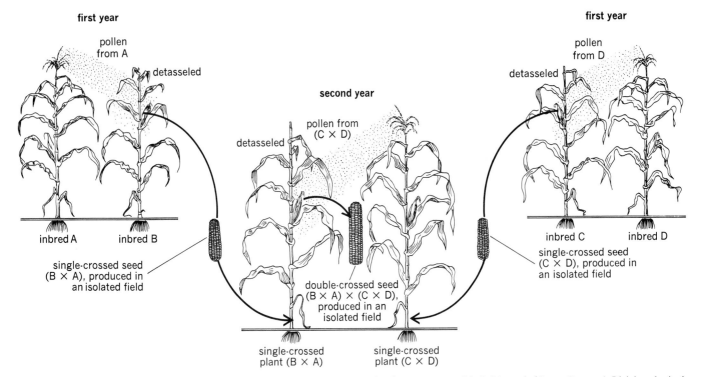

inbred A   inbred B

single-crossed seed
(B × A), produced in
an isolated field

double-crossed seed
(B × A) × (C × D),
produced in an
isolated field

inbred C   inbred D

single-crossed seed
(C × D), produced in
an isolated field

single-crossed
plant (B × A)

single-crossed
plant (C × D)

Sequence of steps in crossing inbred plants and using the resulting single-crossed seed to produce double-crossed hybrid seed. (*Crops Research Division, Agricultural Research Service, USDA*).

inbred lines, which are nevertheless usually of poor vigor and somewhat infertile. Their usefulness lies in the vigor, high yield, uniformity, and agronomic merit of the hybrids produced by crossing different inbreds. Unfortunately, it is not possible from a mere inspection of inbred lines to predict the usefulness of the hybrids to which they can give rise. To estimate their value as the parents of hybrids, it is necessary to make tests of their combining ability. The test that is used depends upon the crop and on the ease with which controlled cross-pollination can be effected.

Tests may involve top crosses (inbred × variety), single crosses (inbred × inbred), or three-way crosses (inbred × single cross). Seeds produced from crosses of this kind must then be grown in carefully controlled field experiments designed to permit the statistical evaluation of the yields of a range of combinations in a range of agronomic environments like those normally encountered by the crop in agricultural use. From these tests it is possible to recognize which inbred lines are likely to be successful as parents in the development of seed stocks for commercial growing. The principal advantages from the exploitation of hybrids in crop production derive from the high yields produced by hybrid vigor, or heterosis, in certain species when particular parents are combined.

Economic considerations. The way in which inbred lines are used in seed production is dictated by the costs involved. Where the cost of producing F_1 hybrid seeds is high, as with many forage crops or with sugar beet, superior inbreds are combined into a synthetic strain which is propagated under conditions of open pollination. The commercial crop then contains a high frequency of superior hybrids in a population that has a similar level of variability to that of an open-pollinated variety. However, because of the selection practiced in the isolation and testing of the inbreds, the level of yield is higher because of the elimination of the less productive variants.

When the cost of seed is not of major significance relative to the value of the crop produced, and where uniformity is important, F_1 hybrids from a single cross between two inbred lines are grown. Cucumbers and sweet corn are handled in this way. By contrast, when the cost of the seeds is of greater significance relative to the value of the crop, the use of single-cross hybrids is too expensive and then double-cross hybrids (single cross A × single cross B) are used, as in field corn. As an alternative to this, triple-cross hybrids can be grown, as in marrow stem kale, in the production of which six different inbred lines are used. The commercial crop is grown from seeds resulting from hybridization between two different three-way crosses.

Recurrent selection. Breeding procedures designated as recurrent selection are coming into limited use with open-pollinated species. In theory, this method visualizes a controlled approach to homozygosity, with selection and evaluation in each cycle to permit the desired stepwise changes in gene frequency. Experimental evaluation of the procedure indicates that it has real possibilities. Four types of recurrent selection have been suggested: on the basis of phenotype, for general combining ability, for specific combining ability, and reciprocal selection. The methods are similar in the procedures involved, but vary in the type of tester parent chosen, and therefore in the efficiency with which different types of gene action (additive and nonadditive) are measured. A brief description is given for the reciprocal recurrent selection.

Two open-pollinated varieties or synthetics are chosen as source material, for example, A and B. Individual selected plants in source A are self-pollinated and at the same time outcrossed to a sample of B plants. The same procedure is repeated in source B, using A as the tester parent. The two series of testcrosses are evaluated in yield trials. The following year inbred seed of those A plants demonstrated to be superior on the basis of testcross performance are intercrossed to form a new composite, which might be designated A_1. Then B_1 population would be formed in a similar manner. The intercrossing of selected strains to produce A_1 approximately restores the original level of variability or heterozygosity, but permits the fixation of certain desirable gene combinations. The process, in theory, may be continued as long as genetic variability exists. In practice, the hybrid $A_n \times B_n$ may be used commercially at any stage of the process if it is equal to, or superior to, existing commercial hybrids.

Asexually propagated crops. A very few asexually propagated crop species are sexually sterile, like the banana, but the majority have some sexual fertility. The cultivated forms of such species are usually of widely mixed parentage, and when propagated by seed, following sexual reproduction, the offspring are very variable and rarely retain the beneficial combination of characters that contributes to the success of their parents. This applies to such species as the potato, to fruit trees like apples and pears that are propagated by grafting, and to raspberries, grapes, and pineapples.

Varieties of asexually propagated crops consist of large assemblages of genetically identical plants, and there are only two ways of introducing new and improved varieties. The first is by sexual reproduction and the second is by the isolation of sports or somatic mutations. The latter method has often been used successfully with decorative plants, such as chrysanthemum, and new forms of potato have occasionally arisen in this way. When sexual reproduction is used, hybrids are produced on a large scale between existing varieties with different desirable attributes in the hope of obtaining a derivative possessing the valuable characters of both parents. In some potato-breeding programs many thousands of hybrid seedlings are examined each year. The small number that have useful arrays of characters are propagated vegetatively until sufficient numbers can be planted to allow the agronomic evaluation of the potential new variety.

Special techniques. So far attention has been concentrated on the general principles of plant breeding and on methods of general applicability. However, there are a few special procedures that should be mentioned.

Cytoplasmic male sterility. In several crop species variants have been found that do not produce fertile pollen. However, pollen fertility can be restored in hybrids that result when the male sterile lines are pollinated by other, so-called restorer, lines. Using crosses between male sterile lines and restorer lines, F_1 hybrid seed supplies can easily be obtained on a large scale. Systems of this kind are used in the commercial production of hybrids in corn, sorghum, sugar beet, and onions. Unfortu-

nately, hybrid corn varieties based on a single cytoplasm, causing male sterility, led to widespread susceptibility to the southern corn blight disease in the United States in 1971. Cytoplasmic male sterility has since been abandoned in the production of hybrid corn. However, the potentialities of using male sterility to produce hybrid wheat are still being explored.

Polyploids. Many crop species are naturally polyploid, and polyploidy can be induced artificially by colchicine treatment and in other ways. Polyploids are often characterized by a more sturdy growth habit and by larger roots, leaves, and flowers than the related diploids. Artificial polyploids are grown commercially in clover, watercress, sugar beet, and forage grasses. In watermelons crosses between normal diploids and artificial polyploids are used to produce hybrids that are sterile and so produce fruit without seeds—obviously a desirable attribute.

Multilinear varieties. Varieties of self-pollinating species like wheat generally consist of genetically identical plants. Multilinear varieties are also made up of genetically similar plants but contain several lines that differ in having genetically different forms of disease resistance. Each component line is produced by backcrossing different forms of resistance into a common recurrent parental variety. The advantage of the multilinear constitution is that, if the resistance of one of the constituent lines breaks down, production will be maintained by the remaining resistant lines.

Haploids. Normally, in the life cycle of higher plants, nuclei of the pollen grains and the egg cells have half the number of chromosomes (the haploid number) of the number in the nuclei of the plant on which they are produced (the diploid number). The diploid number is restored on fertilization by the fusion of egg and pollen haploid nuclei. Means have been discovered of producing essentially normal plants (sporophytes) of several crop species with the haploid chromosome number. The controlled production of such haploids, followed by doubling of the chromosome number using colchicine, enables the immediate fixation of the first products of segregation and recombination. Thus there is a very rapid return to complete homozygosity and homogeneity from hybrids of self-pollinated species. Alternatively, the procedure can give rise to the equivalents of inbred lines in outbreeding species. Haploidy may be induced by the culture on a nutrient medium of anthers or pollen grains (tobacco) by the elimination of the set of chromosomes of one parent in interspecific hybrids (barley and wheat) or by the parthenogenetic functioning of an egg which has not been fertilized by a pollen parent carrying a distinct and dominant genetic marker (corn and potato).

Cell biology. The understanding of methods by which plant cells can be cultured is now considerable. Moreover, unlike animal cells, plant cells in culture can be induced to regenerate into entire organisms. This has made possible the use of cell biological methodology in plant breeding. Two procedures are being explored. First, since very large numbers of cells can be cultured in a relatively small space, and inexpensively, many more potentially distinct genetic variants can be examined than would be the case if entire plants were used.

Cells in culture can be exposed to an environment (say, a drug or an amino acid analog), and only those which are resistant will survive. The survivors can be multiplied and regenerated into entire plants after more rigorous selection than would otherwise have been possible.

The ability to regenerate entire plants from cells has also made it possible to contemplate the fusion of somatic plant cells. Such fusion can lead to the production of hybrids between species that are incapable of sexual hybridization. The first step in this process is the enzymatic degradation of the cellulose, hemicellulose, and pectin walls that surround all plant cells. This releases a naked protoplast; fusion of protoplasts is induced by chemical treatments, such as by polyethylene glycol. Following protoplast fusion, nuclear fusion will occur in some instances. Removal of the wall-degrading enzymes then permits regeneration of the cell wall and the establishment of a culture of hybrid cells which are subsequently induced to regenerate into complete plants. The value of these techniques is not yet fully visualized. The possibility of transfer of genetic material between species and genera is one possibility. It may provide the plant breeder with new reservoirs of genetic variation. Another possibility is in the improvement of asexually propagated crop plants.

[RALPH RILEY]

Bibliography: R. W. Allard, *Principles of Plant Breeding*, 1960; F. N. Briggs and P. F. Knowles, *Introduction to Plant Breeding*, 1967; K. J. Kasha (ed.), *Haploids in Higher Plants*, 1974; A. Müntzing, *Genetics: Basic and Applied*, 1967; R. R. Nelson (ed.), *Breeding Plants for Disease Resistance*, 1973.

Broccoli

A cool-season biennial crucifer, *Brassica oleracea* var. *italica*, of Mediterranean origin, belonging to the plant order Papaverales. Broccoli is grown for its thick branching flower stalks which terminate in clusters of loose green flower buds. Stalks and buds are cooked as a vegetable or may be processed in either canned or frozen form. Cultural practices for broccoli are similar to those used for cabbage. *See* CABBAGE.

New varieties (cultivars) with greater disease resistance and higher quality are continually being developed. Broccoli is slightly tolerant of acid soils and has high requirements for boron and molybdenum. Terminal and axillary clusters are cut 80–140 days after planting. California and Texas are important broccoli-producing states. The total annual farm value in the United States from approximately 40,000 acres is $20,000,000. *See* VEGETABLE GROWING.

[H. JOHN CAREW]

Bromegrass

A common name designating a number of grasses found in the North Temperate Zone that produce highly palatable and nutritious forage. Of these, smooth bromegrass (*Bromus inermis*) is the most important (see illustration). This species was introduced to the United States during the 1880s from central Europe and Russia, where it is native. It proved to be well adapted to regions of cold winters and limited rainfall. Although first widely used

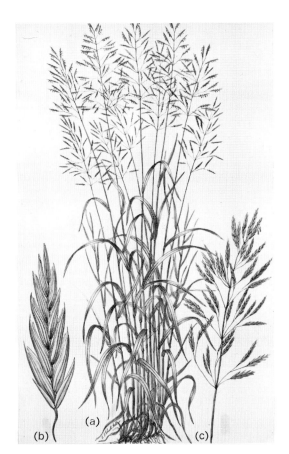

Smooth bromegrass (*Bromus inermis*). (a) Entire plant. (b) Fruit. (c) Inflorescence.

in the eastern Great Plains and western Corn Belt regions, improved strains are now grown extensively for hay and rotation pastures north of the Mason-Dixon line, from the Plains to the Atlantic. Smooth bromegrass is a long-lived perennial, spreads by underground creeping stems, and is fairly deep rooted and drought-tolerant. Top growth is 2–4 ft tall and is used for hay or pasture. Regional strains are available for Canada and the northern two-thirds of the United States. Bromegrass tolerates a wide range of soil conditions, but responds well to higher levels of fertility. Where the moisture supply is adequate, smooth bromegrass grows well in mixtures with alfalfa and red clover. The seeds of bromegrass are large, light, and chaffy, and successful planting requires special seeders. *See* GRASS CROPS.

[HOWARD B. SPRAGUE]

Brucellosis

An infectious disease of animals and man caused by bacteria of the genus *Brucella*. The organisms are *B. melitensis*, found in sheep and goats, *B abortus* in cattle, and *B. suis* in swine. Man becomes infected through direct contact with infected animals or by ingesting their unpasteurized milk. The principal animal reservoirs of the disease are cattle, swine, goats, and sheep. Brucellosis occurs throughout the world and is the most important of the nearly 100 diseases of animals transmissible to human beings.

The brucellae are small, nonmotile, nonsporing, gram-negative coccobacilli. *B. militensis* and *B.*

suis will grow aerobically in trypticase soy broth, but *B. abortus* requires 10% carbon dioxide. Differentiation of the three species is made by biochemical reactions, growth requirements, and serological tests.

Animals. The brucellae localize in the reproductive organs and mammary glands of animals. This makes the disease of serious economic concern to livestock producers and dairymen because it causes abortions and reduces the production of milk. The disease in cattle is known as Bang's disease, or contagious abortion.

Humans. Brucellosis in man, also known as undulant fever or Malta fever, is primarily an occupational disease in which infection through the skin is acquired by contact with the tissues of freshly killed animals, or with the contaminated environment of the animals. The disease is also contracted by drinking unpasteurized milk and by eating fresh cheese prepared from unpasteurized milk.

The acute illness is characterized by chills, fever, sweats, and weakness. Chronic disease results in weakness and mental depression. The usual course of the disease is less than 3 months, but antibiotic therapy (chlortetracycline) reduces the length of the illness. It may also prevent both recurrence and complications, such as osteomyelitis, orchitis, subacute endocarditis, and diseases of the kidney and liver.

Diagnosis. In animals the diagnosis is made by detecting brucella agglutinins in the milk (whey test or ring test) or in the blood. The diagnosis in man is established by the presence of brucella agglutinins in the blood and by isolating brucellae from blood cultures. A standardized brucella antigen is used in tests for brucella agglutinins. The brucella skin test is of doubtful diagnostic value.

Prevention. Human brucellosis can be eliminated only by eradicating the disease in animals. The disease is controlled in cattle by eliminating infected animals. Successful vaccination of cattle against the disease has been achieved with a live brucella culture having stable, attenuated virulence. An effective vaccine has been developed for the protection of sheep and goats, but not for swine.

The incidence of human brucellosis can be reduced by using only pasteurized animal milk for human consumption.

[WESLEY W. SPINK]

Brussels sprouts

A cool-season biennial crucifer (*Brassica oleracea* var. *gemmifera*), which is of northern European origin and belongs to the plant order Capparales. The plant is grown for its small headlike buds formed in the axils of the leaves along the plant stem (see illustration). These buds are eaten as a cooked vegetable. Cultural practices are similar to those used for cabbage; however, monthly mean temperatures below 70°F are necessary for firm sprouts. Brussels sprouts are moderately tolerant of acid soils and have a high requirement for boron. Popular varieties (cultivars) are Half Dwarf and Catskill; however, hybrid varieties are increasingly planted. Harvesting begins when the lower sprouts are firm and 1–2 in. in diameter, usually 3 months after planting. California and

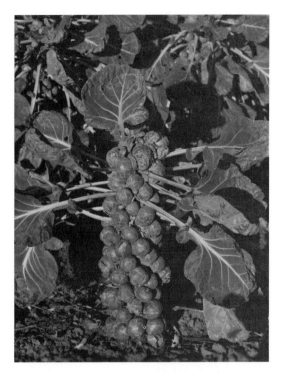

Brussels sprouts (*Brassica oleracea* var. *gemmifera*), Jade Cross (*Joseph Harris Co., Rochester, N.Y.*)

New York are important producing states. The total annual farm value of brussels sprouts in the United States from approximately 6500 acres is $8,000,000. *See* CABBAGE; VEGETABLE GROWING.

[H. JOHN CAREW]

Buckwheat

A herbaceous, erect annual, the dry seed or grain of which is used as a source of food and feed. It is not a true cereal and is one of the very few plants, other than those of the Gramineae family, used for their starchy seed, which is processed as a meal or flour.

Buckwheat belongs to the Polygonaceae family, which also includes the common weeds dock, sorrel, knotweed, bindweed, smartweed, and climbing false buckwheat. Species of buckwheat that have been commercially grown are *Fagopyrum sagittatum* Gilib. (*F. esculentum* Moench), *F. emarginatum* Moench, and *F. tataricum* (L.) Gaertn.

The plant grows to a height of 2–5 ft, with many broad heart-shaped leaves. It produces a single main stem which usually bears several branches, and is grooved, succulent, and smooth except for nodes (illustration *a*). Buckwheat is an indeterminate species in response to photoperiod, and produces flowers and fruits (so-called seeds) until the beginning of frost (illustration *b*).

Species differentiation. *F. sagittatum* and *F. emarginatum* produce flowers that are densely clustered in racemes at ends of branches or on short pedicels that arise from the axils of the leaves. Individual flowers have no petals, but the calyx is composed of five petallike sepals which may be light green, white, pink, or red. Populations include plants typically of two floral types: the pin type which has flowers with long pistils

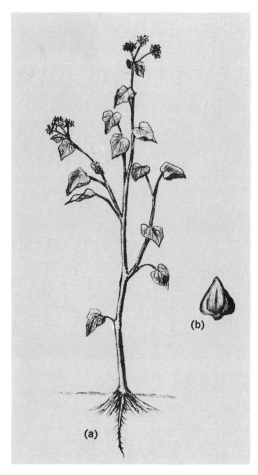

Buckwheat. (a) Mature plant. (b) Seed.

and short stamens and the thrum type which has flowers with short pistils and long stamens. The pistil consists of a one-celled ovary, three-parted style with knoblike stigmas, and eight stamens. Glands (usually eight) which secrete nectar are located at the base of the ovary. Generally, self-fertilization is prevented by a heteromorphic incompatibility system, and seeds are produced only when cross-pollination occurs between the pin and thrum stylar types. The so-called seed of buckwheat (actually a fruit which is an achene) usually has three angles and varies in shape, size, and color.

F. tataricum (commonly known as tartary buckwheat, rye buckwheat, duck wheat, or hulless) differs from the two previously described species. The leaves are narrower and arrow-shaped, and the flowers are smaller with inconspicuous greenish-white sepals. Plants are only of one flower type and are self-fertile.

Cultivation and use. Buckwheat is of minor importance as a grain crop in the United States, and is principally grown in areas of the Northeast where the weather is likely to be moist and cool. It is usually grown on land too rough or poor for other grain crops or, since it matures within 10–12 weeks, as an emergency crop where previous crops have failed. The crop is also used to smother weeds, as green manure, and as food and cover for various game birds and wildlife. Buckwheat is often used as bee pasture, and is the source of a dark, strong-flavored honey which is now so uncommon that it commands a premium price.

[H. G. MARSHALL]

Processing. Buckwheat milling is similar to wheat milling in principle. The grain is cleaned and crushed between a series of steel rolls, and the flour and feed by-products are separated by sieving. On the average 100 lb of dry buckwheat will yield 60–75 lb of flour, 4–8 lb of middlings, and 18–26 lb of hulls. *See* WHEAT.

When buckwheat is received at the mill, it is passed over sieves and subjected to aspiration and scouring to remove all foreign material. If the grain possesses high moisture, it is dried. The grain is cracked to loosen the hull by passing it through the first-break rolls, and the stock is dried in a revolving cylinder where heat can be applied. After drying, the cracked grain is sieved to separate the flour from the hulls, this operation being repeated until the desired product is produced. Some buckwheat is milled to fine flour. Often, however, the particles are not reduced as much as possible, and both middlings and particles of bran are present, especially in dark flour. Buckwheat flour, because of the nature of the grain and the way it is processed, generally is not as highly refined as wheat, rye, or corn flour. It is gritty, not soft and smooth.

Buckwheat flour is used almost exclusively in pancakes or as one of the ingredients in prepared pancake flour. Sometimes buckwheat flour is milled for groats. Two types of food products are made from buckwheat groats, roasted kernels and a farina, or granular product, used in soup. Occasionally groats are used in breakfast foods. Buckwheat was once of interest as a source of flavonol glycoside, known as rutin, used in the treatment of high blood pressure in man, but better sources of that drug have been found. *See* FOOD ENGINEERING.

[JOHN A. SHELLENBERGER]

Bibliography: W. R. Coe, *Buckwheat Milling and Its By-Products*, USDA Circ. no. 190, 1931; H. K. Wilson, *Grain Crops*, 2d ed., 1955.

Budding

A vegetative method of propagation in which a single bud (often a bud sport or bud mutation) serves as a scion and is grafted laterally upon a stock. Bud grafting may be performed throughout the growing season when the bark of the stock is soft and loose, but summer or early fall is usually the most satisfactory time. Success depends upon joining the vascular cambia of the stock and scion. This requires genetic compatibility of stock and scion, pressure to hold the scion firmly against the stock, and protection from desiccation.

Methods of budding used are T or shield (see illustration), patch or flute, hinge, Nicolieren, and chip. The T or shield method is most widely used. A T-shaped cut is made through the outer tissues (bark) of an internode of the stock and the bark separated from the xylem along the cambium. On the scion a thin cut into the wood is made down-stem from an inch above the bud. The wood behind the bud is removed, and the bud is forced into

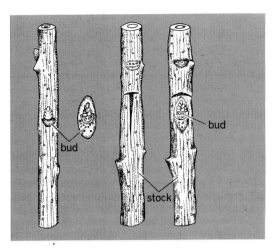

T or shield method of bud grafting.

the incision and held in place by rubber strips or raffia. *See* GRAFTING OF PLANTS.

[JAMES E. GUNCKEL]

Butter

A food fat product made exclusively from milk or cream or both, with or without common salt, NaCl, and added coloring. Butter contains not less than 80% milk fat. It is the second most important food fat, with an annual world production of about 8,800,000,000 lb. The United States produces about 1,200,000,000 lb and has a per capita consumption of about 4.4 lb (fat-content basis). As a spread for bread, in baked goods, and in confections, butter is prized for the flavor that comes from the action of selected microorganisms on cream. *See* MILK.

This article considers butter manufacture, butter oil, ghee, and butter microbiology.

Manufacture. On the farm, processing is carried out by natural ripening of the cream, churning, and manually working to the desired consistency. Country butter is more variable in flavor then is creamery butter.

At the creamery, cream having a fat content of 30–40% is skimmed from milk by centrifuging. Pasteurization and spraying, or stripping, under vacuum remove undesirable flavors and odors and reduce action of microorganisms. Butter may be made from sweet or ripened cream. Ripening is carried out at 50–70°F (10–21.1°C) by introduction of a starter prepared from a bacterial culture and pasteurized milk. Usually about 5% of starter is added. After ripening overnight, color is added. In the batch process sweet or ripened cream is agitated in large rotary churns, 3–10 ft in diameter and 5 or more feet long; this action converts the emulsion from water in oil to an oil-in-water type and coalesces the fat globules. The temperature of churning usually ranges from 48 to 60°F (8.9 to 15.6°C), depending upon the season of the year and the hardness of the butter fat (it is softer in summer).

Churns revolving at 25–30 rpm have internal baffles which lift and drop the contents to provide agitation and splashing. One gallon of 35% fat cream will produce 3.6 lb of butter. After churn-ing to the desired consistency, the buttermilk is drawn off and the butterfat quickly washed with water. The butter is then worked between grooved rolls or with augurs which impart a kneading action. Salt is added during working, and the moisture content is adjusted to produce butter with 80% fat content. After it is worked, the butter is packaged or formed into prints and wrapped.

Butter contains 80–81% fat, 1–3% salt, 1% milk solids, and water. Butter is graded according to a flavor score, usually falling in the range of 89 to 93; the higher the score, the better the flavor.

Continuous processes. At least six different continuous processes for butter manufacture are available, each of which utilizes specialized processing equipment and technology. Continuous processes for making butter generally are economically advantageous and are finding increasing use.

The Swiss Senn and German Fritz processes involve intense mechanical treatment of cream containing up to 40–50% fat. In the Senn process the cream is subjected to rapid agitation at 1500 rpm, decreasing to 20 rpm in the presence of 2–4 atm of carbon dioxide. The mass is deeply cooled and the buttermilk drained from the butter granules, which are sprayed and washed with water, dried in a centrifugal drying machine, sprayed with salt or brine, and worked with a worm gear. In the Fritz method the cream is fed continuously to a cooled horizontal cylindrical tank, where it is distributed in a film over the inner surface and beaten by blades at 3000 rpm, converting it into butter grains and buttermilk. This mass falls into a sloping trough equipped with two worms turning in opposite directions. The buttermilk drains off while the butter moves upward, is forced through two sets of perforated plates, is kneaded with paddles, and leaves the machine as a square tape or may be run directly into the packaging machine. There are also variations of the Fritz process for continuous butter-making by using equipment of Simon, Westfalia, or Silkehorg manufacture.

In the German Alfa and the American Cherry-Burrell, Creamery Package, and Kraft processes, the cream is specially treated to increase its fat content to a high level (78–99.5%). This is done by heating the cream at temperatures of 45–100°C, followed by centrifugal separation. In some cases mechanical force or pressure is also used to aid in breaking or inverting the emulsion. In the Alfa method the high-fat cream (about 78% fat) is run through a special cooler consisting of three cylinders, on the inside of which cooled spiral-ribbed rollers turn. The temperature in each cylinder is carefully controlled. The high-fat cream is converted into butter through the combined action of cooling and mechanical treatment.

In the Cherry-Burrell process high-fat cream (85–95%) is pasteurized in a Vacreator at 88°C. cooled to 45°C, and collected in vats, where color and salt are added and the fat content is reduced to about 80%. It is then pumped continuously through a chiller that agitates and cools the fat to 5–15°C, followed by a texturator, in which the cooled fat is forced through flat, perforated plates. The butter is discharged as a continuous ribbon.

The Creamery Package method treats cream of

75–85% fat content in an emulsion breaker and separates butter oil of 98% fat content from the serum, which is recycled. Salt (brine), water, coloring, skim milk, and a portion of unbroken 80% cream are added to the butter oil in a series of three tanks to adjust to the desired composition. This mixture is continuously pumped through a cylindrical agitated chiller, crystallizer, and extruder, during which the temperature drops from 110 to 40°F and then rises to about 50°F.

In the Kraft process the cream is heated to 99°C and centrifugally treated in two stages to yield a butter oil of 99.5% fat content. This is mixed with 20% acidified milk containing the desired flavoring substances, and the mixture is pumped through a continuous freezer.

Powdered product. A powdered, free-flowing butterlike product has been developed in Australia, and is prepared by homogenizing cream or butterfat with nonfat milk solids and spray-drying under carefully controlled conditions. The small fat droplets are encased with the milk solids. Such products may contain emulsifiers and additives to increase the pH and aid retention of volatile flavorful fatty acids. The product has good storage stability when stored under conditions normally observed for milk powders. It is particularly suitable for use in prepared cake mixes. On addition of water, the butter fat is released to perform its normal function in baking.

Butter oil. This product is made by heating butter to break the emulsion and settling or centrifuging to separate the milk serum from the fat. It may also be prepared by deemulsifying cream. Moisture is reduced to a low level by drying, the butterfat content being over 99%. Although little butter oil is produced in the United States, it is of importance in Australia and New Zealand. It is usually canned, is much more stable than butter, and does not require refrigeration. Because it is practically anhydrous, spoilage by hydrolysis and microbiological action is eliminated. Butterfat consists principally of mixed glycerides of saturated and unsaturated fatty acids in approximately the following percentages: butyric, 3.5; caproic, 1.4; caprylic, 1.7; capric, 2.6; lauric, 4.5; myristic, 14.6; palmitic, 30.2; stearic, 10.5; longer-chain saturated, 1.6; decenoic, 0.3; dodecenoic, 0.2; tetradecenoic, 1.5; hexadecenoic, 5.7; octadecenoic, 18.7; octadecadienoic, 2.1; and longer-chain unsaturated, 0.9.

Ghee. A common food fat in India, ghee is produced from boiled buffalo milk. Its manufacture is similar to that of butter oil. It can be kept for months, or years, without refrigeration but has a more intense flavor than butter or butter oil.

[FRANK G. DOLLEAR]

Microbiology. Seven major groups of microorganisms may be found in dairy products: bacteria, molds, yeasts, viruses, rickettsiae, algae, and protozoa. Only the first three are significant for butter. Discussion of this subject will be under the headings of public health, defects, palatability development, and control.

Public health. The almost complete conversion from farm to factory manufacture of butter has all but eliminated public health hazards. All commercial butter is produced from pasteurized cream. When properly performed, pasteurization destroys

all pathogens. Postpasteurization carelessness is, therefore, the only avenue for infection.

Pathogenic organisms which could, under some circumstances, enter and exist in butter include *Micrococcus pyogenes* var. *aureus* (which produces a toxin that survives pasteurization), some genera of Enterobacteriaceae (*Proteus* and *Salmonella*), *Clostridium, Corynebacterium diphtheriae, Brucella abortus* (undulant fever), *Mycobacterium tuberculosis,* and *Coxiella burneti* (Q fever).

Defects. Proper pasteurization destroys upward of 99.9% of all ordinary organisms present in milk or cream. The minimum recommendations for pasteurizing cream for buttermaking include heating to not less than 165°F (73.9°C) for at least 30 min in an approved vat pasteurizer equipped with a space heater, or to not less than 183°F (83.9°C) for at least 30 sec in an approved high-temperature, short-time pasteurizer equipped with a flow-diversion valve. Other temperature and time combinations may be used if they give equivalent results.

Microbiologically induced flavors, developed prior to pasteurization, may carry over into butter. Attempts to minimize this carryover include the use of soluble food additives (illegal in the United States on the basis of the definition of butter by Act of Congress in 1923) which are largely removed in the buttermilk, or by treatment at less than atmospheric pressures during pasteurization. Neither method is completely effective.

Organisms responsible for flavor defects originate from dirty utensils, or from water and air (indirectly from soil or plants). The name of an organism is often indicative of the flavor it produces. Among the organisms most responsible for flavor and other defects in butter are *Pseudomonas putrifaciens; P. nigrifaciens; P. fragi* and *P. fluorescens* (hydrolytic rancidity); acid-producing types; *Streptococcus lactis* var. *maltigenes;* such yeasts as *Saccharomyces, Candida mycoderma,* and *Torulopsis holmii;* and the molds *Geotrichum candidum, Penicillium, Alternaria,* and *Cladosporium.* Molds are responsible for musty flavors but they, as well as some yeasts and *Pseudomonas nigrifaciens,* may also cause color defects.

All of the *Pseudomonas* groups found in butter are psychrophiles; that is, they grow well at refrigerator temperatures of about 42°F (5.5°C). They may cause putrid or lipolytic flavors in from 5 to 10 days.

Factors responsible for inhibiting the development of microbiological flavor defects in butter include common salt, pH, butter structure, and storage temperatures.

Butter with 2% salt and 17% water has an overall brine concentration of 10.5%, which is inhibitory to some organisms. The growth of psychrophiles is inhibited by a lower pH. In properly worked (mixed) butter, fat is the predominantly continuous phase and surrounds the tiny moisture droplets. Unless the water used in the manufacture of butter is contaminated, the water droplets are overwhelmingly sterile. Also, their size is such that growth of bacteria is impossible. Only molds whose mycelia can penetrate the fat phase can reproduce. Where the interval between manufacture and sale is less than 4–6 weeks, the butter is maintained at 35–55°F (1.7–12.8°C); hence some growth of organisms may be expected to continue, but where storage is from a month to a year or more, temperatures range from 0 to −15°F (−17.8 to −26.1°C) and growth ceases. The number of living organisms may actually decrease.

Palatability development. Not all nationalities prefer butter of the same flavor intensity. Butter made from sweet pasteurized cream is bland but may have a slight nutty or boiled-milk flavor. In general, Americans, Australians, and New Zealanders prefer this flavor. Europeans, Latin Americans, and some Asiatics prefer a more intense flavor. The desired flavor can be developed by the use of milk cultures of certain organisms. These cultures are referred to as starters. They may be added to the pasteurized and cooled cream at temperatures of 72°F (22.2°C) or less, or to the butter at about the time of salting. The latter practice is more economical and facilitates flavor control. The presence of citrates or citric acid is necessary for the development of diacetyl, $CH_3COCOCH_3$, recognized as the chief compound responsible for butter aroma (see illustration). Most unsalted butter is made by the use of starters because they tend to inhibit the growth of psychrophiles.

The organisms present in the starter determine how the flavor compounds develop, and their quantity and intensity. For use in buttermaking, a mixture of two or more of the following organisms is desirable: *Streptococcus lactis, Leuconostoc citrovorum, L. dextranicum,* and *S. diacetilactis;* in recent years the latter has been used alone or in combination with *S. lactis.* In some areas of Europe, *Candida krusii* (a yeast) has been tried in mixed cultures.

Starter distillates, made by steam distillation of starter cultures, are commercially available. Their advantages are economy, convenience, and uniformity. Their disadvantages are lack of delicate flavor and aroma and failure to inhibit the growth of some undesirable bacteria. Addition of lactic or other food-grade acids or of synthetic flavoring compounds could compensate for the latter disadvantage; however, such additions may not comply with the legal definition of butter.

Control. Standards and procedures for controlling the quality of butter have been developed collectively by the butter industry, dairy schools and experiment stations, the U.S. Department of Agriculture, and state regulatory agencies. By education, inspection, and the use of various tests standardized by the American Public Health Association for the maintenance of quality, butter has been greatly improved since the early 1940s.

Procedures for ascertaining the numbers of psychrophiles (as represented by *Pseudomonas putrifaciens*) and for yeasts and molds are especially important because they are, to a great extent, an indication of postpasteurization handling practices.

The introduction of all-metal (mostly stainless steel of the 304 or 316 type) churns and the use of metal in all other equipment have eliminated many flavor problems—especially those due to yeasts and molds. The newer practice of all-welded pipelines and cleaning in place, when combined with the proper use of cleaners and sanitizers, likewise has been an important factor in the production of high-quality butter. *See* FOOD ENGINEERING;

INDUSTRIAL MICROBIOLOGY.   [L. C. THOMSEN]

Bibliography: American Public Health Association, *Standard Methods for the Examination of Dairy Products*, 13th ed., 1972; E. M. Foster et al., *Dairy Microbiology*, 1957; B. W. Hammer and F. S. Babel, *Dairy Bacteriology*, 4th ed., 1957; R. Jenness and S. Patton, *Principles of Dairy Chemistry*, 1959; F. H. McDowall, *The Buttermaker's Manual*, 1953; D. Strobel, W. Bryan, and C. Babcock, *Butter Oil: A Review of Literature*, U.S. Department of Agriculture, 1954; D. Swern (ed.), *Bailey's Industrial Oil and Fat Products*, 3d ed., 1964; U.S. Department of Agriculture, *Minimum Standards for Milk for Manufacturing Purposes and its Production and Processing*, 1963; U.S. Department of Health, Education, and Welfare, Public Health Service, *Grade "A" Pasteurized Milk Ordinance*, 1965; G. H. Wilster, *Practical Buttermaking*, 1969.

Cabbage

A hardy, cool-season crucifer (*Brassica oleracea* var. *capitata*) of Mediterranean origin and belonging to the plant order Capparales. Cabbage is grown for its head of overlapping leaves (see illustration), which are generally eaten raw in salads, cooked fresh, or processed into sauerkraut. Because it normally produces seed the second year, cabbage is considered to be a biennial by most authorities. Others regard it a perennial because it will remain vegetative unless subjected to cold weather.

Chinese cabbage is a related annual of Asiatic origin. Two species are grown in the United States, pe-tsai (*B. pekinensis*) and pakchoi (*B. chinensis*).

Propagation of cabbage is by seed planted in the field, or in greenhouses and outdoor beds for the production of transplants. Field spacing varies; plants are usually 8–18 in. apart in 30–36-in. rows.

Cool, moist climate favors maximum yields of firm heads. However, exposure of young plants to prolonged low temperatures favors seed-stalk for-

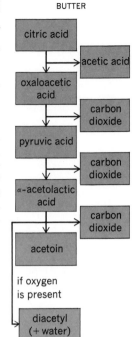

BUTTER

Decomposition of citric acid to diacetyl, chief component responsible for butter aroma.

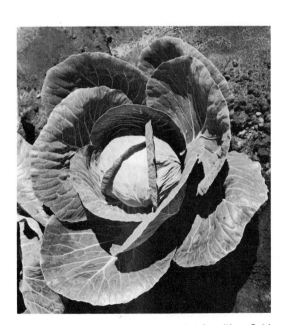

Cabbage (*Brassica oleracea* var. *capitata*), cultivar Golden Acre 84. (*Joseph Harris Co., Inc., Rochester, N.Y.*)

mation without production of normal heads.

Varieties. Cabbage varieties (cultivars) are generally classified according to season of maturity, leaf surface (smooth, savoyed, or wrinkled), head shape (flattened, round, or pointed), and color (green or red). Round, smooth-leaved, green heads are commonest. Popular varieties are Golden Acre and strains of Danish Ballhead; hybrid varieties are increasingly planted. Principal varieties of other types are Chieftain (savoy), Jersey Wakefield (pointed), Red Danish (red), and Wong Bok (Chinese cabbage). Strains of Danish Ballhead are also used for sauerkraut manufacture and for late storing. Varieties differ in their resistance to disease and in the tendency for heads to crack or split in the field.

Harvesting. Harvesting of fresh market varieties begins when the heads are hard enough to be accepted on the market, generally 60–90 days after field planting. Buyer preference for heads weighing no more than 2–3 lb has encouraged close spacing and early harvesting. In the northern states production of cabbage for winter storage has declined as the Texas and Florida winter areas have expanded production, providing green cabbage as competition on the market for the white stored heads.

Texas and Florida are important winter crop producing states; Georgia, Mississippi, and North Carolina produce large acreages in the spring; and New York, North Carolina, and Wisconsin are important for the summer and fall crops.

[H. JOHN CAREW]

Cabbage and cauliflower diseases. Cabbage and other crops of the same species, such as cauliflower, brussels sprouts, and collards, are subject to more than 50 diseases, of which only a few are widely destructive. These include clubroot (*Plasmodiophora brassicae*), blackleg (*Phoma lingam*), yellows (*Fusarium oxysporum* f. *conglutinans*), black rot (*Xanthomonas campestris*), and several virus diseases. *See* BRUSSELS SPROUTS; CAULIFLOWER; COLLARD.

Clubroot and yellows. These diseases are similar in that the pathogens, once introduced into the soil, remain there almost permanently. Neither disease is seed-borne, but both are often carried from place to place in infected transplants or soil.

Yellows (*Fusarium oxysporum* f. sp. *conglutinans*) infects through the roots and becomes systemic, causing leaves to turn yellow and leathery; later they drop off. Xylem vessels turn brown and plants die or fail to produce good heads. The disease is most destructive in warm weather. Yellows of cabbage may be prevented by growing resistant varieties which are commonly available. This is an outstanding example of disease control by growing resistant varieties. Yellows is of minor importance on other crucifers.

Clubroot (*Plasmodiophora brassicae*) infects roots, causing them to swell. There may be many infections on a single root system, preventing proper absorption of water and minerals from the soil and causing stunting of the plant. The disease is favored by wet, acid soils. Infestation of the soil (usually by diseased transplants) should be avoided. Once present, clubroot can sometimes be reduced by liming; however, soil applications of pentachloronitrobenzene appear to be more successful. Clubroot-resistant cabbage has been produced by breeding, but not on wide scale.

Blackleg and black rot. Both of these diseases are seed-borne and the pathogens persist in the soil for as long as 3 years. Spattering rain causes secondary spread of both, especially in seedlings.

Black rot, caused by *Xanthomonas campestris*, a bacterial disease, can cause spots on the leaves but may also become systemic, causing yellowed leaves and blackened vessels, similar to cabbage yellows. Affected leaves drop, and infection of heads is often followed by soft rot.

Blackleg, caused by *Phoma lingam*, causes gray, dead spots on leaves and stems, extending to the roots, which are often destroyed, killing the plant.

Black rot and blackleg can largely be avoided by a 3-year rotation in fields and seed beds, and by using disease-free seed, which is generally available from the Puget Sound area. If seed is infected, hot-water treatment is very effective. No resistant varieties of practical value are known.

Virus diseases. Four or more distinct viruses infect crucifers. Symptoms include mottling, ringlike dead spots, stunting, and black spotting in the tissues. Some viruses affect various other crops and certain weeds, and most are spread by plant lice. These diseases may be reduced by planting seed beds away from infected weeds and other plants. No resistant varieties are available. *See* PLANT DISEASE; PLANT VIRUS.   [CARL J. EIDE]

Cacao

The plant *Theobroma cacao*, also known as the chocolate tree, a small tropical tree of the sterculia family (Sterculiaceae). It bears flowers and fruits throughout the year. The fruits are fusiform capsules containing a mucilaginous pulp and 40 or more seeds. The pods are picked by hand and opened with a knife. The pulp and seeds are removed, cured, and usually fermented. The beans are then cleaned, sorted, and roasted in iron drums. After roasting, the beans are passed through corrugated rollers to break the shells, which are removed by winnowing. Then the seeds or nibs are ground, producing an oily paste which, when cooled and hardened, is the bitter chocolate of commerce. Sugar is added to produce the sweet chocolate. If the oily paste is put through a hydraulic press, a white or yellowish fat, cocoa butter, is obtained. Having the odor and flavor of chocolate, cocoa butter is used to some extent in making chocolate, but it is used mainly in cosmetics and perfumes. After two-thirds of the fatty oil has been expressed, the residue is powdered to make the commercial cocoa. The shells are used for making beverages, to adulterate cocoa and chocolate, as cattle food, and for fertilizer. A native of tropical America, the chocolate tree was cultivated by the Aztecs long before the conquest of Mexico by Cortes. *See* COCOA POWDER AND CHOCOLATE.

[PERRY D. STRAUSBAUGH/EARL L. CORE]

Caffeine

An alkaloid found in a large number of plants used throughout the world in beverages, such as tea, coffee, cocoa, and maté. Caffeine was first isolated by F. Runge in 1820, and was later synthesized by a variety of methods. Caffeine is readily obtained by the extraction of tea dust and as a by-product in the manufacture of decaffeinated coffee.

Wherever caffeine-bearing plants are indigenous, natives use their aqueous extracts as beverages. Legends telling of their discovery indicate that the stimulant action of the plant's constituents has been appreciated for many centuries. This stimulant action is the chief basis for the popularity of caffeine-containing beverages.

Caffeine possesses other pharmacological properties useful in therapy. It is often employed as an ingredient of mixtures for treating headaches. It is also useful as a diuretic drug and as an effective antidote against poisoning by narcotics, such as morphine.　[S. MORRIS KUPCHAN]

Calorie

A unit of the energy used to maintain vital metabolic processes and to support other physiological activities of the body, such as work and exercise, growth, lactation, and maintenance of body temperature. The body's need for energy, measured in kilocalories (1 kcal is the amount of heat necessary to raise 1 kg of water from 15 to 16°C, and is equal to 4186 joules), is a major nutritional priority. The established energy conversion factors of 4 kcal/g of food carbohydrate or protein and 9 kcal/g of food fat are used to estimate the energy content of diets. Since alcohol is a frequent contributor to energy intake, its caloric value is calculated separately at 7 kcal/g. Calorie requirements are influenced by age, sex, body size, level of activity or work, and certain physiological functions such as growth and development, pregnancy, and lactation. The principal impact of climate, that is, heat or cold, on energy requirements appears to be indirect, such as an increased metabolic rate associated with shivering and other voluntary or involuntary movements in cold temperatures and a general tendency to avoid activity and energy expenditure at high temperatures.

In general, there is a remarkably close relationship between individual energy needs or requirements and energy consumption. It is evident that this "calorie-stat" is remarkably effective in a majority of people. However, an excessive intake of calories is metabolically converted to fat and stored. When this process is continued, obesity develops with all of its hazards to health. *See* OBESITY.

When supplies of food and energy are limited, such as in starvation, a significant physiological adaptive mechanism conserves energy through a reduction of metabolic rate and physical activity. Such adaptation permits reasonable function and survival for short periods of time. *See* STARVATION.

Age factor. Infants and children require two to three times more energy per unit of body weight than adults. During the first year of life, energy allowances are reduced from about 120 kcal/kg at birth to 100 kcal/kg near the end of the first year. At that point energy needs for children of both sexes decline to approximately 80 kcal/kg through 10 years of age. This decline proceeds slowly to about 45 kcal/kg for adolescent males and 38 kcal/kg for adolescent females. Naturally there is a wide variation in physical activity of young people, which helps to explain why inactive children are often obese while very active children are usually thin.

As individuals age, there is a progressive decline in basal metabolic rate of about 2% each decade. Also, perhaps more importantly, there is a reduction in work and physical activity. Activity patterns for men in light occupations appear to be reasonably constant between the ages of 20 and 45, but activity tends to decrease about 200 kcal/day from ages 45 to 75 and by about 500 kcal/day after age 75.

Body size. Energy requirements, including basal metabolic rates, are influenced proportionately by body size and, more specifically, by surface area of the body. Height is more influential in determining surface area than weight; in other words, the tall, thin individual has more surface area than the short, squat person who may actually be heavier. Obese individuals expend energy much more inefficiently, but may compensate for their increased energy costs by a decrease in activity. However, the energy needs of underweight individuals may be underestimated unless their ideal weight is used for the calculation instead of their actual weight.

Level of activity. In modern society, work is often sedentary and physical activity generally light. Ever fewer people engage in heavy work. Energy expenditure for work at various levels of activity can be expressed in kilocalories per kilogram of body weight per hour, ranging from a low of 1.5 and 1.3 for men and women, respectively, for very light work, and increasing to 8.4 and 8.0 for very heavy activity. In order to maintain a stable and desirable weight, it is important to balance energy intake with energy expenditure, which is influenced significantly by the level of activity.

Variations in souce of energy. It is generally agreed that the average American diet contains too many calories derived from fat, particularly saturated fat. The health of most individuals could be improved if total fat calories did not exceed 35% of total caloric intake and if the ratio of polyunsaturated fat to saturated fat ranged from approximately 1:1 to 2:1. Such modification would help to reduce total caloric intake and quite possibly might result in a lowering of blood cholesterol with the ultimate benefit of a reduction in atherosclerotic coronary heart disease.

Concern is expressed over the ever-increasing intake of calories from simple sugars, particularly sucrose, which now averages over 100 lb (45 kg) per capita per year, representing about 20–24% of average total caloric intake for the adult. In addition, alcohol calories for adults average 10–12% of total calories. Neither sucrose nor alcohol contributes to the nutritional quality of the diet, and nutritional adequacy becomes increasingly difficult to achieve when these substances are used excessively.　[WILLARD A. KREHL]

Cantaloupe

In the United States, the name "cantaloupe" is applied to muskmelon cultivars belonging to *Cucumis melo* var. *reticulatus* Naud. of the family Cucurbitaceae. The fruits of var. *reticulatus* weigh 2–4 lb (lb = 0.45 kg) and are round to oval; the surface is netted and has shallow vein tracts (see illustration). The flesh is usually salmon-colored, but it may vary from green to deep salmon-orange. When mature, the melon is sweet, averages 6–8% sugar, and has a very distinct aroma and flavor. The flesh is high in potassium, is rich in vitamin C, and,

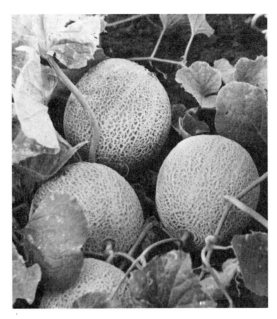

Cantaloupe (*Cucumis melo*) with fruits near maturity.

when deep orange, is also rich in vitamin A. The vines usually bear andromonoecious flowers, and the fruit generally separates from the stem when mature. The use of the name "cantaloupe" to indicate these medium-sized, netted melons has become firmly embedded in American culture. For this reason, little can be done to correct this usage except to point out that "cantaloupe" is a misnomer.

The word "cantaloupe" should be applied to cultivars of *Cucumis melo* var. *cantalupensis* Naud. The fruits of this group are rough and scaly, with deep vein tracts and a hard rind. Cultivars of var. *cantalupensis* are grown in Europe and Asia, but they are seldom grown in the United States.

Because of the continued reduction in available labor, cantaloupes will have to be mechanically harvested if they are to survive as a prominent commercial crop. The present situation in mechanical harvesting may be summarized as follows: Selective harvesting is possible but uneconomical; a satisfactory once-over mechanical harvester is available that will recover marketable fruits without loss; considerable progress has been made in developing a short-internode "bush" cantaloupe with a concentrated fruit set adapted to once-over harvest; and the use of new ripening agents may raise the concentration of mature fruits at harvest to a sufficiently high level to make once-over mechanical harvesting feasible.

With increasing centralization of the crop in the West because of favorable environment and improved transportation, California, Arizona, and Texas produced about 84% of the total cantaloupes harvested in 1968–1973, of which California produced more than 53%. About 6400 tons (1 short ton = 0.9 metric ton) were harvested annually during those years from about 105,100 acres (1 acre = 4047 m²). Annual average yields per acre have increased gradually from 4.0 tons in the 1940s to 6.2 tons in 1970–1973. Per capita consumption remained fairly constant during the 1960s and early 1970s, averaging 8.4 lb. The farm value of the crop in 1973 was about $91,000,000. *See* MELON

GROWING; MUSKMELON.   [F. W. ZINK]

Bibliography: G. N. Davis, T. W. Whitaker, and G. W. Bohn, *Muskmelon Production in California*, Circ. Calif. Agr. Exp. Sta. no. 536, 1965; M. O'Brien and J. C. Lingle, Mechanical harvesting of cantaloupes, *J. Amer. Soc. Agr. Eng.*, 46:74–77, 1965; M. O'Brien and M. Zahara, Mechanical harvest of melons, *Trans. Amer. Soc. Agr. Eng.*, 14: 883–885, 1971; T. W. Whitaker and G. N. Davis, *Cucurbits*, 1961.

Caraway

An important spice from the fruits of the perennial herb *Carum carvi*, of the family Umbelliferae. A native of Europe and western Asia, it is now cultivated in many temperate areas of both hemispheres. The small, brown, slightly curved fruits are used in perfumery, cookery, confectionery, in medicine, and for flavoring beverages. *See* SPICE AND FLAVORING.

[PERRY D. STRAUSBAUGH/EARL L. CORE]

Carbohydrate

A term applied to a group of substances which include the sugars, starches, and cellulose, along with many other related substances. This group of compounds plays a vitally important part in the lives of plants and animals, both as structural elements and in the maintenance of functional activity. Plants are unique in that they alone in nature have the power to synthesize carbohydrates from carbon dioxide and water in the presence of the green plant chlorophyll through the energy derived from sunlight, by the process of photosynthesis. This process is responsible not only for the existence of plants but for the maintenance of animal life as well, since animals obtain their entire food supply directly or indirectly from the carbohydrates of plants. *See* PHOTOSYNTHESIS.

The carbohydrates as a group are comparable in importance with the proteins and fats. Cane or beet sugar, D-glucose, D-fructose, starch, and cellulose may be cited as typical representatives. A number of members of this group are of great industrial importance. Among the undertakings dependent on carbohydrate materials are the cotton industry, certain branches of explosives, brewing, and the manufacture of alcohol.

The term carbohydrate originated in the belief that naturally occurring compounds of this class, for example, D-glucose ($C_6H_{12}O_6$), sucrose ($C_{12}H_{22}O_{11}$), and cellulose ($C_6H_{10}O_5)_n$, could be represented formally as hydrates of carbon, that is, $C_x(H_2O)_y$. Later it became evident that this definition for carbohydrates was not a satisfactory one. New substances were discovered whose properties clearly indicated that they had the characteristics of sugars and belonged in the carbohydrate class, but which nevertheless showed a deviation from the required hydrogen-to-oxygen ratio. Examples of these are the important deoxy sugars, D-deoxyribose, L-fucose, and L-rhamnose, the uronic acids, and such compounds as ascorbic acid (vitamin C). The retention of the term carbohydrate is therefore a matter of convenience rather than of exact definition. A carbohydrate is usually defined as either a polyhydroxy aldehyde (aldose) or ketone (ketose), or as a substance which yields one of these compounds on hydrolysis. However, included within this class of compounds are substances also containing nitrogen and sulfur.

The properties of many carbohydrates differ enormously from one substance to another. The sugars, such as D-glucose or sucrose, are easily soluble, sweet-tasting and crystalline; the starches are colloidal and paste-forming; and cellulose is completely insoluble. Yet chemical analysis shows that they have a common basis; the starches and cellulose may be degraded by different methods to the same crystalline sugar, D-glucose.

Classification. The carbohydrates usually are classified into three main groups according to complexity: monosaccharides, oligosaccharides, and polysaccharides.

Monosaccharides. These simple sugars consist of a single carbohydrate unit which cannot be hydrolyzed into simpler substances. These are characterized, according to their length of carbon chain, as trioses ($C_3H_6O_3$), tetroses ($C_4H_8O_4$), pentoses ($C_5H_{10}O_5$), hexoses ($C_6H_{12}O_6$), heptoses ($C_7H_{14}O_7$), and so on. A monosaccharide may be an aldose or a ketose, depending on the type of carbonyl group (C=O) present. This system gives rise to such names as aldotriose, aldotetrose, aldopentose, and aldohexose for the aldose forms and by such names as ketopentoses and ketohexoses when the ketone group is present. More recently the tendency is to indicate the presence of a ketone group by the ending "ulose" in names such as pentuloses, and heptuloses. *See* MONOSACCHARIDE.

Oligosaccharides. These compound sugars are condensation products of two to five molecules of simple sugars and are subclassified into disaccharides, trisaccharides, tetrasaccharides, and pentasaccharides, according to the number of monosaccharide molecules yielded upon hydrolysis.

The sugars which include the monosaccharides and oligosaccharides are mostly crystalline compounds. The monosaccharides and disaccharides have a sweet taste. Products obtained from hydrolysis of higher molecular weight polysaccharides and consisting of compound sugars that contain as many as nine monosaccharide units are also termed oligosaccharides. However, these higher members are not crystalline compounds. The disaccharides and other groups of oligosaccharides are subclassified into reducing and nonreducing sugars, depending on whether or not the sugar has a functional carbonyl group. In a nonreducing oligosaccharide, the carbonyl groups of the constituent monosaccharide units are involved in glycosidic linkage. The compound sugars are in reality sugarlike polysaccharides, but the prefix "poly" is reserved for carbohydrates which consist of large aggregates of monosaccharide units. *See* OLIGOSACCHARIDE.

Polysaccharides. These comprise a heterogeneous group of compounds which represent large aggregates of monosaccharide units, joined through glycosidic bonds. They are tasteless, nonreducing, amorphous substances that yield a large and indefinite number of monosaccharide units on hydrolysis. Their molecular weight is usually very high, and many of them, like starch or glycogen, have molecular weights of several million. They form colloidal solutions, but some polysaccharides, of which cellulose is an example, are completely insoluble in water. On account of their heterogeneity they are difficult to classify. One common system of classification is based primarily upon the class of monosaccharide yielded on hydrolysis. Thus a polysaccharide that yields hexose monosaccharides on hydrolysis is called hexoglycan ($C_6H_{10}O_5)_n$, where n represents the number of monosaccharide units present. A polysaccharide yielding a pentose sugar is called pentoglycan ($C_5H_8O_4)_n$. Each major class is further subdivided according to the particular hexose or pentose produced. Thus, a polysaccharide composed of the hexose sugar D-glucose is called glucan; those composed of the pentose sugars D-xylose and L-arabinose are called xylan and araban, respectively.

Some polysaccharides, however, yield both hexose and pentose sugars on hydrolysis and are classed as mixed hexosans and pentosans; others, in addition to hexoses and pentoses, frequently on acid hydrolysis yield the uronic acids, D-glucuronic, D-galacturonic, or D-mannuronic acid. Such polysaccharides are frequently referred to as polyuronides. *See* POLYSACCHARIDE.

Reducing and nonreducing sugars. The sugars are also classified into two general groups, the reducing and nonreducing. The reducing sugars are distinguished by the fact that because of their free, or potentially free, aldehyde or ketone groups they possess the property of readily reducing alkaline solutions of many metallic salts, such as those of copper, silver, bismuth, mercury, and iron. The most widely used reagent for this purpose is Fehling's solution, in which the oxidizing agent is the cupric tartrate ion, formed in a strongly alkaline solution of copper sulfate and a salt of tartaric acid. The nonreducing sugars do not exhibit this property. The reducing sugars constitute by far the larger group. The monosaccharides and many of their derivatives reduce Fehling's solution. Most of the disaccharides, including maltose, lactose, and the rarer sugars cellobiose, gentiobiose, melibiose, and turanose, are also reducing sugars. The best-known nonreducing sugar is the disaccharide sucrose. Among other nonreducing sugars are the disaccharide trehalose, the trisaccharides raffinose and melezitose, the tetrasaccharide stachyose, and the pentasaccharide verbascose.

The alkali in the Fehling solution, or other such reagents used for the determination of reducing sugars, causes considerable decomposition of the sugar molecule into reactive fragments which may also reduce the metal ions. Thus, while the total reduction for a given sugar may be constant under carefully controlled conditions and can therefore be used for quantitative purposes, it is impossible to write a balanced equation for the reaction in terms of the simple oxidation of the sugar and reduction of the metal ion.

Analysis. Carbohydrate analysis involves separation of the carbohydrate mixtures, identification of the individual carbohydrates, and estimation of their quantities.

Separation and identification. Sugars, in most cases, occur in living tissues as mixtures. Before a sugar can be identified, it must be isolated in pure form, preferably as a crystalline substance. The pure crystalline compound is readily identified by its melting point, optical rotation, and x-ray diffraction pattern. Preparation of certain crystalline derivatives facilitates isolation and identification of reducing sugars. The phenylhydrazone and phenylosazone derivatives of these sugars are especially useful, chiefly because of their ease of preparation. The phenylosatriazoles, benzimidazoles, and diothioacetal acetates are more advantageous for the purpose of identification.

Application of chromatographic technique provides a useful and rapid method for the separation and identification of sugars. The great advantage of this process lies in the fact that it can be applied to minute amounts as well as to relatively large quantities. For micro amounts chromatography on filter paper is used. The mixed sugar solution is applied as a spot on the narrow edge of a strip of filter paper. The sugars are then separated by using a mixture of water and a partially immiscible organic solvent, such as *n*-butanol or phenol. The paper is then dried and sprayed with coloring reagents, such as *p*-anisidine hydrochloride or aniline hydrogen phthalate, which show the location of the individual sugars. For separation of larger quantities of material, column chromatography is used. In this method the proper choice of solvents and absorbents is important. The solvent is passed through a column containing powdered cellulose, silicic acid, alumina, clay, carbon, or other adsorbent by gravity, suction, or pressure. After sufficient development to form the different zones, the products may be eluted from the column in successive batches.

Color tests. There are a number of color tests which are helpful in the identification of carbohydrates. These tests are based on the condensation of various aromatic amines or phenolic substances with the degradation products of sugars. The Molisch test is used for the general detection of carbohydrates. In this test a purple color is produced when the solution containing carbohydrate is treated with strong sulfuric acid in the presence of α-naphthol. In the Tauber test pentose sugars produce a cherry-red color when heated with a solution of benzidine in glacial acetic acid. Another test for pentoses and uronic acids is based on the fact that a violet-red color develops when these sugars are treated with hydrochloric acid and phloroglucinol. Seliwanoff's test is used for ketoses, which give a red color with resorcinol in hydrochloric acid. The Tollens naphthoresorcinol and the Dische carbazole tests are used for the detection of the uronic acids, D-glucuronic acid, D-galacturonic acid, and D-mannuronic acid. The polysaccharide, starch, produces a blue color when treated with a dilute solution of iodine in potassium iodide, while glycogen gives a reddish-brown color with this reagent.

Paper chromatography and color tests only indicate the probable presence of a particular carbohydrate. For unequivocal proof it is necessary to resort to isolation procedures.

Estimation. The reducing properties of aldoses and ketoses are most frequently utilized for the quantitative analysis of these sugars. A nonreducing sugar such as sucrose or raffinose, or a polysaccharide such as starch, must be first hydrolyzed with acid or with an appropriate enzyme to its constituent reducing monosaccharide units before it is analyzed. Upon heating the reducing sugars with Fehling's solution, containing copper sulfate, tartrate ion, and sodium hydroxide, a brick-red color develops, a result of the formation and precipitation of cuprous oxide.

The quantity of the cuprous oxide precipitate is a measure of the amount of reducing sugar present. Several modifications of this reaction have been used for the quantitative determination of reducing sugars. The estimation of sugar by the Benedict method involves the determination of the reduced cuprous ions colorimetrically after treatment with phosphomolybdic acid. In the Somogyi-Shaffer-Hartmann method, the sugar is estimated by iodometric titration of reduced copper. Several other quantitative methods for the determination of sugars are based on the reduction of ferricyanide ions in an alkaline solution. These reactions can be applied to micro quantities of sugars. There are also spectrophotometric methods, devised by Dische, which are based on light absorption by the reaction products resulting from treatment of sugars with carbazole or cysteine-carbazole in sulfuric acid. Sugars can be accurately identified and determined by their specific optical rotations, provided they are available in sufficient quantities and that no other interfering optically active materials are present.

Stereoisomerism. The sugars consist of chains of carbon atoms which are united to one another at a tetrahedral angle of 109°28'. A carbon atom to which are attached four different groups is called asymmetric. A sugar, or any other compound containing one or more asymmetric carbon atoms, possesses optical activity; that is, it rotates the plane of polarized light to the right or left. The specific rotation of a substance possessing optical activity is the rotation expressed in angular degrees which is afforded by 1 g of substance dissolved in 1 ml of water in a tube 1 dm in length. It is usually given for the sodium D line at a definite temperature, for example, 20°C, and is designated by $[\alpha]_D^{20}$.

The triose glycerose, or glyceraldehyde, has one asymmetric carbon atom and therefore exists in two optically active forms, one dextrorotatory and the other levorotatory (Fig. 1).

The D and L forms of glycerose are related to each other as the right hand is to the left hand, being similar, but not identical. One may not be superposed upon the other. If one model is held

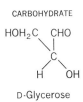

CARBOHYDRATE

D-Glycerose

L-Glycerose

Fig. 1. Spatial arrangement of the groups around the asymmetric carbons of the two isomers of glycerose.

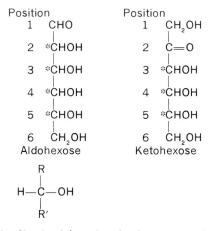

Fig. 2. Structural formulas showing asymmetric carbons (asterisk) for an aldohexose and a ketohexose. Detail of carbon at position 2 in aldohexose is shown where R = CHO and R' = everything below carbon atom 2.

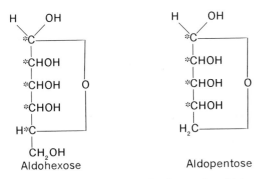

Fig. 3. Structural formulas for ring forms of an aldohexose and an aldopentose. Asymmetric carbons are marked by an asterisk.

before a mirror, the image in the mirror corresponds to the arrangement of the other model. The two compounds whose molecules are mirror images of each other are called optical antipodes or enantiomorphs.

It is difficult to represent stereochemically the more complex sugars having several asymmetric carbon atoms. An examination of the formula for an aldohexose (Fig. 2) reveals that it contains four different asymmetric carbon atoms, that is, each of the atoms marked with an asterisk, at positions 2, 3, 4, and 5, carries four different groups or atoms. The ketohexose contains three

asymmetric carbon atoms, at 3, 4, and 5 (Fig. 2).

As the number of asymmetric carbon atoms in the sugar molecule increases, from the trioses to the higher monosaccharides, the number of stereoisomers increases in accordance with the van't Hoff formula 2^n, where n represents the number of asymmetric carbon atoms.

Thus the possible number of stereoisomers of an aldohexose, such as glucose or galactose, when written in open-chain form, is 2^4 or 16 (eight enantiomorphous pairs). In the ketose sugars, there is one less asymmetric center than in the aldoses of equal chain length; therefore the number of isomers is reduced by a factor of 2. The possible number of stereoisomers of a ketohexose, exemplified by fructose or sorbose, is 2^3 or 8 (four enantiomorphous pairs). Eight stereoisomers, consisting of four pairs of enantiomorphs, are possible for an aldopentose like xylose or arabinose. If, as seen in Fig. 3, the formulas of these sugars are represented in ring form, the first carbon atom in the monosaccharide chain becomes asymmetric because of formation of a cyclic hemiacetal with a new OH group and another center of asymmetry at carbon atom 1. The possible isomers for a cyclic aldohexose therefore become 2^5 or 32, and for an aldopentose 2^4 or 16.

The spatial arrangement of the groups around the asymmetric carbon atom of the dextrorotatory form of glyceraldehyde (glycerose) is arbitrarily called the D configuration, while that of the levo-

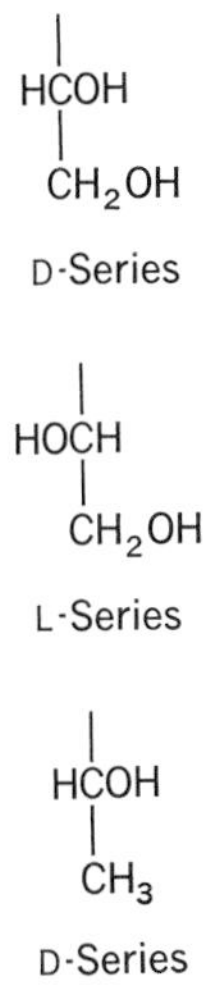

CARBOHYDRATE

```
      |
    HCOH
      |
    CH₂OH

   D-Series


      |
    HOCH
      |
    CH₂OH

   L-Series


      |
    HCOH
      |
    CH₃

   D-Series
```

Fig. 4. Spatial configurations of D and L series showing reference carbon attached to the terminal group.

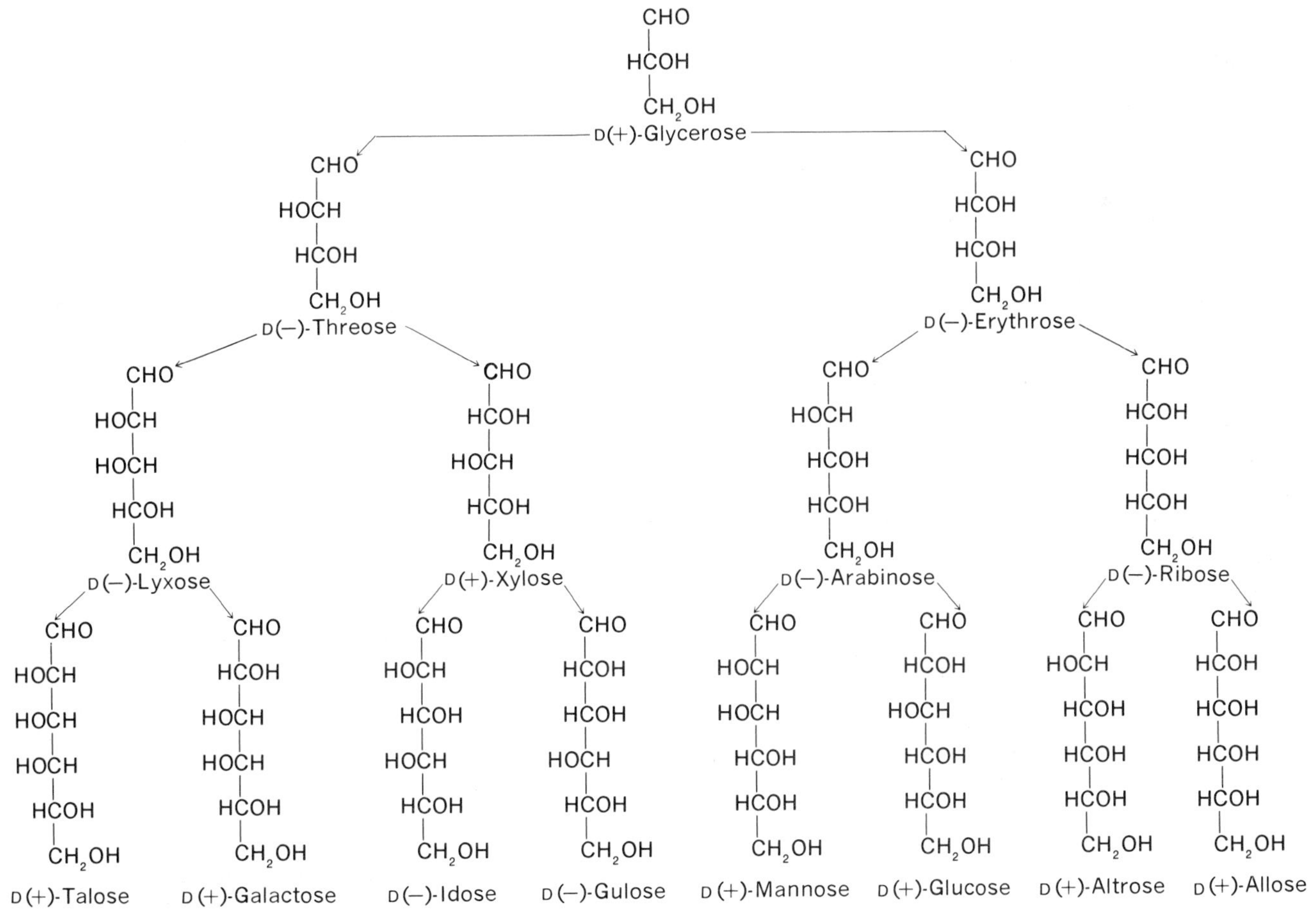

```
                              CHO
                              |
                            HCOH
                              |
                            CH₂OH
                        ─── D(+)-Glycerose ───
```

Fig. 5. The D-series of aldose sugars as related to D-glycerose.

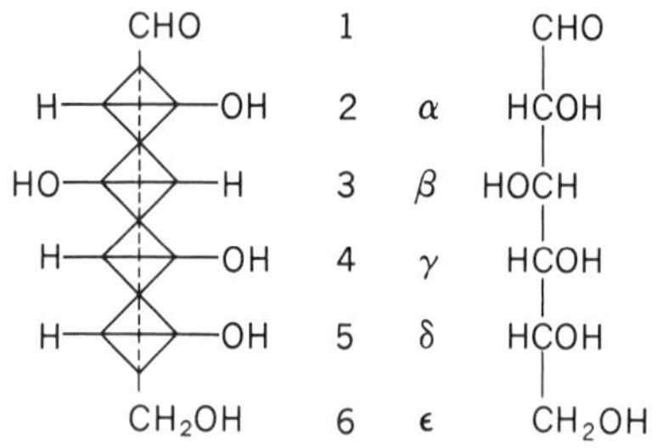

$$
\begin{array}{cccc}
\text{CHO} & 1 & & \text{CHO} \\
\text{H——OH} & 2 & \alpha & \text{HCOH} \\
\text{HO——H} & 3 & \beta & \text{HOCH} \\
\text{H——OH} & 4 & \gamma & \text{HCOH} \\
\text{H——OH} & 5 & \delta & \text{HCOH} \\
\text{CH}_2\text{OH} & 6 & \epsilon & \text{CH}_2\text{OH}
\end{array}
$$

Fig. 6. Projection formula for the aldohexose D-glucose.

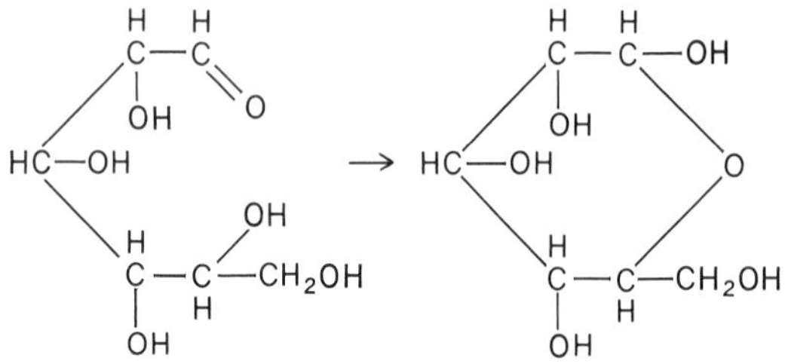

Fig. 7. Six-carbon chain forming hemiacetal ring.

rotatory form is called the L configuration. This connotation of the D and L refers to spatial configuration only and is not an indication of the direction of rotation of the plane of polarized light by the sugar. The reference carbon atom regarding D or L configuration is, for sugars containing more than one asymmetric carbon atom, the asymmetric carbon atom furthest removed from the active, that is, the aldehyde or ketone, end of the molecule and adjacent to the terminal group (Fig. 4).

Rosanoff, who introduced this criterion for designating the D and L form of sugars, regarded all sugars of the D-series as built up, in theory, from D-glycerose, and those of the L-series from L-glycerose. Although not accomplished in practice throughout the series, such a process is rendered possible without interfering with the original asymmetric carbon atom by the stepwise addition of the repeating unit CHOH through the Kiliani cyanohydrin synthesis. It must be emphasized that Rosanoff's representation of the D and L forms of sugar is merely a convention and has no relation to their direction of rotation. If it is desired to indicate the direction of rotation of the compound, the symbols (+), meaning dextrorotatory, and (−), meaning levorotatory, are used. Thus a dextrorotatory sugar with the D configuration is indicated by the symbol D(+), while a levorotatory sugar of the same configuration is represented by D(−). Figure 5 shows the relationship of D-glycerose to the D-trioses, D-tetroses, D-pentoses, and D-hexoses.

Formulation. Thus far the monosaccharides have been considered as open-chain compounds, designated by projection formulas. The projection formula, introduced by Emil Fischer, is based on the convention that tetrahedrons, representing individual asymmetric carbons of a sugar, viewed as though supported by their carbon to carbon bonds with the hydrogen and hydroxyl groups extending outward, are projected upon the depicting plane. This formula is quite convenient, because the relationship between various sugars is easily demonstrated. Its numbering begins at the terminal position associated with the carbonyl group; in

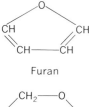

CARBOHYDRATE

Furan

Pyran

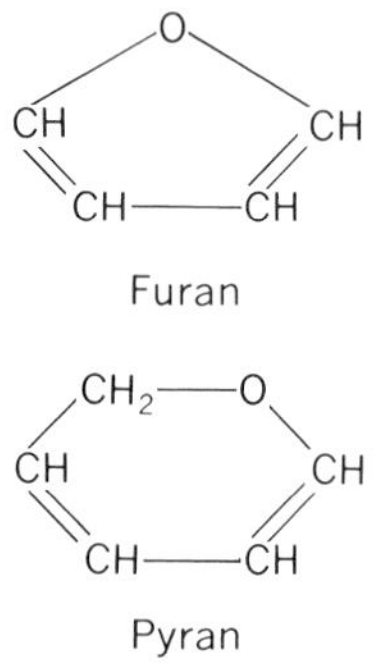

Fig. 8. Structural formulas for furan and pyran.

ketoses the carbonyl group is in carbon atom 2 position. When Greek letters are used, as in the older literature, the carbon next to the —CHO group is called the α-carbon atom.

Although an aldohexose such as D-glucose or an aldopentose such as D-xylose exhibits many of the properties of common aldehydes, its reactivity, when compared with acyclic hydroxyaldehydes such as glycolic aldehyde or glyceraldehyde is not as great as would be expected if the sugar possessed the simple aldehydic projection formula (Fig. 6). Furthermore, the cyanohydrin reaction proceeds with difficulty, and sugars fail to give the Schiff test for aldehydes. Thus, the straight-chain aldehydic projection formula does not represent the essential features of the sugar molecules, particularly their tendency to form five- and six-membered rings. In reality, because of the tetrahedral angles between bonds of the carbon atoms, the chain tends to form a ring. Thus, the ends of a six-carbon chain approach each other as shown in Fig. 7, permitting a reaction between the carbonyl group and a hydroxyl on the fourth or fifth carbon atom and forming a hemiacetal.

The reaction is analogous to the formation of hemiacetals from simple aldehydes and alcohols. Admixture of an aldehyde and an alcohol produces first a hemiacetal. Long standing in an excess of alcohol in the presence of an acid catalyst converts the hemiacetal into a complete acetal, as shown in the equation below.

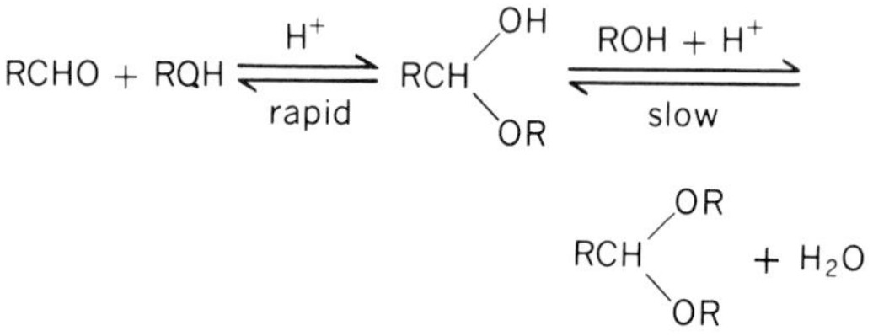

$$
\text{RCHO} + \text{RQH} \underset{\text{rapid}}{\overset{\text{H}^+}{\rightleftharpoons}} \text{RCH}\begin{smallmatrix}\text{OH}\\\text{OR}\end{smallmatrix} \underset{\text{slow}}{\overset{\text{ROH} + \text{H}^+}{\rightleftharpoons}}
$$

$$
\text{RCH}\begin{smallmatrix}\text{OR}\\\text{OR}\end{smallmatrix} + \text{H}_2\text{O}
$$

Such a reaction occurs not only with aldose but also with ketose sugars. Formation of a hemiacetal in a hexose monosaccharide from a reaction between carbon atom 1 and the OH group of carbon atom 6 is not likely, because this would produce a strained seven-membered ring. Six- and five-membered rings are more easily formed because there is very little distortion of the bond angles. Rings of four carbon atoms or less do not form easily.

There is abundant evidence that sugars actually exist as cyclic compounds. Most decisive proof is furnished by the phenomenon of mutarotation, by the existence of two isomeric methylglycosides, and by Haworth's methylation experiments, in which he was unable to demonstrate open-chain structure.

In the older literature the six-membered ring structure of the aldohexoses in which the first carbon atom is linked to the fifth carbon atom through an oxygen atom had been named amylene oxide or δ-oxide configuration. The five-membered rings in which carbon atom 1 is linked to carbon atom 4 had been termed butylene oxide or γ-oxide configuration. In 1927 W. N. Haworth suggested that the five-atom ring sugars should be regarded as derived from furan and the six-atom ring configuration from pyran (Fig. 8).

Thus a sugar containing a γ-oxide or 1,4-oxide ring is called a furanose sugar, and if it is present

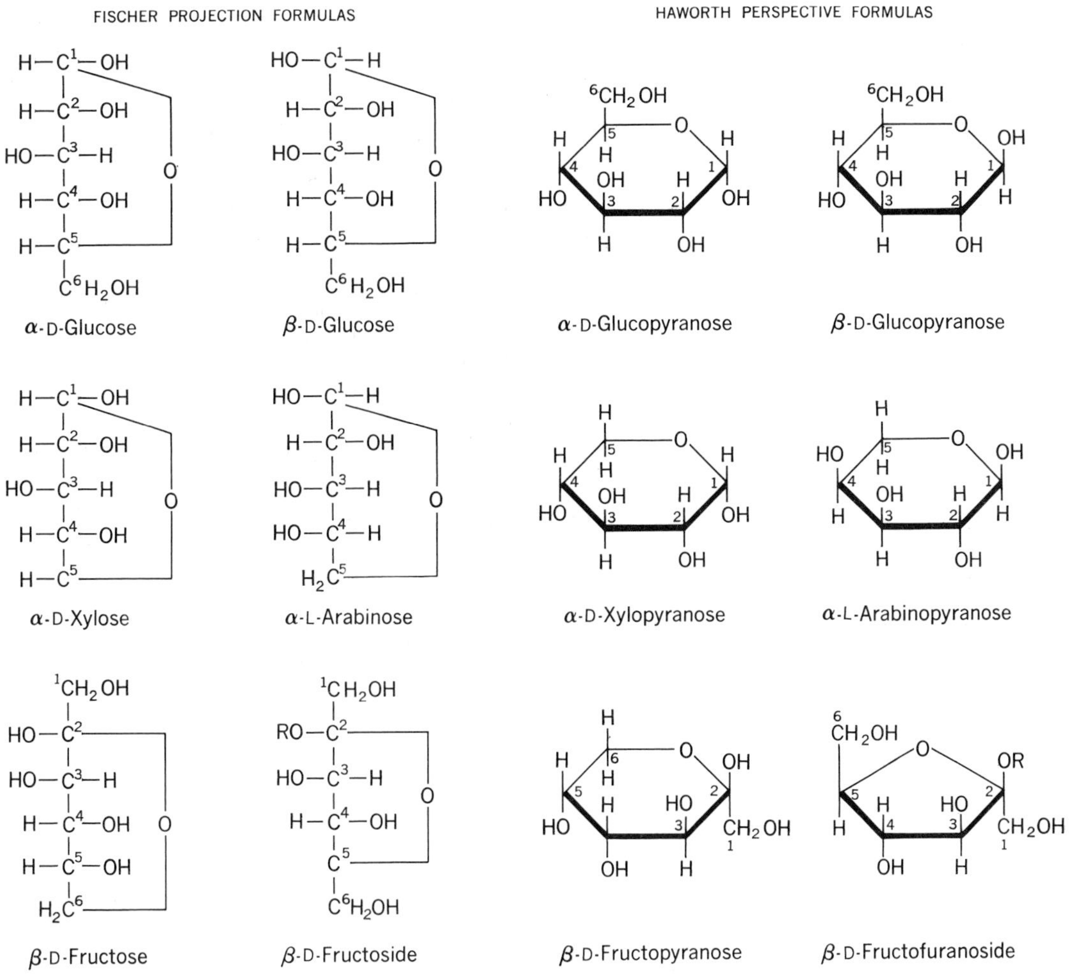

FISCHER PROJECTION FORMULAS

HAWORTH PERSPECTIVE FORMULAS

Fig. 9. Fischer projection formulas and Haworth perspective formulas.

as a glycoside, it is described as a furanoside. It must be noted, however, that unsubstituted furanose sugars have never been isolated, although they do exist in small proportion in solution. Although the 1,4 ring is stable and the 1,5 ring is relatively unstable in the sugar lactones, the reverse is true for the sugars and glycosides. Furanose structures are therefore found either in substituted sugars such as 2,3,5,6-O-methyl-D-glucose, where there is no free hydroxyl on carbon atom 5, or more commonly, when the monosaccharide (D-fructose or L-arabinose) is a constituent of complex sugars, the oligosaccharides or polysaccharides. Similarly the names pyranose and pyranoside are applied to the sugars and sugar derivatives having the six-membered, δ-oxide, or 1,5 rings.

In the Haworth perspective formulas, carbon atoms 1–5 and the ring oxygen are represented in a single plane projecting from the plane of the paper on which it is written. The valences of the carbon atoms not involved in ring formation are situated above or below the plane of the ring. The thickened lines at the bottom of the ring formulas represent the sides of the hexagon nearest to the observer.

When the carbon atoms in the ring are numbered clockwise, as in α-D-glucopyranose, the groups that are written on the right-hand side in the projection formula are represented as project-

ing below the plane of the ring, and the corresponding groups on the left-hand side are projecting above. However, there is a discrepancy in the relative positions of the substituent groups on carbon atom 5 in that the H atom appears in the perspective formula below instead of above the plane of the ring. This apparent anomaly is the result of torsion required to effect ring closure. In forming a ring from the straight-chain aldehydic form, the fifth carbon atom must be rotated so that the oxygen atom in the OH group on this carbon atom is brought into the plane of the first five carbon atoms. Consequently, the H atom attached to carbon atom 5 is now shifted to the other side of the chain, because this carbon atom has been rotated through more than a 90° angle.

The projection and perspective formulas for the α- and β-isomers of D-glucose and for α-D-xylose, α-L-arabinose, and β-D-fructose are shown in Fig. 9.

Since free D-fructose primarily exists in the pyranose configuration, the furanose ring structure of this sugar is shown with the active hydrogen of the potential reducing group substituted. The substituent R may be a D-glucopyranosyl unit as in the disaccharide, sucrose, or a chain of other fructofuranosyl units as in the polysaccharide, inulin.

Mutarotation. Two forms of glucose are known. The α-form is obtained by dissolving the sugar, D-glucose, in water and allowing it to crystallize

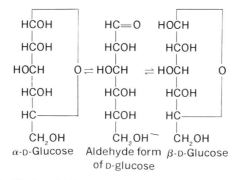

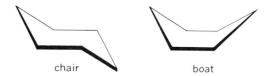

α-D-Glucose   Aldehyde form   β-D-Glucose
                of D-glucose

Fig. 10. Possibilities during mutarotation of D-glucose.

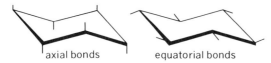

chair   boat

Fig. 11. Conformations of a cyclohexane.

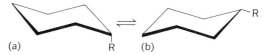

axial bonds   equatorial bonds

Fig. 12. Geometrical arrangements of carbon-hydrogen bonds on the chair form of a cyclohexane.

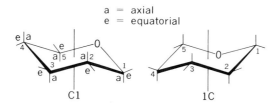

(a)   R   (b)

Fig. 13. Interconversion of (a) axial and (b) equatorial positions for R group of a cyclohexane derivative.

a = axial
e = equatorial

C1   1C

Fig. 14. Interchangeable conformations of a pyranose sugar, designated as C1 and 1C.

through evaporation of the solvent. The β-form is obtained by crystallizing D-glucose from pyridine or acetic acid. The products are not merely different crystallographic forms of the same substance, because they have different properties when dissolved. At 20°C a freshly prepared solution of α-D-glucose has a specific rotation, $[\alpha]_D^{20}$, of +113°, and a freshly prepared aqueous solution of β-D-glucose at the same temperature has a specific rotation of +19°. Upon standing, both solutions gradually change in rotatory power. The optical rotation of the α-D-form decreases and that of the β-D-form increases until they reach the same equilibrium value of $[\alpha]_D +52.5°$, which corresponds to a mixture of 37% α and 63% β. This phenomenon of change in its optical property is called mutarota-

tion. It is displayed not only with glucose but with all crystalline sugars that have a free or potentially free aldehyde or ketone group in the molecule. To account for the existence of two structures, it is assumed that the monosaccharides exist in the form of cyclic hemiacetals rather than in open-chain form (Fig. 10).

The process of mutarotation is due to the labile nature of the hemiacetal linkage and the interconversion of the α- and β-forms through the acyclic aldehyde form which exists in solution to a very small extent (about 0.1%). Mutarotation is catalyzed by both acid and base, with the base being by far more effective.

The α- and β-sugars are stereoisomeric, but they are not mirror images. They are known as anomers, differing from each other only in the positions of the atoms or groups attached to the terminal asymmetric carbon atom.

To avoid confusion in the matter of new isomers or anomers, a convention was proposed by C. Hudson which is generally accepted. This states that for pairs of α- and β-isomers of the D-series, the one with the higher rotation in the positive sense shall be called the α form, whereas the isomer with the lower rotation is designated as β. The reverse holds good for the L-series, the enantiomorph of α-D-glucose being α-L-glucose with a lower specific rotation of $[\alpha]_D -113°$ than β-L-glucose, $[\alpha]_D -19°$. In the α-anomer of D-glucose the OH group attached to the aldehydic carbon atom and the OH group on the adjacent carbon atom are on the same side of the ring (cis position). In the β form these hydroxyl groups are on opposite sides of the hemiacetal ring (trans position).

Sugar conformations. Although the Haworth formulas are an improvement over the Fischer formulas, they still represent an oversimplification of the true configuration of the monosaccharides in space. While the five-membered furanose ring of a sugar is almost planar, a strainless six-membered pyranose ring is not. A nonplanar arrangement of the molecule must be adopted to maintain the normal valency angles in the pyranose ring. The term "conformations" was coined for the various arrangements of atoms in space that can arise by rotation about single bonds.

Since the only difference between a pyranose ring of a monosaccharide and that of a cyclohexane is the presence of an oxygen in the ring of the former compound, there is a close similarity between the molecular geometries of the two types of rings. The concepts developed for the cyclohexane ring can, therefore, be applied to the sugars containing the pyranose rings.

Results obtained by several investigators show that arrangements of cyclohexane which are free from angle strain are either of the "chair" conformation or the "boat" conformation (Fig. 11).

Examination of the chair form of cyclohexane shows that its carbon-hydrogen bonds can be divided into two geometrically different types. Six of them are perpendicular to the plane of the ring and are termed axial (a) bonds, while the other six radiate out from the ring and are termed equatorial (e) bonds (Fig. 12). Because of the staggered arrangements of the hydrogen atoms, the chair conformation (which minimizes repulsions between them) has a lower energy content and is thus more stable than the boat form. Consequently, cyclohexane and most of its derivatives tend to assume the chair conformation.

In cyclohexane derivatives, the group R is axial in one conformation but is readily convertible into the equatorial position (Fig. 13).

Similarly, pyranose sugars can exist in two interchangeable conformations, designated by R. E. Reeves as C1 and 1C (Fig. 14).

The greatest nonbonded interactions in a sugar are due to the hydroxyl groups. In considering preferred conformational stability for any sugar, conformations with large axial substituents should be avoided. In the absence of large polar interactions in the pyranose series, that chair conformation in which the largest number of the bulky groups are in equatorial position is the most stable one. In this connection it should be noted that the CH_2OH group is bulkier than the hydroxyl.

The relationship between the Haworth formulas and the two chair forms for the pyranose sugars is shown in Fig. 15. In each of the pyranose sugars in the illustration there are fewer axial hydroxyl groups and fewer repulsive interactions in the C1 conformation, which is the preferred form.

In conformational formulas, direction of bonds is determined by the tetrahedral valencies of the carbon atoms (Fig. 16).

The application of conformational analysis in carbohydrate chemistry is useful in many cases in predicting relative rates of reactions and the extent to which some reactions will proceed. As an example, the greater proportion of β-D-glucose (in which all hydroxyls are equatorial) in the equilibrium mixture compared with α-D-glucose (which has an axial hydroxyl at carbon atom 1) can be explained. Similarly, the equilibrium between α-D-galactose 1-phosphate (axial hydroxyl at carbon atom 4 in C1 conformation) and α-D-glucose 1-phosphate, which has an equatorial hydroxyl at C=4, resulting in smaller nonbonded interactions, favors the glucose derivative.

Methyl glucosides. When a solution of glucose in cold methanol is treated with dry hydrogen chloride as catalyst, an acetal is formed. Such a compound formed from glucose is called a glucoside (Fig. 17); if the sugar galactose were used, the acetal would be called a galactoside. Methyl glucoside is perhaps the simplest example of a large group of substances in which the hydroxyl of the hemiacetal group at carbon atom 1 of an aldose monosaccharide has been condensed with the hydroxyl group of an alcohol.

In aqueous solution D-glucose exists chiefly as D-glucopyranose. However, a small proportion of this sugar exists in the furanose as well as in the open-chain aldehyde forms, the last in a minute amount. Since the furanose structure reacts more rapidly to form the glucoside than does the pyranose configuration of the sugar, a considerable amount of labile methylglucofuranoside is formed in the first few hours. On prolonged standing or heating, the more stable methyl α-D-glucopyranoside and methyl β-D-glucopyranoside appear. Thus it is evident that when glucose is treated with methanolic hydrochloric acid, the yield of methylglucoside of a particular configuration has little bearing on the structure of the original sugar; that is, the structure of the glucoside may or may not correspond to the structure of the crystalline sugar. However, a relationship in this case can be estab-

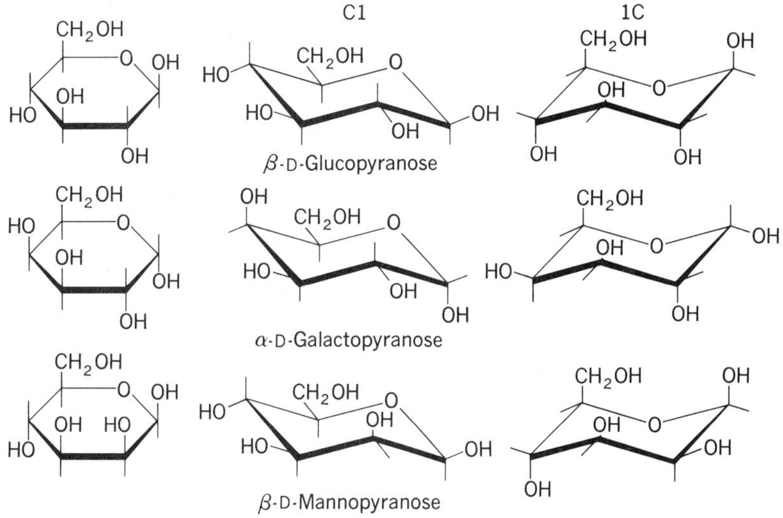

Fig. 15. Relationship between Haworth formula and chair forms for pyranose sugars.

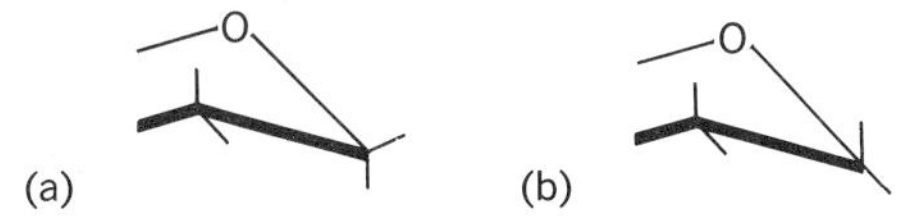

Fig. 16. The glycosidic carbon links in the C1 conformation must be as in (a) not (b).

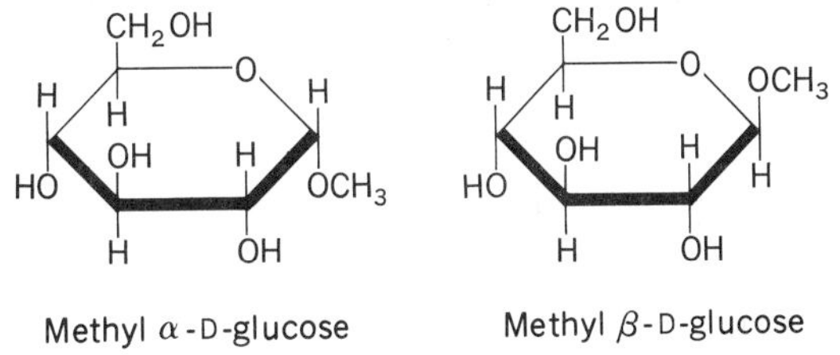

Fig. 17. Formulas for α and β forms of methyl D-glucose.

lished through hydrolysis of a methylglucoside. When pure methyl α-D-glucoside is hydrolyzed, the subsequent mutarotation of the hydrolysis product is found to be in the same direction as that of pure α-D-glucopyranose. It is therefore concluded that α-D-glucose and α-D-glucoside have the same configuration about the first carbon atom.

The α- and β-methylglucosides are crystalline compounds. They may be separated by fractional crystallization or through the agency of enzymes. The enzymes maltase and emulsin act selectively upon the two glucosides, the former hydrolyzing the α-form only and the latter acting upon the anomeric β-compound. The specific rotation of methyl α-D-glucopyranoside is +159°, while that of methyl β-D-glucopyranoside is −33°.

[WILLIAM Z. HASSID]

Bibliography: E. A. Davidson, *Carbohydrate Chemistry*, 1967; R. D. Guthrie, *Guthrie and Honeyman's Introduction to Carbohydrate Chemistry*, 4th ed., 1974; E. G. V. Percival and E. Percival, *Structural Carbohydrate Chemistry*, 1962; W. W. Pigman and D. Horton, *The Carbohydrates*, 2d ed., 1974; J. Staněk et al., *Monosaccharides*, 1964; J. Staněk, M. Černý, and J. Pacák, *Oligosaccharides*, 1965.

Carbohydrate metabolism

The fields of biochemistry and physiology deal with the breakdown and synthesis of simple sugars, oligosaccharides, and polysaccharides, and with the transport of sugars across cell membranes and tissues. The breakdown or dissimilation of simple sugars, particularly glucose, is one of the principal sources of energy for living organisms. The dissimilation may be anaerobic, as in fermentations, or aerobic, that is, respiratory. In both types of metabolism, the breakdown is accompanied by the formation of energy-rich bonds, chiefly the pyrophosphate bond of the coenzyme adenosinetriphosphate (ATP), which serves as a coupling agent between different metabolic processes. In higher animals, glucose is the carbohydrate constituent of blood, which carries it to the tissues of the body. In higher plants, the disaccharide sucrose is often stored and transported by the tissues. Certain polysaccharides, especially starch and glycogen, are stored as endogenous food reserves in the cells of plants, animals, and microorganisms. Others, such as cellulose, chitin, and bacterial polysaccharides, serve as structural components of cell walls. As constituents of plant and animal tissues, various carbohydrates become available to those organisms which depend on other living or dead organisms for their source of nutrients. Hence, all naturally occurring carbohydrates can be dissimilated by some animals or microorganisms. *See* CARBOHYDRATE; GLYCOGEN; STARCH.

Dietary carbohydrates. Certain carbohydrates cannot be used as nutrients by man. For example, the polysaccharide cellulose, which is one of the main constituents of plants, cannot be digested by man or other mammals and is a useful food only for those, such as the ruminants, that harbor cellulose-decomposing microorganisms in their digestive tracts. The principal dietary carbohydrates available to man are the simple sugars glucose and fructose, the disaccharides sucrose and lactose, and the polysaccharides glycogen and starch. Lactose is the carbohydrate constituent of milk and hence one of the main sources of food during infancy. The disaccharides and polysaccharides that cannot be absorbed directly from the intestine are first digested or hydrolyzed by enzymes secreted into the alimentary canal. The nature of these enzymes, known as glycosidases, will be discussed later. *See* FRUCTOSE; LACTOSE.

Intestinal absorption and transport. The simple sugars, of which glucose is the major component, reach the intestine or are produced there through the digestion of oligosaccharides. They are absorbed by the intestinal mucosa and transported across the tissue into the bloodstream. This process involves the accumulation of sugar against a concentration gradient and requires active metabolism of the mucosal tissue as a source of energy. The sugars are absorbed from the blood by the liver and are stored there as glycogen. The liver glycogen serves as a constant source of glucose in the bloodstream. The mechanisms of transport of sugars across cell membranes and tissues are not yet understood, but they appear to be highly specific for different sugars and to depend on enzymelike components of the cells.

Dissimilation of simple sugars. The degradation of monosaccharides may follow one of several types of metabolic pathways. In the phosphorylative pathways, the sugar is first converted to a phosphate ester (phosphorylated) in a reaction with ATP. The phosphorylated sugar is then split into smaller units, either before or after oxidation. In the nonphosphorylative pathways, the sugar is usually oxidized to the corresponding aldonic acid. This may subsequently be broken down either with or without phosphorylation of the intermediate products. Among the principal intermediates in carbohydrate metabolism are glyceraldehyde-3-phosphate and pyruvic acid. The end products of metabolism depend on the organism and, to some extent, on the environmental conditions. Besides cell material that is formed through various biosynthetic reactions, the products may include carbon dioxide (CO_2), alcohols, organic acids, and hydrogen gas. In the so-called complete oxidations, CO_2 is the only excreted end product. In incomplete oxidations, characteristic of the vinegar bacteria and of certain fungi, oxidized end products such as gluconic, ketogluconic, citric, or fumaric acids may accumulate. Organic end products are invariably found in fermentations, since fermentative metabolism requires the reduction as well as the oxidation of some of the products of intermediary metabolism. The energy available from the complete oxidation of 1 mole of glucose with molecular oxygen is approximately 688,000 cal, while that which can be derived from fermentation is very much less; for example, alcoholic fermentation yields about 58,000 cal. In aerobic metabolism, a great deal of the available energy is harnessed for the needs of the organism as energy-rich bonds primarily in ATP through the process known as oxidative phosphorylation. In fermentation, a much smaller amount of ATP is produced. Hence, the amount of biosynthesis and mechanical work that an organism can do at the expense of a given amount of sugar is many times greater in respiration than in fermentation. *See* FERMENTATION.

Glycolysis. The principal phosphorylative pathway involved in fermentations is known as the gly-

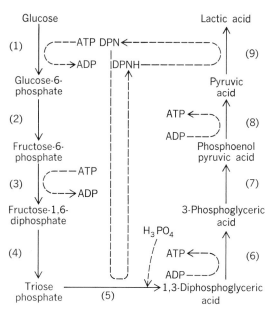

Glycolysis in lactic acid fermentation.

colytic, hexose diphosphate, or Embden-Meyerhof pathway (see illustration). This sequence of reactions is the basis of the lactic acid fermentation of mammalian muscle and of the alcoholic fermentation of yeast. Its main features may be summarized as follows:

1. Glucose is phosphorylated to yield glucose-6-phosphate by the enzyme hexokinase with the conversion of a molecule of ATP to adenosinediphosphate (ADP).
2. Glucose-6-phosphate is epimerized to fructose-6-phosphate by phosphoglucoisomerase.
3. Fructose-6-phosphate is phosphorylated with ATP to yield fructose-1,6-diphosphate. This reaction is catalyzed by phosphofructokinase.
4. Fructose-1,6-diphosphate is split to two molecules of triose phosphate (dihydroxyacetone phosphate and glyceraldehyde phosphate) by aldolase.
5. Both molecules of triose phosphate, which are interconverted by triose phosphate isomerase, are oxidized to 1,3-diphosphoglyceric acid by triose phosphate dehydrogenase. Inorganic phosphate is esterified in this reaction, and the coenzyme diphosphopyridine nucleotide (DPN) becomes reduced to DPNH.
6. 1,3-Diphosphoglyceric acid reacts with ADP to yield ATP and 3-phosphoglyceric acid in the presence of phosphoglycerate kinase.
7. 3-Phosphoglyceric acid is converted to 2-phosphoglyceric acid by phosphoglyceric acid mutase, and the product is dehydrated to phosphoenolpyruvic acid by enolase.
8. In a reaction catalyzed by pyruvic kinase, phosphoenolpyruvic acid reacts with ADP to give pyruvic acid and ATP.
9. Pyruvic acid is converted to the various end products of metabolism. In the lactic acid fermentation, it is reduced to lactic acid with the simultaneous reoxidation of DPNH, which had been formed in step 5, to DPN. In alcoholic fermentation, pyruvic acid is decarboxylated to yield CO_2 and acetaldehyde, and the latter compound is reduced to alcohol with DPNH.

For every molecule of glucose fermented through the glycolytic sequence, two molecules of ATP are used for phosphorylation (steps 1 and 3), while four are produced (steps 6 and 8). Thus, fermentation results in the net gain of two energy-rich phosphate bonds as ATP at the expense of inorganic phosphate esterified in step 5. The excess ATP is converted back to ADP and inorganic phosphate through coupled reactions useful to the organism, such as the mechanical work done by the contraction of muscle or biosynthetic reactions associated with growth.

Oxidative mechanisms. The oxidative or respiratory metabolism of sugars differs in several respects from fermentative dissimilation. First, the oxidative steps, that is, the reoxidation of DPNH, are linked to the reduction of molecular oxygen. Second, the pyruvic acid produced through glycolytic or other mechanisms is further oxidized, usually to CO_2. Third, in most aerobic organisms, alternative pathways either supplement or completely replace the glycolytic sequence of reactions for the oxidation of sugars. Where pyruvic acid appears as a metabolic intermediate, it is generally oxidatively decarboxylated to yield CO_2 and the

two-carbon acetyl fragment which combines with coenzyme A. The acetyl group is then further oxidized via the Krebs cycle.

The principal alternative pathways by which sugars are dissimilated involve the oxidation of glucose-6-phosphate to the lactone of 6-phosphogluconic acid and are known as the hexose monophosphate pathways. In the best-known hexose monophosphate pathway, 6-phosphogluconic acid is formed from its lactone by hydrolysis and is oxidatively decarboxylated to yield CO_2 and the five-carbon sugar, ribulose-5-phosphate. Ribulose-5-phosphate is then converted to glucose-6-phosphate through a series of reactions in which phosphorylated sugars containing three, four, five, six, and seven carbon atoms are formed as intermediates. The principal enzymes involved in these transformations are transaldolase, transketolase, and epimerases. Since the glucose-6-phosphate that is produced from ribulose-5-phosphate is oxidized by the same sequence of reactions, the cyclic operation of this mechanism results in complete oxidation of glucose. Some of the enzymatic steps involved in this pathway provide the pentoses necessary for the synthesis of nucleotides and participate in the photosynthesis of green plants.

Simple sugars other than glucose. The metabolism of simple sugars other than glucose usually involves the conversion of the sugar to one of the intermediates of the phosphorylative pathways described for glucose metabolism. For example, fructose may be phosphorylated to fructose-6-phosphate, which can then be degraded via the glycolytic pathway or converted to glucose-6-phosphate and oxidized through the hexose monophosphate pathway. Similarly, mannose may be phosphorylated to mannose-6-phosphate, which is then transformed to fructose-6-phosphate by phosphomannose isomerase. Alternatively, in some bacteria, mannose is epimerized to fructose before phosphorylation. The principal mechanism for galactose metabolism requires the phosphorylation of the sugar to galactose-1-phosphate and the conversion of this ester to glucose-1-phosphate through the mediation of uridine diphosphoglucose. Glucose-1-phosphate is then converted to glucose-6-phosphate by phosphoglucomutase. The pentoses may be metabolized via their phosphate esters, which are converted to glucose-6-phosphate as described in the discussion of the hexose monophosphate pathway.

Disaccharides and polysaccharides. The dissimilation and biosynthesis of the oligosaccharides are effected through the enzymatic cleavage or formation of glycosidic bonds between simple monosaccharide constituents of the complex carbohydrates. The principal types of enzyme which split or synthesize glycosidic bonds are the hydrolases or glycosidases, phosphorylases, and transglycosylases. The enzymes are generally highly specific with respect to the glycosidic portion, or moiety, and the type of linkage of the substrates which they attack. For example, the glycosidic moiety may be glucosidic or galactosidic and the linkage may be α or β. The essential function of all three types of enzymes is the transfer of the glycosyl moiety of the substrate, which may be designated as the glycosyl donor, to an appropriate glycosyl acceptor, with the liberation of the aglycone. The different types of enzymes generally require

CARDAMON

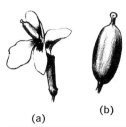

(a)   (b)

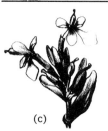

(c)

Cardamon (*Elettaria cardamomum*). (*a*) Flower. (*b*) Fruit. (*c*) Branch tip with flowers and fruits.

different types of acceptors for the transfer reactions, but some enzymes can use a variety of acceptors and can act in more than one capacity. For example, an enzyme can act as a phosphorylase, transglycosylase, or hydrolase for the same substrate.

Hydrolytic cleavage is an essentially irreversible process and hence is used mostly in dissimilative metabolism. Phosphorylases and transglycosylases, on the other hand, may function in biosynthesis as well as the degradation of oligosaccharides.

The glycosidases or hydrolytic enzymes use preferentially the hydroxyl ion of water as the glycosyl acceptor. The aglycone is liberated after combining with the remaining hydrogen ion.

Lactases, for example, are β-galactosidases, and they combine the β-galactosyl portion of the disaccharide lactose with hydroxyl ion of water to yield galactose, liberating glucose. These enzymes can also hydrolyze methyl- or phenyl-β-galactosides with the formation of galactose and methanol or phenol, respectively.

Maltases are α-glucosidases which can hydrolyze maltose to two molecules of glucose.

Sucrases or invertases are enzymes which hydrolyze sucrose to yield glucose and fructose. The typical yeast invertase is a β-fructosidase, specific for the β-fructosyl portion of sucrose. The sucrase found in the human intestinal mucosa, on the other hand, is an α-glucosidase.

Amylases or diastases are enzymes which hydrolyze (digest) starch. The α-amylases, such as the human salivary and pancreatic amylases, split starch to smaller polysaccharide units, known as dextrins, and the disaccharide maltose. The β-amylase of malt, on the other hand, produces maltose as the main product of hydrolysis.

The phosphorylases catalyze the reversible phosphorolysis of certain disaccharides, polysaccharides, and nucleosides by transferring the glycosyl moieties to inorganic phosphate. The breakdown of glycogen and starch by the enzymes known as amylophosphorylases is an example of biologically important phosphorolytic reactions. α-D-Glucose-1-phosphate, which is the product of this process, can be metabolized after conversion to glucose-6-phosphate. Starch and glycogen can be synthesized from glucose-1-phosphate by the reverse reaction. The polysaccharide chain acts as either donor or acceptor for glucosyl groups, inorganic phosphate being the alternative acceptor. The reversible synthesis of sucrose, sucrose phosphate, and cellulose from uridine diphosphoglucose is similar to the phosphorolytic reactions, with the uridine compound serving as glucosyl donor.

The transglycosylases interconvert various disaccharides and polysaccharides by the transfer of glycosyl groups. For instance, dextrins can be synthesized from maltose in a reversible reaction catalyzed by the bacterial enzyme, amylomaltase:

$$n\text{C}_{12}\text{H}_{22}\text{O}_{11} \rightleftharpoons (\text{C}_6\text{H}_{10}\text{O}_5)_n + n\text{C}_6\text{H}_{12}\text{O}_6$$
Maltose   Dextrin   Glucose

Many glycosidases have marked transglycosylase activity.

[MICHAEL DOUDOROFF]

Cardamon

For centuries this plant has been an important spice in the Orient. The plant, *Elettaria cardamomum* (Zingiberaceae), a perennial herb 6–12 ft tall, is a native of India (see illustration). The small, light-colored seeds, borne in capsules, have a delicate flavor. They are used in curries, cakes, pickles, and in general cooking, as well as in medicine. In India the seeds are a favorite masticatory. *See* SPICE AND FLAVORING.

[PERRY D. STRAUSBAUGH/EARL L. CORE]

Carrot

A biennial umbellifer (*Daucus carota*) of Asiatic and Mediterranean origin belonging to the plant order Umbellales. The carrot is grown for its edible roots which are eaten raw or cooked.

Propagation is by seed planted directly in the field. Spacing varies; plants are usually planted 1/2 to 2 in. apart in rows of 18 to 24 in. Temperature and soil moisture affect root color and shape; 60 to 70°F is optimum for high yields of long, deep-colored roots.

Exposure of the young carrot plants to prolonged cold weather (40 to 50°F for 15 or more days) favors seed-stalk formation. Misshapen roots commonly result from nematodes, aster yellows disease, or compacted soils. Most commercial plantings are weeded chemically.

Varieties (cultivars) are classified according to length of root (long or short or stump-rooted) and use (fresh market or processing). Popular varieties for fresh market are Imperator and Gold Pak; for processing, Red Cored Chantenay and Royal Chantenay.

Harvesting of carrots for fresh market begins when the roots are 3/4 to 2 in. in diameter, usually 60 to 90 days after planting. Harvesting by machine is common. Marketing in bunches is declining; most carrots are sold in plastic bags with the foliage removed. Carrots for canning generally have shorter roots and are grown to a larger diameter.

Texas, California, and Arizona are important producing states. The total annual farm value in the United States from about 80,000 acres is approximately $60,000,000. *See* VEGETABLE GROWING.

[H. JOHN CAREW]

Casein

The principal protein of milk. It is present in milk as calcium caseinate and amounts to 80% of the milk protein. When casein is separated from the other constituents and washed free of impurities, it has certain industrial uses, such as in the manufacture of brush bristles, buttons, billiard balls, jewelry, paper, glue, paint, sodium caseinate, and protein hydrolyzates. The competition from synthetic plastics has reduced the demand for casein for some of these uses. *See* MILK.

Casein is made by either of two methods, coagulation by rennet or precipitation by acid. The rennet method is used for producing casein for the plastics industry. The acid precipitation method is used for casein production for other commercial uses, including the food industry. Dilute hydrochloric acid is added to skim milk having a temperature between 35 and 46.1°C. When the pH is brought to a range between 4.8 and 4.0, the casein is precipitated in a coagulated mass or curd. The whey is drained from the curd, and the curd is washed with water until it is relatively free of impurities. When a premium grade is desired, the curd is further washed with water five or six times, starting with water at the same temperature as the whey and using a final wash with water at 15.6°C. The whey, which is drained from the curd, contains about 5% lactose, 0.85% protein, and 0.75% ash, as well as a high percentage of the water-soluble vitamins in the original milk. The curd is pressed, dried with hot air in a tunnel, ground, packed in bags, and stored. *See* FOOD ENGINEERING. [PAUL H. TRACY]

Bibliography: C. H. Eckles et al., *Milk and Milk Products*, 4th ed., 1951; L. M. Lampert, *Modern Dairy Products*, 1970; B. H. Webb and E. O. Whittier, *By-products from Milk*, 2d ed., 1970.

Cashew

A medium-sized (20–30 ft high), spreading evergreen tree (*Anacardium occidentale*) native to Brazil, but now grown widely in the tropics for its edible nuts and the resinous oil contained in the shells. The fruit consists of a fleshy, red or yellow, pear-shaped receptacle, termed the apple, $2-3\frac{1}{2}$ in. long, at the distal end of which is borne a hard-shelled, kidney-shaped ovary or nut about $1\frac{1}{2}$ in. long (see illustration). The shell of this nut is about $\frac{1}{8}$-in. thick and consists of a smooth, relatively thin outer layer (exocarp) and an inner hard layer (endocarp). Between these is a porous layer (mesocarp), filled with a caustic black liquid which blisters the skin and makes the processing of the nut difficult.

Although cashew trees are spread throughout the tropics, commercial production is centered in India, which handles 90% of the world trade. The trees, mostly seedlings, grow on wastelands with a minimum of care, reach full bearing at 8 years of age, and may continue for 25 years or more. Usually the fruits fall from the trees when mature and are gathered by local labor; the nuts are separated from the apples by hand. Some of the apples are marketed locally but most are wasted.

Processing the nuts is a difficult operation because of the caustic liquid in the shells. In 1968 there were about 250 processing factories in India to handle the local crops and, in addition, large quantities of raw nuts from East Africa. The nuts are dried in the sun, cleaned, moistened, and kept for 12 hr in heaps or silos to soften the shells. They are then roasted at 350–400°F. In the roasting process the cashew shell liquid is released and collected as a by-product. The kernels are extracted from the shells, heated to remove the enclosing membrane (testa), graded, and packed in tin cans for export.

Shelled cashew nuts plus cashew shell liquid are second only to jute in India's exports. More than half of these go to the United States; Europe and the Soviet Union are heavy importers also.

Cashew nut kernels are eaten as nuts and used extensively in the confectionery and baking trade. The cashew shell liquid is a valuable by-product, containing 90% anacardic acid and 10% cardol, and is used in the varnish and plastic industries.

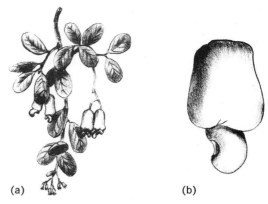

(a)   (b)

Cashew (*Anacardium occidentale*). (a) Branch with leaves, fruits, and nuts. (b) Fruit with nut.

The cashew apples are too astringent for eating without being processed, but when processed may be used for jams, chutney, pickles, and wine. In India much attention is being given to extending and improving the cashew industry. *See* NUT CROP CULTURE.

[LAURENCE H. MAC DANIELS]

Cassava

The plant *Manihot esculenta* (family Euphorbiaceae), also called manioc. It is one of the 10 most important food plants, and the most important starchy root or tuber of the tropics. It originated in Central or South America, possibly Brazil, and was domesticated and widely distributed well before the time of Columbus. Subsequent distribution has established cassava as a major crop in eastern and western Africa, in India, and in Indonesia. Brazil continues to be the world's largest producer. Annual world production is about 100,000,000 metric tons.

The cassava plant is a slightly woody, perennial shrub reaching 10 ft (3 m) in height. The leaves are deeply palmately lobed; the flowers are inconspicuous, and the prominent capsules are three-seeded and explosive at maturity. The roots (see illustration) are enlarged by the deposition of starch and constitute the principal source of food from the plant. Normal yields are about 10 lb (4.5 kg) per plant. The leaves are also eaten (after cooking), and are noteworthy for their high protein content.

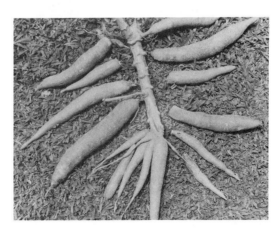

Tuberous roots from a single cassava plant.

The plant is propagated from mature stems which are planted without special treatment. Tuberization occurs gradually; about 10 or 12 months from planting to harvest is normal. Cassava can be grown for 2 or more years, however, and thus is a food that can be used at any season. Once it is harvested, however, the roots deteriorate within a few days.

The chief use of cassava is as a boiled vegetable. It is also a source of flour, called *farinha* in Brazil and *gari* in western Africa, and of toasted starch granules, the familiar tapioca. It can be processed into macaroni and a ricelike food. In the form of dried chips, cassava root is an important animal feed in the international market and is used extensively in Europe. In spite of its popularity, however, cassava root is a poor food. Its protein content is extremely low, and its consumption as a staple food is associated with the protein deficiency disease kwashiorkor. In addition, all parts of the plant contain glucosides of hydrocyanic acid, substances which on decomposition yield the poisonous hydrocyanic acid (HCN, prussic acid). Chronic diseases including goiter are common in regions where cassava is a staple food.

Cassava is under study at international institutes to eliminate its weakness, improve its culture, and foment its utilization. It has a bright future as an industrial starch crop, as food and feed crop, and as a substrate for the production of protein by yeast and fungal fermentations.

[FRANKLIN W. MARTIN]

Bibliography: D. L. Jennings, *Field Crop Abstr.*, 22(3):271–275, 1970; W. O. Jones, *Manioc in Africa*, 1959; F. W. Martin, *Proceedings of the International Symposium on Tropical Root and Tuber Crops*, vol. 1: *Tropical Tuber and Root Crops Tomorrow*, 1970; B. Nestel and R. MacIntyre (eds.), *Chronic Cassava Toxicity*, International Development Research Centre, Ottawa, 1973; T. P. Phillips, *Cassava Utilization and Potential Markets*, International Development Research Centre, Ottawa, 1974

Castor bean

The plant *Ricinus communis*, a member of the spurge family (Euphorbiaceae). It is a coarse, erect, annual herb in temperate regions, and a treelike perennial up to 40 ft tall in warmer climates (see illustration). When ripe, the prickly seed pods separate into three parts, each containing a seed, the castor bean. These seeds contain a thick, colorless or greenish, nondrying oil. After this oil is pressed out of the seeds, boiled with water, and filtered to remove mucilage and proteins, it is the commercial castor oil used medicinally, in soap, as a lubricant, and as a leather preservative.

[PERRY D. STRAUSBAUGH/EARL L. CORE]

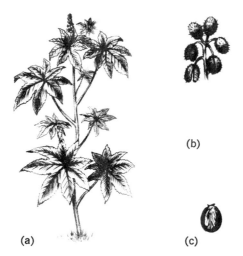

Ricinus communis, castor bean plant. (*a*) Entire plant grows 3–40 ft high. (*b*) Pods of the fruit cluster liberate (*c*) smooth, distinctively marked seeds.

Cattle production, beef

Raising of cattle for meat. The flesh from cattle over 6 months of age is beef and from younger cattle is veal. Beef is a nutritious food analyzing approximately 25% protein and is rich in essential amino acids, B vitamins, and minerals. It is the preferred meat of the world and accounts for approximately 53% of the consumption of red meat.

Cattle belong to the zoological family Bovidae and are ruminants because they have a four-compartment stomach and chew a cud. Most domestic breeds common to the temperate zone originated from European *Bos taurus* ancestry, whereas Zebu or Brahman originated from Asian *B. indicus*, indigenous to the tropics.

World beef production. World cattle numbers in January 1974 were estimated at an all-time record of 1,300,000,000, which is an approximate increase of 11% since 1964. Countries or areas showing greatest percentage increases include Japan, 24%; Western Europe, 10%; United States, 6%; Mexico, 5%; and Canada and Central America, 2% each. Beef cattle numbers have increased in almost all geographic areas since 1964, while total dairy numbers have declined. Further but slower annual increases in beef will likely parallel population growth. The major cattle countries and per capita beef consumption are shown in the table.

The United States, with 122,000,000 cattle (beef and dairy), is the major beef producer. The cattle of India, regarded as sacred, are unimportant as edible beef in world trade. In 1974 Australia and Argentina were the leading beef exporters, but New Zealand, Mexico, and Brazil also exported large amounts. *See* CATTLE PRODUCTION, DAIRY.

World beef production is based largely on the use of grass and harvested roughages. The major phases of beef production in the world are cow herds for raising calves, stockers, and feeders for growing and fattening. Calves are generally allowed to nurse their mothers on pasture for 6–7 months before weaning. Under good management weaned calves average 400 lb at 7 months and with extra creep grain average 500 lb. In some countries, after weaning, calves are grown as stockers on grass or winter roughages until yearlings or 2-year-olds. The pampas of Argentina provides year-round grazing and produces slaughter beef directly from grass at 2 years of age. Many Australian, New Zealand and Argentinean cattle are marketed from pasture alone, while many cattle in the United States, Canada, and England are grain-fed. With increased grain costs, the trend may be to feed grain for shorter periods and fatten more cattle on grain crop silage or on grass.

United States beef production. Approximately 3% of United States beef cattle are in purebred

Estimated cattle numbers and beef consumption in the world, 1973*

Countries and continents	Cattle, 10^6	Per capita beef consumption, lb
India	205.8†	—
United States	122.0	116
Soviet Union	104.0	49
Brazil	95.3	39
Argentina	52.3	137
Australia	29.0	90
Mexico	26.8	24
France	21.9	65
Columbia	21.4	51
Turkey	14.3	11
West Germany	13.9	55
United Kingdom	13.8	54
Canada	12.7	93
Republic of South Africa	10.2	51
Italy	8.6	45
New Zealand	8.2†	105
Netherlands	4.1	41
Japan	3.1†	7
Denmark	2.9	45
Belgium and Luxemburg	2.8	63
Asia	488.0	
South America	204.0	
North America	189.6	
Africa	155.1	
Europe	133.0	
Oceania	40.9	
Australia	29.0	
New Zealand	8.2	

*From *World Agricultural Situation* and *Foreign Agricultural Service.*
†1968 estimates.

registered herds which supply bulls for commercial herds. The rank of the six leading purebred breeds are Hereford (Fig. 1), Angus (Fig. 2), Charolais (Fig. 3), Simmental (Fig. 4), and Shorthorn. In the Gulf area Brahman (Fig. 5) or breeds with Brahman blood such as Santa Gertrudis, Brangus, and Beefmaster are more tolerant of humidity, heat, and insects. A systematic cross of two or three breeds is finding favor with producers because hybrid vigor results in lower mortality and in improved growth and efficiency. Beginning in the late 1960s, many commercial producers seeking greater size and improved gains have included one or more of the European exotic breeds of Charolais, Simmental, Limiosin, Maine Anjou, Chianina, Beef Fresian, and others in their crossing systems. The rough topography and limited rainfall of the Rocky Mountains and sections of the central and western plains adapt these areas to production of feeder calves, yearlings, and some 2-year-olds. In the range areas of the Nebraska Sandhills, Kansas, and Oklahoma Flint Hills, approximately 8–15 acres of grass are required annually for a cow and calf, while in more arid areas of Arizona and New Mexico 150–200 acres are needed per cow and calf. The Corn Belt, areas of the South, and the Pacific Coast produce surplus grain and forage for feedlot fattening.

Feeding beef cattle. Feed is the major cost item of beef production. It is estimated that roughages furnish 80% of the total feed for cattle. The mature cow is physiologically well adapted to utilize, in addition to quality feeds, salvage roughages such as straws, corn stover, cottonseed hulls, and byproducts of the sugar and canning industries. The rumen compartment of a mature bovine stomach can hold 40–60 gal and has millions of microorganisms, such as bacteria, yeasts, and protozoa, to aid roughage digestion. The rumination processes of cud chewing, regurgitation, and rumen microbial fermentation aid in the release of digestible energy in the form of glucose and acetic and propionic acids from the fibrous cellulose stems of roughage. Cattle have an advantage over the monogastric single-stomach swine or poultry because they synthesize their necessary B vitamins and essential amino acids. The nutrient requirements of cattle are water, proteins, carbohydrates, fats, minerals, and vitamins. Energy from carbohydrates and fats along with proteins are of major dietary and cost importance. Quality forages and good pastures, except in soil-deficient areas, can furnish adequate nutrients for maintenance, growth, and reproduction.

With population increases and greater human consumption of concentrate grains, more research effort will likely be directed to maximizing use of corn and milo stovers and by-product straws of grain harvest in beef rations. Treatment of these roughages with alkalies, pressure, and moisture has markedly improved availability and digestibility of energy of these roughages.

Mature cattle eat about 2 lb daily for each 100 lb

CATTLE PRODUCTION, BEEF

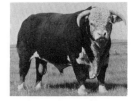

Fig. 1. Hereford bull. (*American Hereford Association*)

CATTLE PRODUCTION, BEEF

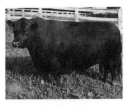

Fig. 2. Angus bull. (*American Angus Association*)

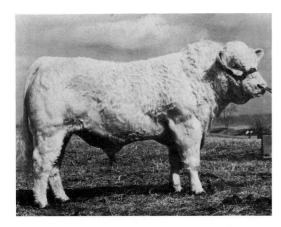

Fig. 3. Charolais bull. (*American International Charolais Association*)

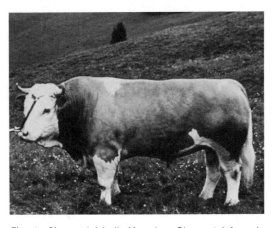

Fig. 4. Simmental bull. (*American Simmental Association*)

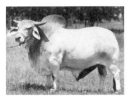

Fig. 5. Brahman, tolerant of humidity, heat, and insects. (*American Brahman Breeders Association*)

of their weight, and younger cattle eat 2.5–3.0 lb of air-dry feed per hundredweight (cured forages and grains of approximately 10% moisture).

The National Research Council gives the maintenance requirement of cattle as 0.75 lb of total digestible nutrient (TDN) energy per 100 lb liveweight. The TDN of a feed is the sum of all digestible organic nutrients, protein, fiber, carbohydrate, and (fat × 2.25). The National Research Council also expresses energy requirements as digestible energy, with 1 lb of TDN equivalent to 2000 Calories (large calories) or 2 therms (1 therm = 1000 Calories) of digestible energy. One pound of gain requires 3.53 lb of TDN above maintenance. Air-dry grains, such as oats, barley, corn, and milo, vary in energy but average 72–80% TDN, and cured roughages, such as straw and hays average 40–50% TDN. Balanced grain rations have more digestible energy and produce larger daily gains. Energy utilization of grains is improved by steaming and rolling or flaking. The average daily gain of calves (over 6 months), yearlings, and 2-year-old steers fed a full feed of 1.75 lb grain per hundredweight are about 2.10, 2.25, and 2.50 lb, respectively. Compared to steers, heifers make 5–10% slower and bulls 5–10% faster gains. Efficiency of gains (energy per pound of gain) favors calves over yearlings and yearlings over 2-year-olds. Estrogenic hormones, such as stilbestrol, synovex, and melangesterol (for heifers), fed or implanted under the skin increase gains and efficiency 12–18%. *See* ANIMAL-FEED COMPOSITION.

The recommended crude protein percent of fattening rations is approximately 12, 11, and 10%, respectively, for calves, yearlings, and 2-year-olds and is somewhat greater for breeding bulls, lactating cows, and very young calves. Digestible protein needs are 75% of crude protein. Grains and many hays and straws are low in protein and are oftentimes supplemented with soybean, linseed and cottonseed oilmeals or both. Green pastures and legume hays are good sources of protein.

Nonprotein nitrogen sources, such as urea, biuret, and starea (supplements synthetically crystallized from nitrogen in the air), are finding wide use as cheap protein substitutes for oilmeals. The rumen microorganisms combine nonprotein nitrogen with carbohydrate and mineral elements into essential amino acids of protein for use by cattle.

Ensiling is preserving of grass forages with 40–50% (haylage) or grain forages (silage) with 60–70% moisture in airtight structures. The exclusion of air and fermentation of carbohydrates in the forages produces preserving lactic and acetic acids. Silages are palatable and are widely used because they reduce curing losses and provide more nutrients per acre.

Low-level feeding (75 mg daily) of the antibiotics aureomycin and terramycin improves roughage utilization, and they are included in finishing rations to minimize disease. Cubing of hay and pelleting of rations by pressure and steam is gaining popularity because compressing facilitates handling and storing, reduces dust, and often improves gain efficiency.

Marketing and grading. Cattle of varying weights, ages, and sexes, of both dairy and beef breeding are slaughtered annually. For clarity of market reporting, cattle are classified as steers, heifers, cows, bulls, stags, veals, and slaughter calves. In 1973 a bullock market class was included for slaughter bulls under 2 years of age, since research shows that young bulls, compared to similar-age steers, gain faster and more efficiently and yield leaner carcasses.

Consumers prefer beef from young grain-fed cattle averaging 900–1200 lb alive. Steer beef from males castrated at a young age is generally the highest priced. Young fat heifers, if not pregnant, yield carcasses comparable to steers; however, heifers mature and fatten sooner and are sold at lighter weights. Pregnancy reduces carcass yield and so heifers undersell steers $1–3 per hundredweight. Cows (mature females) yield more angular carcasses and less tender beef. Bulls (uncastrated males) and stags (late-castrated males) yield coarser-textured meat. A veal is a fleshy young calf averaging 150–300 lb, while those older and heavier up to 550 lb are slaughter calves. The meat of young cattle has more moisture and has a lighter-colored lean. Some use is being made of sterilizing very young bulls by forcing the testes into the abdomen by placing a rubber band on the scrotum. The treated male is unfertile but retains the growth advantage of a bull.

Slaughter cattle are purchased primarily on carcass quality, probable dressing percent, and lean yield and are graded according to government standards in descending value as prime, choice, good, standard, commercial, utility, cutter, and canner. Thickness of muscling (conformation), condition (fattiness), and quality of lean (marbling) are the major factors in grading standards. Dressing percent is the carcass yield based upon liveweight (liveweight ÷ carcass weight) and varies from 65% for prime cattle to 40% for cutter cattle. Fat increases dressing percent whereas water, feed fill remaining in the paunch, coarse bone, and heavy hides reduce dressing percent. An ideal carcass is muscular in the loin, round, and rib; is young and straight-lined; carries a smooth, firm uniform covering of white fat; and shows a cherry-red, fine-textured, well-marbled lean. Grades lower than prime result from a lack of one or more of these desired carcass traits. Marbling, an interspersion of fat with lean, contributes to flavor, whereas texture (diameter of muscle fibers) and youth ensure tenderness. Young carcasses have softer, red-colored bones with cartilage tips on the vertebrae as contrasted to flinty white bone of older beef. Meat from older cattle is less tender due to intermuscular collagen and connective tissue. To ensure tenderness, the better grading carcasses are aged from 10 days to 3 weeks at temperatures of 34–38°F. Papaya enzymes can be added during cooking to tenderize meat. Since tenderizing enzymes also attack other tissues than collagen, overuse during cooking may cause the meat to be too soft. A United States packer suggests that his copyrighted practice of injecting the enzyme into the blood system of cattle prior to slaughter is a more effective tenderizing method than application during culinary preparation. Provisioners are attempting to improve retail efficiency and reduce transportation costs by boning and trimming carcasses at slaughter sites. Some also are packaging portion control beef cuts in airtight cryovac plastic film.

Slaughter. In slaughtering, carcasses are split through the backbone into sides. For wholesale trade, sides are divided between the 12th and 13th ribs into fore- and hindquarters and then retailed primarily as steaks and roasts. The major forequarter cuts are chuck and rib; the hindquarter cuts are loin and round.

Approximately 75% of fresh beef is merchandised by large grocery chains and is mostly choice and good grade. The emphasis for lean, marbled beef has resulted in further scoring carcasses within grades for cutability with 1 as top yield and 5 as the poorest. Cutability or lean yield is determined by measuring the lean area and fat thickness over the longissimus rib-eye muscle exposed between the 12th and 13th ribs, plus accounting for kidney fat.

An attempt is made to utilize all offal of slaughter. Edible offal, such as heart, liver, and tongue, are called meat specialties. The hide, used as leather, represents about 8% of liveweight. Use is made of inedible offal for production of bone meal, blood meal, and meat scraps for livestock feeds; organs and glands for pharmaceutical products; hooves and horns for glue and fertilizer; and intestines for sausage casings.

Reproduction. Cattle are polyestrous, or breed at all seasons. Heifers reach puberty or sexual maturity, depending upon nutrition, at about 5–12 months of age. The estrous period or acceptance of the male averages about 18 hr and the estrous cycle occurs at intervals of 18–24 days. Well-grown heifers can be bred to calve at 2 years of age, but some cattlemen prefer to calve later at $2\frac{1}{2}$–3 years. Average gestation or pregnancy is about 283 days. Twin births occur about 1 in 200 and other multiple births are less common. A heifer born twin to a bull is usually unfertile and is called a freemartin. Young bulls are virile at about 8 months and should be used sparingly until a year old. In range areas one active bull over 2 years is kept for 20–30 cows. Artificial insemination (AI) is not used as extensively with beef as with dairy cattle but is increasing. Some beefmen are researching the idea of synchronizing or controlling estrus by feeding or injecting progesterone hormones. Estrous synchronization permits breeding of many cows (mostly by AI) close together and results in more uniform age calves. Paralleling AI use, the techniques of fertilized ova transplants and hormonal superovulation have proved fairly successful. These techniques permit annual multiple-offspring production from superior genetic cows through surgical transfer of fertilized ova to compatible recipient mothers.

Progressive cattlemen are using performance tests to select cows that will wean 500–600-lb calves at 7 months and feeders that will gain $2\frac{1}{2}$–3 lb daily and weigh 1000–1100 lb at 1 year. Rate of gain and efficiency are highly correlated and heritable, which means that fast-gaining parents should produce fast- and efficient-gaining offspring. *See* BREEDING (ANIMAL).

Diseases. Cattle are afflicted with only a few serious diseases. Competent veterinarian diagnosis and treatment are important. The most universally destructive diseases are tuberculosis, brucellosis or abortion, foot-and-mouth disease, anthrax, and blackleg.

Tuberculosis (TB) is highly contagious and is transmissible to man through milk. TB is caused by a specific bacterium that may attack all parts of the body but particularly the lymphatic glands. There is no specific treatment, but the identification by an annual tuberculin skin test and disposition of reactors has markedly reduced TB.

Contagious abortion, brucellosis or Bang's disease, is a serious reproductive disease caused by *Brucella abortus*. Bang's disease causes birth of premature or dead calves. It has been reduced by blood-testing females (agglutination test) annually and slaughtering carriers. Calfhood vaccination of heifers between 4–8 months can provide immunity. *See* BRUCELLOSIS.

Other reproductive diseases, such as leptospirosis, vibriosis, and trichomoniasis, are prevalent but can be minimized by testing, immunization, and good health management.

Foot-and-mouth disease is caused by a virus and produces blister lesions on the feet and in and on the mouth. The disease is more debilitating than fatal and causes great economic losses due to weight reductions when cattle cannot or refuse to eat. A 1947 outbreak in Mexico was eradicated through inspection, vaccination, quarantine, and slaughter. Outbreaks in Europe and particularly in England in 1967 have banned European cattle imports into the United States. Outbreaks of the disease in Argentina and other countries have limited imports to only canned beef from South America. *See* FOOT-AND-MOUTH DISEASE.

Anthrax (splenic fever) is very infectious and usually fatal. The anthrax organism, a bacillus, can live many years and is transferable to other species and to man. Diagnosis can be made by microscopic examination of a blood sample for the specific bacillus. *See* ANTHRAX.

Blackleg is an acute disease of young cattle. Annual calfhood vaccination is practiced in areas where the disease prevails. When outbreaks occur, the best preventive measures for blackleg and anthrax are burning or deep burial of infected carcasses and prompt vaccination with antiserum. *See* BLACKLEG.

Bloat is a digestive disturbance which causes a loss of millions of dollars annually. Bloat is recognized by distention of the animal's left side due to excessive gas formation in the rumen. Pasture forages such as alfalfa, clover, and other legumes eaten wet oftentimes produce heavy fermentation. A gradual change from dry roughage to legume pasture, as well as feeding hay on pasture, may help minimize bloat. The administration of miscible oils in the drinking water or sprayed on the forage has helped reduce bloat. A chemical feed, Poloxalene, developed in 1966 shows promise in preventing bloat. Poloxalene blocks flavored with molasses to encourage daily consumption are placed in areas of the pasture where cattle gather.

Feedlot health. To reduce shipping fever (hemorrhagic septicemia flu), incoming feedlot cattle are fed for 2 weeks after arrival daily high levels (300–500 mg) of antibiotics. New feeder cattle are usually wormed, sprayed for lice and grubs, and vaccinated for leptospirosis, infectious bovine rhinotracheitis (IBR), and bovine virus diarrhea (BVD). A program of preconditioning feeder cattle on ranches for parasites and feedlot disease immunity is occurring. Foot rot or foul foot, common in wet feedlots, is controlled by low levels of antibiotics and iodine compounds in rations or in salt-mineral mixtures. Vitamin A deficiencies in feedlot cattle are prevented through intramuscular injections of vitamins A, D, and E or by supplemental mixes in the rations. *See* AGRICULTURAL SCIENCE (ANIMAL).

[W. W. ALBERT]

Bibliography: H. M. Briggs, *Modern Breeds of Livestock* 3d ed., 1969; E. W. Crampton and L. E. Harris, *Applied Animal Nutrition*, 2d ed., 1969; L. A. Maynard and J. K. Loosli, *Animal Nutrition*, 6th ed., 1969; National Research Council, *Recommended Nutrient Allowances for Beef Cattle*, 1970; V. A. Rice et al., *Breeding and Improvement of Farm Animals*, 6th ed., 1970; J. R. Romans and P. T. Ziegler, *The Meat We Eat*, 10th ed., 1974; USDA, *Foreign Agricultural Service*, FLM, 1973; USDA, *Official United States Standards for Grades of Carcass Beef*, Title 7, Ch. I, pt. 53, July 1973; USDA, *World Agricultural Production and Trade*, WAS 4, 1973.

Cattle production, dairy

This section of animal agriculture is concerned with the production of milk and milk products. The mammary gland in mammals was developed for the nourishment of their young. Over the centuries man has selected some mammals, especially the cow, goat, and water buffalo, for their ability to produce quantities of milk in excess of the requirements of their young. At the same time man has improved the management and nutrition of the animals so that they can produce milk more efficiently. The production of milk includes selection of animals, breeding, raising young stock, feed production, nutrition, housing, milking, milk handling, sanitation, disease control, and disposal of milk, surplus animals, and manure.

The cattle industry dates back many centuries. In Libya, Africa, friezes dating back to 9000 B.C. show domesticated cows. Written records as far back as 6000 B.C. of Old Mesopotamia (now Iraq) indicate that dairying was very highly developed at that time. These people were the first to make butter. Egyptian records show that milk, butter, and cheese were used as early as 3000 B.C.

Dairy development in America. Dairying in the United States had its principal origin from northern Europe. The first cattle were brought to the West Indies by Columbus in 1495. The first importations to the United States were made to Jamestown, Va., in 1611, and the Plymouth Colony in 1624.

In the United States up to 1850 most families kept a cow and the milk and its products were consumed by the family. Excess milk was used for cheese and butter, but little was sold since transportation was by horse and wagon and no refrigeration was available.

After 1850 dairying became an industry as a result of several major factors. In 1841 the first regular shipment of milk by rail was made from Orange County, N.Y., to New York City. The first cheese factory was built in 1851 in Oneida, N.Y. In 1856 Gail Borden invented the condensed milk process. The first butter factory was started in

New York State in 1856, and the first creamery was established in Iowa in 1871. The separator was invented by Gustav DeLaval in 1878, and in 1890 the Babcock test (to determine fat content) was introduced, which allowed for the impartial buying of milk. The first pasteurizing machine was introduced in 1895, and the first compulsory pasteurization law was passed in Chicago in 1908. Refrigeration came into use in 1880. Contributing to the development of the dairy industry was the establishment of experiment stations, which conducted research on feeding, breeding, and management of cattle. This was accompanied by the organization of the agricultural extension service and other educational facilities to carry information to the dairy farmers. Artificial insemination was introduced in 1938 and is now an important segment of the dairy cattle industry.

World dairy production. The leading milk-producing countries in the world are given in Table 1. Figures are not available for most of the Asian countries, which include the mainland of China and India. Most of the leading milk-producing countries are located in the temperate regions. Dairy cattle numbers and milk production are somewhat more limited in the tropical and semitropical regions. Some countries, namely, New Zealand and Denmark, are not listed among the 10 top countries for milk production but are major export countries because of their large per capita production in comparison to consumption.

Dairy production in United States. Figures on milk production in the United States are given in Table 2. The income from milk accounts for about 10% of the total farm income in the United States, indicating that it is one of the most important agricultural industries. The five leading dairy states in the United States and their annual milk production are Wisconsin, 18,362,000,000 lb; California, 10,601,000,000 lb; New York, 9,822,000,000 lb; Minnesota, 9,382,000,000 lb; and Pennsylvania, 6,971,000,000 lb. The major milk-producing areas are the Midwest and Northeast.

Some marked changes which have taken place in the dairy industry since 1940 are shown in Table 2. Even though there has been a marked decrease in the number of milk cows, the annual milk production has increased because of the marked increase in production per cow. A marked decrease in the number of dairy farms producing milk has been accompanied by an increase in the number of cows per farm and in the number of cows handled by each dairyman. Smaller ineffi-

Table 1. Leading milk-producing countries in the world in 1974

Country	Annual milk production, 10^9 lb
Soviet Union	200.2
United States	115.4
France	67.8
West Germany	47.7
Poland	32.9
United Kingdom	30.4
Netherlands	21.9
Italy	19.8
East Germany	17.2
Canada	17.0

Table 2. Changes in milk production and consumption in United States

Year	Milk cows, 10⁶	Total milk production, 10⁹ lb	Annual production per cow, lb	Per capita consumption, lb
1940	23.6	109.4	4622	819
1950	22.0	116.6	5314	740
1955	21.0	122.9	5842	706
1960	17.5	123.1	7029	653
1965	15.0	124.2	8304	618
1970	12.0	117.0	9747	561
1974	11.2	115.4	10,286	543

cient producers are being forced out of the dairy industry, and only the larger, more specialized farms are remaining.

Milk is used for many products. Approximately 43% goes into fluid milk and cream. In 1974, 16.7% of the milk was used for butter and 22.3% was used for cheese. The other 18% was used for other products, with frozen dairy products being the most important. *See* BUTTER; CHEESE; ICE CREAM; MILK.

Dairy breeds. Most of the milk produced in the United States is by five major dairy breeds: Ayrshire, Brown Swiss, Guernsey, Holstein-Friesian, and Jersey. Approximately 10% of the dairy cattle are registered purebreds. The first breed registry association was organized by the Jersey dairymen in 1868, and all breeds had registry associations by 1880. The purposes of these organizations are to preserve the purity of the breed through registration; to keep official records of the breed; to improve the breed through production testing programs, type classification, and dairy cattle shows; and to promote the breed.

The introduction of the dairy herd improvement associations (DHIA) in 1905 to measure the production of cows greatly aided the improvement of breeds, especially nonpurebred animals. These testing programs produced the needed data for the selection of replacement animals and for culling low-producing animals. The principal features of each of the five dairy breeds are listed in the following paragraphs.

Holstein-Friesian. This is the largest breed in number and in body size. A mature dairy cow weighs about 1500 lb and the bull 2200 lb. The breed was developed in the North Holland and West Friesland provinces of the Netherlands. Holsteins were first imported to the United States in 1621 and 1625 by the Dutch settlers; however, there are no descendants of these animals in the country. In the mid-1850s cattle were imported into Massachusetts from which descendants are now present. Importations in large numbers were made up to 1905.

The Holstein is a distinct black and white, is noted for its rugged conformation, and has a decided advantage in the production of beef and veal, as well as milk. The breed produces the largest volume of milk with the smallest milk fat percentage, averaging about 3.5%. Since the late 1940s the percentage of Holstein cattle in the United States has increased, because the milk-pricing systems have favored breeds that produce large volumes of milk with relatively low butterfat. One of the outstanding cows in the breed (see illustration) was classified Excellent with 97 points, has four re-

cords of over 23,000 lb of milk on twice-a-day milking, and has a lifetime production of over 138,000 lb of milk.

Jersey. The Jersey is the smallest of the dairy breeds. The mature cow weighs about 1000 lb and mature bull 1500 lb. The Jerseys were developed on the Island of Jersey, one of the Channel Islands between France and England. The breed was first imported into the United States in 1850, with large importations occurring between 1870 and 1890. The percentage of Jerseys has been decreasing primarily due to the milk-pricing systems and a decreased consumption of butter. The Jersey ranges from a light fawn to black; some animals have white markings. The breed has the highest milk-fat content, averaging 5.3%, and a high solids-not-fat content. The milk is notably yellow, which is due to a high carotene content.

Guernsey. The Guernsey breed is slightly larger than the Jersey and has many of the latter's common characteristics. The mature female weighs 1100 lb and mature bull 1700 lb. The Guernsey varies from an almost red to a very light fawn, with various sizes of light markings. The breed was developed on the Island of Guernsey, another Channel Island. They were first imported into the United States in 1830; while some importations still occur, they have decreased in numbers. The Guernseys average 4.9% milk fat and have a high solids-not-fat content. The milk also is a deep yellow due to the high carotene content.

Ayrshire. The Ayrshire breed was developed in the County of Ayr in Scotland around 1750. The mature cow weighs approximately 1200 lb and the bull 1850 lb. The Ayrshire is red and white and noted for its general beauty, straightness of top line, symmetry of udder, ruggedness, and excellent grazing ability. The Ayrshires were first imported from Scotland to Massachusetts in 1837, with frequent importations made until 1860.

The average milk-fat content of the Ayrshire is 4.0%. The breed is known for its longevity and lifetime production rather than for its high lactation records.

Brown Swiss. The Brown Swiss is one of the larger breeds with the mature cow weighing about 1400 lb and the mature bull 2000 lb. The Brown

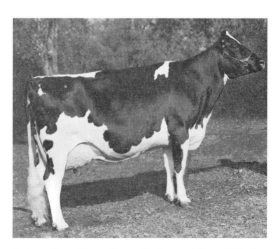

A champion milk producer, Harborcrest Rose Milly, the all-time, all-American Holstein-Friesian aged cow. (*Owned by Paclamar Farms, Louisville, Colo.*)

Swiss varies from a light fawn to almost black, with a mouse color predominating. Brown Swiss have a quiet temperament but a tendency to be stubborn. It is the slowest-maturing breed and is noted for its longevity. Because of size and ruggedness, they are well adapted for beef and veal purposes.

Brown Swiss is one of the oldest breeds. It was developed in the mountain territory of northeastern Switzerland, where in the winter the cows are housed in valleys and barns and in the spring are pastured on mountain slopes. This developed the ruggedness and excellent grazing ability. The cattle (less than 200) were first imported into the United States in 1869. The milk averages 4% milk fat and is well adapted to market milk, condensed milk, and cheese.

Dairy cattle feeding. Research on dairy cattle feeding has provided information on feeding animals according to their requirements to the dairyman, who is interested in meeting nutritional needs at a minimum cost. The nutrient requirements of the dairy cow depend upon a daily maintenance need, milk production and milk-fat test, pregnancy, and growth. The two most important requirements to be met are energy and protein. Various energy standards are used, but the commonest ones in the United States are the total digestible nutrient (TDN) and net energy (NE) standards. The dairyman must also be concerned about the mineral requirements of the cow, particularly calcium, phosphorus, sodium, chloride, and iodine. The other minerals and vitamins are found in sufficient quantities in the feeds.

The main components of the dairy ration are hay, silage, pasture, and grain. Grain is the most expensive portion of the ration and is fed according to the milk production of the cow. Hay and silage are usually fed to the cows free-choice, and a cow consumes daily about 2 lb of hay or 6 lb of silage per 100 lb of body weight. This provides enough energy and protein to meet the maintenance requirements of the cow plus 10–20 lb of milk each day. The rest of the energy and protein must come from grain. Grass and corn are used as silage. *See* ANIMAL-FEED COMPOSITION.

Dairy cattle breeding. The breeding program involves two major aspects. One is the selection and breeding of cows to be used in the dairy herd. The second is reproduction and maintenance of a regular calving interval for maximum milk production. Many commercial dairymen place most emphasis on production in the breeding program and select for type only if the conformation of the animal presents management problems, such as a poorly attached udder. Some purebred dairy cattle breeders who sell replacement stock emphasize the overall type of animal.

To make progress in a breeding program, the dairyman must use records. DHIA records are most commonly used for the selection of milk production. Selection for type is based on official classification scores conducted by the breed associations or the dairyman's own appraisal. Most selection in the breeding program is done at two times. One occurs in the selection of the bull or bulls to be used to breed cows for development of future herd replacements; the second is selecting animals to be culled and replaced by new animals.

Approximately 25% of the cows leave the herd each year, because of disease, reproductive difficulties and low production. With the advent of artificial insemination (AI) and the use of sire proving programs by AI associations, desirable proven bulls are available to almost every dairyman. Approximately 49% of dairy cows in the United States are bred by artificial insemination. *See* BREEDING (ANIMAL).

Maintaining a good breeding program requires that cows calve at regular intervals. Most dairymen try to have a 13- to 14-month calving interval. The ideal is 1 year; however, this is usually not possible. Cows calving at 13- to 14-month intervals produce more milk during their lifetimes than cows calving at wider intervals.

Dairy cattle management. Almost all cows in the United States are milked by machine. Since the late 1950s there has been a marked increase in the number of cows milked in a milking parlor. The recommended milking procedure involves a series of steps based upon the physiology of the cow, as well as the production of clean milk and disease control. The usual recommended steps in a milking operation are: Wash the cow's udder with a disinfectant solution and a paper towel, use a strip cup to detect abnormal milk, apply the milking machine 1–2 min after the cow's udder has been washed, machine-strip by applying pressure on the teat cup claw and massaging the udder when the cow is nearly milked out, remove the machine as soon as milk flow stops, and dip the teat ends in a disinfectant solution. Good milking procedures are required to maintain a low incidence of mastitis, which is the most costly dairy cattle disease. *See* AGRICULTURAL SCIENCE (ANIMAL); DAIRY MACHINERY.

[G. H. SCHMIDT]

Bibliography: J. R. Campbell and R. T. Marshall, *The Science of Providing Milk for Man*, 1975; H. H. Cole, *Livestock Production*, 2d ed., 1966; R. C. Foley et al., *Dairy Cattle: Principles, Practices, Problems, Profits*, 1972; G. H. Schmidt and L. D. Van Vleck, *Principles of Dairy Science*, 1974.

Cauliflower

A cool-season biennial crucifer (*Brassica oleracea* var. *botrytis*) of Mediterranean origin. Cauliflower belongs to the plant order Capparales. It is grown for its white head or curd, a tight mass of flower stalks, which terminates the main stem (see illustration). Cauliflower is commonly cooked fresh as a vegetable; to a lesser extent, it is frozen or pickled and consumed as a relish. Cultural practices are similar to those used for cabbage; however, cauliflower is more sensitive to unfavorable environment. Strains of the variety (cultivar) Snowball are most popular; purple-headed varieties are less common. Cauliflower is slightly tolerant of acid soils and has high requirements for boron and molybdenum. A cool, moist climate favors high quality. Harvest is generally 3–4 months after planting. California and New York are important cauliflower-producing states. Annual farm value in the United States from approximately 26,000 acres is $20,000,000; annual production is usually over 120,000 tons. *See* CABBAGE; VEGETABLE GROWING.

[H. JOHN CAREW]

CAULIFLOWER

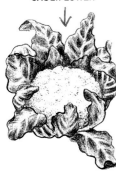
Cauliflower (*Brassica oleracea* var. *botrytis*).

Celery

A biennial umbellifer (*Apium graveolens* var. *dulce*) of Mediterranean origin and belonging to the plant order Umbellales. Celery is grown for its

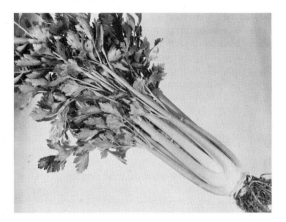

Celery (*Apium graveolens* var. *dulce*, cultivar Greenlight). (*Joseph Harris Co., Inc., Rochester, N.Y.*)

petioles or leafstalks, which are most commonly eaten as a salad but occasionally cooked as a vegetable (see illustration). Celeriac or knob celery (*A. graveolens* var. *rapaceum*) is grown for its enlarged rootlike stem and is commonly eaten as a cooked vegetable in Europe.

Propagation of celery is by seed planted in the field or sown in greenhouses or outdoor beds for the production of transplants. Field spacing varies; plants are generally grown 6–10 in. apart in 18–36-in. rows. Celery requires a long growing season, cool weather, and unusually abundant soil moisture. It has a high requirement for boron, a deficiency of which results in "cracked stem." Exposure to prolonged cold weather (40–50°F for 10–30 days) favors "bolting" or seed-stalk formation.

Varieties (cultivars) are classified primarily according to their color, green or yellow (self-blanching). The most popular green variety is Utah, of which a large number of strains are grown, such as Summer Pascal and Utah 52–70H. The acreage of yellow celery has been declining. Pink and red varieties are grown in England.

Harvesting begins generally when the plants are fully grown but before the petioles become pithy, usually 3–4 months after field planting. In periods of high prices, earlier harvesting is often practiced.

California, Florida, and Michigan are important producing states. The total farm value in the United States from approximately 31,000 acres is approximately $63,000,000. *See* VEGETABLE GROWING.

[H. JOHN CAREW]

Cereal

Any member of the grass family (Gramineae) which produces edible grains usable as food by humans and livestock. Common cereals are rice, wheat, barley, oats, maize (corn), sorghum, rye, and certain millets. Triticale is a new man-made cereal derived from crossing wheat and rye and then doubling the number of chromosomes in the hybrid. Occasionally, grains from other grasses (for example, teff) are used for food. Cereals are summer or winter annuals. Corn, rice, and wheat are the most important cereals. Today, as in ancient times, cereals provide more food for human consumption than any other crops.

Cereal grains have many natural advantages as foods. They are nutritious. One kind or another can be grown almost anywhere on Earth. The grains are not bulky and therefore can be shipped inexpensively for long distances and stored for long periods of time. They are readily processed to give highly refined raw foods.

Preference for a cereal depends on the form and flavor of the food made from it, the amount of nourishment and contribution to health, its cost, its availability, and the food habits of a people.

Food products. Four general groups of foods are prepared from the cereal grains. (1) Baked products, made from flour or meal, include pan breads, loaf breads, pastries, pancakes, flatbreads, cookies, and cakes. (2) Milled grain products, made by removing the bran and usually the germ (or embryo of the seed), include polished rice, farina, wheat flour, cornmeal, hominy, corn grits, pearled barley, bulgor (from wheat), semolina (for macaroni products), prepared breakfast cereals, and soup, gravy, and other thickenings. (3) Beverages are made from fermented grain products (distilled or undistilled) and from boiled, roasted grains. Beverages, such as beer and whiskey, made from cereals are as old as recorded history. (4) Whole-grain products include rolled oats, brown rice, popcorn, shredded and puffed grains, breakfast foods, and home-ground meals made from wheat, corn, sorghum, or one of the other cereals.

Breeding. The long evolutionary development of the cereals has resulted in a wide array of genetic types. These and new mutants have been used to breed varieties that differ in adaptation, productivity, resistance to disease and insect pests, physical properties, composition, and nutrients.

Nutritional value. All cereal grains have high energy value, mainly from the starch fraction but also from the fat and protein. In general, the cereals are low in protein content, although oats and certain millets are exceptions. High-protein genetic types have been found, and, from their use in breeding, new varieties have been developed that possess a higher percentage of protein. Likewise, a better balance has been found among the amino acids in the protein in some lines of corn, barley, and sorghum, and research with wheat is promising. Also, the nature of the starchy fraction can be altered to give products with different physical properties. *See* GRAIN CROPS; GRASS CROPS.

[LOUIS P. REITZ]

Cereal chemistry

The applied branch of biochemistry concerned with the analysis, characterization, processing, and uses of cereals and their constituents. In practice, cereal chemistry is related most often to the processing, uses, and quality control of grains, such as wheat. Cereals may be divided broadly into food grains, such as wheat and rice, and feed grains, such as corn (maize), grain sorghum, oats, barley, rye, and millet, although all cereals can serve either as human food or as animal feeds. Until late in the 19th century, the processing of cereals was essentially the same as that used in Biblical times, namely, grinding between stones. With the introduction of modern roller mills, the physical and chemical properties of the cereal grains became important, and fractions of the cereal grains became available for special uses. Chemists determined the composition of the fractions, to establish specifications for those most useful and to devise processes leading to better food, feed, or industrial use. *See* BARLEY; CORN; MILLET; OATS; RICE; RYE; SORGHUM; WHEAT.

Since starch is the largest component of all cereals, much attention has been given to the chemistry of starch in the major crops wheat and corn. Protein, the next largest component of cereals, is especially important in wheat because wheat gluten is unique in producing bread of good texture. Oil is present in relatively small amounts in cereals, and only corn oil is produced in important amounts. Wheat germ oil is sold for pharmaceutical purposes in relatively small amounts. *See* FAT AND OIL, EDIBLE; PROTEIN; STARCH.

Milling. Dry milling is applied to most cereals to refine or to separate them into fractions or constituents, such as starch, germ, and bran. Only with corn has an extensive wet-milling industry developed. Kernel moisture relationships are important for certain types of dry-milling operations, and controlled use is made of roll pressure, sieve size, and air velocity in classifying particles. Fine grinding with impact mills and use of high-velocity airstreams can separate particles that differ only slightly in density, but differ in protein content. Flours of unusually high protein content can be manufactured. Cereal particles can be agglomerated to reduce dustiness, change bulk density, and improve flowability. In wet milling, corn is steeped in dilute sulfurous acid solution to loosen the hull and soften the gluten. Subsequent operations result in more complete fractionation into starch, gluten, fiber, and oil than is possible with dry milling. For example, 1½ lb of oil may be recovered in the wet milling of corn, whereas only ½ lb of oil would result from dry milling the same sample. *See* FOOD MANUFACTURING.

Chemistry. Much of the knowledge of the chemistry of wheat has come from several state agricultural experiment stations and universities, cereal industry–sponsored research laboratories, and the four wheat-quality laboratories of the U.S. Department of Agriculture at Manhattan, Kans., Pullman, Wash., Wooster, Ohio, and Fargo, N.Dak. Outside the United States, important contributors have been the Grain Research Laboratory, Winnipeg, Canada; the Flour Milling and Bakery Research Association, Chorleywood, England; the Institute for Cereals Flour and Bread, Wageningen, Netherlands; and the Federal Research Institute of Cereal Industry, Detmold, Germany. Utilization of cereals for food and industrial purposes is studied at the Northern and Western Regional Laboratories of the U.S. Department of Agriculture in Peoria, Ill., and Albany, Calif., and by university and private research laboratories. The American Association

of Cereal Chemists, founded in 1914, publishes two journals, *Cereal Science Today* and *Cereal Chemistry*; a book of analytical methods now in its seventh edition; and a monograph series, the most recent being *Wheat Chemistry and Technology* (1964). The International Association for Cereal Chemistry was founded in 1955 with headquarters in Vienna, Austria.

Although the largest uses of cereals are for food and feeds, industrial uses, particularly of corn products, are important. However, cereals have been almost completely displaced by petrochemicals in many former industrial uses. Organic solvents (ethanol, butanol, and acetone) were formerly largely derived by fermentation of grains. Beverage alcohol must still be made from agricultural products, but for industrial use vast quantities of solvents are synthesized from oil, gas, or coal sources. *See* INDUSTRIAL MICROBIOLOGY.

Starch as such or slightly modified by oxidation has found chief industrial use in sizing of paper and sizing and finishing of textiles. Degradation of starch with heat, acid, or both produces dextrins, whose chief uses are as adhesives either alone or in combination with other materials. Because starch contains very large molecules varying widely in molecular size and configuration, widely varying properties are found in starches produced under different conditions and from different sources. Although cornstarch is the cheapest and most abundant, wheat starch is said to have especially desirable properties as a laundry starch and warp size in textile manufacture. Many specialty starches are marketed to meet definite specifications and are designed for specific uses, ranging from ingredients of oil well–drilling muds to dusts for surgical gloves.

The starch granule of ordinary corn contains two types of molecules, a straight-chain glucose polymer called amylose (27%) and a branched, higher-molecular-weight polymer called amylopectin (73%). Waxy corn has nearly 100% amylopectin and is grown and processed for food starch uses. Geneticists, with the help of cereal chemists, have succeeded in breeding corn whose starch contains as much as 80% amylose. If starches containing even higher amylose content can be produced, they can be used to make superior self-supporting films for packaging and paper coatings with wide application. *See* CARBOHYDRATE.

[JOHN A. SHELLENBERGER]

Bibliography: D. W. Kent-Jones and A. J. Amos, *Modern Cereal Chemistry*, 1967; S. A. Matz, *Cereal Science*, 1969; S. A. Matz, *Cereal Technology*, 1970; D. F. Miller, *Composition of Cereal Grains and Forages*, Nat. Res. Counc.–Nat. Acad. Sci. Publ. no. 585, 1958.

Cheese

There are many varieties of cheese, all produced in the following general manner. Raw or pasteurized milk is clotted by acid, rennet, or both. The curd is cut and shaped into the special form of the cheese with or without pressing. Salt is added, or the cheese is brined after pressing.

Acid is produced during manufacture of cheese by fermentation of the milk sugar, lactose. This fermentation is initiated by the addition of a culture of specially selected acid bacteria (starter culture) to the milk. Acid production in cheese curd retards growth of bacteria that cause undesirable fermentations in cheese. Moreover, it favors the expulsion of the whey and the fusion of the curd particles. Fresh cheese (cottage or cream cheese) does not require any ripening, and it is sold soon after it is made. Other varieties of cheese are cured or ripened to obtain the desirable consistency, flavor, and aroma. The flavor and aroma of cheese are obtained by a partial breakdown of milk proteins and fat by the action of microbial, milk, and rennet enzymes. In hard varieties (Chedder, Gouda, Edam, Emmentaler or Swiss, and Provolone) this is done by the microorganisms in the interior of cheese; in semisoft or soft types (Limburger, Camembert, and Roquefort) by the organisms on, or in contact with, the surface of cheese. *See* MILK.

CHEESE MICROBIOLOGY

Microorganisms are essential to the manufacture of cheese, imparting distinctive flavor, aroma, consistency, and appearance.

Starter cultures. Lactic acid starter cultures are important in making cheese. Different types of lactic acid bacteria (*Streptococcus lactis*, shown in Fig. 1, *S. cremoris*, *S. thermophilus*, and homofermentative lactobacilli) are used, depending upon the kind of cheese desired. The starter (both single and mixed strains of bacteria are used) must convert all milk sugar left in the curd into lactic acid within a reasonable time. Several factors may prevent this: the occurrence of natural inhibitors in milk, antibiotics, and bacteriophages.

Some antibiotics (such as nisin) which affect the activity of the starter may be produced by microbes in the milk. Others may be excreted into the milk by cows treated for a particular disease; this happens if penicillin is used to treat mastitis.

Bacteriophages, or phages, are viruses which lyse sensitive bacterial cells and produce new phage particles. Phage particles may get into the milk with infected starter cultures or through contamination with phage-carrying dust particles. Phage particles slow down or totally inhibit the activity of the starter culture, causing insufficient souring and spoilage of cheese. Phage multiplication is influenced by temperature, pH, and calcium content of the medium. Phage outbreaks cause serious economic losses. They can be controlled by rigorous hygienic handling of starters, by culture rotation, or by culturing starters in calcium-free media. Attempts to isolate phage-resistant strains have not met with success.

Flora of cheese. Cheeses of the hard type contain lactic acid streptococci and other bacteria present in the starter. Moreover, they contain all the microorganisms originally present in the raw milk or pasteurized milk. The types of bacteria most important for curing are the streptococci, lactobacilli, micrococci, and propionic acid bacteria. They, together with the enzymes of rennet and milk, break down the proteins to peptides and amino acids, hydrolyze the milk fat to fatty acids, and frequently produce carbon dioxide gas which causes the holes in cheese (Fig. 2). The structure of cheese is greatly changed during ripening.

In semisoft and soft cheeses the lactic acid originally produced by the starter is broken down afterward by molds, yeasts, and bacteria on the sur-

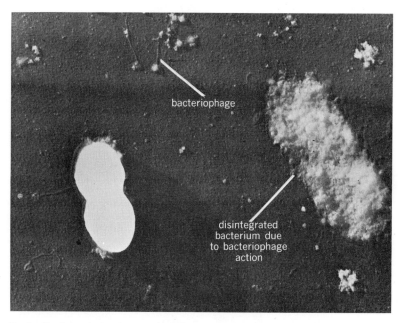

Fig. 1. Electron photomicrograph of *Streptococcus lactis* attacked by phages.

face. The same flora decomposes the protein and the fat to a much greater extent than in hard cheeses. As a result, strong flavors are produced and the structure of the cheese becomes much softer. For the production of blue-veined cheese, needles are pushed into the interior to bring *Penicillium roqueforti* or the other molds, added during the manufacturing of the cheese, into contact with air they need for growth. The blue color is the color of the mold spores. The red color on the surface of some soft cheeses is caused by *Brevibacterium* (*Bacterium*) *linens* and micrococci. For good surface growth, soft cheeses must be cured in high-humidity air (caves or air-conditioned rooms).

Defects of cheese. In hard cheeses an abnormal gas formation is a problem. It can occur at almost any stage of manufacture or ripening. Early

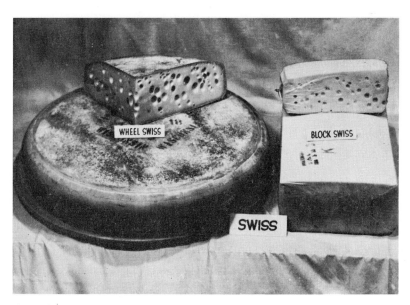

Fig. 2. Swiss cheese with normal eye formation.

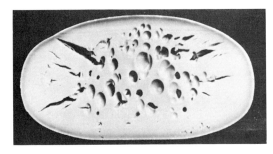

Fig. 3. Late blowing in Gouda cheese.

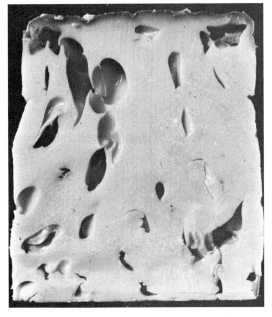

Fig. 4. Evidence of late gas production during the cheese ripening process.

gas production can be caused by coliform bacteria or heterofermentative lactic bacteria. Gas production during cheese ripening (late gas, as in Figs. 3 and 4) may be caused by certain spore-forming bacteria, propionic acid bacteria, *Leuconostoc* species, and *S. diacetilactis*. The use of *S. diacetilactis* and *S. lactis* as lactic starter cultures can cause fruity flavors, as well as gas formation, in Cheddar cheese. Other defects of hard cheese include insufficient or excessive acidity, various off flavors, and discoloration. Soft cheeses may be spoiled by gas production, excessive acidity, improper development of surface flora, and contamination with atypical molds.

Process cheese. Cheeses of different ages are blended. The mixture, melted with the aid of emulsifying salts (citrates and phosphates), is packed in sealed containers (tins, paperboard, foil, or plastic). Few bacteria other than spore-formers survive the heat treatment. No substantial growth of the flora takes place in well-preserved process cheese, but spoilage by anaerobic spore-formers may occur. *Clostridium sporogenes* causes putrefaction and slit openness and *C. tyrobutyricum* causes blowing of tins and packages. Acidity, salt content, and temperature of storage are important in controlling spoilage.

[NORMAN OLSON]

CHEESE MANUFACTURE

Because of different environmental conditions, various methods of making cheese have developed. There are about 18 distinct varieties of cheese and over 400 different names. The commonly recognized varieties are brick, caciocavallo, Camembert, Cheddar, cottage, cream, Edam, Emmentaler, Gouda, Gruyere, Limburger, Neufchâtel, Parmesan, Provolone, Romano, Roquefort, sapsago, and Trappist.

Ripened cheese. In commercial manufacture in the United States, a culture of the desired bacteria is added to clarified pasteurized milk. Usually rennet extract is introduced to facilitate whey separation. It also functions during the ripening of the cheese. Curd shrinkage and its separation from the whey are due to the developed lactic acid, the action of the rennin enzyme, and use of heat. For low-moisture cheese, the curd is cut into small cubes and acid is developed early in the process; the curd is heated to a fairly high temperature and is subjected to a relatively high pressure during processing. The opposite of these conditions will produce high-moisture cheese.

All varieties of cheese are salted. Salt may be added by applying directly to the curd or by floating the fresh cheese in a brine solution, depending on the variety being made.

Ripening, a critical part of cheese making, results in breaking down the rubbery texture of the fresh curd to a softer, smoother, and less plastic body. During ripening, the desired flavor characteristics of a particular variety are developed. Composition of the curd and conditions under which it is held determine the nature and extent of the enzymic action responsible for body and flavor changes.

The chemical changes taking place during cheese ripening have to do in part with a breakdown of the lactose to lactic acid, volatile acids, and alcohol. From lactic acid are formed acetic acid, propionic acid, and carbon dioxide. The protein in the cheese is hydrolyzed to form proteoses, peptones, peptides, and amino acids. The amino acids may be broken down to amines and carbon dioxide. The extent of protein breakdown determines the character and nature of the cheese. In fully ripened Limburger it is nearly complete, but in Cheddar only about one-third of the protein is changed.

Hydrolysis of cheese fats may yield volatile butyric, caproic, caprylic, and capric acids. In making Roquefort cheese, the molds introduced into the curd produce lipase, which hydrolyzes the fat. The fatty acids are further oxidized by the molds, in part to methyl ketones, substances responsible for the flavor and aroma of this cheese.

For ripening most hard cheeses, the desired environment favors activity of the microorganisms and enzymes within the cheese itself and discourages surface growth. For soft cheese varieties, such as Limburger, the growth of organisms at the surface is encouraged. Semisoft cheeses, such as Roquefort and brick, are ripened by a combination of the two methods. Hard cheeses, such as Cheddar, that do not require surface ripening are usually protected against surface evaporation and contamination by a coating of paraffin or plastic.

Unripened cheese. Cheeses such as cottage and cream are made by curdling the milk with acid developed by the growth of starter and by adding rennet. The curd is separated from the whey by cooking and then is drained and salted.

For cottage cheese an attempt is made to retain the curd in the form of small uniformly sized aggregates. In cream cheese the curd is processed so that the particles lose their identity and produce a smooth firm body. Pimentos or fruit, such as pineapple, may be added.

These cheese-making processes are completed within 24 hr. Creamed cottage cheese usually contains 4% fat. Cream cheese contains a minimum of 33% fat and a maximum of 55% moisture. A small amount of gum is sometimes added to cream cheese to improve the body. These cheeses contain about 1% salt.

Cream cheese. The cold-pack method of manufacturing cream cheese follows.

1. Milk is standardized with cream to a fat content of about 11%, pasteurized by heating to 65.5°C for 30 min, cooled to 48.9°C, and homogenized at 1500 lb pressure. About 2% of a good starter is added to 1000 lb of milk.

2. When the pH is 4.4–4.5, the curd is stirred and heated to 52–55°C in 45–60 min.

3. Heated curd is poured into muslin bags and stacked in stainless steel vats for drainage.

4. After sufficient drainage the curd is dumped into a mixer and 1% salt is added.

Cheddar cheese. Cheddar cheese was originally made from raw milk. The more modern procedure involves the use of pasteurized milk.

1. The milk is set at 30°C with 0.5–1.0% starter. A small amount of cheese color is added.

2. Usually after about 45 min the acidity test shows an increase of 0.01%, and 2.5–4.0 oz of rennet per 1000 lb milk is added to firm the curd in 25–30 min.

3. When properly firmed, the curd is cut into 0.25-in. cubes and heated slowly to 37.8–38.9°C. The combined effect of heat, acid, and rennin determines the rate at which the whey separates from the curd. Slow stirring is continued for 30 min after the maximum temperature is reached to prevent the curd from matting. When the curd is properly firmed, the whey is removed.

4. As the whey drains away, the curd begins to mat. The two long slabs of curd, one on each side of the vat, are cut into blocks and occasionally turned to facilitate draining. When the whey has reached an acidity of 0.45–0.55%, the curd is ready to be milled.

5. The matted curd is cut with a curd mill into pieces about 2 in. long and 1/2 in. square. After milling, 1.5% salt is added.

6. The salted curd is placed in metal hoops and put in a cheese press under pressure to cement the small particles together.

7. After removal from the hoops, the cheese is placed in a cool, dry room for 3 or 4 days to form a surface rind. It is then dipped into melted paraffin and placed in the curing room.

Most Cheddar is made with a plastic film coating instead of a rind. Cheese treated in this manner is made into rectangular blocks and prepared in small packages for consumer use.

The cheese may be cured at 0–4.4°C for 3–4 months and then placed at a lower temperature for further curing. Ordinarily a minimum of 6 months is required to develop the flavor and body characteristic of good Cheddar cheese.

In the United States the Federal standard for Cheddar cheese is a minimum fat content of 50% of solids and a maximum moisture content of 39%.

Swiss cheese (wheel). The Federal standards for Swiss cheese specify a minimum of 43% milk fat in the dry matter and a maximum of 41% moisture. To obtain the desired fat to total milk solids ratio, it is usually necessary to standardize the fat by removing a portion of cream from the whole milk to be used.

1. Special copper kettles holding 2500 lb of milk are used for setting the milk. A small amount of starter is added to each kettle as follows: 0.5–2 lb of *Lactobacillus bulgaricus*; 0.5–2 lb of *Streptococcus thermophilus*; and 0.5–2 oz of *Propionibacterium shermanii*.

2. The milk is warmed to 31.1–34.4°C, and 1.5–3.0 oz of rennet, diluted 40 times with cold water, per 1000 lb of milk is added. The curd should be firm enough to cut in about 20 min. Movement of the milk in the kettle is stopped as soon as the rennet is mixed with the milk.

3. The curd is cut with a special device called a Swiss-cheese harp. Within 5 min after the curd is cut, it is "harped" by moving the harp to and fro with an elliptical motion. This is continued until the particles are slightly larger than a grain of wheat. This is usually completed in 15 min from the time of cutting.

The curd is then "foreworked" by operating the mechanical stirrer for 30 min or less. This causes the curd particles to shrink as the whey is expelled and to become firmer.

4. After foreworking, the curd is slowly cooked in the kettle to 48.9–53°C. Usually 30 min is required for this step. The curd is stirred constantly during cooking and for about 1 hr after the steam is turned off in the kettle. This is termed "stirring out." When the curd is sufficiently firm and crumbly, it is ready to be dipped.

5. For dipping the curd, a large coarsely woven cloth supported at the edge with a flexible steel strip is used. The cloth is passed under the entire mass of curd without breaking the curd or turning it over.

The metal strip is then removed, and the edges of the cloth are brought together and tied. The bag of curd is hoisted free of the kettle and the whey is permitted to drain into the kettle.

6. The drained bag of curd is lowered into a circular stainless steel hoop on a drain table. The curd is forced gently into the hoop, and the edges of the cloth are folded over the top. Pressure is applied from above by a screw press. In about 5 min the curd is ready to be dressed.

7. At definite intervals the cheese is redressed and turned. This requires about 9 hr. Then the cheese is left in the press overnight without dressing except for a layer of burlap on top and bottom.

The temperature in the manufacturing room is kept at 21.1–23.9°C to prevent the interior of the cheese, which at time of dipping is 48.9–50°C, from cooling too rapidly.

8. After remaining in the press overnight, the cheese is removed from the hoop and placed in a

brine tank in a 12.8°C room in which the relative humidity is 80–85%. The brine is a 23% solution of sodium chloride in water. After 2–3 days the cheese is placed on a shelf in the cold room for 7–10 days.

9. To cure the cheese, the wheels, each weighing about 175 lb, are placed in a warm room (20–23.3°C, 80–85% relative humidity). Two or three times a week, the cheese is turned over and salt is rubbed into the surface. As ripening progresses, the eye formation typical of Swiss cheese begins. The rate of eye formation, indicated by the amount of bulging, can be regulated to some extent by the shelf location in the curing room and the amount of salt worked into the surface of the cheese. If the curing proceeds too rapidly, the wheel is kept on the cooler lower shelf and more salt is applied. To the discriminating cheese buyer the size and distribution of the eyes are very important.

After 4–6 weeks the cheese will have risen sufficiently and the wheel is returned to the cold room, graded, and sold. At least 6 months is necessary to develop the desired Swiss flavor. During this time a thick rind forms on the surface.

Several modifications of the traditional procedure have been developed. These involve such changes as setting the cheese in rectangular vats and processing the curd into small square blocks and curing it without rind.

Limburger cheese. Limburger is usually made from pasteurized milk. A small amount of lactic starter, 0.7–1.0% of the volume of milk, and rennet sufficient to set the curd in 40 min are added. The setting temperature is 30–32°C. The curd is cut into $\frac{1}{4}$-in. cubes, heated, stirred for a short time, and placed in perforated rectangular metal hoops for pressing and draining. When sufficiently firmed, the curd is cut into 1- to 2-lb blocks.

Salt is rubbed into the surface of the curd, and the blocks are stored at 15.6–20°C, 90–95% humidity. They are rubbed daily with dry salt to close openings on the surface and to distribute evenly the ripening microorganisms, which are added to the surface. A reddish slime soon develops on the surface. After about 2 weeks, the blocks of curd are wrapped in parchment and foil and stored at 10°C, and the ripening is continued. The cheese is ready for market in 6–8 weeks.

The Federal standard in the United States requires a minimum of 50% fat in the solids and a maximum moisture content of 50%. The finished cheese will contain 1.8–2.2% salt.

Blue cheese. The original of the blue-cheese group is probably Roquefort, which is made from sheep's milk in southern France. The use of the term Roquefort is copyrighted by French manufacturers. A similar type of cheese is made from cow's milk and called by different names, such as blue, bleu, Stilton (English), and Gorgonzola (Italian). The English and the Italians sometimes use goat's milk in making blue cheese.

The composition of these cheeses varies, but in general they contain 30–32% fat, 41–43% water, and 4–5% salt. In the United States the Federal standard is a minimum fat content of 50% of the solids and a maximum moisture content of 46%.

Manufacturers of the various types of blue cheese have different methods of processing. In the United States pasteurized homogenized milk is ordinarily used. From 2 to 3% lactic culture and from 3 to 4 oz rennet per 1000 lb milk are added. The setting temperature is 30°C. When the curd reaches the proper firmness in 1–2 hr, it is cut, separated from the whey, salted (1.0–1.5%), and put into metal hoops $8\frac{1}{2}$ in. in diameter and $3\frac{1}{2}$ in. high. The time of adding the spores of *Penicillium roqueforti* varies. Some cheese makers mix them with the curd when filling the hoops, and a few add the mold to the milk before curdling.

The spores are prepared by growing the mold on cubes of sterile whole wheat bread. After the mold growth is sufficiently developed, the bread cubes are dried and powdered. The amount needed for inoculation is 2–4 g/1000 lb of milk.

The hoops are placed on a draining rack without pressure and are turned occasionally to facilitate drainage of the whey and matting of the curd. The drainage takes place at room temperature. The next day the cheese is removed from the hoops and salted in a 8.9°C room with a relative humidity of 80–90%. The salting is done either by dipping in brine or by the application of dry salt and is continued for about 1 week or 10 days.

After drying for 2–3 days, the cheese may be paraffin-coated and then punctured with long needles to admit the air needed for mold growth and to permit carbon dioxide to escape. Cheese not coated with paraffin develops a slimy surface growth which must be removed occasionally. This results in a loss of about 7–8% of the cheese. The cheeses are stored on their sides at a temperature of 8.9–12.2°C and 95–98% humidity.

After about 3 months, the cheeses are cleaned, wrapped in foil, and stored for an additional 1–2 months, or until the desired flavor and body are obtained. The proteinase formed by *P. roqueforti* is active at pH 5.3–7.0 with its optimum activity at about pH 6.0.

Process cheese. Process cheese is a term applied to those cheese products that have been blended, heated, and packed into sealed containers. The term unqualified by any variety name is understood to mean process Cheddar cheese.

A wide variety of materials can be used in making the cheese. Usually, aged and unaged cheeses of the same or different varieties are blended to obtain a mild but distinct flavor. The cheese is trimmed, comminuted, and then heated. The mixture is heated to at least 72–74°C for 10 min and run into glass tumblers, plastic containers, or foil-lined cartons which are sealed to exclude air.

Sodium citrate and disodium phosphate are added to dissolve the protein and emulsify the fats. High-test sweet cream, nonfat dry milk solids, and water may be added to produce a cheese with a desired total solid to fat ratio.

Packaging processed cheese while it is hot increases its keeping time. Blending cheeses of different ages results in a more uniform product. Mixing different cheese varieties provides an almost limitless number of blends. Additional substances, such as fruits and spices, may be added at the time of mixing, and pathogenic microorganisms may be destroyed during the heating process.

The following standards in the United States have been established for pasteurized process cheese products: (1) In pasteurized process cheese made of cheese, cream, emulsifying material, salt, and acid, not more than 40% moisture and not less than 50% fat must be present; (2) in pasteurized process cheese food, in which additional solids from milk, skim milk, cheese whey, or whey albumin are used, the moisture content must not exceed 44%; (3) in pasteurized process cheese spread, which contains the same basic ingredients as pasteurized process cheese, sweetening agents, and not more than 0.8% of stabilizer, the moisture content must not exceed 60% and the fat content must be at least 20%.

[PAUL H. TRACY]

Bibliography: E. M. Foster et al., *Dairy Microbiology*, 1957; F. V. Kosikowski, *Cheese and Fermented Milk Foods*, 1966; G. P. Sanders, H. E. Walter, and R. T. Tittsler, *General Procedure for Manufacturing Swiss Cheese*, USDA Circ. no. 851, 1955; M. E. Schwartz, *Cheese-making Technology*, 1974; A. L. Simon, *Cheeses of the World*, 1956; U.S. Agriculture Research Society, *Cheeses of the World*, 1972; L. L. Van Slyke and W. V. Price, *Cheese*, 1949.

Cherry

The two principal cherries of commerce are the sweet cherry (*Prunus avium*) and the sour cherry (*P. cerasus*). Both are of ancient origin and seem to have come from the region between the Black and Caspian seas. They were probably carried into Europe by birds before humans were there. The cherry was mentioned in 300 B.C. by the Greek botanist Theophrastus. It was taken to America from Europe.

Cherries of minor importance are the dwarf or western sand cherries (*P. besseyi*) of the plains region of North America; the Duke cherries, which are supposedly natural hybrids between the sweet and sour cherry; and the Padus cherries, which bear their small fruits in long clusters or racemes rather than in short fascicles.

Types and varieties. Sweet cherries may be divided into two groups, firm-fleshed types known as Bigarreaus, represented by the Napoleon (also called the Royal Anne), and soft-fleshed types known as Hearts, represented by the Black Tartarian. Sour cherries may also be divided into two groups, clear-juice or Amarelle types, represented by the Montmorency, and colored-juice or Morello

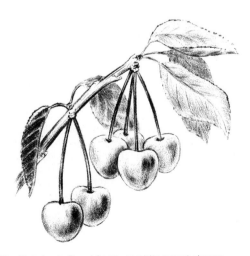

The Napoleon, Royal Anne, or white sweet cherry.

types, represented by the English Morello.

In North America the principal sweet commercial varieties are the Napoleon (white) (see illustration), Bing, Lambert, Van, Schmidt, and Windsor (dark). The principal commercial variety of sour cherry is the Montmorency.

Propagation and culture. Trees are propagated by budding into seedlings of the wild sweet (Mazzard) cherry or of *P. mahaleb*, commonly called the perfumed cherry of southern Europe. The former is best suited to the sweet cherry, and the latter to the sour cherry. *See* BUDDING.

The sweet cherry is somewhat hardier than the peach, and the sour cherry is hardier than the sweet cherry. Wild sweet cherries may grow 100 ft high (1 ft = 0.3 m), and the trees may reach an age of 200 years. Cultivated varieties are usually planted 25–30 ft apart and allowed to grow to heights of only about 15–20 ft for ease of culture and harvest. Sour cherry trees may reach 30–40 ft but are kept at 15–20 ft and planted 18–22 ft apart. Cherry trees do best in well-drained sandy loam soils. They will not tolerate wet soil. Sweet varieties require cross-pollination; common sour varieties are self-fruitful (self-pollinated).

Production and economic importance. The average commercial production of sweet cherries in the United States during the 5-year period 1970–1974 was 132,444 tons (1 short ton = 0.9 metric ton), of which Washington produced 34,520, Oregon 33,880, California 29,080, and Michigan 22,800. In 1974, 45% of the crop was sold fresh, 13% canned, 7% frozen, and 35% brined (mostly for maraschino or confectionary use). The 5-year average (1970–1974) commercial production of sour cherries (also designated "tart" cherries in commerce) was 125,842 tons, of which Michigan produced 89,800. In 1974, 2% of the sour cherry crop was sold fresh, 35% canned, 60% frozen, and 3% for juice, wine, or brine. The 1974 farm value of the United States sweet and sour cherry crops was $114,000,000. *See* FRUIT, TREE.

[R. PAUL LARSEN]

Cherry diseases. Leaf spot, a serious fungus disease caused by *Coccomyces hiemalis*, affects sweet and sour cherries. Diseased leaves drop prematurely, tree growth is retarded, and the cherries are reduced in size and number. This disease may be controlled by spraying trees with lime sulfur solution, copper compounds, or ferbam, an organic fungicide. Black knot, a fungus disease characterized by the development of rough, black swellings on the branches, is prevalent on neglected trees. It may be controlled by removing diseased branches and spraying the tree with a copper compound to prevent further infections by spores of the causal agent, *Dibotryon morbosum*. *See* FUNGISTAT AND FUNGICIDE.

Other fungus diseases are mildew, which covers the leaves with a weblike mass of fungus filaments, and bitter rot and brown rot which destroy the fruit. Brown rot is particularly destructive to sweet cherries growing under humid conditions.

Sour cherry yellows, ring spot, and little cherry are virus diseases that reduce fruit size and ultimately make the trees unfruitful. Control of these diseases is achieved by propagation of virus-free nursery stock, or in the case of little cherry, by removal of all diseased trees to prevent further spread of the virus. Many cherry trees die from too low temperatures or excessive soil moisture. *See* FRUIT (TREE) DISEASES; PLANT DISEASE CONTROL; PLANT VIRUS.

[JOHN C. DUNEGAN]

Bibliography: W. H. Chandler, *Deciduous Orchards*, 1957; N. F. Childers, *Modern Fruit Science*, 1973.

Chicle

A gummy exudate used in the manufacture of chewing gum. It is contained in the bark of a tall evergreen tree, *Achras zapota* (see illustration), belonging to the sapodilla family (Sapotaceae). The species is a native of Mexico and Central America. The latex (secretion) is collected and carefully boiled to remove excess moisture. When the water content is reduced to 33%, the chicle is poured off and molded into blocks. Crude chicle contains resin, arabin, gutta, sugar, calcium, and different soluble salts. For refining, it is broken up, washed in strong alkali, neutralized with sodium acid phosphate, rewashed, dried, and powdered. The resulting product is an amorphous, pale-pink powder, insoluble in water, and forming a sticky paste when heated. In the manufacture of chewing gum, the chicle is cleaned, filtered, and sterilized, and various flavoring materials and sugar are added.

[PERRY D. STRAUSBAUGH/EARL L. CORE]

Chicory

A perennial herb, *Cichorium intybus* (Compositae), with a long taproot, a coarse branching stem, and a basal rosette of numerous leaves. Although the plant is a native of Europe, it has become a common weed in the United States. It is used as a salad plant or for greens. The roasted root is also used as an adulterant of coffee. *See* SPICE AND FLAVORING.

[PERRY D. STRAUSBAUGH/EARL L. CORE]

Cinnamon

An evergreen shrub or small tree, *Cinnamomum zeylanicum*, of the laurel family (Lauraceae). A native of Ceylon, the plant (see illustration) is now in cultivation in southern India, Burma, parts of Malaya, West Indies, and South America. In cultivation the trees are cut back and long, slender suckers grow up from the roots. The bark is removed from these suckers, dried, and packaged for shipping. Cinnamon is a very important spice for flavoring foods. It is used in confectionery, gums, incense, dentifrices, and perfumes. Cinnamon oil is used in medicine and as a source of cinnamon extract. *See* SPICE AND FLAVORING.

[PERRY D. STRAUSBAUGH/EARL L. CORE]

Citron

Citrus medica, a species of true citrus. The plant has a long and interesting history, being the first contact between citrus, which came from the Far East, and western Judaeo-Christian civilization. A citron, the Etrog, was the "hadar" or "goodly fruit" offering at the ancient Jewish Feast of the Tabernacles. At the time of the first Jewish revolt against Rome in A.D. 66–70, the rebels minted their own coins with the Etrog substituting for Nero's imperial visage.

Commercially, citrons are still grown almost

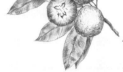

CHICLE

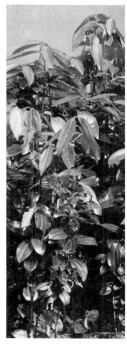

Fruit of *Achras zapota*. (*From L. H. Bailey, The Standard Cyclopedia of Horticulture, vol. 3. Reprinted with permission of Macmillan Publishing Co., Inc. Copyright 1915 by Macmillan Publishing Co., Inc.; renewed 1943 by L. H. Bailey*)

CINNAMON

Cinnamon (*Cinnamomum zeylanicum*). (*USDA*)

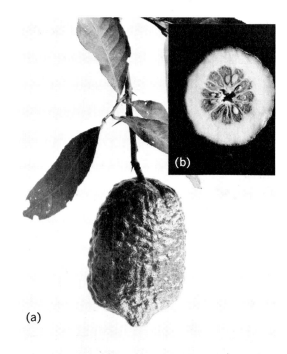

Commercial citron (*Citrus medica*), approximately one-half natural size. (*a*) Foliage and fruit. (*b*) Cross section of fruit. (*From The McFarland Co.*)

exclusively in the Mediterranean area, principally in Italy, Sicily, Corsica, Greece, and Israel. The tree is evergreen, as are all citrus, and frost-tender. It is thorny, straggly, shrubby, and tends to be short-lived.

The fruit is scarcely edible fresh, having a very thick skin with little flesh and that lacking in juice (see illustration). However, it is very fragrant and was valued in ancient times for its aroma and its fragrant peel oil, used in perfumes and as a moth repellent. Later, when the citron was the only known citrus fruit, it was very highly valued. Today, it is grown commercially only as a source of candied peel for use in cakes and confections. The actual candying is usually done in the importing country, the citron peel being exported in brine. Traditionally the fruit was halved and held in large unsealed casks in sea water, a mild fermentation taking place for a week or more, after which additional coarse salt was added and the casks sealed. Today brining is more typically done in a 15% salt solution to which about 2000 parts per million (ppm) of SO_2 has been added as a preservative and 1% $CaCl_2$ to firm the tissues. The candying process involves first leaching out the brine with boiling water and then transfers through successive syrups of increasing strength up to about 75%.

Confusion sometimes arises due to the name "citron" also being used for a small, wild, inedible melon in the United States and for lemons (*C. limon*) in France. *See* FRUIT, TREE.

[WILLIAM GRIERSON]

Citronella

A tropical grass, *Cymbopogon nardus*, from the leaves of which oil of citronella is distilled. This essential oil is pale yellow, inexpensive, and much used in cheap perfumes and soaps. It is perhaps best known as an insect repellent. A large acreage is devoted to the cultivation of this grass in Java and Ceylon.

[PERRY D. STRAUSBAUGH/EARL L. CORE]

Citrus flavoring

Food flavoring derived from the aromatic principles of fruit of the citrus family. Important members of the family for flavoring purposes include orange, lemon, lime, tangerine, and grapefruit. Citron is seldom used. Flavoring is compounded from the oils of citrus fruits, coloring, and synthetic flavor.

Citrus oils. These are found in the skin of the fruit, and the usual commercial source is from canning or processing by-products. Citrus oils occur in oval, balloon-shaped sacs located in the outer rind of the fruit. The percentage present, based on fruit weight, is usually 0.11–0.58%.

Citrus oils are high in terpenes. A member of this family which occurs heavily in the citrus group is *d*-limonene, whose formula is shown below. In

$$\underset{\text{\it d-Limonene}}{}$$

d-Limonene

general, *d*-limonene is subject to an undesirable change in the presence of air and light, resulting in a turpentinelike odor and flavor. This is called "terpeniness" by the industry. The change is best avoided by excluding light and air, and occasionally chemical materials called antioxidants are added which greatly delay its development.

The characteristic odor of most citrus oils is due to oxygenated compounds, especially citral, whose alpha form is shown below. Since these com-

α-Citral

pounds are present at a low level of 2–5%, and since the terpenes are unstable, it is common practice to remove the terpenes to produce terpeneless oils. Terpenes are removed either by fractional vacuum distillation, selective solvents, or a combination of both.

Distilled oil is also obtained as a by-product of the citrus juice operation. In juice manufacture there is an upper limit of oil content for desirable juice. Surplus oil is removed in a deoiler, essentially a vacuum still operating at 54–80°C.

Citrus flavors, usually compounded from the above oils, with synthesized flavor and color additives, are used extensively in the food industry. Primary outlets include candy and carbonated beverage industries, as well as the baking and ice

cream trades. A large market also is found in the detergent field—citrus aromas make washday more pleasant.

Methods of extracting oil. These include Pipkin roll, screw press, Fraser-Brace extractor, and Pipkin juice extractor. All methods give a water-and-oil emulsion which is separated by a two-stage centrifugation to yield a clear, polished oil. The oil is then stored in steel tanks at 0–4°C to allow waxy materials to separate out. This process is called winterizing.

The Pipkin roll method passes fruit peel through two striated rollers rotating in opposite directions. The roller distance is carefully adjusted to remove oil without rasping the peel. Striations in the rollers extract the oil without further contact with the peel, lest it be reabsorbed.

The screw-press method squeezes the crushed peel against a perforated screen, thereby forcing out the oil. Screws may be vertical or horizontal, and water may or may not be added.

The Fraser-Brace extraction utilizes a machine which is basically an abrasive peeler. Abrasive carborundum rollers rasp the peel from the fruit under a water spray. The water and peel mixture is screened and settled to allow oil separation.

The Pipkin juice extractor is used where both oil and juice are required. Whole fruit is fed into cups that exert a squeezing action to extract juice and oil which are caught in separate troughs.

[ROY E. MORSE]

Bibliography: J. B. S. Braverman, *Citrus Products*, 1949; E. Guenther, *The Essential Oils*, vols. 1–6, 1948–1952; J. W. Kesterson and R. Hendrickson, *Essential Oils from Florida Citrus*, Univ. Fla. Agr. Exp. Sta. Bull. no. 521, 1953; J. Merory, *Food Flavorings*, 2d ed., 1968; J. L. Simonsen et al., *The Terpenes*, 5 vols., 2d ed., 1947–1958.

Clove

The unopened flower bud (see illustration) of a small, conical, symmetrical, evergreen tree, *Eugenia caryophyllata*, of the myrtle family (Myrtaceae). The cloves are picked by hand and dried in the sun or by artificial means. The crop is uncertain and difcult to grow. Cloves, one of the most important and useful spices, are strongly aromatic and have a pungent flavor. They are used as a culinary spice for flavoring pickles, ketchup, and sauces, in medicine, and for perfuming the breath and the air in rooms. The essential oil distilled from cloves by water or steam has even more uses. The chief clove-producing countries are Tanzania with 90% of the total output, Indonesia, Mauritius, and the West Indies. *See* SPICE AND FLAVORING.

[PERRY D. STRAUSBAUGH/EARL L. CORE]

Clover

A common name used loosely to designate the true clovers, sweet clovers, and other members of the plant family Leguminosa. This article discusses true clovers, sweet clover, and clover diseases.

TRUE CLOVERS

The true clovers are plants of the genus *Trifolium*, order Rosales. There are approximately 250 species in the world. Collectively they represent

CLOVE

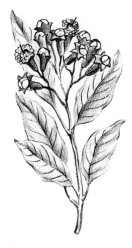

Closed (cloves) and open flower buds on a branch of the evergreen tree *Eugenia caryophyllata*.

the most important genus of forage legumes in agriculture. Different species constitute one or more crops on every continent. As indicated by the number of species and their ecotypes (subspecies) that have been collected and described, the center of origin appears to be southeastern Europe and southwestern Asia Minor. Many species are found in countries that border the Mediterranean Sea. About 80 species are native to the United States, most of them occurring in the general regions of the Rocky and Cascade mountains and the Sierra Nevada. Although these native clovers are not used as crop plants, they contribute to the range for grazing and wild hay and also supply nitrogen to associated grasses. Of those that are now named, it is possible that many are variants of other species. Only a few are native to the humid Eastern states. Most clovers are highly palatable and nutritious to livestock. The name clover is often applied to members of legume genera other than *Trifolium*.

Characteristics. The true clovers are herbaceous annual or perennial plants. However, many perennial species behave as biennials or annuals under attacks of disease or insects, unfavorable climatic or soil conditions, or improper management. In general, clovers thrive under cool, moist conditions although one native species, desert clover (*T. gymnocarpum*), tolerates semiarid conditions. Annual species usually behave as winter annuals where winter conditions are not severe, and as summer annuals at northern latitudes and high altitudes. Clovers grow best where adequate supplies of calcium, phosphorus, and potassium are naturally present in the soil, or where these elements are applied in limestone and fertilizers. They grow from a few inches to several feet tall, depending on the species and the environmental conditions. The leaves have 3–5 roundish to spearlike leaflets. The florets, ranging from 5 to 200 in number, are borne in heads. Colors include white, pink, red, purple, and yellow, and various mixtures. The basic haploid chromosome numbers of the species are 6, 7, and 8. Somatic chromosomes range from 12 to about 130, forming diploids, tetraploids, and polyploids. The flowers of some species are self-sterile and must be cross-pollinated before seed will form; the flowers of other species may be self-fertile and capable of self-pollination; others are self-fertile but do not set seed unless the flowers are tripped and the pollen scattered onto the stigma. Cross-pollination and tripping of flowers are effected principally by bees that visit the flowers for nectar and pollen. Seed color ranges from yellow to deep purple, some being bicolored. There are approximately 60,000–700,000 seeds per pound.

Uses. Clovers are used for hay, pasture, silage, and soil improvement. Certain kinds may be used for all purposes whereas others, because of their low growth, are best suited for grazing. All kinds, when well grown in thick stands, are good for soil improvement. Thoroughly inoculated plants add 50–200 lb of nitrogen per acre when plowed under for soil improvement, the amount added depending on growth, thickness of stand, and length of growing season. Clovers may be grown alone, in combination with grasses and other legumes, or with small grains. In the humid states, or where

irrigated, clovers are sown most frequently with small-grain companion crops. In the Corn Belt they are generally spring-seeded, whereas in the Southern states and in the West Coast region they should be seeded in the fall for best results.

Important species. All the clover species of agricultural importance in the United States are introduced (exotic) plants. Figure 1 shows some of the species most widely used: red clover (*T. pratense*), alsike clover (*T. hybridum*), white clover (*T. repens*), crimson clover (*T. incarnatum*), subclover (*T. subterraneum*), strawberry clover (*T. fragiferum*), persian clover (*T. resupinatum*), and large hop clover (*T. campestre*, or *procumbens*). Other clovers of regional importance, mostly adapted to specific environmental conditions, are rose clover (*T. hirtum*), berseem clover (*T. alexandrinum*), ball clover (*T. nigrescens*), lappa clover (*T. lappaceum*), big-flower clover (*T. michelianum*), and arrowleaf clover (*T. vesiculosum*).

Species characteristics. The following sections discuss the characteristics of the most important species.

Red clover. Red clover is composed of two forms, medium and mammoth, producing two and one hay cuts, respectively. The large purplish-red flower heads are round. An upright-growing perennial, red clover generally persists for 2 years in the northern United States, but behaves as a winter annual in the South. When planted alone or with small grain, seeding rates are 10–15 lb per acre. When seeded with grass and other mixtures, 4–8 lb is sufficient. Under favorable growth conditions, seed yields average 70 lb per acre; in the West under irrigation they may reach 600–800 lb. There are several varieties and strains of red clover such as Kenland, Pennscott, Lakeland, Dollard, and Chesapeake. These produce higher yields of forage and are more persistent than common red clover.

Alsike clover. Alsike clover is an upright-growing species that behaves like a biennial. The growth pattern, seeding methods, mixtures, and uses are similar to those of red clover. The flower heads are much like those of white clover in shape and size, but are slightly more pinkish. Alsike clover is more tolerant of wet, poorly drained soils than red clover and occurs widely in mountain meadows of the West.

White clover. White clover, an inhabitant of lawns and closely grazed pastures, is the most important pasture legume in the humid states. The flowers are generally white, but sometimes they are tinged with pink. The stems grow on the soil surface and root at the joints (nodes) as the plant spreads. There are three main types, large, intermediate, and small, with all gradations between. Ladino is the best-known and most widely seeded variety of the large type, and Louisiana S1 represents the intermediate type. The small type is found principally in pastures that are continuously and closely grazed. All types are nutritious and are relished by all classes of livestock and poultry. The protein content ranges from 15 to 30%, depending on plant age and the succulence of growth. Ladino white clover is sometimes used for silage and hay. White clover is mainly grown with low-growing grasses, not being tolerant of the tall-growing kinds. Seeding rates vary from $\frac{1}{2}$ to 2 lb per acre

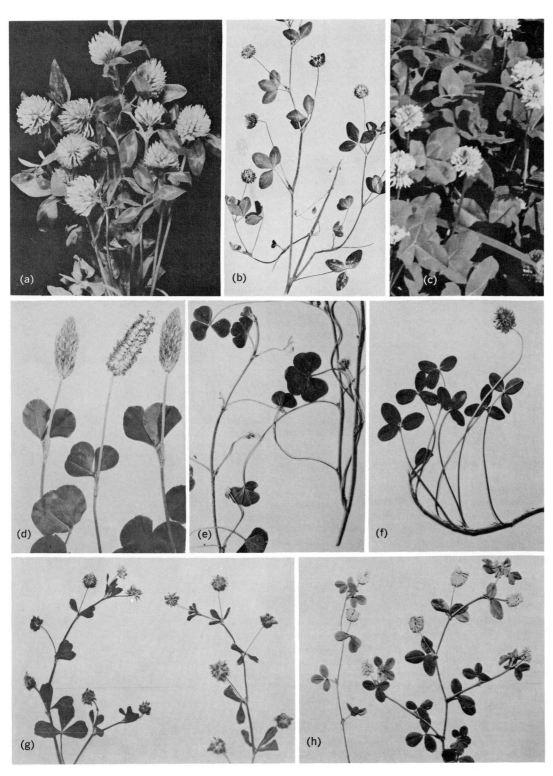

Fig. 1. Important clovers. (a) Red clover (*Trifolium pratense*). (b) Alsike clover (*T. hybridum*). (c) White clover (*T. repens*). (d) Crimson clover (*T. incarnatum*). (e) Sub- clover (*T. subterraneum*). (f) Strawberry clover (*T. fragiferum*). (g) Persian clover (*T. resupinatum*). (h) Large hop clover (*T. campestre* or *procumbens*). (*USDA*)

depending on the seed mixture. For successful growth, it is important to use the variety or strain best adapted to the particular climatic and soil conditions. Limestone and fertilizer must usually be used to get a thick stand and good growth. Spring seeding is recommended for the Northern states and fall seeding for regions having mild win-

ters. For best growth of the clover, grass-clover mixtures should be grazed or cut frequently.

Crimson clover. Crimson clover is used principally as a winter annual for pasture and as a soil-improving crop from the latitude of the Ohio River southward, and along the West Coast. The yellow seed, approximately 120,000 per pound, are planted at the rate of 15–20 lb per acre during the late summer and fall months in a prepared seedbed or on grass which is closely grazed or cut. The seedlings make a rosette of leafy growth during the winter months. With the advent of spring, growth is rapid; the plant reaches 1½–3 ft in height and the flower stems elongate, terminating with pointed crimson flower heads in late spring or early summer. The plant dies when the seed matures. Seed yields average about 250 lb per acre even though large quantities are lost by shattering. Crimson clover is seeded alone, with small grains and grasses, or on grass turf. During the winter it may be grazed when growth reaches 4 in., although if it is too heavily grazed, regrowth is slow. The greatest return for soil improvement is obtained when the largest growth is plowed under. There are several varieties of crimson clover, including Dixie, Auburn, Autauga, Chief, Talladega, and many local strains. When conditions are favorable, all of these will reseed, forming volunteer stands in the fall from seed shattered the previous spring. Common crimson clover does not reseed. When used with Bermuda or other perennial summer-growing grasses, the fall growth of the grass must be closely grazed or clipped.

Subclover. Subclover, a winter annual extensively used for grazing in the coastal sections of the Western states, is the basic pasture crop of the sheep and cattle industry of Australia. The seed are blue-black and the largest of any clover species (about 60,000 per pound). The flower heads on decumbent stems are inconspicuous. As the seed develop, fishhook-shaped appendages are produced which, by their twisting action, pull them into the soil, and hence the name subclover. Seed production is large, but the seed are difficult to harvest. When once established, fall stands develop from seed produced the preceding months. The Australian varieties Mount Barker, Tallarook, and Nangeela have proved to be best adapted to most conditions in the United States. Subclover appears to have considerable promise as a pasture legume under many conditions in the southern United States, but better adapted varieties are needed.

Other clovers. Strawberry clover, a perennial, is a nutritious pasture plant similar in growth habit to white clover, for which it is frequently mistaken. The pinkish flower head looks like a strawberry, and hence the common name. It is highly tolerant of the wet, salty soil common to the Western states.

Persian clover is a winter annual used mostly for pasture and soil improvement but is also an excellent silage plant. It is particularly adapted to the wet, heavy soils of the lower southern part of the United States. The flowers are light purple, and the mature seed are enclosed in balloonlike capsules that shatter easily, float on water, and are readily blown about by the wind. Persian clover is relished by all classes of livestock.

Large hop clover and small hop clover, widely distributed as winter annuals in the Southern states, are used in pastures. They are more tolerant of low soil fertility than the other species and less productive, but are highly palatable to livestock. The flower heads are bright yellow and, when mature, look like the flowers of the hop plant. The two species are similar.

Rose clover is a relatively new winter annual and appears to be best adapted to the foothill rangelands of California.

Berseen is the least tolerant of the clovers to winter freezing and is grown only in limited amounts in southern California and Arizona.

Other recently introduced species are ball clover, lappa clover, big-flower clover, and arrowleaf clover, all winter annuals. Lappa clover grows best in the heavy dark marl soils of the South, whereas ball, big-flower, and arrowleaf clovers appear to be more widely adapted. All are used for pasture, although big-flower and arrowleaf clovers may also be used for hay.

Seaside clover (*T. willdenovii*), white-tipped clover (*T. variegatum*), and long-stalked clover (*T. longipes*) are the most widely distributed of the native western species. All produce thick stands and good growth under varying conditions. *See* LEGUME FORAGES.

SWEET CLOVER

Sweet clover is the common name for all but one species of legumes of the genus *Melilotus*, order Rosales. The exception is sour clover (*M. indica*).

CLOVER

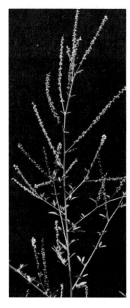

Fig. 2. White sweet clover (*Melilotus alba*). (USDA)

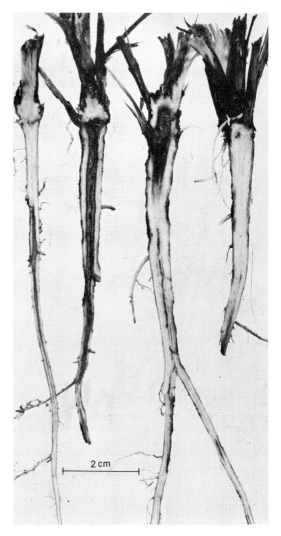

2 cm

Fig. 3. Red clover roots cut longitudinally to show type of injury caused by crown and root rot organisms.

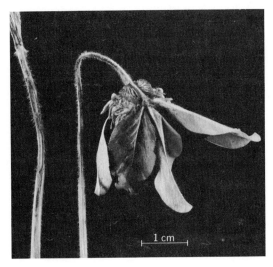

Fig. 4. Northern anthracnose lesions on stems and leaf petiole of a red clover plant.

Origin and distribution. There are approximately 20 species of sweet clover. Some of the biennial species have an annual form. The roots of the biennials develop crown buds from which the second-year growth arises; the roots of annuals do not develop crown buds. Sweet clovers are native to the Mediterranean region and adjacent countries, but several are widely scattered throughout the world, generally by chance introduction. None is indigenous to the United States. White sweet clover (*M. alba*) and yellow sweet clover (*M. officinalis*) are important forage and soil-improvement plants in the United States and Canada and are found growing along roadsides and in waste places in every state (Fig. 2). Sour clover, a yellow-flowered winter annual, is of some value for soil improvement only along the Gulf Coast and in southern New Mexico, Arizona, and California. Improved varieties of white and yellow sweet clovers, with many desired characteristics, are available for farm use.

Uses. Sweet clover is used as a field crop in regions of the United States and Canada where the rainfall is 17 in. or more during the growing season, where the soil is neutral, or where limestone and other needed minerals are applied. It is most extensively grown in the Great Plains and Corn Belt, either alone or in rotations with small grains and corn, and is used for grazing, soil improvement, and hay. Except for those of certain improved varieties, the plants are somewhat bitter because of the presence of coumarin. External and internal bleeding of animals may result from feeding spoiled sweet-clover hay or improperly preserved silage containing sweet clover, a decomposition product of coumarin (4-hydroxycoumarin, commonly called dicumarol), which develops during spoilage, being the toxic principle. Research has led to its use in medicine and for making warfarin, a rodenticide.

[EUGENE A. HOLLOWELL]

CLOVER DISEASES

Clovers may be attacked separately or simultaneously by bacteria, fungi, nematodes, and viruses. Clover diseases are best controlled by growing adapted varieties that tolerate some of the important pathogens.

Fungus diseases. Fungi, such as species of *Pythium*, *Fusarium*, and *Sclerotinia*, produce root and crown rots. They are important in the establishment and persistence of clovers. These fungi can attack plants at any stage of their development and either kill or weaken them so that they die during periods of drought or low winter temperatures (Fig. 3).

Leaf and stem pathogens usually do not kill plants but produce lesions that reduce the functional leaf surface or girdle stems. When abundant, however, they cause defoliation or death of shoots, reducing yield and quality of forage (Fig. 4).

Virus diseases. Most clovers are susceptible to destructive virus diseases that produce leaf mottling and distortion, stunt the plants, and reduce vigor. Some viruses infect not only clovers but also other legumes and nonlegumes. The viruses are initially spread by insects, but some may also be spread by mowing.   [KERMIT W. KREITLOW]

Bibliography: J. G. Dickson, *Diseases of Field Crops*, 2d ed., 1956; A. Stefferud (ed.), Plant diseases, *USDA Yearb. Agr.*, 1953.

Coca

A shrub, *Erythroxylon coca* (Erythroxylaceae), native to Peru and Bolivia, from which the alkaloid cocaine is obtained (see illustration). The leaves of coca, either alone or mixed with lime and the ashes of some plant such as quinoa, are chewed by the natives. Coca used in moderation enables the user to resist fatigue, and thus it is possible for him to endure long periods of labor without either food or drink. Coca chewing becomes a habit which leads to weakness, sickness, and even death. Cocaine is used for local anesthesia and as a tonic in digestive and nervous disorders. It is habit-forming and should be used only by order of a physician. Coca is cultivated extensively in South America, Ceylon, Java, and Formosa. *See* COLA.

[PERRY D. STRAUSBAUGH/EARL L. CORE]

Cocoa powder and chocolate

The seeds of the cacao tree are known in commerce as cocoa beans. When harvested, these seeds have no chocolate flavor, and processing is needed to develop it. *See* CACAO.

Fermentation or curing is carried out in the country of origin immediately after harvesting. The pulpy mass containing the seeds is placed in boxes or baskets and permitted to ferment for 3–9 days. The temperature may go as high as 50°C during this period. The seed is killed, and enzymes activated by the heat catalyze reactions which produce the precursors responsible for chocolate flavor that appears later in the roasting process. The color of the seed changes from purple to brown, and the shell is loosened from the cotyledon.

After fermentation the beans are sun-dried and packed in jute or sisal sacks, containing from 120 to 180 lb, according to the customs in the country of origin. The normal moisture content is in the range of 6–8%. Each seed is enclosed in a hard shell, making up 10–14% of the total weight. The cotyledon is 50–55% fat, 9–14% protein, 20–25% starch, and 10–15% other carbohydrates.

COCA

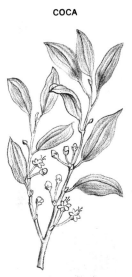

Flowering branch of coca (*Erythroxylon coca*).

Processing technique. The beans are first cleaned in machines known as stoners to remove stones and other tramp materials. The cleaned beans are then roasted, in either batch cylinder roasters or continuous roasters (Fig. 1). Roasting develops chocolate flavor, not present in the raw bean, and also loosens the shell and reduces moisture content to the range of 1–2%. A temperature of 137.8–146°C is reached inside the bean, according to individual flavor requirements.

A development in roasting employs fluidized bed techniques. Roasting in such a bed not only gives a more uniform degree of roast, but permits the use of higher temperature differentials which loosen the shell more fully, thus simplifying its removal in the winnowing process which follows and providing better control over product flavor.

To remove the shells, roasted beans are crushed and winnowed with equipment known as the cracker and fanner. The cleaned broken pieces of cotyledon are known as cocoa nibs. United States government standards of identity for cocoa nibs limit the shell content to a maximum of 1.75% by weight.

For some uses the nibs are treated at this point with alkali to neutralize the natural acids present and enhance color. The alkali is applied in water solution; time is allowed for absorption and penetration, then the nibs are dried or roasted to 1–2% moisture. This is known as Dutch processing.

The roasted or dried nibs are then ground to produce chocolate (Fig. 2). Many types of mills are used, the most common being stone disks and steel roll refiners. The heat of grinding melts the fat, and the ground cell walls are suspended in this fat to produce a slurry. The liquid coming from the mills is known as chocolate liquor or bitter chocolate. United States government standards require a minimum of 50% fat content. Liquor is used directly for flavoring other foods and as a base for the manufacture of cocoa powder, sweet chocolate, and milk chocolate.

Cocoa powder manufacture. The liquor is then passed through special filter presses provided with hydraulic rams to squeeze out additional fat from the cake. The resulting presscake is cooled, pulverized, and sifted to make cocoa powder. While some manufacturers still use silk bolting cloth for the sifting operation, the majority employ wind sifters or classifiers, which make possible the production of a finer powder.

United States government standards classify three types of powder on the basis of fat content: Breakfast cocoa must have a minimum of 22% fat, cocoa is within the range of 10–22% fat, and low-fat cocoa has less than 10% fat.

In Dutch processing, United States government standards permit the use of a maximum of 2.91% potassium carbonate or its neutralizing equivalent of other permitted alkalies, such as the carbonates or hydroxides of sodium, potassium, ammonium, and magnesium.

Cocoa powder is used to flavor candy, baked goods, ice cream, dairy drinks, and syrups.

Cocoa butter. The fat removed by pressing is filtered and is known as cocoa butter. It has a melting point of 33.3–34.4°C, a yellow color, and a slight chocolate flavor and aroma. It is widely used in the pharmaceutical and cosmetic industries because of its melting point, being solid at room temperature but liquid at body heat. The United States Pharmacopoeia has a standard for it. However, the major use for cocoa butter is in the manufacture of milk chocolate and sweet chocolate.

Sweet chocolate. Sweet chocolate is made from chocolate liquor by adding sugar and cocoa butter. The ingredients are mixed in either melangeurs or paste mixers and then refined by passing the resulting paste over steel roll refiners, which grind the sugar to a maximum particle size of 0.0004–0.0016 in. according to the quality desired. The ground material is then combined with additional cocoa butter and worked to a smooth and viscosity-stable paste in machines known as conges. The functions of this operation are to wet all dry sugar surfaces with fat, to obtain maximum surface exposure to permit volatilization of undesired flavors, to permit oxidation of astringent substances, and to permit flavor development through heat processing.

A revolutionary improvement has been made in the conging process. Formerly, the ground material from the roll refiners was added to the conging machine with enough cocoa butter to form a heavy paste immediately, then processed in semiliquid form. However, a dry conge has been developed, capable of working the refined material without the

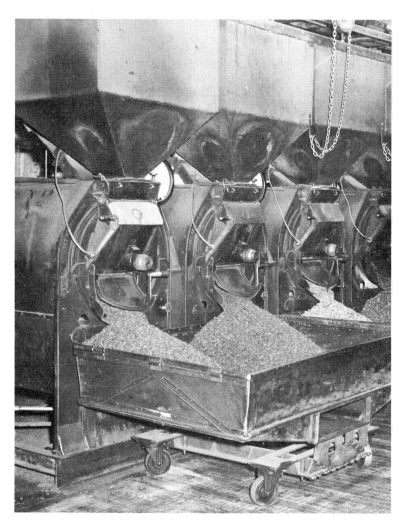

Fig. 1. Roasting cocoa beans. (*Hershey Chocolate Corp., Hershey, Pa.*)

addition of fat. This permits rapid evaporation of surface moisture on the dry solids before they are covered with fat. When liquid fat is added, the absence of surface moisture reduces the interfacial tension between the solids and the fat, and a paste is more readily formed. Addition of the balance of the fat produces finished chocolate. This shortens the processing time and also reduces the amount of fat needed to bring the product to the desired fluidity for use. As cocoa butter is the most expensive ingredient of the mix, there is a substantial economic advantage in the use of this process.

The final sweet chocolate is cast into bars or used in bulk as a coating for confections, baked goods, and the like. United States government standards require that sweet chocolate contain a minimum of 15% chocolate liquor and prescribe the flavoring materials permitted.

Milk chocolate. Milk chocolate is sweet chocolate containing dried milk solids. Because these products have a continuous fat phase, moisture must be removed from the milk before incorporating it in chocolate products. While roller-dried and spray-dried milk are frequently used, the industry also dries milk in combination with sugar to produce a crumb. This permits variations in flavor development, such as partial hydrolysis of the milk fat to intensify the milk flavor.

The dried milk is incorporated with the liquor and sugar in the paste mixer and ground on roll refiners like sweet chocolate. The conging process is used to develop variations in milk chocolate flavor.

United States government standards require a minimum of 10% liquor and 12% whole milk solids in milk chocolate. As much as 22% whole milk solids is sometimes used in milk chocolate designed for eating as such. It is also widely used to coat confections.

Confectioner's coatings. Many confectioners and biscuit manufacturers have turned to chocolate substitutes made with fats other than cocoa butter. This has been done for economic reasons as well as to obtain special effects in their products. The fats employed have melting point ranges which fit the particular needs of the product. By United States government standards sweet cocoa and vegetable fat coating contains fat with a higher melting point than cocoa butter. Sweet chocolate and vegetable fat coating has a fat with a lower melting point than cocoa butter. The latter product is used to coat ice cream.

Application of coatings to centers. Because of the polymorphism of cocoa butter, great care is needed in applying melted coatings to candy or biscuit centers. All but one of the polymorphs are unstable, with a maximum life of 1 month, after which they revert to the most stable form. Therefore the coatings must be applied and frozen in such a way that most of the fat crystallizes initially in the stable form. Otherwise, changes in structure take place which detract from the appearance of the coating while in storage.

Fortunately, the stable form has the highest melting point of all the polymorphs, making it possible to "seed" the liquid coating with crystals of this form and to apply at a temperature which will destroy the lower melting types, thus encouraging stable crystallization throughout.

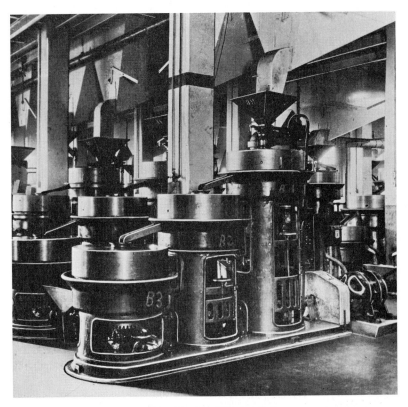

Fig. 2. Liquor mills. (*Hershey Chocolate Corp., Hershey, Pa.*)

When an unstable polymorph experiences a changeover from one form to another, the process is accompanied by a release of latent heat, as well as a contraction in the crystals. The change in appearance known as "fat bloom" is an indication that unstable crystals were originally present. In changing over, a combination of heat release and crystal contraction forces some of the newly formed crystals above the surface of the coating, producing the bloom. *See* FOOD ENGINEERING; FOOD MANUFACTURING.   [NORMAN W. KEMPF]

Bibliography: N. W. Kempf, *The Technology of Chocolate*, 1964; B. W. Minifie, *Chocolate, Cocoa and Confectionery: Science and Technology*, 1970; H. Wieland, *Cocoa and Chocolate Processing*, 1972.

Coconut

A large palm, *Cocos nucifera*, widely grown throughout the tropics and valuable for its fruit and fiber. Usually found near the seacoast, it requires high humidity, abundant rainfall (60 in.), and mean annual temperature of about 85°F. Southern Florida, with mean temperature of 77°F, is at the limit of successful growth. The origin of the coconut has been in dispute, but strong evidence points to southern Asia with wide dispersal by ocean currents and human migrations.

The fruit, 10 in. or more in length, is ovoid and obtusely triangular in cross section (see illustration). The tough, fibrous outer husk (exocarp) encloses a spherical nut consisting of a hard, bony shell (endocarp) within which is a 1/2-in. layer of fleshy meat or kernel (endosperm). The meat is high in oil and protein and, when dried, is the copra of commerce.

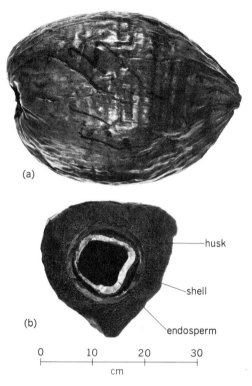

(a)

(b)

husk

shell

endosperm

```
0        10        20        30
|————————|————————|————————|
            cm
```

Coconut. (a) Fruit. (b) Cross section of fruit showing husk, shell, and endosperm (meat).

Production and culture. World production was reported as 29,000,000,000 nuts in 1964 with commercial copra estimated as 3,354,000 metric tons. Principal commercial producers are the Philippines, Indonesia, Malaya, Ceylon, and Oceania. Although many trees grow along the seashore and in native villages without special care, the crop lends itself to plantation culture with control of weeds, fertilization, and protection from diseases, insects, and animal pests.

Palms begin to bear nuts the sixth year after planting and reach full bearing about the eighth year. Individual nuts mature about a year after blossoming and normally fall to the ground. In plantation culture, clusters of mature nuts are cut from the trees with knives on long poles just before maturity. Picking individual nuts by climbing the trees is sometimes practiced.

Processing and products. The thick husks are removed from the nuts, which are then split open with a heavy knife and partially dried to loosen the meat. This is pried out of the shell and dried to about 7% moisture either in the sun, if conditions are favorable, or in kilns with additional heat often furnished by burning the husks and shells.

The oil from the dried coconut meats, or copra, is widely used for margarine, soap, and industrial purposes. High-quality copra may be shredded for confectionery and the baking trade. The residue, after oil removal, is used for animal feed.

Coconut husks are an important source of fiber called coir. In coir production, mostly limited to India, the nuts are harvested about a month before maturity and the husks retted in brackish water for 8–10 days to rot away the soft tissues between the fibers. The fiber is cleaned and washed by hand and dried. In recent years the industry has become partially mechanized. The various grades of coir are used for ropes, mats and matting, and upholstery filling.

In the tropics of both the Orient and the Occident the coco palm is the most useful of all plants to the native population. An important source of food and drink, it also furnishes building material, thatch, hats, dishes, baskets, and many other useful items. *See* NUT CROP CULTURE.

[LAURENCE H. MAC DANIELS]

Diseases. Several diseases attack the coconut plant. Diseases in wild palms adjoining the plantations add to the difficulty of maintaining healthy cultivated stock.

Bud rot, caused by *Phytophthora palmivora*, is controlled to some extent by spraying, fertilizing, and hygiene. Insects and poor nutrition also cause bud failure. Deficient nutrition is associated with four diseases: tapering stem or pencil point, bronze leaf wilt, bitten leaf, and little leaf. Palms weakened by the last three often have odd symptoms when infected by such fungi as *Diplodia*, *Pestalotia*, and *Ceratocystis*. Stem bleeding occurs when *Ceratocystis* enters growth cracks resulting from unbalanced nutrition. This and other fungi such as *Ganoderma*, *Fomes*, *Rhizoctonia*, and *Fusarium* may also cause root rot. Thread blight, *Corticium*, also attacks leaves of vigorous palms.

Cadang-cadang, a serious disease in the Philippines, results from a virus. In the West Indies is another virus disease known as lethal yellowing. Red ring, caused by a nematode, *Aphelenchoides cocophilus*, spreads easily and may be fatal, but it can be stopped by sanitation measures. *See* PLANT DISEASE; PLANT VIRUS.

[FREDERICK L. WELLMAN]

Coffee

Commercially, coffee is the most important caffeine beverage plant in the world. Arabica coffee is a shrub or small tree of the genus *Coffea* (Rubiaceae) and a native of Abyssinia. There are 59 species, but only 4 are of commercial importance. Nine-tenths of the world supply of coffee is obtained from the Arabian species, *C. arabica* (Fig. 1), of which there are about 15 varieties. Coffee is strictly a tropical crop requiring a moderately cool climate that is moist but not wet. The fruit, called a cherry, is a small spherical drupe containing two seeds, the coffee beans. In the wet method the cherries are picked by hand, then pulped and allowed to ferment, and thus the membranes are removed. In the dry method cherries are harvested and allowed to dry, and the exocarp is milled off. The coffee beans are then graded and packed in burlap bags. Finally, the beans are roasted to develop the aroma, flavor, and color desired.

[PERRY D. STRAUSBAUGH/EARL L. CORE]

Diseases. There are more than 350 known diseases of coffee, and new ones are still being discovered on *C. arabica*, *C. canephora*, *C. liberica*, and *C. excelsa*, in widely separated tropical lands. Probably no crop grows under more varied conditions or is subjected to so many unknown diseases.

The leaf rust (*Hemileia vastatrix*), one of the great plagues of man's crops, at first eliminated coffee from many Eastern countries. However, it never became established in the Occident. In Africa and the Orient, control is now obtained by

COFFEE

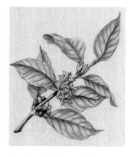

Fig. 1. *Coffea arabica.*

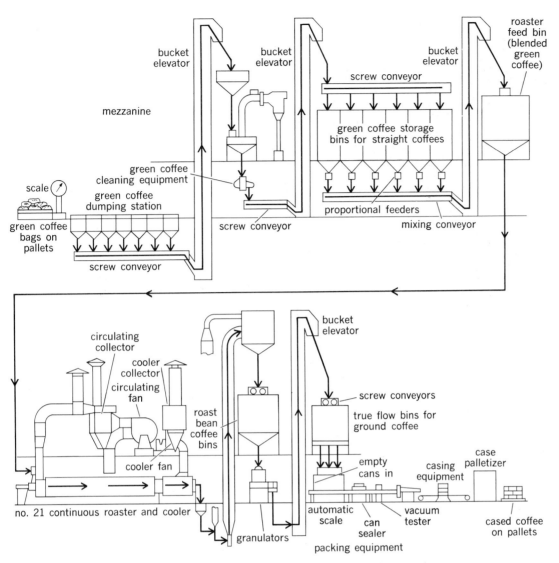

Fig. 2. Modern continuous roasting plant for processing coffee. (*Jabez Burns and Sons, Inc.*)

sprays, and there are new plants selected for resistance. American leaf spot (*Mycena citricolor*) is very serious but it is found only in the Americas, whereas *Cercospora* leaf spot and the leaf rot *Pellicularia koleroga* occur in both hemispheres. The latter are controlled by spraying.

Fruit, stem, and branch infections are injurious. Wilts and trunk cankers, caused by *Gibberella*, *Nectria*, and *Ceratocystis*, are troublesome. Probably six *Rosellinias*, a few *Fusaria*, two *Armillarias*, and fungi like *Fomes*, *Ganoderma*, and *Polyporus* attack roots. Root and trunk infections are reduced by good cultural practices. Coffee is also affected by a half-dozen viruses, two bacteria, and numerous parasitic mistletoes. *See* PLANT DISEASE CONTROL; PLANT VIRUS.

[FREDERICK L. WELLMAN]

Processing. Coffee is the beverage prepared by controlled extraction from ground roasted beans with hot water. Beans are produced in tropical or subtropical climates.

Blending. Green beans are packed and transported in hemp bags. The commercial unit is 60 kg, about 132 lb. On arrival at the roasting plant, beans from many sources are crudely blended to achieve a particular flavor.

Cleaning. The beans are cleaned both before and after roasting. Pneumatic separators remove dust, lint, strings, hulls, and other light material from the green beans. Batches of 12 bags or about 1500 lb are fed through the cleaner and the beans are completely mixed. One modern unit will handle 5000 lb an hour.

Roasting. Roasting is the most important operation in coffee processing because it develops the flavor. Modern automatic control makes possible precise transfer of energy from a source to the beans. To roast 1500 lb of beans, approximately 525,000 Btu must be delivered in 54 min.

Systems now employ externally heated gases of combustion, mainly nitrogen, carbon dioxide, and water vapor, circulated at extremely high velocities to scrub off insulating gas films and permit rapid heat penetration. In batch roasters, energy at relatively low temperatures, 800–900°F, develops fine flavor and a uniform brown color in about 12 min. In continuous roasters, energy is transferred even more efficiently (Fig. 2). Temperature is reduced to about 500°F and roasting time to about 5 min.

Light roasts are attained at bean temperatures of 380–390°F; medium roasts, 400°F; and dark roasts, 425–430°F. At 450°F excessive decomposition of fiber and oils occurs.

At the end of batch roasts, water at the rate of 1 gal per 100 lb is sprayed onto the beans to check or quench the roast, after which the beans are dumped and rapidly air-cooled. Beans roasted continuously are only air-cooled.

Stoning. The second cleaning operation is called stoning. Roasted beans have only half the density of green beans (20 versus 40 lb/ft³) and are lifted by air currents away from heavy material, stones, and other debris. The beans are deposited in specially designed bins which prevent segregation as the beans pass to the grinders.

Grinding. There are two types of grinding mills, the plate or compactor, and the roll or granulator. The plate mill tends to crush particles and yield a higher proportion of fine material than does the granulator with its cutting action. Most grinds contain particles ranging in size between 0.023 and 0.055 in.

Packaging. Can packs, in which the initial vacuum is about 29 in., retain flavor for many months. Some can packs are pressurized with inert gas for flavor retention. Flexible containers made of paper laminated with plastic film or aluminum foil are not vacuumized nor are they gas tight, so storage life is much shorter.

Instant coffee. Soluble or instant coffee manufacturing now utilizes about 20% of the green beans imported.

Preliminary processing is the same as for regular coffee. The roasted beans, however, are equilibrated to a higher moisture content, 7–10%, and ground very coarsely to eliminate fines.

Liquid coffee is made by passing water at temperatures up to 300°F through ground beans in a series of extracting towers (as many as eight) with at least one stage of partial hydrolysis under pressure. This yields an extract containing about 30% solids. From 30 to 35% of the grounds is removed.

After filtration the extract is usually spray-dried in systems that yield hollow beads of solids. But the extract also can be dried in a low temperature vacuum system or it can be freeze dried. The moisture content is reduced to less than 3%. *See* DRYING.

The product is hygroscopic and must be held and packaged under conditions of low humidity. Manufacturers are attempting to return the aroma lost during processing and much research is under way.

Decaffeinated coffee. Decaffeinated coffee, both regular and instant, is prepared from green beans that have been softened by steam, extracted with low-boiling chlorinated solvents, then steamed again to remove residual solvent, and dried.

[ERNEST E. LOCKHART]

Bibliography: A. E. Haarer, *Coffee Growing*, 1963; M. Sivetz and H. E. Foote, *Coffee Processing Technology*, 2 vols., 1964; F. L. Wellman, *Coffee*, 1961.

Cola

A tree, *Cola acuminata*, of the sterculia family (Sterculiaceae) and a native of tropical Africa. Its fruit is a star-shaped follicle containing eight hard seeds, the cola nuts of commerce (see illustration).

These nuts are an important masticatory in many parts of tropical Africa. They have a caffeine content twice that of coffee. The nuts also contain an essential oil and a glucoside, kolanin, which is a heart stimulant. Cola nuts, in combination with an extract from coca, are used in the manufacture of the beverage Coca-Cola. Cola is now cultivated in West Africa, Jamaica, Brazil, India, and other parts of tropical Asia. *See* COCA.

[PERRY D. STRAUSBAUGH/EARL L. CORE]

Colchicine

An alkaloid contained in the corm (underground stem) of the autumn crocus (*Colchicum autumnale*) (see illustration) of the lily family (Liliaceae). In medicine the drug is used principally in the treatment of gout. Colchicine has a specific influence on the division of plant chromosomes, and has been much used by geneticists and plant breeders to bring about doubling of chromosomes, thus producing tetraploid plants. Most colchicine comes from the Netherlands, Italy, Yugoslavia, and Hungary.

[PERRY D. STRAUSBAUGH/EARL L. CORE]

Cold storage

The storage of perishables at low temperatures, usually above freezing, by the use of refrigeration to increase the storage life. In general, the lower the temperature, the longer the storage life. If temperatures are maintained below the freezing point of the product stored, it is called freezer storage. Most fruits and many other products, however, are damaged by freezing and cannot be stored in freezer storage. A cold-storage plant is a large insulated building, with its attendant refrigeration equipment, for storage of commodities at low temperatures. Facilities are often included for quick-freezing fruits, vegetables, meats, and a variety of precooked foods and bakery products for the consumer convenience market. *See* FOOD PRESERVATION.

[CARL F. KAYAN]

Collard

A cool-season biennial crucifer, *Brassica oleracea* var. *acephala*, similar to nonheading cabbage. Collard is of Mediterranean origin and is grown for its rosette of leaves, which are cooked fresh as a vegetable (see illustration). Kale and collard differ only in the form of their leaves; both have been referred to as coleworts, a name taken from the Anglo-Saxon term meaning cabbage plants.

Propagation is by seed. Cultural practices are similar to those used for cabbage; however, collards are more tolerant of high temperatures. Georgia and Vates are popular varieties (cultivars). Collard is moderately tolerant of acid soils. Harvesting is usually 75 days after planting. Important production centers are in the southern United States, where collards are an important nutritious green, especially during winter months. *See* CABBAGE; KALE; VEGETABLE GROWING.

[H. JOHN CAREW]

Corn

Zea mays occupies a larger area than any other grain crop in the United States, where 60% of the world production is grown. Production is widely

COLA

(a)   **(b)**

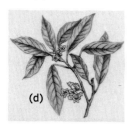

(c)

(d)

Cola (*Cola acuminata*). (a) Seed. (b) Section of fruit showing seed. (c) Fruit. (d) Branch of tree.

COLLARD

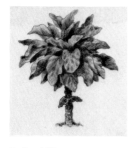

Collard (*Brassica oleracea* var. *acephala*).

distributed throughout the United States, but it reaches its greatest concentration in the states of Iowa, Illinois, Indiana, Ohio, Nebraska, Minnesota, Wisconsin, Michigan, and Missouri. This area, called the Corn Belt, is characterized by moderately high temperature, fertile, well-drained soils, and normally adequate rainfall. The Corn Belt accounts for approximately 80% of corn production in the United States. The average corn acreage for the period 1970–1973 was slightly in excess of 60,000,000 acres (1 acre = 4047 m²), with production in excess of 5,000,000,000 bu (1 bu = 0.03524 m³). Although corn is grown in the United States primarily for livestock feed, about 10% is used for the manufacture of starch, sugar, corn meal, breakfast cereals, oil, alcohol, and other specialized products. In many tropical countries, corn is used primarily for human consumption.

Origin and description. From its presumed origin in Mexico or Central America, corn has been introduced into all the countries of the world that have suitable climatic conditions. However, the corn of today is far different from the primitive types found in prehistoric sites excavated in Arizona, Mexico, and Peru. The origin of corn is still unsettled, but the most widely held hypothesis assumes that corn developed from its wild relative teosinte (*Z. mexicana*) through a combination of favorable mutations, recognized and selectively propagated by early humans. Corn migrated from its center of origin and was being cultivated by the Indians as far north as New England when the first European colonists arrived, whose survival was due largely to the use of corn as food.

Botanically, corn is a member of the grass family. Certain seed types within the species *Z. mays* were given subspecific rank by early investigators. Among these types are the dents (*indentata*), flints (*indurata*), soft or flour (*amylaceae*), sweet (*saccharata*), pop (*everta*), and pod (*tunicata*). Each form (botanical variety) is conditioned by fairly few genetic differences, and each may exhibit the full range of differences in color, plant type, maturity, and so on, characteristic of the species. All types have the same number of chromosomes (10 pairs), and all may be intercrossed to produce fertile progeny. Dent corns are the most important in the United States. Kernel texture is less homogeneous in other areas of the world. Soft types tend to predominate at higher elevations, flint types at lower elevations. This pattern is due, in part, to differences in methods of food preparation, but it has also been influenced by the greater resistance of flint types to stored-grain insect pests, which are more prevalent at lower elevations. Sweet corn is grown more extensively in the United States than in any other country. It is eaten as fresh corn or canned or frozen. In other countries, flint, dent, or flour corns may be eaten fresh, but at a much more mature stage than the sweet corn eaten in the United States. The commercial production of popcorn is almost exclusively American. Pod corn is grown only as a genetic curiosity.

Varieties and types. Corn is a cross-pollinated plant, the staminate (male) and pistillate (female) inflorescences (flower clusters) are borne on separate parts of the same plant (Fig. 1). Plants of this type are called monoecious. The staminate inflorescence is the tassel; it produces pollen that is

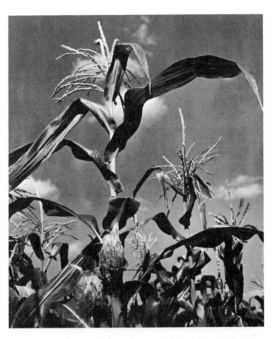

Fig. 1. A corn plant in full tassel (above) and silk (below). The tassel produces pollen that is blown by wind to the silks. (*Courtesy of J. W. McManigal*)

carried by the wind to the silks produced on the ears. Natural cross-pollination permits maintenance of a high degree of genetic variability. As corn was carried by the Indians to different environments in North, Central, and South America, a large array of varieties ultimately was developed. Many of these primitive varieties still exist today. Extensive efforts have been devoted to the collection, classification, and maintenance of this valuable reservoir of genetic variability. Settlers migrating westward took with them their corn seed (botanically fruits). In time, by both planned and natural selection, a large number of varieties and local strains became established and adapted to the new ecological conditions. These strains varied in color of grain, plant, and ear characteristics, and in length of time required to reach maturity. Because of the variability associated with cross-pollination, corn is a highly plastic species, and varieties have been developed that are well adapted to a frost-free growing season of less than 90 days or, in contrast, grow 12–15 ft (1 ft = 0.3 m) tall and require more than 200 days to reach maturity, as in certain areas in Guatemala.

Hybrids. The development of varieties and strains of corn made possible the extension of its culture under diverse soil and climatic conditions. However, modern research methods, used for its further improvement, led to the present widespread use of hybrid corn. Today essentially all of the corn grown in the United States is planted to hybrid seed, and this technology is being adopted in other areas of the world as rapidly as suitable hybrids are developed. *See* BREEDING (PLANT).

Hybrid corn is the first generation of a cross involving inbred lines. Inbred lines are developed by controlled self-pollination. When continued for several generations, self-pollination leads to reduction in vigor but permits the isolation of types which are genetically pure or homozygous. Intense selection is practiced during the inbreeding phase to identify and maintain genotypes having the desired plant and ear type and maturity characteristics, and relative freedom from insect and disease attacks. After the inbred lines have become fairly pure, they are further evaluated in hybrid combinations. Crosses involving any two unrelated lines will exhibit heterosis, that is, yields above the means of the two parents. Only a very few combinations, however, exhibit sufficient heterosis to equal or surpass hybrids in current commercial use. Hence large-scale experimental testing is required to identify new useful combinations.

The first commercial hybrids were double crosses produced by crossing two single crosses, each, in turn, having been produced by the crossing of two inbred lines. Hybrid seed for commercial planting is produced in special crossing blocks (isolated fields). The field is planted with the parents (inbred lines or single crosses) in alternating groups of rows.

The plants in blocks to be used as female parents are detasseled before silk emerges. Thus all seed produced will be pollinated by the male parent. After drying, sizing, and treatment, the seed harvested from the female rows becomes the hybrid seed of commerce. Since the early 1960s the use of single-cross hybrids has been increasing, and in the Corn Belt today probably accounts for 80% or more of the seed used.

Several techniques have been used to control pollination. Initially, manual removal of the tassels was used exclusively. Then cytoplasmic male sterility was used. This type of male sterility is transmitted only through the cytoplasm of the female parent. Since no fertile pollen is produced, no detasseling is required. With this system, pollen production in the farmers' fields is provided either by blending (artificial mixing of sterile and fertile types) or by the use of genetic fertility-restoring factors introduced through the male parent. In 1970 possibly 90% of the hybrid seed used in the United States utilized a single type of cytoplasmic sterility: the Texas type. This cytoplasmic type proved to be susceptible to a new mutant race (race T) of one of the leaf-blight fungi, *Helminthosporium maydis*, and thus the use of this type of sterility was discontinued. Investigations of other types of cytoplasmic sterility are under way. Machines which cut or pull tassels in the seed fields have been developed and are being used extensively. Other types of genetic control of pollen production have been developed, and some attention is being given to the possible use of chemical sterilants.

Companies specializing in hybrid seed production now produce and market the entire seed supply — more than 10,000,000 bu annually. Gains from the use of hybrid seed have been spectacular. The shift from open-pollinated varieties to hybrids, beginning in the 1930s, accounted for a yield increase of 25%. In succeeding years these first hybrids have been replaced by newer, higher-yielding types which have greater disease and insect resistance. Hybrid succession is a continuing process; few hybrids have a commercial life of more than 5 years. The per-acre yield of corn has increased about threefold since the first introduction and use of hybrid seed.

Planting. Planting dates depend upon temperature and soil conditions. Germination is very slow at soil temperatures of 50°F (10°C), and seedling growth is limited at temperatures of 60°F (16°C) or below. Because of these temperature relations, planting begins in Florida and southern Texas in early February and is completed in New York and New England by late May or early June. Planting rates are influenced by water supply, soil type, and fertility and by the maturity characteristics of the hybrid grown. Planting rates for full-season hybrids may vary from 8000 to 12,000 plants per acre in eastern Texas to 20,000 to 24,000 in the central Corn Belt. Check-planting, with hills and rows spaced 38–42 in. (1 in. = 2.5 cm) apart, has been almost completely replaced by drilling. With planting rates above 16,000 plants per acre, drilling in rows 24–36 in. apart has become common practice. The use of nitrogen fertilizer has increased greatly; lesser amounts of phosphorus and potash are applied as needed. Soil tests and experience provide useful guides to economic rates of fertilizer use under different environmental conditions.

Since 1950 there has been a marked trend toward reducing the amount of tillage in seedbed preparation. The variations in the planting systems used are influenced by soil type and topography, amount of crop residues on the soil surface, and the weed-control system to be employed. The use of the minimum tillage system, in which all soil preparation as well as planting is performed in one passage across the field, is increasing. This system, and less extreme modifications of the conventional system, reduces total energy costs.

Weed control. Weed control may be effected by cultivation or herbicides or both. With minimum tillage planting methods, weed control may be more difficult than with conventional seedbed preparation because of crop residues left on or near the surface. Weeds are easiest to control mechanically when they are small, preferably be-

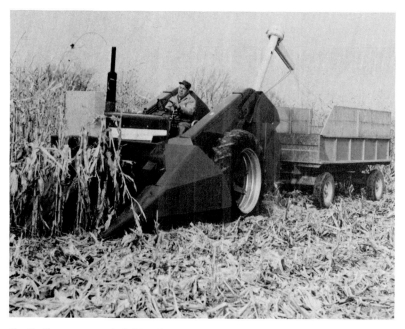

Fig. 2.   Two-row mounted picker for harvesting corn.

fore they emerge. The most efficient and economical tool for killing weeds at this stage is the rotary hoe. Unfortunately this or other mechical cultivation systems are relatively ineffective during extended periods of rainy weather. Disk or shovel cultivators are used after the corn is 6–8 in. (15–20 cm) in height.

Increasing use is being made of selective herbicides. Most broadleaf and grassy weeds may be controlled without damage to corn. Herbicides may be applied either "preplant" or "preemergence." If applied prior to planting, herbicides may be left on the soil surface or incorporated into the soil. Preemergence applications may be made as the seed is planted, or at any time prior to crop emergence. The choice of the many herbicides available is dependent upon many factors, including the type of weeds to be controlled and the farming system used. Under unfavorable early-season weather conditions, neither mechanical nor chemical control nor their combination may be completely effective, and sizable yield reductions may result. *See* HERBICIDE.

Harvesting. Harvesting of corn has undergone a major revolution since 1930. In the 1930s most corn was husked by hand, and the ears were stored in slatted cribs. Harvesting began when the moisture content of the grain had been reduced, by natural drying, to 20–24%. The mechical picker supplanted hand harvesting. The mechanical picker, in turn, has been replaced by the picker-sheller or corn combine, which harvests the crop as shelled grain (Fig. 2). Labor needs for hand harvesting were well over 100 man-hours per 100 bu of corn in the 1930s. Currently, the most efficient farmers spend little more than 1 man-hour per 100 bu. Energy requirements, however, have increased materially. When harvested as shelled grain, at a relatively high moisture content (20–30%), the grain must be dried artificially for safe storage. High-moisture corn to be used for livestock feed may be stored in airtight silos or may be treated with certain chemical preservatives such as propionic acid. Corn stored under either of these systems is not suitable either for industrial processing or for seed. *See* AGRICULTURAL SCIENCE (PLANT); AGRICULTURE, MACHINERY IN.

[G. F. SPRAGUE]

Diseases. Worldwide, more than 112 diseases of corn are known. All do not occur in any one area or time and individual diseases seldom become so severe that a grower is forced out of production. Losses, however, are estimated at 7–17% of the crop, which represents approximately $500,000,000 loss in the 12 leading corn-producing states. It is possible that corn disease loss may become more severe because of wider adoption of continuous cropping, increased fertilization, high plant populations, and uniformity of type.

Many corn diseases, such as corn smuts, are easily recognized, but others are not so evident and are identified only by exacting diagnostic techniques. Many disease losses go undetected, or they may be blamed on unfavorable climatic or soil factors.

Seedling diseases. Seed decay and seedling blights caused by seed or soil-borne *Fusarium* (*Gibberella*) sp., *Diplodia zeae*, *Penicillium* sp., or *Pythium* sp. are troublesome when seed is planted

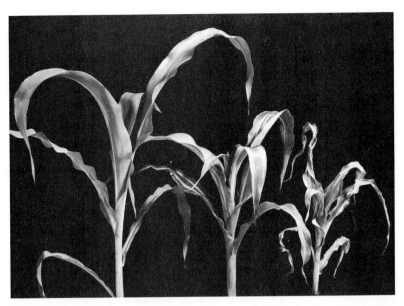

Fig. 3. Bacterial wilt, or Stewart's disease. Corn plant on left is healthy. (*Ohio Agricultural Research and Development Center*)

in cool, moist soil. Planting sound, mature, and chemically treated seed reduces these problems.

Foliage diseases. Of the approximately 25 leaf blights, only a few are important in the United States. Northern corn leaf blight, caused by *Helminthosporium turcicum*, is the most destructive. This disease is common in humid regions and appears to be favored by moderate temperatures and heavy dews. Resistant hybrids are used for control. Of several bacterial leaf diseases known, only one, bacterial wilt or Stewart's disease, caused by *Xanthomonas stewartii*, is of major concern (Fig. 3). This bacterium causes a severe wilt of sweet corn and a leaf blight on dent corn. The best control is resistant varieties, but insecticides can be used to reduce the corn flea beetle which overwinters and spreads the causal bacterium.

Rust and smut. Common or boil smut, caused by *Ustilago maydis* (Fig. 4), is found wherever corn is grown, but losses seldom exceed 2% over any area.

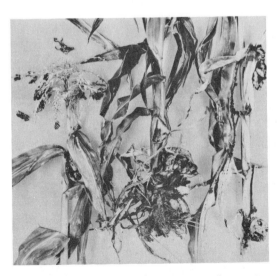

Fig. 4. Corn smut on various parts of plant. (*University of Minnesota Agricultural Experimental Station*)

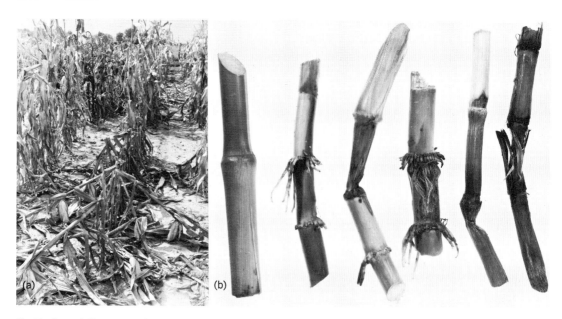

Fig. 5. Corn stalk rot, one of the most widespread corn diseases. (*a*) Corn lodged from stalk rot. (*b*) Bacterial stalk rot, with healthy corn stem on left. (*Ohio Agricultural Research and Development Center*)

Galls may appear on any plant part, and they are usually most prevalent on vigorous plants in soil high in organic material and nitrogen, and increase with mechanical injuries. Control is to plant hybrids with some resistance. The small cinnamon-brown to black particles of common corn rust, caused by *Puccinia sorghi*, on leaves are almost universal where corn is grown. Most widely used varieties have good field resistance.

Stalk and root diseases. Stalk and root rots, primarily caused by *Gibberella zeae, Diplodia zea, Marcrophomina phaseoli,* and *Fusarium moniliforme,* are the most serious and widespread diseases of corn, with annual losses as high as 8–10% for a state and 25% for localized areas (Fig. 5). Conditions favoring disease development may cause plants to die before maturity. This results in poorly filled ears, but the greatest loss may be from stalk lodging, resulting in harvest difficulties and loss of ears on the ground. Many factors affect stalk rot: unbalanced fertility, high plant populations, dry weather in early summer followed by wet weather after silking, leaf damage, delayed harvest, and perhaps continuous cropping. No specific control measures are available other than selection of a locally adapted variety or hybrid with good performance.

Ear diseases. A number of ear rots occur in the field and storage (Fig. 6). Field ear rots increase when humidity and rainfall are high in fall months, by insect and bird damage, by early frosts, and on fallen stalks. Principal pathogens are the fungi *Fusarium (Gibberella), Diplodia, Nigrospora,* and *Cladosporium.* Storage rots, primarily caused by *Aspergillus* and *Penicillium* fungi, can be controlled by proper drying of corn and proper aeration and temperature while in storage. Rotted grain not only causes loss of quality, but may cause digestive disturbances, estrogenic problems, and other illnesses when fed to animals.

Virus diseases. Prior to 1963 viruses were not a factor in corn production, except in localized areas outside the United States. That year maize dwarf mosaic virus (MDMV) (Fig. 7) and corn stunt virus (CSV) appeared in economic proportions in the United States. Both viruses have caused almost complete destruction of susceptible corn in some areas. MDMV has been identified in 15–20 states, in the Corn Belt as well as eastward and southward. CSV is believed to be primarily confined to the Deep South. Aphids are the insect vectors of MDMV and three species of leafhoppers are known to transmit CSV. Resistant corn hybrids

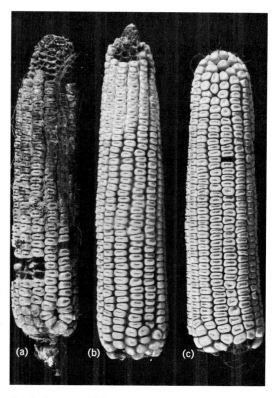

Fig. 6. Ear rots. (*a*) Storage rot. (*b*) Field rot. (*c*) Healthy ear. (*Ohio Agricultural Research and Development Center*)

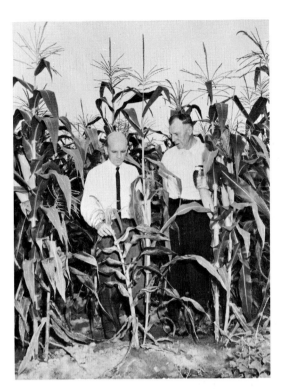

Fig. 7. Corn plant infected with maize dwarf mosaic virus. (*Ohio Agricultural Research and Development Center*)

are used to control MDMV. Wheat streak mosaic virus (WSMV) has been found in certain inbred lines and hybrid corns in some Corn Belt states. The mite vector of WSMV, *Aceria tulipae*, has been determined as causing kernel red streak of corn grains, presumably by the excretion of a phytotoxin while feeding. This disease first appeared in portions of Indiana, Michigan, and Ohio and spread to other areas. Sugarcane mosaic, maize leaf fleck, cucumber mosaic, barley yellow dwarf, barley stripe mosaic, and bromegrass mosaic viruses can infect corn. Some of these have not been found in corn in nature, and one of them has caused serious economic losses. *See* PLANT DISEASE; PLANT DISEASE CONTROL; PLANT VIRUS.

[LANSING E. WILLIAMS]

Processing. Corn may be processed for three general purposes: animal feed, human food, or industrial uses. For animal feed, it may be cracked or ground by a variety of methods, including hammer, burr, or roller mills. For human consumption, cornmeal is produced by grinding either between millstones or with steel rolls. Millstones, which grind slowly at low temperature, are commonly used by small mills, especially in the South. The steel roller system is used by larger corn millers.

Four main parts of the corn kernel are hull, germ, gluten, and starch. The object of milling is to separate these components which, on a moisture-free basis, constitute the following percentages of the entire corn kernel: hull, 6%; germ, 11%; gluten, 11%; endosperm, 70%. The products from milling are corn flour, cornmeal, and feed by-products. Dent corn, either white or yellow, is preferred to flinty varieties for manufacturing cornmeal.

In processing corn two systems are used: dry milling and wet milling.

Dry milling. Shelled corn is passed over magnetic separators to eliminate foreign material and then through scourers to remove the tip cap from the end of the kernel. The cap is often dark and may produce black specks in the finished meal. If the shelled corn is higher than 12% moisture, it may be dried to about that percentage before cleaning and grinding operations. In the process of tempering or conditioning, water is added to toughen the bran before milling. The corn needs to be somewhat dry at the start so that moisture added during tempering will loosen the bran and germ. Water often is added in stages to bring the moisture content to more than 20%; the corn then is allowed to stand several hours. Warm water and steam may be utilized for this purpose prior to milling.

Degermination is accomplished in a machine which contains a horizontal, revolving, cone-shaped drum, covered with small metal projections. This drum is in a housing also studded with metal projections and having small perforations. As the corn passes through the machine, the bran and germ are, to a large extent, pulled from the kernel, and the endosperm is broken into several large pieces. The fine particles of hull and germ pass through the perforations and are thus separated from the endosperm. The stock passes to grading reels where the different-sized particles are separated. From the grading reels, the particles are sent to centrifugal aspirators which remove loose bran. The various grades of aspirated corn fragments are gradually reduced to coarse, medium, and fine grits as they pass between corrugated rolls, with sifting and bolting operations in the same sequence as in wheat milling. The flow sheet for corn milling, though simpler, is similar to that of wheat milling.

Grits intended for industrial use are generally flaked. This is accomplished by steaming the grits before they pass between heavy-duty, heated rolls, operating at approximately the same speed. The heat of pressing between heated rolls causes partial gelatinization of the starch.

Wet milling. Wet-process corn milling is used to separate the various components of the kernel for industrial purposes. The industrial use of corn to manufacture starch, dextrin, and dextrose (glucose) uses as much as 100,000,000 bu per year. In addition, oil is recovered from the germ and fiber, as well as gluten for use in animal feeds. Some corn is utilized for industrial fermentations, especially in time of warfare when the demand often exceeds the supply obtainable from molasses. *See* GLUCOSE; STARCH.

In the wet milling process, which uses in excess of 200,000,000 bu per year, clean corn is steeped from 36–48 hr in diluted sulfurous acid solution to loosen the hull and soften the gluten. At the end of the steeping period, the corn contains 40–50% moisture. The wet corn is passed through a special type of attrition mill consisting of studded rotary plates which turn in opposite directions and tear the kernel apart. This makes possible the separation of the germ, hull, and disintegrated endosperm. Separation is accomplished by passing the material through long tanks as a slurry. Here the germ rises to the surfaces, and the particles of endosperm settle to the bottom. The settlings are separated from the liquid by passing through reels, then they are reground on burr mills to permit the separation of starch, gluten, and hulls. The discharge from the burr mill goes through a series of reels and shakers which permit the starch and gluten, but not the particles of hull, to pass through the bolting cloth. The suspension of starch and gluten flows slowly down slightly inclined, flat-bottomed troughs called "tables." The starch settles on the tables while the gluten passes along with the solution. In some plants, centrifuges separate starch from gluten. Starch collected from the tables is given a series of washings before it is dried in rotary vacuum driers. From there, the product can be further processed into corn sugar (dextrose), corn syrup, or corn starch.

The corn germ is kiln-dried, preheated, and the oil extracted by either pressure or solvent. The oil cake is ground and marketed as oil cake meal for animal feed. The gluten tailings from the tables are concentrated in settling tanks, filtered, and pressed to become a feed by-product. Corn containing 16% moisture will yield about 66% starch, 30% feed material, and 3% oil.

In addition to the usual dry milling operation, corn grits can be further processed into various kinds of breakfast foods. Corn grits are steam-cooked, flavored in various ways, sweetened, combined with other ingredients, processed for careful moisture control, and passed through flaking rolls. The flakes are then toasted. *See* FOOD ENGINEERING; FOOD MANUFACTURING.

[JOHN A. SHELLENBERGER]

Bibliography: W. C. Galinat, The origin of maize, *Annu. Rev. Genet.*, 5:447–478, 1971; A. L. Hooker, *17th Annu. Hybrid Corn Ind. Res. Conf.*, vol. 17, 1962; M. B. Jacobs (ed.), *The Chemistry and Technology of Food and Food Products*, 1951; M. A. Joslyn and J. L. Heid, *Food Processing Operations*, vol. 3, 1964; R. H. Moll and C. W. Stuber, Quantitative genetics: Empirical results relevant to plant breeding, *Advan. Agron.*, 26:277–322, 1974; L. R. Nault et al., *Phytopathology*, vol. 57, 1967; M. C. Shurtleff et al., *N. Cent. Reg. Ext. Publ.*, no. 21, 1967; G. F. Sprague and W. E. Larson, *Corn Production*, U.S. Dep. Agr. Handb. no. 322, 1975; W. N. Stoner and L. E. Williams, *47th Annu. Rep. S. Seedsmen Ass.*, 1965; A. J. Ullstrup, *USDA Agr. Handb.*, no. 199, 1961; R. L. Whistler and E. F. Paschall, *Starch: Chemistry and Technology*, vol. 2, 1967; L. E. Williams et al., *Plant Disease Rep.*, vol. 51, 1967.

Cover crops

Crops grown for the express purpose of preventing and protecting a bare soil surface. Many crops serve this purpose, and some give a high direct economic return. Other crops of lower return value are mainly important as a part of a system of good soil and water conservation and soil productivity maintenance, and it is these that are ordinarily considered cover crops.

Basic benefits of cover crops are in the prevention of soil detachment by wind, rainfall, and splash erosion (Figs. 1 and 2) and in the return of cover crop roots and tops to replenish and add to the supply of soil organic matter.

Permanent cover. Cover crops can be readily grown in humid climates and in arid and semiarid

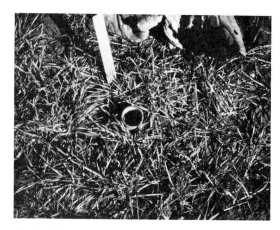

Fig. 1. Soil splash container in a representative location of domestic ryegrass (mixture of *Lolium perenne* and *L. multiflorum*) cover located in cabbage field. This level of cover almost eliminates soil splashing by raindrops.

climates where irrigation provides sufficient water so that cover crops do not rob the soil of needed moisture. Reseeded rangeland is an outstanding example of the use of cover crops. Long-lived grasses such as blue gramma *(Bouteloua gracilis)*, buffalo grass *(Buchloë dactyloides)*, and the bluestems *(Andropogon* sp.) have been widely seeded upon many different soil conditions in the Great Plains. When properly managed, these supply excellent ground cover and grazing for livestock. *See* GRASS CROPS.

Many special areas such as road banks, ditch banks, and recreation areas need the protection of permanent vegetative cover of high quality. A variety of grasses and legumes may be used, depending upon soil and climatic conditions. Crown vetch *(Coronilla varia)* provides a luxurious cover for many road bank conditions. Reed canary grass *(Phalaris arundinacea)* and tall fescue *(Festuca elator)* have been widely and successfully utilized to stabilize ditch banks and waterways. In the northern United States, Kentucky bluegrass *(Poa pratensis)* provides cover for many recreation areas, while in the southern United States Bermuda grass *(Cynodon dactylon)* serves the same purpose.

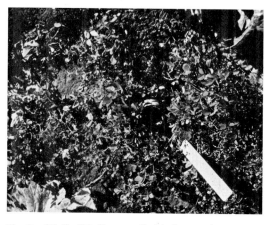

Fig. 2. Alfalfa *(Medicago sativa)* being used as a cover crop. Less effective in preventing splash erosion than domestic ryegrass, it does fix nitrogen from the air.

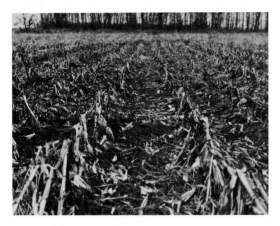

Fig. 3. Early spring view of rolling corn field protected by stalk residues and domestic ryegrass cover.

Management considerations. With the development of low-cost nitrogen fertilizer and more efficient herbicides and insecticides, cover crops now require special management. Low-cost commercial nitrogen has tended to replace man's dependence on the nitrogen produced by leguminous cover crops. Efficient herbicides, such as atrazine, when sprayed over a row crop area will destroy not only all broadleaf and grass weeds but also most seeded cover crops, making it impossible to use domestic ryegrass or other cover crops between crop rows. The use of herbicide in bands, directly over the rows of the main crop, enables the grower to cultivate the row crop and to seed the cover crop between the rows.

Annual winter legumes. A wide range of possibilities exist for the use of cover crops, especially where growers wish to maintain and improve soil productivity. In some areas the so-called naturally reseeding annual winter legumes can be utilized in the row crop each year. Once these plants have matured in a field, there are usually enough hard-coated seeds to establish in the autumn after having remained dormant during the dry summer period. Thus, provided enough seed is scattered to maintain the hard seed supply, one can obtain seed, grazing plants, or hay from a cultivated field plus a normal row crop such as corn or cotton. With this system soil fertility has been known to improve year after year under a system of dual harvests. This system of cover-cropping use still needs intensive study and development.

In general, these kinds of cover crops are restricted to the southeastern United States, where the growing season is long and the winter is mild. Varieties of vetch, most of which are annual legumes, are utilized, including hairy vetch (*Vicia villosa*) and smooth vetch (*V. villosa* var. *glabrescens*), the two commonly grown. Crimson clover (*Trifolium incarnatum*), rough pea (*Lathyrus hirsutus*), button clover (*Medicago orbicularis*), bur clover (*M. arabica*), and black medic (*M. lupulina*) are also used as naturally reseeding legumes.

Spring crops. Many ordinary spring-sown crops can be advantageously used as cover crops. Spring oats (*Avena sativa*) sown in the fall are killed by cold weather but provide excellent ground cover during the fall and winter. Buckwheat (*Fagopyrum esculentum*) can be used as a cover crop to protect

the soil and as a smother crop to control weeds, and at the same time can be turned under for soil improvement. Cereal rye (*Secale cereale*) is widely seeded as a cover crop following the harvest of the main crop.

Advantages. In northern areas it is not unusual for a cover crop like domestic eyegrass to return 4 or more tons of roots and tops to the soil (Figs. 1 and 3). In warmer climates more is produced. Where a legume is utilized, the added benefit of nitrogen fixation is also obtained (Fig. 2). As compared to an annual splash loss of 5 tons of soil per acre per year on bare land, cover-cropped areas suffer little or no splash erosion. They also provide better support and traction for harvesting equipment. *See* AGRICULTURE, SOIL AND CROP PRACTICES IN; NITROGEN FIXATION (BIOLOGY); SOIL CONSERVATION.   [PAUL J. ZWERMAN]

Bibliography: S. R. Aldrich and E. R. Leng, *Modern Corn Production,* 1966; H. Kohnke, *Soil Physics,* 1968; J. H. Martin and W. H. Leonard, *Principles of Field Crop Production,* 1967; L. C. Pearson, *Principles of Agronomy,* 1967.

Cowpea

Vigna unguiculata ssp. *unguiculata,* a legume of such ancient cultivation that its country of origin, either in Asia or Africa, is uncertain. Large-scale production occurs mainly in the southern United States, Africa, the Mediterranean region, and Australia. It was cultivated as early as 1714 in North Carolina. Cowpeas are grown primarily in the United States as a vegetable crop and are also known as southern peas and blackeye peas, the

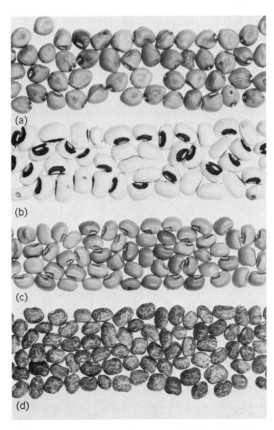

Fig. 1. Four seed types of cowpea. (*a*) Brown Crowder; (*b*) California Blackeye No. 5; (*c*) Dixielee; (*d*) New Era.

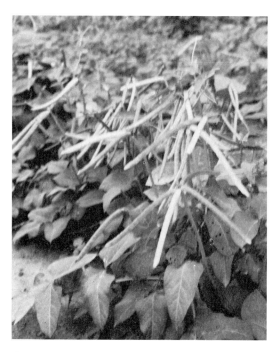

Fig. 2. Cowpea variety grown for processing. Pods are borne above plant.

latter referring to a group of varieties. It is also grown as a hay and forage crop but to a much less extent than in the past. In the tropics and subtropics, cowpeas provide food for millions of people and feed for a large number of livestock. It is cultivated extensively in western Africa and is the principal source of dietary protein in Nigeria.

Varieties. There are at least 200 varieties in the United States, but only about 20 of these are of commercial and home garden importance. All varieties have been arranged in groups based on seed size, shape, color, and color pattern, and on pod color and plant type, either upright or vining (see Figs. 1 and 2).

Cultivation. Cowpeas are grown commercially in the southern United States for fresh market, canning, freezing, and also in home gardens. Soil type is not usually a limiting factor as they grow well on most soils, require very little fertilizer compared with most vegetable crops, and withstand short periods of drought. Seeds are planted when the danger of a killing frost is over. Plantings are made in rows 3 to 3½ ft (0.9 to 1 m) apart with seeds spaced 3 to 4 in. (8 to 10 cm) apart. Two cultivations are generally required during the season.

Harvesting. Depending on variety, from 60 to 75 days are required to reach maturity. Pods are harvested before the seeds become dry, although some blackeye varieties are marketed as dry, mature seeds. Almost all of the commercial acreage for processing is harvested with machines that remove the pods from the vines and shell them in one operation. With other machines, the pods are harvested and shelled in the processing plant. The use of cowpeas as a vegetable crop has increased steadily since 1965. Plant breeders continue to develop more productive, disease-resistant varieties with improved nutritive values. *See* Legume forages.

[BLAKE B. BRANTLEY, JR.]

Diseases. Wilt caused by *Fusarium oxysporum* f. *tracheiphilum*, and root knot caused by nematodes (*Meloidogyne* sp.) are destructive diseases of cowpeas. They are most injurious on sandy soil and often occur together. Three parasitic races of the fungus causing wilt are recognized. Mississippi Crowder is a vegetable-type cowpea highly resistant to race 1 wilt and tolerant to races 2 and 3.

Bacterial canker caused by *Xanthomonas vignicola* attacks the stems and leaves. Cowpea varieties that are resistant to canker include Iron, Brabham, Victor, Groit, New Era, and Brown Sugar Crowder.

Numerous leaf spots occur on cowpeas as minor diseases caused by a variety of microorganisms. These include zonate spot caused by *Aristastoma aeconomicum*, target spot caused by *Corynespora cassiicola*, and bacterial spot caused by *Pseudomonas syringae*.

Fungi that rot the pods are *Choanephora cucurbitarum* and *Botrytis cinerea*.

Diseases that attack the roots and basal portion of the stem are sclerotial blight caused by *Sclerotium rolfsii*, charcoal rot caused by *Macrophomina phaseoli*, sore shin caused by *Rhizoctonia solani*, and cotton root rot caused by *Phymatotrichum omnivorum*.

Cowpea mosaic, a virus disease, is characterized by chlorotic leaves and stunted growth. It is one of the few plant virus diseases reported to be transmitted by a beetle (*Ceratoma trifurcata*). *See* Plant disease; Plant virus.

[HOWARD W. JOHNSON]

Cranberry

The large-fruited American cranberry, *Vaccinium macrocarpon*, a member of the heath family, Ericaceae, is a native plant of open, acid peat bogs in northeastern North America. Selections from the wild have been cultivated since the early 19th century. It is an evergreen perennial vine producing runners and upright branches with conspicuous terminal flower buds (see illustration).

Cultivation. A cranberry bog is made by removing the vegetation on a maple, cedar, or brown-brush swamp, draining it by cutting "shore," "lateral," and "main" ditches, spreading 2 or 3 in. (5 or 8 cm) of sand over the leveled peat, and inserting cuttings of the selected variety of vines through the sand into the peat. Rooting occurs readily within a month, but 3 or 4 years of growth and care are required before the first commercial crop is produced. Care includes frost protection in spring and fall, now largely provided by solid-set, low-gallonage sprinkler systems which effect protection much quicker and with only a tenth of the water formerly required with flood frost protection. Flooding is used in winter to protect the cranberry vines, not from cold but from desiccation when the root zone is frozen. Early-season floods are used for the drowning of pest insects.

Because well-tended cranberry bogs continue to produce annual crops for a century or more without replanting, a half-inch (1.3 cm) layer of sand is spread every 3 or 4 years over the vines (by spreading on winter ice when thick enough) to cover the accumulating cranberry leaves on the soil surface where the cranberry girdler insect would otherwise breed and multiply.

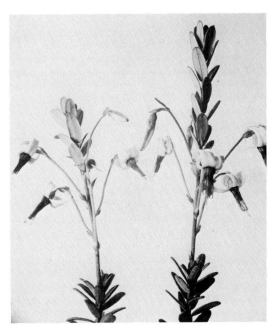

Cranberry uprights in full bloom.

Harvesting. Commercial cranberry growing is confined to Massachusetts, New Jersey, Wisconsin, Washington, and Oregon and to several provinces in Canada. The North American crop annually exceeds 200,000,000 lb (90,000,000 kg) with a raw fruit value to the grower of approximately $25,000,000, but a wholesale product value of nearly $150,000,000, for juices, sauces, relishes, pie fillings, and other uses. Only 40,000,000 or 50,000,000 lb (18,000,000 or 22,500,000 kg) of the cranberries continue to be sold as fresh fruit, and most of these are dry-harvested by machines. Most of the processing fruit is harvested in flood waters, either by machines which pick and deliver the fruit into towed plastic boats or by water reels which detach the berries to float and be driven by wind to shore where they are elevated into bulk trucks. Berries for juice manufacture are usually vine-ripened and deep-frozen for a month or more prior to thawing and extraction. The older form of hand harvest with wood-toothed scoops is now nearly gone, the scoops sometimes being used for ditch-edge picking.

Good-quality fresh cranberries can be stored for several months, refrigerated, with very little loss to decay. Good-quality cranberries can be kept in deep-freeze storage for several years with only minor moisture loss. Frozen berries on thawing are soft and juicy, unlike the firm fresh berry, and must be utilized promptly.

Cranberry bogs in full bloom in early July are a sight to remember because they have 40,000,000 to 50,000,000 white or pink flowers per acre, each of which must be visited by pollinating honeybees or bumblebees to set the berries. The control of frost and winter injury, the control of weeds, insects, and diseases, and the development of more efficient harvest techniques have seen productivity rise from 2000 to over 12,500 lb/acre (2250–14,063 kg/hectare) in the last 50 years. Commercial acreage nationally is stable at about 23,000 acres

(93 km²). Supplies of the fruit are ample to satisfy both domestic and export demand.

The special requirements of the cranberry plant for low fertility, acid soil, and winter protection make it a poor choice for home garden cultivation. *See* FRUIT GROWING, SMALL.

[CHESTER E. CROSS]

Cress

A prostrate hardy perennial crucifer of European origin belonging to the plant order Capparales. Watercress (*Nasturtium officinale*) is generally grown in flooded soil beds and used for salads and garnishing. Propagation is by seed or stem cuttings. High soil moisture is necessary. Leafy stems are cut usually 180 days after planting. Virginia is an important producing state.

Garden cress (*Lepidium sativum*) is a cool-season annual crucifer of western Asian origin grown for its flavorful leaves. Propagation is by seed, and leaves are harvested approximately 2 months after planting.

Upland or spring cress (*Barbarea verna*) is a biennial crucifer of European origin, grown and harvested similarly to garden cress but of lesser commercial importance. *See* VEGETABLE GROWING.

[H. JOHN CAREW]

Cubeb

The dried, nearly ripe fruit (berries) of a climbing vine, *Piper cubeba*, of the pepper family (Piperaceae). This species is native to eastern India and Indomalaysia (see illustration). The

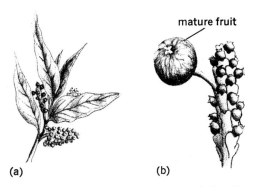

Cubeb (*Piper cubeba*). (a) Leaves and fruit spikes. (b) Spike showing a mature fruit with long pedicel.

crushed berries are smoked, and the inhaled smoke produces a soothing effect in certain respiratory ailments. Cubebs are used in medicine as a stimulant, expectorant, and diuretic. Medicinal properties of cubeb are due to the presence of a volatile oil which formerly was thought to stimulate healing of mucous membranes.

[P. D. STRAUSBAUGH/EARL L. CORE]

Cucumber

A warm-season annual cucurbit (*Cucumis sativus*) native to India and belonging to the plant order Campanulales.

Production. The cucumber is grown for its immature fleshy fruit which is used primarily for pickling and for slicing as a salad. The develop-

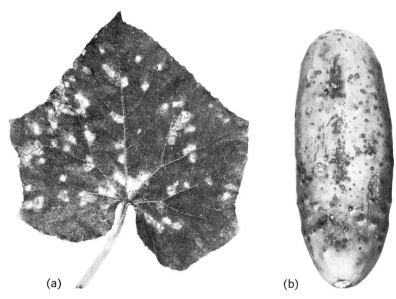

(a)   (b)

Fig. 1. Angular leaf spot disease of cucumber caused by bacterium *Pseudomonas lachrymans.* (a) Leaf spots. (b) Fruit lesions. (*Courtesy of J. C. Walker*)

ment of gynoecious (bearing only female flowers) and hybrid varieties (cultivars) with increased disease resistance is resulting in a continuing change in the varieties of both pickling and slicing cucumbers. In addition, the advent of mechanical harvesting and chemical weed control for pickling cucumbers is altering traditional methods of culture, for example, higher plant populations per acre and single harvests instead of multiple pickings. Important cucumber-producing states are Florida and South Carolina for fresh market and Michigan and Wisconsin for pickling. The total

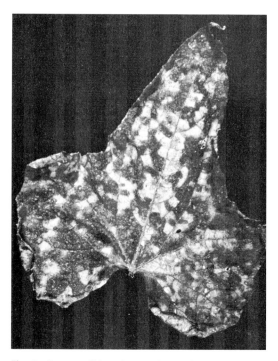

Fig. 2. Downy mildew of cucumber leaf showing yellow angular blotches induced by *Pseudoperonospora cubensis.* (*Courtesy of D. E. Ellis*)

annual farm value in the United States from approximately 170,000 acres is approximately $65,-000,000. *See* SQUASH; VEGETABLE GROWING.

[H. JOHN CAREW]

Diseases. Diseases of cucumbers reduce plant growth, fruit yield, and product quality in both field and greenhouse plantings. Because cucumbers are grown all months of the year, it is necessary to guard against seeding in unfavorable environments and to control seed decay and seedling blight.

Bacterial diseases. Bacterial wilt is a serious disease in the midwestern, north-central, and northeastern regions of the United States, but it is not important in the South or West. Plants infected with the causal bacterium *Erwinia tracheiphila* first show a wilting of a single leaf which remains green, but later all the leaves wilt and the plant dies. A white, stringy, viscid bacterial ooze shows in freshly cut wilting stems. Bacteria-infested spotted and striped cucumber beetles infect the plant while feeding upon it. The bacteria multiply in the plant and become distributed throughout the vascular system. The bacteria overwinter in the body of the insect. Because the only way in which the plants can become infected is through the feeding of the cucumber beetles, control depends upon early and prompt destruction of these pests by insecticides.

Angular leaf spot, incited by the bacterium *Pseudomonas lachrymans,* causes water-soaked spots on leaves and bordered, circular lesions on fruits. The lesions later develop into a brown firm rot extending into the flesh (Fig. 1). The causal bacterium overwinters on infected vine refuse, is seedborne, and is spread by rain and surface water. Control consists of using California seed, which is low in infection, soaking it for 5 min in a mercuric chloride solution (1 part in 1000 parts of water), rinsing the seed in water, and planting promptly.

Fungus diseases. Downy mildew is a destructive disease in the eastern and southern states where the weather is warm and moist, is less damaging in the north-central states, and rarely occurs in the Southwest. It is incited by the leaf-inhabiting fungus *Pseudoperonospora cubensis,* which causes angular, yellowish spots; the spots later turn brown when the leaves shrivel (Fig. 2). The loss of foliage interferes with normal flower set and fruit development. Maturing fruits fail to color properly, are tasteless, and are usually sunburned. Planting of resistant varieties, such as Ashley, Palmetto, Palomar, Santee, and Stono, and treating plants with copper fungicides will provide maximum protection from downy mildew.

Scab is a serious disease in the northern and northeastern states, especially during cool moist weather. The causal fungus, *Cladosporium cucumerinum,* produces small, circular, halo-bordered, water-soaked lesions on leaves and stems. The greatest damage is to the fruit and appears as sunken, dark-brown spots on immature fruit and as rough corky lesions on mature fruit. Control is achieved by planting resistant varieties, such as the slicing variety Highmoor or the pickling varieties Wisconsin SR 6 and SMR 12.

Virus diseases. The cucumber mosaic virus causes mottling of terminal leaves and dwarfing of vines, as well as mottling and varying malformations of the fruits. The virus is harbored in a number of perennial hosts and is spread by aphids. The best means of control is provided by planting resistant varieties, such as the slicing varieties Burpee Hybrid, Niagara, Ohio MR 200, Sensation Hybrid, Shamrock, and Surecrop Hybrid, and pickling varieties Ohio MR 17, Ohio MR 25, Wisconsin SMR 12, and Yorkstate. *See* PLANT DISEASE; PLANT VIRUS.

[JOHN T. MIDDLETON]

Cumin

Aromatic fruits which were highly prized by the ancients. The plant, *Cuminum cyminum* (Umbelliferae), is an attractive little annual herb, now cultivated extensively in southern Europe and India. The fruits are used in soups, curries, bread, cake, cheese, and pickles. The oil is used in perfumery and for flavoring beverages. *See* SPICE AND FLAVORING.

[PERRY D. STRAUSBAUGH/EARL L. CORE]

Currant

A shrubby, deciduous plant of the genus *Ribes*, order Rosales, related to the gooseberry. The fruits are berries, borne in clusters (Fig. 1).

Varieties. The black currant (*R. nigrum*), popular in Europe, is not cultivated in the United States. Red currants are derived from five species, mostly European. There are also white currants which are variants of the red type. Only the red varieties are produced commercially. Currants are grown in home gardens throughout most of the central and northern part of the United States. The greatest commercial production occurs in the states of New York, Washington, and Michigan, but production has been declining in recent years. *See* GOOSEBERRY.

[J. HAROLD CLARKE]

Currant and gooseberry diseases. The diseases of currants and gooseberries are similar and are rather generally distributed throughout the areas in which these crops are grown.

Anthracnose (*Pseudopeziza ribis*) first produces numerous small brownish spots thickly scattered over the upper surfaces of the leaves (Fig. 2). As the disease progresses, the leaves turn yellow and drop, and in severe cases the entire plant may become defoliated. Anthracnose is controlled by applying a commercial lime-sulfur spray while the plants are dormant, followed by sprays with cop-

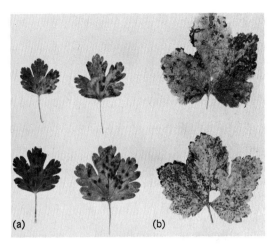

Fig. 2. Anthracnose disease on (*a*) gooseberry (small leaves) and (*b*) currant (large leaves).

per or dithiocarbamate fungicides during the growing season.

American powdery mildew (*Sphaerotheca morsuvae*) first appears as a white powdery growth on the young leaves, shoots, and fruits, and eventually forms a thin felty reddish-brown coating over the affected tissues. This mildew is favored by cool humid weather. It is most damaging on gooseberries, especially those of European origin. The disease is difficult to control, but clean culture and spraying with sulfur usually are effective.

Some species of currants and gooseberries are alternate hosts for the white-pine blister rust (*Cronartium ribicola*), a destructive disease of five-needle (white) pines in Europe and America. The common black currant is the favored host of the fungus. Because the white pines are among the most valuable timber trees in the United States, the black currant has been declared a menace and eradicated in most areas. Other important diseases of currants and gooseberries are leaf spot (*Mycosphaerella ribis*) and cane blight (*Botryosphaerea ribis*). *See* FRUIT GROWING, SMALL; PLANT DISEASE. [EDWARD K. VAUGHAN]

Curry

A mixture of plant spices used with meats and fish and other seafoods, each requiring its own specific curry. One recipe calls for a mixture of turmeric, coriander, cinnamon, cumin, ginger, cardamon, cayenne pepper, pimiento, black pepper, long pepper, cloves, and nutmeg. See separate articles on each of these spices. *See* SPICE AND FLAVORING. [PERRY D. STRAUSBAUGH/EARL L. CORE]

Cysteine

An amino acid. The amino acids are characterized physically by the following: (1) the pK_1, or the dissociation constant of the various titratable groups;

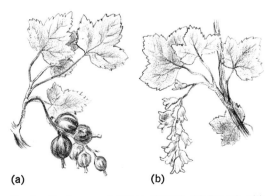

Fig. 1. Black currant (*Ribes nigrum*). (*a*) Branch with cluster of fruits. (*b*) Branch with flowers.

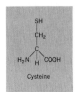

Physical constants of the L isomer at 25°C:
pK_1 (COOH): 1.96 (30°C); pK_2 (NH_3^+): 8.18; pK_3 (SH): 10.28
Isoelectric point: 5.07
Optical rotation: $[\alpha]_D(H_2O)$: −16.5; $[\alpha]_D$(5 N HCl): +6.5
Solubility (g/100 ml H_2O): very soluble

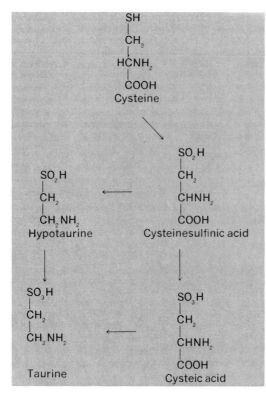

Fig. 1.   Metabolic degradation to taurine.

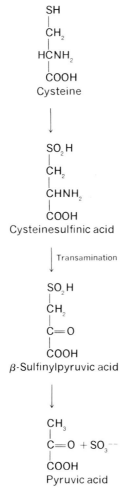

Fig. 2.   Metabolic degradation to pyruvate and sulfite.

(2) the isoelectric point, or pH at which a dipolar ion does not migrate in an electric field; (3) the optical rotation, or the rotation imparted to a beam of plane-polarized light (frequently this beam is the D line of the sodium spectrum) passing through 1 dm of a solution of 100 g in 100 ml; and (4) solubility.

Cysteine forms a red-brown color with 1,2-naphthoquinone-4-sodium sulfonate in a highly alkaline reducing medium (Sullivan reaction). A blue color is formed when cysteine is heated with p-aminodimethylaniline in acid solution, in the presence of ferric ammonium sulfate.

In microorganisms, cysteine probably is formed from serine and inorganic sulfate or sulfide. In animals, cysteine is formed by transsulfuration of serine with the homocysteine from dietary methionine. A variety of metabolic degradation pathways are known, of which the principal ones are the following:

1. Degradation to pyruvate, hydrogen sulfide (H_2S), and ammonia (NH_2).

2. Oxidation to cysteic acid and decarboxylation of this compound to taurine; an intermediate is cysteinesulfinic acid. Alternatively, cysteinesulfinic acid can be decarboxylated to hypotaurine (Fig. 1).

3. Transamination (as cysteinesulfinic acid) with α-ketoglutarate to form β-sulfinylpyruvate, which breaks down spontaneously to pyruvate and sulfite (Fig. 2).

Cysteine furnishes the sulfhydryl group of coenzyme A and, in microorganisms, of homocysteine, the precursor of methionine. It is a constituent of the tripeptide coenzyme, glutathione, and of the amino acid cystine. See AMINO ACIDS; CYSTINE; METHIONINE.   [EDWARD A. ADELBERG]

Cystine

An amino acid. The amino acids are characterized physically by the following: (1) the pK_1, or the dissociation constant of the various titratable groups;

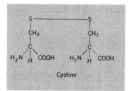

Physical constants of L isomer at 25°C:
pK_1 (COOH): 1.00 (30°C); pK_2 (COOH): 1.7
pK_3 (NH_3^+): 7.48; pK_4 (NH_3^+): 9.02
Isoelectric point: 4.60
Optical rotation: $[\alpha]_D$ (5 N HCl): −232
Solubility (g/100 ml H_2O): 0.011

(2) the isoelectric point, or pH at which a dipolar ion does not migrate in an electric field; (3) the optical rotation, or the rotation imparted to a beam of plane-polarized light (frequently the D line of the sodium spectrum) passing through 1 dm of a solution of 100 g in 100 ml; and (4) solubility.

Cystine after reduction gives the specific reactions for cysteine. Cystine can be reversibly reduced to cysteine. It is formed biosynthetically from cysteine, by oxidation. In addition to the metabolic degradation pathway of cysteine, cystine may also be oxidized directly to cystine disulfoxide, which is decarboxylated and then further oxidized to taurine.

[EDWARD A. ADELBERG]

Cytokinins

Chemical substances which elicit a certain array of plant growth and development responses. Before being classified as a cytokinin, a substance must

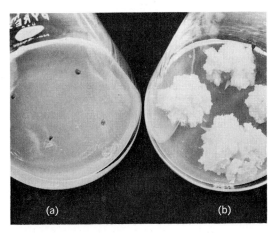

Fig. 1. Cultures of soybean tissue on complete media demonstrating the effects of kinetin on plant growth. (a) Medium without kinetin. (b) Medium with $2 \times 10^{-6}\ M$ kinetin after 5 weeks of growth.

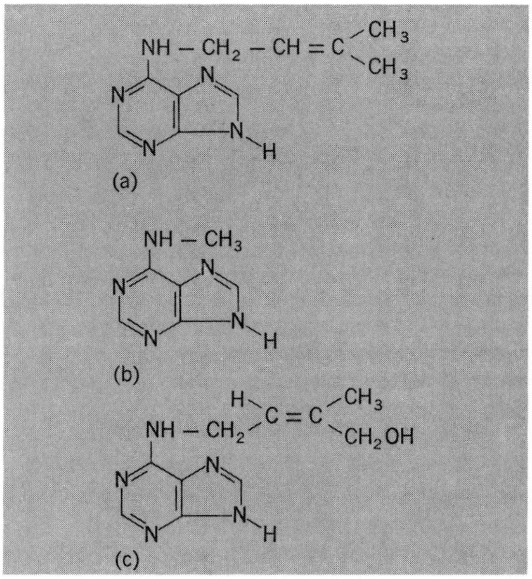

Fig. 3. Structural formulas for three cytokinins: (a) isopentenylaminopurine, (b) methylaminopurine, and (c) zeatin (hydroxyisopentenylaminopurine).

be tested under very particular conditions since other classes of plant growth substances (especially auxins and gibberellins) may promote some similar responses. An especially clear-cut criterion for a cytokinin is the requirement that a compound promote cell division in excised tissues grown on standard media containing auxins as well as vitamins, mineral salts, and sugar. Tissues derived from tobacco stem, soybean cotyledons (Fig. 1), and carrot roots have been used most frequently, and have yielded essentially the same qualitative and quantitative results. These cell division tests have delimited a group of compounds, the most potent of which not only elicits all of the other growth effects previously observed with kinetin but also resembles kinetin in terms of chemical structure. *See* AUXIN; GIBBERELLIN; PLANT GROWTH.

Structural characteristics. Kinetin was the first of the very active cytokinins to be recognized and identified. It may be regarded as a derivative of adenine, a purine compound which plays several extremely important roles in all living things. Adenine is 6-aminopurine, whereas kinetin is 6-furfurylaminopurine (Fig. 2). The furfuryl group of kinetin may be replaced by numerous groups, biological activity being retained although perhaps quantitatively modified. Among other active compounds are the isopentenyl- (Fig. 3a), hydroxyisopentenyl- (Fig. 3c), phenyl-, benzyl-, n-hexyl-, n-pentyl, n-butyl-, and even methylaminopurines (Fig. 3b) with the indicated substituent being attached to the amino group at the 6 position of the purine ring. In many tests 6-benzylaminopurine seems to be more active than kinetin. In the cell division tests the hydroxyisopentenyl derivative (zeatin, Fig. 3c) is the most active of all known naturally occurring compounds.

Effectiveness of the *n*-alkyl analogs is decreased as the chain length is shortened from five or six carbons down to one or as the chain length is increased to above six carbons. These alkyl derivatives attract attention because they are the simplest of the purine cytokinins, and their structures suggest that fat solubility is an important factor in cytokinin action. The purine ring itself is a part of the most active defined compounds, but at least some changes can be made in the ring without nullifying completely the effectiveness in biological tests. Thus replacement of the carbon in the 8 position by a nitrogen atom yields the still active 8-*aza*-kinetin, and addition of an amino group on the 2 position lessens but does not eliminate activity. Addition of groups such as ribose, ribose phosphate, or tetrahydropyrine at the 9 position may alter but not destroy activity in cell division tests; the possibility exists, however, that the cell removes such groups and then uses the free cytokinin.

A group of synthetic substances, including *sym*-diphenylurea (Fig. 4) and many related compounds along with thiourea derivatives, display cytokinin activity in at least some of the biological tests. The effectiveness of these compounds seems generally to be less than that of the more potent purine compounds.

Biological effects. Cell division in cultured tissues may be promoted by some cytokinins at very low concentrations. The effect of zeatin, for example, can be detected at a concentration as low as

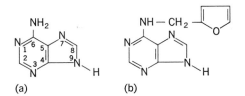

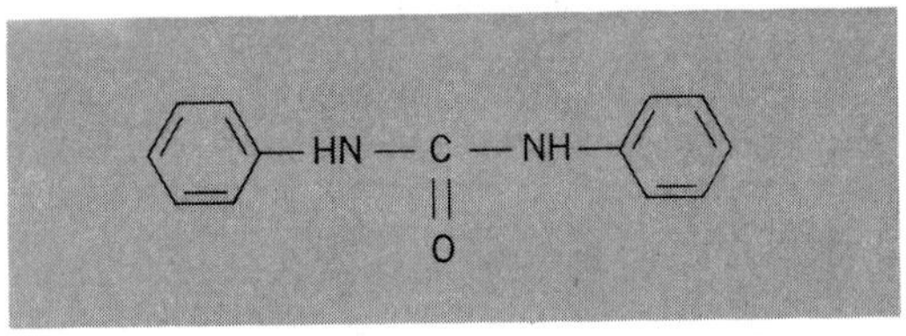

(a)   (b)

Fig. 2. Structural formulas for (a) adenine and (b) kinetin, the type compound for cytokinins.

Fig. 4. Structural formula for diphenylurea, a synthetic compound with cytokinin activity.

5×10^{-11} M, which is about 0.00001 mg/liter. Most other cytokinins are less effective than zeatin, but still may be needed by the cells at concentrations less than 1 mg/liter (that is, less than 1 part per million).

Another effect frequently studied is the preservation of chlorophyll in detached leaves or in pieces of leaves such as those of barley, oats, cocklebur, and tobacco. In many species a leaf begins losing its chlorophyll very soon after being detached from the plant, but treatment with a cytokinin slows this loss. Associated with the chlorophyll loss is the lowering of protein and ribonucleic acid levels; these decreases also may be retarded by cytokinin treatments. This information applies to many detached vegetable materials, and the use of cytokinins to maintain quality during shipping and marketing of vegetables has possibilities.

Expansion of young leaves, such as those of bean and radish, may be promoted by the cytokinins. Of extreme interest is the ability of cytokinins to promote the formation of new shoots in tissue cultures or parts of plants. Examples of this effect include promotion of leafy shoot formation, which has been observed in cultures of pith from tobacco, cotyledons, hypocotyls, roots and leaf fragments of lettuce, pieces of begonia leaves, African violet leaves, and the protonemata of several species of mosses. Cytokinins at very low concentrations also may promote root formation in species such as tobacco and soybean, but inhibit the process at slightly higher concentrations. The outgrowth of the lateral buds is stimulated by cytokinins, thereby overcoming the dominance which is exerted by the apical buds.

Other effects include promotion of seed germination, breaking of dormancy of some buds, stimulation of the mobilization of various metabolites to the point at which the cytokinin has been applied, retardation of senescence, increased anthocyanin or flavonoid synthesis, stimulation of the opening of stomates, increased resistance to heat shock and gamma radiation, both inhibition and enhancement of cell enlargement (depending on the plant material), and acceleration or retardation of flowering. A few effects on viruses, bacteria, fungi, algae, and animal cells have been reported, but no consistency is apparent as yet.

Occurrence. Kinetin, the type compound, was first obtained from heated preparations of deoxyribonucleic acid and has not been found to occur naturally. Zeatin, or its derivatives, has been isolated and chemically identified from several sources including young kernels of maize, coconut milk, young plums, chicory roots, several mycorrhizal fungi, and from crown gall tumors of *Vinca rosea*. Its ribose nucleoside and ribose phosphate nucleotide forms, with the substituents at the 9 position, have been identified both from green plant and fungal sources. Isopentenylaminopurine is produced by the bacterium *Corynebacterium fascians*. It is of interest that this bacterium invades green plants and, apparently by secreting the compound, produces cytokinin effects; especially obvious is the outgrowth of lateral buds to such an extent that the plant may become a thick mass of very short stems. A dihydroderivative of zeatin has been isolated from lupin plants; this compound differs from zeatin only in that the double bond of the side chain has been saturated with hydrogen. 6-Methylaminopurine, naturally occurring in many organisms, displays low cytokinin activity.

Metabolic action. Compounds having cytokinin activity occur in certain ribonucleic acids. Both zeatin and isopentenylaminopurine have been identified in certain transfer ribonucleic acids which combine with amino acids before the amino acids are incorporated into proteins. That this represents the mode of action of the cytokinins is open to speculation; if so, responsive tissues would be expected to incorporate supplied cytokinins into the ribonucleic acid. Considerable evidence has been obtained that the incorporation does occur to a small extent. This mode of action could explain directly several cytokinin effects — especially those effects on ribonucleic acid, protein, and chlorophyll levels — and indirectly perhaps most of the growth effects. There are several facts which do not fit the proposal, but these will perhaps in time be accommodated by elaborations of the idea.

Of course, it may be that the cytokinin effects will eventually be explained by entirely different mechanisms. Regardless of the mechanism, a complete explanation of cytokinin action hopefully will clarify the means by which cytokinins and auxins interact in so many expressions of growth and development. The two types of substances act together in some situations, such as in promotion of cell division, but seem to oppose each other in the control of other phenomena, such as lateral bud outgrowth. The interaction always seems to be quite strong in either case. There are reports of modifications by cytokinins of glucose utilization, respiratory rates, flavonoid synthesis, and enzymatic activities, but the information does not afford as yet any explanation of cytokinin effects on growth and development. *See* PLANT HORMONES; PLANT PHYSIOLOGY.

[CARLOS MILLER]

Bibliography: C. B. Crafts et al., Detection and identification of cytokinins produced by mycorrhizal fungi, *Plant Physiol.*, 54:586–588, 1974; R. H. Hall, Cytokinins as a probe of developmental processes, *Annu. Rev. Plant Physiol.*, 24:415–444, 1973; J. P. Helgeson, The cytokinins, *Science*, 161: 974–981, 1968; H. Kende, The cytokinins, *Int. Rev. Cytol.*, 31:301–338, 1971; D. S. Letham, Regulators of cell division in plant tissues; V: A comparison of the activities of zeatin and other cytokinins in five bioassays, *Planta*, 74:228–242, 1967; C. O. Miller, Ribosyl-*trans*-zeatin, a major cytokinin produced by crown gall tumor tissue, *Proc. Nat. Acad. Sci. USA*, 71:334–338, 1974; T. Murashige, Plant propagation through tissue cultures, *Annu. Rev. Plant Physiol.*, 25:135–166, 1975; F. Skoog et al., Cytokinins, *Annu. Rev. Plant Physiol.*, 21:359–384, 1970.

Dairy machinery

Equipment used in the production and processing of milk and milk products, including milking machines, cream separators, coolers, pasteurizers, homogenizers, butter-making equipment, evaporators and dryers, and related items of equipment. The equipment must be easy to clean and designed to prevent contamination of the milk or milk products from dirt, oil, soluble metals, insects, and other foreign materials.

Construction and design. Stainless steel, an alloy of chromium and steel, is widely used and is highly satisfactory for direct contact with milk and other food products. If properly used, stainless steel does not affect the flavor and is corrosion-resistant to food products. However, corrosion of stainless steel may be caused by prolonged contact with food or by removal of the protective oxide layer, which must be maintained to provide corrosion resistance. The layer is removed by prolonged contact with chlorine. Stainless steel surfaces must be cleaned regularly after use with detergent solutions, and should be sanitized before, rather than after, use so that excessive chlorine contact will be avoided. Surfaces are sanitized by using a hypochlorite solution of approximately 200 ppm of available chlorine.

Most modern dairy equipment is designed to be cleaned-in-place (CIP), without disassembly, by pumping detergents and cleaning solutions through the entire system. Equipment is specially designed to avoid pockets, to provide smooth surfaces, and to avoid burning-on or buildup of the product on food-contact surfaces.

Certain standards of design, construction, operation, and sanitation of milk and food equipment, known as the 3-A standards, have been established; they were developed by three associations and are widely used throughout the industry. The 3-A standards specify such items as composition of the material, thickness of material (gage), surface finish, design of corners and joints, size, power requirements, and method of utilization.

The science of hydraulics is basic to the fluid-flow processes of pumping, piping, agitating, mixing, centrifuging, and homogenizing.

Electric motors are used to supply power for these processes. Electricity is used for heating for small equipment and for instrumentation and control of processing equipment. Boilers furnish hot water and steam for cleaning (equipment and plant) and pasteurizing operations. Steam is the principal utility used for heating. Heating is a major utility necessary for pasteurization, sterilization, sanitation, and production of evaporated and dried milk. Refrigeration is provided through direct-expansion systems, by sweet water (cooled tap water) systems, or with brine systems for cooling of incoming product, storage, ice cream production, and for control of plant environment.

Refrigeration and heating require the major portion of the energy in dairy and food plants. In a medium-size plant the following basic utilities are required per 1000 gal of processed product: 130 kwhr of electricity, 72 ton-hr of refrigeration, 350 lb of steam, and 8000 lb of water.

Milking machines. These units extract milk from the cow's udder and deliver the milk to an adjacent container or, for a pipeline milking system, directly to a central cooling tank. Teat cups extract milk by intermittent vacuum action on a flexible inner wall called an inflation. A strip cup should be used before milking to check the condition of the milk. Machine milking requires $3\frac{1}{2}-5$ min, which is less time than for hand milking. A milking machine consists basically of a unit for providing a vacuum with a power unit, pipes or

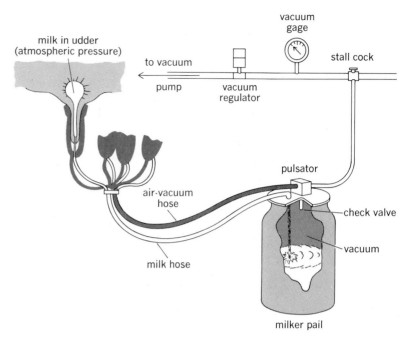

Fig. 1. Arrangement of the component parts of a milking machine.

hoses to the animal, a device for providing pulsations, and a container for collecting the product.

A piston or vane-type pump, usually driven by an electric motor, is used for developing a vacuum of 10–15 in. mercury; a vacuum storage tank next to the outlet of the vacuum pump reduces the fluctuations of the piston. Intermittent action of 45–55 cycles/min is secured by the pulsator unit. Milk may be pumped or transferred to a central point by pipeline using a vacuum.

Types. Milking machines can be classified as portable and pipeline units. The motor and vacuum pump of the portable unit can be either a part of the milker head or on a cart which is moved along behind the cows. The pipeline type can include either a pipeline for the air supply from the vacuum pump to the milker head or a pipeline from the cow to the milk house for transport of milk. With the latter type, there is usually a separate air line. About 1.5 kwhr per cow per month (3–5 cents) is required for electricity for milking using a portable unit.

Operation. Two hoses go to the teat-cup units. One hose, called the air hose, extends from the pulsator, which alternately provides air at atmospheric pressure and vacuum (low pressure) to the teat cups. The other hose is the milk hose, which is under vacuum and moves the milk, caused to flow from the udder at atmospheric pressure, from the teat cups to the milker pail, which is under vacu-

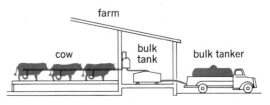

Fig. 2. Handling of milk from cow to tanker.

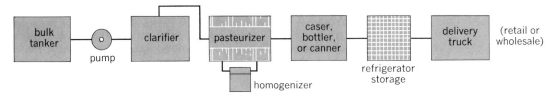

Fig. 3. Processing plant operations.

um, or to the pipeline for a pipeline milking machine (Fig. 1). The rubber inflation surrounds the teat and provides the action for milking by the air-vacuum relationship set up by the pulsator. The rubber inflation is set in the metal cup, and the space between the inflation and the metal cup is alternately connected to air and vacuum, thus resulting in a massaging action. The space inside the inflation is always under vacuum when the teat cups are attached to the cow. The uniform vacuum on the inside of the inflation holds the teat cups in place.

Sanitization. Thorough cleansing of all equipment parts in contact with milk is essential to the production of milk of acceptably low bacteria count. Washing should be done immediately after using by first rinsing with cold water, then hot water using a wetting agent, rinsing with boiling water, and dismantling of equipment. A sanitizing solution may be run through the reassembled equipment just before milking. Local and Federal public health ordinance requirements must be met for equipment and for the milk house.

Farm milk coolers. Milk must be rapidly cooled after production to avoid rapid growth of microorganisms in the product. Milk is normally about 93–95°F as it leaves the cow. Most ordinances require that milk be cooled to 45–55°F within 2 or 3 hr after milking.

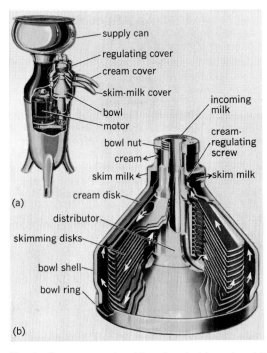

(a)

(b)

Fig. 4. Cream separator driven by electric motor. (a) Entire unit. (b) Cross-sectional view of the separating bowl. (*De-Laval Separator Co.*)

Surface coolers may be used for cooling the milk coming from the cow before it is put in the tanker. The surface cooler may be supplied with cool well water with the final cooling done by mechanical refrigeration. For milk which has been cooled over a surface cooler, the cans may be placed in refrigerated storage to maintain the temperature. Can coolers may be used for cooling the milk coming from the cow to below 50°F. Water is sprayed over the surface of the can or the can is immersed in cold water to provide the cooling. Bulk milk coolers are now widely used for refrigerating and holding milk on farms. Tanks meeting 3-A standards cool milk to 50°F within 1 hr and to 40°F within 2 hr after milking. The temperature of the product should not rise above 50°F when warm milk is added. The milk is normally held at 40°F or below. Milk is normally held 1 or 2 days in the farm bulk tanks (Fig. 2).

Bulk milk tankers. Tankers for bulk milk have insulated cylindrical tanks mounted in a horizontal position, as a trailer or on a truck, and are used for pickup of bulk milk. The tanker driver is responsible for sampling, weighing, checking quality and temperature, and handling the milk. Tolerances for measuring the quantity of product have been established by National Bureau of Standards. The milk is pumped from the farm bulk tank to the tanker to be delivered to the processing plant. At the plant, a pump is usually used for emptying the tanker so that the milk can be transferred from the bulk tanker to a storage tank in the plant. The principal operations in the processing plant are shown in Fig. 3.

Clarifier. A clarifier removes foreign particles from milk by centrifugal force. A filter is sometimes used for this operation but is less efficient than a clarifier. In appearance and operation the clarifier is similar to a separator, but instead of a cream spout, which is on a separator for removal of a portion of the product, the clarifier accumulates the sediment in the bowl. The sediment must be removed periodically in order to maintain product flow.

The milk is normally clarified before homogenization and pasteurization; the process eliminates sediment that may occur before homogenization in the bottled product and prevents the pasteurized product from becoming contaminated. Clarification may be at temperatures of 50–95°F. Generally, a lower temperature of clarification is desired to avoid possible foaming from incorporation of air, to eliminate extraneous material before it is dissolved in the milk, thereby preventing off-flavors, and to reduce removal of components of the product and buildup of sediment in the centrifugal bowl.

Separator. Mechanical centrifugal devices used to extract fat from milk are called cream separators. Milk normally contains 3–6% fat in the form of globules which are lighter in density than the fluid skim milk. These particles rise to the surface when fresh milk is allowed to stand quiescent for several hours and form a layer of cream which may be skimmed from the surface.

In the centrifugal cream separator (Fig. 4), milk is moved into the bottom of an airtight bowl turning at 6000–10,000 rpm, which subjects the milk to radial centrifugal forces up to 500 *g*. The bowl contains stacked disks in the form of inverted cones which divide the milk into thin layers and provide the fluid friction necessary to bring the milk to the needed rotational speed. The angle of the inverted cone is such that the lighter cream particles tend to be forced up the center, where they are removed, and the heavier skim milk flows down the outside of the bowl and into the top, where it is collected. An efficient separator will leave no more than 0.1% fat in the milk.

The usual method of centrifugally separating the cream from the milk is to heat the milk to at least 90°F and as high as 160°F. As the temperature of the milk increases, the viscosity decreases and more efficient separation is obtained. Separators specially designed for efficient separation of cold milk have been developed.

Homogenizer. A homogenizer is a high-pressure pump, which is adjustable in pressure, with three or five pistons, and which forces the milk through small openings to break up and reduce the size of the fat globules. The size of the particles is regulated in general by adjusting the pressure of the valve. One- or two-stage units can be used, with the product passing through one or two homogenizing valves. Pressures from 2000 to 2500 lb per square inch are normally used for single-valve milk homogenizers.

Milk must be heated before homogenization to inactivate lipase activity and to provide efficient breakup of the fat particles. The homogenizer may also be used as a pump.

Pasteurizer. This type of equipment is used to heat milk to a predetermined temperature and hold it at that temperature long enough to kill the pathogenic organisms that may be present, and, equally important, to inactivate enzymes. Satisfactory pasteurization can be obtained at various time-temperature combinations, ranging from at least 30 min at no less than 145°F, for batch pasteurization, to at least 15 sec at no less than 161°F, for high-temperature short-time (HTST) systems. Flash pasteurization at 230°F, followed by discharge into a vacuum chamber for rapid cooling, is also used. This procedure is also termed the vacuum process. Batch-type pasteurizers are heated externally with hot water and require thorough agitation of the milk to heat the milk uniformly. Continuous-flow pasteurizers of the HTST type use regeneration as a means of increasing thermal efficiency by transferring heat from the hot outgoing milk to the cool incoming milk (Fig. 5). Cream and milk products to which sugars or other materials have been added must be given a higher temperature or longer time of pasteurization.

The trend is to higher temperatures and shorter times. Sterilized milk not needing refrigeration is now being produced. Sterilizing milk followed by aseptic packaging provides a means of

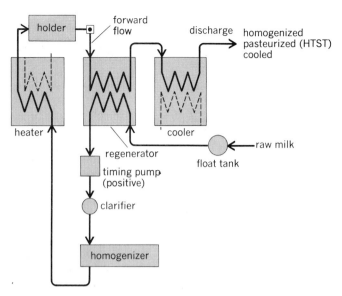

Fig. 5. Schematic representation of pasteurization processes. Details of bypass, relief lines, equalizer, and check valves are not included.

minimum heat treatment and maximum product quality as contrasted with sterilization in the can.

Pasteurized products are placed in glass, metal, paper, or plastic cartons. Some products are placed in bulk containers which are usually placed in cases that are stacked automatically and moved by conveyor into storage. The storage is maintained at 40°F or less. Milk products are often stored in the cooler, in truck lots, so that the retail or wholesale delivery trucks can rapidly make up their loads from the cooler storage. Automatic equipment for stacking and unstacking of cases, for emptying and filling cases with bottles or cartons or both, and for inspecting the cleanliness of containers is used.

Milk is submitted to a vacuum treatment to maintain a uniform flavor and odor by removal of low-boiling-point volatile components. Feed flavors and variation of product throughout the year, which often are caused by volatiles, are removed by submitting the product to a vacuum of 10–20 in. Hg in one or two units. If used, this equipment is normally a part of the overall system of milk pasteurization.

Evaporator and dryer. Water is removed from milk to reduce the bulk and decrease the cost of transportation and storage.

Evaporator. Evaporated milk is produced by removing water to condense the product to 3:1 or 2:1 volume ratios. Condensed milk is often treated by adding sugar. A vacuum pan is operated at a temperature of 130–140°F or at 25 in. Hg vacuum. For large operations, multiple-effect evaporators with one, two, or three stages of moisture removal are used. Decreased steam cost can be obtained with multiple-effect evaporators, a reduction that must be balanced against increased equipment cost. Evaporation usually precedes drying operations. The cost of removing water from the product is less in the evaporator than in the dryer.

Dryer. Dryers are generally of two types: the drum, or roller, dryer and the spray dryer (Fig. 6). The drum dryer is less expensive for moisture removal but has a greater heat effect on the product.

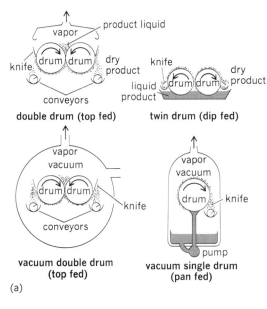

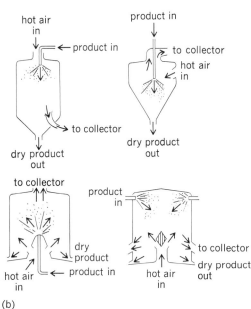

Fig. 6.   Types of milk dryers and method of operation. (*a*) Drum dryers. (*b*) Vertical chamber spray dryers.

With the drum dryer a thin film of product is moved over the steam-heated drum. As the drum turns, moisture is removed and a knife scrapes the product from the drum.

The spray dryer has an atomizing nozzle or a centrifugal device that breaks the product into small droplets. Heated air is forced around the atomizing head and evaporates moisture from the droplets. The dry product is then removed from the dryer. The spray-dried product has better solubility and provides, in general, a more satisfactory product for food. Instantizing equipment provides a procedure whereby dry particles are wetted slightly and agglomerates of particles formed. These agglomerates are then dried. The agglomerates have much more rapid solubility than the nonagglomerated products and provide many products that are known in the trade as instant

products or instant powders. Improvements in methods of processing and drying milk have led to rapid increase in utilization of spray-dried and instantized products for the beverage milk industry. This practice will lead to wide distribution of milk products throughout the United States and the world. *See* BUTTER; CATTLE PRODUCTION, DAIRY; CHEESE; ICE CREAM; MILK.   [CARL W. HALL]

Bibliography: A. W. Farrall, *Engineering for Dairy Food Products*, 1963; C. W. Hall, *Processing Equipment for Agricultural Products*, 1963; C. W. Hall and T. I. Hedrick, *Drying of Milk and Milk Products*, 2d ed., 1971; C. W. Hall and G. M. Trout, *Milk Pasteurization*, 1968; U.S.D.H.E.W., *Grade "A" Pasteurized Milk Ordinance*, 1965.

Dallis grass

A general term for a genus of grasses of which the most important species is the deeply rooted perennial *Paspalum dilatatum*. Dallis grass is widely used in the southern United States, mostly for pasture, and remains productive indefinitely if well managed. Dallis grass does best on fertile soils and responds to lime and fertilizer. On heavier soils it remains green throughout the winter unless checked by heavy frosts. Seed production is hampered by infection with ergot, a fungus that invades developing seeds and produces purplish-black horny bodies. Ergot-bearing seed heads are very toxic to livestock, whether in pasture or in hay, and Dallis grass must be so managed as to prevent consumption of infected heads by livestock. *See* FERTILIZER; GRASS CROPS; PLANT DISEASE.   [HOWARD B. SPRAGUE]

Dasheen

Common name for the plant *Colocasia esculenta*, including the variety *antiquorum* (taro). These plants are among the few edible members of the aroid family (Araceae). Native to southeastern Asia and Malaysia, the plants supply the people with their most important food. The edible corms (underground stems) support a cluster of large leaves 4–6 ft long. A main dish in the Polynesian menu is poi, a thin, pasty gruel of taro starch, often fermented, which is frequently formed into cakes for baking or toasting. The raw corms are baked or boiled to eliminate an irritating substance present in the cells. *See* ARALES.

[PERRY D. STRAUSBAUGH/EARL L. CORE]

Date

The fruit of the evergreen date palm (*Phoenix dactylifera*), a dioecious (each sex on separate plant) species. Pollen, borne only on male palms, must be transferred by hand to inflorescences on female palms to induce fruit production. Date fruits are dry, semidry, or soft, depending on the moisture content at maturity of the particular variety. Soft types tend to spoil or sour more readily ¸than dry types. Most varieties contain about 65% sugar as glucose or fructose. One variety, Deglet Noor, grown primarily in California, contains only sucrose sugar. Palms are propagated by offshoots or suckers and are grown mainly in the semiarid and desert regions of Asia and Africa. Commercial date culture in the United States is limited to areas of high heat (100–120°F; 38–49°C) and low atmospheric humidity, such as the low-elevation deserts of

California and a small part of Arizona. *See* FOOD ENGINEERING; FRUIT, TREE.

[CHARLES A. SCHROEDER]

Defoliant and desiccant

Defoliants are chemicals that cause leaves to drop from plants; defoliation facilitates harvesting. Desiccants are chemicals that kill leaves of plants; the leaves may either drop off or remain attached; in the harvesting process the leaves are usually shattered and blown away from the harvested material. Defoliants are desirable for use on cotton plants because dry leaves are difficult to remove from the cotton fibers. Desiccants are used on many seed crops to hasten harvest; the leaves are cleaned from the seed in harvesting.

True defoliation results from the formation of an abscission layer at the base of the petiole of the leaf. Most of the chemicals bring about this type of defoliation, and the leaves abscise and drop from the plant. Certain fortified oil-emulsion contact herbicides will kill plant leaves at a low application cost, but usually such killing does not result in abscission. *See* ABSCISSION.

The most common agency of defoliation in nature is frost; frosted leaves dry up and fall off after a few days.

Many years ago it was found that a dust of calcium cyanamide applied to cotton plants would result in defoliation. For success, however, it was necessary that the plants be wet with dew and that the humidity remain high for a period of several days and nights.

Because of the advantages of defoliation, much effort has gone into the search for other chemical defoliants. Improved formulations containing calcium cyanamide have been produced; borate-chlorate combinations have proved to be good defoliants; and 3,6-endoxohexahydrophthalic acid (endothall), aminotriazole (ATA), ammonium thiocyanate, magnesium chlorate, arsenic acid, diquat, paraquat, cacodylic acid, tributylphosphorotrithioate, and hexachloroacetone in oil have been used. A new compound, sodium *cis*-3-chloroacrylate, defoliates at 0.5–2.0 lb/acre; desiccation requires up to 5.0 lb/acre.

Alfalfa, clovers, soybeans, field beans, and a good many flower and nursery crops are now defoliated. Other crops such as rice and grain sorghums are sprayed with contact herbicides to prepare them for timely harvest. The term preharvest desiccation is used to describe this process. Since the Pacific campaigns of World War II, work has been going on to discover defoliants for use in jungle warfare. In the war in Vietnam, chemical defoliation of trees became an essential feature of the military effort to prevent ambush and to combat guerrilla methods. Since 1962, millions of pounds of chemical compounds, principally esters of 2,4-D and 2,4,5-T, cacodylic acid, and picloram, have been used in this way. Twin-engined C-123 cargo planes, fitted with 1000-gal tanks and spray booms, carried out the defoliation assignments. Strips bordering highways and waterways were defoliated, as well as borders around military installations, airfields, ammunition dumps, and villages. Defoliants and desiccants were also used to destroy crops. It was in an effort to find such chemical agents that 2,4-D was discovered in 1942 by

E. J. Kraus of the department of botany, University of Chicago. More than 20 years later 2,4-D and 2,4,5-T were the principal compounds used for crop destruction in Vietnam.   [ALDEN S. CRAFTS]

Derris

A genus of tropical shrubs belonging to the legume family (Leguminosae). These plants, with their long branches climbing over other vegetation, occur as members of the jungle undergrowth in Malaysia. Extracts of the roots of *Derris elliptica* have long been used by the natives as an arrow poison and to stupefy fish so they can be caught more easily. Derris root is an excellent insecticide, being harmful to both chewing and sucking insects, but not poisonous to human beings. The insecticidal ingredient of derris root is a white, crystalline substance, which is called rotenone.

[PERRY D. STRAUSBAUGH/EARL L. CORE]

Digestive system

The system consisting primarily of a long tube, the alimentary canal, which includes the mouth, pharynx, esophagus, stomach, small and large intestines, rectum, and anal canal (Fig. 1). In this tube the complicated foodstuffs are progressively split

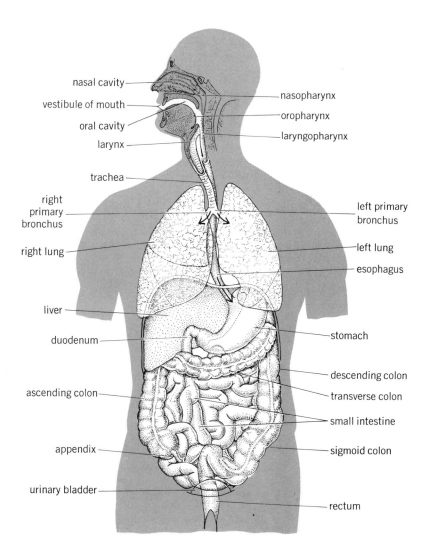

Fig. 1. A schematic representation of the digestive system. (*From G. Wolf-Heidegger, Atlas of Systematic Human Anatomy, vol. 11, Phiebig Publishers, 1971*)

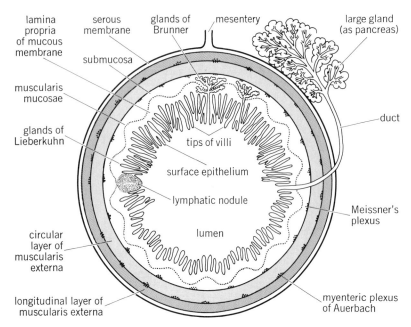

Fig. 2. Cross section of intestinal tract. In the upper half the mucous membrane is depicted with glands and villi as in the small intestine; in the lower half it contains only glands as in the colon. *(From W. Bloom and D. W. Fawcett, Textbook of Histology, 9th ed., Saunders, 1968)*

up into smaller and simpler constituents, which pass through the wall of the canal and are absorbed into the bloodstream. During its passage the food is acted on by secretions of numerous glandular cells which lie in the wall of the canal. The accessory organs of the digestive system lie outside the tube and pour secretions into it by means of ducts.

HISTOLOGY

Nearly all the organs of the alimentary tract have a basic organization of tissue in their walls. There are four layers throughout, but details and degree of development vary in the different parts. These four layers are described below, from inside out (Fig. 2).

Mucosa (mucous membrane). This layer consists of three layers: epithelium, lamina propria, and muscularis mucosae. The lamina propria is a relatively loose connective tissue containing blood vessels, some lymphoid tissue, and usually glands. The muscularis mucosae is a thin layer of smooth muscle that separates the mucosa from submucosa.

Submucosa. This is a layer of loose connective tissue containing blood vessels, lymphoid tissue, and sometimes glands. The plexuses of Meissner (nerve fibers and cells) are found in this layer.

Muscularis. Typically, the mucularis consists of two layers of smooth muscle that are responsible for the movements in the canal. The inner layer is circularly arranged, and the outer layer longitudinally arranged. Between the two layers is scattered the myenteric plexus of Auerbach, which controls the activity of smooth muscles and secretory cells.

Serosa (adventitia). Surrounding the gastrointestinal tract is a layer of connective tissue. Serosa refers to the layer of connective tissue and epithelium that covers most of the organs in abdominal

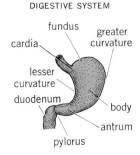

DIGESTIVE SYSTEM

Fig. 3. Gross anatomy of the stomach. *(From W. F. Ganong, Review of Medical Physiology, Lange, 1975)*

and pelvic cavities; adventitia refers to a layer of connective tissue that is continuous with the deeper fascia. Organs (trachea and esophagus) in the thoracic cavity are covered by adventitia (fibrosa).

MOUTH, PHARYNX, AND ESOPHAGUS

The mouth, or oral cavity, is bounded by the teeth and gums anteriorly and laterally, the hard and soft palates superiorly, the tongue inferiorly, and the oropharynx posteriorly. The hard palate is formed by the palatine processes of the maxillary bones and the palatine bones. The soft palate is a posterior extension of the hard palate, but it is chiefly muscle and has the uvula suspended from it in the midline. Together the hard and soft palates separate the oral cavity from the nasal cavity. The mouth opens posteriorly into the pharynx, which serves as a passage for both the digestive system and the respiratory system. The pharynx can be divided into three portions, the nasopharynx, oropharynx, and laryngopharynx. The nasopharynx lies behind the nasal cavity and above the soft palate and uvula. The oropharynx lies behind the oral cavity. The laryngopharynx opens inferiorly into the larynx (anterior) and esophagus (posterior). The mucous membrane of the pharynx is lined with stratified squamous epithelium. Beneath the mucous membrane are a number of skeletal muscles whose contractions are essential for swallowing.

The process of digestion begins in the mouth. Food is mechanically subdivided by teeth and mixed with saliva through the action of the tongue. Saliva contains a considerable quantity of mucus and an enzyme called ptyalin (salivary amylase) which converts starch into sugar. About 1500 ml of saliva are secreted per day.

The esophagus, about 10 in. (25 cm) in length, is a narrow muscular tube which conducts food through the neck and thorax down to the diaphragm, which it penetrates on the left side of the body, to enter the stomach. The esophagus is lined by stratified epithelium and has a thickened circular layer of muscle, the cardiac sphincter, at the esophagogastric junction. This sphincter normally prevents regurgitation of food from the stomach back into the esophagus.

THE STOMACH

The stomach is a large distensible tube that has been bent to one side. The upper and lower curved borders are called lesser and greater curvatures, respectively. The stomach consists of cardia, body (main portion), fundus, and pylorus (Fig. 3). The mucous membrane lining the stomach is thrown into longitudinal folds, called rugae, which allow it to distend. The lumen is lined with a simple columnar epithelium which dips down into frequent openings known as gastric pits. Many long tubular gastric glands empty their secretions into the bottoms of the pits. The surface and neck mucous cells produce mucus over the entire luminal surface. The chief cells of the gastric gland produce a digestive enzyme, pepsin, while the parietal cells produce hydrochloric acid. Pepsin in an acid environment can cleave some of the peptide linkages of protein to form polypeptides of various sizes.

The control of gastric secretion is complicated,

and is exerted through extrinsic nerves, intrinsic nerves, and hormones. It occurs in three phases: cephalic, gastric, and intestinal.

The cephalic phase occurs when food is seen, smelled, or tasted. Impulses pass from the brain to the stomach over the vagus nerves; about 50–150 ml of juice is produced by this phase.

The gastric phase occurs while food is in the stomach. A hormonelike substance, gastrin, is released from the gastric mucosa into the bloodstream when the products of protein digestion, alcohol, or caffeine reach the pyloric portion. Gastrin stimulates the gastric mucosa to secrete gastric juice. Simple mechanical distention of the stomach, as by filling, also causes the release of gastrin.

The intestinal phase occurs when the digesting food mass (chyme) enters the duodenum of the small intenstine. The intestinal mucosa also produces a hormone called enterogastrone which inhibits gastric secretion as well as gastric motility, allowing longer time for gastric digestion of proteins.

The major functions of the stomach are the churning and mixing of food with gastric juices due to muscular movement; production of gastric juices; and absorption of some medicines and alcohol.

The principal components of gastric juice are hydrochloric acid, mucus, proteolytic enzymes, pepsin, rennin, cathepsin, and lipase, gastric intrinsic factor, water-soluble blood groups, and electrolytes. Pepsin in the acid medium converts protein into smaller molecules known as proteoses and peptones. The digestion of carbohydrates and fats is very limited in the stomach. Hydrochloric acid kills many of the ingested bacteria. Gastric intrinsic factor is essential for the absorption of cyanocobalamin (vitamin B_{12}) from the small intestine.

SMALL INTESTINE

The small intestine, a long narrow muscular tube about 10–12 ft (3–3.6 m) long, is divided into three parts on the basis of functional and structural differences.

Divisions. The duodenum, the first 10–12 in. (25–30 cm) of the small intestine, forms a C-shaped bend at the back of the abdomen. The head of the pancreas is located in the curve of the duodenum. A few centimeters distal to the pyloric sphincter, the common bile duct and pancreatic duct (which usually join together to form the ampulla of Vater) empty bile and pancreatic juices into the intestinal lumen. At the ligament of Treitz, the duodenum becomes the jejunum, the second part of the small intestine, measuring approximately 3–4 ft (0.9–1.2 m). The last part of the small intestine is the ileum, measuring about 6 ft (1.8 m).

At the entry of the ileum into the large intestine (cecum) is the ileocecal valve. This is not a true sphincter, but two flaplike folds of tissue which form a one-way valve permitting ready passage from the ileum to the cecum. The ileum and jejunum, unlike the duodenum, are not bound to the body wall. Rather, they are suspended in the mesentery, a fold of peritoneum extending from the posterior abdominal wall. The arrangement allows

the small intestine a considerable range of movement and displacement.

The luminal surface of the small intestine is greatly increased by the formation of grossly visible circular folds, the plicae circulares or valves of Kerckring, and by countless fingerlike processes of microscopic dimensions, the intestinal villi. These villi cover the entire surface of the mucosa and give it a characteristic velvety appearance. At their bases are simple tubular invaginations which form the intestinal glands or crypts of Lieberkühn. Simple columnar epithelium covers the villi and lines the intestinal glands. Scattered among the epithelial cells are mucus-secreting goblet cells, which increase in number toward the lower end of the small intestine. The mucosa of the small intestine also contains solitary lymph nodules, especially in the ileum, and aggregated lymphatic nodules (Peyer's patches) along the antimesenteric border.

Functions. The functions of the small intestine include mixing of chyme, digestion and absorption, secretion, and immunologic functions.

Mixing. The small intestine acts to mix and churn the intestinal contents (chyme) and propel them toward the large intestine.

Digestion and absorption. Nutrients, including fat, carbohydrate, protein, vitamins, and minerals, are absorbed through the wall of the small intestine.

1. Fat absorption. The average American consumes a diet containing 60–100 g of fat per day, mostly neutral fat (triglycerides). Most of the fat is hydrolyzed in the proximal small intestine by pancreatic lipases, forming free fatty acids and glycerol. Salts in the bile juice within the intestine act like detergents and make the breakdown products water-soluble. This enables their passage through the epithelium of the mucosa by passive diffusion. They are conjugated with proteins to lipoprotein (chylomicrons), which readily enters the lymphatics (lacteals) and is transported into the bloodstream. *See* LIPID METABOLISM.

2. Carbohydrate absorption. American diets contain an average of 350 g of carbohydrate per day, consisting of 60% starch, 30% sucrose, and 10% lactose. Conversion of carbohydrate to monosaccharides is necessary for normal absorption. Salivary and pancreatic glands produce a group of enzymes called amylases which convert carbohydrate to intermediary sugars (maltose, sucrose, and lactose) and simple sugars (glucose, fructose, and galactose). These monosaccharides are transported from the intestinal lumen across the brush border into the epithelial cells by a carrier, requiring an expenditure of energy by the cells. *See* CARBOHYDRATE METABOLISM; MONOSACCHARIDE.

3. Protein absorption. The average American dietary intake of protein is 70–90 g per day. The mechanism of digestion and absorption is more complex than for fats and carbohydrates. A much larger group of enzymes is involved to reduce native proteins to their amino acid components. This process begins in the gastrointestinal lumen by pepsin and numerous proteases, which differ in topographical activities and amino acid specificity. Protein digestion occurs sequentially at different sites of action. *See* AMINO ACIDS; PROTEIN METABOLISM.

The manner in which peptides cross the cell

membrane is unknown. Some amino acids are released into the lumen in free form, whereas others enter the cell as dipeptides or polypeptides, later to be digested to amino acids.

4. Vitamin absorption. The absorption of vitamins is poorly understood. Vitamin B_{12} and folic acid are absorbed only in the terminal ileum, whereas fat-soluble vitamins (A, D, E, and K) generally are absorbed throughout the small intestine simultaneously with lipid absorption. Water-soluble vitamins have been little studied. *See* VITAMIN.

Secretory function. Water, hormones (secretin, enterogastrone, glucagon, cholecystokinin, and others), and some enzymes (disaccharidases) are secreted by the intestinal mucosal cells.

Immunologic function. The gastrointestinal tract is an immunologically competent tissue, producing IgA as its predominant immunoglobulin. The intestinal immune tissue is thought to provide the body's first line of defense against the microorganisms contained within the lumen of the bowel.

LARGE INTESTINE

The large intestine, about 5 ft (1.5 m) long, consists of the cecum, appendix, colon, rectum, and anal canal (Fig. 4).

Structure. Most of the large intestine has a wider diameter than the small intestine, but the appendix is an exception, and the pelvic colon may also be relatively narrow. The cecum gives place to the ascending colon, which runs vertically on the right side of the abdomen and turns just below the liver (hepatic flexure) to the left as the transverse colon. It then turns downward near the spleen (splenic flexure) as the descending colon and curves posteriorly along the floor of the pelvic cavity as the sigmoid colon, which leads to the rectum and anal canal.

In most of the large intestine, the longitudinal muscle fibers form three separate strips called taeniae which appear to bunch up the gut into sacculations (haustra). The rectum lacks haustra and has longitudinal rectal columns containing hemorrhoidal blood vessels. The anus is surrounded by an internal sphincter of smooth muscle and an external sphincter of skeletal muscle.

Function. In general, the large intestine has no digestive function. Its main function is to absorb water and inorganic salts, converting 10–17 oz (300–500 ml) of isotonic chyme entering it each day from the ileum to about 5.3 oz (150 g) of semisolid feces. It contains a large flora of microorganisms, which help digest some of the food particles and produce vitamins K and B_{12} and amino acids; these in turn are absorbed by the host. There are no villi on the mucosa. The colonic glands are short. Solitary lymph follicles are present, especially in the cecum and appendix. The movements of the large intestine include intrinsic tonus changes and segmentation contractions like those occurring in the small intestine. These movements mix the contents of the colon and, by exposing more of the contents to the mucosa, facilitate absorption. Some drugs may be absorbed from the colon.

ACCESSORY ORGANS

The major salivary glands, the liver, and the pancreas are the principal organs in this category.

Salivary glands. There are three pairs of salivary glands. The largest is the parotid gland, which lies in the angle between the ear and jaw and has a duct (Stensen's) which enters the mouth opposite the second upper molar tooth. The submandibular (submaxillary) gland lies beneath the base of the tongue and has a duct (Wharton's) penetrating the floor of the mouth to open into the oral cavity under the tongue. The sublingual gland lies anterior to the submandibular gland under the tongue and empties its secretions into the oral cavity through a number of small ducts. Salivary secretion is under neural control. Stimulation of the parasympathetic nerve supply causes profuse secretion of watery saliva with a relatively low content of organic material. The effect of stimulation of the sympathetic nerve supply varies from species to species. In humans, it causes release of small amounts of saliva rich in organic constituents, from submaxillary glands, but has no effect on parotid secretion. Food in the mouth causes reflex secretion of saliva. Salivary secretion can be easily conditioned. In humans, the sight, smell, and even thought of food causes salivary secretion.

Liver. The liver is the largest gland in the body, weighing about 3.3 lb (1500 g). It is located under the right side of the diaphragm, is divided into a larger right lobe and smaller left lobe, and is fixed into position by several ligaments (Fig. 5). The functional unit of the organ is the hepatic lobule, a polyhedral prism of tissue approximately 0.08 in. (2 mm) long and 0.03 in. (0.7 mm) wide, containing anastomosing plates of parenchymal cells and a labyrinthine system of blood sinusoids. The blood supply to the liver is double: the hepatic arteries bring oxygen-rich blood to the sinusoids, and the portal vein brings nutrient-laden blood from the intestine to the sinusoids. The blood in the sinusoids moves slowly toward the central veins. The outgoing blood empties via the hepatic vein into the inferior vena cava.

Between adjacent liver cells are very small channels called bile canaliculi. Bile produced by the parenchymal cells is secreted into these canaliculi, through which it moves toward the bile ducts

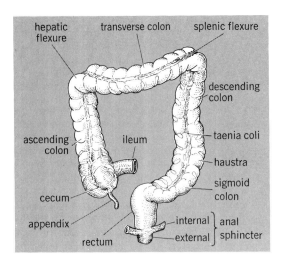

Fig. 4. Human colon. (*From W. F. Ganong, Review of Medical Physiology, Lange, 1975*)

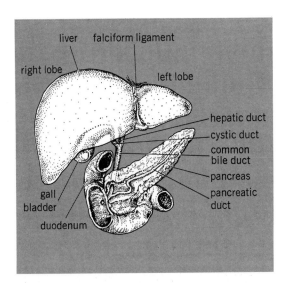

Fig. 5. Relationship of the duodenum to the pancreas and liver. (From B R. Landau, Essential Human Anatomy and Physiology, Scott Foresman, 1976)

at the periphery of each lobule. These interlobular bile ducts form a richly anastomosing network that closely surrounds the branches of the portal vein. At the transverse fossa of the liver, the main ducts from the different lobes of the liver fuse to form the hepatic duct, which after joining the cystic duct continues from the gall bladder to the duodenum as the common bile duct.

There are no digestive enzymes in bile, but bile salts help reduce the surface tension of the duodenal contents, allowing enzymes from the pancreas and intestinal wall better access to the foodstuffs on which they work. Absorbed products of digestion are taken up and metabolized in the liver or are transformed there and returned to the blood for storage or utilization elsewhere. The liver may also receive toxic substances from the intestine or from the general circulation, and is capable of degrading them by oxidation or hydroxylation or of detoxifying them by conjugation. The products of their degradation or their harmless conjugates are then excreted in the bile. The liver also synthesizes several important protein components of blood plasma (such as albumin, globulin, and fibrinogen), and it exercises an important degree of control over the general metabolism by virtue of its capacity to store carbohydrates as glycogen and to release glucose to maintain normal glucose concentration in the blood.

Pancreas. The pancreas is about 6–8 in. (15–20 cm) long and lies almost horizontally across the posterior wall of the abdomen (Fig. 5). It has a head, body, and tail. On the right its head adheres to the middle portion of the duodenum, and its body and tail extend transversely across the back wall of the abdomen to the spleen. It consists of closely packed acini (exocrine portion), which elaborate about 1.27 qt (1200 ml) of digestive juice a day, and small parts of islets of Langerhans (endocrine portion), whose secretion plays an important part in the control of the carbohydrate metabolism of the body.

The exocrine portion secretes the main digestive

enzymes, including trypsin, chymotrypsin, carboxypeptidase, amylase, and lipase. Trypsin, chymotrypsin, and carboxypeptidase further the digestion of protein by converting proteoses and peptones to shorter polypeptides or dipeptides. Pancreatic amylase converts the dextrins of salivary digestion to disaccharides, chiefly maltose, sucrose, and lactose. These disaccharides are further acted upon by disaccharidases (maltase, sucrase, lactase) present in intestinal epithelial cells and are reduced to simple sugars (glucose, fructose, and galactose). Pancreatic lipase hydrolyzes fat into fatty acids and glycerol, both of which can be absorbed from the intestine.   [WEI-JEN CHEN]

Bibliography: W. Bloom and D. W. Fawcett, *A Textbook of Histology*, 10th ed., 1975; W. F. Ganong, *Review of Medical Physiology*, 1975; *Harrison's Principles of Internal Medicine*, 8th ed., 1977; J. R. McClintic, *Basic Anatomy and Physiology of the Human Body*, 1975.

Dill

A small annual or biennial herb, *Anethum graveolens* (Umbelliferae), of high repute among ancient peoples and now cultivated in Europe, India, and the United States. In the United States dill is used mainly as a flavoring for pickles. In France, India, and other countries it is used in soups and sauces, stews, and other dishes. Both the fruits and oil are used in medicine. *See* SPICE AND FLAVORING.

[PERRY D. STRAUSBAUGH/EARL L. CORE]

Distilled spirits

Potable alcoholic beverages, each obtained by distilling an alcohol-containing liquid and further treating the distillate to obtain a beverage of specific character.

Classification. The various distilled spirits are classified according to (1) the raw material which has been fermented and subsequently distilled, such as grain, molasses, and fruit; and (2) the further treatment given the distillate to add specific flavors and aroma. These are referred to as compounded or flavored spirits. Examples of beverages made from grain are whiskeys, vodka, and gin. Some types of vodka and gin are made from potatoes. Molasses is used for the manufacture of rum, and sugar cane juice for the Brazilian cachaça or pinga. Fruits are used for the preparation of brandies, and agave juice for Mexican tequila. The so-called compounded or flavored spirits are made from distilled spirits by the addition of sugar, essential oils, color, herbs, bitters, or other ingredients. Examples are English and Dutch gins, various liqueurs or cordials, absinthe, and aquavit.

Fermentation. When starchy materials are to be fermented, it is necessary to convert the starch to fermentable sugars first. This is done by the addition of amylolytic or diastatic enzymes from malt or certain fungi. Once the starch has been converted to sugar, mostly maltose and glucose, it can be fermented by yeast to alcohol and carbon dioxide. When wine is distilled the fermentation is carried out by various strains of the wine yeast, *Saccharomyces cerevisiae* or its variety *ellipsoideus*. With other sugar-containing substrates, special distillery yeasts may be employed, usually also strains of *S. cerevisiae*, or a natural fermentation by un-

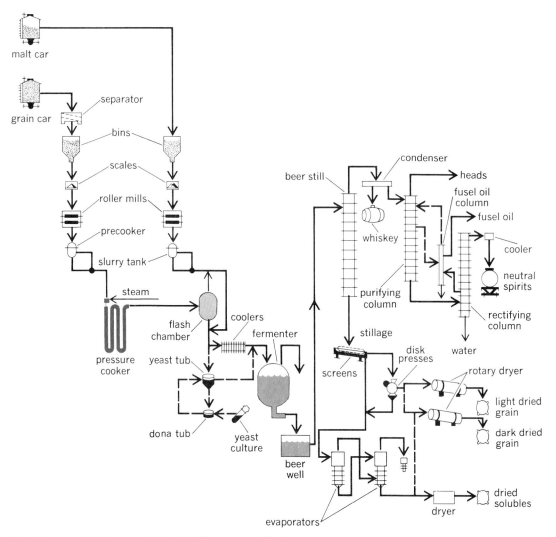

malt car

separator

grain car

bins

scales

roller mills

precooker

slurry tank

steam

flash chamber

coolers

pressure cooker

yeast tub

fermenter

dona tub

yeast culture

beer still

condenser

heads

fusel oil column

fusel oil

whiskey

cooler

neutral spirits

purifying column

rectifying column

stillage

water

screens

disk presses

rotary dryer

light dried grain

dark dried grain

beer well

evaporators

dryer

dried solubles

Flow diagram of whiskey production. (*J. E. Seagram and Sons*)

controlled species of yeast is used. *See* FERMENTATION; WINE.

Distillation process. This is done in stills of various design. In a simple pot still very little fractionation, or rectification, is accomplished. When a still is equipped with a rectifying column, fractions of much higher purity can be collected (see illustration). The batch-type distillation is becoming replaced more and more by continuous stills, especially in the production of grain alcohol or neutral spirits. Normally, three types of fractions are separated. A fraction with a low boiling point, the "heads," is rich in aldehydes and esters. The main fraction is ethyl alcohol and a higher-boiling fraction is rich in so-called fusel oils or higher alcohols. The latter consist of D-amyl- and isoamylalcohol, butyl- and isobutylalcohol, propanol, and others. Isoamylalcohol and amylalcohol are the principal ingredients of fusel oil. The strength of the ethyl alcohol is expressed by the term "proof." In the United States 100 proof spirit is a spirit containing 50% alcohol by volume at a temperature of 60°F. Each degree of proof is equal to 1/2% of alcohol.

Types. The various types of distilled spirits are discussed below.

Brandies. Brandy is a spirit obtained from the distillation of wine or a fermented fruit juice, usu-

ally after aging of the wine in wooden casks. Cognac is a brandy distilled from wines made of grapes grown within the legal limits of Charente and Charente Inférieure Departments, the Cognac region of France. Armagnac is brandy made in the Department of Gers, southeast of Bordeaux. Both types of brandy are aged for many years in oak before bottling. Before bottling, various lots are blended, the alcohol content is adjusted to 42–44% and if necessary, coloring matter such as caramel is added. Brandies distilled from grape pomace of the wine press are called *eau de vie de marc* in France and *grappa* in Italy. Spanish brandies are usually distilled from sherry wines and have a distinctive flavor, quite different from cognac or armagnac. American brandies are primarily products of California and have a flavor different from the European brandies. Whereas in Europe pot stills are most common, continuous stills are preferred in California. Apple brandy is called applejack in the United States and is called calvados in France. It is distilled from completely fermented apple juice and aged in oak barrels for 5–10 years; it has a distinct apple flavor. Other fruits from which brandy is made include black, wild cherries (kirsch or kirschwasser), plums (slivovitz from Hungary or Rumania, and quetsch or mirabelle from France), blackberries, and apricots. When stone fruits are used, some of the stones are broken or crushed and a small amount of the oil is distilled over with the spirit, giving the brandy a more or less pronounced and distinctive bitter almond flavor.

Whiskeys. These distilled spirits are made by distilling fermented grain mashes and aging the distillate in wood, usually oak. Examples are Scotch whisky, Irish whiskey, Canadian whiskey, rye whiskey and bourbon whiskey.

Scotch whisky is made primarily from barley. The barley is converted to malt by allowing it to sprout after which it is dried in a kiln over a peat fire. The malt absorbs some of the smoke aroma which is carried over later with the spirit distilled from it. The drying and roasting of the malt is to a large extent responsible for the flavor of the whisky. After the malt is made into a mash, it is fermented, distilled, and aged in oak casks. These are often casks in which sherry has been shipped. A Scotch blended whisky may contain a certain percentage of grain whisky besides malt whisky.

Irish whiskey is made from malt, unmalted barley, and other grains such as wheat, rye, and oats. The malt used in Irish whiskey is not smoke-cured as in Scotland, and as a result the flavor of the resulting whiskey is different from that of Scotch whisky.

Many types of whiskey are made in the United States. Depending on the principal source of grain, whiskeys are classified as bourbon (corn or grain), rye whiskey (rye), and others. Blended whiskeys are differentiated from straight whiskeys by a certain content of neutral spirits. American whiskeys are aged for a number of years in new charred white-oak barrels. In all types of whiskeys discussed above, the type and quality of the water used in the plant is an important factor in the quality of the finished product.

Gins. These consist essentially of a pure grade of alcohol which has been flavored with an extract of the juniper berry as the chief flavoring agent. The flavor may be imparted by distillation of herbs (distilled gin) or by the addition of essential oils (a compounded gin). There are two principal types of gin: English, or London dry, gin and Dutch gin (jenever).

English gin is made from pure neutral spirits, which are redistilled in the presence of juniper berries and small amounts of other ingredients such as coriander seed, cardamon seed, orange peel, anise seed, cassia bark, fennel, and others. English gin is not aged.

Dutch gin is made of malt. The flavoring ingredients are mixed directly in the mash, after which it is distilled at a rather low proof. Dutch gins are heavier in body and contain more fusel alcohols and other volatile compounds (congenerics) besides ethyl alcohol than does English gin. Some types of Dutch gin are aged. Dutch gin has a pronounced flavor of its own and is consumed straight, whereas English gin is usually used as an ingredient in cocktails.

Rum. The alcoholic distillate from fermented sugar cane juice or molasses is known as rum. Cuban rum is light-bodied and light-colored. The middle fraction of the distillation, known as aguardiente, is used for making rum. The aguardiente is aged in uncharred oak barrels; it is then decolorized, filtered, and supplied with some caramel to give it the proper color. Occasionally some fruit aroma is added. It is then aged for several more years. Jamaica rum is heavier-bodied and contains more congenerics (fusel alcohol, esters, and aldehydes) than Cuban rum. Arak is a rum that comes from the island of Java. It is a dry, highly aromatic rum. A natural fermentation of the molasses by various species of yeast also contributes to the flavor of this drink.

Vodka. A product originally produced in Russia but now popular in many countries, vodka is usually made from wheat. It is highly rectified during distillation and thus is a very pure neutral spirit without a pronounced taste. It is not aged.

Cachaça or pinga. This is a Brazilian spirit made by distilling naturally fermented sugar-cane juice in pot stills. It is high in congenerics and sold at various degrees of proof. It is usually not aged.

Pulque and tequila. Pulque and tequila are of Mexican origin. A sweet sap is obtained from agave (century plant and American aloe) by removing the growing bud from about 3-year-old plants. The sap (aguamiel or honey water) is collected and fermented by natural fermentation and is then called pulque. Distilled pulque is tequila.

Liqueurs. Liqueurs or cordials are alcoholic beverages prepared by combining a spirit, usually brandy, with certain flavorings and sugar. In fruit liqueurs, the color and flavor are obtained by an infusion process using the specified fruit and spirit. Sugar is added after the extraction is complete. Plant liqueurs are made by maceration of plant leaves, seeds, or roots with spirit and then distilling the product. Sugar and coloring matter are added after distillation. A large variety of different liqueurs are marketed. See YEAST.

[EMIL M. MRAK; HERMAN J. PHAFF]

Bibliography: H. J. Grossman, *Grossman's Guide to Wines, Spirits and Beers*, 2d rev. ed., 1974; C. W. Shephard, *Wines, Spirits and Liqueurs*, 1959; L. A. Underkofler and R. J. Hickey (eds.), *Industrial Fermentations*, 2 vols., 1974.

Drought

A general term implying a deficiency of precipitation of sufficient magnitude to interfere with some phase of the economy. Agricultural drought, occurring when crops are threatened by lack of rain, is the most common. Hydrologic drought, when reservoirs are depleted, is another common form. The Palmer index has become popular among agriculturalists to express the intensity of drought as a function of rainfall and hydrologic variables.

The meteorological causes of drought are usually associated with slow, prevailing, subsiding motions of air masses from continental source regions. These descending air motions, of the order of 200 or 300 m/day, result in compressional warming of the air and therefore reduction in the relative humidity. Since the air usually starts out dry, and the relative humidity declines as the air descends, cloud formation is inhibited—or if clouds are formed, they are soon dissipated. The area over which such subsidence prevails may involve several states, as in the 1962–1966 Northeast drought or in the dust bowl drought of the 1930s over the Central Plains.

The atmospheric circulations which lead to this subsidence are the so-called centers of action, like the Bermuda High, which are linked to the planetary waves of the upper-level westerlies. If these centers are displaced from their normal positions or are abnormally developed, they frequently introduce anomalously moist or dry air masses into regions of the temperate latitudes. More important, these long waves interact with the cyclones along the Polar Front in such a way as to form and steer their course into or away from certain areas. In the areas relatively invulnerable to the cyclones, the air descends, and if this process repeats time after time, a deficiency of rainfall and drought may occur. In other areas where moist air is frequently forced to ascend, heavy rains occur. Therefore, drought in one area, say the northeastern United States, is usually associated with abundant precipitation elsewhere, for example, over the Central Plains.

After drought has been established in an area, there seems to be a tendency for it to persist and expand into adjacent areas. Although little is known about the physical mechanisms involved in this expansion and persistence, some circumstantial evidence suggests that numerous "feedback" processes are set in motion which aggravate the situation. Among these are large-scale interactions between ocean and atmosphere in which variations in ocean-surface temperature are produced by abnormal wind systems, and these in turn encourage further development of the same type of abnormal circulation. Then again, if an area, such as the Central Plains, is subject to dryness and heat in spring, the parched soil appears to influence subsequent air circulations and rainfall in a drought-extending sense.

Finally, it should be pointed out that some of the most extensive droughts, like those of the 1930s dust bowl era, require compatibly placed centers of action over both the Atlantic and the Pacific.

In view of the immense scale and complexity of drought-producing systems, it will be difficult for man to devise methods of eliminating or ameliorating them.

[JEROME NAMIAS]

Bibliography: J. Namias, *Factors in the Initiation, Perpetuation and Termination of Drought*, Int. Union Geod. Geophys. Ass. Sci. Hydrol. Publ. no. 51, 1960; W. C. Palmer, *Meteorological Drought*, U.S. Weather Bur. Res. Pap. no. 45, 1965.

Ecology, physiological (plant)

The study of biological processes and growth under natural or simulated environments. This article deals only with the physiological ecology of plants the principal life-cycle processes are germination, growth, photosynthesis, respiration, absorption and loss of water and nutrients, and reproduction. Each of these is a complex series of physical and chemical reactions in cells and tissues of the plant. *See* PHOTOSYNTHESIS; PLANT, WATER RELATIONS OF; PLANT GROWTH; PLANT PHYSIOLOGY.

Scope. Physiological ecology attempts to explain why a certain species of organism is able to grow or survive in a specific environment. This question has not been answered completely for any species. An answer requires a knowledge of the genetic structure of the species and the interactions between the deoxyribonucleic acid (DNA) of the genes and physiological processes in an individual as they operate under the impact of the total environment.

The potential geographical range of a species, both natural and cultivated, depends upon the nature and degree of genetic variation among its individuals, the range of physiological and morphological adaptability within each individual (phenotypic plasticity), and the frequency and extent of occurrence of suitable environments. These three complex variables, operating together, determine the rates of physiological processes and thus the degree of success in growth and reproduction of individuals of a species in a particular environment.

Almost all widespread species are genetically diverse. Within such species, ecological races (ecotypes) have evolved in response to environmental selection of genetic material. Sometimes these races merge gradually with each other to form a genetic gradient (ecocline) of adaptability to an environmental gradient. The races and clines consist of local populations, usually with enough genetic diversity to allow some survival within certain limits of environmental change. Studies of process rates within local populations, ecoclines, and ecotypes provide a measure of the environmental tolerance limits of a species. Such comparative physiological ecology is a relatively new interdisciplinary field. The data which it is providing are improving the understanding of the adaptability of plants and of the evolution of physiological processes.

Such data may be obtained in natural environments under field conditions or in controlled simulated environments. Field measurements are difficult because of logistics and the vagaries of uncontrolled environments but have the advantage of providing realistic values. Measurements under controlled laboratory environments are more precise, but the technical difficulties of reproduction of natural environments are great, costly, and often insurmountable. A research strategy combining both is the future goal.

Field measurements. Genetically determined ecotypes or ecoclines are found by transplanting individuals of a species from different environments to uniform gardens and comparing their growth rates and appearance. Controlled-environment rooms or chambers may be used in place of the uniform garden. Plants may also be started from field-collected seed rather than by transplanting older plants. If inherent morphological and physiological differences exist, they show up rather quickly in the uniform and controlled environments of the garden or growth room.

Physiological rates can be measured in the field if portable instrumentation is available. This can be difficult logistically because of weight of equipment, distances, and environmental severity. Miniaturization of circuits and the use of solid-state components is helping to solve this problem. Mobile laboratories in enclosed trucks or trailers make it easier to get laboratory precision in the natural environment of the plant. The processes most often studied in the field or laboratory are germination, growth, energy exchange and water loss of the leaf, photosynthesis, respiration, and flowering.

Germination and growth. Germination percentages are easy to measure in the field by planting known numbers of seed. Germination is studied in the laboratory in seed-germination chambers or on temperature-gradient bars, usually run under constant light and temperature conditions. However, alternating temperatures result in better germination in many species. Growth may be measured in height, in terms of fresh or dry weight, or in caloric values.

Energy and water relations. The temperature of a leaf is a result of the balance between heat income and heat loss. The measurement of these components of the energy budget of the leaf involves radiation receipts and losses, evaporative losses, convection, net radiation, and metabolism. Detailed techniques for measuring energy budget will not be described here. However, leaf temperatures may be measured by thermocouples, thermistors, or by noncontact infrared thermometers (bolometers). Leaf temperature on a sunny day is largely under the control of transpiration (evaporative heat loss); the effect is greater in a large leaf than in a small one. In turn, leaf temperature affects transpiration rate itself and the important metabolic processes of photosynthesis and respiration. All these processes are influenced by mean wind speed, turbulent variations, and thermal stability of the air.

Transpiration rates of nonwoody plants or young trees or shrubs may be measured by loss of weight of systems consisting of a plant having its roots in a sealed container of moist soil. A plant may be enclosed in a transparent airstream chamber and its water-vapor losses measured by an infrared gas analyzer adapted for the absorption spectrum of water vapor or by the use of electrical humidity-sensing devices, including wet and dry thermocouples. Transpiration rates of large woody plants are difficult to measure directly. Immersing the cut end of a twig in water in a buretlike potometer measures transpiration indirectly through absorption. Another method involves weighing a freshly cut twig with leaves and reweighing after a few minutes; transpiration is equal to loss in weight per unit time. Transpiration rates must be related to leaf surface area, leaf fresh weight, or to soil-moisture tensions.

The ability of a plant to absorb water from the soil is best measured by the water potential in the leaves. Water potential is the difference in free energy or chemical potential (per unit molal volume) between pure water and water in cells and solutions. The potential of pure water is set at zero; the potential of water in cells, solutions, and soil therefore is less than zero, or negative. In rapidly transpiring plants there is a gradient of decreasing water potential from the soil through the roots, stems, and leaves to the air. This causes water to move from the soil through the plant to the atmosphere. In order to absorb water, plants must maintain a water potential lower (more negative) than that of the soil. Leaf water potential can be measured in the field by the Schardakov dye method or with a Scholander pressure bomb. More precise measurements are possible in the laboratory with a thermocouple psychrometer apparatus.

Photosynthesis. Net carbon assimilation may be measured by enclosing a plant or leaf in a sealed transparent chamber, passing air through the chamber, and measuring decrease in carbon dioxide (CO_2) by absorbing CO_2 in potassium hydroxide solution and titrating. A better method employs an infrared gas analyzer adapted for the CO_2 absorption spectrum. The decreased CO_2 content of the air after passing through the chamber can be continuously recorded in either a closed or open system (see illustration). Overheating of the air and leaves within the chamber by radiation is a difficult problem to correct, particularly under remote field conditions. Refrigeration and a relatively high air-flow rate help to keep chamber and leaf temperatures close to that of the outside air. Leaf temperatures should be measured with thermocouples or thermistors. Photosynthesis may also be measured by using radiocarbon as $^{14}CO_2$ in a closed-chamber system for a given amount of time and making subsequent counts of the amount fixed in the leaf or stem tissues. Another field method utilizes measurements of the CO_2 flux within and above wholly unconfined foliage of natural or cultivated vegetation. The rates of photosynthesis and respiration should be related to the leaf area, the fresh and dry weight, or the chlorophyll content.

Respiration. Respiration of leaves, branches, or small individuals may be measured by darkening the chamber by either of the two gas-flow methods and measuring CO_2 production by the plant, but it is not certain whether such results compare with respiration in the light. It may be measured at night in the open-vegetation flux method, or by CO_2 accumulation under strong inversions (chilling of air near the ground). Soil and other respiration factors are then included, and these are difficult to measure independently. The temperature dependence of respiration may be studied further by measuring the temperature relationships of the oxidative rates of the mitochondria.

Productivity. Since photosynthesis is the basic process introducing energy into the food chain, measurements of photosynthesis may be used to estimate net primary productivity in ecosystems. Such productivity may also be measured by peri-

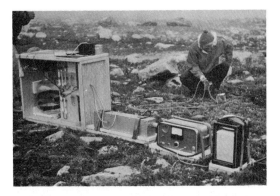

Portable infrared gas analyzer being used to measure photosynthesis of alpine plants at 11,000 ft in Wyoming. The plant is in the small chamber in the right background and is connected by tubing to the pumping and flow-meter apparatus at the left, then to the analyzer, amplifier, and recorder on the right.

odic harvesting of the vegetation and determining the dry weight and caloric value per unit of land surface per unit time.

Flowering and fruiting. These phenomena may be observed in the field as phenological events and correlated with trends in environmental conditions through time. They may also be studied experimentally both in the field and growth chamber by manipulation and control of temperature and photoperiod. *See* PHOTOPERIODISM IN PLANTS.

Measurements in controlled environments. All processes may be measured with greater ease, precision, and environmental variety in controlled-environment facilities. Disadvantages of such facilities are the difficulties of exactly reproducing natural environments, even in small space, and their cost.

Two principal types of controlled environment facilities are in use: (1) relatively small reach-in or walk-in chambers in which thermoperiod, photoperiod, light intensity and quality, and sometimes humidity are controlled, and (2) phytotrons, relatively large air-conditioned buildings in which a variety of controlled environments are available. There are several phytotrons. Among them are one at the Earhart Laboratory at California Institute of Technology (the original "phytotron"), one at Gif-sur-Yvette near Paris, the C.S.I.R.O. phytotron at Canberra, Australia, the North Carolina phytotron at Duke University and North Carolina State University, one at the Royal College of Forestry in Stockholm, and the biotron at the University of Wisconsin. Controlled growth chambers are manufactured by several companies and are available in a variety of models and sizes.

Chambers and phytotrons are valuable tools in physiological ecology because their environments can be controlled and programmed and are reproducible so that an experiment may be repeated. The principal problems in environmental control are in obtaining light intensities and leaf energy budgets approaching those in full sunlight. Humidity control is also difficult.

One important contribution of controlled-environment research is evidence for better germination and growth in many species under cycling temperatures rather than at the constant temperatures of most laboratory experiments. This is in agreement with growth and temperature cycles under natural conditions.

Dependent upon the data of physiological ecology is knowledge of the effects of changing environments on metabolic rates, growth, and reproduction of native and economic plants. This science is also basic to an understanding of primary productivity and efficiency in ecosystems. Physiological ecology, in turn, is dependent upon development of portable and precise field instruments and mobile laboratories, more space in phytotrons, and the training of ecologists capable of adapting physiological methods to field conditions.

[W. D. BILLINGS]

Bibliography: W. D. Billings, Physiological ecology, *Annu. Rev. Plant Physiol.*, 8:375–392, 1957; W. D. Billings, *Plants and the Ecosystem*, 1964; D. M. Gates, Energy exchange and ecology, *BioScience*, 18(2):90–95, 1968; W. M. Hiesey, The physiology of ecological races, *Annu. Rev. Plant Physiol.*, 16:203–216, 1965; P. J. Kramer and T. T. Kozlowski, *Forest Tree Physiology*, 1960; H. A. Mooney and W. D. Billings, Comparative physiological ecology of arctic and alpine populations of *Oxyria digyna*, *Ecol. Monogr.*, 31:1–29, 1961; F. W. Went, *The Experimental Control of Plant Growth*, 1957.

Egg processing

Commercial procedures used in the collection and distribution of shell eggs and the further processing of shell eggs for industrial uses. Eggs commonly used in the United States are considered to be produced exclusively by the domesticated chicken. Table 1 illustrates typical yields or conversions of the basic unit of raw material, the case, into normally encountered items of commerce.

Egg statistics. The per capita consumption of egg products in the United States has been relatively constant since 1960, varying from the equivalent of 27–30 shell eggs per person per year. Approximately 10% of the total eggs produced in the United States are processed into egg products. Annual production of whole, plain, and mixed egg products have fluctuated in the range of 190- to 220,000,000 lb, with liquid egg products accounting for slightly under 10% of the total and frozen egg products the balance. Although distribution shifts considerably from year to year, production of albumin has ranged from 80,000,000 to 150,000,000 lb, mostly frozen; production of yolk has been in the vicinity of 110,000,000 lb, with slightly over 10% liquid and the rest frozen. Thus total annual egg products have been in the vicinity of 400,000,000–450,000,000 lb.

Use of albumin has been shifting from the liquid or frozen form to the dried form. Also, use of plain whole-dried egg has been giving way to use of fortified products. These products (in trade parlance, tex products) often consist of 70 parts whole egg and 30 parts yolk, to which is added a concentrated carbohydrate syrup, which upon drying yields a product containing 70–80% egg solids.

Uses and constituents. Frozen eggs and egg solids are used primarily in bakery goods, doughnuts, noodles, mayonnaise, confectionery items, and prepared mixes. In bakery products eggs are used for their binding, leavening, and emulsifying actions; flavor; color; and nutritive value. Several quality attributes are of utmost importance to the user of egg products, for example, chemical composition, nutritional value, microbiological properties, organoleptic properties, and functional performance. Table 2 is a comprehensive summary of important chemical and nutritive properties of frozen and dehydrated eggs. Data are presented in grams, milligrams, or micrograms per 100 of product, as indicated for each nutrient.

Eggs are an excellent source of nutritional elements, with all vitamins, except vitamin C, present

Table 1. Typical conversion factors for eggs and egg products

1 case = 30 doz = 47 lb total
= 39.5 lb liquid whole egg
= 17.7 lb liquid whites
= 21.8 lb liquid yolk
= 10.8 lb whole egg solids
= 2.8 lb egg white solids
= 8.0 lb egg yolk solids

Table 2. Composition and nutritive values of egg products*

Nutrients per 100 g of product	Whole eggs		Egg white		Egg yolk	
	Fresh or frozen	Solids	Fresh or frozen	Solids	Fresh or frozen	Solids
Calories	163	606	51	412	312	656
Water, g	74.5	5.0	88.6	8.0	55.0	5.0
Protein, g	12.0	44.6	10.0	80.7	14.0	30.0
Amino acids, g						
Arginine	0.80	2.99	0.63	5.08	1.01	2.13
Aspartic acid	0.70	2.59	0.60	4.84	0.77	1.62
Cystine	0.26	0.98	0.25	2.02	0.24	0.51
Glutamic acid	1.48	5.50	1.24	10.01	1.69	3.57
Glycine	0.44	1.65	0.40	3.23	0.49	1.03
Histidine	0.32	1.20	0.27	2.18	0.41	0.87
Isoleucine	0.84	3.12	0.72	5.81	0.97	2.05
Leucine	1.02	3.79	0.85	6.86	1.19	2.51
Lysine	0.82	3.03	0.66	5.33	1.01	2.13
Methionine	0.40	1.47	0.41	3.31	0.34	0.72
Phenylalanine	0.65	2.41	0.61	4.92	0.64	1.35
Serine	0.92	3.43	0.69	5.57	1.25	2.64
Threonine	0.66	2.46	0.52	4.20	0.85	1.79
Tryptophan	0.23	0.85	0.20	1.61	0.25	0.53
Tyrosine	0.55	2.05	0.46	3.71	0.64	1.35
Valine	0.98	3.66	0.88	7.10	1.02	2.15
Lipids, g	11.0	40.8	—	—	28.9	60.7
Cholesterol						
Fatty acids, g	3.6	13.1	—	—	9.7	18.1
Monounsaturated	6.2	22.3	—	—	16.6	30.6
Polyunsaturated	1.4	5.1	—	—	3.8	6.9
Saturated	0.8	2.9	—	—	1.8	3.9
Phospholipids	3.3	12.4	—	—	9.0	20.0
Minerals (ash), g	1.0	3.7	0.7	5.7	1.6	3.4
Calcium, mg	54.0	201.0	6.0	48.4	147.0	309.0
Chlorine, mg	100.0	372.0	131.0	1057.0	67.0	141.0
Copper, mg	0.17	0.63	0.04	0.32	0.25	0.52
Fluorine, mg	0.06	0.22	0.02	0.16	0.12	0.25
Iodine, mg	12.0	45.0	6.8	54.9	16.0	34.0
Iron, mg	2.1	7.8	0.3	0.24	5.6	11.8
Magnesium, mg	9.0	33.5	11.0	89.0	13.0	27.0
Manganese, mg	0.04	0.15	—	—	0.11	0.23
Phosphorus, mg	210.0	781.0	17.0	137.0	586.0	1231.0
Potassium, mg	149.0	554.0	149.0	1202.0	110.0	231.0
Sodium, mg	111.0	413.0	175.0	1412.0	78.0	164.0
Sulfur, mg	233.0	867.0	211.0	1702.0	214.0	449.0
Zinc, mg	1.3	4.8	0.01	0.8	3.8	8.0
Vitamins						
A, IU	1140.0	4240.0	—	—	3210.0	6741.0
B_{12}, μg	0.28	1.04	0.01	0.08	0.83	1.74
Biotin, μg	22.5	83.7	7.0	56.5	52.0	109.0
Choline, g	0.53	1.97	—	—	1.49	3.13
D, IU	50.0	186.0	—	—	150.0	315.0
E, mg	2.0	7.4	—	—	6.0	12.6
Folic acid, mg	9.4	35.0	1.6	12.9	23.2	48.7
Inositol, mg	33.0	122.8	—	—	—	—
Niacin, mg	0.1	0.37	—	—	—	—
Pantothenic acid, mg	2.7	10.0	0.13	1.05	6.0	12.6
Pyridoxine, mg	0.25	0.93	0.22	1.78	0.31	0.65
Riboflavin, mg	0.29	1.08	0.26	2.1	0.35	0.74
Thiamine, mg	0.1	0.37	—	—	0.27	0.57
Carbohydrates, g	0.7	—	0.8	—	0.7	—

*Data were mostly obtained or calculated from values in: USDA, C&FERD, ARS, *Handbook 8*, 1963; USDA, HNRD, ARS, *Home Econ. Res. Rep.*, no. 24, 1964; *J. Amer. Diet. Ass.*, 33:1244–1254, 1957.

SOURCE: Technical Committee of the Poultry and Egg National Board, *A Scientist Speaks About Eggs*, Bull. no. E-26, 1961.

in substantial quantities. The lipids of egg yolk are composed mainly of highly unsaturated fatty acids, containing a large proportion of the essential fatty acid, oleic acid. Egg protein is recognized as a biological standard in nutritional research. *See* NUTRITION.

Commercial egg production. Shifts in egg production have resulted in a decrease in the small farm flock typical of the egg industry in the 1950s to large commercial-type enterprises with 30,000–100,000 laying hens. A few installations have as many as 1,000,000 birds. This shift has not only resulted in improved quality and decreased cost of shell eggs but has significantly altered the geographical production pattern. In the United States large increases in production have taken place in the Southeast, South, and West, with accompanying decreases in the Middle West and New England. The Middle West still remains the center of surplus egg production and is the location of most egg-processing operations.

Shell eggs are sprayed with an edible mineral oil on the farms or ranches to preserve quality. After transport to central locations, eggs are washed under high-speed sanitary conditions, graded for quality by candling, classified as to size, placed in cartons of a dozen, and distributed under refrigeration to retail outlets. Grading and size classification are carried out under U.S. Department of Agriculture or state standards in most plants.

Egg products. Most eggs to be converted to egg products are broken by high-speed mechanical breakers capable of operating at 25–35 cases of eggs per hour. These machines separate the white and yolk or produce whole egg at higher production rates. After thorough mixing and standardizing for solids content or color or both, eggs must be pasteurized prior to being packed for frozen consumption or drying. Whole-egg and egg-yolk products are pasteurized at minimum temperatures of 140°F for 3.5 min to lower the microbiological population and eliminate pathogens. Egg white, being more sensitive to heat, must be pasteurized at lower temperatures or at the higher temperatures after being subjected to stabilizing chemicals such as aluminum sulfate. Hydrogen peroxide is also useful in chemical pasteurization of egg white. Following pasteurization, eggs for freezing are placed in 30-lb tin containers and blast frozen at −20 to −40°F. Distribution of frozen eggs follows normal wholesale food channels, with the bulk of the product going into bakeries, candy manufacturers, and institutions. Egg liquid to be dried is cooled immediately after pasteurization to less than 40°F and either dried on the premises or hauled by insulated tank trucks to centrally located egg-drying plants. Table 4 lists properties of commercial frozen eggs.

Egg-white drying. Prior to drying, egg-white liquid undergoes extensive processing to ensure the retention of its functional and organoleptic properties in the finished product. All egg whites for drying must be pasteurized as described above. A small amount of free glucose must be removed to prevent the Mailliard reaction, which causes brown discoloration and off-odors in the dried product. Glucose is removed by the use of bacteria or yeast capable of utilizing glucose or by enzyme systems capable of converting the glucose to a nonreactive material, such as gluconic acid.

Several whipping aids have been approved by the Food and Drug Administration for addition to egg white to retain the high whipping abilities following drying. The most commonly used whipping aid is sodium lauryl sulfate. Following appropriate adjustment of pH with lactic, citric, or other approved food acids, the liquid egg white is spray-dried in conventional dryers. It is essential that egg-white dryers be provided with dust-collecting systems.

Spray-dried egg-white solids are normally packed in 150-lb fiber drums or 25- to 50-lb polyethylene-lined boxes for shipment to food manufacturers.

Egg white is also air-dried in pan or tunnel systems, in which the egg white is poured in a thin layer on trays. After appropriate liquid treatment as described above, these trays are subjected to temperatures up to 130°F until a pseudocrystalline product is obtained. These crystals, or flakes, are used as such or ground into a fine powder for greater solubility. This type of product is used primarily in the confectionery industry. Typical specifications for egg-white solids are given in Table 3.

Egg-yolk drying. Liquid egg yolk from the breaking plants is collected at drying plants in the manner described for egg white. If not already pasteurized, the egg yolk is held at 140°F for 3.5 min. Egg yolk may be spray-dried directly or it may be subjected to a stabilizing treatment to remove the free glucose, as is necessary with egg white. The glucose-oxidase enzyme system is used for this process almost exclusively.

Egg yolk must be dried to a final product containing 95% egg-yolk solids, many different kinds of spray-drying equipment being suitable for this

Table 3. Specification guide*

	Frozen			Solids				
Category	Whites	Plain yolk	Whole	Angel whites	Flake albumin	Free-flowing stabilized whole	Free-flowing stabilized yolk	Fortified whole-egg (tex) with carbohydrates
Moisture (solids)	11.8% min.	43.0% min.	26% min.	8% max.	14% max.	3% max.	3% max.	4% max.
Fat	0.02% max.	25% min.	11% min.	none	none	40% max.	57% min.	31% min.
pH	—	—	—	7.0±0.5	5.5±0.5	7.5±0.5	6.5±0.5	7.5±0.5
Protein	10.5% min.	16.0% min.	12.5% min.	80% min.	75% min.	44% min.	30% min.	27% min.
Carbohydrate	—	—	—	none	none	none	none	30% max.
Color	—	SOP	SOP	creamy	clear yellow	NEPA 2–4	NEPA 2–4	—
Viable bacteria	50,000/g max.	10,000 max.	10,000 max.	5000 max.	10,000 max.	10,000 max.	10,000 max.	10,000 max.
Yeast	—	10 max.	10 max	10 max.	10 max.	10 max.	10 max.	10 max.
Mold	—	10 max.	10 max.	10 max.	10 max.	10 max.	10 max.	10 max.
Coliform	1000/g max.	10 max.	10 max.	10 max.	10 max.	10 max.	10 max.	10 max.
Salmonella	negative	negative	negative	negative	negative	negative	negative	negative
Granulation	—	—	—	100%		100%	100%	100%
				USBS-80		USBS-16	USBS-16	USBS-16
Additives				SLS 0.1% max.			SS 2% max.	—
Performance	SOP	SOP	SOP	SOP	SOP	SOP	SOP	SOP

*SOP = specified on purchase; SS = sodium silicoaluminate; SLS = sodium lauryl sulfate; NEPA = National Egg Products Association light-to-dark color scale; and USBS = U.S. Bureau of Standards.

process. Egg yolk is commonly converted to a free-flowing powder by the addition of small quantities of such anticaking agents as sodium silicoalumi-nate (less than 2%) or silicon dioxide (less than 1%). Ability to flow freely appears to be of partic-ular importance to mayonnaise manufacturers. Table 4 gives specifications for yolk products.

Whole-egg drying. Whole-egg solids are manu-factured in a similar manner, as are many blends of whole egg, yolk, and added ingredients, to meet specific functional requirements. Common addi-tives are carbohydrate products, which may be derivatives of either sucrose or corn-syrup solids. These carbohydrates, when added prior to spray-drying, help retain the original foaming and emul-sifying abilities of the liquid egg. Whole egg may be converted to a free-flowing product, as de-scribed above for egg yolk. Specifications for whole egg and fortified products are also given in Table 3. *See* FOOD ENGINEERING.

[RICHARD H. FORSYTHE]

Bibliography: E. W. Benjamin et al., *Marketing Poultry Products*, 5th ed., 1960; W. J. Stadelman and O. Cotterill, *Egg Science and Technology*, 1974; Technical Committee of the Poultry and Egg National Board, *A Scientist Speaks about Eggs*, bull. no. E-26, 1961.

Eggplant

A warm-season vegetable (*Solanum melongena*) of Asiatic origin belonging to the plant order Polemoniales (formerly Tubiflorales). Eggplant is grown for its usually egg-shaped fleshy fruit (see illustration) and is eaten as a cooked vegetable. Cultural practices are similar to those used for tomatoes and peppers; however, eggplant is more sensitive to low temperatures. Popular purple-fruited varieties (cultivars) are Black Beauty and a number of hybrid varieties; fruits of other colors,

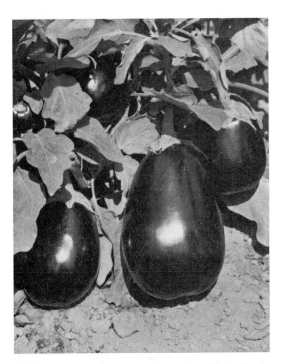

Eggplant (*Solanum melongena*), cultivar Black Magic. (*Joseph Harris Co, Rochester, N.Y.*)

including white, brown, yellow, and green, are used chiefly for ornamental purposes. Harvesting generally begins 70–80 days after planting. Flori-da and New Jersey are important eggplant-pro-ducing states. The total annual farm value in the United States from about 4000 acres is approxi-mately $3,500,000. *See* PEPPER; TOMATO; VEGE-TABLE GROWING.

[H. JOHN CAREW]

Erosion

The loosening and transporting of rock debris at the Earth's surface, aptly described as the wearing away of the land. Agents of erosion include sur-face, ground, and ocean water; ice (especially gla-ciers); wind; gravity; and organisms.

Erosion removes, on the average, 1 ft (vertically) of rock material in the order of thousands of years. From the time it begins until the lowest possible level has been reached, erosion progresses down-ward through topographic stages of gradually di-minishing slope described by W. M. Davis as youth, maturity, and old age, where each stage is characterized by a distinctive group of landforms. According to an alternate description by W. Penck and L. King, erosion progresses by laterally di-rected planation and parallel retreat of slopes.

Erosion is of great concern to man because it may remove the fertile topsoil, change watercours-es and landforms, and cause damage to valuable man-made structures. Erosion has removed valua-ble ore deposits and rendered some land uninhab-itable, but has also stripped off worthless overbur-den, making some mineral deposits available, and smoothed wide areas, making land suitable for ag-ricultural purposes. Quickening of the pace of ero-sion (accelerated erosion), brought about by man, has produced landforms and other abnormal con-ditions that are detrimental to the productivity of the land. *See* SOIL; SOIL CONSERVATION.

[WALTER D. KELLER]

Evapotranspiration

A term applied to the discharge of water from land surfaces to the atmosphere by evaporation from lakes, streams, and soil surfaces and by transpira-tion from plants. The term is applied both to the process and to the quantity of water discharged. On the average, two-thirds of the precipitation is returned to the atmosphere by evapotranspiration, but this ratio varies from nearly 100% in deserts to one-third or less where precipitation is high and evaporation relatively small.

Evaporation and transpiration are considered together because of the great difficulty of measur-ing or estimating them separately. Transpiration is the process by which water is taken in by plant roots, moved up through the stem or trunk, and released as vapor through the leaves. The maxi-mum possible evapotranspiration, termed potential evapotranspiration, is governed by the available heat energy and is taken to equal the evapora-tion from a large water surface. Actual evapotran-spiration is determined by available moisture and is generally much less than the potential evapo-transpiration. Actual evapotranspiration is never greater than precipitation except on irrigated land. For a river system actual evapotranspiration can be approximated as the precipitation over the tributary area less the streamflow leaving the basin. This approximation ignores retention of water in the groundwater or in reservoirs and diversions from the basin.

Local estimates of actual evapotranspiration are made with lysimeters, large tanks of soil with growing plants, for which the gain or loss of water can be determined by weighing or accounting for water supplied to the tank.

Phreatophytes. Evaporation can remove water from only a relatively thin surface layer of soil, but transpiration removes water from the entire root depth of plants. Phreatophytes obtain water from the groundwater or the capillary fringe above the water table and have root systems extending to great depths, for example, mesquite, 60 ft, and alfalfa, 100 ft. In addition to mesquite and alfalfa, typical phreatophytes include salt grass, salt cedar (tamarisk), willow, cottonwood, and greasewood. It has been estimated that 25,000,000 acre-ft (1 acre-ft = 325,400 gal) of water is transpired annually by nonbeneficial phreatophytes in the 17 western states of the United States.

Xerophytes and mesophytes. Xerophytes are plants of desert regions and are adapted to survive for long periods without moisture. However, when moisture is available, they transpire at the same rates as mesophytes, plants of humid regions, that require nearly continuous water supply.

[RAY K. LINSLEY]

Bibliography: V. T. Chow, *Handbook of Applied Hydrology,* 1964; R. K. Linsley, M. A. Kohler, and J. L. H. Paulhus, *Hydrology for Engineers,* 2d ed., 1975; R. C. Ward, *Principles of Hydrology,* 1968.

Farm crops

The farm crops may be roughly classed as follows: (1) food crops—the bread grains (wheat and rye), rice, sugar crops (sugarbeets and sugarcane), potatoes, and dry legume seeds (peanuts, beans, and peas); (2) feed crops—corn, sorghum grain, oats, barley, and all hay and silage; and (3) industrial crops—cotton (lint and seed), soybeans, flax, and tobacco. *See* BARLEY; BEAN; CORN; COTTON; GRAIN CROPS; OATS; PEA; PEANUT; POTATO, IRISH; POTATO, SWEET; SORGHUM; SOYBEAN; SUGAR CROPS; TOBACCO.

Regional cultivation. Crop production is regionalized in the United States in response to the combination of soil and climatic conditions and to the land topography, which favors certain kinds of crop management. In general, commercial farm crops are confined to land in humid and subhumid climates that can be managed to minimize soil and water erosion damage, where soil productivity can be kept at a relatively high level, and where lands are smooth enough to permit large-scale mechanized farm operations. In less well-watered regions, cropping is practiced efficiently on fairly level, permeable soils, where irrigation water can be supplied. The tilled crops, such as corn, sorghums, cotton, potatoes, and sugar crops, are more exacting in soil requirements than the close-seeded crops, such as wheat, oats, barley, rye, and flax. The crops planted in solid stands, mostly hay crops (as well as pastures), are efficient crops for lands that are more susceptible to soil and water erosion.

United States productivity. The United States has the highest production of any area of its size in the world with regard to farm crops, together with pasture and rangelands that support livestock. Productivity per acre has increased tremendously since 1946 because of a combination of factors that have resulted in more efficient systems of farming. These factors include greatly improved use of mechanical and electric power and a high degree of mechanization applied to land and water management, methods of land preparation, planting, crop protection (against insects, diseases, and weeds), harvesting, curing, and storage. There have been marked advances in improving varieties of all crops and in seed technology. The development and application of effective pesticide chemicals and the greatly increased use of commercial fertilizers have been included in the newer farming systems. Soil and water conservation programs are widespread, resulting in better choice of many kinds of crops and of farming practices that are most suitable to the local climatic conditions and to the capabilities of the local classes of soils. Most of the farm crops are grown on about 300,000,000 acres of the 1,450,000,000 acres of privately owned land in the 48 mainland states. *See* AGRICULTURAL SCIENCE (PLANT); AGRICULTURE, SOIL AND CROP PRACTICES IN; FERTILIZING; LAND DRAINAGE (AGRICULTURE).

Farming regions. The major farming regions of the United States are named from the predominant kinds of crops grown, even though there is tremendous diversity within each region. The Corn Belt includes a great central area extending from Nebraska and South Dakota east across much of Iowa, Missouri, Illinois, and Indiana to central Ohio. To the north and east of this region is the Hay and Dairy Region, which actually grows large quantities of feed grains. To the south of the Corn Belt is the Corn and Winter-Wheat Belt, but here also extensive acreages of other crops are grown. The southern states, once the Cotton Belt, now concentrate on hay, pasture, and livestock, with considerable acreages of soybeans and peanuts. The cultivated portions of the Great Plains, extending from Canada to Mexico, with annual rainfall of 15–25 in, are divided into a spring-wheat region in the Dakotas and a winter-wheat region from Texas to Nebraska, with grain sorghum a major crop in all portions of the Great Plains where soil conditions and topography favor tillage. The Intermountain Region, between the Rocky Mountains and the Cascade–Sierra Nevada mountain ranges, is cropped only where irrigation is feasible, and a wide range of farm crops is grown. In the three states of the Pacific Region, a great diversity of crops is grown. Cotton is now concentrated in the irrigated regions from Texas to California.

Marketing. From a world viewpoint, the United States is known most widely for its capacity to produce and export wheat. However, this nation has become a major producer of soybeans for export, and rice exports have become important. The ability to produce feed grains in abundance and at relatively low cost has created a large world market for United States corn, sorghum grain, oats, and barley. Although United States cotton once dominated the world market, its total production is now only about one-quarter of the world cotton supply. Most of the other farm crops are consumed within the United States. Tobacco and sugar crops are high acre-value crops, as are potatoes, peanuts, and dry beans. The production of these high acre-value crops is concentrated in localized areas where soils and climate are particularly favorable, rather than in broad acreages.

[HOWARD B. SPRAGUE]

Fat and oil, edible

One of the three major classes of food products. Along with carbohydrates and proteins, fats and oils supply the energy requirements of man and animals. They consist principally of glyceride esters of fatty acids and are characteristically soluble in organic solvents such as petroleum hydrocarbons, ether, chloroform, and carbon tetrachloride. Fats are usually defined as solid or plastic at ordinary temperatures, but the term may be used for all such compositions regardless of melting point. Oils are liquid at edible temperatures. Fats and oils in the diet serve to increase palatability and enhance the flavor of foods. They provide a lubricating action, increase the satisfaction of eating, and delay the onset of hunger. In a bakery product, fat improves the texture. *See* FOOD.

The two major groups are animal fats and vegetable oils. Animal fats, a product of the meat-packing industry, are obtained by processing the fatty tissue of hogs, cattle, sheep, and fowl. Marine animals such as the whale are also processed to obtain edible fat. Butter is a special type of animal-fat product from milk. The vegetable oils are pressed or extracted from a variety of plant seeds. Of primary importance as sources of edible oil on a world basis are soybeans, cottonseed, peanuts, corn germ, olives, coconut, rapeseed, sesame, sunflower, safflower, cocoa beans, and various oil palms. Major domestic production is limited to the first four of these, but dried coconut meat (copra) is imported and processed domestically, and imported cocoa beans are processed for cocoa butter. *See* BUTTER.

Nutritive value. The nutritive value of fats and oils is characterized by high energy content. They supply about 9.3 cal/g, over twice that of proteins and carbohydrates, and serve as a source of energy as ingested and as stored in the body. Digestibility coefficients, the percentage of ingested fat absorbed, range from 94 to 98%. Fats that melt above 50°C, such as mutton fat, are less completely digested.

Fats and oils serve as carriers for the fat-soluble vitamins A and D, aiding their absorption from the intestinal tract, and are the chief source of vitamin E. They also have a sparing action on some vitamins of the B complex. They are the source of the polyunsaturated or essential fatty acids, required for structural development of tissues and prevention of fat-deficiency disease which in man manifests itself as eczema. Diets with fats containing a high proportion of polyunsaturated fatty acids are reported to lower abnormally high blood cholesterol levels. *See* NUTRITION; VITAMIN A; VITAMIN D; VITAMIN E.

Chemical constitution. Edible fats and oils are basically esters of glycerol, $C_3H_5(OH)_3$, and vari-

ous fatty acids, most of which have an even number of carbon atoms arranged in a long straight chain. They may be represented by structural formula (I), where R, R′, and R″ represent the carbon

$$
\begin{array}{c}
\text{H} \\
| \\
\text{H—C—OOCR} \\
| \\
\text{H—C—OOCR}' \quad \text{(I)} \\
| \\
\text{H—C—OOCR}'' \\
| \\
\text{H}
\end{array}
$$

chains of the fatty acids. The fatty acids may be saturated, that is, each carbon atom in the chain is linked by single bonds to other carbon atoms or to hydrogen atoms, as in palmitic (hexadecanoic) acid, represented by structural formula (II); or they may be unsaturated, having one or more carbon atoms in the chain joined by two bonds as in oleic acid.

$$
\begin{array}{c}
\text{H H H H H H H H H H H H H H H O} \\
| \; | \; | \; | \; | \; | \; | \; | \; | \; | \; | \; | \; | \; | \; | \; \| \\
\text{H—C—C—C—C—C—C—C—C—C—C—C—C—C—C—C—C—OH} \\
| \; | \; | \; | \; | \; | \; | \; | \; | \; | \; | \; | \; | \; | \; | \\
\text{H H H H H H H H H H H H H H H}
\end{array}
$$
(II)

Hydrogen, halogens, and other chemical reagents can be added to the double bonds of unsaturated acids to form saturated acids or derivatives. The most important saturated acids in edible fats are palmitic, with 16 carbon atoms; stearic, with 18 carbon atoms; lauric, with 12 carbon atoms; and butyric, with 4 carbon atoms. Oleic acid, having 18 carbon atoms and a double bond in the 9 carbon atom position, can be represented as structural formula (III). It is the most abundant unsaturated

$$
\begin{array}{c}
\text{H H H H H H H H H H H H H H H H O} \\
| \; | \; | \; | \; | \; | \; | \; | \; | \qquad | \; | \; | \; | \; | \; | \; | \; \| \\
\text{H—C—C—C—C—C—C—C—C—C=C—C—C—C—C—C—C—C—OH} \\
| \; | \; | \; | \; | \; | \; | \; | \qquad | \; | \; | \; | \; | \; | \; | \\
\text{H H H H H H H H H H H H H H H}
\end{array}
$$
(III)

acid. Acids having more than one double bond include linoleic, with 18 carbon atoms and two double bonds in the 9 and 12 positions; linolenic acid, with 18 carbon atoms and three double bonds in the 9, 12, and 15 positions; and arachidonic acid, with 20 carbon atoms and four double bonds in the 5, 8, 11, and 14 positions. The amounts of different fatty acids constituting various fats are shown in the table. *See* LIPID.

Fatty acids are distributed among the glycerides in a complex manner, which accounts for the wide variations in the physical properties of fats. In animal fats considerable proportions of fully saturated glycerides occur. Only in a few oils, such as cocoa butter, are there a limited number of glycerides of specific configuration. Cocoa butter consists almost exclusively of two glycerides, 2-oleopalmitostearin and 2-oleodistearin.

Nonglyceride components, which are not saponified by alkali, constitute from about 0.5 to 2% of most fats. They include sterols, hydrocarbons (such as squalene), carotenoids, and fat-soluble vitamins. The tocopherols (one of which is vitamin E) function as antioxidants and delay the development of rancidity in the fat.

Spoilage factors. Oxidation and hydrolysis are spoilage factors in the production and storage of

Typical fatty-acid composition of animal fats and vegetable oils[a]

	Saturated			Unsaturated		
Type	Pal-mitic	Ste-aric	Other[b]	Oleic	Lin-oleic	Other
Fats						
Lard	29.8	12.7	1.0	47.8	3.1	5.6[c]
Chicken	25.6	7.0	0.3	39.4	21.8	5.9[c]
Butterfat	25.2	9.2	25.6	29.5	3.6	7.2[c]
Beef fat	29.2	21.0	1.4	41.1	1.8	3.5[c]
Cocoa butter	24.0	35.0		39.0	2.0	
Oils						
Corn	8.1	2.5	0.1	30.1	56.3	2.9
Peanut	6.3	4.9	5.9	61.1	21.8	
Cottonseed	23.4	1.1	2.7	22.9	47.8	2.1[d]
Soybean	9.8	2.4	1.2	28.9	50.7	7.0[e]
Olive	10.0	3.3	0.6	77.5	8.6	
Coconut	10.5	2.3	78.4	7.5	Trace	1.3

[a]As weight percentages of component fatty acids.

[b]Butterfat and coconut oil contain saturated fatty acids having 4–14 and 6–14 carbon atoms, respectively. Peanut oil contains several percent of acids of 20 carbon atoms and above.

[c]Mainly hexadecenoic acid; 0.2–0.4% arachidonic acid.

[d]Cottonseed oil contains about 0.5–1% of fatty acids having a cyclopropene ring (malvalic and sterculic acids).

[e]Mostly linolenic acid.

edible fats and oils. Incipient oxidation may produce flavors characterized as grassy, buttery, beany, or fishy. Rancidity is an advanced state of oxidative deterioration. Oxygen from the air first reacts with the unsaturated fatty acids at or adjacent to the double bonds to form hydroperoxides which then decompose to yield aldehydes having the pungent odor and flavor of rancid fats. Oxidation is catalyzed by light and metals such as copper or iron, and is accelerated by heat. Preventive measures include packaging in brown glass or metal containers; use of nitrogen, an inert gas, in processing and packaging and addition of citric acid during processing to inactivate trace metals. Antioxidants are added to control rancidity in fats deficient in naturally occurring antioxidants. Widely used antioxidants include as NDGA (nordihydroguiaretic acid), BHA (butylated hydroxyanisole), BHT (butylated hydroxytoluene), or propyl gallate. The more saturated fats and hydrogenated fats are less subject to oxidative deterioration. In processing or use, fats should never be in contact with equipment or utensils made of copper or copper-containing alloys.

Hydrolytic spoilage results only in fats in contact with moisture. Butter, margarine, and many processed foods contain enough moisture that hydrolysis may be encountered. With most fats hydrolysis does not noticeably affect the flavor, but butter becomes strong and coconut oil develops a soapy flavor. This type of spoilage may be catalyzed by the enzymes present in other components of a processed food product or enzymes liberated by microorganisms.

Testing procedures. Tests used in establishing quality and grade of crude vegetable oils include free fatty-acid content, determined by titration of an alcohol solution of the oil with standard alkali, and refining and bleaching tests. Replicated refining tests on 500-g oil samples are carried out using specified amounts of sodium hydroxide and the refining loss determined by weighing the soapstock and the decanted refined oil. The color of the refined oil, or oil bleached by heating with a stand-

ard bleaching clay, is determined photometrically.

Various characteristics of processed oil and fat products are used in specifications and control. Smoke points are determined on cooking oils by heating in an open cup to the smoking temperature of about 440°F or above. Salad oils must pass at least a 5½-hr cold test during which the oil must not cloud or crystallize when packed in ice.

Unsaturation is measured as iodine value, calculated as the percent iodine absorbed by the fat. As determined by the Wijs method, a weighed sample of fat is dissolved in carbon tetrachloride and 100–150% excess of iodine monochloride in glacial acetic acid is added. After 1/2 hr, potassium iodide is added to convert the unused reagent to iodine, which is then titrated with sodium thiosulfate. Iodine value is related to hardness of a fat and its stability to oxidation. The lower the iodine value the harder and more stable the fat.

Stability to oxidation is measured by accelerated tests at elevated temperatures. In the Schaal test, the fat is heated in an oven at 140°F until rancidity develops. Other tests involve aerating the heated fat under standardized conditions and periodically measuring peroxide formation by iodometric titration or measurement of oxygen absorption of fat held at a constant elevated temperature. With specified fat products these accelerated tests may be correlated with shelf life.

Plastic properties of shortening, margarine oil, and coating fats are important and a number of methods are useful for defining consistency or plastic range. Micropenetration measures in tenths of a millimeter the penetration of a steel needle dropped on fat conditioned overnight by chilling in a refrigerator and then tempering at the temperature of the determination. Measurements at several different temperatures are used to establish the plastic range. Typical micropenetration values at 25°C for shortening, margarine fat, and lard are 10.0, 11.7, and 13.7 mm, respectively.

Plastic properties are dependent upon the content of liquid and solid glycerides. The percentage of solid glycerides at any given temperature may be estimated by measuring the expansion of the fat confined in a dilatometer as the temperature is raised and the volume changes with change of state from solid to liquid.

Other characteristics frequently determined include moisture and volatiles, saponification value, unsaponifiable matter, density, refractive index, melting point, and titer. For shortenings containing emulsifiers, monoglyceride content is determined iodometrically following oxidation with periodic acid.

Fatty-acid composition may be determined by converting the acids to methyl esters and separating them by gas-liquid chromatography (GLC). The most suitable liquid phase is a polyester, such as diethylene glycol succinate (DEGS).

Ultraviolet, infrared, nuclear magnetic resonance, and mass spectroscopy are useful for identification of fatty acids or determination of functional groups.

Production methods. Processing of oilseeds is carried out by pressing, extraction with solvents, or a combination of the two. Preparation of the seed requires cleaning, hulling, and separation of the hulls on shaking screens and by aspiration. The meats are ground or cracked and flaked to a thickness of 0.005–0.010 in. by passing through rolls. Flaked meats are cooked or tempered prior to pressing or extraction.

Pressing of oilseeds is usually done in continuous screw presses. The cracked or flaked, cooked or tempered meats are fed to the screw, which exerts a high pressure and presses the oil out between the bars making up a cylindrical cage or barrel. Oil content of the cake is reduced to about 3–4%. Prepressing requires less power, and 10–15% oil is left in the cake and subsequently extracted with solvent.

Extraction of flaked oilseeds or prepress cake with commercial hexane is the most efficient process, removing all but 0.5–1.0% oil. Several types of extractors are used but most operate on a continuous countercurrent principle with the flakes passing through the extractor in the opposite direction from the solvent. A single extractor processes 100 tons or more of soybeans per day or an equivalent quantity of other oil-bearing materials.

Animal fats are recovered from fatty tissue by the process of rendering. Rendering by the dry process is analogous to frying. Well-hashed stock is heated and stirred in open or closed steam-jacketed kettles at about 230°F. The fat is released as protein is coagulated. The cracklings are strained from the fat and pressed to recover the animal fat. Leaf lard is usually dry-rendered.

Wet-rendering is carried out by cooking in steam autoclaves at pressures of 40–60 psi for 4–6 hr and drawing off the floating fat, which is settled or centrifuged.

The newest rendering process includes comminution of the fat, heating, and centrifuging to remove fat from the tissue.

Refining is the general term used to describe the overall process of purifying fats and oils. Specifically it is the initial process of treating the crude oil with alkali to remove free fatty acids, coloring matter, and mucilaginous gums. The oil is mixed with alkali and heated to about 150°F, when it forms soaps of the free fatty acids. Impurities are adsorbed on the soap, which can be settled out but more frequently is continuously separated by centrifuges. Soda ash and sodium hydroxide are refining agents used in one- or two-stage processes. The refined oil is water-washed in centrifuges and dried under vacuum.

Extracted oils may be refined, or refined and bleached, before removal of the extracting solvent. With cottonseed oil this results in a lighter-colored product.

Bleaching is an adsorption process for removing color. Refined oil is stirred with about 1.0% of bleaching clay at 220–230°F, followed by filtration through a filter press. About 0.1–0.2% of activated carbon may be used with the clay. Bleaching readily removes most of the yellow carotenoid pigments. Special acid-activated clays or carbons are used to remove green pigments present in some oils.

Deodorization is the process of blowing hot oil with steam under a high vacuum to remove traces of volatile materials causing odor or flavor. Temperatures of 400–475°F and a vacuum of 5–6 mm are usually used in batch, semicontinuous, or continuous processes.

Texturization of plastic fats, such as lard or shortening, is a rapid solidification process which produces a fine crystal structure and a smooth firm product. The liquefied fats are continuously cooled and solidified on refrigerated chilling rolls or by passage through Votator units. Air or nitrogen is whipped into the product during the process.

Hydrogenation is a catalytic process of converting liquid oils into more saturated plastic fats by the direct addition of hydrogen. Refined oil and 0.2–0.10% of an active nickel catalyst are charged to a converter maintained under vacuum. The converter is equipped with an efficient stirrer for agitation and gas dispersion and a heating jacket to hold the contents at 200–400°F. Highly purified hydrogen is introduced under pressure maintained at 5–60 psi. Composition and physical characteristics, type and concentration of catalyst, pressure, and agitation or gas dispersion must be carefully controlled to give the desired product. The fat is rebleached and filtered after hydrogenation to remove the catalyst.

Crystallization, or winterization, of cottonseed oil is required for the production of salad oil to prevent solidification or crystallization at refrigerator temperatures. Refined and bleached oil is gradually chilled during a period of about 36 hr to 42°F to crystallize the more solid glycerides. Solids are filtered out and the oil deodorized.

Cottonseed oil is sometimes winterized in the extraction solvent. Crystal inhibitors, such as oxystearin, may also be added to the oil to retard crystallization at refrigerator temperatures. Soybean oil may be winterized to remove a small amount of wax.

Beef fat is crystallized at 85–90°F to separate oleo oil from oleostearin, and lard can be crystallized at 50°F to separate edible lard oil and grease. Separation is accomplished by pressing.

Emulsifiers, for example, mono- and diglycerides, are added to shortening to improve tenderness and increase shelf life of baked products, particularly bread and cakes. Also used as emulsifiers in margarine, they are prepared by reacting fats with glycerol.

Lecithin is a natural emulsifier recovered from crude soybean oil by water-washing. Purified by solvent fractionation, it is widely used as an emulsifier in food products, particularly margarine and chocolate coatings.

Acetoglycerides or acetin fats are modified fat products in which a portion of the fatty acids are replaced by acetic acid either by acetylating monoglycerides or by ester interchange of fats with triacetin. They may be stable liquid oils or flexible solid fats useful as moisture-retentive coatings on foods such as meats, cheeses, nuts, and raisins. Some types also have emulsifying characteristics.

Mayonnaise and salad dressings. These are made from salad oils, eggs or egg yolks, vinegar or lemon juice, seasonings, and sugar. Mayonnaise is a semisolid emulsion that must contain 50% oil, although it usually contains more nearly 70% oil. It is prepared by mixing in high-speed beaters.

Salad dressings are similar in composition to

mayonnaise but contain a cooked starch base and the oil content is usually 40–50% but may be as low as 20%.

Animal fats. These are produced under federal inspection and are classified as edible or inedible depending upon the source of fatty tissue. They are relatively saturated although they contain a small amount of the highly unsaturated arachidonic acid. Advances in processing techniques, particularly interesterification, the rearrangement of glycerides to a random or directed distribution of fatty acids, have greatly increased their utility, so that some shortening products are now mixtures of vegetable and animal fats.

Lard and rendered pork fat are produced domestically to the extent of about 2.2×10^9 lb annually. Lard does not of necessity require processing, aside from texturization. However, it may receive mild processing treatment to improve flavor and an antioxidant may be added to improve stability. Iodine value is 53–77 and melting point is 33–46°C.

Beef fat or tallow is quite hard, having an iodine value of 40–48 and melting point of 40–47°C. Only limited quantities find use in edible fat products.

Chicken fat has an iodine value of 64–76 and melting point of 32–34°C. Small quantities are produced and consumption is limited almost entirely to those of the Jewish faith, who use it as a cooking fat.

Vegetable oils. Vegetable oils account for well over one-half the total of edible fats produced and consumed in the United States.

Olive oil is prized for its natural flavor and is used crude as a salad or cooking oil without processing. The United States imports between 50×10^6 and 60×10^6 lb annually. It has a high content of oleic acid, an iodine value of 80–88, and is liquid at refrigerator temperatures.

Corn oil, produced from corn germ, is a product of the corn-milling industry. Annual United States production is about 450×10^6 lb. Used almost exclusively as a salad or cooking oil, it has a high content of linoleic acid, and an iodine value of 103–128. See CORN.

Soybean oil production has grown tremendously since the introduction of soybeans to the United States from the Orient in the 1920s, and today is 6×10^9 lb, of which 80% is consumed domestically in shortening, margarine, and salad oil. With an iodine value of 120–141, it contains major proportions of linoleic acid and 6–8% of linolenic acid. See SOYBEAN.

Cocoa butter is the fat pressed or extracted from cacao beans; it is not refined. It has the unique property of melting sharply just below body temperature, producing a cooling sensation in the mouth. It contracts upon solidification and the solid breaks with a sharp fracture or snap. Because of its physical properties, resulting from relatively simple glyceride composition, and its compatibility with chocolate liquor, it is used as a coating fat for confections and other foods. It has an iodine value of 35–40 and a melting point of 28–36°C. See COCOA POWDER AND CHOCOLATE.

Coconut oil is a highly saturated fat containing mainly lauric acid, 12 carbon atoms, and other saturated fatty acids of 8–16 carbon chain length. It is extremely resistant to oxidation but develops

an off-flavor upon hydrolysis. Its utility is limited because it is relatively soft and of short plastic range. It is used principally as a cooking oil, for confectionary fats, and in margarine. Iodine value is 7.5–10.5 and melting point 23–26°C.

Cottonseed oil production in the United States averages about $1,500 \times 10^6$ lb per year. Its major fatty acid is linoleic. It is processed for salad oil, shortening, and for use in margarine and mellorine. A stable liquid oil, it has an iodine value of 99–113. See COTTON.

Peanut oil is produced from peanuts surplus to demand for edible peanuts, or of lower grade, to the extent of 150×10^6 lb annually. It is used principally as a cooking oil and has an iodine value of 84–100. See PEANUT.   [FRANK G. DOLLEAR]

Bibliography: K. Bloch, *Lipide Metabolism,* 1960; H. A. Boekenoogen, *Analysis and Characterization of Oils, Fats and Fat Products,* 1960; H. J. Deuel, Jr., *The Lipids: Their Chemistry and Biochemistry,* 3 vols., 1951–1957; E. W. Eckey, *Vegetable Fats and Oils,* 1954; H. G. Kirschenbauer, *Fats and Oils: An Outline of Their Chemistry and Technology,* 1960; K. S. Markley, *Fatty Acids: Their Chemistry, Properties, Production and Uses,* 4 pts., 2d ed., 1960–1967; V. C. Mehlenbacher, *The Analysis of Fats and Oils,* 1960; *Official and Tentative Methods of the American Oil Chemists' Society,* 1946–1967; D. Swern, *Bailey's Industrial Oil and Fat Products,* 3d ed., 1964.

Fennel

The culinary spice and the plant *Foeniculum vulgare* (Umbelliferae), a tall perennial herb native to the Mediterranean region (see illustration). It now occurs in all parts of the world, often as an escape

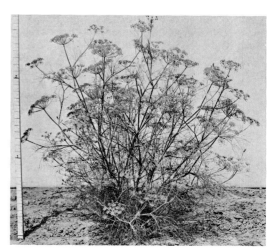

Fennel (*Foeniculum vulgare*). (*USDA*)

from cultivation. The fruits are used in cookery, confectionary, and for flavoring beverages. In modern French and Italian cooking, fennel is indispensable. Oil of fennel is used in medicine, soaps, and perfumes. See SPICE AND FLAVORING.

[PERRY D. STRAUSBAUGH/EARL L. CORE]

Fermentation

A term used since 1600 to denote a decomposition of foodstuffs generally accompanied by the evolution of gas. The best-known example is alcoholic fermentation, in which sugar is converted into alcohol and carbon dioxide. This conversion, described by the equation below, was established by J. Gay-Lussac in 1815.

$$C_6H_{12}O_6 \rightarrow 2CO_2 + 2C_2H_5OH$$
Sugar   Carbon   Alcohol
dioxide

Before 1800 the association of yeast or leaven with fermentation had been noted, but the nature of these agents was not understood. Experiments of C. Cagniard-Latour, of F. T. Kützing, and of T. Schwann in 1837 indicated that yeast is a living organism and is the cause of fermentation. This view was opposed by such leading chemists as J. von Liebig and F. Wöhler, who sought a chemical rather than a biological explanation of the process. The biological concept became generally accepted following the work of Louis Pasteur, who concluded that fermentation is a physiological counterpart of oxidation, and permits organisms to live and grow in the absence of air (anaerobically). This linked fermentation and putrefaction as comparable processes; both represent decompositions of organic matter brought about by microorganisms in the absence of air. The difference is determined by the nature of the decomposable material; sugary substances generally yield products with pleasant odor and taste (fermentation), whereas proteins give rise to evil-smelling products (putrefaction).

Pasteur also discovered the lactic acid and butyric acid fermentations, and from his experiments concluded that each kind of fermentation was caused by a specific microbe. Later work has supported this idea to a large extent, and considerably increased the number of specific fermentations.

During fermentation organic matter is decomposed in the absence of air (oxygen); hence, there is always an accumulation of reduction products, or incomplete oxidation products. Some of these products (for example, alcohol and lactic acid) are of importance to man, and fermentation has therefore been used for their manufacture on an industrial scale. There are also many microbiological processes that go on in the presence of air while yielding incomplete oxidation products. Good examples are the formation of acetic acid (vinegar) from alcohol by vinegar bacteria, and of citric acid from sugar by certain molds (for example, *Aspergillis niger*). These microbial processes, too, have gained industrial importance, and are often referred to as fermentations, even though they do not conform to Pasteur's concept of fermentation as a decomposition in the absence of air. For details of various fermentation processes *see* INDUSTRIAL MICROBIOLOGY.

[CORNELIS B. VAN NIEL]

Bibliography: R. Dubos, *Louis Pasteur, Free Lance of Science*, 1950; J. W. Foster, *Chemical Activities of Fungi*, 1949; H. J. Peppler (ed.), *Microbial Technology*, 1967; S. C. Prescott and C. G. Dunn, *Industrial Microbiology*, 3d ed., 1959.

Fertilizer

Materials added to the soil to supply elements needed for plant nutrition. The principal elements required are nitrogen, phosphorus, and potassium.

Several others—calcium, magnesium, sulfur, boron, iron, zinc, manganese, copper, molybdenum, and chlorine—are needed in lesser amounts. They are supplied in such various ways as materials produced for the purpose, as incidental components of fertilizers supplying other nutrients, and as compounds already present in the soil. *See* PLANT, MINERALS ESSENTIAL TO.

Fertilizers may be products manufactured for the purpose, by-products from other chemical manufacturing operations, or by-product natural materials. By-products, particularly natural organic materials, were important nutrient sources in the early days of the industry. The growing need for fertilizers, however, has outstripped the supply of by-products. Today manufactured materials are the major type by far and by-products have only minor significance.

The fertilizer industry once was mainly a simple materials-handling and mixing technology. However, it has become a major segment of the chemical industry, with giant plants embodying advanced developments in chemical engineering producing very large quantities of fertilizer. Several factors have contributed to its change in status: a maturing in agricultural practice in developed countries, rapidly increasing use of fertilizer in countries that had used little before, and a growing realization that massive production of fertilizer is the first line of defense against the problems of growing populations. The increase in world fertilizer consumption is indicated in the illustration.

Fertilizer types. The nutrient elements cannot be supplied to plants as such; they must be combined with other elements in the form of suitable compounds. Phosphorus, for example, is toxic to plants in the elemental form but is a good fertilizer when combined with oxygen and ammonia to form ammonium phosphate. For each of the elements there are several compounds that can be used. The choice between them, in most cases, is based on economic factors. Material is used that gives lowest cost per unit of nutrient applied to the soil.

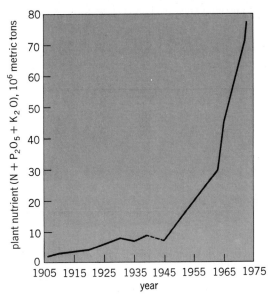

World fertilizer consumption for fiscal years 1906–1973. (*Food and Agriculture Organization*)

Nitrogen, phosphorus, and potassium are called the macronutrients because of the relatively large amounts needed. The usual requirement range per acre per cropping season is 50–200 lb of nitrogen, 10–40 lb of phosphorus, and 30–150 lb of potassium.

Nitrogen is supplied in the ammoniacal (NH_4^+) or nitrate (NO_3^-) form or as urea, (NH_2)$_2$CO. Except in unusual situations, one form is as good as the other because in the soil the ammoniacal and urea forms are rapidly converted by microorganisms to nitrate. The principal fertilizer nitrogen materials are ammonium nitrate, urea, ammonia, ammonium sulfate, and ammonium phosphate.

Phosphorus is supplied mainly as ammonium phosphates and calcium phosphates. Ammonium phosphates are the leader and are increasing in importance. The ammonium phosphates have advantages of higher nutrient concentration and higher water solubility, which favor them in regard to handling and shipping costs and, in some instances, in agronomic value.

Potassium is supplied almost entirely as potassium chloride, a mineral widely available in various parts of the world and usable without altering its chemical structure.

Sulfur, calcium, and magnesium are also essential elements but are needed in lesser quantities than the macronutrients. Therefore they are called secondary nutrients. Typical quantities of the secondary nutrients needed per acre per cropping season are as follows: 5–50 lb of sulfur, 5–25 lb of calcium, 3–30 lb of magnesium. In the past, substantial quantities of the secondary nutrients were supplied incidentally in macronutrient fertilizers, such as from calcium phosphates, from soil minerals, and from power plant emissions of sulfur oxides. However, with the trend to ammonium phosphates and other high-concentration products and to control of stack gas emissions, there is an increasing requirement for specifically formulating secondary nutrients into fertilizer products.

The remaining essential elements are called micronutrients; the amounts required are very small, from a trace to 1 lb/acre. They are usually supplied as cations or anions of salts such as borates or sulfates.

The nutrient amounts given refer to the quantity taken up from the soil by various crops. This does not mean necessarily that such an amount added to the soil will supply the plant adequately; there are many ways in which nutrient can be lost before the plant can take it up. Moreover, some nutrient is obtained from materials already present in the soil. Therefore, the amount of fertilizer actually applied depends on several factors that vary widely. Beyond the factor of plant need, a major consideration is the financial ability and technological status of the farmer; these are major factors in the very wide variation in fertilizer application per acre in various parts of the world. Highly developed and crowded countries use the most; in Belgium, for example, average macronutrient application is about 200 lb/acre. In contrast, less-developed areas, such as India, use as little as 1 lb/acre. *See* PLANT, MINERAL NUTRITION OF.

Nitrogen. This nutrient is required by plants in the largest quantity. Its use is expanding more rapidly than for any of the other nutrients. It has been found that, if adequate amounts of phosphorus, potash, and other nutrients are applied, very large amounts of nitrogen, coupled with high plant population per acre, give yields much higher than those attainable under previous fertilization practice. In 1956 world consumption was higher for phosphate and potash than for nitrogen (tonnage is on the oxide basis, P_2O_5 and K_2O, the common reporting method in the industry). But by 1961 nitrogen had passed both and continues to climb rapidly: in 1972–1973 the estimated world use of fertilizer nitrogen was 36,052,000 metric tons.

The fetilizer nitrogen supply is divided among several materials as shown in Table 1.

Ammonia. The basic nitrogen fertilizer material is ammonia, used both as a primary fertilizer and as the starting material for all the other leading nitrogen fertilizers. Ammonia is also an important general chemical, but its principal use (almost 85% of the total on a worldwide basis) is in the fertilizer industry. In 1974 there were about 91 complexes in the United States, with a production capacity of more than 17,738,000 tons per year.

In past decades the fertilizer industry used large quantitites of natural nitrogen materials, such as animal by-products, ammonia recovered from coal during coke production, and sodium nitrate from localized natural deposits in Chile. Today these sources are inadequate or too expensive; elemental nitrogen, present in inexhaustible quantities in the atmosphere, is the major source by far, accounting for more than 95% of the fertilizer nitrogen used in the United States.

Ammonia production technology changed rapidly in the 1960s. Natural gas became firmly established as the major feedstock, particularly after discovery and development of gas bodies in Europe and Japan. The use of elevated pressure in reforming, that is, reaction of gas with steam to give synthesis gas (hydrogen plus carbon monoxide), added considerable economy to the process. Also, low-pressure shift conversion, that is, reaction of synthesis gas with steam to eliminate carbon monoxide and produce more hydrogen, was widely adopted.

After purification the hydrogen is combined with nitrogen (introduced earlier in the process as air) under pressure (2000 psig or more) and high temperature (425–650°C) in the presence of promoted iron catalyst to form ammonia.

Table 1. Fertilizer nitrogen supplied by various materials

Material	Nitrogen content, %	Supply, 10^3 metric tons of nitrogen*	
		United States	World
Urea	45–46	389	5104
Ammonium nitrate	33.5	986	5513
Complex fertilizers	Varies	—	2332
Anhydrous ammonia (used as such)	82	2431	—
Ammoniated superphosphate	Varies	—	—
Ammonium sulfate	20.5	177	2194
Nitrogen solutions (used as such)	Varies	1030	—
Calcium nitrate	15.5	—	227
Sodium nitrate	16	9	89
Ammonium sulfate nitrate	Varies	—	203
Calcium cyanamide	28	—	130
Ammonium phosphate	Varies	99	243
Other nitrogen fertilizers	Varies	194	7318

*In 1972–1973.

The synthesis step in ammonia production has undergone major changes. Centrifugal compressors, used to compress the nitrogen-hydrogen mixture to synthesis pressure, have reduced plant cost. Single converters produce up to 3000 tons of ammonia per day, and converter design has been simplified to make the large size feasible.

Use of ammonia directly as a fertilizer requires use of pressure equipment since ammonia is a gas at atmospheric pressure. The material is carried in pressure tanks on applicators and injected into the soil through injector knives. Care is necessary to avoid loss by volatilization, and with deep placement, the ammonia is quickly sorbed by the clay and other constituents of the soil.

In 1958 ammonia became the leading nitrogen fertilizer in the United States. Use in other parts of the world, although growing, is relatively small.

Urea. Urea is expected to surpass ammonium nitrate as the world's leading form of nitrogen fertilizer in about 1976 and to continue to gain in importance. This is due to the more favorable economics in producing urea, to its high nutrient content (45–46%), and to its explosive-free properties in comparison with ammonium nitrate. With increasing costs for handling and shipping, the high concentration is assuming more and more importance.

Some urea is used in chemical industry, mainly in plastics production and in animal feeds, but the major proportion by far goes into fertilizers, either for direct application or as a constituent in mixes.

Urea is made by reacting ammonia and carbon dioxide under pressure and at elevated temperature but without a catalyst. The carbon dioxide is readily available because it is a by-product, usually wasted, in manufacture of ammonia from carbonaceous materials. Thus there is little or no cost for the carbon dioxide, but the urea plant must be built close to an ammonia plant.

The urea reaction does not go to completion; the product from the reactor is a solution of urea and ammonium carbamate, an unstable compound of ammonia, water, and carbon dioxide. The solution must be heated to decompose the carbamate and drive off the resulting ammonia and carbon dioxide, which are then recycled back to the reactor. The urea solution is concentrated to a melt containing less than 1% water in an evaporator. Practice differs in the method used for converting the melt to the final solid product. Prilling, which involves solidification of melt droplets by air-cooling in a tall tower, is the most widely used method. There is an increasing trend to granulation of the melt instead of prilling in the United States, because the granules are stronger and larger than prills. Also, air pollution abatement is less difficult for granulation.

Urea processes differ mainly in the method of removing and recycling the unreacted gases and in means of energy recovery. The processes have become increasingly efficient due to innovations for recovery and reuse of process heat for preheating feeds and for generation of steam which is used in the process.

Corrosion is a major problem in urea manufacture. Reactors lined with stainless steel are widely used. Some add air or oxygen to decrease corrosiveness of the stainless steel. A few reactors have been lined with highly resistant materials such as glass or titanium.

Another problem is formation of biuret, $(NH_2CO)_2NH$, during manufacture. Formation can be kept to a minimum by reducing the time during which the urea solution is exposed to elevated temperature. Biuret is harmful to some types of plants.

The use of urea presents the added problem that surface application may result in nitrogen loss because of urea decomposition (by hydrolysis) back to the gases from which it was made. The decomposition is accelerated by high soil temperature, low pH, and an enzyme (urease) found in the soil. By proper attention to conditions of application, losses can be kept to an acceptable level.

Urea is less hygroscopic than ammonium nitrate and gives less trouble with caking. It is also nonexplosive.

Ammonium nitrate. The most important nitrogen fertilizer, from the standpoint of world consumption, is ammonium nitrate. Large tonnages are used directly as a fertilizer, and considerable amounts go into mixtures with other materials. The material plays the somewhat remarkable double role of fertilizer and explosive. The explosive tendency has been somewhat of a problem in handling and shipping for fertilizer use. In modern practice, however, the hazard has been adequately controlled. In some countries ammonium nitrate fertilizer is diluted to a concentration of less than 70% by adding limestone so that the mixture is not detonable.

Ammonia and nitric acid are the raw materials for ammonium nitrate production. Since nitric acid is made by oxidizing ammonia with air, the only basic raw material needed is ammonia. This gives ammonium nitrate some advantage because other major nitrogen fertilizers require some raw material in addition to ammonia.

Nitric acid plants differ mainly in the pressure used at various stages of the process. Ammonia is oxidized catalytically with air by passing the mixture through a platinum catalyst screen at high temperature, after which the product gases are cooled and then passed through a scrubber, where water absorbs the nitrogen oxides to form nitric acid. The absorption and sometimes the oxidation are carried out at pressures up to about 100 psig.

Ammonium nitrate is made by neutralizing nitric acid with ammonia, usually in pressure-type neutralizers so that steam can be recovered from the highly exothermic reaction. The neutralized solution is then concentrated to a melt of low moisture content in an evaporator. Practice differs in the method used for converting the melt to the final solid product. Like urea, most ammonium nitrate is prilled. However, there is an increasing tendency to granulation, primarily to minimize air pollution problems.

Finally, ammonium nitrate is usually conditioned to reduce moisture absorption and caking. The main practice is either to coat with up to about 2% of a parting agent, such as clay, or to add a lesser amount of one of several chemical additives.

Ammonium sulfate. Ammonium sulfate is declining in popularity in relation to urea and ammonium nitrate. A major reason for the decline is the low nutrient concentration of 20–21% for ammonium sulfate versus 33–34% for ammonium nitrate and 45–46% for urea.

Almost all of the ammonium sulfate produced in the United States and much of that in the remainder of the world are from by-product sources. Much of this is derived from coke manufacture (by scrubbing ammonia out of the oven gases with sulfuric acid) and from production of caprolactam. Coke ovens, for example, supply about 750,000 tons of ammonium sulfate annually in the United States. A considerable tonnage is made also by reacting ammonia with sulfuric acid, which often is a by-product from petroleum refining or organic syntheses.

Manufacture of ammonium sulfate is relatively simple. Solution, either by-product or made by neutralizing sulfuric acid, is concentrated and then crystallized in one of several crystallization processes or else compacted into flakes.

Nitrogen solutions. In the United States liquid forms of fertilizer are quite popular because they can be handled and applied with a minimum amount of labor. The use of anhydrous ammonia, already described, is an example of this. Ammonia, however, must be handled under high pressure and must be applied carefully to prevent loss. To avoid these problems a class of products called nitrogen solutions has been developed. These are of various types, but in general they can be classified as water solutions of nitrogen salts (plus ammonia in some), all characterized by low vapor pressure (above atmospheric) or, in some instances, no gage pressure at all. The nonpressure solutions can be handled in ordinary tanks without special precautions and can be sprayed on the soil surface without loss. The pressure type requires some care in handling and must be injected into the soil, but the pressure is so low, only a few pounds, that requirements are much less rigorous than for anhydrous ammonia.

Nitrogen solutions are popular in the United States but are little used in other parts of the world. In 1973–1974 consumption in the United States was more than 4,049,000 tons, or about 1,185,000 tons of nitrogen—second only to anhydrous ammonia.

The leading nitrogen solution is a combination of urea and ammonium nitrate. These two salts are soluble separately only to the extent of about 20% nitrogen, but they have a mutual solubility effect on each other that produces a 32% nitrogen content when the two are dissolved together. About 80 lb of the combined salts can be dissolved by 20 lb of water.

Pressure-type solutions that contain ammonia and urea or ammonium nitrate, or in some products all three together, are also popular. The advantage of the ammonia is that it increases the total nitrogen content of the solution. Several of the pressure solutions contain over 40% nitrogen, with vapor pressures on the order of 10–15 psig.

Aqua ammonia, a solution of ammonia in water, also has the advantage of easier handling than anhydrous ammonia, but nitrogen content must be reduced to about 20% to get a satisfactorily low vapor pressure. Nevertheless, large quantities of aqua ammonia are used (about 724,000 tons in 1973–1974).

Other compounds. Numerous other nitrogen compounds are used as fertilizers, but the amounts are much smaller than for the leading nitrogen fertilizers described and are not expected to gain in the foreseeable future.

Sodium nitrate was once a major fertilizer but in 1972–1973 supplied only about 0.4% of world fertilizer nitrogen. The relative low nitrogen content (16%) is a major disadvantage in view of rising labor and shipping costs. About 10% of the world tonnage is consumed in the southeastern part of the United States, where the use is to some extent traditional.

Calcium nitrate is used mainly in Europe and in 1972–1973 supplied about 1% of world nitrogen. Almost half of the production is in Norway, where the material was made in the past as a method of using nitric acid made by the now-obsolete arc process for nitrogen fixation; production still continues from nitric acid made by ammonia oxidation.

Calcium cyanamide, made from calcium carbide and atmospheric nitrogen, in 1972–1973 made up about 0.6% of the nitrogen supply. Most of the production is in Europe and Japan.

Organic nitrogen materials once were major nitrogen fertilizers but now are estimated to supply less than 1% of the nitrogen. Organics may regain a significant place, however, because of the growing problem in disposing of urban organic waste. When the problem becomes severe enough in a situation to warrant waste processing, fertilizer usually is the most appropriate product to make.

Controlled-release nitrogen materials are not used in large quantities but may become significant in the future. By using a slowly soluble nitrogen compound or depositing an impermeable coating on a soluble one, release of nitrogen in the soil through dissolution of the fertilizer is delayed, thus reducing leaching and other losses that can be incurred with soluble nitrogen materials.

Multinutrient fertilizers supply the remainder of the fertilizer nitrogen, about 11 and 19%, respectively, of world and United States consumption. These are classed with phosphate or mixed fertilizers rather than with nitrogen products.

Phosphate. World consumption of fertilizer phosphate is not as large as that of nitrogen. In 1972–1973 the estimated world usage was 22,595,000 metric tons, with about 20% of the total used in the United States. The principal phosphatic fertilizers and their consumption and phosphate content are listed in Table 2.

Phosphoric acid. Modern high-analysis phosphatic fertilizers, such as ammonium phosphate and concentrated superphosphate, require phos-

Table 2. Fertilizer phosphate supplied by various materials

Material	Phosphate content, %	Supply, 10^3 metric tons of phosphate*†	
		United States	World
Ordinary superphosphate	16–22	32	4109
Concentrated superphosphate	44–47	487	2271
Complex fertilizers	Varies	–	2636
Basic slag	17.5	–	1238
Ground phosphate rock	Varies	1	–
Ammonium phosphate	20–46	181	2992
Other phosphate fertilizers	Varies	60	2742

*As P_2O_5. †In 1972–1973.

phoric acid in their manufacture. The acid in turn is made from phosphate rock, an ore found mainly in the Soviet Union, North Africa, and the United States (principally in Florida).

The leading method for phosphoric acid manufacture involves treatment of phosphate rock with sulfuric acid. The insoluble calcium phosphate in the ore dissolves in the acid, and crystals of calcium sulfate form. After separation of the calcium sulfate by filtration, the acid is concentrated to the level required in making the various fertilizer phosphates. This is called the wet process for phosphoric acid.

In the United States wet-process acid plants, the calcium sulfate is precipitated as a hydrated form called gypsum. The gypsum is discarded in storage piles and becomes a problem because of the large amount produced; the tonnage is larger than that of the phosphate rock used. It is simply not economical to reuse the waste gypsum. In Japan and some European countries, the by-product gypsum is reused to produce building materials, such as wallboard and cement.

Production of phosphate fertilizer uses over half of the sulfur consumed in the United States. In 1973 about 70% of this sulfur was supplied from elemental sulfur mined by the Frasch (hot-water) process and the remainder from sulfur removed from oil and natural gas. The trend is to increasing use of recovered sulfur.

Another method of phosphoric acid production is the electric furnace process. Phosphate rock, mixed with coke and silica, is heated to a high temperature in the furnace to reduce the phosphate to elemental phosphorus. The phosphorus is then burned with air and the resulting oxide absorbed in water to give phosphoric acid. The furnace method is not competitive with the sulfuric acid process for producing fertilizers except in unusual situations involving high sulfur cost and unusually low electrical power cost. The capital investment required for the furnace process is much higher than for the wet process. The furnace process yields a higher-purity product acid, but pure acid is not required for fertilizers.

A major development is superphosphoric acid which contains less water than ordinary phosphoric acid. Superphosphoric acid is made either by concentrating wet-process acid to a much higher concentration than usual (70–72% P_2O_5 versus 54%) or by using less water in the furnace method. The superphosphoric acid has the advantages of higher concentration, lower suspended solids (in the wet-process type), and certain chemical properties which make it preferable for production of some types of fertilizers. The superphosphoric acid is especially desirable for production of liquid products because it provides higher concentration and improved quality.

Ammonium phosphate. Ammonium phosphates are the leading forms of phosphate fertilizer and are gaining in importance. Over half the fertilizer P_2O_5 in the United States is applied in this form. Major reasons for the increasing popularity of the ammonium phosphates include: (1) high nutrient concentration, (2) good storage and handling properties, (3) high water solubility, (4) relative ease of production in large plants, and (5) favorable economics in comparison with competing products.

The most popular ammonium phosphate product is diammonium phosphate, which contains 18% nitrogen and 46% P_2O_5.

Several processes have been developed for making ammonium phosphates. In one of the more popular ones, the acid is treated with part of the ammonia in a tank-type vessel, the partially ammoniated slurry flows onto a rolling bed of solids (solidified ammonium phosphate) in a rotary granulating drum, the rest of the ammonia is injected under the bed of solids, the granules are dried, and the finished product of the desired particle size is screened out. Fine material passing through the screen is recycled to the drum to provide the bed of solids.

Important new products in the ammonium phosphate family include solid ammonium polyphosphate and urea-ammonium phosphate. Urea-ammonium phosphate is made by granulating urea into ammonium phosphate to give very-high-concentration products such as 28% nitrogen and 28% P_2O_5. Ammonium polyphosphate is made in either granular or liquid forms by contacting phosphoric acid and ammonia in a simple pipe reactor to produce a high-temperature, anhydrous melt. This anhydrous melt is either granulated or dissolved in water so as to give products with comparatively high nutrient concentration and good storability.

Superphosphate. The oldest of the phosphatic fertilizers, is normal superphosphate. The manufacturing process is quite simple: Phosphate rock is mixed with sulfuric acid (a smaller amount than in phosphoric acid production), the resulting slurry is held in a container for a few minutes until it solidifies, and the material is removed to a storage pile, where it cures for approximately 3 weeks in order for the reaction between rock and acid to reach completion.

The cured superphosphate is used to some extent as a fertilizer without further treatment, but most of it serves as one of the starting materials in making other fertilizers. The status of the material is declining, mainly because of its low nutrient concentration (about 20% P_2O_5). In the period 1961–1962 through 1972–1973, the percentage of world phosphate supplied by normal superphosphate declined from 49 to 26%.

Concentrated superphosphate (usually called triple superphosphate) is in a much better position because of its higher concentration (about 46% P_2O_5), over twice that of normal superphosphate. Its popularity has been growing in the United States for several years, and in 1964 it passed normal superphosphate, the leader since the beginning of fertilizer history. On a worldwide basis, triple superphosphate has not yet surpassed normal superphosphate in popularity; during 1972–1973 it supplied 14% of the phosphate, and the normal type supplied 26%. However, triple superphosphate is expected to continue to gain in importance.

Triple superphosphate is made by treating phosphate rock with phosphoric acid rather than with sulfuric acid. Therefore there is no sulfate present to dilute the product; instead, the acid supplies more nutrient phosphate than does the phosphate rock, and a very high nutrient content is realized.

Triple superphosphate is manufactured in much

the same manner as the normal type. The rock and acid are mixed, the slurry held in a "den" until it solidifies, and the moist mass transferred to storage for curing. Unlike normal superphosphate, much of the triple is granulated; that is, finely divided material cut from the curing pile is agglomerated to particles of fairly large size, on the order of $\frac{1}{16} - \frac{1}{8}$ in. in diameter. In this form it is easier to handle in direct application and in mixing with other granular materials to make a multinutrient, nondusty fertilizer.

The present trend is to directly granulate triple superphosphate without any denning step. Phosphoric acid and phosphate rock are continuously mixed in tanks to produce a fluid slurry which is then granulated, dried, and screened to give a hard, spherical granular product.

Nitric phosphate. In making ammonium phosphates or the superphosphates, sulfuric acid is required. This can be a major problem during periods when sulfur is in short supply or for countries that have no indigenous sulfur sources. Therefore there is interest in acidulation of phosphate rock with nitric acid, rather than with sulfuric.

Substitution of nitric acid for sulfuric or phosphoric acids, however, causes some special problems. Reactions with phosphate rock gives phosphoric acid plus calcium nitrate, rather than the phosphoric acid–calcium sulfate combination formed when sulfuric acid is used in making phosphoric acid. Calcium sulfate precipitates and can be separated, but calcium nitrate remains dissolved in the acid. If allowed to remain through further processing, it has a diluting effect and, more seriously, makes the product hygroscopic.

Various methods have been developed for coping with the calcium nitrate problem. In Europe it is crystallized out (by cooling the solution) and used directly as a fertilizer. Hygroscopicity is a problem, but with moistureproof bags the poor physical properties can be tolerated. Other acids that give an insoluble calcium salt can be used along with the nitric to convert the calcium nitrate, for example, to calcium sulfate or calcium phosphate.

In a typical process, phosphate rock is treated with 20 moles of nitric acid and 4 moles of phosphoric per mole of calcium phosphate in the rock. The acidulate slurry is then neutralized with ammonia and granulated. The phosphoric acid and ammonia convert the calcium nitrate to dicalcium phosphate and ammonium nitrate, both acceptable products.

In the crystallization version, enough calcium nitrate is crystallized out so that, when the solution is separated and ammoniated, the remaining calcium precipitates as dicalcium phosphate and the nitrate is converted to ammonium nitrate.

One disadvantage to nitric phosphate is reduced nutrient content because part or all of the calcium is left in the product. A typical product contains 20% nitrogen and 20% phosphate; in comparison, complete removal of the calcium would give a product containing about 24% of each nutrient.

Nitric phosphates are popular in continental Europe, but production in other major fertilizer-producing areas, the United Kingdom, the United States, and Japan, is relatively low. These products are most popular in countries that have limited supplies of native sulfur.

Other compounds. A few other phosphates contribute to the fertilizer supply. The most important of these is basic slag, fourth in world phosphate supply but losing ground to the newer highly concentrated materials. Basic slag, which contains only about 17% P_2O_5, is popular because it is a byproduct of steel production in Europe and therefore sells at a relatively low price. Over 1,162,000 metric tons of P_2O_5 was supplied by basic slag in Europe in 1972–1973, but only a minor proportion was made in other parts of the world.

Phosphate rock itself is also a leading phosphate fertilizer. Although the ore is so insoluble that acidulation or other treatment normally is considered necessary to make it usable, there are special soil-crop situations in which finely ground phosphate rock gives enough crop response to make its use justifiable. Although phosphate utilization is much lower than for processed phosphates, elimination of the processing cost makes it economical.

Generally the crop response to ground phosphate rock is better when it is applied to acid soils. Even then, the effectiveness is dependent on the mineral structure of the phosphate, with some types being much more effective than others.

Phosphate rock consumption as a direct fertilizer is quite large, about 1,800,000 metric tons of P_2O_5 in 1972–1973 (world usage). The full amount is not counted when ranking phosphate rock with other phosphate fertilizers, however, because much of the P_2O_5 in the rock is inert and unused.

Thermal phosphates are used to a limited extent, mainly in Germany and Japan. Phosphate rock is heated, usually to fusion, with some solid material that reacts with the rock at high temperature. In Japan, for example, the reactant is a magnesium silicate ore. In Germany soda ash plus silica has been used. The product has low concentration (19–24% P_2O_5) and is declining in popularity.

Bones and other organic sources of phosphate, once the leading type, have little significance in phosphate supply.

Potash. Tonnage of potash is the lowest of any of the macronutrients, estimated at 18,750,000 metric tons (of K_2O) in 1972–1973 as compared with 22,595,000 for P_2O_5 and 36,052,000 for nitrogen. The United States leads in consumption, with France, Germany, and the Soviet Union also major consumers.

The potash industry is quite simple in comparison to the nitrogen and phosphate industries. Atmospheric nitrogen and phosphate rock must be subjected to expensive processing to make them usable as fertilizers, but potash ore is soluble and can be used directly as mined without any treatment other than removing impurities. Hence, potash supply is more of a mining industry than a chemical processing.

The principal potash ore, supplying more than 90% of the world total, is potassium chloride. The natural deposits are tremendous; Canadian reserves in 1972 were estimated to contain about 11,000,000 metric tons of recoverable K_2O.

The Soviet Union leads in potash production, followed by Canada, East Germany, West Germany, the United States, and France. Most of the potash mined, over 90%, is in the form of potassium chloride. Potassium sulfate, also a soluble, readily available material, is the only other potash ore of significance.

Potassium chloride is a high-grade material with more than 60% potassium after impurities are removed. Potassium sulfate is somewhat lower in nutrient content, about 50% K_2O. Both are normally used in fertilizer mixtures without any intended reaction with other constituents, although reaction does occur incidentally in some cases, as in mixtures with ammonium nitrate, in which reaction with potassium chloride produces ammonium chloride and potassium nitrate in the mixture.

Minor quantities of potassium nitrate and potassium phosphate fertilizers are produced by treating potassium chloride with either nitric acid or phosphoric acid.

Mixed fertilizers. Most fertilizers are of the mixed type; that is, they contain more than one nutrient. This is mainly a convenience for the farmer since his soils need nutrients in certain proportions. Although he could buy single-nutrient materials and apply them in the desired ratios, it is more convenient and usually less expensive to buy them already mixed.

A mixed fertilizer may be simply a mechanical mixture, or the constituent materials may be reacted to form a "chemical" mixture. In the early days of the industry, the mechanical mixture was the prevalent type; today chemically reacted products occupy an important place in the industry.

The chemically mixed fertilizers usually are made by processes involving ammoniation of some combination of phosphoric acid, sulfuric acid, and superphosphates. Superphosphates, both the normal and concentrated types, are acidic in nature and will take up a considerable amount of ammonia. Either ammonia or ammoniating solutions may be used. The solutions have the advantage that they supply ammonium nitrate or urea as well as ammonia, and therefore give a higher content of nitrogen in the mix.

Much of the mixed fertilizer is produced in granular form; the powdery, dusty mixtures of the past have met with increasing resistance on the part of farmers. Granulation, usually carried out in a rotary drum or a paddle mixer, is accomplished by moistening the mix with water or with solution until the dry solids agglomerate. The modern practice is to carefully adjust the amount and proportion of soluble materials used (urea, ammonium nitrate, or acids), so that, at the elevated reaction temperature reached in the granulator, the proper proportion between liquid and solid phases will be reached and granulation accomplished at low water content. This method reduces the expense of drying, which is relatively high when water alone is used for granulation.

Trends in granulation are toward prereaction of acids and ammonia in separate tank or pipe reactors before feeding them to the granulation step. Heat and moisture are driven off during the prereaction, thereby decreasing the liquid phase in the granulator. This permits use of high proportions of acids, lowering cost of feed materials. The prereactor also can completely eliminate the need for drying some products.

Liquid mixed fertilizers are also an important fertilizer type. Low handling cost has popularized the liquid type to the extent that 14% of all mixed fertilizers in the United States is supplied in liquid form, and liquids are continuing to gain in popularity. In other parts of the world, however, liquids are not used as extensively.

The basic step in liquid fertilizer production is reaction of phosphoric acid to make an ammonium phosphate solution. Other materials, such as urea–ammonium nitrate solution and potassium chloride, are then added to give the nutrient ratio desired.

Although liquid fertilizers are simple to handle with pumps and through pipelines, they have the drawback that the water required to keep the constituents in solution dilutes the product. Development of polyphosphates has improved this situation; for example, a solution containing 11% nitrogen and 37% phosphate can be made from superphosphoric acid, but with the usual type of acid the contents are 8% nitrogen and 24% phosphate.

The most popular process for producing ammonium phosphate liquid mixtures involves contact of wet-process superphosphoric acid containing about 20% of the phosphate in polyphosphate form in a pipe reactor. The heat of ammoniation drives off more water so that a hot melt with 70–80% of the phosphate as polyphosphate is discharged from the pipe. The melt is caught in a circulating stream of liquid fertilizer and cooled before storing. The increase in polyphosphate content substantially improves the storage and handling properties of the liquid.

However, if the liquid mix contains a large proportion of potash, the polyphosphate is not nearly so effective in increasing concentration. For such products, suspension fertilizers, a relatively new fertilizer type, give a very high nutrient content. Suspensions are made by restricting the amount of water and carrying the resulting crystallized salts in suspension by use of 1% or so of clay as a suspending agent.

Bulk blending. The trend to granulation has brought about a revival of the mechanical-mixing practice prevalent in the early days of the industry, but with the difference that granular rather than powdered materials are used and the product is handled mainly in bulk rather than in bags. The main advantage is that a very simple mixing plant is adequate and the resulting low investment makes small, community-type plants feasible. Materials brought into such a plant do not have to be shipped very far after they are mixed, in contrast to "chemical-mixing" plants, which must be relatively large because of higher investment. Such plants must distribute the product over a larger area, and therefore raw materials may be hauled back over part of the route they traveled initially.

The principal materials used in bulk blending are ammonium nitrate, ammonium sulfate, urea, superphosphate, ammonium phosphate, and potassium chloride—all granular. They should be of uniform size to minimize segregation in handling and shipping.

The favorable economics of bulk blending have caused the practice to grow rapidly. It is estimated that more than one-third of the mixed fertilizer consumed in the United States is in the bulk blend form.

Micronutrients. Supplying micronutrients is not yet a very significant activity in the fertilizer industry. Although such nutrients are as essential as the macronutrients, natural supplies in the soil are adequate in most instances. The number of identified deficient areas is growing, however, and use of micronutrient materials is increasing.

From the standpoint of amount used, the principal micronutrient appears to be zinc, followed by boron, iron, manganese, and copper. Reliable figures on the comparative amounts consumed are not available. The tonnage is low, however, probably not more than 50,000 tons of total material annually in the United States.

Practice is split between "shotgun" and prescription application. Most agronomists and technical people prefer the prescription method, in which soil analysis and crop response are used as the basis for prescribing application in a particular situation. The "shotgun" approach involves mixing small amounts of micronutrient material into standard mixed fertilizers, on the basis that the micronutrient is needed generally as insurance against the development of deficiency.

Micronutrient salts can be incorporated in liquid fertilizers if polyphosphate is a constituent. The polyphosphate sequesters the micronutrient metals (zinc, iron, copper, and manganese), holding them in solution when they would otherwise precipitate.

There are often problems in incorporating micronutrients into solid fertilizers of the bulk blend type. The micronutrient must be finely divided because such a small amount is required; if granules were used they would be too far apart when applied to the soil. Mixing the fine material with granular mixed fertilizer, however, is a problem because the different sizes segregate in handling. Methods have been developed to cause the micronutrient to adhere to the surface of the granules. *See* AGRICULTURE, SOIL AND CROP PRACTICES IN; FERTILIZING.   [C. H. DAVIS]

Bibliography: British Sulphur Corporation Limited, *Phosphorus and Potassium No. 68*, p. 19, November-December 1973; Food and Agriculture Organization, *Annual Fertilizer Review*, United Nations; Statistical Reporting Service, *Consumption of Commercial Fertilizers*, U.S. Department of Agriculture, annual reports; Statistical Reporting Service, *Consumption of Commercial Fertilizers by Class*, U.S. Department of Agriculture, annual reports; Tennessee Valley Authority, *North American Production Capacity Data, January 1975*, National Fertilizer Development Center, Muscle Shoals, AL, Circ. Z-57; Tennessee Valley Authority, *TVA Fertilizer Bulk Blending Conference* (held Aug. 1–2, 1973, Louisville, KY), National Fertilizer Development Center, Muscle Shoals, AL, Bull. Y-62; U.S. Bureau of Mines, *1972 Minerals Yearbook*, vol. 3, U.S. Department of Interior, 1974.

Fertilizing

Addition of elements or other materials to the soil to increase or maintain plant yields. Fertilizers may be organic or inorganic. Organic fertilizers are usually manures and waste materials which in addition to providing small amounts of growth elements also serve as conditioners for the soil. Commercial fertilizers are most often inorganic. Fertilizer analysis and systematic application began about 1850 and marked the beginning of scientific crop production.

Grades. Commercial fertilizers are mainly designed to supply one or more of the three major elements nitrogen, N, phosphorus, P, and potassium, K, in suitable chemical form. The fertilizers are graded in the order N-P-K, the numbers indicating the percentage of the total weight of each of the three components. Hence, the numbers 5-10-10 represent a mixture containing 5% nitrogen, N, 10% phosphorus pentoxide, P_2O_5, and 10% potassium oxide, K_2O.

Physical forms. Chemical fertilizers are marketed in both dry and liquid forms. Dry forms include powdered, granulated, and pelleted fertilizers. Liquid fertilizers are obtainable in high-pressure and low- or nonpressure forms. Mixed fertilizer solutions are usually nonpressure liquids.

Application methods. Methods of applying fertilizers vary widely and depend on such factors as kind of crop and stage of growth, application rates, physical and chemical properties of the fertilizer, and soil type. Two basic application methods are used, bulk spreading and precision placement. Time and labor are saved by the practice of bulk spreading, in which the fertilizer is broadcast over the entire area by using large machines which cover many acres in a short time. Precision placement, in which the fertilizer is applied in one or more bands in a definite relationship to the seed or plants, requires more equipment and time, but usually smaller amounts of fertilizer are needed to produce a given yield increase.

When applied at planting, the fertilizer is usually placed in a single band 1–3 in. (1 in. = 2.54 cm) to

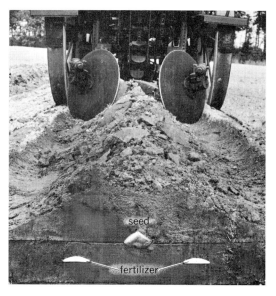

Fig. 1. Safe placement of fertilizer in reference to seed or seed piece is very important. This picture shows an efficient placement of fertilizer for potatoes. Attachments to make fertilizer placement at the time of planting are available on most field row planters. (*USDA, Agriculture Research Service*)

the side of and 2–6 in. below the seed (Fig 1). Care must be taken to have enough soil between the seed and fertilizer to prevent damage to the seed or developing seedlings. For crops highly susceptible to fertilizer injury, only a small amount of starter fertilizer may be applied at planting, with the remainder being applied as a side-dressing after the plants have emerged. Several side-dressings may be applied during the growing season to those crops with a high requirement for nitrogen or other elements which leach easily. Gaseous or volatile liquid fertilizers are applied 5–6 in. deep by using a narrow chisel tool and sealing the opening with a press wheel to prevent losses.

For some deep-rooted plants, subsoil fertilization to depths of 12–20 in. is advantageous. This is usually a separate operation from planting, and uses a modified subsoil plow followed by equipment to bed soil over the plow furrow, thereby eliminating rough soil conditions unfavorable for good seed germination. Top-dressings are usually applied by broadcasting over the soil surface for closely spaced crops such as small grains. Side-dressings for row crops may be placed at depths from surface to 5 in., but care must be taken to avoid damage to plant roots from the plow foot.

Equipment. Since solid fertilizers range from dense heavy materials to light powders and liquid fertilizers range from high pressure to zero pressure, a variety of equipment is required for accurate metering and placement. In addition, application rates may be as low as 50 lb/acre (56 kg/ha) or as high as 6 tons/acre (13.3 metric tons/ha). Large bulk spreaders usually use drag chains or augers to force the material through a gate or opening whose size is varied to regulate the amount passing through and falling on the spreader. One type of spreader consists of rapidly rotating horizontal disks with vanes mounted on their tops. The fertilizer is spread by centrifugal force over widths varying from 10 to 50 ft (3 to 15 m). Although this method is simple, the accuracy of distribution is affected by particle size, wind velocity, and slope of land on which the application is made. Another spreader consists of long perforated tubes through which the fertilizer is moved by augers.

Often the main supply bin contains simple agitators to prevent heavy or damp materials from bridging. The star-wheel metering unit is commonly used on drills and some row-crop fertilizer hoppers. This dispenser operates horizontally, with fingers carrying increments of fertilizer under a shield which is adjustable in height. Some drills have hoppers with rounded perforated bottoms. The hole size is adjustable by a slide, and the fertilizer is forced through by agitators mounted above the bottom of the hopper. Other mechanisms have been used, but basically all regulate the flow by varying opening size or speed of star wheel or agitator.

Liquid fertilizer of the high-pressure type (for example, anhydrous ammonia) is usually regulated by valves or positive displacement pumps. The size of the orifice may be controlled manually or automatically by pressure-regulating valves. Low-pressure solutions may be metered by gravity flow through orifices, but greater accuracy is obtained by using compressed air or other gases to maintain a constant pressure in the tank. This method eliminates the effect of temperature and volume changes. Nonpressure solutions may be metered by gravity or by gear, roller, piston, centrifugal, or hose pumps. The accuracy of the gravity type can be improved by the use of a constant head device by which all air is introduced into the tank at the bottom.

All of the pumps except the piston and hose types must be calibrated at a fixed pump speed since their output is not linear. Therefore, the overall accuracy of placement is dependent upon maintaining a constant driving speed, which is very difficult on rolling terrain. Errors of 15% or higher may be introduced by variations in driving speed. The piston and hose pumps can be driven by a wheel rolling over the ground, making their output proportional to driving speed. The hose pump consists of any number of hoses which are compressed by rollers in a sequential action which squeezes the liquid along the hoses. Since the output is determined only by the speed at which the pump is rotated, no manifolds, valves, or orifices are needed. Nonvolatile fertilizer solutions are often pumped into the supply lines of irrigation systems to allow simultaneous fertilization and irrigation.

With the exception of the bulk spreaders and other broadcasters, most fertilizer application devices are built as attachments which can be mounted in conjunction with planters, cultivators, and herbicide applicators. Often the tanks, pumps, and controls used for liquid fertilizers are also used for applying other chemicals such as insecticides.

[J. G. FUTRAL]

Effect on growth and yield. For plants to develop, all the nitrogen and mineral elements essential for growth must be supplied by way of the root system or, to a limited extent, through the leaves. The total supplies of mineral elements in certain soils are often adequate for many years of crop production, but the rate at which those elements become available for plant use may be too slow. Each nutrient must be in adequate supply in intensity and capacity, and in a reasonably favorable balance with all the others. Hence potassium, phosphorus, and any of several micronutrients may be deficient in rate of supply because of

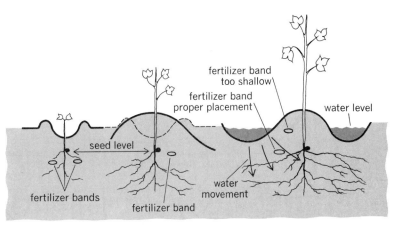

Fig. 2. Relationship of the placement levels of plant food materials to the movement of water. (*From Western Fertilizer Handbook, California Fertilizer Association, 1965*)

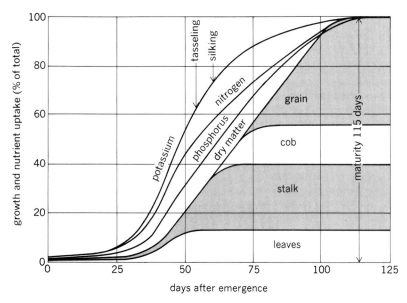

growth and nutrient uptake (% of total)

days after emergence

Fig. 3. Graph showing the growth and the uptake of nutrients in relation to the accumulation of dry matter by corn plants. (*From C. E. Millar, L. M. Turk, and H. D. Foth, Fundamentals of Soil Science, Wiley, 1965*)

fixation or adsorption by the soil; lack of nitrogen may become a limiting factor through adverse microbial conditions or excessive loss by leaching. Moreover, the rate of supply of nutrients must be favorable throughout the various ontogenetic stages of growth.

Desirable characteristics. Fruit or storage organs, rather than merely vegetative yield, are often desired. Further, it is frequently the total content of some substance within the harvested organ that is important rather than the weight or size of the organ alone. Thus the quality of tomatoes or grain or the percentage of sugar in cane or beets is economically important. The mineral supply at later stages of growth may determine the economic value of the crop. For example, high nitrogen acquisition at later stages of development may lead to increased protein but decreased carbohydrate content. Therefore mineral nutrition must be in favorable accord with development of desirable characteristics of vegetative growth and the harvested product.

Nutritional requirements. Plant growth and the quality of the harvested product are dependent on proper nutrition. Mineral materials are usually derived from the soil and, while total supply is important, the rate of effective availability is paramount. Plant and soil form an integrated system, in which the root is the nutrient-absorbing organ. While the type of root development is a species characteristic, its distribution in space may depend on environmental conditions in the medium. Thus it may vary in lateral and vertical disposition and in production of root hairs. Modifications also depend on physical and chemical conditions in the soil. Cultural management, such as cultivation, water, fertilization, spacing (competition), and cropping regime, may be determinative. If rooting into areas of nutrient adequacy is extensive (other factors being satisfactory), additional fertilizer may not be essential. Soil depletion, however, requires resupply to meet plant demand; deficiencies must be corrected for optimum growth. Growth is dependent on nutrient supply. Conversely, since plant need varies with rate of growth and the stage of ontogenetic development, the time, placement, and rate of fertilization are important. Some typical fertilizer placements are illustrated in Fig. 2. Plant growth, nitrogen distribution, and total sorption in corn are shown in Fig. 3 and in the table.

Nonlegumes may require greater nitrogen fertilization than legumes. In this respect, the microbiological population and other soil factors, such as temperature, aeration, pH, and organic matter, are important. Bacterial species and their numbers are an important facet of fertility relations in general, especially insofar as nitrogen fixation and the presence of organic matter are concerned. Pathological disease incidence varies with fertilization. Fertility relations affect evapotranspiration by modifying the ratio of canopy cover to soil surface area, thus determining efficiency of water use. Rate of replenishment of nutrients from the soil or other medium may limit growth, as root sorption may create depletion zones in the rhizosphere of roots. *See* NITROGEN FIXATION (BIOLOGY); SOIL MICROBIOLOGY.

Fertilizers. For improving the mineral nutrition of plants, single materials or favorable combinations of chemicals are compounded and used. Chemical compounds may include all of the miner-

Approximate plant growth, sorption of primary nutrients, and water use for a 100-bu corn crop per acre or hectare*

Plant part	Basis	Dry weight	Nutrient sorption†			Water use‡
			N	P	K	
Shoots	Acre	13,000 lb	155 lb	26.3 lb	104 lb	6.5×10^4 lb
	Hectare	14,600 kg	173.7 kg	29.5 kg	116.5 kg	7.3×10^4 kg
Roots	Acre	5,000 lb	50 lb	8.7 lb	33 lb	2.5×10^4 lb
	Hectare	5,600 kg	56.0 kg	9.7 kg	37.0	2.8×10^4 kg
Shoots and	Acre	18,000 lb	205 lb	35 lb	137 lb	5.5×10^6 lb
roots	Hectare	20,200 kg	229.8 kg	39.2 kg	153.4	6.2×10^6 kg

*From American Potash Institute, *Plant Food Your Corn Absorbs*, 1959; National Plant Food Institute, *Our Land and Its Care*, 1962.

†Apart from certain possible luxury accretion, the total sorption of nutrients represents that necessary during growth. That part in roots is restored to the soil. Therefore the net removal of nutrients is that contained in the shoots, unless stover is returned to the soil.

‡Total water use during growth (5.5×10^6 lb or 6.2×10^6 kg) includes that for growth and that expended in evapotranspiration. The water in shoots is in large part lost to the air on crop maturity; that in roots is largely returned to the soil.

al elements that are essential to growth. Micronutrients, occurring as impurities in fertilizer-grade chemicals, in come cases may be inadequate for maximum plant development and extra supplies may have to be added. Some latitude is permissible in the balance of elements supplied, but both marked deficiencies or marked excesses of any one element must be avoided.

Balanced fertilizers. Commercial fertilizers, manures, lime, or other materials may be added to provide essential mineral elements at required levels of availability or as amendments to make environmental conditions more favorable, improve structure, or enhance microbial activity within the soil so that such factors do not become limiting to growth and development. Sometimes reference is made to the use of balanced fertilizers. The balance that is important is not in the fertilizer but in the soil after the fertilizer has been added and has reacted with the soil. The same fertilizer may produce different effects in different soils. Addition to the soil does not necessarily ensure availability; certain elements, such as potassium, phosphorus, and at least some of the micronutrients, are strongly fixed in some soils. This is especially true where the colloidal clay content of the soil is relatively high. In any case, what is important is the ability of the plant to acquire essential nutrients in proper quantities favorable for the species at any particular time during growth and development, assuming other factors to be optimal.

Soil type and composition. When considering application of fertilizer to soil, general information should be sought regarding the types of soil in the area and their physical and chemical compositions. Crops favorable to the representative soil and climatic conditions should be considered. Local agricultural information on these matters is usually available. "Feeding" zones vary with species and soil management. Shallow-rooted species absorb from and deplete zones different from those of deep-rooted crops. As roots grow, absorb, and die and after root decomposition, minerals may be redistributed thereby in the soil and thus provide a more available source of nutrients for succeeding plantings. Fallowing allows replenishment from parent and residual organic materials. Total salt and pH tolerance of species, as well as the total specific salt content and pH of the soil, must be considered. Protracted applications of single or even some mixed fertilizers may correct unfavorable conditions or cause adverse changes in total salt level, exchangeable ion ratios, or pH of the soil. The nature of the materials and of all interrelated facets of cropping and soil dynamics determine the result. For example, simple leaching may correct total salinity; sulfur, with microorganism activities, may correct alkalinity; lime may correct acidity; and gypsum may correct an unfavorable ion-exchange balance and the soil structure.

Types of fertilizers. Fertilizer materials may be organic (urea) or inorganic (ammonium phosphate, potassium nitrate); natural (Chilean sodium nitrate, calcium sulfate) or synthetic (ammonium sulfate); simple, mixed (two or more), or complete (containing N, P, and K). They may be applied to soil in gaseous (ammonia), liquid (ammonia, or solutions), or solid (rock phosphate) states. Filler or make-weight material may be added to solid concentrates. Numerous factors must be considered in deciding the most productive mode, place, amount, balance, and time of application to fulfill known or anticipated plant needs. Knowledge of specific crop requirements at various stages of development (seedling, vegetative, reproductive), soil and irrigation water analysis, periodic plant tissue tests, and previous growth and harvest results will assist in suggesting management practice.

Maintaining adequate soil conditions. Natural and artificial materials can replenish nutrients as well as improve structure and water-holding capacity of many soils. Temperature, pH, aeration, and activity of microorganisms determine the rate of decomposition and supply or loss of nutrients. Natural manures are good sources of N, P, and K; stubble may be low in N, P, and Ca, but may be supplemented with ammonium sulfate, superphosphate, and limestone. Cover crops, especially legumes, are a means of effectively supplying natural organic matter to soils and favorably altering nutrient availability. Similarly, crop rotation can usefully provide protracted land use while meeting economic supply and demand. It is often necessary on a long-term basis to obviate or correct development of certain soil pathogens. Nurse crops under some conditions, for example, in orchards) can be beneficial. Manures, though beneficial on many soils, are not necessarily indispensable. Fully satisfactory plants or their products can be attained with soilless culture. Although soilless culture cannot supplant usual agricultural methods generally, it can supplement them where mechanics and economics justify such methods.

Choice of fertilizer. The best fertilizers to use depend on the anticipated plant need and interactions with the soil, prior to or during cropping, which may determine availability for plant growth. Organics and many inorganics are useful where suitable. Need must be known, and the appropriate combinations of elements must be applied to favor soil conditions and plant growth. A single inorganic salt or combinations of such salts may accomplish this. The ratios of essential elements in a fertilizer should be considered on their atomic equivalent basis per unit weight, not as the oxides or otherwise, which is the way the plant utilizes them. Further, size of particle and nature of the

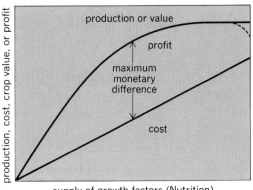

Fig. 4. Representation of the economics of crop production per unit area. Schematic shapes of curves (increases) may vary with conditions.

chemicals should be considered; granules or larger particles and relatively insoluble compounds may dissolve slowly, which may be desirable or disadvantageous. Some applied ions may be fixed on soil colloids (such as K or P) or precipitated (such as Ca, Fe, or P) through chemical double decomposition. Some solubles (such as NO_3) may be leached by excessive amounts of water to subsoil or drainage systems and thus become ineffective or lost.

So-called sustained-release fertilizers are marketed; they are coated particles that release the elements slowly and protractedly. To lessen fixation of micronutrient cations by soil colloids, these metals are effectively supplied in chelated form, which involves weak chemical binding. In this form they may be sprayed upon foliage and thus effectively fertilize the plant. Natural materials may supply micronutrients as an appreciable impurity, though often inadequately.

Soil conditioning. Soil amendments or conditioners are often applied to improve structure for aeration, water penetration, and other soil conditions. Natural organic materials may be helpful, if not supplied excessively. Gypsum can favorably increase granulation and flocculation of soil colloids, being especially useful in nonsaline alkali soils. Some synthetics have been proposed to improve soil structure but thus far are not economically practical. Some have been suggested to decrease excessive evapotranspiration but, here too, further experimental trial is necessary for practical and economic feasibility.

To properly fertilize a crop, the agriculturist should know fairly well the nature and properties of soils, fertilizers, and plants, their many interactions, and the economics of fertilization (Fig. 4). *See* AGRICULTURE, MACHINERY IN; AGRICULTURE, SOIL AND CROP PRACTICES IN; FERTILIZER; PLANT, MINERAL NUTRITION OF; PLANT, MINERALS ESSENTIAL TO; PLANT GROWTH.

[THEODORE C. BROYER]

Bibliography: C. A. Black, *Soil-Plant Relationships*, 1968; H. D. Chapman, *Diagnostic Criteria for Plants and Soils*, 1966; W. H. Garman (ed.), *The Fertilizer Handbook*, 1963; E. J. Hewitt, *Sand and Water Culture Methods in the Study of Plant Nutrition*, 1966; M. H. McVickar, G. L. Bridger, and L. B. Nelson (eds.), *Fertilizer Technology and Usage*, 1963; W. H. Pierre et al. (eds.), *Plant Environment and Efficient Water Use*, 1966; E. J. Shaw (ed.), *Western Fertilizer Handbook*, 1965; H. B. Sprague (ed.), *Hunger Signs in Crops*, 1964; J. F. Sutcliffe, *Mineral Salts Absorption in Plants*, 1962; S. L. Tisdale and W. L. Nelson, *Soil Fertility and Fertilizers*, 1966; A. Wallace (ed.), *A Decade of Synthetic Chelating Agents in Inorganic Plant Nutrition*, 1962.

Fescue

A group of grasses, of which the most important species in agricultural use is tall fescue (*Festuca arundinacea*). Two improved strains that are similar in appearance and value are Alta, produced in Oregon, and Kentucky 31. The leafy and vigorous plants grow to a height of 3–4 ft. Tall fescue has a wide range of soil and climatic adaptation and responds to fertile soils, in which it develops open sods. In mild climates growth continues through-

out winter. Sustained summer growth is usual. Fescue is used for both hay and pasture, although it is sometimes unpopular because of the harshness of the older leaves. Good seed habits, ease of establishment, and high productivity have increased its use for pasture over much of the United States.

Other important fescues are Meadow fescue (*F. elatior*), used to limited extent in pastures and as a shade-tolerant lawn species; red fescue (*F. rubra*), a fine-leaved type (several strains) used almost exclusively for lawns; and Idaho fescue (*F. idahoensis*), sheep fescue (*F. ovina*), and hard fescue (*F. duriuscula*). The last group are all fine- or bristle-leaved types adapted to drier regions and poorer soils. *See* GRASS CROPS.

[HOWARD B. SPRAGUE]

Fiber crops

Many plants are grown as fiber crops because of their content or yield of fibrous material which is used for many commercial purposes and for home industry. The production and use of plant fibers date back many centuries and form the basis for one of the earliest industrial processes. Fibers may be extracted from various parts of different plants.

Long, mutiple-celled fibers can be subdivided into hard, or leaf, fibers that traditionally are used for cordage, such as sisal for binder and baler twine and abaca or manila hemp for ropes; soft, or bast (stem), fibers that are used for textiles, for example, flax for linen, hemp for small twines and canvases, and jute and kenaf for industrial textiles such as burlap; and miscellaneous fibers that may come from the roots, such as "broom" root for brushes, or stems, as Spanish moss for upholstery, or fruits, as coir from coconut husks for cordage and floor coverings.

There are many exceptions to these uses. For example, some sisal near the sources of production is used for bags, and jute is used for cordage. However, the large quantities that enter international trade are used as indicated above.

Short, one-celled fibers come from the seeds or seed pods of plants such as cotton and kapok. Cotton is the world's most widely grown and used textile fiber. Kapok, because of its low tensile strength, goes primarily into upholstery, pillows, and life preservers. Many plant fibers are being replaced wholly or in part by synthetic or man-made fibers. Mixtures of natural and synthetic fibers often exhibit qualities superior to either used alone.

[ELTON G. NELSON]

Fig

A deciduous tree, *Ficus carica*, with a milky juice growing in subtropical regions of Asia, Africa, Europe, and the United States. The fruit, a syconium, consists of a fleshy hollow receptacle lined with pistillate, or female, flowers and with a small opening at the end (see illustration). Most edible types and varieties develop fruit without pollination. Smyrna-type figs require pollination by a small wasp, *Blastophaga psenes*, which lives primarily in the inedible, pollen-bearing caprifig or wild fig. Seedy fruits of the Smyrna-type fig are considered of finer flavor than those fig types without seeds. In the United States figs are grown primarily in California with minor production in Ari-

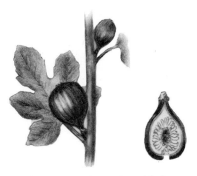

Fig (*Ficus carica*), details of branch and fruit.

zona, Texas, and Florida. The annual crop value is approximately $8,500,000. *See* FRUIT, TREE.

[CHARLES A. SCHROEDER]

Filbert

A nut from any plant in the genus *Corylus;* also called hazelnut. About 15 species are recognized, distributed widely over the North Temperate Zone and ranging in size from shrubs to tall trees. Filberts in commerce are derived mostly from the European species *C. avellana* and *C. maxima.* Hybrids of these with the American species, *C. americana,* are grown sparingly in the eastern United States.

Filberts belong in the birch family (Betulaceae), which produces the staminate (male) flowers in catkins on the previous season's growth and the pistillate (female) flowers, which form the nuts, at the end of the current season's shoots. The wind-blown pollen is shed from the catkins in late winter or early spring, when the pistillate flowers are receptive to fertilization. Cross pollination is necessary to produce a crop of nuts. The round or oval nuts, ½ to ¾ in. (1.3 to 1.9 cm) in diameter, are developed in a leaflike husk, from which they fall at maturity.

Filberts are grown widely in Europe and the Mediterranean basin, where much of the crop is consumed locally. Imports to the United States come mostly from Turkey. In the United States filberts are grown in Oregon and Washington.

American filberts are grown as small trees with single trunks. This requires frequent removal of the sucker shoots, which normally grow from the base and produce a bush. In Oregon harvesting is done with machines which rake the nuts into windrows and pick them up from the smooth-rolled ground.

Filberts are sold in shell, or the kernels are roasted and used in confectionery and baked goods. See NUT CROP CULTURE.

[LAURENCE H. MAC DANIELS]

Fisheries conservation

The term fishery is used in this article to mean the place for taking fish or other aquatic life, particularly in sea waters. The term has various legal connotations depending upon whether the right to take fish is founded on ownership of the underlying soil and therefore exclusive (several fishery), whether the right to fish in public waters is enjoyed in common with others (common fishery), or whether the right is an exclusive privilege, derived from royal or public grant, and independent of the ownership of the underlying soil (free fishery).

A fishery may be operated for pleasure (sport fishery) or for profit (commercial fishery). Fisheries include finny fish; mollusks, such as clams, mussels, and oysters; shellfish, including lobsters, shrimp, and crayfish; aquatic plants; sponges; coral; sea cucumbers; amphibians, chiefly frogs; reptiles such as turtles, alligators, and crocodiles; and mammals, including whales, seals, and walruses. *See* MARINE FISHERIES.

Distribution and types. Fisheries are important for the production of food and of raw materials for industry, and for recreation. They occur in all the many kinds of waters that together compose nearly three-fourths of the Earth's surface. The two principal types are marine (salt-water) fisheries, which annually yield 25,000,000–30,000,000 metric tons of products; and fresh-water (inland, continental), producing annually a recorded catch of 3,000,000–4,000,000 metric tons plus a sporting take of great but unknown magnitude. Both types have potentials far greater than present realizations.

Marine fisheries are mostly commercial and are located predominantly in the Northern Hemisphere. The most important fishery centers and the principal products they yield are the northeastern Atlantic (flatfishes, including halibut and flounder, cod, haddock, coalfish, herring, and shrimp); the northwestern Pacific (salmon, flatfish, herring, crab, shrimp, lobster, squid, and octopus); the northwestern Atlantic (flatfish, cod, haddock, herring, lobster, and crab); and the Indo-Pacific (herring, bonito, mackerel, and shrimp).

The major fresh-water fishing areas and their products are Asia (ayu, salmon, milkfish, carp); Soviet Union (salmon, whitefish); Africa (many kinds of fish); and central and northern North America (trout, whitefish, bass, perch and their relatives). Fresh-water fisheries in the more highly civilized parts of the world are used primarily for sport. However, they are important largely for food in primitive regions, including parts of Africa and South America, and in densely populated lands, especially those on a rice economy, such as India, China, Japan, and the smaller nations of Southeast Asia.

Problems. The major problem in fishery conservation is how to control both man and the aquatic community to ensure the production and the harvest of aquatic crops for the present and for the future when the demand will probably be greater than now. Lack of knowledge or care by fishermen may make their fishing efforts inefficient, their treatment of captured fish wasteful, and their methods of capture destructive to stocks needed as "seed" for future harvests. Handlers, marketers, and consumers may cause waste by careless preservation (refrigeration, salting, and canning) and by inefficient preparation for the table. Lack of information may also be responsible for inadequate harvest of many underexploited or unexploited segments of the resource. Consumers need to be educated away from preferential buying habits that accelerate the demand and price for certain species but lead to the discard of other kinds of aquatic organisms with equally sound food values.

The destruction of the aquatic habitat by man accentuates fishery problems, especially in inland waters. Deforestation and destructive agriculture, resulting in soil erosion and excessive warming of waters, have changed the fish-producing characteristics of many streams, usually for the worse. Sewage and industrial wastes reduce the quality of water suited for desired aquatic life. Organic pollutants such as domestic sewage may remove life-important oxygen from the water (waters generally are undesirable for aquatic life if the dissolved oxygen in them falls below 3 ppm). Pollutants may also be directly poisonous to fish and other water organisms (for example, most chemicals that are poisonous to man, such as cyanides, are also toxic to desirable aquatic life). Habitats may be destroyed by smothering them with silt (washings from mineral refineries such as coal and iron). *See* SOIL CONSERVATION.

Man has likewise created problems for aquatic life in continental waters by changing phases of the water cycles. Deforestation and agricultural land drainage have lowered the ground water table and have lessened stream flows during dry periods. The construction of dams for water storage, power, navigation, industry, flood control, domestic water supply, and irrigation has interfered with the movements (usually for spawning) of native migratory fish. Outstanding problems created by dams are those affecting the migrations of the Columbia River salmon in the western United States and the Atlantic salmon throughout its range in both northeastern North America and Europe. To date there has been little success in developing devices (fish ladders) that enable fish to progress over high dams to upstream spawning areas. Irrigation channels may lead fish to doom by leaving them stranded when the channels are drained, and fish may be destroyed by being jammed against intake screens of power developments. Fluctuations in water level may destroy fish nests by making the water over them too shallow or too deep.

Problems of fisheries conservation also arise from fishing. The greatest problem is that of managing each fishery so as to provide sustained yields of desired species. The solutions of these problems lie in research, public education, legislation and law enforcement, and continuing reevaluation of management procedures. Fishing itself may be destructive; the gear may injure the young while capturing harvestable adults. Fishing may exceed the capacity of a species to maintain itself through reproduction and growth. Although the species may not be exterminated by such overfishing, the fishery may become unattractive economically and for recreation. If it "collapses" entirely, this may bring considerable hardship to the fishermen. Similarly, underfishing is wasteful. In small inland waters, underfishing may destroy the quality of a fishery by leading to overpopulation and thus dense stands of undersized fish, which are unattractive to fishermen. Selective fishing for preferred species, often for predatory ones, may cause coarse, unwanted kinds to usurp the fish-producing capacity of a body of water.

Some problems of fisheries conservation arise naturally. Included are diseases, natural pollution such as "red tide" of protozoa in marine water, parasites, predators, and the gradual evolution of lakes toward ponds and dry land and of streams toward sluggish, base-level waterways.

Management. Laws to regulate fishing are the chief instruments of fishery management. This is particularly true in the commercial fisheries. Commonly, laws control who may fish, as well as where, when, and how they may fish. These laws regulate the kind, size, and amount of fishes that may be taken during a prescribed period. Legal measures such as antipollution legislation also protect the habitat of aquatic organisms. Because of changing conditions, the efficacy of laws should be continually reviewed.

The artificial propagation of fishes and other aquatic organisms, reputedly practiced in China for several centures B.C., is a means of increasing the quantities of preferred species. In Southeast Asia aquiculture combined with rice culture is an important source of fish for human food. Preferred food fishes in Europe (carp, trout) and North America (trout) are also produced for sale at fish farms or hatcheries. In addition, bait fish are propagated (and sold) extensively in North America. Aquatic farm production methods are also applied to oysters (as food or for pearls), frogs, turtles, ornamental fishes (such as goldfish), and water plants (ornamental, as the lotus, or edible, as the water chestnut).

Some artifically propagated fishes are used in the management of sport and commercial fisheries. Many kinds have been established successfully in waters far removed from their native ranges or in newly created water areas. Still others have been stocked successfully to bolster numbers available to sport fishermen. However, countless others have been placed in waters not suited to them and they soon disappeared, or they have been planted where adequate spawning stocks of the species were already present, in which cases they were wasted or they aggravated an already bad situation of overpopulation. In other situations, the artificially stocked fish have increased so rapidly that they have destroyed or seriously menaced desirable species already present.

Aquatic life in continental lakes, ponds, and streams requires a stable supply of water, with chemical and physical factors varying according to species requirements. Consequently, much effort is spent in learning the best conditions for life of preferred organisms and in managing habitat to provide the prescribed conditions. Often the environment can be improved. Starting in the headwaters of a stream system, land-use practices may be adjusted with the water world in mind, for example, by retarding surface runoff and encouraging percolation of water into the ground. In the water area itself, chemical, physical, and biological changes can be made to enhance stability, productivity, and yield to fishermen. Pollution and erosion may be controlled and improvement made in food, feeding, and shelter conditions. Species composition, competition, predation, and fishing pressure can be regulated somewhat.

Ponds have been built for many centuries to provide fish and fishing in areas having few natural surface water bodies. In the middle years of the 20th century, there was a surge of artificial pond or lake construction in the United States and hundreds of thousands of small impoundments resulted from the farm pond program, especially in states not bordering the Great Lakes.

Fishery management measures also include educational programs on fish conservation. They likewise encompass basic and developmental research in government and university laboratories. Moreover, these measures include the training of professional fishery scientists to develop and apply the most effective fishery methods.

In general, governments regulate inland, coastal, and boundary-water fisheries. Fishermen are commonly required to buy licenses to fish. In the United States, regulation is primarily at the state level, with the state retaining ownership of the fishes in public waters. In many international waters, international agreements and treaties are used. Often these are in the form of international commissions such as the North Pacific Fishery Commission, Northwest Atlantic Fishery Commission, and the International Great Lakes Fishery Commission.

There are numerous governmental aids to the conservation of fisheries at the local, national, and international levels. Educational programs constitute one of these. Another aid is in the form of exploration for new stocks and the development of more effective gear and methods for handling, storing, manufacturing, shipping, and marketing the products. There is also direct Federal aid to states for research and the development of fishing. This is particularly true in the United States, where certain taxes are earmarked for the purpose. The Food and Agriculture Organization of the United Nations, as well as certain individual nations, extends international aid and mutual assistance in conservation.

[KARL F. LAGLER]

Flax

The flax plant (*Linum usitatissimum*) is the source of two products: flaxseed for linseed oil and fiber for linen products. Plants with two distinct types of growth are used for seed and fiber production (Fig. 1), but fiber is sometimes a by-product of linseed production, and seed is an important by-product of fiber flax. Flax is an annual plant with a stem size that varies between about 1/16 and 1/4 in. in diameter. The flax flower has five petals, which are blue, white, or pale pink (Fig. 2). The color of the flower depends on the variety. Seeds of most varieties are varying shades of brown and yellow. Flax must be grown in rotation with other crops and not planted on the same land more frequently than once every 4 to 6 years; otherwise disease-producing organisms build up in the soil and yields may be greatly reduced unless resistant varieties are grown. *See* SEED (BOTANY).

Flax for fiber. Flax for fiber requires fertile, well-drained, and well-prepared soil and a cool, humid climate. It is planted in the early spring at 80 lb/acre or more. The high rate of seeding provides a dense stand of slender stems that branch only at the very top. Some chemical weed control may be necessary. A few weeds such as wild oats, cereal crops, perennial thistles, or morning glories will destroy the value of the crop for fiber, and all fields badly infested with weed seeds of any kind must be avoided for planting fiber flax. *See* AGRICULTURE, SOIL AND CROP PRACTICES IN; HERBICIDE.

Harvesting. When about half the seed pods (bolls) have turned yellow, harvesting must be started. If the bolls are allowed to reach full maturity before harvesting, quality is greatly reduced.

Fiber flax is harvested by a machine that pulls it out of the ground and ties it in bundles. Some flax is still pulled by hand. Stems are kept parallel while the seed is removed; bundles of the straw are then packed vertically in concrete tanks and covered with warm water to ret, a process in which bacterial action loosens the fiber in the stem. The bundles of wet, retted straw are set up with the tops held together and the root ends spread out so the bundles form "gaits" or "wigwams" to dry in the sun. The dried flax is retied in bundles and stored under cover until it is scutched, a process in which the straw is first crushed to break the woody portion of the stem into small pieces (called shives) and is then subjected to a beating operation that removes the outer bark and the woody parts from the line (long parallel) fiber. During the beating operation, short tangled fiber called tow also comes out of the line fiber with the shives and must be further cleaned. In Western Europe the scutching operation is mechanized. There, the straw is spread in a thin layer, held near the center by a gripping device on a narrow belt, and carried between fluted rollers to break the woody parts into shives. The shives are then beat out of one end, device grips the cleaned portion, and the other end is cleaned, leaving long (40–100 cm) strands. *See* AGRICULTURE, MACHINERY IN.

Uses. The best-known use for flax fiber is in the manufacture of fine linen fabrics; other uses are linen thread, linen twine, toweling, and canvas. Seed from fiber flax is used for replanting and for oil. The major producer of flax fiber is the Soviet Union, but the world's best fiber comes from Belgium and adjoining countries. Most Irish linen is manufactured from fiber produced in Belgium. The United States production of flax for fiber has dwindled from about 18,000 acres in 1942 to none since 1958.

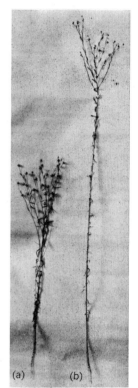

Fig. 1. Types of flax plant. (*a*) Seedflax. (*b*) Fiber flax. (*USDA*)

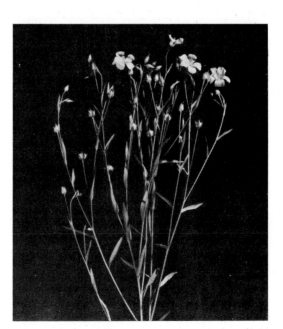

Fig. 2. Flowering top of flax plant showing buds and seed capsules. (*USDA*)

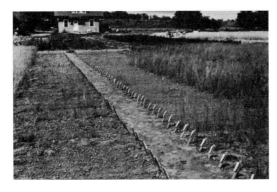

Fig. 3. Wilt resistance plot in Minnesota. Each stake marks a line of flax. On the left most of the plants were killed by wilt, whereas those on the right are resistant. (*Minnesota Agricultural Experiment Station*)

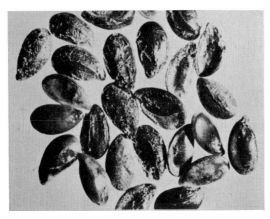

Fig. 4. Blight of flaxseed caused by several fungi. (*Minnesota Agricultural Experiment Station*)

Flax for seed. The sowing rate for seedflax is lower than for fiber flax, about 40–50 lb/acre. The varieties used produce short straw and a relatively high yield of seed with 35–44% oil. Machines used for planting and harvesting cereals are also used for flax for seed. Planting is usually done in the early spring on a well-prepared seedbed on land relatively free from weed seeds. A small acreage of flax is sown in the fall in Texas. Herbicides may be used to control weeds.

The world's major producers of flaxseed are Argentina, Canada, India, the Soviet Union, and the United States. In 1973 about 99% of the flaxseed acreage in the United States was in Minnesota, North Dakota, and South Dakota.

The principal uses of linseed oil are in the manufacture of protective coatings—paint, varnish, and lacquer. It is also used in linoleum, printer's ink, and patent and imitation leathers, and as core oil for making sand forms in metal casting. Uses that promise to become of great importance are as antispalling compounds for concrete highway construction and as curing agents for concrete.

The linseed cake remaining after the oil is extracted is used as a high-protein livestock feed. Large quantities of clean (weed-free) straw from seedflax are used in the production of a high-grade paper. This product is used to make cigarette and other fine papers.

[ELTON G. NELSON; JOSEPH O. CULBERTSON]

Diseases. Of the diseases of flax, the more common are: rust, *Melampsora lini*; wilt, *Fusarium oxysporum lini*; pasmo, *Mycosphaerella linorum*; browning or stem break, *Polyspora lini*, seedling blight and root rot caused by many species of fungi that belong to the genera *Alternaria, Aphanomyces, Colletotrichum, Fusarium, Phoma, Pythium, Rhizoctonia, Thielavia*, and others; viruses such as aster yellows and curly top; and nonparasitic diseases induced by heat, mineral deficiency, and toxic substances. *See* PLANT, MINERAL NUTRITION OF; PLANT VIRUS.

The importance of these diseases varies greatly with cultural practices, cropping sequence, environmental conditions, quality of seed, and varieties grown. Diseases that are destructive in one region may be of minor importance in another. Thus, pasmo is a major problem in the upper Mississippi Valley, but is of minor importance in California, and it is unknown in Mexico. Likewise, stem break is a troublesome disease in many parts of Europe, but it is of little importance in the United States.

At the beginning of the 20th century, flax wilt was the limiting factor in flax production in the United States. At this time it was discovered that this disease was caused by a fungus, *Fusarium* sp., and that it was possible to select wilt-resistant lines of flax, if the selections were made on infested, "wilt sick," soil. As a consequence, wilt disease is now controlled by growing resistant varieties (Fig. 3).

Rust is the most conspicuous and potentially the most dangerous disease of flax; it occurs throughout the important flax-growing regions of the world. This fungus comprises numerous distinct parasitic races and no variety of flax is resistant to all of them; hence rust must be controlled by growing varieties of flax that are resistant to the races of rust that are prevalent in a given region at a given time.

Pasmo was introduced into the United States from Argentina about 1915, but it did not become destructive in this country until about 30 years later. At present no varieties of flax are resistant to this disease, but varieties differ considerably in their susceptibility to it.

Damage of various kinds to seed bolls is common and is induced by many agents, such as fungi, viruses, insects, and hail. This damage is often associated with infected or shriveled seed (Fig. 4). Damage to the seed coat during harvest is common, especially when the seed is dry; sometimes more than 75% of the seed may be cracked. These cracks, although frequently microscopic in size, serve as avenues of entrance for many species of fungi. Seed rot and seedling blight are usually associated with damaged seed (Fig. 5). Stands usually are greatly improved if damaged seed are treated with an appropriate fungicidal chemical. *See* FUNGISTAT AND FUNGICIDE.

Most of the flax diseases can be controlled, or materially reduced, by planting sound and disease-free seed, treating seed with a suitable fungicide,

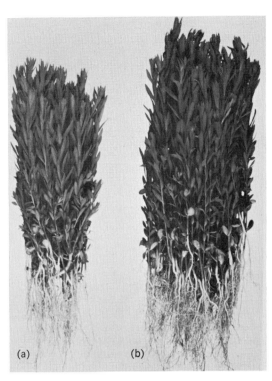

Fig. 5. Effect of the treatment of seed on the control of seedling blight in flax. (*a*) Nontreated seed. (*b*) Seed treated with an organomercuric compound. (*Minnesota Agricultural Experiment Station*)

using good cultural practices including early planting, practicing sanitation and a good cropping sequence, and growing disease-resistant varieties. *See* PLANT DISEASE CONTROL.

[MILTON F. KERNKAMP]

Bibliography: See AGRICULTURAL SCIENCE (PLANT); PLANT DISEASE.

Floriculture

The segment of horticulture concerned with commercial production, marketing, and retail sale of cut flowers and potted plants, as well as noncommercial home gardening and flower arrangement.

Florist crop production. Commercial crops are grown in greenhouses in every state, but during summer in northern states and throughout the year in southern California, Florida, and other southern states asters, chrysanthemums, peonies, stocks, and gladiolus are grown outdoors. The wholesale value of floriculture crops grown in the United States in 1975 was nearly $500,000,000. Important commercial floriculture states are California, Florida, Colorado, Pennsylvania, New York, Massachusetts, Illinois, Ohio, Michigan, and New Jersey.

Greenhouse crop culture is intensive agriculture with annual production costs of $100,000–200,000 per acre of growing area per year, depending upon the specific crop. Automation is being expanded.

The grower manages the environment (temperature, light, photoperiod, nutrients, water, and atmosphere) to meet the needs of the particular crop. Carnations are grown in cool temperatures (50°F at night), and roses at warmer temperatures. The photoperiod (length of day) is controlled automatically by artificial light and black cloth covers to initiate flowers, such as chrysanthemums, so they can be produced every day of the year. Soil is treated with steam or special gases to kill weed seeds, diseases, and soil insects. Soluble fertilizers injected into watering systems supply nutrients to plants grown in well-prepared soils, or substitutes such as peat and vermiculite, or peat and sand. Carbon dioxide is injected into the greenhouse atmosphere to increase photosynthesis. Automation is used in automatic watering, ventilation control, greenhouse air conditioning, machines for mixing soils and filling flats, conveyors for potted plants and cut flowers, and so forth. Insects and diseases are controlled by spraying, by fumigating with aerosols, by root-absorbed chemicals, and by resistant cultivars (varieties).

Wholesale marketing. Most cut flowers are sold through wholesale markets, with large quantities shipped by jet airline, especially from California, Colorado, and South America, to all parts of the country. Many cut flowers and nearly all potted plants are transported by truck.

Retail floriculture. The usual retail florist shop prepares arrangements of cut flowers and potted plants for all occasions for local use and also sends orders by telegraph and telephone for delivery throughout the world. Other outlets such as garden centers, department stores, variety stores, and supermarkets sell increasing quantities of floriculture products for home use.

Home gardening. Gardening for recreation and home beautification is an American tradition. Bedding plants, geraniums, and other landscape plants grown by florists and nurserymen make the home property attractive. Garden flowers, commercial cut flowers, and decorative foliage plants are used in the home for enjoyment. *See* PHOTOPERIODISM IN PLANTS; PLANT GROWTH.

[JOHN G. SEELEY]

Bibliography: F. B. Hillier, *Basic Guide to Flower Arranging*, 1974; A. Laurie, D. C. Kiplinger, and K. S. Nelson, *Commercial Flower Forcing*, 1968; K. S. Nelson, *Flower and Plant Production in the Greenhouse*, 1966; P. B. Pfahl, *Retail Florist Business*, 1968.

Folic acid

A yellow vitamin, slightly soluble in water, which is usually found in conjugates containing varying numbers of glutamic acid residues. It is also known as pteroylglutamic acid (PGA), and has the structural formula shown in the illustration.

It is known that vitamins M and B_c, factors R, S, and U, the *Lactobacillus casei* factor, and a number of others are pteroylglutamates. Folic acid is usually assayed microbiologically by the use of *L. casei* or *Streptococcus faecalis*. Because of the various forms in which the vitamin appears in nature, some having different activity for the two organisms, and because of the difficulty in hydrolyzing the PGA conjugates, it is extremely difficult to determine absolute amounts of the vitamin.

Biochemistry. Biologically active forms of folic acid occur as tetrahydrofolic acids. Four of these, N^5-formyltetrahydrofolic acid (the citrovorum factor, folinic acid, or leucovorum), N^{10}-formyltetrahydrofolic acid, N^5,N^{10}-methenyltetrahydrofolic

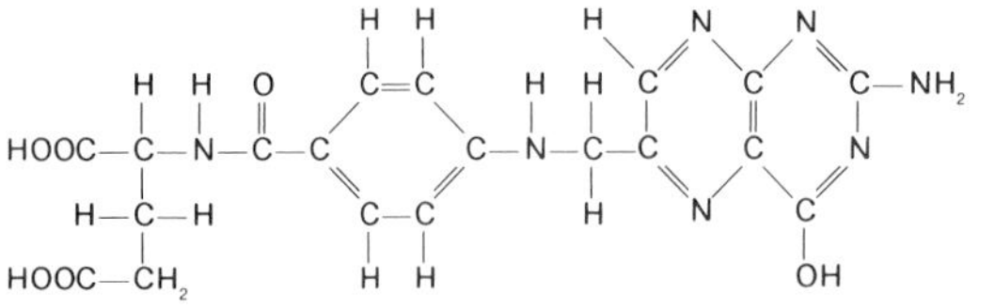

Structural formula for folic acid (pteroylglutamic acid).

acid, and formiminotetrahydrofolic acid have been found in natural products. Liver and kidney enzymes which catalyze the conversion of folic to tetrahydrofolic acids have been obtained. Ascorbic acid appears to be involved in some of these conversions. Folic acid enzymes are biological carriers of 1-carbon fragments shown below:

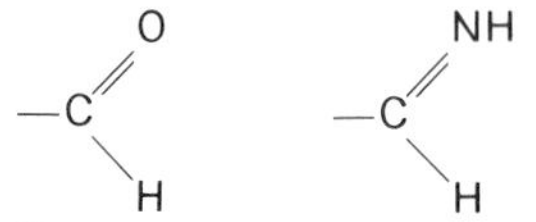

Formyl   Formimino

—CH$_2$OH   —CH$_3$
Hydroxymethyl   Methyl

These groups are important in the synthesis of purines and pyrimidines, which are components of nucleic acids; in the synthesis of the methyl group of methionine; and in the metabolism of some amino acids, including glycine, serine, histidine, glutamic acid, and phenylalanine.

Nutritional requirements. Folic acid is required by a large number of animals and microorganisms. Many animals obtain enough folic acid from intestinal synthesis so that a dietary source is not necessary. In these species, the feeding of antibiotics or sulfa drugs can precipitate deficiency signs. Folic acid deficiency is usually accompanied by poor growth, anemia and other blood dyscrasias, and gastrointestinal disturbances.

Folic acid is so widespread in nature and intestinal synthesis is so great that a folic acid deficiency in humans because of low dietary intake is probably not very common. With improved diagnostic methods an increasing number of folic acid deficient patients have been discovered. Deficiencies of other nutrients (particularly iron, ascorbic acid, or vitamin B$_{12}$) leading to impaired folic acid metabolism, difficulties in hydrolysis of folic acid conjugates by intestinal enzymes, or poor absorption may lead to a number of clinical conditions in which folic acid deficiency is involved. These include various nutritional macrocytic anemias, sprue, idiopathic steatorrhea, and pernicious anemia. The daily requirement of humans for folic acid is unknown, but on the basis of food analyses and therapeutic experience, it appears to be about 0.1 mg for the normal adult.

The anemia of pernicious anemia may be prevented by giving a person more than 0.1 mg of folic acid per day, although the neurological manifestations of this disease may progress. Sale without prescription of vitamin preparations recommending more than 0.1 mg folic acid per day has been prohibited by the Food and Drug Administration. *See* VITAMIN.

Folic acid antagonists such as aminopterin, which inhibits the conversion of folic to folinic acid, have been used in the treatment of leukemia

and have in many cases brought about temporary remissions.

[STANLEY N. GERSHOFF]

Industrial production. Folic acid is produced commercially by the simultaneous reaction of 1,1,3-tribromacetone with 2,5,6-triamino-4-hydroxypyrimidine and *p*-aminobenzoylglutamic acid. Dibrompropionaldehyde, with the assistance of an oxidizing agent, is sometimes used as a substitute for tribromacetone. Although various by-products are produced in such a reaction, selected conditions of pH and temperature give a reasonably good yield of crude folic acid. Purification of the crude folic acid through the zinc and magnesium salts gives a golden product essentially free of impurities.

Various processes can be used to make folic acid, but this one has been given because of its relative simplicity. The intermediates can be made readily by standard and familiar techniques. Most of the other processes are based on a stepwise conversion of the pyrimidine to the pteridine ring, along with additions to the benzoylglutamic molecule. Folic acid is then produced in a two-component condensation, rather than a three-component condensation.   [RICHARD J. TURNER]

Food

The material that enables man to grow and to maintain and reproduce himself. Food is composed of chemicals (natural or synthetic) in various combinations and is as essential to life as water and oxygen, which are also important constituents of foods.

The growth of modern urban civilization and an expanding world population have led to the development of new and revolutionary methods in agriculture. With the aid of mechanical equipment, better seed, and improved techniques, one farm worker in the United States can supply enough food for 40 persons. The lengthening of time and distance between production and consumption of food has necessitated development of new and improved methods of processing, packaging, and distributing foods. A vast industry has grown up to meet this need effectively. In the United States the food industry accounts for $100,-000,000,000 per year.

Food scientists, technologists, and engineers are concerned with the many-faceted problems of transfer of food from field to consumer in the most wholesome and palatable condition possible. Their concern involves such problems as freshness, appearance, stability, avoidance of contamination,

Table 1. Essentiality of amino acids

Essential or indispensable	Partially essential or partially indispensable	Nonessential or dispensable
Isoleucine	Arginine	Alanine
Leucine	Cysteine	Aspartic acid
Lysine	Cystine	Glutamic acid
Methionine	Histidine	Glycine
Phenylalanine	Tyrosine	Hydroxyproline
Threonine		Proline
Trytophane		Serine
Valine		

and prevention of spoilage, as well as development of new products from food components. In particular, they are responsible for the maintenance or enhancement of the palatability and nutritional value of the product through various processing procedures. Food additives, which play so large a role in solving these problems, are discussed more fully later in this article.

In any dietary regimen minimal amounts of three types of materials must be provided: energy-producing compounds, structure-producing compounds, and compounds necessary to energy-exchanging reactions. These three types include proteins, carbohydrates, fats, vitamins, and mineral elements, which constitute the classes of chemical compounds used to describe the composition of any particular food. Water may be considered essential for their utilization.

ESSENTIAL COMPONENTS

Energy for the various life processes is supplied by carbohydrates, fats, proteins, vitamins, and minerals.

Energy requirements. Age, sex, and activity of an individual are the primary determinants of energy requirements. Strenuous activity requires more calories per day than does sedentary work; for example, 4500 Calories (Cal) as compared to 2400 Cal for a 70-kg male. A 16-year-old boy needs 3400 Cal per day, whereas a 65-year-old woman needs only half as much. [A large Calorie (Cal) equals 1000 small calories (cal) or one small kilocalorie (kcal).] Energy values have been calculated to be about 4.1 kcal/g for carbohydrate, 4.1 kcal/g for protein, and 9.3 kcal/g for fat. *See* CALORIE.

Carbohydrates. Generally carbohydrates are sweetening agents but are not limited to this function. Carbohydrates include glucose, fructose, maltose, lactose, sucrose, glycogen, dextrin, starch, and cellulose. The body uses them chiefly as sources of heat and energy. The carbohydrate cellulose is utilized mainly as roughage. *See* CARBOHYDRATE.

Proteins. Nitrogenous material necessary for structure is provided by the proteins, which are large molecules composed of amino acids joined in peptide linkage. Proteins function in tissue growth and repair; formation of antibodies, enzymes, some hormones, and hemoglobin; maintenance of acid-base balance; and formation of hereditary material. At least eight amino acids are considered essential for adult man. The amino acids listed in Table 1 may be obtained from hydrolysates of various proteins. *See* AMINO ACIDS; PROTEIN.

Fats. Fats are esters of numerous fatty acids with various alcohols. Knowledge of human requirements for fatty acids is still far from complete, but three—linoleic, linolenic, and arachidonic—are considered essential or indispensable. Essential or indispensable implies that the body either cannot synthesize these fatty acids at all or cannot synthesize them rapidly enough for independence of a dietary source; therefore the component must be supplied in the diet. *See* LIPID.

Chemical balance. In addition to requiring food in sufficient quantity to provide body structure and dissipable energy, man needs food in sufficient variety to maintain the body chemistry in equilibrium.

Vitamins. Vitamins are organic chemical compounds necesary for normal nutrition and health and must be supplied in the diet. Many vitamins serve to activate enzymes.

Others have functions not fully clarified, but all serve some function in cell chemistry. Requirements vary with age, sex, and occupation. Vita-

Table 2. Known vitamins

Letter	Name	Function
Fat soluble		
A	Axerophthol	Important to vision and general health
D_2	Calciferol	Antirachitic factor
E	Tocopherol	Antisterility factor
K	Phylloquinone	Antihemorrhagic factor
Water soluble		
C	Ascorbic acid	Oxidation-reduction systems in cells, antiscorbutic factor
H	Biotin	Probably acts as a coenzyme
	Choline	One of an essential methyl transfer group
B_{12}	Cyanocobalamine	Antipernicious anemia extrinsic factor
	Inositol	Related to metabolism of glucose
	Niacin	Coenzymes I and II (pellagra preventive)
B_3	Pantothenic acid	Related to acetyl coenzyme A
	p-Aminobenzoic acid	A component of the folic acid group
M,Bc	Folic acid (pteroylglutamic acid)	Necessary for normal functioning of hematopoietic system
B_6	Pyridoxine	Coenzyme metabolism of amino acids and of fats and fatty acids
B_2,G	Riboflavin	Coenzyme systems involved in phosphorylations (respiratory enzymes)
B_1	Thiamine	Involved in oxidative decarboxylations (cocarboxylase)

Table 3. Minerals needed by the human body

Name	Function
Calcium	Catalyst, enzyme activator, milk production
Phosphorus	Metabolism, acid-base regulation, vitamin and enzyme activity
Magnesium	Protein formation from amino acids
Sodium	Regulator of neutrality, balances basic ions, muscle contraction
Potassium	Muscle function, nerve excitability, carbohydrate metabolism
Manganese	Enzyme activator, affects thiamine utilization, related to reproduction physiology
Iron	Catalyst
Copper	Catalyst
Cobalt	Found in vitamin B_{12}
Iodine	Constituent of thyroxin
Sulfur	Part of amino acids
Zinc	Carbon dioxide metabolism, functioning of pancreas

Table 4. Daily dietary allowances[a]

Age[b], years	Weight, kg	Weight, lb	Height, cm	Height, in.	kcal	Protein, gm	Vitamin A activity, IU	Vitamin D, IU	Vitamin E activity, IU	Ascorbic acid, mg	Folacin[c], mg	Niacin, mg equiv.[d]	Riboflavin, mg	Thiamin, mg	Vitamin B6, mg	Vitamin B12, µg	Calcium, g	Phosphorus, g	Iodine, µg	Iron, mg	Magnesium, mg
Infants																					
0–1/6	4	9	55	22	kg × 120	kg × 2.2[e]	1500	400	5	35	0.05	5	0.4	0.2	0.2	1.0	0.4	0.2	25	6	40
1/6–1/2	7	15	63	25	kg × 110	kg × 2.0[e]	1500	400	5	35	0.05	7	0.5	0.4	0.3	1.5	0.5	0.4	40	10	60
1/2–1	9	20	72	28	kg × 100	kg × 1.8[e]	1500	400	5	35	0.1	8	0.6	0.5	0.4	2.0	0.6	0.5	45	15	70
Children																					
1–2	12	26	81	32	1100	25	2000	400	10	40	0.1	8	0.6	0.6	0.5	2.0	0.7	0.7	55	15	100
2–3	14	31	91	36	1250	25	2000	400	10	40	0.2	8	0.7	0.6	0.6	2.5	0.8	0.8	60	15	150
3–4	16	35	100	39	1400	30	2500	400	10	40	0.2	9	0.8	0.7	0.7	3	0.8	0.8	70	10	200
4–6	19	42	110	43	1600	30	2500	400	10	40	0.2	11	0.9	0.8	0.9	4	0.8	0.8	80	10	200
6–8	23	51	121	48	2000	35	3500	400	15	40	0.2	13	1.1	1.0	1.0	4	0.9	0.9	100	10	250
8–10	28	62	131	52	2200	40	3500	400	15	40	0.3	15	1.2	1.1	1.2	5	1.0	1.0	110	10	250
Males																					
10–12	35	77	140	55	2500	45	4500	400	20	40	0.4	17	1.3	1.3	1.4	5	1.2	1.2	125	10	300
12–14	43	95	151	59	2700	50	5000	400	20	45	0.4	18	1.4	1.4	1.6	5	1.4	1.4	135	18	350
14–18	59	130	170	67	3000	60	5000	400	25	55	0.4	20	1.5	1.5	1.8	5	1.4	1.4	150	18	400
18–22	67	147	175	69	2800	60	5000	400	30	60	0.4	18	1.6	1.4	2.0	5	0.8	0.8	140	10	400
22–35	70	154	175	69	2800	65	5000	—	30	60	0.4	18	1.7	1.4	2.0	5	0.8	0.8	140	10	350
35–55	70	154	173	68	2600	65	5000	—	30	60	0.4	17	1.7	1.3	2.0	5	0.8	0.8	125	10	350
55–75+	70	154	171	67	2400	65	5000	—	30	60	0.4	14	1.7	1.2	2.0	6	0.8	0.8	110	10	350
Females																					
10–12	35	77	142	56	2250	50	4500	400	20	40	0.4	15	1.3	1.1	1.4	5	1.2	1.2	110	18	300
12–14	44	97	154	61	2300	50	5000	400	20	45	0.4	15	1.4	1.2	1.6	5	1.3	1.3	115	18	350
14–16	52	114	157	62	2400	55	5000	400	25	50	0.4	16	1.4	1.2	1.8	5	1.3	1.3	120	18	350
16–18	54	119	160	63	2300	55	5000	400	25	50	0.4	15	1.5	1.2	2.0	5	1.3	1.3	115	18	350
18–22	58	128	163	64	2000	55	5000	400	25	55	0.4	13	1.5	1.0	2.0	5	0.8	0.8	100	18	350
22–35	58	128	163	64	2000	55	5000	—	25	55	0.4	13	1.5	1.0	2.0	5	0.8	0.8	100	18	300
35–55	58	128	160	63	1850	55	5000	—	25	55	0.4	13	1.5	1.0	2.0	5	0.8	0.8	90	18	300
55–75+	58	128	157	62	1700	55	5000	—	25	55	0.4	13	1.5	1.0	2.0	6	0.8	0.8	80	10	300
Pregnancy					+200	65	6000	400	30	60	0.8	15	1.8	+0.1	2.5	8	+0.4	+0.4	125	18	450
Lactation					+1000	75	8000	400	30	60	0.5	20	2.0	+0.5	2.5	6	+0.5	+0.5	150	18	450

[a]The allowance levels are intended to cover individual variations among most normal persons as they live in the United States under usual environmental stresses. The recommended allowances can be attained with a variety of common foods, providing other nutrients for which human requirements have been less well defined. See text for more detailed discussion of allowances and of nutrients not tabulated.

[b]Entries on lines for age range 22–35 years represent the reference man and woman at age 22. All other entries represent allowances for the midpoint of the specified age range.

[c]The folacin allowances refer to dietary sources as determined by *Lactobacillus casei* assay. Pure forms of folacin may be effective in doses less than 1/4 of the RDA.

[d]Niacin equivalents include dietary sources of the vitamin itself plus 1 mg equivalent for each 60 mg of dietary tryptophan.

[e]Assumes protein equivalent to human milk. For proteins not 100% utilized, factors should be increased proportionately.

SOURCE: National Academy of Sciences – National Research Council, *Recommended Dietary Allowances*, 7th ed., 1968.

mins have been classified on an alphabetical basis, a fat- or water-soluble basis, and with the establishment of chemical structure, by specific chemical title (Table 2). The absence of a vitamin from the diet leads to deficiency symptoms that can be relieved by administration of adequate amounts of the vitamin in question. Fortunately, the American diet generally provides all the vitamins necessary for normal human needs. The strength of vitamin preparations usually is stated in international units based on the activity of a standard preparation: milligrams or micrograms. *See* VITAMIN.

Minerals. Small amounts of certain inorganic chemical compounds, known as mineral elements, are essential to good health. Mineral requirements appear to be associated with the state of vitamin nutrition and with endocrine activity. The needed minerals are listed in Table 3.

Minerals such as aluminum, bromine, fluorine, selenium, and silicon appear to be necessary, but their exact function is not clear.

Table 4 lists recommended dietary allowances compiled by the Food and Nutrition Board.

STAPLE FOODS

The staple foods form the basis of the dietaries of civilized man and may be classified by origin (Table 5).

Plant origin. The first step in the natural synthesizing of chemical elements into food molecules takes place in plants. The plant concentrates the foods so produced in seeds and nuts (less so in fruits) and stores them in leaves and stems. These basic plant processes give rise to the wide variety of cereals, vegetables, and other plant foods.

Cereals. Cereals are universally considered essential. They contain carbohydrates, proteins, some mineral salts, and fat. Cereals are easily dried, take up little moisture, and keep well in the natural state. The following cereals are of particular interest.

Wheat is an ancient and highly respected food material; it grows in regions of relatively low rainfall and wide extremes of temperature. A number of varieties are grown, depending on cultivation in winter or spring. Crops are subject to rusts and damage from insects. Wheat yields flours of different grades, and its largest use is in the manufacture of baked products. *See* WHEAT.

Corn, or maize, is the most valuable cereal crop of the American continent. Corn is used as green corn; as the raw material for other products such as cornmeal, hominy, and cornstarch; and in the manufacture of breakfast foods such as cornflakes and puffed corn. It is also used in fermentations as basic raw material for grain alcohol and distilled beverages, butyl alcohol, and acetone; and for manufacture of glucose, syrups, oil, and other products. The greatest use of corn, however, is as cattle feed. *See* CORN; DISTILLED SPIRITS.

Rye is an extremely hardy plant. It is used as a grain crop for animal feed; raw material for the manufacture of distilled liquors, particularly rye whiskey; and flour in certain types of bread. *See* RYE.

Barley is a cereal that is a food for man and animals and a source of malt for brewing. Barley malt is used for breakfast foods and special food preparations; for malt syrups which may find use in baking industries; for flavoring foods or for medicines; in brewing beverages; as a diastatic or desizing agent in textile processing. *See* BARLEY.

Oats is an excellent food for animals; it is eaten by humans in the form of oatmeal, rolled oats, or other breakfast foods. *See* OATS.

Rice grows in many varieties and is a nutritious and easily digested food. When polished, the essential vitamin, thiamine, is lost. This leads to a high incidence of beriberi, because rice constitutes the main source of food for one-third of the world's population. *See* RICE.

Food-processing operations in the form of milling are applied to many cereals. Milling includes various operations involved in the transformation of cereals, particularly wheat, into flour. These are largely mechanical in nature (grinding, reduction, bleaching by chemical means, and grading) and depend on a reduction in size of the components making up the wheat kernel, with a subsequent separation of particles by size and composition.

Sugars and syrups. Sugarcane is crushed, the juice clarified, the raw sugar crystallized and separated from the molasses, and further refined by a series of treatments. Sugarbeet processing differs somewhat in that the sugars are removed initially by repeated diffusion of the ground beets with water. Syrups, of which maple and cane are representative, result from the concentration of all the sugar of the original sap or juice. *See* SUGAR.

Sugar industries of the United States constitute an important segment of the food industry. Large quantities of raw sugar are imported and then refined as a supplement to native sugar production. Sugarbeets grow best in temperate climates, whereas sugarcane requires subtropical conditions. In Europe and the United States sugarbeets are an important source of sugar. Beet pulp residues and beet tops and crowns are dried and used as a valuable stock fodder.

Vegetables. A great variety of plant products are eaten raw as greens and salad materials; many others are boiled, baked, or cooked in conjunction with meats or other food materials.

Extensive year-round use of vegetables in the diet has largely resulted from the development and improvement of preservation processes. Cultivation, harvesting, packing, storage, and shipment involve many problems. Among these are soil, climate, growth, physiological and microbiological damage, insect attack, plant diseases, bruising or injury during handling, and ventilation and tem-

Table 5. Staple foods classified by origin

Plant origin	Animal origin
Cereals: wheat, corn (maize), rye, barley, oats, rice	Meats: beef, pork, mutton, poultry
Sugars: sugarcane, sugarbeets	Eggs
Vegetables: potatoes, sweet potatoes, cassava, peas, beans, onions, tomatoes, soybeans	Dairy products
Fruits: banana, citrus, plantain, apples, berries	Fish and marine products
Nuts: groundnuts (peanuts), coconuts, various seeds	
Microbes: molds, mushrooms, yeast	

peratures while the vegetables are in storage.

Potatoes, used also as flour and starch, are the most valuable vegetable crop in the world, being used for human food, stock feed, fermentations, and for industrial ethyl alcohol. Ranking next in importance to potatoes, tomatoes are high in water content and contain sugar, malic acid, and heat-stable vitamins; they are an important source of vitamin C. Carrots, beans, and onions also are widely grown and eaten raw or cooked. Soybeans are a highly valued crop, furnishing cooking oil, high-quality protein, and fermented sauces, as well as being an auxiliary flour source.

Fruits. Fruits are a source of sugar, organic acids, mineral salts, and vitamins. They are uniformly high in moisture and low in starch.

Apples are used as fresh fruit, for cooking in various ways, and for canning. Apple juice is a source of cider and vinegar. Pectin is an apple by-product used in the manufacture of jellies.

The principal citrus fruits of the United States are oranges, grapefruit, and lemons. Limes, tangerines, and kumquats are also of commercial interest. Citrus fruits are used as fresh fruits, fresh and frozen juices, and as a source of pectin, citric acid, and ascorbic acid (vitamin C). See articles on individual citrus fruits.

Other fruits of commercial importance are grapes, strawberries, pears, peaches, bananas, and cranberries. See articles on individual fruits.

Nuts. Included in this category are groundnuts, or peanuts, coconuts and other tree nuts, and various seeds. Nuts and seeds are high in fat and protein and contain fair amounts of carbohydrates. Their oils are converted into fats by hydrogenation to provide important components of spreads and for cooking. *See* FAT AND OIL, EDIBLE.

Microbes. Molds, yeasts, and mushrooms have increased in importance as foods. Yeasts have been used since primitive times; newer culture methods for yeasts and mushrooms have extended their marketability. *See* YEAST, INDUSTRIAL.

Animal origin. These foods are composed predominantly of protein, are low in carbohydrate content, and contain varying amounts of fat. Of the many animal foods, milk most nearly approaches the perfect food, containing proportionately significant amounts of all nutrients except iron. Milk by-products are cheese and butter.

Meat and poultry products. Beef, mutton and lamb, and pork are the principal meat products. By-products are lard from hog fat; stearin and tallow from beef fat; sausage, made of a number of meat products; gelatin from hides and trimmings. *See* AGRICULTURAL SCIENCE (ANIMAL).

Poultry includes domestic birds, alive or dressed, which have been raised for eating purposes and egg production. These birds are chickens, domestic fowls, duck, geese, turkeys, and pigeons. Birds are killed by bleeding, the feathers and the contents of the body cavity are removed, and the birds are immediately chilled by one of several methods. *See* POULTRY PRODUCTION.

Eggs. With proper humidity, adequate ventilation, and freedom from odors, eggs may be stored successfully for periods of 9 months or longer if kept at a temperature slightly above their freezing point. Eggs may be cleaned by sandblasting or washing. The egg contents may be frozen, dehydrated, or freeze-dried. *See* EGG PROCESSING.

Dairy products. Fluid milk for commercial distribution is usually pasteurized, that is, subjected to a temperature of 143°F (61.7°C) for at least 30 min or 161°F (71.7°C) for 15 sec, and then cooled and bottled. The importance of safety and cleanliness is stressed in the dairy industry. Milk may also be condensed or evaporated, dried, powdered, or separated into skim milk and cream. *See* MILK.

Butter is churned from cream and is usually salted. Margarines are spreads similar to butter but made of hydrogenated fats, usually vegetable in origin, with added butter-type flavors and coloring. *See* BUTTER.

Ice cream is the frozen product made from a combination of milk products (cream, butter, or milk—either whole or evaporated, condensed, skimmed, or dried) and two or more of the following ingredients: eggs, water, and sugar, with harmless flavoring and coloring matter, and with or without stabilizer or emulsifier or both. In the manufacture of ice cream, freezing is accompanied by agitation of the ingredients to avoid crystallization and to incorporate air for proper texture. *See* ICE CREAM.

Cheese is defined as the product made from curd obtained from the whole, partly skimmed, or skimmed milk of cows or other animals, with or without added cream. Curd is made by coagulating the casein with rennet, lactic acid, or other suitable enzyme or acid. The separated curd is used with or without further treatment by heat or pressure, or by means of ripening ferments, special molds, or seasoning. *See* CHEESE.

Fish and fish products. Fish and fish products are cooled by ice or refrigeration until port is reached. Further preservation methods for longer periods of time include freezing, canning, salting, drying, and smoking. Shellfish are subjected to special chlorine treatment.

PROCESSED AND REFINED FOODS

Processed foods are intentionally subjected to special treatment to extend storage life before consumer purchase. A refined food is not necessarily a complete food, but rather an ingredient or supplement in the diet or in manufactured foods. The distinction between processed and manufactured foods is not sharp; for example, canned whole-kernel corn might be considered a processed food and cornflakes a manufactured food.

Food technology. Modern food processing combines unit engineering operations with basic scientific principles by bringing together the essential knowledge of the chemistry, microbiology, and nutritional qualities of foods and the engineering skill to apply and control various operations in manufacturing treatments that yield commercial foods. In food processing, contamination by biological or chemical agents (microorganisms, insects, pests, trace metals, or container odors) must be avoided, and care taken to preserve nutrient materials and to prevent changes in palatability attributable to modifications in odor, flavor, and texture and other organoleptic characteristics. Consumer acceptability of a quality product is the final test of processing treatment.

Foods and their varieties differ in suitabilities for processing. A process useful for one food may be quite unsatisfactory for another food. Methods of processing include: (1) drying, or dehydration; (2) salting or use of other preservatives; (3) freezing; (4) vacuum freeze-drying; (5) heating, as in pasteurization and sterilization; (6) ionizing radiation; and (7) treating with antibiotics.

Concurrent with the development of processing methods has been the growth of packaging (metal cans, glass and plastic containers, and flexible wrappings) and refrigeration industries.

Food spoilage. All foods are subject to spoilage, the extent of which depends upon a number of factors. Among these are the number and kind of microorganisms present, the number and kind of enzymes present, whether the food has been pretreated or not by sulfur dioxide, germicidal vapors, or rays of various kinds. Among environmental factors affecting keeping quality are the temperature and humidity at which the food is held; whether the food has been frozen, heated, moistened, or dried; and the particular nature of the food itself, its composition or structure.

A food thought fit to eat by one person may be quite unattractive to another. In general, acceptability of a food is determined by its state of development or maturity, absence of contamination in processing, and presence or absence of microbial or enzymatic action. Causes of spoilage may be microorganisms, insects or other pests, enzyme activity, natural metabolic reactions, and environmental effects, such as freezing, burning, drying, oxidation, and so forth. *See* FOOD SPOILAGE.

Spoilage classification. A three-part food-spoilage classification may be set up as follows: relatively stable, protectable, and perishable.

Staple foods are relatively stable; they do not perish or spoil unless handled carelessly. These foods include sugar, flour and cereal grains, and dry beans.

Protectable or semiperishable foods remain unspoiled for fairly long periods with proper care. These are potatoes, certain varieties of apples, nut meats, onions, dried fruits, and other dehydrated foods.

Perishable foods spoil readily without special preservative methods. In this class are meats, fish, most fruits and vegetables, poultry, eggs, milk and milk products, and shellfish.

Spoilage is any change in the natural state of the food that lessens its desirability, either for esthetic or health reasons. In general, these changes are of a biological nature brought about by growth of microorganisms, or are autolytic changes brought about by enzymes produced within the tissue itself. In some cases changes result from oxidation. These factors may act alone or in combination. Microorganisms may synthesize compounds that alter the flavor, color, or odor of the food.

Microbial decomposition products. The products formed by microbial decomposition of fat, carbohydrate, and protein may be alcohols, aldehydes, aliphatic acids, carbon dioxide, fatty acids, glycerol, hydrogen, ketones, methane, amines, amino acids, ammonia, polypeptides, proteoses, peptones, or aromatic acids. Decomposition of proteins results in the splitting of the protein molecule into constituent groups and is usually associated with the liberation of odoriferous compounds.

Many microorganisms contain lipolytic enzymes that hydrolyze fats into fatty acids and glycerol and may also produce rancidification. Further breakdown of the fatty acid portions may occur through oxidation, with the formation of shorter-chained acids, aldehydes, ketones, and peroxides.

Microbial action on carbohydrates produces acid and gas; the general action is known as fermentation. If air has free access to the food, such acids will be unstable. The higher carbohydrates may undergo some changes due to microbial action; for example, the conversion of starch sugars and acids.

Spoilage causes. For some particular food products, the causes of spoilage are as given below.

Moisture content determines the extent of microbial spoilage of bakery products, grains, and meals and flours made from them. Molds can grow at fairly low moisture levels, while at higher moistures microbial growth takes place. If dry foods are prepared with a low moisture content and properly packaged, no growth occurs in them.

In sugars and sugar products, spoilage is limited to those microorganisms that are able to grow in concentrated sugar solutions, among which are certain yeasts and molds.

Fruits and vegetables are spoiled by plant pathogenic microorganisms and rots of various kinds.

Raw meat may be spoiled by microbial activity, surface slime and molds, enzymatic autolysis, and fat oxidation. The physiological state of the animal at killing, the method of killing and bleeding, and the rate of cooling determine to a large degree how extensively microorganisms will develop and spoil the meat.

Fish is spoiled chiefly by microbial growth but also by autolysis and oxidation when processed and stored.

Undesirable changes in eggs, poultry, and milk are brought about by the growth of microorganisms. Bacteria are common agents of spoilage, unless refrigeration is carefully utilized.

The prevention or retardation of these spoilage effects is a primary aim of the food-processing industries. *See* FOOD PRESERVATION.

Nonmicrobial spoilage. Oxidation in fatty foods is a serious source of spoilage. It can be largely controlled through packaging such foods under vacuum or an inert gas or by addition of an antioxidant. Naturally occurring enzymes can produce changes under proper conditions. A dried product blanched (heated) before drying will keep, whereas an unblanched one spoils because of enzyme activity.   [JOHN H. NAIR/BERNARD E. PROCTOR]

FOOD ADDITIVES

Food additives are substances added to foods during processing to retain or improve desirable characteristics or quality.

The increasing urbanization of the Western nations and the inevitable lengthening of the time lapse between harvest or slaughter and the consumption of foods at table, together with the rapid increase in the variety and types of manufactured foods, have created a need for substances known as food additives. The Food Protection Committee of the Food and Nutrition Board of the National Research Council describes food additive in their 1959 publication as "a substance or mixture of substances, other than a basic foodstuff, which is present in food as a result of any aspect of production, processing, storage, or packaging. The term does not include chance contaminants."

Use of food additives has extended beyond mere preservation to include all stages of production, processing, and distribution of food. Additives may enhance flavor, improve texture, heighten color, better the appearance, or retain or increase nutritive value; facilitate mass production of products of uniform quality and properties; prevent microbial spoilage or oxidative changes (especially during transportation and distribution); increase effectiveness of sanitary packaging and protection of foodstuffs for retail sale; or add to ease, rapidity, and uniformity of preparation in the home.

General definitions. The Food, Drug and Cosmetic Act, as amended Sept. 6, 1958, defines a food additive as "any substance the intended use of which results or may reasonably be expected to result, directly or indirectly, in its becoming a component or otherwise affecting the characteristics of any food (including any substance intended for use in producing, manufacturing, packing, processing, preparing, treating, packaging, transporting or holding food; and including any source of radiation intended for any such use), if such substance is not generally recognized, among experts qualified by scientific training and experience to evaluate its safety, as having been adequately shown through scientific procedures (or in the case of a substance used in food prior to January 1, 1958, through either scientific procedures or experience based on common use in food) to be safe under the conditions of its intended use; except that such term does not include—

"(1) a pesticide chemical in or on a raw agricultural commodity; or

"(2) a pesticide chemical to the extent that it is intended for use or is used in the production, storage, or transportation of any raw agricultural commodity; or

"(3) any substance used in accordance with a sanction or approval granted prior to the enactment of this paragraph pursuant to this Act, the Poultry Products Inspection Act or the Meat Inspection Act of March 4, 1907 as amended and extended."

Although insecticides, fungicides, rodenticides, and other pesticidal agents used in agricultural technology may remain in foods as residues, these are regarded as incidental or unintentional and are not classified as food additives. They are subject to separate regulatory control under the Insecticide, Fungicide and Rodenticide Act and other provisions of the Food, Drug and Cosmetic Act. Chemicals used in the manufacture of packaging materials such as paper products, plastics, or can enamels may become incidental additives if they migrate into foods packed in contact with such containers. Prior to their use it must be demonstrated that, if these chemicals do migrate, they are either harmless of themselves or are present in such infinitesimal amounts as to be negligible.

Functional classification. Some additives serve more than one function when present in certain foods. However, they may be classified according to their intended purpose as described below.

Flavoring agents. Flavoring agents make up the largest and most important group of food additives.

Many of the most familiar of these are the natural spices and essential oils and extracts, such as clove, ginger, citrus oils, and vanilla. Equally important, though less well known, are such synthetic aromatic chemicals as aldehydes, esters, and alcohols, which may be used to impart to foods such flavors as strawberry, cherry, pineapple, walnut, wintergreen, and many others. Other compounds, of which monosodium glutamate and sodium inosinate are examples, serve as flavor enhancers in meat products. Soft drinks, confectioneries, baked goods, and gelatin desserts are typical of foods owing much of their appeal to added flavoring agents. The number of natural and synthetic flavorings approved as safe for use in foods runs into many hundreds. *See* MONOSODIUM GLUTAMATE.

Nutrients. Minerals and vitamins are added to foods to restore nutritional values lost in processing or to supplement natural content of nutrients. Iodine in the form of iodized table salt was the first nutritional supplement to be added to a food; its use in the Great Lakes area and the Pacific Northwest has caused practically complete disappearance of goiter, formerly so prevalent in these areas. Vitamin D added to fluid milk has made rickets rare in this country. After dietary studies revealed that many Americans received inadequate intakes of iron, thiamine, riboflavin, and niacin, the Food and Nutrition Board of the National Research Council recommended enrichment of flour and bread with minimum and maximum levels of these substances. Such additions are practically universal in the United States today. Calcium as carbonate or phosphate is added to special dietary foods. Sodium fluoride and silicon fluoride are introduced into water supplies deficient in fluorine in order to improve dentition. Addition of thiamine to polished rice has greatly reduced the incidence of beriberi in some Asiatic countries. Pellagra, traceable to nicotinic acid deficiency in diets high in cornmeal, has been almost eliminated in the southern United States through vitamin fortification.

Preservatives. Palatability and wholesomeness of many foods reach a peak at harvesttime. Other foods are most appetizing when they come from the end of the production line in the food-processing plant. During storage and distribution, undesirable changes occur in flavor, color, texture, and appetite appeal. The food producer uses various preservatives to delay these changes.

Antioxidants. Oxygen in the air may cause off-colors or undesirable flavors; for example, browning of apple or peach slices or rancidity in lard. Antioxidants are used to retard such effects. Dipping of fresh fruit in ascorbic acid solutions (vitamin C) prevents enzymatic browning. Sodium ascorbate retards oxidation of cooked, cured, and comminuted meat products. Off-flavors in frozen fish are retarded by dipping in ascorbic acid. Its compounds are also used in beer, flavoring oils and emulsions, and in confectionery.

Off-flavor development in lard, vegetable oils, hydrogenated shortening, crackers, biscuits, breakfast cereals, dry cake mixes, and soup mixes due to oxidation is safely retarded by addition of butylated hydroxyanisole, butylated hydroxytoluene, lecithin, and tocopherols. Sometimes these are added in combinations with citric or ascorbic acids to produce a more active synergistic effect. Sulfur dioxide and sulfites are useful antioxidants for wine and beer, sugar syrups, and cut, peeled, or dried fruits and vegetables.

Antimicrobials. Molds, bacteria, and yeasts produce another kind of food spoilage, but good sanitary practices in the modern food-processing plant, together with additives effective in controlling such spoilage organisms, keep losses to a minimum. Common table salt (sodium chloride) has been used for centuries to keep meat and fish from spoiling. High concentration of sugars helps preserve fruit jams and jellies, as well as canned and frozen fruits, against microbial spoilage. Chlorine and hypochlorites control microorganisms in public water supplies. Sorbic acid and sorbates inhibit mold in cheese wraps, pie fillings, and fruit syrups. Benzoic acid and sodium benzoate have long been used as safe preservatives in pickles, catsup, relishes, soft drinks, jellies, jams, and preserves. Bread no longer becomes moldy or ropy quickly in hot weather because the baker adds calcium propionate or sodium diacetate to the dough. Antibiotics such as chlor- or oxytetracycline help keep dressed poultry and fresh fish in a marketable condition 7–10 days longer than if they were not present. They are quite safe because they decompose harmlessly during cooking.

Emulsifiers. Desirable consistency in many foods is difficult to achieve or maintain unless an emulsifying agent is added. These surfactants facilitate and stabilize oil-in-water (or water-in-oil) dispersions. The most important emulsifiers are the mono- and diglycerides of various fatty acids and their derivatives. Other surface-active chemicals are used as emulsifiers in foods, for example, sorbitan and polyoxyethylene sorbitan derivatives of fatty acids. They maintain mixtures of oil and vinegar in salad dressings long after agitation stops. They are widely used in bread, baked goods, and cake mixes to improve handling characteristics of batters and doughs, improve loaf volume and uniformity, and yield finer-grained goods.

In chocolate and confectionery emulsifiers keep cocoa fat in a stable emulsion and thus retard bloom, or surface whitening. Emulsifiers help disperse insoluble essential oils and flavors in such food products as beverages, pickles, and candy. Uniformity of texture in ice cream and frozen desserts is increased through addition of small amounts of emulsifiers, which likewise are useful in pressure-dispensed toppings. Lard, margarine, and other shortenings are improved by the addition of surfactants.

Thickeners. The appetizing mouth feel of many foods, as well as their flavor appeal, is traceable to smooth, uniform texture derived from added stabilizers or thickeners. Chocolate milk retains particles of cocoa in suspension because the milk has been thickened with a stabilizer. Such agents impart body or viscosity to fluids or emulsions. They include glycerol, sorbitol, gelatin, pectin, vegetable gums (alginates, carrageenin, and karaya), and cellulose gums (carboxymethylcellulose). They are used in processed cheese and salad dressings; in ice cream and frozen desserts they help prevent formation of large, coarse ice crystals. Also, they prove useful in preventing evaporation of flavor from cake mixes, gelatin desserts, and puddings.

Added pectin gives desirable thickness to jellies and jams when the fruit lacks sufficient natural pectin to form a gel.

Acidulants. Some foods lack sufficient tartness or acidity to give the greatest flavor intensity. Organic acids, such as malic, citric, acetic, fumaric, tartaric, and adipic, are used to provide the requisite tartness. The soft-drink industry is the greatest user of acids and employs phosphoric acid for much of its production. Gelatin desserts, jellies, jams, and preserves rely on added acid for accentuating fruit flavors.

Leavening agents. Doughs and batters that are not fermented are rendered light and porous through addition of leavening agents. Yeast, which produces carbon dioxide through fermentation, was used almost exclusively before the chemical reactions of leavening were understood. Sodium bicarbonate constitutes the major source of carbon dioxide in baking powders and is combined with an acid (alum, monocalcium phosphate, potassium acid tartrate, or sodium acid pyrophosphate) or acid-producing compounds (glucose-delta-lactone) and starch (to absorb moisture). Release of carbon dioxide may be slow or rapid, depending on the acid used. Special acid salts are employed in mixes such as pancakes, muffins, biscuits, cakes, and self-rising flour to stabilize the leavening agent for long periods.

Coloring agents. Appeal to the eye heightens enjoyment of foods. For this reason coloring agents are often employed to improve food appearance. Since addition of color to margarine became legal in the United States, use of margarine as a spread has quadrupled until it has largely replaced butter. Coloring agents may be of natural origin, such as turmeric, annatto, caramel, carmine, and carotene; or they may be one of the synthetic certified food colors. Since 1960 all color additives are subject to Federal pretesting and certification. They are widely used in foods to compensate for color changes occurring during processing or to give the appetizing color expected by consumers. Principal uses are in soft drinks, confectionery, icings, jellies, baked goods, fillings, cake mixes, cereals, popcorn, packed fruits, cheese, butter, margarine, and meat products.

Bleaching agents. The yellow color of freshly milled flour gradually disappears on aging as a result of oxidation. This maturing makes flour satisfactory for baking. Bleaching with chemical agents accelerates this process and produces uniformity in color. For this purpose oxides of nitrogen, chlorine, chlorine dioxide, nitrosyl chloride, or ammonium persulfate are employed. Benzoyl peroxide is used to whiten blue cheese made from cow's milk. Another effect of these oxidizing agents in wheat flour is to produce more stable, elastic, and uniform doughs.

Anticaking agents. Some powdered foods tend to lump or cake on storage. Anticaking agents or desiccants prevent this occurrence in table salt, confectioner's sugar, malted milk powder, onion or garlic salt, and meat-curing mixes. Among the chemicals used as anticaking agents are calcium phosphate, magnesium carbonate, calcium or magnesium silicate, silica gel, talc, and starch.

Sequestrants. The presence of minute amounts of certain metals such as copper or iron can adversely affect the color, clarity, flavor, or stability of many foods. Sequestrants are agents that separate out or set aside these trace elements. Citric acid and citrates and phosphoric acid and phosphates have long been employed for this purpose. Calcium and sodium salts of ethylenediaminetetraacetic acid (EDTA) are effective in wines, vinegar, and soft drinks to give clarity. Those oils and fats that contain traces of iron or copper oxidize rapidly to become rancid, because these metals catalyze or hasten the reaction. Citrates and phosphates are effective here as sequestrants. Phosphates prove useful in processed cheese and evaporated milk as sequestrants.

Humectants. Humectants absorb or retain moisture. They include glycerol, propylene glycol, and sorbitol. A major use is in shredded coconut, but the confectionery and dried-fruit industries find humectants advantageous.

Clarifying agents. Fruit juices, vinegar, wine, beer, and soft drinks frequently exhibit turbidity, damaging the appearance of the liquids. A variety of compounds are used as clarifying agents to improve quality. These include tannin, gelatin, albumin, methyl cellulose, pectinases, and proteinases (papain, bromelin, and fungal enzyme preparations).

Firming agents. Firming agents are employed to impart firmness to or improve texture in processed foods. Alums have long been used in converting cucumbers into pickles. Salts of calcium ensure firmness in canned tomatoes, potatoes, and apples; these salts also aid in the coagulation of certain cheeses. Magnesium chloride ensures firmness in canned peas.

Artificial sweeteners. Nonnutritive sweeteners, such as saccharin, impart sweetness to foods without adding calories. Their sole use is in low-calorie or diabetic foods, such as beverages, canned fruits, and desserts. Before they were banned (Feb. 1, 1970) because of possible harmful side effects, the cyclohexylsulfamates, or cyclamates, (calcium or sodium salts) were widely used as artificial sweeteners.

Foam regulators. Food processors use foam regulators either to stabilize foams or to depress them. Dextrins, peptones, and cellulose gums are added to pressure-packed toppings so that they will be propelled from the containers fully foamed. They ensure that beer and root beer will produce a head when dispensed.

Foaming in the boiling of syrups and jellies and in the fermentation of wines proves objectionable. Dimethyl polysiloxane prevents this. When added to orange juice prior to filling the containers, it eliminates foaming and enables the consumer to get full measure.

Conditioners. Commercial bakers need doughs that ferment vigorously and evenly; to assure this action, they employ yeast foods or conditioners. Such chemicals improve elasticity and stability of doughs and facilitate baking of products to uniform quality. For this purpose bakers add mixtures of potassium bromate and iodate; calcium peroxide; ammonium chloride, sulfate, and phosphates; calcium carbonate, lactate, sulfate, and phosphates; and sodium chloride.

Aerating agents. Carbonated beverages depend on carbon dioxide, added under pressure, for their flavor appeal. Cream is dispensed from pressur-

ized containers charged with nitrous oxide or food-grade Freon.

Inert gas. For packaging purposes a number of foods require an inert atmosphere to retain good flavor. This atmosphere is provided by evacuation of the air and its replacement with nitrogen, carbon dioxide, or a mixture of the two. Whole milk powder is so packed normally. The U.S. Armed Forces require similar treatment for most foods which are shipped overseas to military units in the field.

Buffering agents. With many processed foods, quality depends on adjusting and stabilizing pH (hydrogen ion concentration) to an optimum value. This adjustment is accomplished by means of buffering agents. Sodium salts of acetic, citric, phosphoric, and pyrophosphoric acids are employed for this purpose. They are used in confectionery, jellies, jams, preserves, soft drinks, prepared cereals, meat cures, and evaporated milk. Lactic, citric, and acetic acids serve to adjust pH to the desired end point in processed cheese, pickles and brines, canned vegetables, and some kinds of confectionery.

Enzymes. In various food processing operations, enzymes also serve as valuable additives. In practice, enzymes are permitted to react only to an established optimum condition and are then inactivated by heat. Their function is to effect hydrolysis of such food components as proteins, carbohydrates, and hemicelluloses. Proteases of plant (papain, bromelin, ficin), animal (pepsin, trypsin, pancreatin), or microbiological (fungal or bacterial) origin serve as meat tenderizers or clarifying agents for fruit juices. Amylase and invertase are utilized in the manufacture of glucose, invert sugar, and cocoa syrups. Pectinase clarifies beverages and fruit juices. Glucose oxidase prevents the browning reaction (sugar–amino acid reaction). Carotenase is useful in bleaching flour.

Other additives. Among additives of lesser importance are clouding agents used to impart turbidity to beverages; coating agents for glazing oranges and chocolate confectionery and for facilitating removal of baked goods from pans or confectionery from slabs; hydrolytic agents to effect cleavage of proteins, carbohydrates, and cellulosic materials; and growth stimulators, such as antibiotics or phenylarsonic acid to promote rapid growth of poultry and livestock.

Legal aspects. Under the Food Additives Amendment of 1958, all additives in use prior to Jan. 1, 1958, and not deemed by qualified experts to be safe on the basis of either appropriate scientific tests or experience in common use in foods are subject to approval (or exemption) by the Food and Drug Administration. Petitions for a regulation governing the conditions under which a food additive may be used must contain full information concerning its identity, composition, proposed use and effect, analytical determinations, and toxicity. Unless exempted from regulatory control, the use of an additive is subject to a regulation that will prescribe the food or classes of food in which it may be safely used; a specified maximum limit of use; the manner of addition or use; directions, labeling, and packaging requirements; and other conditions of use.

[JOHN H. NAIR]

Materials transferred to foods by contact, such

as ingredients of packaging or of equipment surface coatings and similar trace materials, are considered indirect additives and are subject to the same regulatory requirements as direct additives. Chemicals used in processing transiently are considered incidental additives and are similarly regulated, but do not have to be declared on the label as ingredients of the food (nor do indirect additives). This consideration holds equally for diatomaceous earths, carbon for decolorizing or filtering purposes, or solvents volatilized during processing, because these leave only minute traces of residue. To the extent that the administration of drugs or growth stimulants (such as antibiotics and hormones) to livestock or poultry may, intentionally or otherwise, leave residues in meat, milk, or eggs, they are regarded as food additives and so regulated (but need not be declared on the label).

No fundamental distinction can be made between food additives of natural origin and those produced synthetically, and a substance can legally be both a food and a food additive. All food additives must be proved safe for their intended use unless they are generally recognized as safe by experts qualified by scientific training and experience to evaluate safety (mostly materials in the food supply prior to 1958). *See* FOOD ENGINEERING.

[VIRGIL O. WODICKA]

Bibliography: W. R. Aykroyd, *Food for Man*, 1964; Code of Federal Regulations, 21 CFR 1.17, 1.18, 125.1, and 125.5; R. W. L. Goodwin (ed.), *Chemical Additives in Food*, 1967; F. L. Gunderson et al., *Food Standards and Definitions in the United States: A Guidebook*, 1963; F. L. Hart and H. J. Fisher, *Modern Food Analysis*, 1969; J. L. Heid and M. A. Joslyn, *Fundamentals of Food Processing Operations*, 1967; M. B. Jacobs (ed.), *The Chemistry and Technology of Food and Food Products*, 3 vols., 2d ed., 1951; National Academy of Sciences, *Recommended Dietary Allowances*, 1974; *Nat. Acad. Sci.—Nat. Res. Counc. Publ.*, no. 398, 1965; *Nat. Acad. Sci.—Nat. Res. Counc. Publ.*, no. 750, 1959; H. O. Triebold and L. W. Aurand, *Food Composition and Analysis*, 1963; U.S. Department of Agriculture, *Food: The Yearbook of Agriculture*, 1968.

Food engineering

The technical discipline involved in food manufacturing and refined foods processing. It encompasses the practical application of food science in the efficient industrial production, packaging, storing, and physical distribution of nutritious and convenient foods that are uniform in quality, palatable, and safe. Controlled biological, chemical, and physical processes and the planning, design, construction, and operation of food factories and processes are usually involved. *See* FOOD MANUFACTURING.

Food engineering is the food industry equivalent of chemical engineering. Food science in industry converts agricultural materials into products that are marketable because they meet a consumer need and can be profitably sold at reasonable prices by virtue of being economically produced, packaged, and distributed.

Food engineering is a vital link, therefore, between farms and food stores in the lifeline of modern civilization. Without it, food would be available only at farms, in forms produced by nature, and only in season.

Many natural foods must be preserved in order to be stored and shipped long distances to population centers. To provide a varied, nutritious diet, many raw food materials must be refined, and others combined with various ingredients and processed to produce food in new forms, such as bread, cheese, ice cream, frankfurters, soft drinks, cake and dessert mixes, candy, many breakfast cereals, ketchup, and salad dressings.

Because food engineering is applied in food manufacturing and refined foods processing, it requires a knowledge of unit operations and processes such as cleaning, separating, mixing, forming, heat transfer, moisture removal, fermenting, curing, packaging, and materials handling. This requirement to a large extent differentiates food engineering from food science. Yet these operations involve applied food science, just as chemical engineering encompasses chemistry. That is why the food engineer must have a working knowledge of food chemistry, bacteriology, and industrial microbiology, as well as of physics, mathematics, and basic engineering disciplines.

Food engineering should be differentiated from food technology. In teaching technology, some schools include considerable engineering in the curriculum to train students in the practical application of food science. Graduates of these schools are in reality food engineers. Other schools emphasize food science, and qualify graduates primarily for research and quality control work. The food technologists from these schools actually are food scientists.

Students interested in research select a curriculum which emphasizes food chemistry, bacteriology, and microbiology. Those interested in food manufacturing and processing choose a curriculum with less emphasis on food science and more on mathematics, physics, engineering principles, and unit operations and processes.

Food engineers are hired not only by commercial food manufacturing and processing firms, but also by food machinery and ingredient companies, makers of containers and packaging materials, government food control and research agencies, food laboratories, and schools teaching food engineering, technology, and science while conducting research on food and nutrition.

Food engineering has contributed to ever-accelerating progress in the food manufacture beyond the pot and kettle stage of batch operations of large-scale kitchen techniques. It has developed many automatically controlled, continuous processes which are more efficient, provide better quality control, and are more sanitary. It has developed food manufacturing and processing into a highly technical industry.

The food industry faces the challenge of practically taking the homemaker out of the kitchen by providing economical products that require almost no effort or time in preparation. Products which can be made ready to eat by being heated in their packages go a long way toward attaining this goal.

Some outstanding achievements in food engineering include continuous bread-dough making and forming, manufacture of low-cost, high-quality prepared mixes, development of instant coffee and tea processes, dehydration of potatoes to produce the instant mashed product, production of pre-cooked frozen convenience foods, continuous butter churning, freeze-drying or sublimation, final dehydration of solid foods after puffing to open the structure, preservation of beer and wine by micropore filtration to remove yeasts and spoilage bacteria, pneumatic bulk handling of dry and liquid raw materials, aseptic filling of packages, and automatic control of processes.

Promising projects under development are preservation of foods by nuclear or electronic radiation, heat processing by high-frequency electromagnetic waves, and foam-mat drying (dehydration of fluids in foamed state). In development, too, is the use of membrane processes such as reverse osmosis and electrodialysis to concentrate or demineralize liquid foods.

FOOD REFINING

Refining of foods through processing is a large, important commercial business, vital to the food supply. Refining involves operations which convert raw materials into forms more suitable as food, with longer storage and shelf life.

Sugar, for example, is obtained by refining. Cane sugar is produced by squeezing the juice from the cane by the mechanical pressure of huge steel rolls; the juice is clarified and concentrated in big vacuum evaporators; crystals are formed in the concentrate, separated from the liquor by centrifuging, and then dried and sometimes pressed into cubes. The refining operation has merely extracted naturally occurring sugar from its source to make it usable in convenient form. See SUGAR.

Milk is clarified and pasteurized to make it safe to drink; it usually is vitaminized to improve its nutritive value. Soybeans must be refined to yield edible oil; corn to yield oil, starch, sugar, and syrup. Wheat is refined by milling to make flour. Similar processes apply to a long list of common foodstuffs. See MILK; SOYBEAN.

In addition to producing consumer items, refiners supply large quantities of their products in bulk to food manufacturers to be used as ingredients in manufactured foods.

Examples of refined foods are dried and frozen eggs, spices and flavorings, edible fats and oils, sugar, syrup and molasses, honey, starch, gums, gelatin, cocoa, coffee, tea, milk, flour, rice, and oat cereal. See EGG PROCESSING; STARCH.

Food refining and manufacture together constitute not only a vital industry but one of the largest ones in the United States. Food science, technology, and engineering have made refining operations highly technical and efficient, and are accelerating progress. A wide variety of continuous, automatically controlled unit operations and processes is employed to save labor, improve quality, and reduce costs.

An example of significant advance is impact-in-air milling of wheat, in which the grain is disintegrated by high-speed revolving blades. The different fractions of the grain are then separated by air classification to yield flour with special baking properties. Another example is the tailoring of shortening to specific uses by modifying the molecular structure through chemical processing.

Many food refining plants are located near the area in which the raw material is produced, such as the soybean plants in Illinois, the cane sugar

factories in Louisiana, and the flour mills in Minneapolis. Milk pasteurizing plants, however, are near their customers, because the milk is bottled immediately after pasteurization. Food manufacturing plants producing highly perishable items, such as bread, usually are near their market. Those turning out long-life items, such as preserves, are more often near the raw material supply. Perishability of the raw material, as with fruits and vegetables for canning and freezing, often dictates that the food plant be close to where the food is grown. See BARLEY; BUCKWHEAT; COCOA POWDER AND CHOCOLATE; COFFEE; OATS; PEANUT; RICE; RYE; TEA; VINEGAR; WHEAT.

UNIT OPERATIONS AND PROCESSES

Unit operations in food factories are the mechanical manipulations and handling employed to change the physical form or composition of the food, to move it from one operation or process to another, and to package it.

Unit processes are the methods used to change the chemical or biological characteristics of the food, to preserve it, as in curing meat; to make it more palatable, as in aging cheese; or to develop special qualities, as in fermenting wort to produce beer by developing alcohol and carbon dioxide.

In the food industry, the two terms often are loosely employed to designate steps in the processing and manufacture of food.

A typical food factory performs a series of unit operations and processes in refining a raw material or in producing a fabricated food item. The combination of operations and processes is different for the various branches of the industry, but many of the individual operations and processes are employed in several branches of food treatment.

Washing, separating, mixing, scaling, handling, process control, sanitation, waste disposal, and packaging are examples of unit operations found in many types of food factories.

Application of heat, fermenting, curing, and aging exemplify unit processes common to various branches of the industry.

Since the widely used unit operations and processes are technical common denominators of the industry, knowledge of the engineering and scientific principles involved is essential to food engineers and technologists who go into the production phase of the industry.

Significant improvements in many unit operations and processes have taken place since 1945. Most notable is the trend to continuous instead of batch operations and processes, with improved efficiency, capacity, and controllability. Extensive application of automatic control has been part of the trend to continuous methods.

In heat processing, progress has been made through high-temperature, short-time pasteurizing and sterilizing. Not only is capacity increased, but there is less heat damage to flavor and vitamin content.

Notable advancement in handling has been achieved through extensive application of pneumatic conveying of dry materials and pumping of fluid and plastic materials.

Potentially important new processes include (1) freeze-drying, or removal of moisture under high vacuum while the product is in a frozen state, (2) pasteurization and sterilization by irradiation with nuclear rays or electron beams, (3) heat processing with high-frequency radio waves, and (4) membrane separation techniques to remove water or minerals from fluid foods. *See* FOOD SCIENCE; FOOD TECHNOLOGY.

General operations are the processes employed in every type of food processing and manufacturing plant—and in many phases of plant operations—in contrast with specific processes. Handling of materials is an example. No matter what type of plant is involved, this operation is widely utilized. It is necessary to move raw materials, ingredients, and supplies from the receiving dock into plant storage, through the various process operations required to make the finished product, and through the packaging lines. Finally, the packaged product must be transported to the plant warehouse or directly to the shipping platform, and then moved into trucks or railway cars. For efficiency all of this is done mechanically.

Process control, which is treated in detail later in this article, and several other operations are widely employed in food plants. Such operations include sanitation, quality control, and waste disposal.   [FRANK K. LAWLER]

Sanitation. Sanitation in the food industry is the planned control of the production environment, equipment, and personnel to prevent or minimize spoilage, product contamination, and conditions offensive to the esthetic senses of the discriminating consumer, and to provide clean, healthful, and safe working conditions.

To be successful, competent management must plan and execute sanitation controls. The most important contribution of the sanitation program is the recognition and interpretation of potential hazards and their correction or control. The following general categories indicate some of the broad areas of sanitation concern in food industries.

Housekeeping implies orderliness and freedom from refuse in all areas.

Rodent elimination involves knowledge of rodent habits, recognition of problems, and permanent control through structural changes, removal of harborages and food supplies, and supplementary poisoning and trapping.

Insect elimination from food products and ingredients in the factory requires recognition of serious or incipient infestations, identification, and knowledge of habits and ecology. Control methods may involve changes in structure, equipment, or process, and the safe use of insecticidal chemicals.

Microorganisms, the type and significance of which vary with product and type of operation, must often be controlled by process and equipment change, cleaning, and sanitizing chemicals.

Construction and maintenance of buildings and equipment are of major importance in sanitation. New units can be planned to simplify sanitation maintenance, reduce costs, and eliminate the hazards of contamination and spoilage.

Cleaning of plant and equipment involves careful organization, training, work scheduling, and the use of the best available equipment, methods, and materials. The trend is to clean processing equipment in place, without dismantling. This is done by an automatic system that circulates and sprays cleaning and sanitizing solutions inside equipment in timed sequence.

Employee facilities, such as rest rooms, locker rooms, drinking water, eating facilities, and working environment, must be well maintained for the comfort and safety of the workers if they are to remain happy and maintain production efficiency and product quality.

Laboratory tests, of importance to the sanitation program in the food plant, must be understood to be utilized to the best advantage.

Water supply quality and plant distribution systems, as well as waste treatment and disposal, and lighting and ventilation, are often a part of sanitation.

Inspection techniques, tailored to the specific sanitation situation, must be learned, taught, and applied for efficient functioning and adjustment of the sanitation program.

[EDWIN S. DOYLE]

Quality control. Quality control is the evaluation of raw materials, unit operations, unit processes, or finished products and comparison of the results with fixed standards. These standards may reflect the manufacturers' or the customers' viewpoints. They may be based on physical properties, such as size and color; chemical properties, such as acidity; sensory attributes, such as odor and flavor; legal requirements, such as net weight; or on public health standards of microbial content. When possible, quality control depends on objective physical or chemical tests, but for foods these are usually supplemented by a panel of trained tasters. The tests are applied according to a statistical design, following an analysis of the specific problem. Frequency of sampling and analytical accuracy required are related to the degree of quality control desired. Statistical analysis of data previously obtained defines the limits beyond which a product is rejected, an operation readjusted, or a process changed. In addition, good quality control can show trends that indicate changes should be made before any losses have actually occurred. Care should be taken that the quality control program does not become so detailed and costly that it reaches the point of diminishing return. Quality control is essential for the product uniformity that enables mass-produced foods to be advertised, distributed, and sold throughout the world.

[REID T. MILNER]

Waste disposal. Both solid and liquid wastes are encountered in the food industry. The solid wastes are segregated and, in many cases, processed into salable by-products. When solids are composed of materials that are not salable, compacting to ratios of up to 8 : 1 improves handling efficiency and cuts cost of disposal. Liquids may be discharged into streams or municipal sewers, or treated on the premises.

Legislation concerning pollution of surface waters has greatly reduced the quantity of liquids discharged into streams. Discharge into municipal sewer systems offers the best solution and is most often employed.

Fruit and vegetable canneries and freezing plants that have highly seasonal operations use large quantities of water that tend to overload municipal facilities. Many of these plants have found it necessary to install waste-treating systems. Most common methods employed involve screening, lagoons, septic tanks or cesspools, sedimentation, sand filtration, chemical treatment, aeration to oxidize organic material, and spray irri-

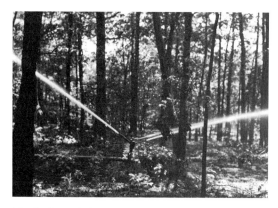

Fig. 1. Spray irrigation system. Screened effluent from vegetable processing plant is spread over forest area, where it is quickly absorbed. Purified water then discharges to stream. (*Food Engineering, Chilton Co.*)

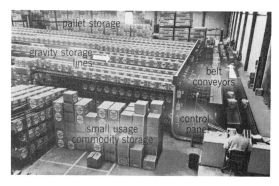

Fig. 3. Gallo wine electromechanical handling.

gation (Fig. 1). Screening is an absolute necessity unless wastes are discharged to lagoons where odors are no problem. Ion exchange is a promising method for treating saline wastes.

Plants for milk processing, brewing, meat packing, and corn products refining and wineries each present special problems. However, good housekeeping practices, recovery of by-products, and reuse of waters can greatly reduce volume and concentration of the waste.

Where discharge to municipal plants is impractical, installation of specially designed primary and secondary treatment systems (Fig. 2) may be necessary. In some cases, adjustment of pH and addition of nutrients and enzymes improve efficiency of bacterial action.

A modular system has been introduced in which oxygen is mixed and dissolved in a turbulent wastewater falls zone. It is said to double or triple the capacity of conventional aeration tanks and to greatly reduce power requirements.

Other systems developed for specific wastes include: (1) combined chemical flocculation and impressed electric current to remove suspended solids from edible-oil wastewaters; (2) fungal synthesis of corn- and soy-processing wastes to reduce biological oxygen demand and to produce marketable by-products; and (3) oil-based evaporative drying of thick sludges or wet powders to make sterile solids that can be burned as boiler fuel.

[ARTHUR V. GEMMILL]

Materials handling. Materials handling is the in-process and in-plant handling or conveyance of raw, semifinished, and finished materials to storage and point of shipment. Improved handling systems present the greatest potential means for cutting production costs, increasing production within present plant areas, and providing a smooth, continuous flow-through process to storage or shipment areas. Depending on the characteristics of a product, it may be conveyed by semimechanical, mechanical, gravity, hydraulic, or pneumatic systems, or a combination of these.

In-process handling systems provide the conveying linkage between the unit operations of a process. With a few exceptions, such as monorail equipment used for meat carcass handling, most systems are designed for mass movement of materials. In all cases, every consideration is given to the characteristics of the product, and systems are designed to handle materials with minimum damage, move them swiftly to minimum distances, and provide sanitary requirements.

In-plant handling systems include the conveyance of raw materials from receiving platform or storage to process, as well as the handling and storage of finished goods (Fig. 3). The mechanized means selected for these purposes also are based on consideration of the characteristics of the raw material and that of the container and shipping package of the finished product.

Flow rate, time, quantity, kind, and direction of flow can be automatically controlled by instruments, electromechanical or electronic devices and systems. The trend is to handle raw materials in bulk and to feed them to the product batch or stream automatically. The movement of finished products into and out of warehouses is being automated.

[CARL R. HAVIGHORST]

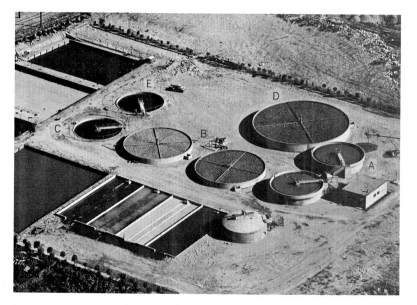

Fig. 2. Brewery waste-disposal system. Since brewery wastes have high biochemical oxygen demand (BOD) and suspended solids, they require extensive treatment. In this installation, liquid waste is pumped to primary clarifiers. A = effluent going through biofilters; B = intermediate clarifier; C = secondary biofilter; D = secondary clarifier; E = stage before discharge. (*Food Engineering, Chilton Co.*)

PROCESS CONTROL

Chemical, physical, and biological changes in food processing are measured and controlled automatically by individual instruments and by integrated systems.

Correctly applied, control instruments and systems are the key to modern-day food processing and increased profits. Automatic control increases operating efficiency, reduces slowdown or stoppages in production, and assists in maximum utilization of equipment and maintaining product uniformity and quality.

Automatic controls and systems reduce the quantity of products which do not meet specifications. They make possible the most effective use of operating utilities—steam, power, and water—and the most economical use of ingredients. Automatic process controls can monitor many different types of variables without interruption throughout the operating day and can reduce costly reruns by sensing and diverting an off-specification product before it reaches a filler bowl or packaging line.

Control loop. A basic, automatic control system is designed to maintain balanced conditions within a process under normal or abnormal conditions. It comprises three elements—a measurement device, controller, and final control element, such as a valve (Fig. 4). The three elements working together are referred to as a control loop. Control is maintained by measuring important variables such as temperature, pressure, flow, level, pH, salt content, Brix (density), and concentration and taking corrective or limiting action when a variable deviates from a predetermined standard. The latter is the commonest type of control used and is called feedback control.

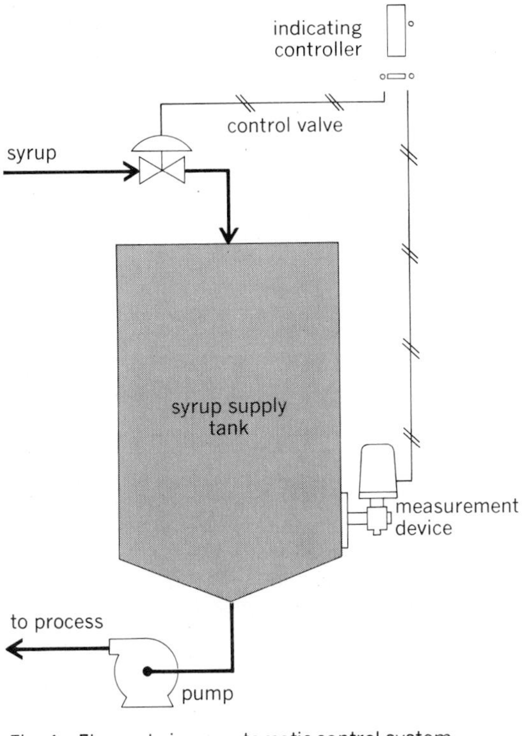

Fig. 4. Elements in an automatic control system.

The measurement may be made continuously or at intervals, depending on the process. Generally, continuous or semicontinuous processes require continuous measurement and control. Batch processes are usually more efficient if continuous measurement and control are used. Instruments in the control loop may be of the electronic or pneumatic variety.

System implementation. Since some processes are more difficult to keep stabilized than others, controllers of different capabilities are necessary. Some controllers simply open or close the control valve with no modulating action. Others maintain the variable at a predetermined point by modulating the valve, and still others maintain the variable within prescribed limits. Satisfactory process stabilization can be achieved on practically any process with the correct controller.

Factors involved in selecting an automatic control system include:

1. Desired results. Some processes require that the measurement be maintained precisely at the desired value, called the set point; others require control within certain limits.

2. Controllability of the process. Many processes that cannot be controlled manually are easy to control automatically. The process determines the type of control required.

3. Valve selection. The control valve should be properly selected and sized for compatibility with the required controller and to meet process demands.

Successful implementation of a complex food process control system depends on sound application engineering. Good engineering practices are essential, especially in applications such as the continuous production of corn syrup, the production of edible oils, and the automatic control of a brew house. Instruments must be selected, installed, and maintained correctly, for they provide the communication link between the operator and a process.

New techniques. Recent technological progress in measurement and control techniques enable the food industry to control more precisely many variables inherent to a particular process. Instruments for continuously measuring refractive index, turbidity, density, viscosity, conductivity, and moisture have joined the ranks of those measuring temperature, pressure, and flow. Electrode systems selective to specific ions are becoming available to industry. Electrodes selective to fluoride ion concentration are now used industrially; sodium, calcium, chloride, and other electrodes have also been developed.

Clean-in-place (CIP) systems are being used in all segments of the food industry. The sanitary construction of many measuring instruments allows process vessels, pipelines, and instruments to be thoroughly cleaned without disassembling. Other instruments measure and control temperature and concentration of the sanitizing solutions as well as the sequence and contact time of the solutions. CIP control systems provide more effective cleaning procedures and reduce the risk of contamination through improper manual cleaning.

Advanced control techniques have gained wide acceptance within the food industry. Feedforward control, digital blending control, and digital computer control have all found acceptance.

In essence, the feedforward system detects variations in the material and heat balance of the process and acts to make changes before the controlled variable is affected.

Feedforward control refers to control action in which information concerning all conditions (for example, concentration variation, steam variations, and feed variations) that can disturb the variable being controlled is converted into corrective action to minimize deviations of that variable.

Feedforward systems can be used to provide optimum throughput of hard-to-control evaporators or to permit drying of various food products without measuring the moisture content of those products. The control of pH and of distillation columns is another area in which feedforward control is being utilized successfully.

Many packaged foods and condiments are blends of several ingredients. Ice cream, candy, soup mixes, and the like require precise proportioning to assure quality. Analog control concepts, electronic and pneumatic, have been applied to measure ingredients and to control them in desired proportions.

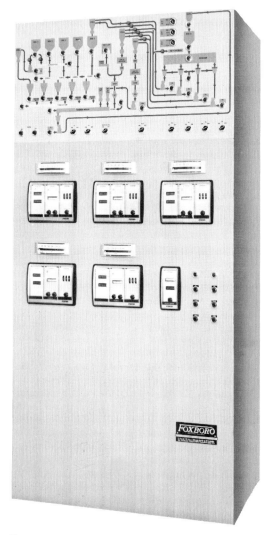

Fig. 5. Semigraphic cabinet which is used for control of blending. (*Foxboro Co.*)

Continuous in-line control and mixing of ingredients have been difficult to achieve because of tight tolerances required by food manufacturers. Semicontinuous and batch blending has been widely accepted because of the limitations of proposed continuous systems and because in-line mixing devices could not provide desired results.

Technological progress in continuous and batch formulation control techniques, as well as in the design and operation of in-line mixers, has led to an advancement in ingredient blending. Automatic, continuous, in-line digital blending systems currently control flows of both wet and dry ingredients, in exact predetermined proportions, to ensure final or intermediate blends that meet exacting specifications (Fig. 5). Gravimetric feeders with digital or pulse outputs are being used in conjunction with turbine meters, positive displacement meters, or magnetic flow meters to produce the required measurements. For batch control, automated digital batch/weigh systems using load cells and digital control concepts proportion ingredients in desired quantity and sequency.

Punched-card systems are used for both continuous and batch control. Formulations are stored on punched cards which contain all necessary blending information, including ingredients to be used, the quantity of each, the total blend rate, and total batch quantity. In batch systems they also select the sequence of ingredient usage.

Process-control digital computers are a relatively new tool available to the food industry for controlling complex processes. They can provide management with almost instantaneous information concerning the entire process by monitoring any number of variables as well as pump and motor operation. They provide rigid control enforcement and make numerous calculations and decisions in a fraction of a second.

Computers receive inputs (measurements) and dispatch outputs (control signals) to maintain the process variable at the desired value. Because of the speed with which the computer functions, many hundreds of inputs are sampled and acted upon each second, providing essentially continuous control action.

A digital computer control system can be programmed to provide, among other benefits, an optimizing routine, continuous or demand printout of information, advance control techniques, formulation control, inventory maintenance, and a record of any slowdown or failure.

Computers are firmly entrenched in formulation control in bakeries. The industry uses computers for monitoring and controlling a large assortment of variables, and it is apparent that computers have the potential for providing receiving, shipping, accounting, and inventory control functions. Savings are realized in reducing materials waste and "giveaway," and quality control is simplified considerably. Since finished products are more uniform, there is less finished product waste, and machine utilization is greater.

Control center. An important part of any process control system is the control console, or cabinet, which houses the instruments and associated equipment. The modern control center is, in many cases, a complex arrangement of dials, gages, control stations, push buttons, switches,

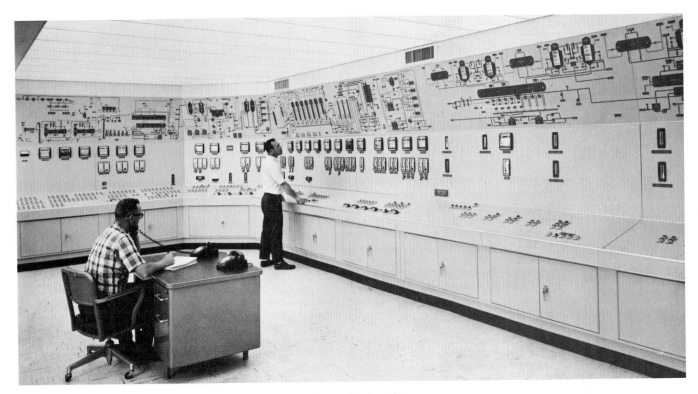

Fig. 6. Control panel with pneumatic instrumentation in a control room. (*Foxboro Co.*)

alarm lights, and graphic or semigraphic displays which show a flow diagram of the process (Fig. 6).

The design of a process-control center depends upon many factors, for the operator must be able to run his process not only under normal, automatic conditions but also under abnormal conditions, when a malfunction has occurred somewhere in the system. He must have the capability of taking over manually any phase of the process at any time. The operator must know where the trouble spot is located, what the trouble is, and which variable to manipulate in order to make corrections. To assist him in this task and to enable him to locate trouble areas at a glance, the graphic display has been devised. The display shows process vessels, various symbols, and color-coded flow lines. Progress lights and alarm lights are often included.

Careful attention must be given to the front-of-panel layouts so as not to confuse the operator and to limit operator fatigue. All components that pertain to a particular loop are clustered so that they are easily accessible in the event of an emergency or during startup and shutdown procedures. The sequence-of-use principle is employed consistently in the design of control cabinets; that is, devices are mounted so that they follow a logical sequence, thereby affording the operator easy access to the process. Closed-circuit television may provide visual information difficult to assess in other forms (Fig. 7).

The content and arrangements of control cabinets vary widely; hence, human engineering concepts provide the most logical configuration and display for a particular process.

New equipment. Manufacturers and designers of instruments and control systems have kept pace with the dynamic growth of food industries by

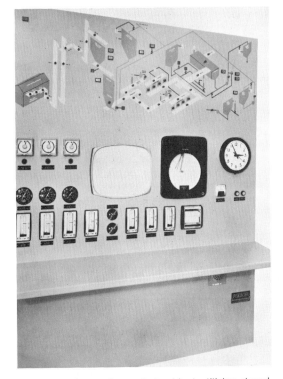

Fig. 7. Example of a control cabinet utilizing closed-circuit television. (*Foxboro Co.*)

providing many new products and systems to solve production problems. Wide acceptance by food processors of time-proved control techniques and advanced concepts such as feedforward control, digital blending, and computer control have led to

significant improvements in process efficiency, production flexibility, and utilization of utilities. To achieve maximum benefits, sound process and instrument application engineering must be the rule.
[GEORGE P. TREARCHIS]

Raw materials preparation. The processes discussed in this section are those operations necessary to make natural food materials from the farm ready for marketing or for further processing.

Citrus fruit, for example, may be washed, sorted for size, inspected, waxed, and even colored before it is shipped to fresh-fruit markets. Much fresh produce is cleaned, inspected, sorted, trimmed, and prepackaged for retail sale. This assures better quality, reduces waste, is sanitary, enhances sales appeal, and saves labor in food stores.

Citrus fruit also may be cited as an example of a raw material that is prepared for processing. The fruit is inspected, cleaned by a washing operation, and sorted into size classifications before the juice is extracted, concentrated, and frozen.

Unit operations employed in raw materials preparation include cleaning, separating, draining, trimming, peeling, dehusking, hulling, shelling, pitting, coring, stemming, silking and size reduction, centrifuging, dressing, filtering, solvent extraction, and rendering.

These operations do not change the basic characteristics of the food material. This is in contrast with raw materials conversion, which does change the nature of the material.   [FRANK K. LAWLER]

Cleaning. The cleaning operation consists of the removal of soil, dust, spray residues, insects, superficial rots, and other contaminating substances. This is accomplished by tank soaking, pressure sprays, brush and shaker washers, and detergents. Even acids and alkalies have been used for removing spray residues from fruits and vegetables. The United States Food and Drug Administration considers that commercial cleansing methods should be fully as effective as good home kitchen practice. Both blowers and vacuum suction are used to remove debris, dust, and insects from dry or semidry food materials such as cereals. Magnets placed in the processing lines are commonly used to remove metallic objects from such dry materials as beans, rice, and cereals.

Separating. Separating is a unit operation used to classify products as to color, size, weight, shape, and texture. There are a number of separators, one of which is the gravity type which depends upon the flow of dry materials on an inclined plane. Size separations are easily made by passing peas, for example, down an inclined plane fitted with openings of several sizes. Another is the quality-gravity pea separator which separates peas on the basis of weight; the more mature peas, being heaviest, sink. Photoelectric devices will separate and discard dark-colored particles, as in breakfast foods, or discolored grains in rice or cereals. The so-called squirrel cage washer and separator consists of an inclined rotating and sometimes vibrating screen which separates peas into four or five sizes.

Roller sorters are accurate and fast and do not injure soft fruits such as pears and apples. Roller conveyors with a fixed space between the rolls will remove debris such as stones, soil clumps, and leaves. Weight sorters have been perfected to the point where they are reasonably fast and accurate

and operate without injury to soft fruits such as tomatoes, pears, and apples. By far the most common separators for grains are the several vibrating screen devices, often fitted with gravity flow and air blasts. Screens in series and with different sized perforations are often used. So-called fanning mills for small seeds fall into this class.

Centrifuges are used to separate fat from milk or other emulsions. They are also used to remove sediment or precipitates from liquids such as fruit juices. Cyclone air separators for fine particles such as flour, meals, small seeds, and powdered foods are used in many designs. In discussing the separating operation it must be kept in mind that several types of separation are normally used in the processing of a single food.

Flotation is a physical principle often used in separating products of different specific gravity. Examples are the quality-gravity separation of peas and lima beans in standardized brines. Flotation is also used to clean vegetables; the light trash floats, while soil clumps, pebbles, and heavy particles sink to the bottom. After crushing, apricot hulls may be separated from the pits by flotation in running water. Frozen citrus fruits can be detected from sound fruit by flotation. Brine flotation methods are useful in separating bone and cartilage from the poultry meat in boning machines. The extracted mixture passes through brine flumes fitted with baffles, and a good separation is obtained. In machine-extracted crab meat a good separation of chitinous materials and shell from the meat is obtained by brine flotation.

Draining. In the preparation of fruit, vegetables, meat, and seafood for canning and freezing, careful and consistent draining is required so that excess water is not transferred to the can or package. Food laws severely restrict the quantity of water so transferred. Thus peach, apricot, and pear halves are always placed cup down on belts to drain before filling. Cherries, berries, and other foods which absorb water easily must be well drained on vibrating screens or belts to remove excess moisture. Only by using fruit of a constant moisture content can the syruping operation be accurate, that is, the maintenance of desired sugar concentration, or Brix, in the consumer product. If oysters and clams are not drained carefully, it is impossible to secure the required drained weights in the can. On the other hand, in a product such as tomatoes, draining can be excessive and much of the juice which is an integral part of the tomato may be lost. Care must be taken in the blanching operation to avoid undue loss of moisture from such vegetables as spinach, broccoli, and snap beans.

Trimming. Trimming is a simple operation usually performed in one of two stages during the preparation of vegetables or fruit for processing. Crude or preliminary trimming is often done before the product is washed. It is a part of the sorting operation and consists of discarding culls and misshapen, discolored, semidecayed specimens. The tops of vegetables, as well as discolored and slightly decayed portions, are removed by hand trimming. More careful trimming is done on a conveyor belt after the fruits or vegetables have been carefully sorted and cleansed. Here, surface blemishes, immature or bruised portions, and pieces of skin are removed. Such trimmed produce is often consigned to a lower grade, but it is still sound food and need not be discarded in spite of its poorer quality and sale value. Mechanical devices perform standardized trimming operations, such as cutting tips from beans and stems from mushrooms.

Peeling. Peeling is done both by hand and mechanically. Hand peeling has been largely replaced by steam, abrasion, gas flame, or lye treatment to remove the peel. Some fruits, such as plums, figs, cherries, berries, and apricots, are not peeled at all. Although there are no standardized methods of removing the peel from such dissimilar foods as pineapples, grapefruit, apples, pears, peppers, and sweet potatoes, equipment is available for handling each product. Hot lye (sodium hydroxide) solution is used for peeling peaches, pears, sweet potatoes, carrots, and peppers. A low concentration of 1.5–3% is used for fruit, while 5–15% is used for vegetables. The albedo, or rag, of peeled grapefruit is usually removed by a spray or a dip in lye solution, the lye being promptly removed by a water spray or dip. There is little or no residue of the lye on products that have been treated with it. Since lye tends to discolor peaches and some other foods, acid washes are sometimes used to preserve the natural color. The most recent lye peeling technique is the so-called dry caustic technique that reduces the amount of water in the plant's waste effluent. Steam peeling is used generally for white potatoes and some other vegetables since it is a less costly method for large quantities. It also gives the highest percentage recovery of edible portion. Hand trimming is usually necessary to remove minor defects. Abrasive-type peelers are used today mainly in restaurants and institutions since they are wasteful and leave an undesirable rough texture. Roasting by gas flame is an unusual method which is sometimes used for peeling sweet peppers and pimientos.

Dehusking, silking, and cutting. These operations are largely confined to sweet corn. Until recently, these were hand operations but now all the larger canning and freezing plants use efficient and speedy mechanical huskers, silkers, and cutters. Huskers consist of a pair of rapidly revolving rubber or milled-steel rolls which catch the husks much as a clothes wringer does wet clothes. The rolls can spread apart sufficiently to allow the husks to pass between them, but powerful springs return them at once to their normal position. Single machines operate at the rate of 60–70 ears a minute, and the twin-type machines double this capacity. Most corn factories use a desilker which consists of a series of revolving rolls and brushes which remove the silk before the corn is cut from the cob. Final desilking takes place in the flotation separator following the cutting operation. There are several types of corn cutters. The husked and trimmed ears are fed through curved knives that accommodate themselves by springs to the size of the ear. For cream-style corn, scrapers remove the remainder of the kernel still clinging to the cob after the first cutting process. Some packers pulp or "Creamogenize" a portion of the corn and return it to the canned product to improve its consistency. The present trend is a preference for whole-kernel canned and frozen sweet corn. The whole kernels are removed from the cob by spe-

cially designed cutting knives. The kernels are carefully inspected on a conveyor belt and the silk and debris are removed by a flotation separator. A dewatering vibrating screen removes excess moisture before the kernels pass to the filling machine.

Shelling. Shelling is an operation limited to raw foods such as dry corn, beans, dry peas, peanuts, pecans, and walnuts. Corn is readily shelled in one of several types of contact shellers. Often the process includes air-blast cleaning to remove adhering chaff and dust. For grinding, shelled corn should contain not over 14% moisture. Hulled corn or hominy is made by treating shelled corn with lye to loosen the hull, leaching out the lye, and cooking the greatly enlarged kernels until tender. Hulled corn was a very important colonial food.

Fresh peas, chick peas, and browneye peas are shucked by threshers or viners located either in the fields or at the processing plant. The viners simply beat out the peas from the pods. Both peanuts and walnuts are shelled by passing the nuts between carefully adjusted rollers which crush the shell but do not break the meats. Popcorn is normally dried to a moisture content of 13–14% before shelling. This is the moisture content which

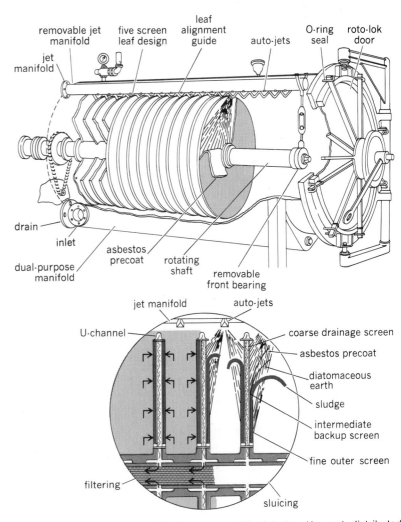

Fig. 8.   Vertical leaf pressure filter. Slurry enters side of shell and is evenly distributed to the leaves, where solids are deposited. Filtrate moves to center shaft and is discharged. For cleaning, water is sprayed on slowly rotating leaves from header in top of shell. (*Food Engineering, Chilton Co.*)

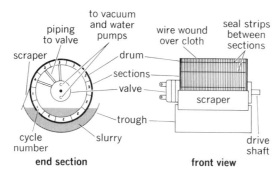

Fig. 9. Vacuum filter. Vacuum filter comprises compartmented drum rotating in trough. Slurry is fed to trough and picked up by drum. Liquid portion is drawn through filtering media and discharged at center. Solids are deposited on surface of drum and removed by scraper.

gives maximum popability.

Stemming and pitting. Stemming and pitting are necessary for some fruits, especially cherries. While cherries are usually stemmed by hand, machines are available which save time. Blueberries harvested with scoops contain stems which are difficult to remove. The use of vibrating screens helps to remove many stems but no method has been found to be fully effective. Blanching blueberries for 10–30 sec helps to remove the stems and also tenderizes the skins for freezing. Gooseberries may be passed through a machine resembling a bean snipper to remove stems and floral cups.

Sweet cherries are not usually pitted. Sour or pie cherries, and to some extent dates, olives, and raisins, are pitted by forcing a three-pronged plunger through firmly held fruit. Raisins are steamed before seeding. Machines greatly speed the pitting of apricots and peaches.

Coring. Coring is limited to such fruits as apples and pears. Apples are usually run through a combination peeler-corer and seed-cell remover,

an ingenious combination of three machines. Manual trimming is necessary after machine peeling and coring no matter whether the apples are to be canned, frozen, or used in applesauce. Seed cells constitute a serious defect and must be removed. Pears are cored either by hand or by one of several types of mechanical corers. A special contour-bladed knife is used in hand coring. Because of the peculiar shape of the pear, considerable hand trimming is needed. [CARL R. FELLERS]

Filtering. This technique separates liquids and solids by means of a pressure differential which may be created either by vacuum on the underside of filtering media, or by external force applied on the upstream side. The technique is largely used in breweries, wineries, fruit-juice plants, and vegetable-oil and sugar refineries.

Pressure filters employ papers or cloth supported on horizontal or vertical leaves, or fine metal screens with 2500 or more openings per square inch. These are usually precoated with nonfibrous materials, such as diatomaceous earth (Fig. 8).

One development employs sheets or pads of high-quality asbestos and cellulose fibers intimately blended and interlocked to form a filter matrix of controlled porosity and high wet strength. These remove and retain solids, semisolids, colloidal contaminants, and microorganisms. Incorporation of activated carbon enables removal of color and odor.

Vacuum filters are of two fundamental designs: (1) compartmented drums covered with wire cloth, perforated metal, cotton, wool, or synthetic materials and (2) totally enclosed cylindrical units with plates or disks mounted on vertical or horizontal hollow shafts.

In the compartmented drum filters (Fig. 9), the drum is rotated in a tank containing slurry to be filtered. Vacuum, applied to the inside of the drum, picks up slurry and deposits solids on the filter media. The filtrate discharges through a valve in the axis. As the drum rotates, the cake may be washed and partially dried by vacuum before it is removed by a scraper.

The cylindrical units employ direct or precoat filtration. Slurry is fed into the cylindrical housing, passes through the plates, and discharges through the central shaft. Cleaning may be manual or automatic by centrifugal spinning of the disks to ensure complete removal of filter cake.

For slimy materials, drums are precoated before operation, and, as they rotate, a moving knife continuously shaves off deposited solids plus a small amount of the filtering media. The latest advance is the use of micropore filters in commercial-scale processing to remove yeast and bacteria from beer and wine to avoid spoilage. Air for aseptic filling enclosures is filtered to take out bacteria.
[ARTHUR V. GEMMILL]

Dressing. Slaughter and dressing are generally a continuous process, except where animals are frozen prior to dressing. Dressing includes all operations required to prepare the hot carcass for chilling (to remove body heat) and subsequent breakdown.

The degree of dressing depends upon the type of animal, market requirements, local preference, and custom. Dressing on the rail is the most modern procedure employed today.

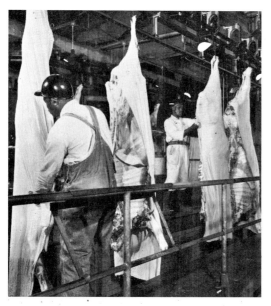

Fig. 10. Beef carcasses shrouded with a muslin cloth as they leave dressing floor en route to the cooler. Shroud helps to smooth and whiten the fat. (*Armour and Co.*)

Shipper beef is eviscerated, hide removed, head and feet dropped, split into sides, and shrouded for chilling (Fig. 10).

Dressing of sheep is quite similar; calves, however, are dressed and chilled with the hide on or off.

Hogs are scalded and singed to remove hair prior to evisceration and splitting (Fig. 11).

Fish may be completely dressed, scaled, and eviscerated, or may only be eviscerated.

Most poultry is plucked and eviscerated, and wing joints, feet, and head are removed.

Expressing. Expressing is a mechanical process for separating the liquid and solid components of a substance by the use of pressure. The process is widely used in separating the oil from such oil-bearing material as oilseeds, nuts, fruits, and fatty animal tissue and to a lesser extent in the separation of juice from such foods as citrus fruit, grapes, pineapples, apples, and tomatoes.

A great variety of equipment, both batch and continuous, is used in expressing. Pressures ranging up to 40,000 psi are applied mechanically, hydraulically, or centrifugally.

Materials to be expressed are normally pretreated, ground, and heat-treated in the production of oil. Juice fruits are ground or crushed.

Solvent extraction. This is a process for separating one component of a substance by use of a solvent in which the component is soluble.

The process is widely used in separating oil from oil-bearing material, principally and most practically when the oil content is low, as in soybeans. Solvent extraction is also used commercially in processing cottonseed, flaxseed, corn germ, wheat germ, animal fat, castor beans, soybeans, and cocoa, and for the extraction of essential oils (Fig. 12).

After pretreatment (expressing, grinding, crush-

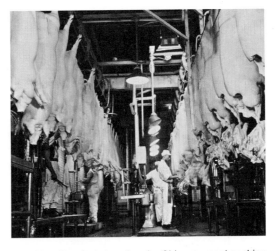

Fig. 11. Hog-dressing line in Chicago meat-packing plant. (*Armour and Co.*)

ing, roasting, or flaking), materials to be extracted are brought in contact with a solvent in either batch or continuous processing equipment. Solvents normally used are low-boiling hydrocarbons or chlorinated hydrocarbons. The solvent extract or miscella is distilled to remove the solvent. The extracted cake is also desolventized. Solvent-extraction milling of rice to recover high-quality rice oil and bran has been developed.

Rendering. Rendering is a process employing heat for separating oil and fat from animal tissue. Heat is applied principally to coagulate cell proteins, permitting release of the oil. Rendering is universally used in the production of lard and tallow from meat fats.

Dry rendering is carried out either in open agi-

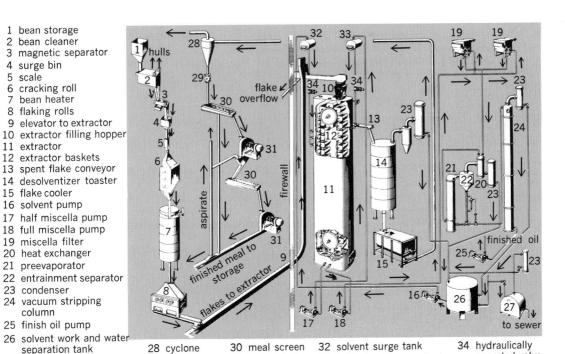

1 bean storage
2 bean cleaner
3 magnetic separator
4 surge bin
5 scale
6 cracking roll
7 bean heater
8 flaking rolls
9 elevator to extractor
10 extractor filling hopper
11 extractor
12 extractor baskets
13 spent flake conveyor
14 desolventizer toaster
15 flake cooler
16 solvent pump
17 half miscella pump
18 full miscella pump
19 miscella filter
20 heat exchanger
21 preevaporator
22 entrainment separator
23 condenser
24 vacuum stripping column
25 finish oil pump
26 solvent work and water separation tank
27 waste water evaporator
28 cyclone
29 rotary valve
30 meal screen
31 meal grinder
32 solvent surge tank
33 half miscella surge tank
34 hydraulically operated valve

Fig. 12. Soybean preparation—solvent extraction and recovery and meal grinding. (*French Oil Mill Machinery Co.*)

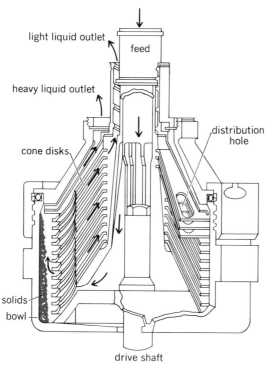

Fig. 13. Example of a settling centrifuge. (*Food Engineering, Chilton Co.*)

tated kettles or in closed vessels under vacuum. Wet rendering is conducted in open kettles at low temperatures with added water, or at high temperatures under steam pressure. The type of oil or fat product desired usually determines the type of process used. The latest process is continuous rendering in a closed process. Chopped fat is heated, finely comminuted, and centrifuged to separate liquid fat from solid cell-wall material.

[CLARENCE K. WIESMAN]

Centrifuging. Centrifuging is a technique for separating solids from liquids, or liquids from liquids, by application of centrifugal force. It is widely used in the food industry for clarifying fruit and vegetable juices, milk, and oils; separating fat from milk and starch from gluten; dewatering crystals; reclaiming meals and oils from meat and fish wastes; and removing sludge from hot wort.

Two basic types of unit are employed in the operation, settling machines and filtering centrifuges. In settling machines the mixture of liquids, or of liquids and solids, is stratified by centrifugal force. The separated components are either drawn off continuously, or one settles on the inside of the bowl and is removed intermittently (Fig. 13). Machines currently are made with split bowls which open automatically to discharge solids.

In filtering centrifuges, solids are collected on the surface of a perforated basket, while the liquid passes through the accumulated mass and is caught in an annular casing which diverts it to a discharge point (Fig. 14). Provision is made for purifying the separated crystals by washing. Solids may be discharged from the basket intermittently or continuously.

[ARTHUR V. GEMMILL]

Raw materials conversion. This is the processing of natural foods from the farm to preserve them, change them into a more useful form, or combine them with other materials and ingredients to produce manufactured foods. Examples are milling wheat into flour, fermenting cabbage to make sauerkraut, smoking meat, and making bread.

Additional examples of conversion operations include size reduction (such as cutting and grinding), mixing (to combine various materials and ingredients), forming into a particular shape and size (such as fishsticks), heating (as in cooking preserves), freezing, and dehydrating.

[FRANK K. LAWLER]

Size reduction. The mechanical size reduction of materials to facilitate processing by the production of slurries, pastes, and particles with distinct size or shape characteristics (for example, by grinding, cutting, comminuting, disintegrating, pulping, pureeing). The mills used are of sanitary design, with product contact surfaces and even entire units fabricated of stainless steel. Some have jacketed feed-throats and milling chambers for chilling or heating heat-sensitive or low-melting-point materials. The airstream may be tempered to regulate final product temperatures or moisture levels; facilities for milling in an inert atmosphere may be separate or in conjunction with these special effects. Some processes use a prebreaker, before the mill, to reduce materials to acceptable size.

Grinding is done in modern attrition mills (plate, stone, stone-composition, or roller) which are mechanical descendants of old stone mills, but are now so refined that their end products, capacities, and efficiencies are highly improved. One such mill uses rotating (5400–7400 rpm) carborundum plates, grinds materials to smooth (0.0025- to 0.005-in. particle size) texture. A roll-type coffee mill,

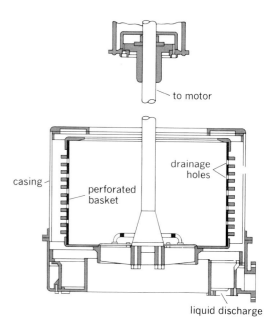

Fig. 14. Filtering centrifuge. Perforated baskets are employed. Crystals are deposited on inside, liquid moves through openings, and is discharged from casing. (*Food Engineering, Chilton Co.*)

adaptable to multiple-unit sequential grinding, employs micrometric roll adjustment in increments of 0.002 in. New grain milling principles include fluid-energy, turbo milling, and impact milling. Employing the principle of fluid-energy attrition, material is injected into a cylindrical reduction chamber of irregular, oval shape. It is entrained in a pressurized stream of fluid, air, or gas moving at supersonic velocities. Violent jet action shatters the grains by impact and abrasion. Centrifugal force shifts large particles to the outer periphery; smaller ones drift to the inside of the cylinder and, as they are reduced to submicron size, exit in the spent stream. An inclosed vertical rotor with radial blades segmented to its shaft provides an air-vortex principle for ultrafine grinding. The rotor turns at 1500–2500 rpm, creating air vortexes between blades of 30,000-fpm peripheral speed. Particles of 1-micron (μ) size result from impact, in air, against walls, and from interparticle abrasion and attrition in air vortexes. In impact milling of whole-grain flour, grain is batched into a horizontal, clockwise revolving drum (140 rpm); centrifugal force holds it against the inner periphery until it strikes a diversion bar. This hurls it into a gang of saws revolving counterclockwise (2400 rpm), which splits the grain. The number of passes determines particle size.

Cutting is another method for reducing materials to desired configurations by halving, slicing, cubing, chopping, or comminuting. Halving, for example, of cling peaches is done by high-speed halving-pitting machines. One of these automatically positions peaches so that halving knives divide them at the fruit's suture, then by torque action twists the halves apart, simultaneously releasing the pit from the flesh. Finer honing and induction hardening of knife edges allow high-speed, simultaneous, transverse-longitudinal cutting, producing cube shapes as small as 3/8 in. An example of reducing material to pulp by cutting is the silent cutter in which a rotating bowl passes sausage meat under a rotating circular knife.

Comminuting-disintegrating machines have in common the mechanical principle by which they achieve size reduction. Swing hammers or knives are attached to a rotor which revolves at high speed within a chamber. Some units operate on horizontal axes; others are vertical or set at decided angles (Fig. 15). Fine particles are separated, and desired particle sizes are discharged through classifying screens, mechanical or air-separation devices. Coarse particles are recycled. Crystalline, granular, soft, or fibrous materials are reduced to the following sizes: coarse (20–80 mesh); fine (80–300 mesh); superfine (200–400 mesh); and ultrafine, down to $3–5\ \mu$.

Pulping mechanically reduces materials such as meat, fruits, or vegetables to a moist, undissolved mass; and pureeing reduces materials of high moisture content such as fruits or vegetables to a pumpable slurry. These results may also be achieved by boiling. Often a unit process is composed of one or more of the preceding size reduction unit operations; for example, size reduction by special machine and then sieving the undesirable pulp from puree, or liquid from pulp. A familiar process is that used for tomato products in which

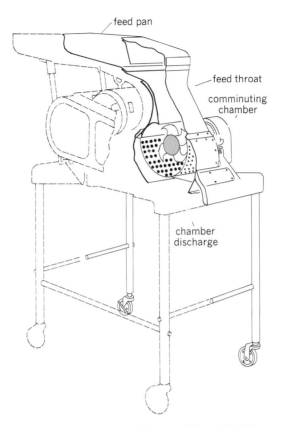

Fig. 15. Comminuting machine. (*W. J. Fitzpatrick* Co.)

a combined chopper-pump, or a comminuter, reduces whole tomatoes to make the hot-break process possible.   [CARL R. HAVIGHORST]

Food mixing. Food mixing is a key unit operation involving instrumented blending of dry and liquid ingredients with or without heat (cooking) and on a batch or continuous basis.

An automatic system of making bread dough, supplanting operations of three bakery departments, has an hourly capacity of 4000–6000 loaves (Fig. 16). The initial ingredients are agitated in a tank, in which yeast activity is simulated. Flour is

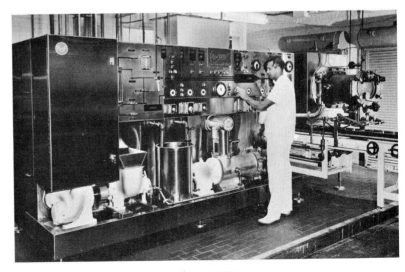

Fig. 16. Continuous bread-dough system. (*AMF Inc.*)

added, and the liquid sponge, or mix, is pumped to agitator-equipped holding tanks. The sponge is then pumped to a continuous horizontal mixing trough into which liquid sugar is metered. It is finally pumped to a dough-development system, where dough pieces are extruded into pans that are conveyed to final proofer and oven.

Another example is the two-step, continuous blending of mayonnaise and cake batters. Solids and liquids are metered into a bowl-type preblender with twin-disk impeller. The blend proceeds to a postblender, which is equipped with rotating and stationary toothed disks and a compressed gas inlet. In producing mayonnaise, the final mixing with vinegar is done in nitrogen atmosphere. By providing starch-vinegar cooking facilities, the system also produces salad dressings.

Ultrasonics is offering rapid mixing, emulsifying and homogenizing of mayonnaise, dressings, cheese spreads, margarine, soups, sauces, ice cream, and peanut butter, with improved smoothness and stability.

Modern colloid mills now mix, mill, and homogenize, in single pass, to offer stable emulsions and uniform size reduction of such items as dressings, meats, fish pastes, cheese, and chocolate.

Dry or semidry mixes, such as chocolate, powdered milk, and bakery premixes, are uniformly blended by a high-speed paddle-type unit that breaks up and disperses agglomerates. The unit can handle 3000–10,000 lb/hr.

Machines can automatically proportion ingredients into a dough mixer that extrudes and cuts macaroni, spaghetti, and noodles to lengths at a capacity of 1000 lb/hr.

A new conical mixer requires little power and employs a precessional motion of the rotating screw for rapid blending of dry materials and wetting or dissolving of solids.

A heated, rotating double-cone unit blends and dries products under vacuum. Another high-capacity rotary dry blender (four-way action unit) assures high mix uniformity.

High-volume blenders now speed the uniform mixing of dry materials and the dispersion of liquids, regardless of viscosity. Rotating twin-shell

units (50 ft³) have been modified for a liquid feed operation like blending melted shortening into dry mixes, and spices or flavoring emulsions into granular bases in 10–15 min.

Two novel German mixing machines are gaining wider commercial use. One uses compressed air to agitate and intermingle dry free-flowing materials. The other sprays fluid, such as shortening fat, onto powder as the fat is dispersed pneumatically.

Another blender flows dry material over a conical surface in a thin layer as a second dry or fluid substance is added to it.

Still more recent is a mixer with two cones rotating in opposite directions at high speed. Two materials (dry or liquid) flowing over the cones are thrown together and thoroughly interspersed at the periphery of the mixer. Yet another innovation is the mixer in which fine dry materials move up vibrating inclines and spillover to effect blending.

An advanced starch-gum jelly process employs mixer-heat-exchanger assembly for continuous cooking and cooling of starch-sugar slurry at the rate of 2500 lb/hr. Before the cooked product goes into the cooling section, the flavor-color solution is introduced.

A simplified aerating process for making foamy marshmallow and nougats consists of (1) mixing air and liquid by jetting, (2) further mixing by mechanical impingement at high velocity against a fixed target from which the product is deflected with turbulence, and (3) straining and diffusing through a porous medium.

In fluid mixing, propeller- or turbine-type units do an efficient job with most liquids when impeller size, speed, and mounting are properly specified.

Food forming. Food forming is the mechanized shaping of products to precise shape and size. Basic techniques include extruding (spaghetti); sheeting between rolls, cutting into strips, and crosscutting into slices or bars (cheese and candy); sheeting and die-cutting (cookies); stuffing into casing (sausage); molding in metal or starch cavities (candy); depositing metered portions onto belt (chocolate bits); dividing into portions and rounding by rolling over rotating metal surface (bread dough); rounding by rotating portions between belts traveling in opposite directions (meat balls); twisting (dough); layering by depositing one sheet on top of another (candy); layering by multiple folding (pastries); puffing by vacuum (candy), by sudden pressure release (cereals), or by formation of gas or vapor in processing (potato puffs); tableting by compacting powdered or granular material in dies by plunger action (confections); agglomerating powdered material (to form larger, more soluble particles) by intermingling in humid atmosphere (instant dry milk).

Cutting into slices, strips, or cubes (straight or corrugated) is forming in a sense. Some innovations are as follows.

1. With continuous extrusion of dough in the automatic production of white bread, a machine with only two operators can extrude 70 loaves (1 lb each) per minute (Fig. 17).

2. In those food industries requiring a product in individual pieces, a precision rotary unit can vacuum-form 2500 lb of product per hour. This permits continuous operation into a fryer, enrober, or freezer.

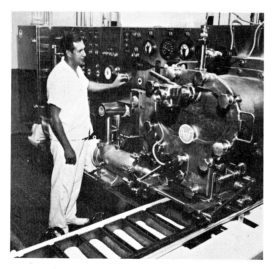

Fig. 17. Forming bread loaves by continuous-extrusion process. (*AMF Inc.*)

3. Mint creams are deposited onto a continuous belt and proceed directly to cooling and chocolate coating units.

4. Modern equipment hopper-feeds confections through sheeting rolls onto belts traveling through a chilling tunnel and then slits the sheet of multi-layer confection into continuous strips that are cut into bars for chocolate coating. Cookie batter is similarly sheeted through rolls, with the sheet cut into shape. The batter may be hopper-fed through forming dies.

5. An air-operated unit can shape 400 link-type skinless sausages per hour. The machine also produces other meat emulsions in desired forms.

6. There is a machine that forms a wide range of products in chub-shaped packages by shaping and sealing roll-fed plastic film around a tube into which the product is metered; package ends are sealed with metal clips.

7. Mold-type chocolates such as tablets, solid bars, and filled confections may be produced at the rate of 800/min.

8. New equipment cuts fruits, vegetables, and meats into various forms such as strip, slice, dice, quarter, crinkle-cut, or french-fry.

9. An automatic molder-twister-panner twists and joins dough pieces at a rate of 90/min.

10. A machine extrudes 1000 lb of dough per hour to form macaroni, spaghetti, and noodles.

11. There is a process for dry or press coating tablets as a substitute for costly pan-coating operations.

12. Meat emulsions can be stuffed into casings in making frankfurters and other sausage products. Another more continuous sausage process consists of grinding meat, mixing in spices, and then pumping to a comminutor, which feeds to receiving tanks and stuffing nozzles.

13. A cooker-extruder gelatinizes starchy material with heat, mixes it with added ingredients, and extrudes the product through forming dies of various shapes. This system produces snack foods very efficiently.   [JOHN V. ZIEMBA]

Heat treatment. The heat treatment of food is one of the important processes for the conditioning of food for preservation. This treatment accomplishes many objectives, including inactivation of microorganisms, enzymes, or poisonous compounds and production of desirable chemical or physical changes in foods.

When compared to typical engineering material such as metals or minerals, food is relatively susceptible to thermal degradation. Therefore, to produce nutritionally sound and microbially safe food products, heat treatment should be accurately controlled in order to accomplish its objectives. To assist in this control, the temperature responses of foods subjected to heat treatments are frequently estimated by using empirical or theoretical heat-balance equations.

Heat treatment follows different patterns. It may involve application of heat indirectly, as in a tubular heat exchanger, or it may be accomplished through the direct contact of the heating medium with the food, as in the baking of bread in a hot-air oven. The principal operations involving heat treatment of foods are blanching, preheating, pasteurization, sterilization, cooking, evaporation, and dehydration.

Blanching is a hot-water or steam-scalding treatment of raw foodstuffs to inactive enzymes which might otherwise cause quality deterioration, particularly of flavor, during processing or storage. Most vegetables and some fruits are blanched before canning, freezing, or dehydrating. The commonly used types of equipment are rotary perforated drums, rotary screw conveyors or troughs, and pipe flume blanchers. Water is the predominant heating medium in drum and flume blanchers; steam is used in the screw-type blancher. Temperature is usually 100°C or slightly lower. The length of treatment, when preceding freezing, varies from 50 sec to 10 or 11 min.

Preheating is a treatment used immediately before canning to ensure the production of a vacuum in the sealed container. When the product cools, the headspace vapor condenses. Foodstuffs of liquid or slurry type are usually preheated in tubular heat exchangers which are equipped with screw conveyors if necessary. Foods of particulate type, submerged in a brine or syrup in the open-top container, are passed through a heated chamber, known as an exhaust box, in which steam is the usual heating medium.

Pasteurization is relatively mild heat treatment of food and involves the application of sufficient thermal energy to inactivate the vegetative cells of microorganisms, molds, yeasts, or enzymes that are harmful to human beings or to food quality, or both. The inactivation of bacterial spores, which are extremely resistant to heat, is not required, since pasteurized food is usually stored at refrigerator temperatures or the chemical composition of the food prohibits the germination of bacterial spores. Typical heating times and temperatures for pasteurization are 30 min at 65°C or 15 sec at 72°C. Heat sterilization requires more thermal energy than pasteurization does and is usually accomplished by heating food which is packed and sealed in containers made of metal, glass, or plastic film laminated with aluminum foil. One heat sterilization or pasteurization treatment is divided into heating and cooling phases. During the heating phase, the food is heated for the proper time by applying the heating medium, usually saturated steam or hot water maintained at the appropriate temperature. The cooling phase begins immediately following the heating phase. Since the temperature is at its maximum, or almost maximum, level at the end of the heating phase, it should be lowered as quickly as possible to avoid any unnecessary thermal destruction of the nutritional or organoleptic quality of the food.

There are batchwise and continuous heat-sterilization processes which are currently in commercial use, and the general trend is toward continuous processes. They are more economical in terms of heat energy, labor, and time than batchwise processes are, but the cost of equipment for continuous processing is generally greater. The continuous food sterilizing system, which is one of the most widely used in the United States, requires only 50% as much steam and 15–40% as much labor per unit of food processed as conventional batchwise systems need (Fig. 18).

The hydrostatic system (Fig. 19), which originated in Europe, uses approximately 25% less

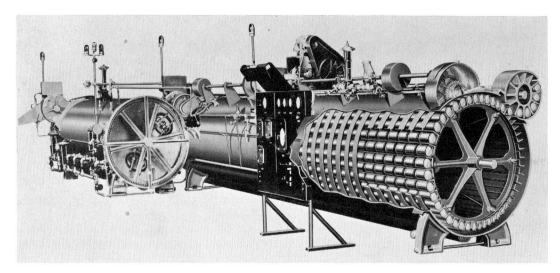

Fig. 18. Cutaway view showing a continuous-pressure food sterilizing system which is of the reel and spiral type. The smaller tank at the left is a continuous pressure cooler. (*FMC Corp.*)

steam and water per unit of food processed than the conventional batchwise system of processing does.

A continuous sterilizing process in which cans of food are heated as they are rolled over a series of gas burners has been developed in France.

The temperatures to which food is heated in conventional sterilization processes are dependent on the acidity of the food. A normal temperature range for the heat sterilization of low-acid food is 105–120°C.

Some heat sterilization methods are called high-temperature short-time (HTST) processes. An HTST process usually consists of two separate

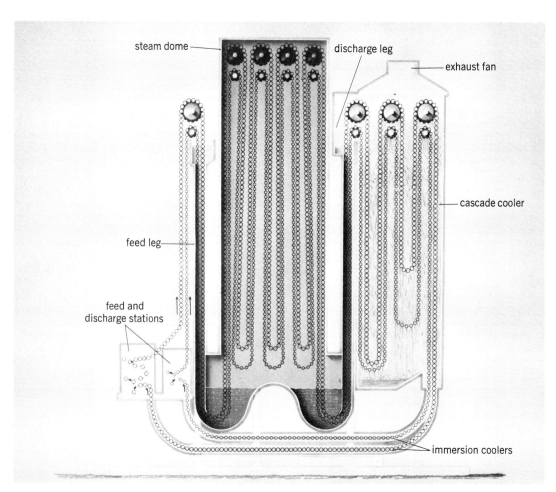

Fig. 19. Hydrostatic system of sterilizing food in sealed containers. (*FMC Corp.*)

heat treatments applied in sequence. The purpose of the first treatment is to inactivate enzymes by heating food for 5–10 min at 65–85°C, the second to inactivate microorganisms by heating food for 3–30 sec at 125–150°C. There are sound reasons for the requirement of two heat treatments in HTST processes. The rate of thermal inactivation of a biochemical or biological factor increases as the heating temperature increases. High temperatures have a great influence on microbial inactivation; but, in contrast, enzymes are less sensitive to thermal inactivation at temperatures above 120°C. Therefore, the first low-temperature and second high-temperature heatings are required for enzymic and microbial inactivations, respectively. In HTST processes, food is usually heat-sterilized before being placed into appropriate containers. The commercial application of these processes is mostly limited to liquid food since it is difficult to heat particulate foods quickly to the desired high temperatures. However, there have been a few trials of HTST processes with liquid-particulate mixtures by using scraped-surface heat exchangers (Fig. 20).

The table gives examples of commercial heat treatments whose major objectives are the physical or chemical modification of food rather than the inactivation of microorganisms or enzymes.

Microwave energy has been used for heat treatments of several foods, for example, finish-drying of potato chips after deep-fat frying and drying of noodles. Microwaves (which are electromagnetic waves) of 2450-MHz frequency are most often used for food processing. This frequency is one of those set aside for industrial, scientific, and medical use. Microwave energy can be used to heat any substance in which there are free polar molecules, and most foods contain free water molecules, which are polar. When food is subjected to these waves, each water molecule rotates rapidly around its axis since it aligns with the alternating electric field produced by the waves. Since this electric field changes at extremely high rates (for example, there are 2,000,000,000 alternations in 1 sec), frictional heat is generated. Food is fairly uniformly heated with microwave energy, and there have been several experimental trials on sterilizing food by this method. *See* MICROWAVE.

Cooling of foods. This phase of processing involves two types of techniques, applied to two categories of food.

The first type of technique is used for meats, dairy products, fruits, and vegetables which are marketed in the fresh state. To avoid serious loss of these products through decay, they are substantially reduced in temperature, either before shipment begins or during the first part of the transport period, and are held at a temperature between 0 and 4.4°C throughout their transport period.

Meat is cooled by refrigeration of carcasses immediately after slaughter. Milk is cooled by refrigeration immediately after production, and milk products are similarly cooled as the last step in the manufacturing process. Packing fruits and vegetables with ice when loading for transport is still widely practiced in some localities.

Two systems of precooling, or cooling prior to shipping, which are generally regarded as improvements over the old ice-packing method for fruits

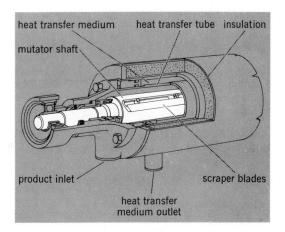

Fig. 20. Votator scraped-surface heat exchanger. (*Chemetron Corp.*)

and vegetables, are hydrocooling and vacuum cooling. Hydrocooling consists of spraying continuously cooled water onto the product, which is placed in wholesale-size containers, and recirculating the water. The water generally contains salt in solution to lower its freezing point and may also contain a fungicide or a bactericide, in which case the process is usually called stericooling. In vacuum cooling (Fig. 21), water is forced to evaporate from the surfaces of vegetables or fruits by a vacuum of 29.7 in. (100,292 N/m²) or more created around the product. This system is especially good for products such as lettuce and spinach which have large surfaces in relation to volume.

During transport, the temperature of cooled fresh meat, dairy products, vegetables, and fruit is maintained by mechanical refrigeration, solid carbon dioxide, liquid nitrogen, or bunker ice in the car or van. In cooling and storing fresh produce, sufficient cooling capacity must be used to lower the temperature, counteract heat access by radiation, and counteract the vital heat (heat of respiration) of the product. To illustrate, a carload of tomatoes of specific heat 0.95 and weighing 20,800 lb (12,960 kg) must lose 19,760 Btu (1 Btu = 1055 J) per degree of cooling. Under average condi-

Commercial heat treatments for physical or chemical modification of food

Process	Heating medium	Sample food	Heating-medium temperature, °C
Baking	Direct heating with air and radiative heating with oven walls	Breads, biscuits	120–150
Deep fat frying	Direct heating with oil	Potato chips, noodles, doughnuts	160–185
Drum drying	Indirect heating with steam	Bananas, potato whey	135–145
Evaporating	Indirect heating with steam	Tomato paste	100–110
Forced-air drying	Direct heating with air	Vegetables	60–95
Freeze-drying	Indirect heating with heat-exchange fluid or direct heating with thermal radiation	Fish, meat	40–80 (fluid)
Spray-drying	Direct heating with air	Instant coffee, milk powders	205–310

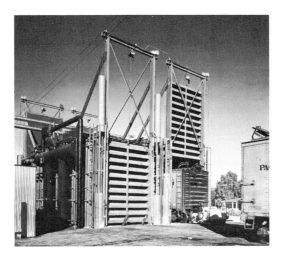

Fig. 21. A vacuum cooler of railroad-car size. (*Gay Engineering Corp.*)

tions, heat penetrating from outside the car amounts to approximately 3000 Btu per degree of temperature differential; and the vital heat per carload of ripe tomatoes, at 26.7, 21.1, 15.6, or 10°C, is approximately 103,000, 73,000, 54,000, or 34,000 Btu per day, respectively.

Approximately 14% more heat is evolved from mature green tomatoes than from ripe tomatoes. Most fruits evolve heat at a higher rate than tomatoes do, and vegetables as a class evolve heat more rapidly than fruits do.

The second category of foods includes those that are heat-treated during processing and are commercially distributed in ways other than through restaurants. Only a minute percentage of these foods is sold to consumers in the hot state. Therefore, most foods distributed commercially are cooled. Foods that are sterilized by heat are cooled after sterilization either by cooling the sealed containers with cold water or by passing the bulk food through water-cooled or refrigerant-cooled heat exchangers, depending upon whether the sterilization is accomplished by conventional means or by a system in which the food is sterilized before it is packaged. Foods pasteurized by heat are similarly cooled, either in the closed container or by heat exchanger. Cooling in closed containers may be achieved by a continuous, automatic operation, but more often a batchwise operation is used. Cooling of bulk material is carried out predominantly by continuous operation.

Foods that are heat-treated for purposes other than sterilization or pasteurization and that are cooled by a continuous operation as a step in processing include starch jelly confections, cooled from 140.5 to 97.8°C by being spread on the surface of a cooled cylinder; chocolate, which, during the pulverizing operation, is subjected to circulating air at 10°C to keep its temperature below 46.1°C; converted rice, which, after a pressure steam treatment, is cooled in circulating air; citrus concentrate, which is prepared by freezing out the water; butter, which is chilled to 4.4°C in ammonia-cooled cylinders; and foods of many varieties which are packed in cartons, including ice cream, and which are frozen in numerous types of continuous systems.

[KAN-ICHI HAYAKAWA; C. OLIN BALL]

Freezing. This is the use of subzero temperature for the freezing-preservation of foods, which thereafter are stored in low-temperature environment until consumed. Freezing is achieved by automatic plate freezers, continuous and batch air-blast units, direct- and spray-immersion freezers, and continuous freezers for liquid and semiliquids; examples are the double-contact pressure plate, tray cart in air-blast tunnel, and air-blast room freezers.

Cryogenic freezing with a spray of liquid nitrogen as the food moves through a tunnel on a conveyor has found limited commercial use, principally for shrimp but also for other products that are high-priced or have low moisture content. Much research on this technique is under way.

One superfast freezing medium, liquid food-grade Freon, is reported to be less expensive than liquid nitrogen because most of the evaporated refrigerant is recovered by condensing.

Moisture removal. The preservation of foods by sun-drying, the oldest known food process, is still practiced. However, modern principles of evaporation as applied to semisolid and liquid food materials, new thermodynamic techniques, and new unit operations are utilized to produce a number of new liquid, solid, or powdered foods.

Evaporation or boiling down, the classic batch method of concentrating material, has in most cases been replaced by vacuum evaporators (Fig. 22). Typical products are concentrated (frozen) orange juice; other juices such as tomato, apricot and peach; milk; and tomato sauce and paste. Some products lend themselves to concentrations as high as 50% solids without any depreciation of quality.

In most evaporators the liquid product flows down the inside walls of vertical heat-exchange tubes. One, however, has plate heat exchangers.

Types of units used range from single to multiple effects and, depending largely on product characteristics, utilize single-pass or recirculation flow principles with high temperatures (ordinarily steam) or low temperatures (provided by a heat pump). Efficient utilization of the heat pump is achieved by using heat from the cooling water of the compressor to heat the product and refrigeration to chill water for the barometric condenser. Some units are equipped with fractionating columns to recover product essence, often lost in discharged vapors, which subsequently is combined with evaporated material to recapture its natural flavor. Some plant wastes, for example, whey from cheese manufacture, or sardine stickwater, now are recovered by evaporation and used as feed. All modern evaporation units are highly automated by instrumentation to conserve labor costs and assure uniform quality of end products. All product-contact surfaces are of stainless steel.

The trend is to single-pass short-time high-temperature evaporation. One type of evaporator system generates the heat by mechanical compression of the vapor between stages.

For high-viscosity concentrates there are evaporators with devices that scrape the heating surface. The removal of water from wine and juices by reverse osmosis under high pressure is being developed. In limited use is freeze-concentration, water in the fluid food being crystallized into ice and separated by centrifuging.

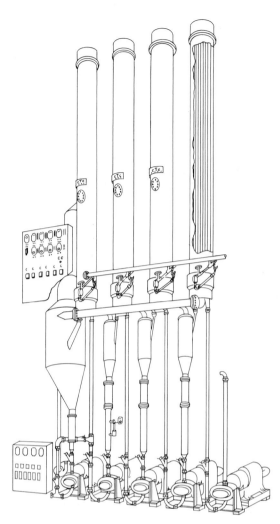

Fig. 22. Thermovac, four-stage, single-pass, highly automated evaporator. Temperatures and velocities are minutely, accurately, and automatically controlled in all four phases of the process.

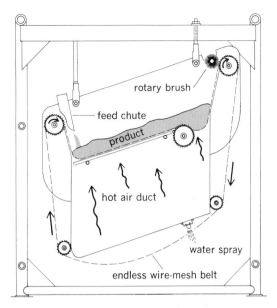

Fig. 23. Belt-trough drier. A spiral movement is imparted to the product to gain drying efficiency.

Drying and dehydration is done either in a batch-type or continuous operation. Batch-type drying using cabinets or trays on mobile racks that are moved through tunnels by chain or hydraulic ram are typical but less efficient than continuous belt-type dryers. The continuous-type unit employs through-product, heated-air circulation. It provides means for better control of moisture-humidity, and permits deeper product beds, thus increasing production capacity while conserving labor and steam.

High ratio of heating surface to product volume is achieved with the drum dryer. A thin layer of product is spread on the surface of an internally heated, rotating hollow cylinder or pair of cylinders. The product, dried to a 1–4% moisture in one revolution, is then removed from drum by a scraper or "doctor knife."

A belt-through dehydrator, originally designed for dehydration of food particles as part of the dehydrofreezing process, is also used as a drier (Fig. 23). Its inclined, moving belt imparts a foldover, spiral movement to the product and achieves high and uniform drying efficiency.

Spray driers were developed especially to convert milk to a readily reconstituted dry powder.

Materials such as solutions or slurries are introduced into the drying chamber either by high-speed centrifuges (6000–20,000 rpm) or high-pressure nozzles (2000–10,000 psi) into a heated atmosphere (137.8–148.9°C) moving at high velocity. Evaporation from the atomized mist takes a fraction of a second, with overall drying time usually under 30 sec. The largest volume of dried product ($1-3\frac{1}{3}\%$ moisture) falls to the bottom of the chamber and is continuously removed. The fine particles entrained in exhaust air are recovered by cyclone collectors.

Continuous vacuum dehydrating occurs in a vacuum chamber, where the concentrate (for example, orange juice of 58% total solids) is transferred from a feed trough, by a roller, to an endless, stainless belt, powered by two drumlike pulleys. One drum heats the belt, the other cools it. Complete dehydration takes place as the film-covered belt moves from the feed roller across the heating drum to the cooling drum, where a doctor knife scrapes off the crystalline powder.

Freeze-drying is ordinarily done in a vacuum cabinet with heating and cooling facilities. This process has been used for over 30 years in the biological sciences for preservation of unstable materials. Fundamentally, it consists of water removal under high vacuum by sublimation from the solid phase, ice, to the gaseous phase, water vapor. Various types of cabinets or refrigerated ovens are used. All produce vacuums of 300–700 millimicrons. Materials dried by this method range from semisolids for meats to powders for juice concentrates. Low product temperatures, retention of size and shape of product pieces, and porous structure for quick rehydration are benefits. One commercial application of freeze drying is the production of instant coffee.

Dehydrofreezing is a dual process which involves partial dehydration followed by freezing. A quality product of light weight is produced. Pimientos were used in the first commercial application of the process and were followed by peas.

[CARL R. HAVIGHORST]

In limited use is puff-drying of vegetables. After partial drying in a hot-air tunnel, the product pieces are expanded to make them more porous by sudden release from a pressure chamber, or gun. This facilitates the escape of moisture in the final conventional drying operation. The dry porous product rehydrates quickly, too.

Another recent development is foam-mat drying. Here fluid material is whipped into foam with the aid of a chemical stabilizer. Then foam is dehydrated in perforated trays or on a metal belt and mechanically disintegrated to a porous powder that rehydrates readily.

Foam spray drying involves injection of gas into a liquid, such as milk, before it is discharged from the nozzles. The gas expands the sprayed droplets to form porous dry particles.

Irradiation. This is one of the newest methods of preserving foods. The method of treating raw materials by irradiation to extend the storage period commonly refers to the use of ionizing radiations.

In this category are the penetrating radiations such as γ- and x-rays, and those less-penetrating radiations such as cathode rays or β-particles.

Gamma rays arise from the nuclei of radioactive isotopes during their decay processes, whereas x-rays are produced by man-made accelerators. Both have the same properties at the same energy levels.

Cathode rays, electrons, or β-particles are synonymous in terms of physical characteristics and effects. Cathode rays are streams of electrons accelerated by a high-voltage potential. Beta particles are actually electrons emitted from the nuclei of radioactive atoms during their decay processes.

These ionizing radiations have been used for extension of storage life, or pasteurization, and for sterilization in recent experiments.

Radiopasteurization may be accomplished by surface treatment, in which case low-energy irradiation is used. An example is the extension of the storage life of frankfurters by reducing the mold and bacterial formation on the surface.

Reduction of the total microbial flora throughout a product by substerilization doses of 1,000,000 radiation absorbed doses (rad) or less describes the process of penetrating radiopasteurization. An example is the extension of the storage life of hamburger by treatment with doses of 500,000 – 1,000,000 rad, thereby reducing the bacterial load from 10^6 bacteria per gram to less than 10^3 bacteria per gram with resultant increase in storage life at 7.2°C from 1 week to 1 year.

Sterilization refers to the utilization of doses high enough to result in the conventional type of commercial sterilization considered in terms of thermal processing. In this case, depending on the type of spoilage organisms, doses of 10^5 to 5×10^6 rad are required. Irradiation also kills insects and larvae in grain, prevents onions from sprouting in storage, and speeds rehydration of dehydrated vegetables.

Antibiotic treatment. Certain antibiotics, such as tetracyclines, at one time were approved by the U.S. Food and Drug Administration for use in dilute solutions into which eviscerated poultry was dipped to expand its storage life under refrigeration about two weeks. In Canada and other countries, dilute solutions can be used to make ice for refrigerating fish. While antibiotics kill surface spoilage bacteria, such treatment may possibly have undesirable long-term side effects.

Fermentation. Fermentation is a means of preserving foods or developing new foods by the conversion of various carbohydrate materials through the use of microorganisms. Examples of fermentation in the production of foods are the following: the conversion of lactose to lactic acid with the resultant end product of fermented milk, such as yogurt, or the resultant end product of cottage cheese or other cheeses; the conversion of flour by yeasts to break down the sugars into carbon dioxide, thus producing a fluffy loaf of bread; the conversion of sugars in cabbage and cucumbers to produce sauerkraut and pickles. *See* CHEESE; FERMENTATION; INDUSTRIAL MICROBIOLOGY.

In the Far East, a number of soybean products are produced by fermentation processes. An example is the Japanese product miso, produced by the action of *Aspergillus*, a mold, on cooked soybean.

The fermentative processes take place through enzyme reactions. The enzymes, produced by the microorganisms in their growth and metabolism, in turn convert the various raw materials cited above.

Pickling, curing, and aging. The processes of pickling, curing, and aging refer mainly to applications in the meat industry and to a lesser extent in the fish and dairy industries. Various meats such as pork shoulders, hams, and briskets of beef are soaked in brine solutions containing sugar and spices. Included in the pickling solution are sodium nitrite and sodium nitrate, which produce the typical pink coloration of pickled meats. Quick curing now is achieved by pumping the solution into pork bellies through 100 or more hollow needles.

Following the pickling process some of the meats, such as hams, may be smoked. Others like corned beef are not smoked.

The addition of pickle results in longer shelf life due to the increase in salt in the food product.

Curing generally refers to the storage of products like cheddar cheese for a period of time under controlled environmental conditions in order to develop taste, aroma, and proper texture. The changes that take place in the curing process are a result of the enzymes from the microorganisms. The temperatures for curing usually range from 0 to 4.4°C and the time required is from 3 to 12 months.

Aging refers generally to cheese and other food products and in particular to alcoholic beverages, which are also one of the most important industrial examples of fermentations.

During the aging process various harsh-flavored materials, such as the fusel oils, are converted to more mildly flavored materials. The aging process may continue for a period of a few months to several years. During this time, changes take place in the solids, esters, acids, and aldehydes, as well as fusel oil, with a resultant better-flavored product.

Smoking. Smoking is a method for enhancing flavor and extending shelf life of products. This is accomplished by volatilization and redeposition of certain components of hardwoods in smokehouses. The smokehouses are generally built of sanitary stainless steel with excellent temperature and humidity control (Fig. 24). The substances volatilized and redeposited are pleasantly flavored in addition to possessing bacteriostatic properties.

Although many methods of smoke application have been used, the ones of prime importance are burning of hardwood sawdust; destructive distillation of hardwood chips; friction-plate generation of smoke from hardwood logs; and electronic smoking consisting of imposing one electrical charge on the smoke particles and the opposite charge on the product, thus causing rapid deposition and penetration of smoke particles. One recent innovation consists of vaporization of liquid wood distillate.

Time, temperature, and relative humidity are carefully controlled during the smoking process; these conditions are varied according to the type of product being smoked.

Churning. Churning is a mechanical mixing process used essentially to separate the fat phase from a fat-water system. The process is universally used in the manufacture of butter. Churning and modifications of churning are also employed in the production of margarine.

The first step of a churning operation converts an oil-in-water emulsion (O/W) to a water-in-oil emulsion (W/O) through agitation and the incorporation of air. Once this conversion has been attained, with continued mixing the fat will agglomerate from the aqueous phase. After removal of the aqueous phase, churning is continued to incorporate salt and moisture and to standardize the composition of the butter.

Churning as conventionally done is a batch process carried out in horizontal rotating cylindrical vessels with baffles or vanes for improving agitation and working of the contents.

Continuous methods for making butter which replace churning are being increasingly used. *See* BUTTER; MARGARINE.

Deodorizing. Deodorizing is a steam distillation process for the removal of small amounts of volatile odor and flavor substances (Fig. 25). The process is routinely used in the preparation of fats and oils for the manufacture of shortenings and margarine. Off-flavors are occasionally removed from cream by deodorization.

Deodorizing is carried out in batch and in continuous equipment. In both, the material to be deodorized is heated under reduced pressure and treated with steam to strip out the volatile components.

Plasticizing. Plasticizing is a mechanical process employing rapid chilling, agitation, and gas incorporation for improving the texture and consistency of a fat or fat product.

Most fats, when cooled slowly from the liquid state, form large crystals and produce a grainy product. When they are cooled rapidly, the crystal size is small and the texture is smooth. Additional working of the chilled fat and the incorporation of gas into it improve its plasticity.

Good plasticity is vital to the functional properties of a fat, directly affecting the shortening, creaming, and volume-producing characteristics of fats used in baked products and the spreadability of margarine.

Plasticizing is carried out continuously in chill roll equipment or in closed systems employing concentric-tube heat exchangers equipped with agitation and gas-incorporation devices.

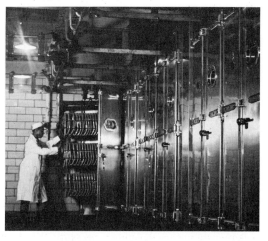

Fig. 24. Smokehouse provided with automatic temperature and humidity controls.

Hydrogenating. This is a chemical process for converting liquid fats into solid or semisolid fats. It is a catalytic process which adds hydrogen to ethylenic or double bonds in the fatty acid chains of the fat.

Hydrogenated fats have higher melting points and more plasticity than nonhydrogenated fats, and are also more suitable for the manufacture of "solid" shortenings and margarine. Hydrogenation also removes undesirable odors and colors from fats and increases their stability. The process, however, increases the degree of "saturation" of the fat.

Hydrogenating is normally carried out batchwise in 10- to 20-ton capacity agitated converters equipped for heating and cooling. Refined oil, containing a dispersed catalyst (usually nickel), is heated to reaction temperature and hydrogen is admitted to the converter. The reaction is exothermic, and once it has begun cooling is necessary to remove the excess heat. When the reaction has proceeded to the extent desired, the fat is cooled, filtered to remove the catalyst, and deodorized.

The properties of the hydrogenated fat can be partially controlled by the manner in which the reaction is carried out. The degree of hardening, as well as the course of reaction, is influenced by time, temperature, pressure, the type of catalyst used, and the concentration of the catalyst.

Decolorizing. Decolorizing is a mechanical separation process for the removal of naturally occurring undesirable color bodies. Decolorizing, or bleaching, is an adsorption separation in which the impurities are selectively adsorbed on an activated surface.

The process is used primarily in the refining of fats, oils, and sugar. Adsorbents used are normally bleaching clays or earths and carbon.

Decolorizing is performed in batch and continuous equipment. A filtration step follows the decolorizing process to remove the adsorbent.

[CLARENCE K. WIESMAN]

Puffing. A process that expands foods to several times their original volumes is called puffing. It is a key operation in converting cereal grains and cooked doughs into palatable dry breakfast foods, such as puffed wheat and puffed rice.

FOOD ENGINEERING

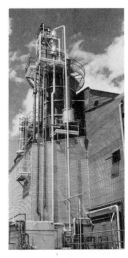

Fig. 25. A continuous vegetable oil-deodorizing unit. (*Blaw-Knox Co.*)

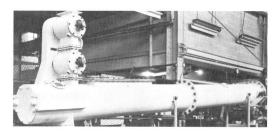

Fig. 26. Vacuum puffing unit which expands confections, such as mints and malted centers, up to 30 times original volumes, while evaporating 1–3% of product moisture. At feed end (left), double vacuum locks are shown. (*Stokes Equipment Div. of Pennwalt Corp.*)

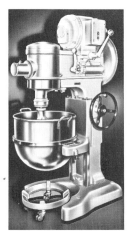

Fig. 27. Bakery whipping unit. Beater has sanitary, open-rim bowl that fits on four-caster dolly. (*Hobart Manufacturing Co.*)

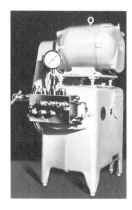

Fig. 28. Homogenizer. A three-cylinder pump with a minute adjustable orifice through which the product is forced under high pressure. (*Cherry-Burrell Corp.*)

Moist grains are heated (with or without added steam) in an enclosed, sanitary pressure chamber where, almost instantly, accumulated pressure is released by opening a large, quick-acting valve (Fig. 26). Resultant expansion of vapor within the grain or dough explodes the product. Process variables such as product moisture content, pressure, and temperature must be carefully regulated.

In one process, partially dehydrated vegetables are puffed by discharge from pressure "guns" to speed final drying.

Powdered citrus juices and other dehydrates are also puffed, in this case during vacuum drying, to increase their solubilities. Candy pieces are puffed by vacuum. Some foods are puffed by gas or vapor generated in processing.

Whipping. Whipping incorporates gas (usually air) into relatively viscous liquids, and is essential in the production of ice cream, mayonnaise, and marshmallow. Agitators employed for whipping are of three general types: (1) beaters that fold gas into the liquid (Fig. 27); (2) shaft-mounted propellers that rapidly draw liquid between the blades; and (3) toothed disks that rotate between toothed stators. The last two units cause churning.

In the manufacture of ice cream, the mix is frozen while a definite volume of air, called the overrun, is incorporated by a specially designed dasher. Mayonnaise is whipped in the rotating-disk unit, generally with nitrogen instead of air to minimize the oxygen-induced rancidity of fats.

Deaeration. Deaeration is the removal of air from foods and beverages either to curb oxygen-induced spoilage or to reduce the volume of a powdery product.

Bulk liquids are deaerated by being subjected to vacuum, usually with application of heat. Packaged carbonated beverages such as beer are deaerated by mechanically striking the container. This causes foaming that eliminates the air in the headspace before closing the container.

Powders are deaerated by vacuum processing; the evacuated air may be replaced by an inert gas, such as nitrogen. This practice greatly extends the keeping quality of products such as dried whole milk, soluble coffee, and powdered fruit juices. Oxygen-sensitive fluid products, such as juice concentrate, often are deaerated by purging the air out with nitrogen by sparging.

Crystallization. Crystallization is the separation of relatively pure solute from a saturated solution as it is evaporated or cooled. Since the precipitated crystals may entrain some of the impurities of the mother liquor, they generally are centrifuged and recrystallized from pure solvent to obtain a pure product.

A major refining step in the processing of sugar, salt, and monosodium glutamate, crystallization is usually carried out in vacuum pans which are large single-effect evaporators. It may occur spontaneously as the solution becomes progressively supersaturated, or can be induced by seeding the boiling solution. Precise control of evaporator temperature, vacuum, and feed rate is essential for maximum yield of proper-sized crystals.

Emulsifying and homogenizing. These are techniques for producing substantially nonseparating mixtures of insoluble materials by mixing and particle-size reduction. Typical emulsions and suspensions thus manufactured include dairy products, mayonnaise, and fruit juices.

Homogenizers exert intense shearing action on the particles of a mixture as they are pumped at high pressure through minute orifices (Fig. 28). A similar effect is achieved with colloid mills, which employ closely spaced high-speed rotors and stators.

Ultrasonics offers another rapid and efficient means of stabilizing food mixtures. Vibrations with frequencies in excess of 18,000 Hz are transmitted to the product. Ultrasonically homogenized peanut butter, for example, is now being produced.

Coatings. Coatings are generally applied to baked goods, ice cream novelties, and confections to enhance the taste and the attractiveness of these products.

Rectangular and round cakes are iced by a machine which deposits the frosting in a sheet. Sweet rolls, buns, and Danish pastry are iced by high-speed continuous units as they are conveyed under print rollers that give the icing a hand-finished appearance.

Confections such as hard candies, nuts, and chewing gum are sugar-coated in heated pans that slowly rotate at an angle of about 60° to the horizontal. Successive portions of supersaturated sugar solution, containing flavoring and color (if required), are added and evaporated from the product surface. This builds up the coating by depositing thin layers of sugar.

Chocolate-coated products, such as ice cream and candies, generally are coated by enrobers. However, hand-dipping is still practiced. In machine operation, products are first bottom-coated as they are conveyed (on a wire belt) over a shallow layer of molten chocolate. For top coating, they pass through curtains of molten chocolate that cover them completely (Fig. 29). The coating is set in a cooling tunnel.   [LEONARD TRAUBERMAN]

FOOD PACKAGING

Food packaging is a total system which assures separation of the contained product from the environment and protection against external chemical, physical, and biological influences. As a system, it provides protection, containment, communication, and unitization while affording sanitation, retention of product quality, and consumer convenience.

Food packaging should be regarded as a total system designed to be a basis for distribution from processing site to consumer. Capacities, opera-

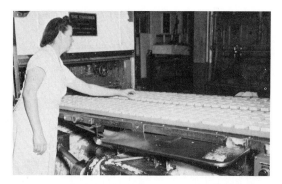

Fig. 29. Enrober. Enrobing unit receives candy bars on a plastic conveyor belt, coats them with tempered chocolate. The chocolate is piped to the machine from the melting kettles. (*National Equipment Co.*)

tional speeds, costs, and functional requirements must be matched within the system and must be integrated with requirements of the product, processing plant, warehouse, transportation, retailer, and consumer.

Food packaging might be categorized by several schemes, such as by materials (metal, glass, paper, plastic, and composites); package form (can, bottle, pouch, bag, wrap, carton, and case); packaging process (canning, bottling, pouching, bagging, overwrapping, collating, filling, closing, labeling, coding, and casing); food product; or packaging level (primary, secondary, tertiary, and quartiary). Each method of classification has its merits and disadvantages, and none is without considerable overlap into other categories.

Among the most prominent external forces that have had a powerful influence on food packaging since the early 1960s have been legislative acts on labeling; regulations on nutritional labeling; enforcement of regulations on indirect additives which might be derived from packaging materials; concern over solid-waste disposal, litter, and environmental insult; the limitations placed on the packaging industry by the energy problem; depletion of natural resources; shortages of capital; fear of permanent damage to life; good manufacturing practices regulations; and the retailers' desire for electronic-machine-readable coding. A discussion of a few of these follows. No one can yet fully assess the beneficial effects of these actions. However, the direct and indirect costs to the consumer have amounted to hundreds of millions of dollars.

Labeling. The "Truth in Labeling" Act instituted in the mid-1960s stipulated that all food packages bear a uniform and accurate representation of the weight, volume, or count of the package contents. The law further provided for more accurate graphic depiction of the nature of the contents. Thus, descriptions of the product upon the package were to be accurate statements of both the quality and quantity of contents. Accompanying the mandate were provisions encouraging food packagers to voluntarily reduce the number and variety of sizes made available to consumers.

Indirect additives. The 1958 Delaney Amendment to the 1938 Food, Drug and Cosmetic Act stated that any chemical additive capable of causing cancer was specifically prohibited from food products. This amendment is the basis for the so-

called zero tolerance rule in that it stipulates any additive in any quantity capable of causing cancer. Chemical additives are defined as any compounds which enter the product intentionally or unintentionally, or are entered directly or indirectly. Since many packaging materials are in intimate contact with the foods contained, components of the materials may be extracted into the food. These components or indirect additives may be compounds having a functional value in food packaging or may be compounds which are present incidentally. The measurable presence of such compounds which have demonstrated carcinogenic activity naturally triggers prohibition in the packaging materials. Analytical techniques have become so sophisticated that compounds may be detected and identified even when they are present in only parts-per-billion quantities.

Manufacturing practices. In the making for some years and certain to be expanded in the future are the Food and Drug Administration Good Manufacturing Practices, which define operations within food plants which are conducive to the safety of packaged foods. These regulations are prepared through joint efforts of industry and government and are designed as common-sense tuidelines to attempt to ensure safety. The concept was initially instituted because a small minority fo food packagers had failed to adhere to technical guidelines which did not have theforce of law and which represented the most effective means of ensuring the safety of the food supply for consumers.

Package disposal. While consumer safety and intersts have been the justification for regulations dealing with additives and Good Manufacturing Practices, concern over the environment and solid waste are matters of much less direct immediate benefit to consumers. Like the safety issues, however, concerns for the effect of packaging on the environment have arisen suddenly with surprising, unexpected secondary ripple effects.

Increasing amounts of waste are generated with increases in population and the standard of living. Highly visible to consumers are the mounting quantities of packaging materials discarded. Since the advent of convenience or nonreturnable bottles and cans for beverages in the early 1960s, consumer acceptance has grwon dramatically; and consequently, the amount of beverage packaging materials being handled by conventional solid-waste disposal systems has also increased. Since the basic solid-waste-handling systems remain assembly at the usage site followed by vehicular pick-up and ultimately dumping into the ground, increases in volume quantity have severely taxed the unimproved systems. Because of the visibility of food, and especially beverage, packaging in the solid-waste stream, environmentalists began campaigns in 1970 to reduce the quantities of nonreturnable packaging. Their special targets included soft-drink and beer cans which together constitute 40% of all cans manufactured and used in the United States, nonreturnable soft-drink and beer bottles, and paperboard milk cartons.

Degradable packaging. The issue of litter has stimulated many studies in the development of biodegradable packaging, that is, packaging that would disintegrate to invisible components as a result of exposure to natural elements. Biodegradable packaging would be counter to the need for stable waste required for sanitary landfill. For effective use of solid-waste dumps, it is necessary that the waste be resistant to the elements so that the recovered land does not collapse due to biodegradation. Further, biodegradability contradicts the concept of the protective value of packaging.

Yet another direction or research has been to find better means of ultimate useful degradation of packaging, as in incineration. Much of the packaging which is functionally effective does not burn well when it is being destroyed or being used to provide thermal energy to, say, generate electrical power. Among the problems encountered are that glass and metal must be separated out as nonburnable, and that some plastics such as PVC might possibly emit quantities of corrosive HCl.

Universal Product Code (UPC). In a long-sought answer to the problem of improving productivity in retail food store operations, a Universal Product Code was created to appear on all food packages. This code, designating the manufacturer, brand, product, and package size, was designed to be read by electronic reading devices, thus eliminating the need for package price marking and for manual checkout procedures in retail stores. These electronic devices scan the code and transmit their reading to a computer memory which records the item and price and totals the purchase automatically.

Packaging materials. A broad spectrum of materials is employed for packaging, depending upon the ultimate package configuration and upon economics. Immediately containing the food product is the primary package, which is no longer a simple material. In a continuing effort to provide the most cost-effective functional package, developments have been directed to combining materials to provide an optimum synergy of the desired attributes of the basic materials. For example, in a glass package, the glass would contribute impermeability, rigidity, inertness in contact with the food, and vertical stacking strength in distribution. In the same glass package, drawn aluminum with a plastic core would provide the closure, paper and adhesive the label, and a thin plastic coating protection to the glass surface to minimize the potential hazard from breakage.

Primary packages might be generally classified as cans, bottles and jars, bags and pouches, wraps and cartons. Secondary packaging is usually composed of paperboard cartons or wraps, but considerable quantities of plastic unitizers are being increasingly employed. Tertiary packaging is usually the corrugated shipping container, but can also be paperboard or plastic wrap. The selection of the best combination depends upon the food product being contained, the marketing objective, the distribution system available, and the degree of protection demanded during the distribution and use cycle.

Metals. By far the largest use of metals in packaging is in making cans to contain carbonated beverages, including beer, and food that is heated within the can to effect preservation through commercial sterilization. The most widely used metal is steel which, in the past, was traditionally coated and later electroplated with tin to protect against corrosion. The tin was further protected on the interior with organic coatings to minimize interaction of food with the steel through microscopic imperfections in the tin.

Since 1965, tin-free steel, or steel coated with very thin coatings of chomium, has largely displaced tin-plated steel for beverage cans, which constitute the largest single application for rigid metal cans. Tin-free steel is also coated to minimize the possibility of corrosion or adverse flavor interactions between product and metal.

Tin-plated cans continue to be used for food products. Tin-plated cans are formed in three pieces, a body and two ends. The body is formed from a flat sheet into an open-ended cylinder which is joined by mechanical locking and soldering. Since 1955, the weight of metal used has been significantly reduced through developments in metallurgy.

Tin-free steel cans are also formed from flat blanks which are turned into cylindrical shapes and joined by either heat-activated adhesive or by welding. The overlap at the seam or joint is smaller in tin-free than in tin-plated cans, and so a smaller quantity of flat plate is employed to fabricate the same size of cans, thus reducing the cost.

Under development are "black-iron" cans, or cans which are formed from steel which has no metallic coating but an integral organic plastic coating. Many such cans have already entered the marketplace with apparently successful results.

Can ends are formed from flat sheet which is fabricated into discs. Around the rim of the disc is inserted a plastic material which effects the final closure when the end is mechanically clinched to the cylindrical body. The can maker forms the cylinder and end, and attaches one end, called the can-maker's end, to the body. More and more, large-size food packagers are fabricating their own cans in-plant and, through a surge storage, sending the open-ended cans to the packaging line. In the packaging operation, the product is filled into the can-end material to take advantage of its relative which is also mechanically clinched into position using a highly sophisticated and reliable high-speed double-seaming operation.

In the mid-1960s, aluminum entered the scene as a can-making material, initially solely as a can-end material to take advantage of its relative ease of scoring and tearing. Integral-rivet half-depth scored ends with tabs and loops became rapidly accepted as convenience or easy-opening ends for beverage cans. Such ends were virtually interchangeable with previously more conventional tin-plated or tin-free steel.

Taking greater advantage of the formability of aluminum, the metal was drawn into the shape of a cup or can body to create the two-piece aluminum can. With two fewer seams than a steel can, there was significantly less probability of a leaker, especially from pressurized contents. With no long seam, the can could be printed fully in the round, thus eliminating an unsightly unprinted area. Further, aluminum cans are lighter weight than steel. The advantages of aluminum coupled with a price equivalent to that of steel has led to a significant employment of aluminum for beer and carbonated beverages. Due to the relatively thin walls and the possibility of paneling or wall collapse due to the difference of pressure from the atmosphere to the can interior, relatively few two-piece aluminum cans are used for other foods.

Drawing techniques are being employed for tin-plated steel to produce two-piece steel cans having the advantages of aluminum plus, in theory, better economics. Taking the process a step further, "black-iron" or steel with no further metallic coating is also being drawn into two-piece cans used for beer and carbonated veberages. Organic coatings wholly replace the metallic coatings.

As a result of vigorous competitive activity, the once prosaic and relatively simple three-piece tin can is now but one type in a broad spectrum of cans available and commercially used for food and beverage packaging.

In foil form, aluminum is used to make semirigid containers for specialty foods, frozen precooked foods, and bakery products; as wraps for candies and cheese; and as overwraps for cartons and frozen-food trays.

Aluminum foil in combination with paper and plastic films and heat-seal coatings is employed as carton overwraps, direct wraps, shipping case liners, labels, bags, pouches, brown-and-serve trays, ice cream containers, carton liners, and canister liners. Thickness ranges from 0.00025 to 0.006 in.

Glass. Glass is suitable for foods because it can be molded into various shapes and is inert and transparent. Despite its advantages, glass has not grown as rapidly as have the plastic bottles which have replaced it.

Glass is molded into containers of innumerable shapes and sizes, large or small, tall or squat, and narrow- or wide-mouthed, and used for liquids, solids, and semisolids. Because glass is inert, it does not add anything to or take anything from a product, and due to its transparency, it displays foods in their natural color and shape. Further, it is impermeable and has high vertical stacking strength. With integral plastic film coatings made from PVC or ionomer, brittleness is somewhat reduced; moreover, the plastic film will contain any fragments arising from breakage. The foamed polystyrene wraps so visible on many glass containers have very little physical advantage, but improve the label appearance markedly.

Modern machines turn out glass containers much faster than old-time blowers, and also make them lighter, stronger, more suitable, and more uniform in color. Improvements in closures and production methods have also increased their popularity. Probably the most significant improvement in glass since the mid-1960s has been the reduction in weight to contain equal volumes. This benefit has arisen from coatings placed on the glass as it is formed and later as it is annealed, which increase the surface strength.

To data, line speeds run 350 containers per minute and up. Baby-food jars are being run at more than 500–1000 per minute. Beer and carbonated beverage lines run at speeds in excess of 800 packages per minute, with one experimental line now rated in excess of 1500 packages per minute.

At one time, cork was almost the only closure used for bottles. Numerous types of gaskets, suitable for a variety of products, have been developed by closure manufacturers. With proper gaskets and high-speed machine application, lug and screw caps are suitable for almost all products.

Closures for glass containers are mostly made of metal or plastic, though paper is used in the dairy industry for glass and paper containers to hold liquids. Aluminum roll-on-closures have largely displaced crown closures for beverages.

Major closure types include crown, vacuum, rolled-on, screw cap, lug cap, tamper-proof, snap-fit, and press-on, the newest being press-on twist-off.

Since 1958, many kinds of easy-to-open closures have been adapted, not only for glass but for other types of containers.

Paper. This basic packaging material is modified or combined with other materials to offer many product protection features. Among other properties, paper is designed and coated or constructed to be impervious to gas, grease, water, or moisture vapor; to resist insect penetration, corrosion, and mold growth; and to withstand impact, tear, puncture, water penetration, and embrittlement. It is also fabricated to be nontoxic, odorless, and tasteless.

Protective papers include plain kraft (from sulfate pulp); laminated (asphaltic) kraft (used largely for industrial applications); coated (heat-sealable polyethylene) kraft; waxed paper (thin-calendered wax-coated paper); wet-strength (added resin) paper; vegetable parchment (acid-treated cellulose); greaseproof paper (dense, uncalendered paper from hydrated pulp); and glassine (dense, supercalendered paper from highly refined special pulp).

Paper's principal attribute is as a strong and reliable substrate for materials that impart other properties such as gas or water vapor impermeability. Although paper is printable and can be made greaseproof, its major virtues are strength, ease of formation, and economy.

Glassines may be plain, lacquered (coated with heat-sealable resinous materials), wax-coated, or laminated (several plies of glassine with wax laminant). Glassines are among the few papers used as direct packaging materials without further coating or converting, particularly for confectionery. Coated glassines are used for snack food packaging.

Paperboard is paper with a gage above 0.010 in. and is employed to make cartons and other types of semirigid packaging. Paperboard containers comprise liquid-tight containers, composite paper cans, set-up boxes, and folding cartons.

Lightweight, liquid-tight containers are essentially used for dairy products, frozen foods, and delicatessen items. They are of either the nested type, made of virgin sulfate or sulfite stock and treated with wax or plastic or untreated; or of canister shape (conical, cylindrical, or rectangular), of manila stock, plain or lined with sulfite or sulfate. For specific uses, canisters may be lined with glassine, cellophane, plastic, or parchment, and they may be treated with wax or plastic formulas or untreated. Most liquid-tight paperboard cartons are, however, formed from polyethylene-coated semibleached sulfate in a flat scored and die-cut blank. The blanks are erected on the same machine on which the carton is filled and sealed closed. In the United States, most such cartons have a gable-shaped top. In other parts of the world, roll-stock paperboard is used, and a block or brick shape is formed.

The composite paper or fiber can is a rigid, multi-ply paper body with metal or paper ends. The all-paper type is cylindrical, while the composite type, made of a paper body with metal ends, may be round, square, oval, oblong, or rectangular. The body wall is generally fabricated from chip, box, or sulfate boards, while combinations of these and kraft, jute, foil, glassine, aluminum foil, and others may also be employed. A wide range of adhesives is used for multi-ply-constructed bodies that are usually wax- or plastic-coated on the inside. Easy-opening aluminum, tin plate, or lacquered blackplate are used in the metal ends, which are affixed by double seaming.

Set-up boxes are of a rigid type, made from paperboard and delivered ready for use. Generally, they consist of top and bottom but they vary widely in type and shape. They are used for confections, baked goods, and certain prestige items to create impulse buying and protect products in storage and distribution. Because of the space volume occupied, set-up boxes have been declining in importance for food packaging.

There is an almost endless variety of folding-carton structural styles formed from flat blanks. However, carton constructions are classified as tray or tube type. The tray type is an unbroken paperboard bottom panel, with each side and end wall panel connected to its adjacent wall by a glued flap, a hook-engaging slit in the wall, or some other connection. These may be of two-piece construction—base and cover with or without transparent window. The tube type contains a seam or flap glued by the carton maker. Styles include the seal-end carton with one end closed, the tuck-end construction with one end closed, a combination tuck-end and lock-end closure, and a lock-bottom construction.

Plastics. Plastics are made from synthetic organic resins or polymers or natural polymers. Nearly all used for food packaging are thermoplastic and so are sealable by heat and pressure. They can be modified for certain applications. They possess many types of protective properties, in addition to being attractive and highly durable. Basically, they include the following types:

Polyethylene is characterized by extreme toughness and rubberiness. Polyethylenes are generally divided by resin density imparted by chemical formation. Low-density polyethylene is highly branched and is usually used for films and coatings; high-density is molded into semirigid bottles. It is formed from resin into film by extruding into a sheet form. Polyethylene has found increasing applications because of its excellent physical and protective qualities and relatively low cost: polyethylene is by far the most widely used plastic packaging material.

Polyethylene extrusion is used for coating paper, paperboard, and various other films and is used as one of the plies in a range of laminated combinations (for example, extrusion-coating it directly onto cellophane). Polyethylene imparts moisture resistance, tear strength, and heat sealability.

Pliofilm, one of the earliest packaging plastics, is a rubber-hydrochloride, heat-sealable film that is available in several basic types and grades. Various types are modified with stabilizers and plasticizers to produce films that excel as a barrier to gas and water vapor, are tough and flexible, and serve for heavy-duty special purposes. Relatively little rubber hydrochloride is now used for packaging.

Vinyls are resins of vinyl chloride or blends of vinyl chloride, vinyl acetate, and other resins. These materials, blends of polyvinyl chloride, and other materials have been the center of considerable controversy due to the potentially hazardous nature of the components. Thus, while clear, tough films may be cast, or good impermeable sheet may be formed by calendering, or clear, impermeable bottles may be blow-molded, relatively little is used for food packaging. The largest application today is for wrapping fresh meat in retail stores, where appearance, toughness, and ability to transmit oxygen are key factors.

Saran is a polyvinylidene chloride (PVDC) film with such outstanding properties as water and gas impermeability, strength, cling, and high temperature resistance. It has some significant limitations, however, since problems are encountered in heat sealing and machine handling. Nevertheless, Saran is the most widely used plastic material to impart barrier properties to plastic and near-plastic materials.

Polyester is an exceptionally tough film made from a polymer of ethylene glycol and terephthalic acid. The film is finding use as a transparent window material for cartons, bags, and wraps. Its initial success was as a laminant for cook-and-serve packages. Its most common use is as a thermoformable component for processed meat packaging.

The polyolefin, polypropylene, is being used in increasing quantities in plastic film making. Polypropylene, which may be formed by casting or extrusion, usually followed by stretching to orient the material and thus improve its properties, is clearer than polyethylene, and has similar water-vapor-barrier characteristics. Its gas-barrier properties are, however, significantly better than virtually any commercial plastic film except PVDC. Polypropylene was, at one time, regarded as the coming replacement for cellophane, but it does not have the same machineability characteristics as cellophane and so has not yet achieved its predicted potential. Nevertheless, polypropylene is widely used as a laminating plastic and unsupported as an overwrap material for candy and such.

Polystyrene is a polymeric plastic whose principal attribute in film form is clarity and sparkle. Because it is gas-permeable, polystyrene is used to wrap fresh produce which must have access to atmospheric oxygen and egress for carbon dioxide produced during respiratory processes. In heavier gages, however, polystyrene is an inexpensive, easily formed material which has widespread use as a container for refrigerated dairy products such as yogurt and cottage cheese.

Ionomer resins, such as Surlyn A, were commercially introduced in the early 1970s and have made giant strides toward use as packaging films and coatings. These thermoplastic materials, closely related to polyethylene, are extremely versatile. They have properties of both cross-linked and non-cross-linked hydrocarbon polyolefinic polymers. Solid-state properties stem from the cross-linked, and melt-flow from the non-cross-linked. Through molecular manipulating, a unique combination of properties can be tailored for food packagers.

Moreover, cross-linking is thermally reversible to provide really thermoplastic resins.

As for ionomer applications, converters have been test-mating ionomer films with polyethylene, cellophane, and so forth. The broad heat-seal range of ionomers is used in combination with oriented polypropylene films for packaging cheese, coffee, and other products. Ionomer films are utilized in skin packaging, where resistance to puncturing is desirable.

Ionomer coatings offer improved grease and abrasion resistance. They can be applied to foil, plastic, and paperboard. They have found use in the packaging of granular dried-food items such as coffee. Use of ionomers as an adhesive and heat-seal coating improves the durability of paper-foil pouches and thermoformed plastic packaging. Other uses include vacuum packaging, where deep-draw properties are required; ionomer sheet-formed containers, as for frankfurter, sliced luncheon meat, cheese, margarine, and peanut butter packs; blow-molded, clear, tough plastic bottles; and tough, transparent closures.

Cellulosic films. Although the first of the so-called plastic packaging materials were derived from cellulosic materials, these are not truly plastics. Thus, somewhere between paper and true hydrocarbon plastics are the cellulosic films, of which cellophane is the most important both from a commercial and a historical standpoint.

Cellophane is a transparent, versatile film composed of a plasticized base sheet of regenerated cellulose, which is essentially greaseproof, and can be made moisture- and vapor-proof through coatings, primarily PVDC and nitrocellulose. Its functional properties are utilized in such applications as direct wraps, overwraps, bags, pouches, window cartons, and laminations.

Cellophane is available in many different grades and types, with a type for almost every conceivable application. Basically, it comes in four forms: uncoated, intermediate moisture-proof, moisture-proof, and water-resistant. Thickness ranges from 0.0008 to 0.0017 in.

Cellulose acetate, which differs from cellophane in that the acetate base is water-insensitive and soluble in certain solvents, is used for packaging fruits and vegetables because of insensitivity to water softening and high rate of gas and water vapor transmission, for window material in cartons, and for rigid transparent containers.

Laminated materials. Two or more plies of similar or dissimilar film gage materials are made into a single sheet. An endless variety of laminated materials are tailor-made to meet requirements of specific packaging problems. Selection of materials influences properties desired, as uniting decorative appeal of aluminum foil with the mechanical strength and greaseproof quality of glassine to produce an excellent candy wrapper.

It has become possible to extrude two or more plastic materials into a single integral sheet, deriving the desirable characteristics of each in the optimum quantity. These coextrusions are now widely used for snack food and confectionery packaging. Once believed to be a major means for marrying a multiplicity of properties, the application of coextrusion has been limited by difficulties in bonding even similar plastic materials.

Lamination or actual adhesive bonding of plastic to paper, foil, or plastic remains the principal means of combining two or more flexible materials to obtain a final material having a suitable combination of properties.

Semirigid plastic containers. With the development of the polyethylene squeeze bottle in the late 1940s, plastic resins became a very important part of the semirigid package market, intruding in a major way into the formerly exclusive province of glass.

Polystyrene and high-density polyethylene vie for market leadership in this category, with both more heavily employed for nonfoods than for foods due to their relatively poor gas permeability properties. Polystyrene has excellent clarity and, with rubber modifiers, good impact strength. Polyethylene has better permeability properties and strength.

Most semirigid plastic packages are made by taking advantage of their thermoplastic properties. The resin is melted and then forced into a mold, where it is chilled and thus set into the desired shape.

For bottle manufacture, a tube or parison is extruded and then air-blown in a mold into a bottle shape. The liquid resin or melt may be directly injected into a mold, which would lead to an injection-molded bottle. Injection molding is more expensive than blow molding due to the higher costs of molds and the greater quantities of materials employed. Both injection and blow molding may be combined to produce injection-blow-molded bottles.

The thermoplastic resin may be extruded into a sheet which may then be reheated and pressure- or vacuum-formed into a cup shape.

These techniques have been applied not only to basic polystyrene and polyethylene materials, but also to other plastic materials such as polypropylene, which has excellent contact clarity. Polyvinyl chloride (PVC) has been limited in the United States by its implied toxicity problems and so has limited use despite the best combination of properties of the major commercial plastics. In Europe and elsewhere, PVC is widely used for semirigid packaging of water and of edible oil.

Among the newer plastics for food containers is acrylonitrile butadiene styrene (ABS). It incorporates toughness, chemical resistance, high-gloss appearance, and low-temperature impact strength into an opaque rigid container. It can be electroplated and embossed.

ABS is a terpolymer—a combination of three monomers. Because of this, molecular weight and branching, as well as other aspects of the terpolymer, can be readily altered to give desired properties. For example, the acrylonitrile monomer imparts chemical resistance. Butadiene gives it flexibility, impact strength, and low-temperature resistance. Styrene makes it free from odors and adds tensile strength.

When used to package soft margarines, ABS containers offer high-gloss appearance, high grease resistance, rigidity, printability, and good release properties. ABS containers cannot be hot-filled because they heat-distort at temperatures of 180–250°F (81–121°C).

Adaption of a conventional metal-drawing machine for cold-forming ABS sheet into plastic containers has promised new packaging innovations. Without heating, the plastic in 0.015-in. gage may be cold-stamped into rectangular containers without noticeable thinning at the corners. A single metalworking-type die could produce up to 50 containers per minute. Successive stampings produce draws of several inches.

Probably the most discussed plastic materials of the 1970s have been those used for soft-drink bottles. Acrylonitriles have long been employed for fiber production, and their high gas impermeability has been well known. In the near-pure form, however, acrylonitriles are very brittle and virtually unmanageable. When combined or copolymerized with acrylics or polystyrene, however, the resulting resin has excellent gas-barrier properties and fairly good strength. The strength may be later improved by orientation during formation or by adding modifiers such as rubber compounds to the formulation. Bottles injection-blow-molded from acrylonitrile copolymers have excellent oxygen- and CO_2-barrier properties and so are suitable for carbonated beverage packaging. Consequently, they are being evaluated commercially for these applications. Similarly, bottles formed from polyester are in the commercial marketplace.

Neither allows the shelf life permitted by glass, but both plastics have sufficient properties for commercial distribution.

Packaging methods. The selection of machinery and packaging lines is influenced by the type of product and package handled. Packages are fed to the line for product filling, sealing, labeling or overwrapping, coding, and packing into shipping cases that are sealed.

It is very important to differentiate among primary, secondary, and tertiary packaging since primary packaging involves bringing together product and package, while tertiary consists of unitizing a number of primary or secondary packages. In general, primary packaging is conducted at high speed and, as the level pf packaging changes, the speed decreases. Due to the speed and the difference between food product and packaging material, primary packaging is generally more complex than secondary or tertiary.

Primary packaging may be performed starting with fully preformed packages requiring only filling and closing, or may begin with packaging materials that are formed in-line with the filling and closing operations. In the extreme, dry granular plastic resin may be inputted to blow-mold a bottle which is filled and closed in the mold, a European method for forming polyethylene milk bottles. Between the extremes of starting with preforms or with packaging raw materials is a full spectrum of combinations of the two.

The important concept of packaging equipment is that it be integrated into a total system, that is, it be matched in speed and capacity with both the food product and the packaging material entering, and the capabilities of the downstream secondary and tertiary packaging equipment.

Primary equipment. Preformed package lines consist of package infeeds, fillers, closers, and unitizers. The infeed section of the equipment is designed to align and clean the preformed packages and thus ready them for subsequent packaging operations.

Cans and glass containers may be automatically unloaded from shippers or from bulk truck or rail cars and dumped in helter-skelter fashion onto an unscrambler for single-file delivery onto the line, right side up, for filling. Palletized shipments are now matched to infeeds so that tiers may be neatly, quickly, and accurately removed from pallets and aligned into the infeed section of packaging lines. Obviously, pallet unloaders are most suitable for high-volume operation.

Unloaders for smaller-volume operations handle many cartons of empty packages per minute. One type conveys cartons upside down as containers drop onto the unscrambler after carton flaps are opened. Another employs vacuum cups to engage the bottoms of bottles (packed upside down), lift them from cartons, and invert them for feeding to the unscrambler. Still another uses mechanical fingers to grip and unload narrow-neck bottles, and still another unloads metal cans by electromagnetic pick-up.

Unscramblers are required even after removal from bulk pallet unload systems. Unscramblers of the rotary and straight-line types employ disks, belts, gates, and reverse-flow principles. A noiseless, gentle-handling, walking-beam type unscrambles 500 containers per minute.

Accumulators serve as a temporary surge or storage area for the steady flow of containers to the packaging line in the event of shutdowns or variations in line-machine speeds. One type employs a revolving disk, another a trough or conveyor-belt-fed table area.

Cleaners are used for all types of lines to remove foreign matter and debris. Air cleaning may be used for cans. Simple inverting is sometimes adequate, although water cleaning is more desirable. Bottle cleaners for new bottles are of water-rinsing and air-cleaning types. One automatic rinser feeds bottles into carrier-mounted pockets, alternately subjecting them to air jets, water-conditioning spray, prerinse, draining, and right-side-up transfer onto conveyor. An air cleaner receives bottles from the conveyor and injects air while the starwheel discharges them onto the conveyor.

Equipment for handling preformed plastic bottles or cups is not unlike that for glass or cans. Paperboard cartons, on the other hand, are generally received as precut flat or glued blanks which must be formed or set up. Equipment ranges from that which applies adhesive to flat blanks, brings together corners or edges and forms an open-top or open-ended container, to that which snaps open a preassembled paperboard carton which has been flattened for simplified storage and shipment.

Moving up the levels of complexity, paperboard cartons may be set up with internal flexible packaging material liners, as in dry cereal cartons. The paperboard imparts rigidity, while the flexible liner provides the moisture barrier impossible with paperboard due to as yet unsolved problems with passage of gases through adhered edges and flaps. The equipment may form a pouch which is inserted into the carton shell, or may literally form the liner and carton shell simultaneously around the same mandrel, discharging the interconnected combination to the subsequent filling station.

Flexible pouches may be formed in a converter's plant and received in stacked form; but more commonly, pouches are formed in-line with filling from flat roll stock. Two basic types of form-fill equipment are employed, vertical and horizontal. In the vertical type, the roll stock is unwound and turned over a tube where a long seam is heat-sealed together. While in the vertical attitude, a cross heat seal is made at the base, the product filled, and a cross heat seal made at the top. These machines operate at up to 30–40 cycles per minute, with the speed limited by the velocity with which the product may flow vertically past the cross seal. Vertical form-fill-seal machines are widely employed for snack foods, crackers, coffee, and fluid condiment foods.

Horizontal form-fill-seal equipment also begins with roll-stock flexible packaging material but unwinds in a horizontal attitude to form a three-side seal pouch with an upward-facing opening. The open-top pouch may then be filled by conventional means and heat-seal-closed by applying heat and pressure after filling. Speeds of several hundred packages per minute may be achieved by modularizing the operation—that is, performing several functions in multiples. Output of vertical form-fill-seal equipment is increased by adding machines.

Both systems represent efficient means of providing economical flexible packaging. Vertical systems are used for plastic and paper/plastic packaging while horizontal systems are employed when aluminum foil is required since horizontal systems treat the materials very gently and do not damage their integrity. Thus, horizontal systems are used to package dehydrated soups, drink mixes, and condiment and sauce mixes, all of which require the moisture-barrier protection of aluminum foil.

Many variations on these basic systems exist for special applications. For example, by using two-roll infeed, the effect of horizontally formed flat pouches may be achieved in a multiple-lane vertical attitude. In yet another variant, the product may be power-fed into a tube formed horizontally, with the actual formation and closure of the material accomplished in the same manner as on vertical equipment but turned 90°.

As may be inferred, a very broad range of equipment has been designed to handle the many different product-package requirements in existence today.

As a general rule, the highest speed–output combinations are achievable by starting with preformed containers, since a unit operation has been removed from the system. On the other hand, a few very-high-speed outputs of up to 1000 per minute may be achieved with horizontal pouching in portion control sizes, as for granulated sugar.

Filling components must be designed and built for specific categories of food products—that is, there are no universal fillers. Fillers are designed for dry, liquid, and viscous products. Dry fillers may have speeds of up to 350 packages per minute, while liquid fillers may fill at up to 2000 packages per minute.

Basic types of filling machines include (1) net weighers to scale the product and fill the weighed charge into the package (Fig. 30), (2) gross weighers to scale the product and package (both of the above now use electronic sensing and analog feedback for control); (3) volumetric fillers to measure out the product with a rotating plate containing calibrated pockets; (4) metering fillers to establish

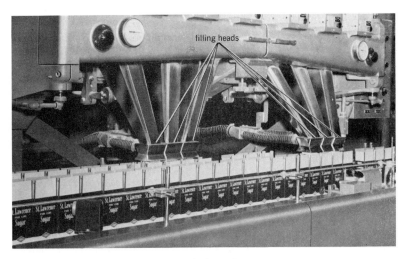

Fig. 30. Six-head carton filler. (*Pneumatic Scale Corp.*)

a standard rate of product flow for filling into containers at specific time intervals; and (5) auger-type feeders to deliver the measured amount of product.

Filling speeds may be increased by increasing the speed of an individual filler, a procedure which, of course, has a finite upper limit, or by using multiple fillers. With the latter technique, the multiple units may function in parallel or in sequence. In sequential operation, each event in the filling occurs at a different time on a different filler, while the package remains on a single filler head during the entire sequence. Thus, liquid fillers may have up to one hundred heads in order to achieve package outputs of up to 2000 cans per minute. Naturally, filler speeds of this order of magnitude must be matched to empty-can input speed, product flow, and capabilities of downstream secondary and tertiary packaging components of the system.

Liquid filler operations are speeded through improvements in machine design such as wider nozzle openings, positive displacement, positive nozzle shut-off between events, and by smooth and efficient handling of the metal and glass containers being filled and closed. Examples of production rates per minute are 1050 soft-drink bottles (12 oz), 700 bottles of ketchup (14 oz), 800 cans of juice (6 oz), and more than 900 jars of baby food.

Liquid fillers for containers with cavity openings below 38 mm cover those operating on the principles of (1) gravity filling, liquid flowing by gravity from an overhead surge tank through filling valves and cutting off at a predetermined level in the container; (2) gravity vacuum, gravity filling in a closed-vacuum system; (3) pressure gravity, using a booster pump to produce pressures of 10–20 psi to increase the speed of gravity filling of heavy viscous liquids; (4) vacuum, evacuating air from the container to force liquid into it from a reservoir below; (5) pressure-vacuum, employing modification of standard vacuum filler with pressure feeder; and (6) volumetric, utilizing a filler tank with an accurately controlled liquid level and measuring cups to deposit a premeasured amount into the container (see Fig. 31).

Fillers for viscous products in general use are of two basic types, straight-line and rotary plunger. The difference is that straight-line fillers operate

FOOD ENGINEERING

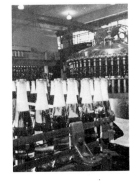

Fig. 31. Beer filling line. (*Miller Brewing Co.*)

intermittently on a given number of containers, while rotary plunger fillers fill and discharge containers continuously. Both employ cylinders and pistons for accurately measuring and forcing the product into containers. Positively controlled inlet and outlet valves are necessary components to assure that the pistons draw in the required quantity of product, and discharge fully, cleanly, and precisely into the package. Such fillers are used for products such as cottage cheese, juice concentrate, and meat paste.

Manual and mechanically assisted manual fill is still widely employed for products that are not readily handled by other means (whole hams, fresh meat cuts, broccoli spears, fish fillets, and so on).

Closing equipment employed is influenced by the type of package being handled. Bags or pouches formed from or having in their constructions thermoplastic material are generally sealed by application of heat and pressure. Heat sealers include roller, band, jaw, high-frequency, or impulse types for sealing unsupported films, coated materials, laminations, and combinations of coated and laminated materials. Cartons are conveyed from the filling machine past the glue applicator, flap closer, and compression belt. Cans are sealed by rotary seamers that apply and mechanically crimp the top lid to the can body.

For sealing glass bottles and cans, rotary or straight-line automatic capping machines are employed to handle lug-type caps, side-seal closures, and continuous-thread caps.

In recent years, a large number of cans and increasingly large numbers of glass packages have been predecorated or labeled during converting operations. Nevertheless, most packages are still designed to accept labels after closing. Labels made from paper or paper compositions are applied by machine to cans, package overwraps, jars, or bottles, either from roll-fed stock or from stacks. Cans are usually horizontally fed through a wrap-around labeler, where a moving belt carries them past the glue applicator and under the horizontal label stack. Pressure-sensitive labels are applied either mechanically or by air-feeding from roll-fed stock onto wrapped packages.

The widest diversity of machine types and applications exists in the labeling of bottles and glass jars. Machines range from simple table-model hand-operated gummers to fully automatic units capable of bringing together, in an assembly operation, the container and various combinations of labels numbering as many as four to a container. Plain labels are glue-applied, and thermoplastic labels are heat-applied to the containers. They are applied to the front or simultaneously to the front and back body of the containers, as well as to the neck and body of bottles. Speeds run up to 800 glass packages per minute, and the new rotary machines literally wipe the label onto the curved surface of the bottle. Labels may also be applied by decal or screening, both procedures which are common for plastic bottles which are molded with extensive flat faces for label acceptance.

After primary packaging, some packages are wrapped to add further protection. The use of wrapping for protection is decreasing as more barrier properties are built into the primary package.

On the other hand, wrapping in preprinted flexible materials is still common for large products such as cakes or fresh meats or cheeses.

Wrapping machines perform their operations in many ways. In one machine, the package is lifted by a reciprocating elevator through the time sequence of positioning and wrapping. Lengthwise wrapper overlap is sealed against the bottom of the package, with end folds turned under the package and sealed against the bottom or folded and sealed against the end panels.

Other wrappers achieve similar results without an elevator through the use of intermittently rotating pockets, where several folding operations are performed. In others, the package is carried through all operations in a horizontal plane and past an L-shaped folding line that wraps, folds, and seals two ends and one edge of the package.

Typical speeds are 180 cartons of frozen food and 1200 chewing gum sticks per minute.

Semirigid plastic materials may be thermoformed in-line for packaging processed meats, cheeses, jams, jellies, and dairy products. Plastic sheet is unreeled, heated, formed into a shallow cavity, filled, and then closed using heat-sealing methods. For processed meats and cheeses, further preservative properties are imparted by depleting the oxygen through vacuum or vacuum-plus-gas-flush operations between filling and final sealing.

Packages and shipping containers should be and now are largely mandated to carry markings indicating the code date, batch number, lot number, and other identification legends. Markings are machine-applied to packages by inking, notching, perforating, indenting, or embossing. Imprinting attachments are employed for wrapping, bag-making, and bundling machines which handle material in roll form.

Coding, marking, and imprinting machines are available as attachments for other packaging or conveying equipment; there are also in-line units that fit along with machines for filling, capping, sealing, cartoning, and casing, as well as independent units.

Imprinting has advanced from the use of raised type to newer noncontact electrostatic methods which are higher-speed than mechanically actuated systems.

Secondary equipment. Secondary and subsequent downstream equipment is designed to accumulate and unitize primary packages in order to assure that they are further protected and may be handled as a single unit and thus more efficiently and economically. In a few instances, secondary or multiple packaging is an inherent integral part of the primary packaging operation. In most equipment, however, the secondary packaging is an integrated module downstream from the primary packaging.

In one of the few instances of a wholly integrated primary-secondary multiple packaging machine, for dry-soup or dry-drink pouching, the product is packaged and unitized on a complete, automatic packaging line. The system starts with roll-fed, sealable flexible material which is formed into pouches, filled with products, and sealed. The machines print and code pouch material or insert one, two, or three pouches into preglued paperboard cartons. Some seal pouches with vacuum or inert gas. Speeds are up to 500 or more multiple packages per hour.

In the more common downstream packaging operations, however, the system is designed with modular unit operations and intermodular surge areas to ensure total system performance.

In bundling operations, packages are conveyed from canning, bottling, wrapping, or carton filling-sealing machines to the bundler, which assembles them into units of predetermined count and pattern. The patterned bundle is then machine-wrapped in paper, film, paperboard, or corrugated board. The bundler, using glue, heat, or mechanical locking, may apply separate end seals from roll or magazine for identification or appearance, may imprint wrappers with a mounted imprinter, and may apply easy-opening devices.

Casing and bundling machines are used to accumulate cans, cartons, and glass containers or multipacks of cans, glass, or cartons automatically for semiautomatic or automatic leading into corrugated shipping cartons which are then glue-, tape-, or staple-sealed.

The most common method is glue, which is both the cheapest and strongest.

Case loaders include (1) gravity roll-in types, in which cans are tiered (by rolling) to a proper pattern as the operator places the shipping container on a loading horn, releasing a plunger to insert the cans into a container; (2) offset-conveyor-feed type, in which cartons are elevated and grouped by an offset infeed conveyor; the container is manually placed on a loading horn and loaded with accumulated cartons; (3) elevator-feed type, in which cartons are fed into the case loader via the single- or multiple-lane infeed belt and mechanically elevated until a prescribed pattern is formed; and (4) case feeder, former, positioner, loader, and sealer machine that collects cartons from 10 wrappers and accumulates, groups, and finally loads 30 cartons into an end-loading, preformed shipping container.

Corrugated cases are now being increasingly made by wrapping a flat blank around the accumulated unitized primary packaged product. Wraparound casing provides a tighter and hence more stable pack, and is less expensive than inserting into preglued knocked-down cases.

Another means of improving packaging value effectiveness is inserting the primary package into a corrugated tray which is later further bound tightly with a plastic shrink film.

During the early 1970s, notable gains were made with wrapping individual and collated packages with a skin of drum-tight shrinkable film.

Shrink-wrapped corrugated-tray shippers are especially suited for mass retail displays. They help to assure in-stock condition and significantly reduce retail handling as well as tertiary packaging material costs.

The first of the widely used tray-overwrapping shrink films was 1.5-mil, oriented cast polyvinyl chloride (PVC). Newer and less costly is a 1.5 mil, one-way (mono-oriented) PVC that heat-shrinks only around the girth of a tray.

The most common shrink film used today, however, is low-density polyethylene, which is inexpensive, tough, and very machinable. Even though it lacks clarity, this attribute is not necessary for distribution packaging.

The shrink-wrapping concept has carried over from tray-packed canned goods to similarly packed glass and paperboard-carton-filled foods. Even individually packed products are now shrink-wrapped. A case in point is the shrink wrapping of difficult-to-package baked goods in both round and rectangular foil pans and paperboard trays.

Equipment for shrink packaging is usually intermittent motion, permitting speeds of up to 25 packs (of up to 24 primary packages) per minute. In western Europe where the concept is widespread, however, continuous-motion equipment functioning at 40 to 60 packs per minute is in commercial use, and prototype equipment capable of up to 100 packs per minute has been demonstrated.   [AARON L. BRODY]

Nutrition labeling. This is a standardized way to tell the consumer through labeling the chief nutritional characteristics of foods. The nutritional properties stated are based on a serving of the food. The size of the serving in common household units is stated on the label and also, for packaged foods, the number of servings in the package. The label then states the number of calories and the number of grams each of protein, carbohydrate, and fat in the serving of food. If so desired, the purveyor may further qualify the declaration of fat by saying how much of it is saturated and how much is polyunsaturated (only for significant sources of fat). The amount of cholesterol present may also be stated if the food is a significant source.

The next section of the label sets forth the content of protein (restated in different units) and micronutrients per serving. Each nutritionally labeled product must declare the amount of vitamins A and C, thiamine, riboflavin, niacin, calcium, and iron. Optionally, it may also declare vitamins D, E, B_6, and B_{12}, folic acid, phosphorus, iodine, magnesium, zinc, copper, biotin, or pantothenic acid.

In this section, the nutrient levels are declared as percentages of the United States Recommended Daily Allowances (RDA). These United States RDAs are based on but not quite identical to the Recommended Daily Dietary Allowances of the Food and Nutrition Board of the National Research Council (NRC). The RDA values are chosen on the generous side of the NRC values to be safe, because the label values constitute a much reduced and simplified set. In order to be practical for labeling, the large number of base values supplied by the NRC table could not be used. Accordingly, the United States RDA used for labeling supplies only four sets of values: one for infants, one for children under 4 years of age, one for pregnant and lactating women, and one for adults and children over the age of four. Except for foods for special dietary use, it is seldom necessary, therefore, to use more than two columns to state micronutrient content, and most foods manage with one.

Protein is restated in this section as a percentage of the United States RDA in order to give some cognizance to the varying biological value of proteins, based on their amino acid balance. This is done by setting the United States RDA for protein for adults at 45 g if the protein efficiency ratio (PER) of the protein is equal to or greater than that of casein, and at 65 g if it is less. If the PER is less than 20% of that of casein, the protein may not be listed in this section.   [VIRGIL O. WODICKA]

Bibliography: American Meat Institute Committee on Textbooks, *By-products of the Meat Packing Industry*, rev. ed., 1950; J. A. Azoub, Continuous microwave sterilization of meat in flexible pouches, *J. Food Sci.*, 39:309–313, 1974; A. E. Bailey, *Industrial Oil and Fat Products*, 2d ed., 1951; C. O. Ball and F. C. W. Olson, *Sterilization in Food Technology*, 1957; A. L. Brody, *Flexible Packaging of Foods*, 1970; A. L. Brody (ed.), *The Last Frontier for Cost Reduction: Physical Distribution Packaging*, 1975; C. Butler, J. W. Slavin, and F. B. Sanford (eds.), *Refrigeration of Fish*, pts. 1–5, U.S. Fish and Wildlife Service, Fishery Leaflet numbers 427–431, 1956; S. E. Charm, *Fundamentals of Food Engineering*, 1963; W. V. Cruess, *Commercial Fruit and Vegetable Products*, 4th ed., 1958; A. W. Garrall, *Engineering for Dairy and Food Products*, 1963; A. Griff, *The Plastic Can*, 1974; R. C. Griffin and S. Sacharow, *Principles of Package Development*, 1972; J. F. Hanlon, *Handbook of Package Engineering*, 1971; F. L. Hart and H. J. Fisher, *Modern Food Analysis*, 1970; K. Hayakawa, Estimating temperature of foods during various heating or cooling treatments, *ASHRAE J.*, 14: 65–69, 1972; J. L. Heid and M. A. Joslin (eds.), *Food Processing Operations*, vols. 1 and 2, 1963, and vol. 3, 1964; G. W. Irving, Jr., and S. R. Hoover (eds.), *Food Quality: Effects of Production Practices and Processing*, AAAS, 1965; M. B. Jacobs, *The Chemistry and Technology of Food and Food Products*, 3d ed., 1958; E. A. Leonard, *Economics of Packaging*, 1974; A. Levie, *The Meat Handbook*, 1963; A. Lopez, *A Complete Course in Canning*, 10th ed., 1975; J. Milgrom and A. L. Brody, *Packaging in Perspective*, 1974; B. E. Moody, *Packaging in Glass*, 1963; G. J. Mountney, *Poultry Products Technology*, 1966; F. A. Paine, *Packaging Materials and Containers*, 1967; M. E. Parker, E. H. Harvey, and E. S. Stateler, *Elements of Food Engineering*, vol. 2, 1954; N. Potter, *Food Science*, 1973; B. E. Proctor and S. A. Goldblith, Preservation of foods by irradiation, *Amer. J. Public Health*, 47:439–445, 1957; G. F. Reddish (ed.), *Antiseptics, Disinfectants, Fungicides, and Chemical and Physical Sterilization*, 2d ed., 1957; S. Sacharow and R. C. Griffin, *Food Packaging*, 1970; S. Sacharow and R. C. Griffin, *Basic Guide to Plastics in Packaging*, 1973; W. A. Simms (ed.), *Modern Packaging Encyclopedia*, 1974; C. M. Swalm, *Chemistry of Packaging Materials*, 1974; U.S. Department of Agriculture, *Food for Us All*, The Yearbook of Agriculture, 1969; W. B. Van Arsdel and M. J. Copeley, *Food Dehydration*, 2 vols., 1963, 1964.

Food manufacturing

The commercial production and packaging of food products that are fabricated by processing or combining various ingredients or both. Manufactured foods are basically different from any found in nature, but they are fabricated principally from natural ingredients, and often include small quantities of chemical food additives to improve nutritive value, taste, color, shelf life, and convenience in use. A limited quantity of simulated meatlike foods has been fabricated from soya protein and other ingredients, and significant increase in this business is expected. Much development is being done on the production of intermediate-moisture foods for human consumption, using a process similar to the one for making intermediate-moisture pet foods.

Mechanical manipulation, chemical treatment, biologic processes, heat treatment, or freezing may be involved. For example, bread is manufactured by combining flour, shortening, yeast, and other minor ingredients to make dough. Kneading and fermentation of the dough change the characteristics and develop flavor. The dough is formed into loaf-sized pieces, put into bake pans, proofed, and baked to form bread, which is sliced and wrapped.

Some foods, however, are prepared for consumption by refining processes which do not essentially change the nature of the material. Milk, for example, is clarified by centrifuging and pasteurized by heat treatment to kill pathogenic organisms. This treatment makes it safe for human consumption, but does not change it basically.

Food manufacturing and processing involve many unit operations, such as separating, mixing, forming, application of heat or refrigeration, packaging, materials handling, and process control. These are carried out in some 38,000 plants in the United States, ranging in size from small retail bakeries to a processing plant covering 35 acres. Of these plants, more than 14,700 have over 20 employees and account for 92% of the industry's total value added by manufacture. The food industry has 1,600,000 employees, more than any other industry. It spends some $1,600,000,000 a year for modernization and expansion, purchases huge quantities of raw materials from farmers and ingredient manufacturers, uses some $13,500,000,000 of packaging materials and containers, and produces more than $74,000,000,000 a year of finished foods for consumption in homes and mass-feeding institutions and for export.

Originally an enlarged version of a kitchen, the typical food factory has been developed through engineering into a highly efficient, technical industrial plant. Many processes have been converted from batch to continuous methods and put under automatic control. Materials and finished products are handled with high efficiency and little labor, with the aid of bulk pneumatic conveyors, pumps, mechanical conveyors, and lift trucks. Modern food factories are built with sanitary floors and walls of tile and brick, and much of the equipment is made of stainless steel. Most of the newer plants are in suburban areas on attractively landscaped plots. Aside from being built with sanitation in mind, many modern plants are showplaces through which visitors are taken on regular tours as a public relations operation.

Food factories are inspected by Federal health authorities if they do interstate business, and by state and municipal authorities when they do business locally. Health agencies also require that additives and packaging materials used in food manufacturing be approved as safe before they may be employed.

Manufacturers usually sell their products to retail stores through wholesalers, though some sales are made direct to large chain-store organizations. Many dairies and bakeries also deliver directly to the home. Sale of processed and manufactured foods to restaurants and caterers is a rapidly growing business; and so is sale of convenience products via vending machines.

Major branches of the food manufacturing and refining industry are those producing bakery products; flour and cereal products; milk and other dairy products; canned, frozen, and dehydrated fruits and vegetables; fruit and vegetable juices; preserves; meat; poultry; fish; soft drinks; beer and ale; wine; confections; coffee; tea; spices and condiments; sweeteners; syrups; baby foods; dessert mixes; roasted nuts and nut butters; oleomargarine; shortenings and edible oils; and mayonnaise and salad dressings. *See* FOOD; FOOD ENGINEERING; FOOD SCIENCE; FOOD SPOILAGE.

[FRANK K. LAWLER]

FOODS INTENDED FOR HUMAN CONSUMPTION

As indicated above, foods that are destined for human consumption are manufactured under closely controlled and carefully inspected conditions of cleanliness and acceptable hygienic practices.

Bakery products. These foods are made from flour by moistening, processing, and baking. Baked bread is one of the oldest products produced by man from naturally occurring raw materials, using invented processes. In its basic ingredients, processes, and characteristics, bread has changed little since the Stone Age. However, close control of processes produces a more uniform product, and enrichment of materials results in a more nutritious product. Moreover, time has brought other innovations in baking which have led to numerous other baked goods, including cakes, pies, and cookies.

Bread and bread types. Bread is manufactured by mixing together and kneading into a homogeneous mass flour, water, salt, and yeast. Other added ingredients are classified as optional and are added according to their function and to the characterization of the finished product. Wheat protein when mixed with water forms a spongy mass known as gluten. The two main proteins comprising gluten are gliadin, which gives gluten its elas-

ticity, and glutenin, which gives gluten its strength. With the unique properties of these two gluten-forming proteins and with the production of carbon dioxide gas and alcohol during a fermentation period, yeast-leavened products can maintain this gas production, thereby making a product with a predetermined volume as desired.

Bread varies according to customer demand for different richnesses in formula and physical make-up of the dough pieces. White open or round-top pan bread is the most popular and accounts for approximately 82% of all bread produced in the United States. The remaining 18% consists of hearth-type bread (baked directly on the hearth or tray of the oven without pans), rolls (hamburger, hot dog, and hard), rye bread, and other varieties, in which the formula meets customer demand. Bread doughs are also made up into various forms, packaged, and frozen as convenience foods to be baked by the customer immediately before serving. Partially baked rolls for finish-baking before serving also are produced.

Loaves are classified as bread or rolls according to size. Dough weighing over 8 oz is classified as loaf bread, when baked, while dough weighing less than 8 oz is classified as rolls. These two products may be made from the same dough.

Bread and rolls are further classified according to the type of leavening agents used to acquire the desired volume. Quick breads are leavened by a chemical leavening agent, such as baking powder. This type of bread or roll does not require a fermentation period and can be made up into the desired product as soon as the dough is mixed. Other characteristics of quick breads are denseness, course grain, and crumbly texture. Corn bread and baking-powder biscuits are typical examples of chemically leavened quick breads.

Yeast-leavened breads are leavened by carbon dioxide gas produced during the fermentation period. The dough mass goes through further changes during the fermentation period; these changes in turn make the final product more palatable, larger in volume, closer grained, with thinner cell walls, and of a more silky texture than is characteristic

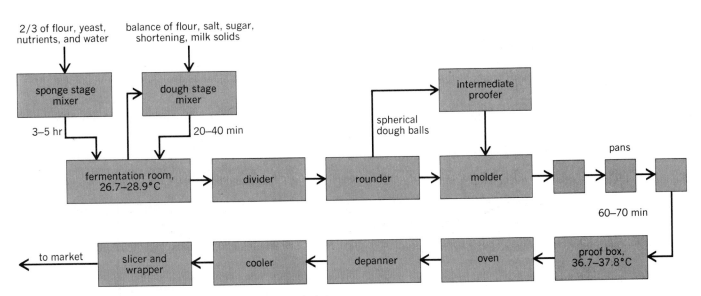

Fig. 1. Flow chart for conventional batch, or sponge-and-dough, bakery process.

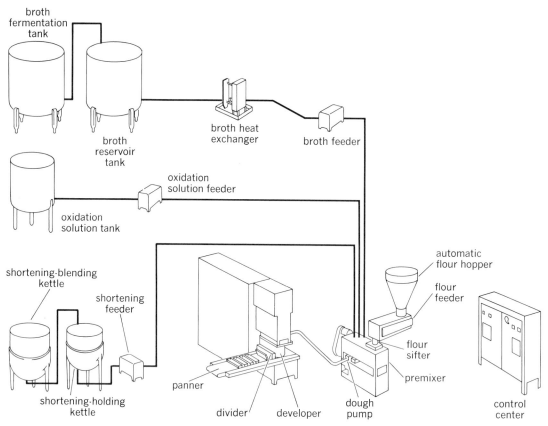

Fig. 2. Flow chart for continuous-mix bakery process. (*Wallace & Tiernan Div. of Pennwalt Corp.*)

of the chemically leavened quick breads.

Basically there are three methods employed in the manufacture of yeast-leavened breads. Choice is governed by the product desired and by customer acceptance.

1. In the batch, or sponge-and-dough, method a sponge is mixed and fermented for approximately 3–4 hr (Fig. 1). The sponge is placed in the dough mixer, where the balance of flour and other ingredients are added and mixed into a dough. The dough is given a short fermentation period (known as floor time), after which it is run through the balance of the makeup equipment.

2. The straight-dough technique differs from the sponge-and-dough method in that all ingredients are added at one time and that there is only one mixing stage and one fermentation period. The fermentation period for a straight dough is approximately 2–3 hr. After fermentation is complete, the dough enters the divider and continues through the same makeup equipment as for the sponge-and-dough method.

3. The continuous-mix method is a recent development in the manufacture of bread and is characterized by use of highly specialized equipment (Fig. 2). This equipment provides continuous operation from the weighing of ingredients until the developed dough is deposited in the pans for final pan-proofing and baking. From the oven on, equipment is the same as in the sponge-and-dough method. Preparation steps are, however, greatly different. Conventional equipment such as mixers, fermentation rooms, divider, and molder are eliminated. More skilled but fewer operators are re-

quired. Floor space is greatly reduced; units manufacturing 6000 lb of dough per hour require only 800 ft² of floor space.

Nearly all bread and roll products manufactured in the United States are sold in sealed wrappers or bags, the latter increasingly so. Plastic film and wax paper are the packaging materials most commonly used.

The baking temperature of bread is approximately 450°F (235°C). When the bread emerges from the oven, the interior temperature is near the boiling point of water 212°F (100°C). The temperature must be reduced to approximately 100°F (40°C) to render the loaf suitable for slicing and wrapping or bagging.

Other products. Cake production is a simpler operation than bread making. Cakes differ widely in characteristics but, since they are made without yeast, no fermentation periods are involved. Instead of doughs, batters are used for cake production, the basic difference between the two being the thinner consistency of batter due to the higher liquid content. Cakes may be divided into foam and shortening types. In the shortening type, the leavening action comes from the reaction of sodium bicarbonate and an organic acid. These may be added as separate ingredients or in combination as baking powder. In the foam-type cakes, a high proportion of egg white is used, which aids the batter in retaining the air incorporated during the mixing operation. The expansion of this air during the baking operation normally gives all the needed volume without the use of any chemical leavening. Handling methods are essentially the same for all types of cakes. The batter is mixed and deposited in pans by mechanical means, which go directly to the oven for the baking operation. Cakes are then transferred to racks for cooling and are wrapped on machines specially designed for that purpose.

This usual method of cake production is a batch operation as far as mixing is concerned. Other mixers are now also in use to which ingredients are continuously proportioned and which deliver an uninterrupted stream of batter into the cake pans.

Doughnuts are made in bakeries but are fried in fat instead of being baked. Some doughnuts make use of yeast and a fermentation reaction for lightness, while cake types are chemically leavened. Special machines are used for scaling off the desired weights, shaping the pieces, and depositing them into the frying fat.

Most cookies are chemically leavened and so are similar to cakes except for adjustments necessary because of differences in shape and size. Ordinary crackers are made from yeast-fermented doughs and with the use of relatively low-protein flours. An adjustment of the developed acidity by the addition of soda produces the type of cracker that is most common.

Pies make up a considerable proportion of the output of some bakers, especially retail ones. Pies may have only a bottom crust or also a second one over the filling. A large number of fruit and other fillings are used. Pie crusts can best be made from relatively low-protein flours and must contain a high fat percentage to have the desired tenderness.

Amounts produced. Table 1 gives information on the size of the baking industry in terms of poundage produced. The source is the U.S. Bureau of the Census 1966 compilation. Other surveys have indicated no appreciable change in production figures during recent years, so the data can be accepted as accurately reflecting current production of the baking industry, exclusive of retail, single-shop bakeries. The latter are not a major factor in the production of white bread and other items on the list.

Standards. Definitions and standards for bakery products are covered under the Federal Food and Cosmetic Act, U.S. Department of Health, Education, and Welfare, Food and Drug Administration,

chapter 21, part 17. Enriched bread, rolls, and buns are required to carry on their label a statement of optional ingredients. Such enriched food, to be so identified, is also required to contain in each pound of bread not less than 1.1 mg and not more than 1.8 mg of thiamine, not less than 0.7 mg and not more than 1.6 mg of riboflavin, not less than 10.0 mg and not more than 15.0 mg of niacin or niacinamide, and not less than 8.0 mg and not more than 12.5 mg of iron.

Enrichment of white bread with three B vitamins was inaugurated in the United States in 1941 at the National Nutrition Conference for Defense as a medical measure to improve the health of the population by using a common food as a carrier for essential nutrients. Standards for enrichment were carefully determined to meet known deficiencies in the average American diet. It has been estimated by the U.S. Department of Agriculture that the enrichment program has added one-third more thiamine, one-fifth more iron and niacin, and one-tenth more riboflavin to the general diet than would be available if bread and other cereal foods were not enriched. Enrichment of bread is a major factor in the control of deficiency diseases and the improvement of health. *See* FERMENTATION.

[TEMPLE MAYHALL]

Cereal products. Cereal preparations consist of breakfast foods, coffee substitutes, and specially processed grains for domestic and export consumption. Examples of the latter products developed for use mainly in less-developed countries are bulgur, a partly debranned, parboiled wheat, and pearled wheat, which is a more refined bulgur. Wheat gluten alone or gluten mixed with whole-kernel cooked wheat can be made into a meatlike product. New kinds of cereal breakfast foods are being developed frequently which have a variety of product size, color, and flavor. Some require cooking but others, such as cornmeal, rolled oats, farina, germ, bran, and cracked wheat, can be eaten uncooked. The more popular breakfast foods are sold already cooked or require minimal cooking before serving. The manufacture of ready-to-serve breakfast foods is a relatively new industry, developed largely since 1910.

There are two classes of ready-to-serve cereal breakfast foods: those made from entire grains or their milled products, and those made from fabricated cereal products. Both types are found on the consumer market in the form of flaked, puffed, shredded, or granulated breakfast foods. There are considerable variations within each type in regard to the cereals employed, the amount and kind of cooking, and the flavoring used. Flaked products may be made from corn, rice, or wheat. The most popular breakfast food of this type is flaked corn, which is manufactured from corn grits or hominy. Hominy for flaking is cooked in rotary steam cookers for 2–3 hr and is flavored with sugar, salt, malt, honey, or other ingredients while in the cookers. The cooked grits are broken up, cooled, dried to a moisture content of about 15% and then held in tempering bins for 6–8 hr to equalize moisture distribution. After the tempering process, the material is passed through heavy-duty flaking machines. The flakes thus produced go to special-type ovens for toasting, after which they are cooled and placed in storage bins until packaged. Vita-

Table 1. Annual baked goods production (not including retail single-shop bakeries)*

Product	Thousand pounds
White pan bread	8,861,343
White hearth bread	426,998
Whole wheat and other dark wheat breads	643,216
Rye breads	509,545
Raisin and other specialty breads	419,506
Rolls—bread type	2,063,124
Sweet yeast goods	875,053
Doughnuts—cake type	388,269
Soft cakes	1,122,242
Cookies	1,930,797
Crackers	1,369,194
Pretzels	139,380
Pies	694,402

*U.S. Bureau of the Census.

mins may be added just before packaging.

Puffed-type breakfast foods were among the first developed. Originally only rice and wheat were puffed, but the process has been extended to many other grains such as corn, barley, millet, beans, peas, and soybeans. Puffed breakfast cereals are also produced from cooked doughs. Puffed cereal products are prepared by placing the material in pressure cookers or puffing guns. There the vapor pressure is gradually increased to a predetermined level, then pressure is suddenly released. This allows the water vapor to expand, puffing the product. With wheat and rice, as much as a tenfold volume increase can be obtained. The expansion for other materials is less.

Shredded breakfast food is generally prepared from wheat. Clean wheat is agitated in pressure cookers until the starch is gelatinized completely without disintegrating the kernel. The cooked wheat is cooled and placed in bins for conditioning before going to the shredding machine. Shredding is done by rolls; one roll is smooth and the other has about 20 circular grooves per linear inch cut in the surface. The cooked wheat is forced under pressure between the two rolls, which rotate toward each other. This forms the material into slender strands, which are carried along on a moving belt, where successive layers of strands are added until the desired thickness has been obtained. The shreds are cut to designated size by flat-edged knives operating from both above and below the flow of material. The cut pieces are placed in baking pans and heated at about 260°C for approximately 20 min. After cooling, the product is ready for packaging.

The preparation of granular-type ready-prepared breakfast cereals is a rather complicated procedure. The flow sheet for production of this type of breakfast food is shown in Fig. 3.

A common type of granulated breakfast cereal is prepared from long-extraction wheat flour made into a dense, close-grained type of bread by conventional baking methods. The loaves are broken to produce a crumbled product, which is again baked and then crushed between coarsely corrugated rolls. The ground material is graded to secure a fairly uniform granulation size and is packaged for use.

Roasted cereals have been commonly used for a long time as substitutes for coffee. The manufacture of coffee substitutes starts with the careful roasting of whole wheat, which is then granulated and combined with a mixture of roasted bran and sugarcane molasses. The color of the product is used as a guide in judging the length of the roasting period. When the material is removed from the rotary roasters, it is rapidly cooled in pan coolers. Products made in this manner are about 50% water-soluble. For the preparation of more water-soluble products, the roasted granulated material is percolated with hot water and the solution is clarified, concentrated in vacuum, and finally dried in vacuum drum driers. The dried extract is in brittle sheets, which are ground to the desired particle size and packaged for distribution. Besides wheat, roasted barley, rye, and bran are also used for coffee substitutes. *See* CEREAL.

[JOHN A. SHELLENBERGER]

Chewing gum. This is a kind of confection that contains gum base, a masticatory material that does not dissolve in saliva when the gum is chewed. American gum averages in content 20% gum base, 16% corn syrup, 63% sugar, and less than 1% flavoring, such as mint, fruit, and spice.

Chicle, from Central America, was the principal gum base component in 1910. By 1940 jelutong, a more elastic material from Indonesia, was used to a greater extent. Chicle again became the major component during Japanese occupation of the East Indies, with greatest use in 1944. Since then sorva, from South America, has displaced much chicle and jelutong. These three gum bases represent

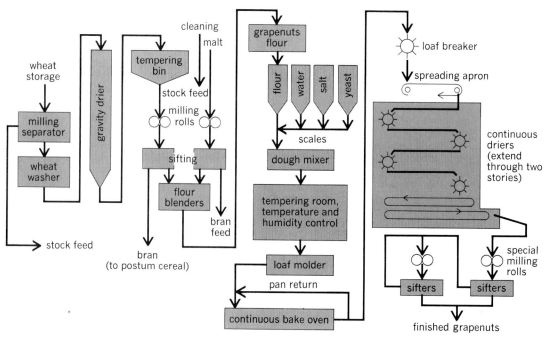

Fig. 3. Flow sheet for manufacture of granular-type cereal breakfast food. (*General Foods Corp.*)

dried latexes from trees. Progressively more and more domestic ingredients, such as resins and waxes, are replacing the imported products. Calcium carbonate, which is a component of most base formulas, neutralizes traces of acid forming on the teeth from fermented food residues and so tends to reduce dental caries. Whatever ingredients are used in a gum base, they are blended together hot. *See* CHICLE.

The melted gum base is cleaned and mixed with syrup, sugar, and flavor; the resulting chewing gum is shaped by extrusion and rolling. Additional powdered sugar is used on the surface to prevent adhesion to wrappers. A hard sugar coating can be built up on shaped pieces of gum in a tumbling pan by alternate wetting with a sugar solution and evaporating the added water in a dry air blast.

[HERBERT W. CONNER]

Condiments. These are agents used to enhance the flavor of a food, to alter or supply a distinctive flavor when none exists, and to change the appearance of foods by giving color (such as paprika or curry powder). Condiments may include many varying types of materials: (1) spices such as pepper, mustard, ginger, and nutmeg; (2) herbs such as basil, marjoram, tarragon, and parsley; (3) seeds such as poppy, anise, and dill; (4) chemicals such as sodium chloride and monosodium glutamate; and (5) sauces made from cooking wines, vinegars, and relishes.

Properties of most condiments are distinct because of their volatile characteristics or the substances of definite chemical composition therein.

Standards have been promulgated by the Federal Food and Drug Administration for the more important spices, herbs, and seeds as listed above. These consist of specifications for percentages of crude fiber, total ash, volatile oils, starches, and other basic constituents of each specific item. The purpose of such standards is for the maintenance of uniformity of product, the insurance of freshness, and the provision of proper quality control for the consumer. *See* SPICE AND FLAVORING.

[ALFRED J. FINBERG]

Confections. The per capita annual consumption of confections is 18 lb. The confectionery industry manufactures annually over 2,000,000,000 lb of carbohydrates, with a value of more than $1,000,000,000. There are more than 2000 varieties of confections and most of these have hundreds of different variations. For example, there are as many as 500 different formulas for nougats.

About 70 farm products of varying carbohydrate content furnish more than 90% of all the raw materials for the over 2000 varieties of confections. Common sweeteners used in confections are refined crystalline cane or beet sugar, brown sugar, liquid sugar, corn syrup, dextrose, sorbitol, starch, molasses, honey, and maple sugar. More emphasis is being placed on the addition of vegetable and animal proteins in confections, such as soya proteins, zein, yeast, gelatin, and pulverized dried beef. Also available are improved vegetable and animal fats. Fats and oil are important in fudge and nougat types of confections.

Usage factors. The major factors considered by a candy technologist in determining sweetener usage are differences in physical and chemical properties of various sweeteners, their relative prices, in some cases restrictions imposed by Federal or state regulations, and to a lesser extent advertising and sales programs, in-plant handling problems, consumer preference, and psychological factors.

The most important physical and chemical properties, considered in their order of relative importance to the candy industry are (1) relative sweetness; (2) solubility and crystallization characteristics; (3) density of liquid sweeteners and moisture content of solid sweeteners; (4) hygroscopicity; (5) flavor; (6) fermentation and preservative properties; and (7) molecular weight, osmotic pressure, and freezing-point depression.

Proteins and fats also vary considerably with respect to the above properties. Requirements also vary widely, according to the qualities desired in the particular type or class of confection. The large variety of products turned out by the confectionery industry require a remarkable flexibility from the carbohydrates which serve as major constituents of these products.

Confections are divided into three categories: hard candies or high-boiled sweets, chewy confections, and aerated confections. The second and third categories are further subdivided into two classes, where the sugar solution is supersaturated (grained) or unsaturated (nongrained). Candies that grain are of crystalline structure and include the fondant types, such as cream centers, crystallized creams, fudge, pulled-grained mints, rigid-grained marshmallows, and soft- and hard-type pan centers. The nongrained candy group consists of marshmallows; taffies; chewy candies, such as nougats, caramels, and molasses kisses; jellies; and gums. There are many intermediate or hybrid types of confections combining the characteristics of both the grained and nongrained candies. Sugar is the universal graining agent. The regulators are corn syrup, invert sugar, sorbitol, and others that retard or prevent sucrose crystallization.

Sugar, or sucrose, has the highest rate of solution, and the smaller the crystal size the more rapid the solution. It forms highly supersaturated solutions which withstand supercooling. Most important of the chemical reactions of sugar is its ability to hydrolyze to produce invert sugar. The color developed in sugar solutions is a function of the pH, and color cannot be formed unless inversion has first taken place. Invert-sugar syrups are known for being hygroscopic and retarding the crystallization of concentrated sugar solutions. *See* SUCROSE; SUGAR.

Corn syrups are noted for retarding and controlling the crystallization of concentrated sugar solutions. For practical purposes regular corn syrup, high-conversion corn syrups, and enzyme syrups have equal effects and can be used interchangeably on a solids basis to control sugar crystallization in such products as fondant, fudge, or other grained confections. Total solubility of the many sugars found in corn syrup and moisture present in the confection minimize the crystallization of the sucrose. Singly, each sugar increases the tendency to crystallization, but this factor of total solubility in the liquid phase overbalances any such tendency. Dextrins add viscosity, which increases the body of nongraining confections.

Dextrose, or glucose, possesses the ability to change solubility characteristics and modify the relative sweetness of confections. Dextrose also tends to crystallize more slowly than sucrose and the solution at the same concentration is less viscous. Sorbitol, derived from dextrose, is a sugar alcohol and seems to have plasticizing properties in confections. Besides having a narrow humectant range, it has an effect on the sugar crystal, which results in keeping candies soft for extended periods of time. It appears to be gaining in favor as a softening agent for both grained and nongrained confections. *See* GLUCOSE.

Hard candies. Hard candies or high-boiled sweets are essentially a highly supersaturated, supercooled solution of sucrose containing 1% or less of moisture. This solution, which may be likened to glass, is usually prevented from crystallizing by the addition of invert (or of invert formed in the batch) or corn syrup or both, depending upon the properties desired. They are usually compounded in the ratio of 70 sugar/30 corn syrup for open-fire cooking, and 60 sugar/40 corn syrup in vacuum-processed batches. If the hard candy is to be relatively slow dissolving, a larger proportion of corn syrup is used, as in a banana caramel; if a quicker-dissolving product is wanted, such as a clear mint, smaller amounts of corn syrup are used. Corn syrup controls sweetness and reduces friability of hard candies. These are susceptible to fracture from mechanical shock, because of internal stresses induced by unequal cooling. Syrups of high dextrin content and low dextrose and maltose fractions are used to control hygroscopic properties. Formulations and processing techniques in the manufacture of hard candy confections are designed to make a product of low hygroscopicity and different degrees of sweetness which is ungrained, dense, and brittle in texture.

Chewy confections. Chewy confections of the nongraining type, such as kisses, caramels, gums, and jellies, are formulated with sucrose, corn syrup, fat, and milk solids. The ratio of sugar solids to corn syrup solids, plus 12–15% of moisture, is such that the carbohydrates remain in solution. The dextrins impart body or chewy texture, and in caramels the milk solids contribute flavor and texture. Natural and artificial flavors are accentuated by the sugar, invert sugar, and corn syrup. Fats, which are usually of the vegetable type because of their excellent shelf-life properties, are added to impart body and lubricating qualities. Emulsifiers such as lecithin, monoglycerides, sorbitan monostearate, and polyoxyethylene sorbitan monostearate, are added to make the product more palatable. Standard 42 dextrose equivalent (DE) corn syrup has widest application, because it contributes the desirable chewy characteristic without danger of excessive hygroscopicity.

Gums and jellies may be subdivided into two classes on the basis of the gelling agent, those utilizing starch and those utilizing pectin. Starch gums employ about 10% thin-boiling starch which is gelatinized during processing by the free water in a sucrose-corn syrup solution that is cooked with it. It is essential to use excess water at the beginning of cooking to ensure complete gelatinization—that is, about 1 gal of water for every pound of starch in the batch. No excess water is necessary, however, in a continuous method. Sucrose and corn syrup are present in approximately equal proportions and are concentrated to about 76% solids before being cast into a corn-starch molding medium. On cooling, a firm, resilient, transparent gel results. Crystallization is prevented because of the high solubility of mixed sugar present and the gelatinized starch. Although standard 42 DE corn syrup is most commonly used for gum work, the enzyme-converted 53 DE type has advantages due to its humectant properties and extra sweetness. Up to 25% of the total sweetener may also be in the form of refined corn sugar, which promotes sweetness and reduces viscosity of the batch, enabling faster moisture evaporation and prolonging shelf life because of its hygroscopic character. However, a high ratio of dextrose to sucrose may cause graining in the piece due to the relatively low solubility of dextrose.

Pectin and low-methoxyl pectin jellies are compounds of sucrose, corn syrup, pectin, citric acid, water, and a buffer salt, concentrated by heat to a solids content of about 75%, which is necessary for proper gel formation. A 50:50 mixture of sucrose and corn syrup is conventional practice. This ratio effectively inhibits graining and gives the minimum difficulty from excess moisture absorption on the surface. Because the pH of pectin jellies must be adjusted to between 3.45 and 3.55 for proper setting of the pectin gel, significant quantities of invert sugar are formed from the sucrose, giving rise to possible subsequent sweating problems. Accordingly, a corn syrup of relatively low dextrose equivalent is the logical selection to avoid undue amounts of hygroscopic sugars in the mixture. Sorbitol appears to be effective in all pectin jellies, whereas the MYRJ emulsifiers are more beneficial in starch gum confections.

Aerated confections. Aerated confections are of two basic types: those made from unsaturated solutions and those made from supersaturated solutions which give graïned confections. Aerated, unsaturated solutions, such as frappés and marshmallows, are not necessarily chewy. Both of these products are formed with sugar and corn syrup rarely in excess of 45 and 55%, respectively, combined with water and an aerating agent, usually albumin or soybean protein for frappés and gelatin for marshmallows. A diffusion method for continuous production of foam candy results in longer shelf life because of smaller uniform air cells, while less gelatin or other whipping agent is required because of lessened fatigue in process. Because of the high proportion of corn syrup and the protection afforded by the protein colloids, the system remains unsaturated with respect to sucrose. Concentration of the total solids, without incurring supersaturation, to a level safe from microbiological spoilage is made possible with the corn syrup or invert fraction, which may be either standard 42 DE or special 52 DE type in the case of uncoated goods, or special 52 DE and 63 DE enzyme or invert sugar in the case of coated marshmallow products. Molasses, honey, and maple sugar are used in all types of confections, primarily as a flavoring. Honey has very good humectant properties.

Grained, aerated confections are the supersaturated solutions that form grained confections, such as creams, fondants, nougats, fudges, and grained marshmallow items. Fondants and creams are prepared by concentrating a sucrose, corn syrup, and water solution to about 85% total solids, by use of a ratio of sucrose in excess of that of corn syrup so that precipitation occurs when the supersaturated solution is seeded or when crystallization is induced by mechanical means. This generally implies a proportion of 80:70 parts of sucrose to 20:30 parts of corn syrup. The mixture is usually boiled to 114.4–116.7°C. Agitation or seeding is carried on at reduced temperatures of about 110°F in order that the crystals so formed will be of impalpable size.

Some air is incorporated by the mechanical action of the equipment used in making the fondant. In the case of creams, the fondant is used as a seeding medium and a small percentage of egg or soybean albumin in the form of mazetta is used to impart some air. The functions of the corn-syrup portion are to serve as a humectant that will keep the products soft and palatable and to permit concentration of soluble solids in the liquid phase to a level of about 80%, which will prevent growth of microorganisms. All three types of corn syrups have applications, the special 52 DE and enzyme-converted 63 DE imparting effective humectant properties. Invert sugar in combination with corn syrup gives excellent results. Refined corn sugar may be used in limited amounts, but it is not generally recommended because of its tendency to grain off in coarser crystals. Sorbitol with corn syrup seems to give a more uniform and whiter cream and fondant.

Fudges are similar to caramels, containing sugar, corn syrup, milk solids, and vegetable fats, but are slightly aerated by mechanical agitation with the aid of egg or soybean protein frappés. Soybean proteins are gaining favor because they bring out the color of the cocoa powder or cocoa liquor used in chocolate fudges. The ratio of sugar to corn syrup is higher, enabling precipitation of sugar crystals to form short, crystallized texture. All three types of corn syrup have applications, as in creams. Although the syrups of higher dextrose equivalents are used in chocolate-coated bars, the quartermaster ration chocolate-type covered disks have 10% sorbitol to ensure a shelf life of the product of at least 2 years.

Grained marshmallows are produced with sugar, corn syrup, and an aerating agent such as gelatin or albumin. The corn syrup, invert sugar, or sorbitol serves to retain softness in a supersaturated, aerated sucrose system. Refined corn sugar (dextrose) may be incorporated to 20–25% of the total sweetener because of its hygroscopicity and higher fluidity, which permit faster beating to the desired specific gravity of the product. Standard 42 DE and special 52 DE syrups are preferred for this item. Enzyme-converted syrups or invert sugar, if used, should be used sparingly to avoid excessive softening due to absorbed moisture. What applies for grained marshmallows applies for grained nougats. In this confection, gelatin is seldom used and the aerating agent is usually egg albumin, soybean protein, or a 50:50 mixture of the two. Vegetable fats are used to promote smoothness and palatability to the confection. Since a high percentage of nougat confections is coated with chocolate or chocolate-type coatings, the 63 DE enzyme-converted corn syrups or invert sugar are used.

[JUSTIN J. ALIKONIS]

Dessert manufacture. This is the commercial preparation of sweet foods to be served at the end of a meal. Canned fruits, such as peaches, cherries, and pineapple, are packed either in a sugar syrup or in a sugarless water solution with or without synthetic sweeteners and with or without thickeners to simulate a sugar syrup. The latter variety results from the emphasis on low-calorie and dietetic foods.

Many convenience desserts, such as rice pudding, Indian pudding, and crepes suzettes, are canned for home use. Pie fillings are packed in cans and packages. Frozen desserts include fruits such as strawberries and rhubarb, specialty items such as pies and puddings, and many types of ice cream and related desserts. Among dehydrated

Table 2. World catch of seafood by countries, 1974[a]

Country	10³ metric tons	10⁶ lb
Japan	10,773	23,750
Soviet Union	9,236	20,362
China, Peoples Republic of	6,880[b]	15,168[b]
Peru	4,150	9,149
United States	2,744[c]	6,049[c]
Norway	2,645	5,831
India	2,255	4,971
Korea, Republic of	2,001	4,411
Denmark	1,835	4,045
Thailand	1,626	3,585
Spain	1,511[b]	3,331[b]
South Africa, Republic of	1,415	3,120
Indonesia	1,342	2,959
Philippines	1,291[b]	2,846[b]
Chile	1,127	2,485[b]
Canada	1,027	2,264
Iceland	945	2,083
France	808	1,781
Korea, North	800[b]	1,764[b]
Vietnam, South	714[b]	1,574[b]
Nigeria	685	1,510
Poland	679	1,497
Brazil	605[b]	1,334[b]
Scotland	538	1,186
England and Wales	532[b]	1,173[b]
Germany, Federal Republic of	526	1,160
Angola	470[b]	1,036[b]
Mexico	442	974
Malaysia, West	442[b]	974[b]
Burma	434	957
Portugal	428[b]	944[b]
Italy	425	937
Germany, East	363[b]	800[b]
Senegal	357[b]	787[b]
Netherlands	326	719
Argentina	301[b]	664[b]
Vietnam, North	300[b]	661[b]
All other[d]	6,867	15,139
Total	69,845	153,980

[a]From the Food and Agriculture Organization of the United Nations, *Yearbook of Fishery Statistics*, vol. 38, 1974.

[b]Data estimated by FAO.

[c]Includes the weight of clam, oyster, scallop, and other mollusk shells; this weight is not included in other United States catch statistics.

[d]Residual.

Table 3. World catch of seafood by species groups, 1974*

Species group	10³ metric tons	10⁶ lb
Herring, sardines, anchovies, etc.	13,731	30,271
Cods, hakes, haddocks, etc.	12,697	27,992
Misc. marine and diadromous fishes	9,112	20,088
Fresh-water fishes	9,054	19,960
Redfish, basses, congers, etc.	4,587	10,112
Mackerels, snoeks, cutlassfishes, etc.	3,621	7,983
Mollusks	3,437	7,577
Jacks, mullets, sauries, etc.	3,312	7,302
Salmon, trouts, smelts, etc.	2,449	5,399
Crustaceans	1,937	4,270
Tunas, bonitos, billfishes, etc.	1,875	4,134
Misc. aquatic plants and animals	1,470	3,241
Flounders, halibuts, soles, etc.	1,178	2,597
Shads, milkfishes, etc.	749	1,651
Sharks, rays, chimaeras, etc.	558	1,230
River eels	52	115
Sturgeons, paddlefishes, etc.	24	53
Total	69,845	153,980

*From the Food and Agriculture Organization of the United Nations, *Yearbook of Fishery Statistics*, vol. 38, 1974. Data estimated by FAO.

desserts are found dried fruits (figs, apricots, plums). Gelatin desserts are made by combining sugar, plain gelatin, citric acid, sodium citrate, flavor, and color. Pudding powders, such as chocolate pudding, may be regular (requiring cooking) or instant (requiring mixing only). These contain powdered sugar (dextrose), starches (pregelatinized in instant pudding), flavor, and color.

[ALFRED J. FINBERG]

Fish and seafood products. A great variety of food is prepared from many species of fish (Pisces) and shellfish (Mollusca and Crustacea). Table 2 shows the world catch of seafood by countries, and Table 3 by species groups. Seafood products are preserved by refrigerating, freezing, canning, salting, smoking, pickling, dehydrating, or combinations of these processes (Table 4). In many countries they serve as a principal source of protein and an important source of fat, minerals, and vitamins in the diet.

Fresh seafood products. These are highly perishable. Deterioration proceeds in direct proportion to delay in initial chilling and to storage temperature (degrees above 0°C). Chilling or refrigeration of round and dressed fish usually is accomplished by

surrounding the product with flaked, chipped, or shaved ice, but refrigerated brine systems have been introduced successfully in some fisheries. Fillets, steaks, and shellfish meats are packed into metal or glass containers, plastic bags, or cardboard cartons, which are then surrounded by ice. Some market forms of fish are shown in Fig. 4. Extension of fresh storage life by such chemical preservatives as benzoates, nitrites, and organic chlorine compounds, and by antibiotics such as chlortetracycline and oxytetracycline incorporated into ice has been proposed, but their use has not been widely accepted. Irradiation pasteurization followed by refrigerated storage appears to be a successful method and is being further investigated. *See* CHLORTETRACYCLINE; OXYTETRACYCLINE.

In most countries, strictly enforced regulations control public health problems involved in production and marketing of shellfish. Oysters and clams are marketed in the shell or as fresh meats. Only the adductor muscle of scallops is marketed. Crabs are cooked and sold as whole, eviscerated, and picked meat. The meat is washed in dilute brine to remove shell fragments and may be pasteurized to reduce bacteria count and inactivate enzymes. Most lobsters are marketed alive, although some are sold as chilled boiled lobsters or lobster tails. Prawns usually are beheaded at sea since only the tail portions are edible. Pacific Coast shrimp are shelled by mechanical peelers or by hand, and sold as cooked meats.

Frozen fish and shellfish. The production of these items is increasing throughout the world. In the United States, fillets, blocks, and steaks are of greatest importance.

Whole and packaged seafoods are frozen in sharp freezers with and without air circulation, in plate freezers under pressure, and in air-blast freezers. Freezing at sea by direct immersion of whole fish in refrigerated brine has long been used in the tuna and salmon fisheries. Filleting and freezing groundfish aboard factory ships is becoming increasingly important in Europe.

Adverse changes occurring in frozen fish include dehydration, discoloration due to oxidation and decomposition of blood pigments, rusting due to oxidation of fat, loss of flavor, development of off-flavors, acquisition of undesirable odors, and

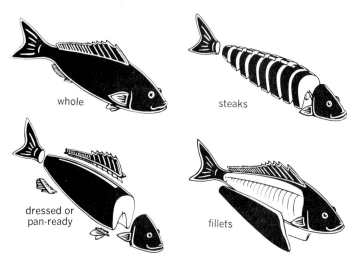

whole   steaks   dressed or pan-ready   fillets

Fig. 4.   Common market forms of fresh fish. (*U. S. Fish and Wildlife Service*)

Table 4. Disposition of U.S. fish catch, 1974 and 1975*

End use	1974 10⁶ lb†	1974 Percent	1975 10⁶ lb†	1975 Percent
Fresh and frozen				
For human food	1,526	30.9	1,548	32.0
For bait and animal food	117	2.4	118	2.4
Total	1,643	33.3	1,666	34.4
Canned				
For human food	817	16.5	813	16.8
For bait and animal food	107	2.2	122	2.5
Total	924	18.7	935	19.3
Cured	74	1.5	69	1.4
Reduction to meal, oil, etc.	2,299	46.5	2,172	44.9
Grand total	4,940	100.0	4,842	100.0

*From the U.S. Department of Commerce, NOAA, National Marine Fisheries Service, *Fisheries of the United States, 1975*, Current Fish. Stat. no. 6900, p. 17, March 1976. Data are preliminary.   †10⁶ lb = 453,600 kg.

denaturation of protein. Their development is inhibited by use of packaging materials with low moisture and oxygen transmission rates, packages without air spaces, vacuum and gas packaging, proper warehousing, control of temperature and humidity, and use of ice coatings or glazes.

For fish of good initial quality, maximum storage limits are 10 months for lean and 6 months for oily fish at the usual commercial storage temperature of −5 to 0°F. Storage life is decreased at temperatures above 0°F and greatly extended at lower temperatures.

Precooked and prepared frozen fishery products have become a major factor in the industry since 1953. While many products (portions, cakes, dinners, main dishes, and pot pies) are available, fish sticks and breaded shrimp are the principal production items (Fig. 5). More uncooked than cooked breaded shrimp are produced.

Canned seafood products. These are seafood products which are packed into hermetically sealed containers and heat-processed to destroy organisms which cause spoilage. The United States canned seafood production is shown in Table 5.

The operations utilized in canning seafoods are like those used for other protein foods. Specific details vary with different species and location. The condition of the raw material (freshness, size, sexual maturity, and substances upon which the animals have been feeding) and the workmanship affect the quality of the canned item. Proper cooling is essential to avoid overprocessing or stack burn.

Discoloration of seafoods and containers is a serious problem. Sulfur, released as hydrogen sulfide, combines with the iron of the can forming black iron sulfide. This may be prevented by the use of parchment liners, increasing the acidity of the product, or enameling the interior of cans with materials containing zinc. Zinc reacts with hydrogen sulfide to form white zinc sulfide. The most common defect in crab is blueing, caused by the reaction of oxidized copper in the hemocyanin in the crab's blood with ammonia in the flesh, resulting in a copper-ammonium complex. Live slaughtering and bleeding of crabs minimizes this defect, while dipping crabmeat in brine containing zinc or aluminum salts inhibits this discoloration. The development of discoloration in canned tuna is caused by abnormal reactions of heme-containing compounds. Occasionally, glasslike crystals of magnesium ammonium phosphate hexahydrate (struvite) are formed in canned seafoods. Their development may be inhibited by the addition of sodium hexametaphosphate.

Cured products. These include seafoods which are processed by drying, salting, smoking, pickling, ripening, and combinations of these. Curing is the most important means of seafood preservation other than chilling in every country except the United States and Canada. Preservation is effected by reduction of moisture, increase in acidity, or by the development of unfavorable temperatures. Throughout the world more herring is cured than any other species.

Drying of seafoods is done by natural or mechanical means. Natural air drying attempts to retain the form of the product. Fish are split, cleaned, boned, and hung on racks to dry. Shrimp, the most important product dried in the United States, is cooked in brine, peeled, and then dried on screens. Dehydrated fish are those which are cooked, flaked, and ground prior to drying by mechanical means. Freeze-drying has been investigated and found suitable for use with seafoods. Drying by sublimation from the frozen state using microwaves as an energy source is a recent experimental innovation.

Salting, the most important method of curing, preserves by extracting water (osmosis) from the product. Purity of salt and maintenance of low temperatures during curing are essential. Dry-salting procedures are used for lean fish such as cod. Cleaned and split fish are piled in alternate layers with salt, and the brine which forms is permitted to drain away (kenching). Fat fish are brine-salted to minimize contact of fish with air. Mild-cured salmon is the most expensive item produced by brine salting.

Spoilage occurs in salted fish when halophilic bacteria cause reddening of the surface of the fish or molds cause dun (chocolate-brown spots) or other colored colonies on the surface. Most salted products must be held under refrigeration.

Smoked seafoods are preserved by salting and drying, although compounds (phenols and formaldehyde) which inhibit spoilage are deposited on the fish from the smoke. Hardwoods are used exclusively. Liquid smoke and salt impregnated with wood-smoke chemicals are sometimes used as flavoring agents. Lightly smoked seafoods, frequently artificially colored, must be maintained under refrigeration or further preserved by canning or freezing. Hard-smoked or dry products are comparatively stable at room temperature. Most spoilage is due to mold growth on surfaces.

Seafoods are cold-smoked (below 32.2°C) and hot-smoked or barbecued (cooked at smoke-house temperatures of 65.6–121.1°C). Herring is the only smoked seafood that is not a luxury. Hard-smoked or red herring are heavily salted and cold-smoked until hard and dry. Bloaters are round herring,

Table 5. Production of canned fishery products in the United States, 1974 and 1975*

Species	1974			1975		
	Standard cases†	Pounds†	Dollars†	Standard cases†	Pounds†	Dollars†
Gefiltefish	300	14,398	6,985	267	12,833	6,396
Herring specialties	115	5,524	2,958	83	3,990	3,334
Mackerel	84	3,779	921	213	9,591	2,578
Roe and caviar	22	1,066	3,893	27	1,314	3,659
Salmon	1,831	87,881	137,290	1,364	65,483	102,645
Sardines, Maine	1,074	25,131	21,745	1,111	26,008	24,917
Tuna	33,390	661,577	824,697	26,811	530,238	651,999
Tunalike fish	394	7,789	5,726	652	12,928	9,956
Other fish	94	4,502	2,099	114	5,440	2,189
Total fish	37,303	811,647	1,006,316	30,644	667,825	807,671
Clams	3,552	96,228	48,354	3,107	81,641	45,130
Crabs	230	4,692	13,783	175	3,585	10,841
Oysters	546	14,603	10,074	478	8,732	7,974
Shrimp	3,320	24,181	45,682	2,030	15,651	27,349
Squid	230	11,060	2,387	190	9,110	1,839
Other shellfish	17	822	819	17	802	807
Total shellfish	7,895	151,585	121,100	5,997	119,521	93,941
Total for human consumption	45,199	963,232	1,127,416	36,641	787,346	901,612
Bait and animal food	12,308	590,774	178,431	10,958	525,989	133,250
Grand total	57,506	1,554,006	1,305,847	47,599	1,313,335	1,034,862

*From U. S. Department of Commerce, NOAA, National Marine Fisheries Service, *Fisheries of the United States, 1975*, Current Fish. Stat. no. 6900, p. 35, March 1976.

†In thousands.

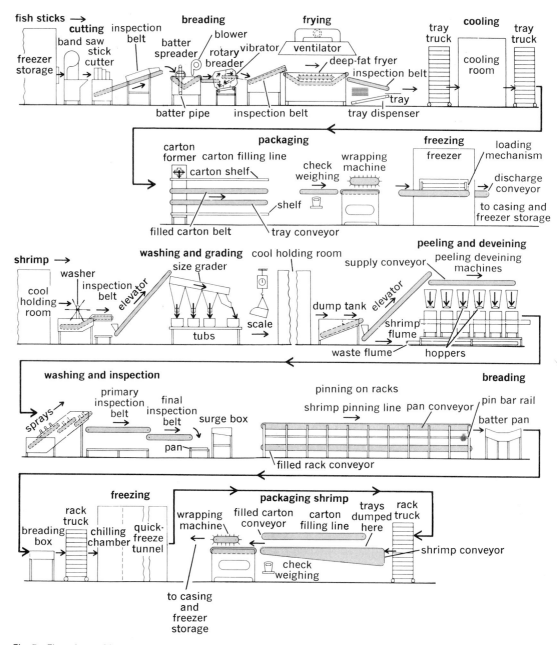

Fig. 5. Flow sheet of fish-stick and breaded-shrimp production lines. *(From Food Eng., 27(2):118–121, 1955)*

lightly salted and cold-smoked for a short time. Kippers are split and eviscerated fish, lightly salted and cold-smoked for a short time. Buckling are large, fat, round herring, lightly salted, cold-smoked a short time, then cooked by hot smoking.

Pickled seafood products are preserved by organic acids either produced by fermentation of the raw material or by addition of vinegar (acetic acid). Added spices exert a slight preservative action. Pickled seafood products are the most important source of animal protein in many Asian countries, of major importance in Europe, but minor in the United States.

Fish meal and oil. These are produced from the inedible portions of fish, though some industrial or scrap fish, menhaden in particular, are caught only for reduction purposes. Table 6 shows the production of fish meal and oil in the United States.

Fish meal is produced by a dry-rendering or batch process and by a wet reduction or continuous operation. Solvent extraction methods are also used. In the batch operation, the ground raw material is dried under vacuum in a steam-jacketed drier equipped with rotating paddles. The dried meal is pressed hydraulically to remove excess oil, which is then purified by use of settling tanks or centrifuges.

The raw material for wet-rendering is ground, cooked by steam injection, and pressed in continuous screw-type equipment to remove most of the water and oil. The meal is dried in direct flame, steam-jacketed, or steam-tube driers. The press liquor is centrifuged to separate the oil from suspended and dissolved protein materials (stickwater), which may be concentrated to 50% solids and sold as condensed solubles or put back in the meal during drying.

Fish meals contain up to 70% protein, less than

Table 6. Production of fish meal, oil, and solubles in the United States, 1974 and 1975*

Product	1974		1975	
	Tons†	10³ dollars	Tons†	10³ dollars
Dried scrap and meal				
Anchovy	14,058	4,188	27,704	6,559
Menhaden	203,859	60,369	191,443	45,993
Tuna and mackerel	48,244	11,603	37,209	6,384
Unclassified fish	25,491	7,303	22,972	5,631
Shellfish	9,062	917	11,012	976
Total	300,714	84,380	290,340	65,543
Solubles				
Menhaden	102,939	8,010	83,624	5,381
Unclassified	34,320	3,720	44,226	3,372
Total	137,259	11,730	127,850	8,753
	10³ lb†		10³ lb†	
Body oil				
Anchovy	5,602	835	12,857	1,547
Menhaden	217,045	46,061	213,271	29,182
Tuna and mackerel	6,819	810	6,444	691
Unclassified	8,514	1,510	13,081	1,183
Total	237,980	49,216	245,653	32,603

*From U.S. Department of Commerce, NOAA, National Marine Fisheries Service, *Fisheries of the United States, 1975*, Current Fish. Stat. no. 6900, p. 37, March 1976.

†1 short ton = 0.9 metric ton. ‡10³ lb = 454 kg.

10% moisture, and less than 15% oil. They are used as supplements in animal feeds as a source of high-quality protein, B vitamins, the animal protein factor, and minerals. Fish meals are used for human consumption in Africa and Asia.

Homogenized condensed fish is a concentrated partial enzymic acid or alkaline hydrolysate produced from fish waste or scrap fish which is used as an animal feed supplement in place of fish meal.

Fish body oils produced during the manufacture of fish meal are highly unsaturated. Industrial-quality oils are used in paints, inks, and for ore flotation. Edible-quality oils are used in margarine and for addition to certain canned seafood items.

Fish liver oils are the principal natural source of vitamin A and contain considerable quantities of vitamin D. They are used in animal feeds, in pharmaceutical preparations, and for fortifying foods such as margarine. Their production has decreased since production of synthetic vitamin A. *See* VITAMIN A; VITAMIN D.

[JOSEPH A. STERN]

Fruit products. Fruits are the ripened ovaries of flowers, the edible portion being the fleshy covering over the seeds. The term fruit generally refers to tree fruits and berries. Being acid, fruits lend themselves to conventional methods of preservation and manufacture.

Canning. Because the main spoilage agents in fruits are non-heat-resistant microorganisms, canning preservation is functional. Exposure of prepared fruit products to temperatures near 93.3°C is generally adequate for their sterilization. The process involves the heating of manufactured fruit products in sealed containers of glass, tin, or plastic in boiling water or steam at atmospheric pressure. One-pound containers of fruit products usually are satisfactorily sterilized by a 20-min treatment.

Freezing. The generally delicate nature of fruits requires rapid freezing techniques for best results, followed by storage of frozen products at −17.8°C or below. Sugar is usually a part of the packing medium, either mixed in dry or added as a syrup. Vitamin C (ascorbic acid) may be added to avoid color changes due to oxidation in ruptured tissues exposed to air. *See* ASCORBIC ACID.

Dehydration. Sun drying is a very widely used method of preserving fruits. Dehydration, or artificial drying, of fruits yields greatly improved products but is more expensive. Successful dehydration involves washing, sorting, trimming, slicing, or dicing fruit, exposure to burning sulfur fumes, or dipping into sulfite solutions, followed by the removal of the water in the tissues with dry hot air. The sulfur treatment is useful in protecting the delicate nature of fruit flavors and preventing discoloration due to oxidation. Dried fruits with moisture contents of less than 20% will usually keep for several years if protected from the elements and insects. Dried fruits with more than 26% moisture will mold and become inedible if not highly sulfured. Drying may be accomplished by exposing the prepared, sulfured fruit to the sun or to drying in tunnels, in cabinet dehydrators, in kiln dryers, in vacuum dryers, or in freeze dryers.

Pickling. Fruits may be pickled by boiling in water until tender and placing in a spiced sugar syrup. The fruits are packaged into glass or tinned containers, filled with hot syrup, and sealed. If the fruit and syrup are above 82.2°C when packaged, no further processing is required. Filled containers should be inverted to sterilize the lids.

Jams, jellies, and preserves. The manufacture of fruit into jellies and preserves is one of the oldest and most important means of using large amounts of sound fruits which may not be well shaped or which for other reasons are unsuited for fresh market outlets.

Jellies are prepared by boiling the fruit, extracting the juice, filtering the juice, adding sugar, concentrating, packaging, and sterilizing.

The requirements of a fruit jelly are that the proper combination of acid, pectin, and sugar in water be reached so that a gel will form. This will occur when the pectin present amounts to 1%, the pH value of the substrate is approximately 3.1, and the concentration of sugar is near 65%. Too high a pectin content results in a very rigid gel, too low a content in a weak gel. If the pH value is below 2.9, a very weak gel forms, and no gel formation occurs above 3.5. Gel formation occurs with more than 60% soluble solids. Too high a sugar content results in a sticky gel. Acid, pectin, and sugar concentrations are interdependent; each must be in balance with the other variables to have acceptable gel formation.

Jams, jellies, preserves, marmalades, and fruit butters are products prepared from fruit juices or fruit with added sugar or both. After concentration by evaporation to a point where microbial spoilage cannot occur, the prepared products can be safely stored. Commercially, the prepared fruit products are filled into containers, usually glass, allowing the mass to set in the container.

A jelly is a semisolid food made from not less than 45 parts of fruit juice by weight to each 55 parts by weight of sugar. This substrate is concentrated to not less than 65% soluble solids. Pectin and acid may be added to overcome deficiencies that might occur in the fresh fruit. A jam has a requirement similar to jelly, with the exception that it is the fruit ingredient that is used rather than the fruit juice. Preserves retain the form of the original fruit and should consist of whole or cut fruit in a clear syrup of high sugar concentration. Otherwise the requirements are similar to those for jams and jellies. Marmalade is a product usually made from citrus fruit and is the jellylike product made from properly prepared juice and peel with sugar. It has the same requirements to achieve a gel structure as jelly. Fruit butter is a smooth, semisolid food prepared from a mixture containing not less than five parts by weight of fruit ingredient to each two parts of sugar, concentrated to not less than 43% soluble solids.

Fruits vary in their jelly-making ability. Crab apples, sour apple varieties which are not overly mature, sour berries, citrus fruits, grapes, sour cherries, and cranberries contain sufficient pectin and acid to yield good jelly naturally. Sweet cherries, quinces, and melons are rich in pectin but low in acid. Strawberries and apricots contain sufficient acid but are low in pectin. Peaches, figs, and pears are low generally in both acid and pectin. Commercially available pectin and edible acids permit a manufacturer to correct these deficiencies in fruits.

Juices. Juices are made from fruit usually lacking good market quality, but of sound character otherwise. Fruits are washed, sorted, trimmed, pulped, and extracted. The juice collected is screened and may be filtered. Some fruit juices are improved in appearance if clarified. This does not apply to juices of citrus, apricot, pineapple, and others which are more popular when cloudy. Apple, cranberry, cherry, and grape juice are examples of clarified juices which have good acceptance. These fruit juices may be preserved by canning, freezing, dehydration, or chemical additives. Sodium benzoate is a preservative permitted by Federal government regulation in fruit juices to the amount of 0.1%. Sorbic acid is another permitted preservative.

Grape juice is prepared from mature grapes which are washed, crushed, and pressed. The juice is pasteurized by heating to above 79.4°C, then stored to permit separation of suspended solids and tartrates at temperatures below 0°C. The settled juice is separated from the sediment, then filtered, bottled, and sterilized.

Apple juice is made from washed apples which are crushed and pressed. The juice is filtered and bottled, with and without clarification.

Orange juice is extracted, and the juice is separated from the oil that may be released from the skin. The juice may be screened and canned, or concentrated in a vacuum system to 60°Brix. The concentrate may then be diluted with fresh juice to 42°Brix, packaged into cans, and frozen rapidly. The frozen concentrated juice is then reconstituted by adding three volumes of clean water.

Purees. Fruit pulp may be concentrated and preserved as such by canning or freezing. Fruit purees are used mainly for manufacturing in the bakery and ice-cream industries, or to reconstitute into fresh fruit beverages and fruit-juice-flavored drinks.

Glacéed fruit. Fruit may be preserved by allowing its slow impregnation with syrup of increasing sugar concentration, developing such osmotic pressures within the tissues that microbial attack is prevented. This candied fruit is then washed, dried, and packaged. Candied fruit may be given a dip into syrup and again dried to develop a thin glaze of sugar coating; this product is called glacéed fruit.   [NORMAN W. DESROSIER]

Meat products. The manufacture of meat products includes those processes which prepare the product for consumption and increase the stability, improve the texture, increase the convenience, or alter the flavor, color, and appearance of various meat items. Various processes are employed, depending upon the desired result. These include cooking, freezing, comminuting, curing, smoking, drying, canning, and packaging. Salt, sugar, sodium or potassium nitrate or nitrite, spices and flavorings, as well as various enzymatic agents and other additives often are used. These are important both to the packer and to the consumer. The packer benefits because of the increased utilization of meat cuts and the greater stability given perishable raw materials. The consumer benefits in having available a greater variety of items at a reasonable price and in a range of textures and flavors.

The manufactured meat products can be grouped as follows: cured and pickled, cured and smoked, tenderized fresh, frozen, and canned.

Cured and pickled meats. Cured meats are those items which have had combined with them salt, sodium or potassium nitrate, and sodium or potassium nitrite. Sugar and spices are optional ingredients. The cure may or may not be added as a water solution.

The salt functions as a preservative, while the nitrate and nitrite combine with the meat pigments to form fairly stable colored compounds.

Cured meats can further be divided into two major categories, those which have been heated or cooked and those which have not. An example of cured meat which has not been heated is corned beef brisket. This item is produced by the use of a liquid curing or pickling solution. The beef brisket may be pumped with the curing pickle by means of a single- or multiple-needle injection device and then be immersed in a pickling solution for a period of 1–7 days.

In the category of cured and smoked meat products is dried beef, which is cured by being immersed in pickling solution and then heated, dried, and smoked for a prolonged period of time.

Cured and smoked meats. In the category of cured, smoked, and cooked meats is a broad line of sausage products, such as frankfurters and bologna, which differ from cured and pickled meats in that they are prepared from finely chopped or comminuted meat to which have been added salt, sugar, spices, and flavorings (Fig. 6). They may also include such items as cereals, milk powders, protein hydrolysates, and other substances.

These products are not pickled since cure penetration is obtained during an extensive mincing or chopping procedure. To secure the low temperatures often necessary for stability during the heating process, suitable amounts of ice are incorporated during the chopping operation. Ice also introduces moisture and thus increases the acceptability of the end product by assuring proper juiciness.

The products are usually heated in the smoke house to approximate internal temperatures of 65.6–76.7°C. Hardwood smoke is introduced, and the products are smoked for a length of time

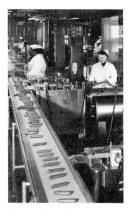

Fig. 6. Frankfurter packaging line. The moving belt carries the product to weighing and packaging operations in rear. (*Armour and Co.*)

sufficient to impart the characteristic smoked flavor. This smoking operation further increases stability of the end products by depositing on the surface a certain quantity of bacteriostatic agents.

Since these items have been heated to temperatures sufficiently high to inactivate many undesirable parasites, they are generally considered suitable to eat without any further heating.

Tenderized fresh meats. Enzyme tenderization of fresh meats, particularly of certain beef cuts, has been a practice of long standing. A proteolytic enzyme such as papaya, in fairly purified form, is usually used. The meat products are dipped in enzyme solutions and then frozen if they are to be sold in interstate commerce. Another tenderizing process involves injecting an enzyme solution into the bloodstream of the animal before slaughtering it.

Frozen meats. Many frozen meats fall in the category of processed meat products since the processes employed in their manufacture increase their utility or convenience. Examples are various breaded items such as veal cutlets, pork chops, meat sticks, and related items (Fig. 7).

The cooking and rapid freezing of certain meat dishes is a well-established practice and an example of manufacturing processes which increase the convenience of meat products for consumer use. In this category are such items as meat pies, precooked meat entrees, and various complete dinners. Generally the precooked meat items hold up better in frozen storage if they are covered with a gravy, since this covering of gravy apparently tends to reduce oxidation.

Canned meats. These are meats that are preserved by heat sterilization while enclosed in cans or glass jars. They may or may not be precooked prior to being placed in the container. If finely divided materials are to be processed and if it is desirable that they remain in this finely divided state, it is necessary that these items be precooked prior to being placed in the container. Such precooking usually is only sufficient to denature the proteins so that they do not exhibit any binding properties.

The containers are processed at 104.4–126.7°C for periods of time sufficient to inactivate most bacteria and to cause the heat-resistant type of bacteria to become dormant. This kind of treatment results in a commercially sterile product. The shelf life of these items is theoretically unlimited, although in practice it seldom exceeds 2 or 3 years.

It is often desirable to use meats which are slightly tough, since high-temperature pressure cooking causes tender meats to fall apart.

Certain canned meats are produced without inducing complete sterility. These include items such as large canned hams, luncheon meat, and spiced ham. These items generally are reacted with curing ingredients and then processed to temperatures of approximately 71.1°C while in the can. Such items generally require storage at refrigeration temperatures of 4.4–10°C and are very stable at these temperatures, having shelf life of approximately 2–3 years or longer.

Fats. These are important by-products of slaughtered livestock and the manufacture of meat products. As raw materials, fats form the base of a great variety of finished fat and oil products.

Heat treatment or rendering separates the fat

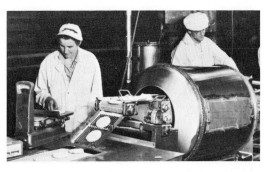

Fig. 7. Stainless-steel breading machine dips frozen veal cutlets in batter, then breads them as they pass through rotating drum. (*Armour and Co.*)

from the fatty tissue on which it is found in the animal. Of the several processes employed for rendering, the choice depends upon the type of fatty tissue to be processed and the character of the fat product desired. Rendering methods in common use include low-temperature dry rendering, high-temperature dry rendering, and steam rendering.

In the manufacture of lard a number of processes follow rendering. These include decolorizing or bleaching, deodorization, chilling, plasticizing, and packaging. In some cases lard is hydrogenated. The catalytic rearrangement of lard molecules has been widely adopted for the purpose of improving functional properties.

Rendered beef or mutton fats are termed tallows or oleo stocks, depending upon the rendering method. Tallow is processed similarly to lard. Oleo stock is grained and pressed to yield oleo oil and stearine. Rendered lard is sometimes grained and pressed, but this procedure is diminishing.

Refined lard enjoys great demand as a shortening and, with edible tallow, is increasing in use as an ingredient in the formulation of compound shortening products. Both lard and oleo products are used in the manufacture of margarine. *See* FAT AND OIL, EDIBLE.   [CLARENCE K. WIESMAN]

Poultry products. Per capita consumption of poultry in the United States amounted to 44.4 lb in 1968. A major portion was fresh (ice-packed) poultry either as whole chickens or cut-up parts. About one-third of this total was delivered to the consumer as frozen whole or cut-up poultry.

Commercial poultry production in flocks of 25,-000–100,000 chickens accounts for most of the production. In modern poultry plants, birds are dispatched humanely and allowed to bleed thoroughly before going to the scald tank to facilitate removal of feathers. Feathers are removed by mechanical equipment with a minimum of handwork required. While suspended from moving sanitary conveyors, the poultry are further processed under close inspection. All viscera are removed, along with head and feet. The eviscerated poultry are cooled to below 1.7°C in less than 2 hr in tanks containing large quantities of cracked ice. After cooling, the poultry are cut into parts and packed into boxes for freezing, packed in ice whole and ready to cook, or frozen for distribution. Poultry to be canned are processed in a similar manner, after which they are pressure cooked. The meat, removed from the bones, is placed in cans and sterilized in the usual manner or used as ingredients in chicken pot pies, turkey pot pies, and so on. Specialty items, such as roast stuffed turkey, precooked fried chicken, and precooked complete dinners, are manufactured by many firms.

[RICHARD H. FORSYTHE]

Sauces. The word sauce is derived from the Latin word salsa, meaning salted or pickled and also tart or pungent. The usage no doubt developed from the ancient practice of preserving foods by salting. Among the early types were fish sauces such as anchovy, which are within the category of salt preservation. Such sauces were followed by acid-type sauces prepared in a vinegar-type brine in which fruits, sugars, and spices had been cooked. However, the purpose of any sauce is to enhance the flavor of the food it graces, not to disguise it.

The complicated formulas of present-day sauces are the achievements of highly skilled cooks who maintain their own secret recipes and methods. Sauces range from the simplest type such as spiced vinegars (tarragon, garlic, and herb) to fruit sauces such as peach, apricot, and date combinations. The two basic types which are served hot are brown sauce and white sauce.

Brown sauce (sauce Espagnole) is the basic sauce from which most dark sauces are derived. The main ingredients from which variations may be made are browned flour, onions, meat stock, butter, spices, fat, and vegetables.

White sauce (sauce Béchamel) is the basic sauce from which most white sauces are derived. The main ingredients from which variations may be made are flour, milk, onions, spices, meat or fish stock, butter, fat, and vegetables.

Sauces which are generally emulsified are mayonnaise, salad dressing, and related dressings. The vegetable oil content of these products ranges from 30 to 85%. The oils used are mainly soybean or cottonseed and are oil-in-water emulsions. They also contain 4–10% egg yolk, with the exception of the pourable types of French dressings, which generally contain a vegetable gum or stabilizer to maintain emulsification. These products are commercially manufactured through the use of mills of colloid or homogenizing types, pressure types of homogenizers, ultrasonic homogenizers, or continuous automatic mixers combined with high-pressure units. The latest development in this field has been the introduction of instantaneous cooking followed by continuous cooling of the starch phases of salad dressings. The average commercial salad dressing contains 30–40% vegetable oil; the average mayonnaise, 75–80% vegetable oil. The difference is made up with cooled starch paste for salad dressings. This "jet-type" handling of starches has effected tremendous economies and streamlining of the entire salad-dressing industry.

The coordination of these developments has resulted in uniform final emulsification by proper dispersion due to particle-size reduction control. New commercial products such as Hollandaise and Béarnaise sauces have been direct results of these applications, together with sterilization procedures.

Improved methods of manufacture have been incorporated into the handling, cooking, homogenizing, and packing of the following types of sauces. Tomato sauce and tomato ketchup are made from tomato pulp strained free of skins and seeds and concentrated with vinegar, sugar, and spices to different solids levels. Chili sauce is tomato pulp with the seeds remaining and concentrated with added sugar, vinegar, and spices to specific solids level. Worcestershire sauce is a combination of vinegar, hydrolized proteins, vegetables, and fruits; these are allowed to age in barrels to develop balanced flavor blend. Soy sauces (chop suey sauce) contain proteins such as wheat, corn, or soybean hydrolized by carefully controlled acid hydrolysis, and may have added condiments, molasses, and caramel color. Pepper or hot sauce is made by concentrating chili or tabasco peppers and adding vinegar and salt. Meat or barbecue sauce is a combination of tomato pulp, soy base, vinegar, and spices. Mustard sauce and prepared mustards are made by grinding or milling mustard seeds and adding vinegar and spices. Applesauce is a combination of cored, sliced apples cooked with sugar, water, and spices. Cranberry sauce is made by cooking cranberries, sugar, and water to

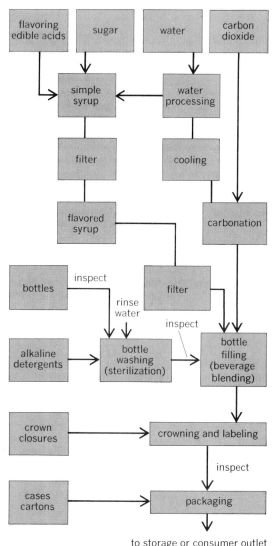

Fig. 8.   Flow diagram of bottled carbonated beverage manufacture. (*National Soft Drink Association*)

specific solids. Then, finally, there are the many types of fruit sauces, mentioned above, made from fruit such as peaches and apricots, which are concentrated, combined with sugar and spices, and packed for use as ham glazes or with meat dishes.

The texture, flavor, appearance, and uniformity have all been appreciably improved by the above developments of stabilization and manufacture. In the words of Auguste Escoffier, the father of modern cookery, "A sauce emphasizes flavor, provides contrast and makes perfection complete." The culmination of this statement is that the true duty of the perfect sauce is to enhance the dish it accompanies without affecting its intrinsic flavor.
[ALFRED J. FINBERG]

Soft drinks. Soft drinks, as the name implies, are beverages which are nonalcoholic. They may be divided into two classes: carbonated soft drinks (sometimes referred to as soda, soda water, and soda pop), and still soft drinks (similar beverages without carbonation). A flow chart of the manufacture of soft drinks is shown in Fig. 8.

The U.S. Food and Drug Administration's standard of identity for carbonated soft drinks defines them as the class of beverages made by absorbing carbon dioxide in potable water. The amount of carbon dioxide used is not less than that which will be absorbed by the beverage at a pressure of 1 atm and a temperature of 60°F. The beverage may contain buffering agents. It either contains no alcohol or only such alcohol (not in excess of 0.5% by weight of the finished beverage) as is contributed by the flavoring ingredient used. Some soft drinks, notably the cola types, are made with kola nut extract or other natural caffeine-containing extracts or both. Such drinks shall contain caffeine in a quantity not to exceed 0.02% by weight. *See* COLA.

The optional ingredients that may be used in such proportions as are reasonably required to accomplish their intended effects include one or more sweeteners; flavoring ingredients; natural and artificial color additives; acidifying agents; buffering agents; emulsifying, stabilizing, or viscosity producing agents, foaming agents, and chemical preservatives.
[HARRY E. KORAB]

Soups. Canned soups are manufactured by conventional canning processes. They may be of the clear, cream, thickened, vegetable, or vegetable-meat types. They are usually concentrates which are cooked in batches. Heat processing may be short or long. The hot batch is filled directly into cans, which are hermetically sealed and sterilized.

Frozen soups are cooked concentrates prepared batchwise in the same way as for sterilized soups. After filling, the cans are chilled and quick-frozen. Storage is at 0°F or lower until distributed. Fish-base soups, in particular, are well-suited as frozen varieties, since conventional sterilization would greatly impair their flavor.

Dehydrated soups are mixtures of dry ingredients with dehydrated stock and either dehydrated or freeze-dried vegetables or meat. After careful blending, the mixes are filled into flexible-wall bags or paper boxes, which are automatically sealed. Modern packaging developments have provided wall structures which satisfactorily protect dehydrated soups from moisture uptake.
[JOHN H. NAIR]

Vegetable products. Vegetables are edible annual plants of which the immature succulent roots, bulbs, stems, blossoms, leaves, seeds, or fruits are eaten. Certain perennial nonwoody plants of which roots, stems, leaf stalks, or leaves are consumed are also classed as vegetables. Fruit vegetables such as pumpkin and tomato are technically fruits which are eaten as vegetables. Vegetables for processing are generally referred to as truck crops.

Canning. Successful canning of vegetable products ensures the destruction of food-spoilage microorganisms and enzymes with moist heat, and the storage in functional containers to prevent reinfection and chemical deteriorations. Both tin and glass containers are satisfactory and some plastic films may be used. The food spoilage organisms associated with vegetables are generally anaerobic spore-forming bacteria able to withstand several hours at boiling water temperatures. Vegetable products are therefore sterilized at temperatures between 115.6 and 121.1°C. In this temperature range, food qualities are successfully retained, and sterilization of 1-lb containers of vegetable products can be carried out in less than 1 hr.

Because most vegetables have pH values ranging between 4.5 and 7.0, there is danger from growth of *Clostridium botulinum*, and heat processes must be such that this organism is destroyed. It is possible to lower the pH value of vegetables to below 4.5, and thereby employ less-severe heat treatments. *See* BOTULISM.

In practice, vegetables for processing are harvested at their peak quality and brought to the canning factory. They are washed, sorted, prepared by such processes as peeling, trimming, cutting, or dicing, packed into containers which are usually filled with a hot dilute salt brine, sealed, given the necessary heat sterilization, cooled, labeled, and stored for subsequent distribution.

Freezing. Because of their high moisture content, vegetables usually freeze between −3.9 and 0°C. The more rapidly vegetables are frozen, the better is the retention of fresh qualities. Storage should be at −17.8°C or lower. The successful freezing process involves a step for inactivation of enzymes in the tissues. The most satisfactory method to date has been by blanching, that is, heating the food to temperatures above 79.4°C. In addition to inactivating enzymes, heating wilts vegetables, facilitates packaging, sets food color, and removes the earthy odors of vegetables. Packaging is necessary to prevent the loss of moisture by sublimation, which causes dehydration of the tissues. In such a condition, termed "freezer burn," the tissues are irreversibly denatured.

Dehydration. For best storage stability, vegetable products must be dried to below 2% moisture content. Dehydration may be accomplished by tunnel, kiln, cabinet dryers, vacuum dryers, and freeze dryers.

Vegetables to be dried are washed, sorted, trimmed, sliced, diced, and prepared for drying. Enzyme inactivation is required, and may be accomplished by blanching in hot water or steam. Prepared vegetable tissue may be given a treatment in dilute sulfite solutions, which protect against scorching damage during dehydration. Sulfites are removed during rehydration and cooking.

Dried vegetables may be compressed in volume and packaged, an important consideration in conserving storage space. Suitable containers are needed to protect the dried tissues from acquiring moisture from the environment, which accelerates deterioration.

Pickling. The fermentation of vegetables involves the conversion of sugars to acid with the aid of selected microorganisms. The addition of salt to the fermentation vat controls and establishes a selection of the organisms capable of growth. The fermented vegetable food products have clean, characteristic flavors and qualities. In combination with canning, fermentation of food products is adequate for preservation. *See* FOOD MICRO-BIOLOGY.

Juices. Vegetables are washed, sorted, trimmed, and pulped. During pulping, stems, seeds, and skins which may be present are removed. The pulp is further screened to yield a homogeneous juice. The tomato is the most widely accepted vegetable juice, and is made by the extraction of juice and substantial pulp from red ripe tomatoes. The juice may have salt added as an optional ingredient. The juices of several vegetables, for example, tomato, carrot, parsley, and onion, may be combined into a vegetable cocktail juice. Canning is the most widely practiced method of preserving vegetable juices, although some juices have been dried successfully.

Purees. The pulped juice from vegetable tissues may be concentrated into puree. Such puree finds use in remanufacture into other food products, for example, tomato puree in the manufacture of bean sauces and in home cookery.

Pickles and relishes. Pickled vegetable products are made from fermented vegetable tissues. The fermented stock is washed free of excessive salt and packaged into containers in a spiced, flavored vinegar solution. The packaged pickles are then preserved by canning.

Pickled vegetables may be remanufactured into various forms of relishes, particularly where the shape and form of the fermented product has been damaged. Spiced, flavored vinegar solutions are added to combinations of pickled vegetables, either in large pieces or in coarse grind. Such relishes are preserved by canning, usually in glass containers.

Ketchup. Ketchup, or catsup, is a popular condiment, made by concentrating the juice and pulp of tomatoes, and adding salt, sugar, vinegar, and seasoning. Pulped tomatoes are concentrated by boiling or in a vacuum concentration unit to the desired consistency and solids content. The condiment is made into several grades, depending upon the concentration made of the tomato solids. Fancy ketchup has more than 32% of total solids present, while standard grade has as little as 25%. The prepared condiment is preserved by canning, usually in glass containers for consumer uses. Chili sauce is a similar product to which the seeds have been returned and which has larger pieces of tomatoes.   [NORMAN W. DESROSIER]

FOOD ANALOGS

Food analogs are foods created by humans from agricultural raw materials which possess the appearance, flavor, and textural qualities of the foods they are designed to simulate. They are sometimes referred to as fabricated foods.

Food analogs are fabricated from lower-cost agricultural raw materials such as grains, legumes, by-products of food processing such as cheese whey, fish muscle of little or no economic importance, and meat by-products such as bone marrow and low-cost organ meats. Such unlikely sources of protein and other nutrients as grasses, waste paper, and blood from animal slaughter have been successfully used.

Food analogs which are being marketed in the United States resemble chicken breast meat slices, beef slices, hamburger, ham slices and cubes, sausage and frankfurters, fish filets, shrimp, and scallops. Many simulated dairy products such as milk powder and cheese analogs are being sold. Over 100,000,000 lb of nonfat dry milk replacers composed of cheese whey and vegetable protein are being sold to the food processing industry, because of the reduced surplus of milk in the United States, resulting from the high cost of feed grains.

Economic and nutritional factors. Margarine was probably the first of the food analogs; it is certainly the best-known. Margarine, produced from lower-cost animal and vegetable fats and milk by-products, was developed as a low-cost replacement for butter.

With advances in science and technology, the quality of margarine advanced to the point where it is virtually indistinguishable from butter. Because of certain improvements over the natural product, such as better keeping and spreading qualities, many people today prefer margarine.

In the advanced countries, such as the United States and those of western Europe, the people have been able to obtain the high-quality protein and many other nutrients required for good nutrition from animal sources such as meat, milk, seafood, and poultry, including eggs and cheese. Other peoples of the world, in less developed countries, have not been able to obtain a plentiful supply of animal-based protein because of climatic, political, or cultural problems and thus have endured severe problems of malnutrition. Malnutrition may be due to either insufficient quantity of protein or the lower quality of vegetable protein.

In recent years, the needs of certain peoples of the world for cereal grains such as wheat and rice has been such that the pressure of demand has caused grain prices to rise astronomically. Since animals must be fed grain, meat prices have risen concurrently. There has, therefore, been a great interest in food analogs for two reasons: (1) to supplement the diets of the populace of the advanced countries since they cannot afford animal protein in the quantities heretofore consumed, and (2) to supply a palatable source of high-quality nutrients for the people of the underdeveloped countries who have never had an adequate supply of nutritive food. There is also a desire for foods designed to alleviate certain medical problems, including foods with lower saturated fat, with lower cholesterol, or free of salt or gluten.

Developing technology. The concept of food analogs is old in the culinary art. Centuries ago, the European homemaker lacking the funds to use much meat learned through the clever use of sauces, flavors, and spices to use lower-cost pro-

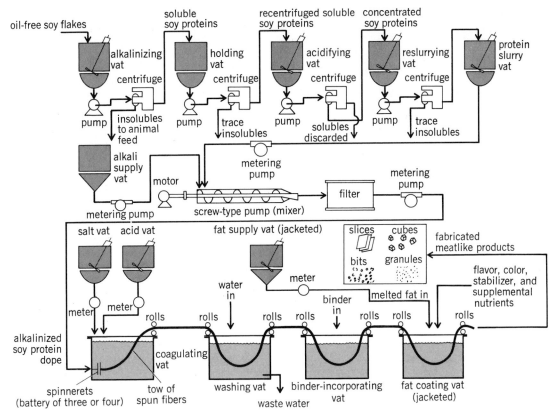

Fig. 9. Flow chart of the fiber-spinning technique. (*From Food Eng., November 1969, and used by N. R. Lockmiller,* *Increased utilization of protein in foods, Cereal Sci. Today,* *18(3):77–81, 1973*)

tein sources such as seafood in soups, stews, casseroles, and the like in such a manner that they were acceptable as "meat" dishes. The Oriental people have used hydrolyzed vegetable protein for centuries to impart a meatlike flavor to their food, predominately vegetable and seafood. Soy sauce is an example.

In more recent years, advances in science and technology have permitted improvement in this technique since the chemistry of food components is now understood more fully. Food analogs are based fundamentally on a knowledge of the chemistry and technology of protein. Protein is the nutrient of greatest importance in food analogs since it is the nutrient in shortest supply. Because of its physical characteristics, it has become the fiber which provides the textural characteristics of the food analog. *See* PROTEIN.

Using the technology developed for the production of synthetic textile fibers, such as rayon and nylon, R. A. Boyer developed in 1954 a process for preparing a synthetic meat from protein fibers. Most of the chewy textured meat analogs produced since have been based on that process.

In 1959 a method for producing meatlike analogs via a direct extrusion process, eliminating the spinning of fibers, was introduced. This method is lower in cost but produced an analog lacking some of the textural qualities of those made from spun fibers. For this reason, the resulting finely divided granules were used as meat extenders by blending with a major portion of meat in comminuted meat products such as hamburger, frankfurters, and bologna. A dual extrusion process, the Wenger Uni-Tex method, has enabled the production of

analogs with the textural characteristics of meat.

Spinning process. In the spinning process (Fig. 9), based on the Boyer process, protein, usually soya, is solubilized in an alkali aqueous media. The viscous gellike mass, called dope, is forced through a spinnerette (die) containing as many as 15,000 fine holes each with a diameter of 4/1000 of an inch. The filaments thus produced are extruded into an acid bath which sets the fiber by coagulating the protein. The fibers, averaging 20 μm in diameter, from a number of spinnerettes, usually three or four, are gathered into a bundle of 1/4-in. diameter and then a number of bundles are assembled into a "tow" of 3- to 4-in. diameter. The tows are fed into a series of baths, going through rollers at each bath, which squeeze out the salt produced by neutralization. The rolls are set successively at greater speed to stretch the fibers, which imparts the degree of tenderness or strength desired. Elongation of the fibers due to stretching is from 50 to 400%, depending on the protein used.

The first bath washes the fibers, the second incorporates binders such as egg albumin or vegetable gums, and the third, primarily for the incorporation of fat, also includes flavor, color, emulsifiers, and nutrients.

The fibers are next cut to size and compressed into the desired shape—a ham slice, chicken slice, beef cubes, and so on.

This process is the basis for most of the meat- or fishlike analogs currently available. These include the breakfast sausages and bacon strips that have gained significant consumer acceptance.

Thermoplastic extrusion process. The second basic process for the production of analogs is the

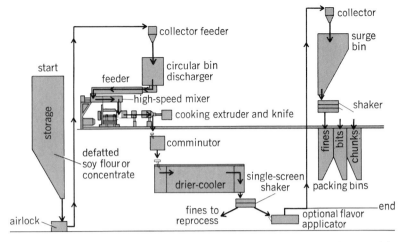

Fig. 10. Typical arrangement of extrusion cooking system for textured soy protein meat extender. (*From O. B. Smith, Textured vegetable proteins, in Lowell D. Hill, ed., World Soybean Research, Danville, IL, Interstate Printers & Publishers, 1976; used by permission*)

thermoplastic extrusion process. Not only is the process itself more economical, but lower-cost protein such as soya flour with 50% protein may be utilized, as opposed to protein isolates of 90% protein content which are required for the spinning process.

The equipment required for this process is essentially that developed for the production of snack foods (Fig. 10). Using this method, a dough is developed containing protein, fat, carbohydrates, flavors, emulsifiers, color, and nutrients. The dough is forced through the extruder/cooker barrel under high temperature and high pressure into atmospheric pressure or reduced pressure, at

which point it expands to provide the lighter density and textural characteristics of the desired analog.

As originally developed, the process produced meatlike particles after cutting and drying of the extrudate which were intended only as meat extenders, such as for addition to hamburger, meat loaf, and frankfurters as a partial supplement, not to exceed about 25% of the total meat on a rehydrated basis.

Dual extrusion process. A third method, the dual extrusion or Unitex process, is an evolution of the second method (Fig. 11). It permits the extrusion of a meat or seafood type of analog. Dies being designed for use in this process will permit the production of such sophisticated analogs as shrimp and crab meat.

During the extrusion/cooking, a number of chemical changes take place in the dough or matrix. Starch granules are gelatinized. Protein, when heated in the presence of water at the proper pH, becomes a thermoplastic gel which then can flow in a laminar fashion, enabling the protein polymers to orient parallelwise, thus providing textural structure. Certain biological growth inhibitors, such as the antitrypsin factor found in raw soya protein, are inactivated. Most importantly, the soluble proteins are denatured so that they are less soluble but digestible.

Volatile phenolic off-flavors which give the raw soybean its bitter beany flavor are flashed off in the escaping steam, rendering the finished product more palatable.

The product produced by the original thermoplastic extrusion process possesses an open, elongated cell structure with a pocketed, somewhat twisted appearance having a density of 10 to 22 lb/ft³. With the advent of the dual extrusion

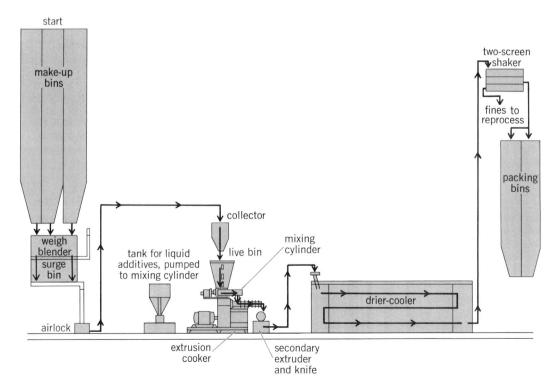

Fig. 11. The Uni-Tex process for production of a new type of meat or seafood analog. (*From O. B. Smith, Textured vegetable proteins, in Lowell D. Hill, ed., World Soybean Research, Danville, IL, Interstate Printers & Publishers, 1976; used by permission*)

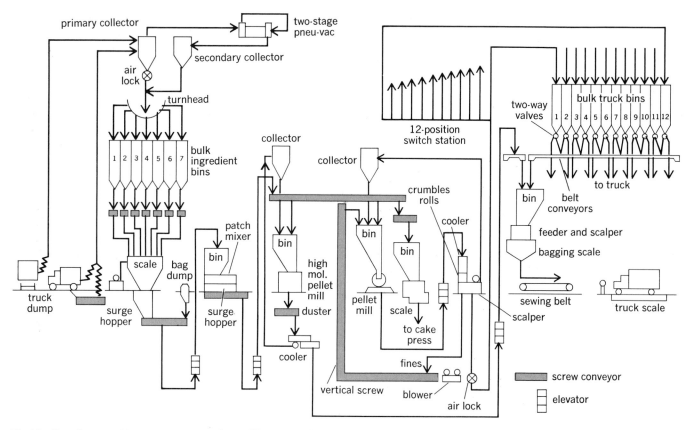

Fig. 12. Flow diagram of formula feed plant. (*Sprout Waldron and Co., Inc.*)

process, a dense product, with even, parallel, rectilinear structures, having a density of 22 to 27 lb/ft³ is produced. The structure is untwisted and devoid of gas pockets, thus lacking the sponginess of the original extruded product and therefore having the chewiness of meat pieces.

Lipton process. A fourth process, known as the Lipton process, was actually designed to restructure meats for dry-soup manufacture. Meat will vary widely in chewiness, tenderness, color, and other physical characteristics. To produce a more uniform meat particle, meat pieces are ground and made up into a dough with a protein source, egg albumin as a binder, and color and other additives. The matrix is then extruded through a hamburger-grinderlike device, cut into small uniform pieces, and dried. There is apparently no application other than dry soup mixes for this type product.   [WILLIAM H. KNIGHTLY]

FOODS INTENDED FOR ANIMAL CONSUMPTION

While for the most part foods processed for consumption by animals are handled with the same care and conditions of hygiene, they are not subjected to the same inspections by governmental agencies as foods intended for human consumption.

Animal feed. Feed processing involves a series of operations requiring considerable equipment, applied skill, and organized effort to procure, grind, and blend the variety of raw materials used in present-day feeds. There are approximately 2000 feed-processing plants in the United States, ranging from large commercial enterprises and large feed lot operations to relatively small units.

Feed ingredients, such as grain, are cleaned to remove foreign material, ground fine in a hammer mill, and stored in bins equipped with feeders for removing known quantities when preparing the feed blend. Approximately 75% of the weight of most finished feed consists of processed cereal grains such as corn, sorghum grain, oats, or barley. Bran, shorts, and red dog (products resulting from the flour-milling industry); distillers' dried grains (by-products of the fermentation industry); soybean oil meal, cottonseed oil meal, or linseed oil meal (by-products of the oil-extraction industries); and dehydrated grasses are common constituents of formula feeds. The by-products and other ingredients are also stored in bins. The remaining 25% of the feed consists of ingredients which add to the basic constituents special nutritional properties, such as extra protein or fat content from either vegetable or animal sources and the essential amino acids, vitamins, disease-preventing drugs, and hormones. *See* NUTRITION.

There are two systems of manufacturing formula feeds: the continuous and the batch methods. In the continuous method, the proportion of each ingredient required in the formula is compounded by percentage feeders continuously metering each required ingredient into a conveyor feeding into a mixer (Fig. 12). The batch system accumulates the feed in a batch scale hopper. Increments by weight of each ingredient are added to the batch, which is discharged to a mixer that distributes the constituents uniformly throughout the mix. The finished formula feed may be packed as it comes from the mixer; or it may have liquids added, such as molasses, fish solubles, and stabilized animal fats; or it may be pelleted with or without added liquids. Pelleting acts to compact and bind all ingredients into small round or rectangular shapes $\frac{1}{8}$–1 in. in cross section. Pellets are considered more palatable and assure the consumption of all constituents of the formula, reducing losses due to wind, dust, or spilling. When pellets are too large or compact, they are crushed with a pair of specially corrugated cracking rolls that break each pellet into two or three parts, called granules or crumbles. *See* ANIMAL-FEED COMPOSITION.

The finished feed, if necessary, may be dried to assure practical, safe storage without development of bacterial damage, or it may be packed in paper or burlap sacks of various sizes. Feed is also handled in bulk for delivery to feed lots in quantities varying from 1 to 50 tons. Bulk shipments are made by truck or rail.   [JOHN A. SHELLENBERGER]

Pet foods. These are usually nutritionally complete products which adequately support growth and life, even if fed exclusively.

Pet foods are made from proper mixtures of meat, fish, fowl, bone, cereal, milk, minerals, and vitamins. The minerals and vitamins are added in quantities necessary to augment the natural foodstuffs. They may be prepared in various finished forms, canned, frozen, or dried.

The canned products are sterilized at high temperatures to permit storage without refrigeration. The frozen variety often is limited to raw meat or seafood. Dry items are stable at room temperature, though usually not as long as canned items.

Those pet foods which include meat contain a fairly large proportion of highly nutritious organ meats as well as other meat products.

The manufacture of the canned variety is fairly standardized in that the grinding, blending, filling, and sterilizing procedures are well known. The dry variety, particularly dry dog food, can be manufactured in a number of different ways, ranging from pelletizing of dry ingredients to hot-air and vacuum drying of moistened, expanded pastes and extrusions. Little or no preparation is needed for the frozen products since these are generally raw.

A significant innovation is intermediate-moisture pet food that keeps without canning or refrigeration. Careful control of amount of "active water" in the product avoids spoilage.

Aseptic canning of certain pet foods appears entirely possible. In this procedure the product is sterilized outside the can and then filled into a sterilized container, whereupon it requires no further cooking and is stable at room temperature for indefinite periods.   [CLARENCE K. WIESMAN]

Bibliography: A. M. Altschul, *Proteins: Their Chemistry and Politics*, 1965; American Meat Institute Foundation, *The Science of Meat and Meat Products*, 1960; A. E. Bailey, *Industrial Oil and Fat Products*, 1964; C. H. Campbell, *Campbell's Book*, 1950; H. F. Conway and R. A. Anderson, Protein fortified extruded food products, *Cereal Sci. Today*, 18(4):94–97, 1973; Feed Production School, Inc., *Feed Production Handbook*, 1961; Food and Agriculture Organization of the United Nations, *Yearbook of Fishery Statistics*, vols. 38 and 39, 1974; B. Graham-Rack and R. Binsted, *Hygiene in Food Manufacturing and Handling*, 1964; F. L. Hart and H. J. Fisher, *Modern Food Analysis*, 1969; A. Heath, *The Book of Sauces*, 1948; M. J. Jacobs, *The Chemistry and Technology of Food and Food Products*, 1951; M. A. Joslyn and J. L. Heid, *Food Processing Operations*, vol. 3, 1964; N. R. Lockmiller, Increased utilization of protein in foods, *Cereal Sci. Today*, 18(13):77–81, 1973; S. A. Matz, *Bakery Technology and Engineering*, 1960; S. A. Matz (ed.), *The Chemistry and Technology of Cereals as Food and Feed*, 1959; G. J. Mountney, *Poultry Products Technology*, 1966; J. Owens, *The Book of Sauces*, 1947; E. Parker and H. Litchfield, *Food Plant Sanitation*, 1962; S. V. Poultney, *Vinegar Products*, 1948; J. Rackis, D. J. Sessa, and D. H. Honig, *Soybean Protein Foods*, ARS 71–35, U.S. Department of Agriculture, 1967; O. B. Smith, in George Inglett (ed.), *Fabricated Foods*, 1975; U.S. Department of Commerce, *Bulletin*, 1967; U.S. Department of Commerce, NOAA, National Marine Fisheries Service, *Fisheries of the United States, 1975*, Current Fish. Stat. no. 6900, March 1976; U.S. Department of the Interior, *Fisheries of the United States–1967*, 1968.

Food microbiology

The branch of biology that deals with the microorganisms involved in the spoilage, contamination, and preservation of food. All kinds of microorganisms can find their way into food through the ordinary routes of contamination, and nearly all of them will find food items suitable media in or on which to grow. Foods handled by people are subject to contamination from all kinds of disease-producing organisms. Food microbiologists must know how to detect the disease-producing organisms, how to prevent their entrance into food, and how to destroy them if they are present. This public health aspect of the subject is very important and involves the use of many special tests and experimental animals. *See* FOOD PRESERVATION.

The extent to which food is contaminated or mishandled is reflected in the number of microorganisms present. Therefore, the food microbiologist must be concerned with the standardization of tests designed to determine the number of organisms and, where possible, the establishment of standards of permissible contamination. With this goes the problem of proper standards of sanitation in the handling of food to avoid unnecessary contamination and growth of microorganisms. It involves an understanding of sanitary engineering practices and equipment design that facilitates adequate cleaning, and a knowledge of how to detect, measure, and reduce contamination.

Another aspect of food microbiology concerns food preservation. Some foods are preserved and desirably flavored by fermentation processes; therefore, the specialist needs to be familiar with the organisms involved as well as their physiology and behavior in fermentation.

Analytical procedures for vitamins and amino acids often use bacteria as assay tools, so that this activity also becomes a concern of the food microbiologist.   [HARLYN O. HALVORSON]

The following sections discuss various aspects of food microbiology concerned with fermented food, fruits and vegetables, eggs, shellfish, meat, and canned foods.

Fermented food. There are a number of foods which acquire their special character (flavor, texture, aroma) by a fermentation process involving the participation of bacteria, yeasts, and molds, singly or in combination. Most commonly the microorganisms cause a transformation of carbohydrates (often to lactic acid) and of proteins. Examples of fermented foods are sauerkraut, fermented pickles, Spanish-type olives, certain dairy products (buttermilk, acidophilus milk, yogurt, kefir, kumiss, leben, and various types of cheese) and certain fermented Oriental foods. In the broadest sense fermented alcoholic beverages, vinegar, and yeast-leavened bread may be included, as well as such products as cocoa, coffee, and tea in which microbes participate in the production of the products of commerce. *See* COFFEE; DISTILLED SPIRITS; MILK; TEA.

Sauerkraut. Sauerkraut is made by adding about 2.5% salt (weight basis) to shredded cabbage. The salt draws out the plant juice, which undergoes a natural lactic acid fermentation because of the presence of sugars. Usually the heterofermentative *Leuconostoc mesenteroides* develops first, producing lactic and acetic acids, ethanol, mannitol, and carbon dioxide, CO_2. It has a low acid tolerance and when the acid content reaches 0.7–1.0%, it is replaced by the homofermentative *Lactobacillus plantarum*. This organism produces only lactic acid. In the last stages of fermentation *Lactobacillus brevis* (heterofermentative) completes the process, bringing total acid content to 1.7–1.8%, of which about a fifth is acetic acid.

Cucumber pickles. There are many kinds of pickles, some of which are made by a fermentation process. The fermentation of cucumbers is somewhat complex because of the different brining procedures in use. In the manufacture of fermented salt stock an initial brine concentration of about 8% is gradually increased to 16–18% over a period of 6 weeks or more. During this period salt-tolerant lactic acid bacteria (*L. plantarum, L. brevis,* and *Pediococcus cerevisiae*) carry out the fermentation. The acid formed is lactic acid and the total amount is usually 0.6–1.0%. When the pickles are packed, much of the salt and acid is leached out and replaced by vinegar, lactic acid, or both, and herbs and spices. In some types of pickles a limited natural fermentation is allowed to proceed in the presence of a low salt concentration (3–5%). Partly fermented dill pickles must be pasteurized to stop the fermentation. They are often referred to as Polish, overnight, or fresh-fermented dill pickles. Innumerable variations in processing techniques are in use.

Spanish-type olives. For Spanish-type olives the particular brine treatment depends on the olive variety. After the olives are treated with lye to remove the bitter glucoside, they are brined and undergo a lactic acid fermentation. Final salt content is usually 6.5% and lactic acid 0.8–1.2%.

Fruits and vegetables. Fruits and vegetables are susceptible to attack by fungi, yeasts, and bacteria. Infection may occur in the field or orchard, in which case plant pathogenic (parasitic) organisms are involved. After harvest and during storage of the fresh product, parasitic organisms may continue their activity, but in addition saprophytic organisms (those that live on dead organic matter) become active by gaining entrance to the plant tissues through damaged areas. After fruits and vegetables are processed by canning, freezing, or dehydration, or made into modified products (juices, purees, syrups), specific types of saprophytic or-

ganisms are encountered as spoilage organisms. *See* PLANT DISEASE; YEAST.

Yeasts and molds are primarily responsible for the spoilage of fruits and fruit products, whereas bacteria are the most common cause of spoilage in processed vegetables. Environmental conditions of storage of fresh as well as processed products determine to a large extent what organisms will develop. These conditions include temperature of storage, presence or absence of oxygen or other gases, humidity, and such intrinsic factors as the pH of the product, its chemical composition, and its moisture content. In any situation all these factors must be considered interrelated to each other.

Cold storage. During cold storage (above −1 to −0.5°C, the freezing point of most fruits and vegetables) the growth of microbes is merely retarded, but not prevented. Those organisms that grow optimally at temperatures below 20°C (psychrophiles) are especially troublesome. In some products, such as bananas and avocados, physiological chilling injury occurs when they are stored below 45–55°F, and with injury microbial development is accelerated. In other products, such as tomatoes and citrus fruits, storage near the freezing point greatly increases their susceptibility to microbial attack upon return to room temperature. Carbon dioxide gas is sometimes used (5–10%) in the atmosphere of cold storage rooms to retard mold development (especially for apples). Periodic exposure to sulfur dioxide has been found beneficial in the storage of fresh California table grapes. While freezing arrests the growth of spoilage organisms, only a limited percentage of the population is killed, so that upon thawing rapid spoilage of the frost-damaged tissues results.

Drying. Preservation by drying is based on creating a product with high soluble solids content. When drying conditions are poor, sun-drying of fruits may result in the development of osmophilic yeast and molds. Spoilage of blanched vegetables has been observed in dehydrators when humidity control was neglected and drying was slow. The spoilage is due to starch fermentation by *Aerobacter aerogenes*.

Canning. In canned vegetables thermophilic sporeforming bacteria from the soil are most troublesome. *Bacillus stearothermophilus* and *B. coagulans* are responsible for flat sour spoilage of canned vegetables. *Clostridium nigrificans* causes sulfide stinkers by producing H_2S. Hard swells are caused by the thermophilic *Č. thermosaccharolyticum*. It produces CO_2 and hydrogen (H_2). Mesophilic sporeformers occur only in underprocessed canned vegetables or in leaky cans. *C. botulinum* originates in the soil and is a serious cause of food poisoning; outbreaks occasionally occur in home-canned vegetables which have a pH higher than 4.5. [HERMAN J. PHAFF]

Eggs. The interior of the freshly laid egg is usually sterile; subsequent microbial quality is determined by sanitation and storage conditions. No definite pattern characterizes the type of contamination that develops in the interior of eggs, since the microbial flora is chiefly a reflection of the environment. Cracks in the shell and high humidity encourage microbial invasion. Elevated temperatures accelerate spoilage. Organoleptically unsound eggs are called rots; black rots result from anaerobic proteolytic bacteria producing hydrogen sulfide. Molds invade shell eggs under storage at high humidity. Commercial dried eggs if properly processed contain fewer microorganisms than the liquid eggs used as raw materials. *See* EGG PROCESSING.

Shellfish. The microorganisms inhabiting both the surface and interior of shellfish are a reflection of the microbial flora of the water from which they are taken. Contamination by sewage-polluted waters is of major concern. Numerous outbreaks of typhoid fever have been traced to contaminated shellfish. However, holding contaminated shellfish for a time in unpolluted water results in natural purification. Numerous organisms may be responsible for the spoilage of shellfish. The specific type of spoilage is largely determined by the water from which the fish are harvested. The speed of spoilage is determined both by the initial level of organisms and by the storage temperature but occurs fairly rapidly.

Meat. Meats are not only stabilized by all common preservation methods, but, in addition, the preparation and merchandizing of many items involve a combination of two or more preservation procedures. Fresh red meats are refrigerated. Cured meats such as ham, bacon, and sausage contain chemical preservatives (salt, nitrate, nitrite) but are, in addition, heat processed and stored under refrigeration. Fresh and cured meats are also canned. With severe heat processing a shelf-stable product is produced; certain cured products, such as hams, are canned with only mild heat processing, and the resulting product is not shelf-stable but must be refrigerated. In certain products stability is attained in part through other processes: fermentation (thuringer), drying (hard sausage), smoking (bacon), and impregnation with vinegar (pig's feet). Each type of meat product has a characteristic microbiological flora; the nature of the flora is determined more by processing methods than by the type of microorganisms which predominate in the raw meat.

Fresh meats. Fresh meats as cut from the chilled animal carcass are contaminated with microorganisms characteristic of the living animal's environment. The living tissues of the animal, with the exception of the gastrointestinal system, are sterile but become contaminated during the slaughtering and dressing operations. While the majority of the contaminants on fresh meats will not grow during refrigerated storage, those that do survive on refrigerated fresh meats consist almost entirely of cold-loving bacteria which are able to grow during refrigerated storage. These organisms grow on the meat surfaces and produce alkaline end products.

Cured meats. These are contaminated by acid-producing bacteria, similar to those which sour milk, that do not require oxygen for growth. The bacteria characteristic of fresh meats are apparently excluded from cured products by the presence of salt, nitrate, and nitrite.

Canned meats. Canned meats are either "commercially sterile" (shelf-stable) or carry a microflora consisting of spore-forming bacteria. In perishable canned meats the surviving spores are prevented from growing by refrigeration. In shelf-stable cured canned meats the surviving spores are kept dormant through heat shock processing combined with residual curing ingredients.

Canned-food spoilage. This may be traced to the growth of microorganisms which survive processing or enter the can through leaks after processing. Spoilage of underprocessed canned foods is almost always due to the growth of heat-resistant spore-forming bacteria. Leaky cans, conversely, show a spoilage microflora reflecting the environment outside the can; usually heat-resistant bacteria are not involved.

Medium- and low-acid foods. Such foods as peas, corn, and milk may exhibit flat-sour spoilage wherein surviving spores germinate and produce acid but no gas during growth, the unopened can appearing normal. Heat-resistant spores capable of growth at elevated temperatures (above 50°C) may cause swelling of cans of low acid food and the appearance of cheesy or sour odors. In other cases putrefactive anaerobic spore-forming bacteria lead to swelling and putrid odors. In still other cases heat-resistant thermophilic spore-forming bacteria produce hydrogen sulfide, H_2S, which imparts a rotten-egg odor to the product.

Acid foods. Such foods as tomato juice and canned fruits receive lower heat treatments and show somewhat different spoilage. Acid-tolerant spore-formers may produce abnormally high amounts of acid without swelling the can. Non-spore-formers, such as yeasts, molds, and lactic acid bacteria, may spoil can contents with or without can swelling.

With the exception of putrefactive spoilage, none of the above abnormalities is a public health hazard. Canned foods are processed in such a manner that chance of contracting botulism, caused by the toxin of a putrefactive bacterium, is lessened. Commercially canned foods have been free of the botulism hazard for over 30 years. *See* BOTULISM.

[JOHN H. SILLIKER]

Bibliography: J. C. Ayres et al. (eds.), *Chemical and Biological Hazards in Food*, 1969; C. L. Duddington, *Micro-organisms as Allies: The Industrial Use of Fungi and Bacteria*, 1961; W. C. Frazier, *Food Microbiology*, 2d ed., 1967; L. W. Slanetz et al., *Microbiological Quality of Foods*, 1963; H. H. Weiser, *Practical Food Microbiology and Technology*, 2d ed., 1971.

Food preservation

The science and art of employing processes which protect food from degradation by rodents, insects, microbes, enzymes, or undesirable chemical alteration. A variety of processes may be used, either alone or in combination, including refrigeration, freezing, canning, drying and dehydration, salting, fermentation, chemical additives, and radiation.

Refrigeration. Modern industry commonly uses cooling as an effective means to extend the shelf life of a variety of perishable foods. Commercial and household refrigeration units effectively maintain low nonfreezing temperatures which preserve the desirable characteristics of perishable foods for reasonable periods of time. The reduced temperature retards the growth of spoilage microorganisms such as bacteria, yeasts, and molds. For good refrigeration the temperature should be lower than 7.5°C but high enough to keep the food from freezing. A special commercial refrigeration technique is "controlled atmosphere," in which the atmosphere of the refrigerated space is altered, the oxygen content is markedly reduced, the carbon dioxide content increased, and the humidity controlled. This procedure effectively maintains the quality of many fruits, such as apples, for as long as a year.

Freezing. Frozen foods are popular items. They keep for long periods of time when properly prepared, packaged, and stored. Microbial action is arrested, but the microbes are not necessarily destroyed. Enzymatic action is markedly reduced but not eliminated. To further reduce enzymatic activity, foods having active enzymes, such as fresh vegetables, undergo a special heat treatment known as blanching. The blanching process consists of quickly heating the product to near boiling temperatures, then cooling it prior to freezing. Modern mechanical refrigeration units maintain the proper temperature during storage, distribution, and marketing of frozen foods. Each food type has its own recommended storage period, after which undesirable off-flavors slowly develop.

Canning. Commercial canning (thermal processing) as a means to preserve foods dates back to the days of Napoleon. Today foods to be canned are placed in hermetically sealed containers and then heat-processed. The heat treatment must be severe enough to destroy the spores of toxigenic organisms that may be present. The thermal process, involving the required time span and temperature of heating, depends on the particular food product and the container size. The equipment may be a pressure container (retort) or a more sophisticated apparatus which allows for a continuous operation. The operator of the thermal processing equipment must possess a certificate showing proper instruction in the use of such equipment. Home canners should always follow approved techniques. Pressure cookers should always be used for vegetables such as peas, beans, and beets. *See* FOOD ENGINEERING.

Drying and dehydration. Drying is one of the oldest methods of food preservation. It is a process copied from nature. Cereal grains and nuts are preserved by natural drying during ripening. Sun drying has been practiced for centuries. The use of heat from an energy source to speed up the removal of water is a more modern application and is referred to as dehydration. The water content of the food is reduced to a critical level below which microorganisms cannot grow. This level is related to the water-binding properties of the food, hence such water does not act as free moisture. Microorganisms need free water in order to grow and multiply. Intermediate-moisture foods are those in which the moisture content is reduced to a level low enough to keep spoilage microorganisms from growing but moist enough for the food to have improved palatability characteristics. Semimoist pet foods are common articles of commerce. Semimoist human foods are now being developed.

Salting. Salt was used in the preservation of food, either alone or in combination with drying, before recorded history. Large quantities of salt are used in the brining of pickles and olives to ensure that proper fermentation develops. Salt and salt solutions serve a variety of functions in a great variety of food processing operations.

Fermentation. Fermentation is a biological process which depends on certain microorganisms to produce chemical substances which inhibit the growth of undesirable microorganisms. One such action is the inhibition of toxin-producing bacteria by the lactic acid produced from carbohydrates in the fermented food. There are three primary examples of food preservation via fermentation by microorganisms: (1) yeast fermentation, resulting in the production of alcohol, (2) the bacterial fermentation of alcohol to acetic acid (vinegar), and (3) the bacterial fermentation of carbohydrates to lactic acid and related by-products. While the natural flora of the product to be fermented has historically been the source of the necessary microorganisms, now in most dairy fermentations and in many pickle and sausage operations, commercial starter cultures are used. Foods involved in lactic fermentation include soured milk, butter, cheeses, pickles, sauerkraut, olives, breads, and sausages. *See* FERMENTATION.

Chemical additives. Food additives are nonnutritive substances added intentionally to food, generally in small quantities, to improve its appearance, flavor, texture, or storage properties. They must meet legal requirements. The uses and compounds are many and varied, but all serve to impart desirable qualities to the food, such as the prevention of rancidity or the inhibition of microbial growth. Butylated hydroxyanisole (BHA) and butylated hydroxytoluene (BHT) are commonly used to prevent rancidity in fatty foods. Benzoic acid and sorbic acid, and their salts or derivatives, are used as antimicrobial compounds. They are most effective in acid or slightly acid foods. *See* FOOD.

Radiation. The potential of using ionizing radiations for the stabilization of perishable foods has been under investigation since the early 1950s. There are a variety of potential applications. Cold sterilization requires a radiation intensity of 2–7 megarads, whereas a dose sufficient to inhibit the sprouting of potatoes in storage is between 6000 and 9000 rads. A dose of 40,000–60,000 rads is used in an insect deinfestation process for white flour. The full potential of ionizing radiations in food preservation is yet to be developed. *See* FOOD MICROBIOLOGY; FOOD SPOILAGE. [Z. JOHN ORDAL]

Bibliography: N. W. Desrosier, *The Technology of Food Preservation*, 3d ed., 1970; J. L. Heid and M. A. Joslyn, *Fundamentals of Food Processing Operations, Ingredients, Methods and Packaging*, 1967; N. N. Potter, *Food Science*, 2d ed., 1973.

Food science

The applied science which deals with the chemical, biochemical, physical, physicochemical, and biological properties of foods. Chemical properties of foods include; (1) composition, that is, constituents, such as proteins, fats, and carbohydrates, which make up food; (2) chemical reactions which occur when foods are processed (canned, frozen, dried, irradiated, and so on), packaged, or stored; and (3) interactions of food constituents with chemical additives, such as bleaching agents and antioxidants. Biochemical properties are related to postharvest (plant) or postmortem (animal) enzymatic activity, and to the presence of physiologically active constituents, such as vitamins and other nutrients which are essential to man or animals. Physical properties include color, specific gravity, refractive index, viscosity, texture, and various thermal constants. Physicochemical properties relate to the behavior of colloids, solutions, crystals, and so on, occurring in foods. Biological properties pertain to the activity of macroorganisms, such as insects or parasites, and microorganisms, including bacteria, molds, yeasts, and viruses, found in foods (which are involved in spoilage and fermentation), as well as the effects of natural or induced toxicants. *See* FOOD MANUFACTURING; FOOD MICROBIOLOGY.

Food science provides the basic knowledge for food technology, which is the application of science and engineering to the research, production, processing, packaging, distribution, preparation, and utilization of foods.

Food science is taught in more than 40 universities in the United States; many offer degrees.

The professional organization for food scientists is the Institute of Food Technologists, with over 9000 members in the United States and abroad. Phi Tau Sigma is the international honor society for food scientists, who may be admitted in recognition of professional achievement in the field.

The Institute of Food Technologists publishes *Food Technology*, where applied research articles and news of the society appear, and *The Journal of Food Science*, which carries more fundamental research reports.

Professionals in food science are employed in university teaching and research; in Federal, state, and municipal inspection and regulatory agencies; and in government and industrial research laboratories. They are also employed in product development, quality control, sanitation, production, packaging, and technical sales and service within companies producing food products or providing ingredients, machinery, packaging materials, and other supplies for food processors.

[GIDEON E. LIVINGSTON; MYRON SOLBERG]

Food spoilage

Foods undergo many different types of spoilage, resulting in abnormal colors, flavors, odors, or in other changes, such as consistency. Spoilage cannot be equated to danger to the consumer; indeed, in most instances, foods which contain poison of either chemical or biological origin show no external evidence of spoilage.

Perishable foods. Fresh meat, vegetables, and fruits have a limited shelf life, after which time spoilage is expected, even though all phases of processing and storage may be optimal. The shelf life of perishable foods is determined by the initial quality of the raw materials, the method of processing, and subsequent handling.

Spoilage of perishable products is usually characteristic, being determined primarily by the chemical nature of the food, the type of microbial contamination it carries, its packaging, and its storage condition. For instance, raw milk sours because of the activity of lactic acid–forming bacteria. Fresh meats develop characteristic slime and off-odors as a result of the growth of bacteria which produce alkaline conditions. Frankfurters and certain other cured meat products develop a surface slime due to the growth of acid-forming bacteria similar to those found in dairy products.

Shelf-stable foods. Canned and dried foods are processed with the aim of producing a food which may be stored for indefinite periods, even at warm temperatures, without undergoing apparent change. Stability is imposed by such factors as heat (canned foods), drying (dried vegetables), and chemicals (addition of acid, such as in mayonnaise).

Spoilage of shelf-stable foods is, by definition, an abnormal and unexpected condition. Underprocessing of canned food leads to unstable products in which the contents of the can undergo putrefaction or fermentation with the development of abnormal odors, consistencies, and flavors. Usually the instability of the product is evinced by the swelling of the unopened can. Insufficient dehydration or improper storage in humid atmospheres leads to off-conditions in dried food products. Failure to add sufficient vinegar to mayonnaise renders the product subject to microbial attack.

Spoilage mechanism. Chemical changes are responsible for spoilage. These changes are brought about through enzyme action. These enzymes may have their origin in the food material or may be elaborated by microorganisms such as yeasts, molds, and bacteria which contaminate the product. In general, enzymes derived from foods themselves are of secondary importance to those elaborated by microorganisms; however, when foods are held under conditions which preclude microbial action, the natural enzymes in the food materials may be the primary reason for spoilage. The fat-splitting enzymes in frozen foods cause this type of spoilage.

Yeast and mold spoilage. This is most characteristic of foods with high acid or sugar content. Molds characteristically grow on the surface; yeasts which are capable of growth in the absence of air may spoil food either by the formation of slime or by fermentation of the entire food mass. Molds occasionally present a spoilage problem in cream, eggs, various sugar products, butter, and cheese. Yeasts are associated with the fermentation of candy, butter, mayonnaise, catsup, syrup, olives and pickles. In certain foods, the addition of benzoic, propionic, and sorbic acids aids in the control of yeasts and molds.

Bacterial spoilage. This type of food-product spoilage is as varied as the capabilities of this large group of microorganisms. The major classes of food substances are all subject to some form of bacterial decomposition, and within each class, there is frequently a major type or pattern of spoilage which is characteristic. The most important determinants with respect to the type of spoilage are the methods of processing and storage. For example, the spoilage of fresh meats is primarily a surface phenomenon involving highly aerobic bacteria. If, however, fresh meats are stored in the absence of oxygen, they will undergo spoilage of a different type, a spoilage brought about by lactic acid–forming bacteria of the same general characteristics as those which spoil fresh milk. The same fresh meat product, if canned, may undergo spoilage, but the bacteria involved are heat-resistant forms which survive processing, the so-called spore-forming bacteria. By analogy, if fresh milk were aerated, the same organisms which spoil fresh meats could be expected to spoil the fresh milk; similarly, spore-forming organisms are involved in the spoilage of canned milk products.

Abnormal or unusual spoilages. Abnormal or unusual spoilages of food products occur periodically. Such spoilage may be seasonal, regional, or entirely haphazard in appearance. In extreme cases a food plant may have to cease manufacture of a product due to contamination with undesirable microorganisms responsible for peculiar spoilage. problems. Examples of such unusual spoilage include green discoloration of milk; gas pockets and in extreme cases the explosion of cheese. In most cases, a particular organism or group is responsible for each of these conditions. *See* FOOD ENGINEERING; FOOD MICROBIOLOGY; FOOD PRESERVATION.

[JOHN H. SILLIKER]

Food technology

The application of science and engineering to the refining, manufacturing, and handling of foods. In this sense it is essentially the same as food engineering. However, many food technologists by training and experience are food scientists rather than engineers. *See* FOOD ENGINEERING.

As defined by the Institute of Food Technologists, "food technology is primarily based on the fundamentals of chemistry, physics, biology, and microbiology, any of which sciences may find an expression through an engineering operation.

"Knowledge of food technology enables its possessor to develop new products, processes, and equipment, to select proper raw materials, to understand and control manufacturing operations, to solve technical problems of food manufacture and distribution, including those involved in plant sanitation, and those affecting the nutritional value and public health safety of foods, and to know the fundamental changes of composition and of physical condition of foodstuffs which may occur during and subsequent to the industrial processing of the foodstuffs."

Degrees in food technology are given by some leading colleges and universities. However, the amount of mathematics, physics, and engineering principles included in the curriculums varies considerably. That is why some food technologists are trained as food engineers, but others are primarily food scientists. The former are best qualified for food manufacturing and processing operations, the latter for research and quality control.

Specialized branches of food technology, science, and engineering are taught in many institutions of higher education, primarily state colleges and universities with agricultural schools. Thus, it is possible to obtain degrees in dairy, cereal, fruit and vegetable, baking, meat, and brewing chemistry or technology.

Specialized phases of food technology, such as food chemistry, bacteriology, and nutrition, are taught in many schools with scientific curriculums.

To the extent that they are applied in developing and growing suitable raw materials for manufacture and processing, horticulture and animal husbandry are food sciences.

[FRANK K. LAWLER]

Foot-and-mouth disease

A highly contagious virus disease of economic importance, infecting cattle, pigs, sheep, and goats. It is characterized by fever, salivation, and formation of vesicles in the mouth and pharynx and on the feet. It may be transmitted to man.

Epizootics may be characterized by high mortality rates. Survivors are poor producers of milk and meat. The infective virus is about 22 mμ in diameter, and is considered a member of the rhinovirus subgroup of picornaviruses. A variety of experimental animals and tissue cultures can be infected.

Diagnosis is by isolation of virus and by serologic tests.

Formalin-inactivated virus vaccines immunize, but only temporarily. Attenuated-virus vaccines have been developed and used in the field with reported success. In serious epizootics all susceptible animals in the area are slaughtered, and strict quarantine is observed. To prevent human infection, boiling or pasteurizing of farm products under suspicion should be adequate.

[JOSEPH L. MELNICK]

Frost

A covering of ice in one of several forms produced by the freezing of supercooled water droplets on objects colder than 32°F. The partial or complete killing of vegetation, by freezing or by temperatures somewhat above freezing for certain sensitive plants, also is called frost. Air temperatures below 32°F sometimes are reported as "degrees of frost"; thus 10°F is 22 degrees of frost.

Frost forms in exactly the same manner as dew except that the individual droplets that condense in the air a fraction of an inch from a subfreezing object are themselves supercooled, that is, colder than 32°F. When the droplets touch the cold object, they freeze immediately into individual crystals. When additional droplets freeze as soon as the previous ones are frozen, and hence are still close to the melting point because all the heat of fusion has not been dissipated, amorphous frost or rime results.

At more rapid rates of condensation, the drops form a film of supercooled water before freezing, and glaze or glazed frost ("window ice" on house windows, "clear ice" on aircraft) generally follows. Glaze formation on plants, buildings and other structures, and especially on wires sometimes is called an ice storm, or a silver frost storm, or thaw.

At slower deposition rates, such that each crystal cools well below the melting point before the next joins it, true crystalline or hoar frosts form. These include fernlike assemblages on snow surfaces, called surface hoar; similar feathery plumes in cold buildings, caves, and crevasses, called depth hoar; and the common window frost or ice flowers on house windows.

So-called killing frosts occur on clear autumn nights, when radiative cooling of ground, air, and vegetation causes plant fluids to freeze. At such times, the air temperature measured in a shelter 5–7 ft above ground usually is at least 5°F below freezing, but such standard level temperatures are poor indicators of frost severity. Air temperature varies greatly with height in the first few feet above the ground, and also with topography and vegetation around the shelter.

When wind is absent, the air layer immediately above the ground, rather than the ground itself, loses the most heat by radiation. Then the lowest temperature is 2–6 in. above, and about 1°F colder than, a bare ground surface. Above this near-ground minimum, an inversion of temperature develops for several to many feet thick. Plants radiate their heat faster than the air or ground, and may be colder than this air minimum temperature.

Frost damage can be prevented or reduced by heating the lowest air layers, or by mixing the cold surface air with the warmer air in the inversion above the tops of plants or trees.

Valley bottoms are much colder on clear nights than slopes, and may have frost when slopes are frost-free. In some notable frost pockets or hollows the air temperature may be 40°F colder than at nearby stations on higher ground, because of cold air drainage and the greater radiative cooling of level areas than of slopes.

[ARNOLD COURT]

Fructose

A sugar that is the commonest of ketoses and the sweetest of the sugars. It is also known as D-fructose, D-fructopyranose, and levulose fruit sugar. It is found in free state, usually accompanied by D-glucose and sucrose in fruit juices, honey, and nectar of plant glands. D-Fructose is the principal sugar in seminal fluid. It can be isolated as crystalline β-D-fructopyranose, melting point (mp) 102–104°C. It is strongly levorotatory in solution, having a specific rotation $[\alpha]_D = -132.2°$, which changes by mutarotation to $-92.2°$ (in water). Its course of mutarotation indicates the presence of an appreciable amount of the furanose form in solution. See CARBOHYDRATE.

The hydrolysis of cane sugar, or sucrose, leads to the production of equilmolar amounts of D-fructose and D-glucose. On the other hand, inulin, a polysaccharide occurring in roots of the dahlia, chicory, and many Compositae, yields D-fructose alone. From the latter sources, it is prepared industrially. See SUCROSE.

As represented in the illustration, fructose normally occurs as fructopyranose, with a 1,5 oxidic ring. In combined form, however, as in sucrose or inulin, the fructose residue contains the 1,4 ring, and thus is of the fructofuranose type.

D-Fructose is more soluble in water than D-glucose and has a much sweeter taste. It is readily fermented by bakers' yeast, resulting in the same products, ethyl alcohol and carbon dioxide, as glucose.

D-Fructose is readily utilized by diabetic animals. In persons with diabetes mellitus or parenchymal hepatic disease, the impairment of fructose tolerance is relatively small and not at all comparable to the diminution in their tolerance to glucose. See METABOLIC DISORDERS; MONOSACCHARIDE.

[WILLARD Z. HASSID]

Fruit, tree

Tree fruits include temperate, subtropical and tropical zone species. Most temperate zone fruits are deciduous, that is, they lose their leaves in the autumn. They are grown principally in regions protected from prolonged summer heat and severe winter cold (above −10 to −15°F or −23 to −26°C). The principal deciduous tree fruits grown in the United States are apple, peach, pear, plum, apricot, sweet cherry, tart cherry, and nectarine. Tree nuts, such as almond, pecan, walnut, and filbert, are sometimes classified as deciduous tree fruit crops.

Most subtropical fruit trees are evergreen. They will withstand temperatures somewhat below freezing during their dormant or semidormant season, but not the extreme temperatures tolerated by the temperate zone crops. Major subtropical fruits in the United States are the citrus group (for example, orange, grapefruit, lemon), olive, avocado, fig, and others of lesser importance. The Japanese persimmon might be considered as a borderline case between the temperate and subtropical zone groups, and avocado is often classed as a tropical fruit.

Tropical fruits are killed or severly injured by temperatures below freezing and some are sensitive to cold temperatures above freezing. For example, papayas will survive in the milder areas of the subtropics but fail to mature fruits of good quality. The principal tropical fruits grown in the continental United States are date and mango, while banana and papaya are important in its island possessions.

Areas of production. California produces over 50% of the total United States deciduous fruit tonnage and is the number one state in production of peaches, pears, plums, apricots, and nectarines, as well as an important producer of apples and sweet cherries. Washington is first in production of apples and sweet cherries, while Michigan ranks first in tart cherry production. California also ranks first in production of lemons, olives, avocados, figs, dates, almonds, walnuts, grapes, and several other orchard crops. Florida is first in production of oranges and grapefruits.

Production, value, and utilization. The annual production and value of the major United States

Production and value of major United States tree fruit crops, 1976

Fruit	Production, 10^3 short tons*	Used fresh, approx %	Value, $10^6
Temperate zone			
Apple	3,115	61	549
Peach	1,398	40	255
Pear	827	42	111
Plum (including prune)	626	24	115
Nectarine	133	100	30
Apricot	129	10	26
Sweet cherry	120	58	62
Tart cherry	73	4	36
Tropical and subtropical zone			
Orange, tangerine, tangelo	11,213	19	791
Grapefruit	2,850	46	150
Lemon, lime	720	62	105
Olive	80	1	24
Avocado†	106	99	64
Fig†	41	12	8
Date†	24	100	6
Papaya	52	81	7

*10^3 short tons = 907 metric tons.
†Average 1974–1975 crop.

tree fruit crops are shown in the table. The production and value of apple, pear, sweet cherry, and nectarine have increased since the mid 1960s, while peach, plum, apricot, and tart cherry have declined in both production and value.

Orange production increased 48% from 1968 to 1976. This is by far the greatest increase of any other tree fruit crop and is due primarily to rapidly expanding sales of frozen concentrate juice from Florida. Grapefruit production increased 38% during the same period.

Banana, although not grown in the continental United States, ranks with or ahead of the apple and orange in United States consumption. In worldwide production the grape ranks far ahead of any fruit crop, largely because of the demand for wine.

Most deciduous fruits are consumed fresh and in various processed forms, including canned, frozen, preserves, juice, and dried. Exceptions are commercial nectarines which are sold primarily as fresh fruit and tart cherries which are nearly all processed. (The nectarine is actually a smooth-skinned peach.) Processed plums are primarily the dried prunes from California plus limited quantities of canned plums.

Processors used 72% of the 1975–75 citrus crop, nearly 100% of the olives, and 94% of the figs. Most of the other tropical and subtropical zone fruits were sold fresh.

Propagation. Nearly all tree fruits, whether deciduous or tropical, are propagated asexually by budding or grafting the desired variety onto the selected rootstock. The rootstock is usually a young seedling or a clonal stock.

Most deciduous tree fruits are grown on seedlings of selected species. Trees grown on seedling stocks attain normal size, as opposed to dwarfing or semidwarfing stocks which are gaining favor, particularly with the apple. Seedlings of peach, apricot, and several plum species (such as mariana and myrobalan) are used as stocks for peach, apricot, and plum. Mazzard and mahaleb cherry seedlings are used for most sweet and tart cherries. Apple and pear seedlings are used for standard-sized trees of these two fruits, while selected dwarfing clones of apple are used for dwarf apple trees, and quince is used as a pear dwarfing stock. Several citrus species are used as rootstocks for the various citrus fruits. *See* separate articles on the common named fruits.

Cultivation. The tree fruit crops are grown commercially in orchards or groves, usually in single rows which permit necessary cultural operations for each tree. Nearly all tree fruit crops have similar requirements of training, pruning, spraying to control diseases and insects, and cultivation or chemical control of weeds. Most tree fruits receive applications of nitrogen and other nutrients as required. In areas of low rainfall, orchards are irrigated.

Most orchard crops are harvested by hand, although mechanical harvesting has been successful for some processing crops, including tart cherries and plums for drying (prunes).

[R. PAUL LARSEN]

Bibliography: N. F. Childers, *Modern Fruit Science*, 1973.

Fruit (tree) diseases

Tree fruits have diseases that may spoil the appearance of the fruits or render them unfit for human consumption; diseases may also lower yield or shorten the productive life of the trees. Most of the tree-fruit diseases are highly specialized, attacking specific hosts. Only infrequently will one tree-fruit disease attack a wide range of fruits.

Temperate-zone fruits. Diseases of temperate-zone fruits (sometimes called deciduous fruits) are due to fungi, bacteria, viruses, and adverse environmental conditions.

Fungus diseases. Fungi are the most frequent causes of temperate-zone tree-fruit diseases. For example, a perennial threat to most commercial and home apple orchards is the apple scab disease (Fig. 1). Caused by the fungus *Venturia inaequalis*, scab may cause premature defoliation, June drop of young fruits, and unsightly blemishes on ripe apples. A similar disease attacks most varieties of pears and is caused by *V. pyrina*.

Stone fruits, such as peaches, plums, cherries, apricots, and nectarines, are frequently damaged extensively by brown rot caused by the fungus *Monilinia fructicola* (Fig. 2). This disease attacks the flowers (causing blossom blight), infects terminals and twigs with twig blight, and is widely recognized by its destruction of ripe fruit at harvest time.

Many diseases caused by fungi attack and destroy leaves of tree fruits: cherry leaf spot, *Coccomyces hiemalis* (Fig. 3); peach leaf curl, *Taphrina deformans*; apple cedar rust, *Gymnosporangium juniperi-virginianae*; leaf blight of pears, *Mycosphaerella sentina*; and apple powdery mildew, *Podosphaera leucotricha*.

Bacterial diseases. Bacteria also attack tree fruits, causing extensive damage in some regions. For example, fireblight of apples and pears, *Erwinia amylovora*, is a common disease of pomaceous fruits in most seasons (Fig. 4). Bacterial leaf spot of stone fruits, *Xanthomonas pruni*, is often the cause of serious damage to leaves, twigs, and fruits of peaches, apricots, almonds, cherries, plums, and nectarines. Crown gall, *Agrobacterium tumefaciens*, may infect tree fruits in the nursery row,

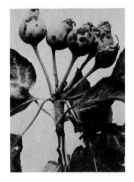

Fig. 1. Apple scab on young fruit.

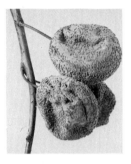

Fig. 2. An example of brown rot on plums.

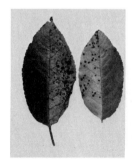

Fig. 3. Cherry leaf spot.

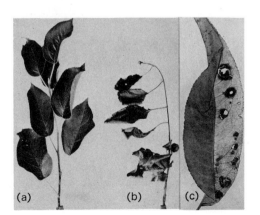

Fig. 4. Several examples of bacterial plant diseases. (a) Healthy apple twig and (b) fireblight-diseased apple twig. (c) Bacterial leaf spot of peach.

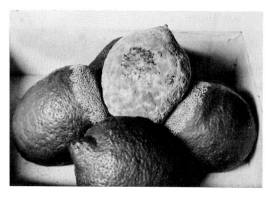

Fig. 5. Blue-green molds (*Penicillium italicum* and *P. digitatum*) which take a heavy toll in storage, transit, and market. The illustration shows how these decay-causing molds can spread by contact from a single infected fruit. (*Photograph by L. J. Klotz*)

causing the formation of large galls on roots and stems of young apple, peach, and pear trees.

Virus diseases. Diseases caused by viruses, such as yellows, rosette, and phony, are especially prevalent on peaches, plums, cherries, apricots, and almonds. *See* PLANT VIRUS.

Effect of environment. The growth of fruit trees and the production of fruit may also be affected by unfavorable environmental conditions such as infertile soil, low temperatures, drought, and poor drainage.

[ERIC G. SHARVELLE]

Citrus diseases. Citrus is subject to a great number of diseases, most of which are distributed throughout the citrus-producing countries of the world. Infectious diseases of citrus are caused by bacteria, fungi, and viruses and may be grouped according to the parts of trees affected, that is fruit, leaves and twigs, and trunks and roots.

Fruit. Numerous rots, internal derangements, and external markings result from fungal and bacterial infections. Fruit decay develops chiefly dur-

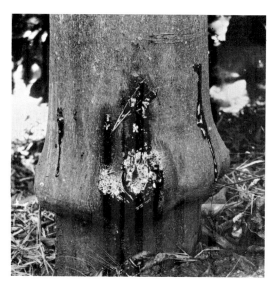

Fig. 6. Gummosis, a disease caused by the fungus *Phytophthora citrophthora*, which damages or kills many citrus trees. Infection by this fungus, a water mold, is favored by excessive moisture. (*Photograph by L. J. Kotz*)

ing storage and transit from infections established largely in surface wounds during growing and from picking, packing, or marketing operations. Citrus fruit requires careful handling to avoid economic loss from decay caused by such fungi as the common green mold, *Penicillium digitatum*; blue mold, *P. italicum* (Fig. 5); brown rot, *Phytophthora citrophthora*; and cottony-rot, *Sclerotinia sclerotiorum*. Some decays are described as contact rots because the causal fungi can spread through an entire box of fruit from one infected fruit.

Leaves and twigs. Some of the fruit-rotting fungi and others cause leaf-blight and dieback of twigs. A bacterium, *Xanthomonas citri*, is the cause of citrus canker which attacks leaves, twigs, and fruits. Introduced on citrus plants sent from Japan to Florida in 1913, it threatened to destroy the citrus industry there. Its eradication, requiring destruction by burning of 4,000,000 orchard and nursery trees, is the most remarkable achievement in plant disease control.

Trunks and roots. Some of the fruit-rotting fungi, particularly species of *Phytophthora* and *Diplodia*, are responsible for root rots and gumming diseases of trees (Fig. 6).

Virus diseases. Citrus is subject to several destructive virus diseases. One of these, psorosis, causes development of bark lesions and eventual death of trees. Since it was learned that psorosis is a bud-perpetuated disease that does not spread naturally, it has been possible to avoid it by propagating from psorosis-free sources. Another virus disease, tristeza, causes rapid decline or death of trees of sweet orange, grapefruit, and tangerine propagated on certain susceptible rootstock varieties. Tristeza virus is known to be spread by three species of aphids. It virtually destroyed the citrus industries of Argentina and Brazil in the 1930s. Damage from tristeza in the United States has been less because more of the citrus is on resistant rootstocks and the two species of the genus *Aphis* that spread it here are less efficient vectors than the one species common in South America.

[JAMES M. WALLACE]

Bibliography: See PLANT DISEASE.

Fruit growing, small

Cultivation of the small fruits which include those commonly known as berries, such as blackberries, dewberries, raspberries, cranberries, blueberries, strawberries, gooseberries, and currants. Grapes are occasionally included with the small fruits in horticultural publications, but more frequently are listed as vine fruits. There is no botanical category which includes all the small fruits because they represent diverse groups of at least three plant families and several genera. They are considered together because of their size similarity of cultural requirements, and the fact that all, except the cranberry, are well adapted to culture in the home garden.

Cranberries are grown extensively in very limited localities in Massachusetts, Wisconsin, New Jersey, Washington, and Oregon, where marshland and cool temperatures are available. Blueberries are confined primarily to limited areas in New Jersey, Michigan, North Carolina, and Washington. They grow best in well-drained, sandy, peat land, somewhat similar to cranberry land, but

Some important small-fruit-producing states

Crop	Producing states
Strawberries	Oregon, California, Tennessee, Michigan, Louisiana, Washington, Arkansas, Kentucky, New York
Raspberries	Michigan, Oregon, New York, Washington, Ohio, Pennsylvania, Minnesota
Blackberries and dewberries	Oregon, Texas, California, Washington, Michigan, Arkansas, Oklahoma, Alabama, North Carolina
Currants and gooseberries	New York, Oregon, Washington, Michigan

there is some commercial production on the sandier mineral soils. The other small fruits are grown on ordinary agricultural soils. Dewberries, a type of blackberry, thrive on soils that are extremely sandy to medium-sandy loams; blackberries, raspberries, and strawberries do well on sandy loam to clay loam, and currants and gooseberries on medium to clay loam. In a few cases growers raise several kinds of small fruit, but usually a grower will produce only one type of berry, frequently as a sideline in addition to other farm crops or tree fruits. One of the major problems associated with the production of all berries except the cranberry is that picking is mostly by hand, which requires a rather large temporary labor force during the harvest season.

Aside from gooseberries, currants, and cranberries, the fruit of many berries is consumed fresh for dessert purposes, hence is sold on the fresh market to the extent that the available demand will absorb it; the remainder, which usually constitutes a major part of the crop, is processed for sale as frozen fruit, or is made into such products as jellies and preserves. The total small-fruits industry of the United States returns about $100,000,000 per year to the growers. Because of the different types of fruit and the scattered location of the plantings (see table), there is no cohesive force to tie all the growers together into a nationwide industry, as there is in certain other branches of agriculture. See separate articles for important small fruits listed under their common names. *See* FRUIT, TREE.

[J. HAROLD CLARKE]

Fumigant

A pesticidal chemical or chemical formulation that functions in a gaseous state. Chemical formulations are designed to increase toxicity, reduce flammability, give off warning odors, and provide for sorption at different rates.

Types. Physical types of fumigants include gases, liquids, and solids. Gases, such as methyl bromide and hydrogen cyanide, exist in a gaseous state at normal room temperatures and pressures and must be stored in cylinders under pressure until used. Liquids, such as the 8:20 mixture of carbon tetrachloride and carbon disulfide, volatilize upon exposure to air. Solids, such as aluminum phosphide and calcium cyanide, produce hydrogen phosphide and hydrogen cyanide upon exposure to moisture in air. Most fumigants except

hydrogen cyanide are heavier than air.

There are several chemical types of fumigants. These include: halogenated hydrocarbons, such as carbon tetrachloride and ethylene dibromide; sulfur-containing compounds, such as carbon disulfide and sulfur dioxide; cyanides, such as hydrogen cyanide and calcium cyanide; and others, such as phosphine and ethylene dioxide. Although many chemicals are registered as fumigants, extensive use is limited to a few.

Properties. In addition to volatility and toxicity to insects, essential properties of fumigants include diffusion and sorption, all of which affect their use. Heavy fumigant gases diffuse more slowly than lighter gases and do not penetrate as well. All gases diffuse more rapidly at higher temperatures. Heavier-than-air gases diffuse by gravity. The gas molecules may adsorb to the surface of commodities such as grain or they may be absorbed or chemisorbed into the commodities. The extent of sorption is determined by weight and volatility of the gas, temperature and moisture of the area or commodity, and the presence of extraneous materials such as dust and chaff. Desorption follows at variable rates. An effective fumigant application occurs when toxic concentrations are maintained long enough to be lethal to the pests.

Uses. Fumigants are used in space fumigations to disinfest food-processing plants, warehouses, grain elevators, boxcars, shipholds, stores, and households, and in spot fumigations within those structures. They are used in atmospheric vaults and vacuum chambers and are applied extensively to stacked bags of grain or stored foods under polyethylene sheets, to trees under tents to control scale insects, and to areas of land to destroy weeds, soil-infesting insects, and nematodes.

Disadvantages. Fumigants have certain inherent disadvantages: Reinfestations may develop as the gas dissipates; off-flavors and odors may result; some are flammable and explosive; some leave toxic residues; certain liquid fumigants are organic solvents; and others are corrosive to metals. All fumigants are toxic to humans; danger exists before, during, and after application. However, fumigants can be applied safely and effectively by trained applicators equipped with safety equipment. For safety reasons, applicators should never work alone.

Action. Fumigant molecules enter the insect's respiratory tubes or penetrate the cuticle and act as respiratory, nerve, or protoplasmic poisons. Some insects close their respiratory tubes after contact with the gas, thus requiring prolonged toxic concentrations. Considerable variability in toxicity exists depending on the fumigant employed and the pest involved. [DONALD A. WILBUR, SR.]

Bibliography: H. A. U. Monro, *Manual of Fumigation for Insect Control*, 2d ed., revised, 1969.

Fungistat and fungicide

Synthetic or biosynthetic compounds used to control fungal diseases in humans, animals, and plants.

Chemotherapy in humans. Cutaneous sporotrichosis is the only mycotic disease of humans for which there is a specific chemotherapeutic drug, potassium iodide. This drug is neither fungistatic nor fungicidal. The mode of action is unknown, but it is thought that the drug alters the tissue response to the etiologic agent in such a manner that factors involved in the host's resistance to *Sporothrix schenckii* may eventually kill the fungus. Potassium iodide is unsatisfactory for the treatment of other forms of sporotrichosis.

Only two drugs are available for the treatment of progressive, life-threatening mycotic diseases. Amphotericin B, a polyene produced by *Streptomyces nodosus*, is used in the treatment of histoplasmosis, blastomycosis, coccidioidomycosis, and disseminated candidiasis, aspergillosis, and sporotrichosis. This drug binds to sterols in the fungal cell membrane and increases the permeability of the cell, resulting in loss of potassium and other essential components. Amphotericin B is administered intravenously since it is poorly absorbed from the gastrointestinal tract. It is nephrotoxic, requiring careful monitoring of kidney function.

Flucytosine (5-FC) is a fluorinated pyrimidine. Its mode of action is thought to be through interference with pyrimidine metabolism of the fungal cells. Flucytosine is used primarily for patients with systemic infections due to *Candida* species and *Cryptococcus neoformans*. It is used occasionally in combination with amphotericin B. The drug is administered orally. Although not as toxic as amphotericin B, kidney and liver function studies are done at regular intervals while the patient is on this medication.

Several drugs are available for treating the dermatophytoses. Miconazole is a synthetic phenylimidazole whose mode of action is not clearly understood. It is thought to affect permeability of the fungal cells in a manner similar to that of some polyenes. Miconazole is available as an ointment. It is used on skin lesions caused by *Trichophyton mentogrophytes*, *T. rubrum*, and *Epidermophyton floccosum*. Tolnaftate and haloprogin are two other fungistatic drugs used topically in the treatment of the dermatophytoses.

Griseofulvin is a fungistatic drug produced by *Penicillium griseofulvum*. Its mode of action is not completely understood, but it apparently interferes with protein synthesis of the fungal cell. It is administered orally, and subsequently is detected in the stratum corneum.

Nystatin is produced by *Streptomyces noursei*. It is used either orally or topically for treatment of candidiasis of the skin, mucous membrane, and gastrointestinal tract. It is ineffectual in the treatment of systemic candidiasis.

Pimaricin is a polyene that is considered to be an excellent antifungal agent for ocular infections, and is especially active against *Fusarium* species. It is not available commercially in the United States.   [LEANOR D. HALEY]

Agricultural fungicides. Chemical compounds are used to control plant diseases caused by fungi. American farmers spend more than $100,000,000 annually to buy and apply fungicides; nevertheless, plant diseases destroy more than $3,500,000,000 worth of crops each year. Fungicides now used include both inorganic and organic compounds. Agricultural fungicides must have certain properties and conform to very strict regulations, and of thousands of compounds tested, few have reached the farmer's fields. Special equipment is needed to apply fungicides. *See* PLANT DISEASE.

Inorganic fungicides. Inorganic fungicides, such as bordeaux mixture and sulfur, are still used in the greatest amounts. Bordeaux mixture is made by mixing a solution of copper sulfate with a suspension of lime (calcium hydroxide). In 1974 about 38,000,000 lb of copper sulfate, worth about $13,000,000, was sold to make bordeaux mixture. In the same year 150,000,000 lb of processed sulfur was sold for use as a fungicide; this quantity of sulfur was valued at about $45,000,000.

Organic fungicides. Organic fungicides have become increasingly important since 1934. Some of the most useful are derivatives of dithiocarbamic acid. Examples are ferbam and ziram, the iron and zinc salts respectively of dimethyldithiocarbamic acid, and nabam, zineb, and maneb, the sodium, zinc, and manganese salts respectively of ethylenebis(dithiocarbamic acid). Another related fungicide of importance is thiram or bis-(dimethylthiocarbamoyl)sulfide. Other representative fungicides which are widely used are captan, N-(tri-chloromethylthio)-4-cyclohexene-1,2-dicarboximide; chlorothalonil, tetrachloro-isophthalonitrile; glyodin, 2-heptadecyl-2-imidazoline acetate; chloranil, tetrachloro-p-benzoquinone; dichlone, 2,3-dichloro-1,4-naphthoquinone; and dodine, n-dodecylguanidine acetate. An organic compound commonly used to control powdery mildews is dinocap, 4,6-dinitro-2-(1-methylheptyl)phenylcrotonate. Cycloheximide, an antibiotic, is used on cherries, ornamentals, and turf. Newer agricultural fungicides are anilazine, 4,6-dichloro-N-(2-chlorophenyl)-1,3,5-triazine-2-amine; fentin hydroxide, triphenyltin hydroxide; and dichloran, 2,6-dichloro-4-nitroaniline.

Requirements and regulations. The stipulations that must be met by manufacturers before they can sell fungicides and other pesticides have been drastically revised. In 1972 the Federal Environmental Protection and Control Act (FEPCA) substantially changed the Federal Insecticide, Fungicide, and Rodenticide Act (FIFRA) of 1947. The FEPCA made the U.S. Environmental Protection Agency responsible for regulating the sale and use of pesticides within the country. The law states that all pesticides shall be classified according to their degree of toxicity to humans and other nontarget organisms: safer materials for "general use," and more toxic materials for "restricted use." All pesticides must still be proven effective before they may be registered for sale, and their labels must state all legal uses and the conditions of use. The law also requires that eventually each state must certify the qualifications of those who apply pesticides commercially. Fortunately, most agricultural fungicides are generally safer than the compounds used as insecticides or herbicides. *See* HERBICIDE; INSECTICIDE; PESTICIDE.

Because fungicides must now be labeled for specific uses on specific crops, the cost of development largely limits their use to such major crops as peanuts, citrus, potatoes, and apples. To fill the gap, the U.S. Department of Agriculture has established the IR-4 program to finance and facilitate label clearance for the use of pesticides on minor crops.

Formulation. The manner in which these compounds are applied, that is, as wettable powders, dusts, or emulsions, is often essential to the success of agricultural fungicides. Raw fungicides must be pulverized to uniform particles of the most effective size, mixed with wetting agents, or dissolved in solvents. These carriers or diluents must not degrade the fungicides or injure the plants.

Foliage fungicides. This type of fungicide is applied to aboveground parts of plants, usually to prevent disease rather than cure it. Because they are intended to form a protective coating on the plant surface that kills fungus spores before infection occurs, foliage fungicides must adhere to foliage despite weathering. Fungicides also must be sufficiently stable chemically to resist degradation by water, oxygen, carbon dioxide, and sunlight. Sometimes, as in the case of zineb, specific chemical changes by weathering are necessary to produce highly fungicidal derivatives. Protective fungicides must be insoluble in water in order to remain on foliage. Certain foliage fungicides, however, are water-soluble. These materials destroy the fungus in disease spots after infection. Fungicides of this type are called eradicant or contact fungicides. An example is dodine, n-dodecylguanidine acetate.

Seed and soil treatments. Seeds and seedlings are protected against fungi in the soil by treating the seeds and the soil with fungicides. Seed-treating materials must be safe for seeds and must resist degradation by soil and soil microorganisms. Some soil fungicides are safe to use on living plants. An example is pentachloronitrobenzene, which can be drenched around seedlings of cruciferous crops and lettuce to protect them against root-rotting fungi. Other soil fungicides, such as formaldehyde, chloropicrin, and methyl isothiocyanate, are injurious to seeds and living plants. These compounds are useful because they are volatile. Used before planting, they have a chance to kill soil fungi and then escape from the soil.

Systemic fungicides. Systemic fungicides are compounds that permeate plants to protect new growth or to eliminate infections that have already occurred. Since the advent of benomyl, methyl 1-(butylcarbamoyl)-benzimidazol-2-yl-carbamate, and of carboxin, 2,3-dihydro-6-methyl-5-phenylcarbamoyl-1,4-oxathiin, other effective systemic fungicides have become available. These three are representative of the newer materials: thiophanate-methyl, 1,2-bis-(3-methoxycarbonyl-2-thioureido) benzene; dodemorph, N-cyclododecyl-2,6-dimethylmorpholine; and ethirimol, 5-n-butyl-2-ethylamino-4-hydroxy-6-methyl pyrimidine.

Application methods. Dusters and sprayers are used to apply foliage fungicides. Conventional sprayers apply 300–500 gal/acre at pressures up to 600 psi. This equipment ensures the uniform, adequate coverage necessary for control. Recent developments in spray equipment are the mist blower and the low-pressure, low-volume sprayer. The mist blower uses an air blast to spray droplets onto foliage. Mist blowers have been successful for applying fungicides to trees but are less satisfactory for applying fungicides to row crops. The low-pressure, low-volume sprayers are lightweight machines that apply about 80 gal of concentrated spray liquid per acre at a pressure of about 100 psi. These have been successfully used to protect tomatoes and potatoes against diseases caused by fungi. The most recent refinement of this method is ultralow-volume (ULV) spraying. With ULV spraying, which employs special spinning cage

micronizers, growers can protect certain crops by applying as little as 0.5–2 gal of spray liquid per acre. Fungicides are also applied from aircraft. [JAMES G. HORSFALL; SAUL RICH]

Bibliography: D. L. Fowler and J. N. Mahan, *The Pesticide Review*, 1975; R. W. Marsh (ed.), *Systemic Fungicides*, 2d ed., 1977; W. T. Thomson, *Agricultural Chemicals*, book IV: *Fungicides*, 1976; D. C. Torgeson (ed.), *Fungicides*, 1967.

Garlic

A hardy perennial, *Allium sativum*, of Asiatic origin and belonging to the Amaryllidaceae family. Garlic is an ancient condiment vegetable popular in many countries. It grows best in a Mediterranean-type climate but will tolerate colder winters. The plant is onionlike except for flat leaves, and the culture is similar to that of onions. The edible bulb is composed of pungent segments called cloves. As with the onion, bulbing is promoted by long days and high temperatures. Cultivars vary in the tendency to produce an infloresence. In those that do, flowers abort in the bud stage so that true seed is never produced, but bulbils often arise in the umbel. Varietal improvement is limited to selection or mutation.

Principal cultivars in the United States are California Late (sometimes called Italian or Pink), California Early (Mexican), and Creole (Texas White). A number of local strains exist. California Late with its attractive, good-keeping bulbs is preferred for fresh market. A type called Tahiti, Greatheaded, or Elephant with large bulbs of few cloves is actually a leek.

The crop is asexually propagated by planting cloves in the fall or early winter. The bulbs are ready for harvest in late spring or summer depending on the cultivar and climate. The plants are pulled after the lower leaves begin to dry and are dried in windrows for 1 to 3 weeks, then tops and roots are removed. For storage, temperatures around 10°C with low relative humidity are desirable. Most of the 10,000-acre (4049 ha) United States crop is grown in California, with scattered acreages elsewhere, producing $12,000,000–18,000,000 worth of garlic. About 70% of the California crop is dehydrated for garlic salt. *See* VEGETABLE GROWING. [PHILIP A. MINGES]

Gelatin

A protein derived from the skin, white connective tissue, and bones of animals. It is composed entirely of amino acids joined in polypeptide linkages to form a linear polymer. It gives typical protein reactions and is readily hydrolyzed to yield its amino acid or peptide components. *See* AMINO ACIDS; PROTEIN.

Manufacturing process. The protein collagen is the precursor of gelatin, and if pretreated with acid yields type A gelatin, which is isoionic at pH 7.0–8.5. Pretreatment with lime yields type B gelatin, which is isoionic at pH 4.7–5.0. Frozen edible-grade porkskins, processed to yield type A gelatin, provide about one-half the total United States production. Calfskin and beefskin pieces, known as splits, after treatment with concentrated lime solution for periods up to 90 days, yield type B gelatin and provide about one-third of the United States total. Bones of the water buffalo and beef cattle, after demineralization by leaching with dilute hydrochloric acid, are known as ossein. This raw material is usually lime-treated to yield type B gelatin and provides about one-sixth of the United States total. After pretreatment with acid or lime, the raw materials are washed, to remove mineral matter and other impurities, and are extracted with warm water several times to remove the gelatin. The solution is filtered, concentrated in vacuum evaporators, filtered again, and is then chilled to form a sheet of jelly. This is dried and then ground to the desired particle size. To hasten drying, the jelly is sometimes extruded through a die to form noodlelike material with a much greater specific surface, thus facilitating the removal of moisture.

Characteristics. The jelly strength of gelatin, expressed in grams, is measured at 6.66% concentration, with the Bloom gelometer, which is a type of penetrometer. Highest grades test 250–325 Bloom, and the weakest grades 50–100 Bloom. Average molecular weight probably varies from a low of 20,000 to a value of 120,000 for the highest grades.

The protective colloidal efficiency, as measured by the Zsigmondy gold number, is 0.009 for type B gelatin and 0.02 for type A gelatin, thus indicating that type B is slightly more effective than type A. The gold numbers are constant over the entire Bloom range for each type. These low gold numbers indicate the high protective colloidal value of gelatin.

Amino acid composition. The approximate amino acid composition of gelatin is shown in the table. Although gelatin is not a complete protein because it lacks the essential amino acid tryptophan, it does supply several amino acids lacking in the protein of wheat, barley, and oats. It thus exhibits a protein-sparing action in diets where the cereal grains are a principal component. Pure gelatin is free from antigens and hence does not cause allergic reactions. Where it is desirable to increase the dietary protein, for growing children, for obese persons, and for geriatric feeding, gelatin is an excellent dietary supplement.

Use in foods. The use of gelatin as a food in the United States increased approximately sixfold from 1933 to 1976. The principal uses are (1) gelatin desserts; (2) meat products, such as canned hams, meat loaves, luncheon meats, headcheese, scrapple, and souse; (3) candy such as marshmallows, circus peanuts, wafers, fondant; (4) ice cream, sherbets, and water ices; (5) canned soups such as jellied consommé madrilene; and (6) such bakery items as icings, frostings, cake fillings, and chiffon pie fillings. United States usage of gelatin was estimated at more than 73,000,000 lb for the year 1976.

Gelatin is used to prolong the flavor-lasting property in chewing gum. Part of the flavor is added as such, and part in particles of gelatin. After the straight flavor has been chewed out, the flavor locked into the gelatin particles begins to be evident. Thus the flavor will last several times as long as with gum containing only ordinary forms of flavor. Similarly, use of a release agent that prevents chewing gum from sticking to artificial dentures can be extended to increase the effective time by more than half an hour.

Flavors that oxidize readily or evaporate easily are encased in gelatin for such uses as dry cake mixes and icing mixes. Orange or lemon oils are so used in considerable quantity. Tiny hollow spheres of gelatin contain the oil or flavor, which is thus protected from evaporation or oxidation.

Nutritionally gelatin is used to counteract fingernail defects, and has been studied together with different diets as affecting nail, hair, and body growth of rats.

Use in drilling and agriculture. Gelatin is used as a protective colloid in drilling muds when deep wells are driven for the petroleum, sulfur, and salt industries. In agriculture gelatin is applied to fertilizers, sprays, and animal feeds.

Use in pharmaceuticals. Principal pharmaceutical uses are in the manufacture of hard capsules, soft elastic capsules, suppositories, pill coatings, pastilles, and emulsions. This grade gelatin also finds use in delayed or depot medication and in cosmetics, where it is valued because it is not an allergen. A special pyrogen-free grade of gelatin serves as a substitute for blood plasma. Gelatin sponges have been developed for use as absorbable sterile surgical dressings.

Millions of pounds of gelatin are used annually in the United States for stabilizing vitamins, enzymes, and vaccines. In this application the unstable biological is emulsified with the gelatin solution so that it is the internal phase, completely surrounded by gelatin (as, on a much larger scale, in a honeycomb the honey is enclosed in wax). The emulsion is then either cast into tiny pellets and dried or flowed into a slab, dried, and ground. Vitamins so stabilized can be blended with minerals and resist oxidation and destruction for many months of storage.

[J. AVERY DUNN]

Bibliography: H. Borginon, Photographic properties of the gelatin macromolecule, *J. Photogr. Sci.*, 15(5):207–214, 1967; F. L. DeBeukelaer, J. R.

Approximate amino acid composition of gelatin

Amino acid	Amino acid content, %	
	Type B gelatin from ossein, splits, or calfskin	Type A gelatin from porkskin
Nitrogen	17.4	18.0
Alanine	8.7	9.2
Glycine	26.9	30.5
Valine*	2.6	2.7
Leucine*	3.1	3.2
Isoleucine*	1.9	1.5
Proline	14.0	16.3
Phenylalanine*	1.9	2.1
Tyrosine	0.14	0.69
Tryptophan*	—	—
Serine	2.9	2.9
Threonine*	2.2	2.2
Cystine	0.05	0.09
Methionine*	0.85	0.80
Arginine*	6.4	8.8
Histidine*	0.63	0.67
Lysine*	5.2	5.1
Aspartic acid	6.9	6.3
Glutamic acid	12.1	11.7
Hydroxyproline	14.4	13.1

*Essential amino acids in human nutrition.

Powell, and E. F. Bahlman, Standard methods for determining viscosity and jelly strength of glue, *Ind. Eng. Chem.*, 16:310–315, 1924; Gelatine symposium, *Biol. Abstr.*, 33:688, 1959; B. Idson and E. Braswell, Gelatin, *Advan. Food Res.*, 7:235–238, 1957; E. M. Marks, Gelatin: A review, in R. E. Kirk and D. F. Othmer (eds.), *Encyclopedia of Chemical Technology*, vol. 10, 2d ed., 1966; M. P. Mohn, Effects of different diets and gelatin on nail, hair and body-growth of rats, *Anat. Rec.*, 139(2):256, 1961; R. E. Neuman, Amino acid composition of gelatins, collagens and elastins from different sources, *Arch. Biochem.*, 24:289–298, 1949; D. A. Sutton, Gelatin and glue research (symposium), *Nature*, 200(4905):412, 1963; R. S. Zsigmondy, Die Hochrothe Goldösung als Regens auf Colloide, *Z. Anal. Chem.*, 40:697–719, 1901.

Gibberellin

A generic term, referring to any member of a family of naturally derived compounds, some of which are plant hormones, all having a specific chemical configuration (a gibbane skeleton) and, usually, a broad spectrum of biological activity.

Discovery. The gibberellins first came to the attention of plant scientists through the efforts of E. Kurosawa, a Japanese plant pathologist working in Formosa on foot rot of rice (the "Bakanae" disease). In 1926 he demonstrated that the medium in which the fungal pathogen *Gibberella fujikuroi* had been growing could produce pronounced stem elongation of rice and maize, identical with the symptoms found when the fungus itself grew on rice. This and subsequent work in Japan led to the isolation and characterization of several compounds which were biologically active. Final elaboration of the structure of gibberellic acid (GA_3) was accomplished by B. Cross and J. Curtis in 1954.

Production. For some time the only source of gibberellins was the fungus, and about a dozen biologically active compounds have been isolated from culture filtrates. Commercial production of gibberellins is still based on fermentation procedures similar to those used for the preparation of many antibiotics. Gibberellins have also been isolated from plants and seeds, and species of *Phaseolus* have been particularly rewarding in this respect. Naturally occurring gibberellins are still being characterized; the number reached 15 in 1968. Not only angiosperms but gymnosperms, ferns, green and brown algae, and possibly bacteria have also been reported as containing gibberellinlike substances. *Gibberella*, however, remains the only fungus known to produce gibberellins. *See* INDUSTRIAL MICROBIOLOGY.

Classification. Nomenclature is based on the gibbane skeleton, and although many of the gibberellins have five rings, some lack the lactonic configuration. The gibberellin GA_3 has been available in greatest quantity, so most of the physiological effects ascribed to the group have been obtained only with this compound. However, the testing of many derivatives on a variety of biological systems has indicated that, although no one structural feature is essential for biological activity, the gibbane skeleton, with proper stereochemistry and a free carboxyl at the C-10 position, seems to be necessary for a high level of activity (see illustration).

Occurrence. In higher plant tissue GA_1 and GA_3 through GA_8 have been identified, and though GA_3 has been thought of as the "type" gibberellin, it is neither the most active nor the most commonly found.

In general, the concentration in plants is low, as would be expected with hormones, but differences in concentration between tissues are common and amounts vary from about 1 to 16,000 $\mu g/kg$ fresh weight. The higher concentrations have been reported from seeds. Glycosides and amino acid conjugates also have been found in some plants, and in other cases proteolytic digestion of tissue has produced extracts with gibberellin-like activity. The biological significance, if any, of these forms of gibberellins is not known.

Bioassay. A variety of bioassays has been developed for the quantitative determination of gibberellins. In general, these tests employ either sections of plant parts (stem sections, leaf disks, cereal endosperm) or seedlings. Somewhat greater sensitivity is achieved with section tests, and with careful control of experimental conditions amounts as small as 10 pg/ml (10^{-11} g/ml) can be reproducibly measured. Some of the tests have indicated pronounced sensitivity to one gibberellin or to a group of gibberellins. Cucumber seedlings, and the Cucurbitaceae in general, are markedly more responsive to gibberellins lacking a hydroxyl group in either the 7 or 8 position, for example, GA_4, GA_7, and GA_9.

Different developmental stages or different organs of the same plant may demonstrate differential responses to the various gibberellins. All of the gibberellins promote stem elongation of *Silene*, but only GA_7 initiates flowering. GA_7 is also the only gibberellin which induces stem elongation of *Lunaria*, and it seems that, with a few exceptions, GA_7 is more consistently high in biological activity than the other extensively examined gibberellins.

Isolation. Chromatographic techniques (paper, thin-layer, and gas-liquid) are used frequently for the separation of gibberellins. Gas-liquid chromatography can be used for both quantitative and qualitative investigations and, when coupled with mass spectrometry, may eventually replace bioassay measurement techniques. Relatively specific colorimetric spray reagents, such as 5% ethanolic sulfuric acid or 20% $SbCl_2$ in chloroform, have been used in conjunction with paper and thin-layer chromatography, but the limit of sensitivity seems to be about 0.01 mg. Also, spectrophotofluorometry provides a fairly specific means of estimating and identifying purified samples of gibberellins, since both activation and emission spectra of derivatives are characteristic.

Biosynthesis. A. J. Birch, R. W. Rickard, and H. Smith demonstrated in 1958 that both acetate and mevalonic acid were incorporated into gibberellins by the fungus, and subsequent work confirmed their postulate that the gibberellin biosynthetic pathway involves the condensation of isoprenoid units, essentially similar to the pathway of cholesterol and steroid biosynthesis. B. E. Cross, working with the fungus, and C. A. West, working with cell-free higher plant enzyme systems, have identified many of the intermediate compounds produced during gibberellin biosynthesis. A cy-

gibbane skeleton

Gibbane skeleton, the basic structure and variations of gibberellins derived from natural sources.

clized diterpene hydrocarbon, (−)-kaurene, appears in both systems to be a close precursor to the gibberellins.

Exogenous biological activity. During the 1950s much of the investigative work on the biological effects of gibberellins was carried out by P. W. Brian and coworkers in England. They, and many others since, recognized that the striking responses of plants elicited by gibberellin were generally accentuations of normal growth patterns rather than alterations to abnormal forms. For example, dwarf varieties of many species, such as peas, corn (maize), beans, and coffee, can be induced to grow as tall as the corresponding tall varieties; other aspects of the induced growth are normal. Rosette plants, in which little or no stem growth occurs during the first year, normally require either a cold temperature period or exposure to particular day-length conditions or both before stem elongation takes place. Treatment with gibberellins can usually replace these requirements, causing rapid, and in some cases prolonged, stem elongation, though, again, other aspects of growth remain normal. *See* PHOTOPERIODISM IN PLANTS; PLANT GROWTH.

Flowering. Another pronounced effect of gibberellin, first reported by A. Lang in 1956, is the promotion of flowering in long-day or cold-requiring plants kept under "noninductive" conditions. This effect is probably an indirect influence resulting from a more direct action on stem elongation, but it established the gibberellins as the only known group of compounds that could consistently and reproducibly cause flowering of higher plants.

Dormancy. An interruption of dormancy in several different kinds of plant tissues is also a characteristic response to gibberellin: Dormant potato tubers undergo vigorous sprouting. In some varieties of seed, such as Douglas fir, sweet cherry, and peach, hormone treatment wholly or partially replaces the cold requirement for germination, while in others, such as lettuce and various grasses, the light requirement is circumvented. Bud and shoot dormancy of many woody perennial plants can be shortened, and the onset of this type of dormancy, involving leaf fall, autumnal coloration, and the cessation of growth, frequently can be delayed by treatment.

Other effects. Gibberellins also have been reported to influence leaf shape and size; stimulate cambial activity; alter geotropic responses of shoots, petioles, and leaves; modify sex expression toward increased male, and in some cases, female expression; induce parthenocarpic fruit growth; change the spectrum and activity of enzymes in several plant tissues; and affect many other aspects of plant growth and development.

Endogenous activity. Perhaps the most investigated and best understood endogenous role of gibberellin is in the germination of cereal grain. The cereal seed is approximately 90–95% stored reserves (starch, protein, lipid, phytic acid, hemicellulose, and other nutrients) and 5–10% embryo. During germination the reserves are hydrolyzed to more mobile constituents, which are used by the embryo as nutrients and energy sources for its early growth. About 12 hr after the start of imbibition, the embryo releases gibberellin into the endosperm. The hormone induces the aleurone layer, which is 1–3 cells thick and surrounds the endosperm, to synthesize hydrolytic enzymes (α-amylase, proteinase, ribonuclease, endo-β-gluconase, and probably others), which are released into the starch cells, where they hydrolyze the stored reserves. The utilization of the contents of these cells thus completes the cycle initiated and controlled by the embryo through the mediation of a gibberellin hormone. The response also has important commercial aspects since, when supplied exogenously, gibberellin drastically shortens the time required for the necessary degree of hydrolysis of endospermal reserves during malting. *See* SEED (BOTANY); SEED GERMINATION.

Commercial uses. In addition to their use during malting, gibberellins hold promise as stimulators of pasture and lawn grass growth during winter. Because gibberellins cause increased stem elongation of sugar cane, more internodes become available for sugar accumulation. Treatment of grapes enlarges berries and lengthens berry pedicels, thus decreasing the loss due to rotting. Other potential uses, such as the prevention of regreening of citrus fruits, increasing the yield of cotton crops, and stimulation of early forest tree growth, are under investigation. The widespread occurrence and pronounced biological effects of the gibberellins leave little doubt about their importance as natural plant-growth regulating compounds. *See* PLANT HORMONES.   [L. G. PALEG]

Bibliography: P. W. Brian, The gibberellins as hormones, *Int. Rev. Cytol.*, 19:229–266, 1966; L. G. Paleg, Physiological effects of gibberellins, *Annu. Rev. Plant Physiol.*, 16:291–322, 1965; F. Wightman (ed.), *Biochemistry and Physiology of Plant Growth Substances*, 1968.

Ginger

An important spice or condiment; also the plant from which it is obtained, *Zingiber officinale*, of the ginger family (Zingiberaceae). The plant is a native of southeastern Asia. It is an erect perennial herb (see illustration) having thick, scaly,

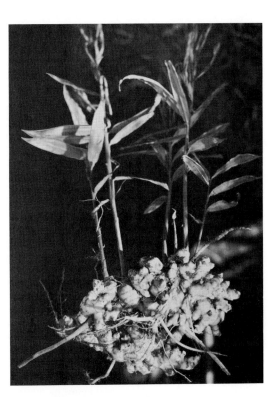

Ginger (*Zingiber officinale*). (*USDA*)

branched rhizomes which contain starch, gums, an oleoresin (gingerin) responsible for the pungent taste, and an essential oil which imparts the aroma. The rhizomes, dug up after the aerial parts have withered, are treated in different ways to produce green ginger or dried ginger. Ginger is used in medicine, in culinary preparations (soups, curries, puddings, pickles, gingerbread, and cookies), and for flavoring beverages such as ginger ale and ginger beer. The plant is grown in China, Japan, Sierra Leone, Jamaica, Queensland, and Indonesia. *See* SPICE AND FLAVORING.

[PERRY D. STRAUSBAUGH/EARL L. CORE]

Glucose

A monosaccharide also known as D-glucose, D-glucopyranose, grape sugar, corn sugar, dextrose, and cerelose.

Occurrence. Glucose in free or combined form is not only the most common of the sugars but is probably the most abundant organic compound in nature.

It occurs in free state in practically all higher plants. It is found together with D-fructose in considerable concentrations in grapes, figs, and other sweet fruits and in honey. In lesser concen-

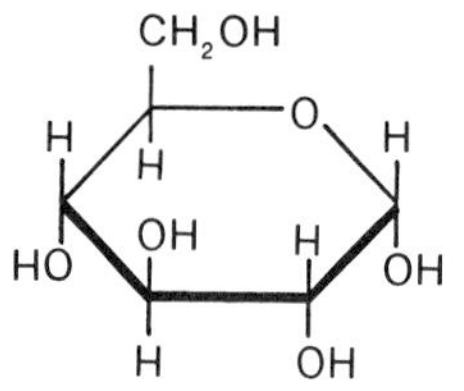

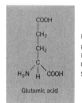

Fig. 1. Structural formula for α-D-glucose.

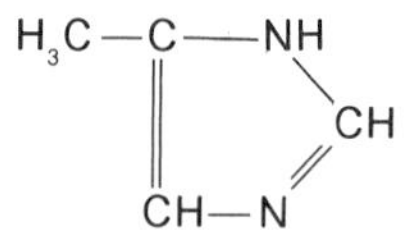

H₃C—C—NH

(structural formula)

Fig. 2. Structural formula for iminazole.

trations, it occurs in the animal body fluids, for example, in blood (0.08%) and lymph. Urine of diabetic patients usually contains 3–5%. *See* FRUCTOSE.

Cellulose, starch, and glycogen are composed entirely of glucose units. Glucose is also a major constituent of many oligosaccharides, notably sucrose, and of many glycosides. It is produced commercially from cornstarch by hydrolysis with dilute mineral acid. The commerical glucose is used largely in the manufacture of confections and in the wine and canning industries. *See* FOOD ENGINEERING; GLYCOGEN; STARCH.

Chemistry. Glucose exists in two modifications (α and β). The sugar crystallizes from aqueous solution at temperatures below 50°C as α-D-glucose monohydrate which has a melting point (mp) of 80°C. At temperatures above 50°C but below 115°C, the stable form is anhydrous α-glucose (Fig. 1), mp 146°C, $[\alpha]_D$ +113°, mutarotating to +52.2° in water. Above 115°C and below its melting point, the β anomer, mp 148–150°C, $[\alpha]_D$ + 19°, mutarotating to +52.2°, is the stable form. β-Glucose can be prepared by crystallization from pyridine or from acetic acid. Ordinary glucose is chiefly the α compound.

Reactions. Glucose undergoes the general reactions of aldoses. On oxidation with bromine, it yields D-gluconic acid, $CH_2OH\cdot(CHOH)_4\cdot COOH$; oxidation with nitric acid produces D-saccharic acid, $COOH\cdot(CHOH)_4\cdot COOH$. On reduction with sodium amalgam or borohydride, D-glucose is transformed into the hexahydric alcohol, sorbitol (D-glucitol), $CH_2OH\cdot(CHOH)_4\cdot CH_2OH$. *See* MONOSACCHARIDE.

Under the influence of dilute alkalies, it undergoes a series of changes and decompositions which leads to the formation of hydroxy acids, such as lactic acid. When treated with ammonia in the form of ammoniacal zinc hydroxide, glucose is converted, even at ordinary temperature, into methyl iminazole (methylglyoxaline) (Fig. 2).

Metabolism. D-Glucose is the principal carbohydrate metabolite in animal nutrition; it is utilized by the tissues, and it is absorbed from the alimentary tract in greater amounts than any other monosaccharide. Glucose could serve satisfactorily in meeting at least 50% of the entire energy needs of humans and various animals.

Glucose enters the bloodstream by absorption from the small intestine. It is carried via the portal vein to the liver, where part is stored as glycogen, the remainder reentering the circulatory system. Another site of glycogen storage is muscle tissue.

The glucose cycle has been depicted by C. F. Cori and G. T. Cori in the diagram below.

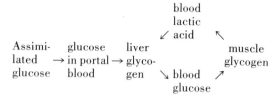

Glucose is readily fermented by yeast, producing ethyl alcohol and carbon dioxide. It is also metabolized by many bacteria, resulting in the formation of various degradation products, such as hydrogen, acetic and butyric acids, butyl alcohol, acetone, and many others. *See* CARBOHYDRATE.

[WILLIAM Z. HASSID]

Glutamic acid

An amino acid. The amino acids are characterized physically by the following: (1) the pK_1, or the dissociation constant of the various titratable groups; (2) the isoelectric point, or pH at which a dipolar ion does not migrate in an electric field; (3) the op-

(structural formula)

Physical constants of the L isomer at 25°C:
pK_1 (COOH): 2.19; pK_2 (COOH): 4.25; pK_3 (NH_3^+): 9.67
Isoelectric point: 3.22
Optical rotation: $[\alpha]_D(H_2O)$: +12.0; $[\alpha]_D$(5 N HCl): +31.8
Solubility (g/100 ml H_2O): 0.84

Glutamic acid

tical rotation, or the rotation imparted to a beam of plane-polarized light (frequently the D line of the sodium spectrum) passing through 1 dm of a solution of 100 g in 100 ml; and (4) solubility.

Glutamic acid forms an alcohol-insoluble calcium salt. The amino acid has many important functions, including the following:

1. It is the principal point by which ammonia enters organic compounds (reductive amination of α-ketoglutarate), and the central distribution point for amino nitrogen by transamination.

2. It is the precursor of glutamine, the added amide group serving as a storage form of nitrogen and as a precursor of certain nitrogen atoms in purines, histidine, and glucosamine.

3. It is the precursor of proline and of arginine.

4. It is incorporated into both glutathione and folic acid.

Glutamine biosynthesis begins by the reductive amination of α-ketoglutarate, catalyzed by glutamic acid dehydrogenase. Depending on the organism, diphosphopyridine nucleotide reduced ($DPNH^+$) or triphosphopyridine nucleotide reduced ($TPNH^+$) may serve as hydrogen donor. During metabolic degradation the most common pathway is through deamination to α-ketoglutarate. A novel pathway exists in the bacterium *Clostridium tetanomorphum*, which ferments glutamic acid to butyric acid, acetic acid, carbon dioxide,

CO_2, ammonia, NH_3, and hydrogen, H_2, by reaction sequence including mesaconic and citramalic acids. *See* AMINO ACIDS; ARGININE; FOLIC ACID; HISTIDINE; PROLINE.

[EDWARD A. ADELBERG]

Glutamine

An amino acid. The amino acids are characterized physically by the following: (1) the pK_1, or the dissociation constant of the various titratable groups; (2) the isoelectric point, or pH at which a dipolar ion does not migrate in an electric field; (3) the op-

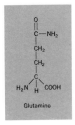

Physical constants of the L isomer at 25°C:
pK_1 (COOH): 2.17; pK_2 (NH_3^+): 9.13
Isoelectric point: 5.65
Optical rotation: $[\alpha]_D(H_2O)$: +6.3; $[\alpha]_D(1\ N\ HCl)$: +31.8
Solubility: (g/100 ml H_2O): 3.6 (18°C)

tical rotation, or the rotation imparted to a beam of plane-polarized light (frequently the D line of the sodium spectrum) passing through 1 dm of a solution of 100 g in 100 ml; and (4) solubility.

Glutamine with its amide group is an important storage form of nitrogen in plants and animals; it also serves as the precursor of certain ring nitrogen atoms in purines and histidine and of the amino group in glucosamine. The biosynthetic pathway for glutamine is from glutamic acid, by the reaction below. Adenosinetriphosphate (ATP) is

Glutamic acid + ammonia + ATP →
glutamine + ADP + phosphoric acid

required in the reaction, and adenosinediphosphate (ADP) is one of the products.

During metabolic degradation glutamine is converted to α-ketoglutarate by either of two pathways: (1) deamidation to glutamic acid, followed by deamination; or (2) transamination of the amide group to a keto-acid acceptor, forming α-ketoglutaramic acid. The α-ketoglutaramic acid is then hydrolyzed to α-ketoglutaric acid and ammonia. *See* AMINO ACIDS.   [EDWARD A. ADELBERG]

Glutelin

A general name for a class of proteins which are insoluble in water, alcohol, or neutral salt solutions but readily soluble in dilute acids or alkali. Glutelins are mixtures of various similar proteins; some of them are denatured on exposure to alkali-hydroxide. The most extensively investigated glutelins are those obtained from the insoluble residue derived from wheat kernel, barley, and rice after the prolamines have been extracted with 70 – 80% alcohol. Examples are glutenin from wheat and oryzenin from rice. *See* PROLAMINE; PROTEIN; RICE; WHEAT.

[GERTURDE E. PERLMANN]

Glycine

An amino acid. The amino acids are characterized physically by the following: (1) the pK_1, or the dissociation constant of the various titratable groups;

(2) the isoelectric point, or pH at which a dipolar ion does not migrate in an electric field; (3) the optical rotation, or the rotation imported to a beam of plane-polarized light (frequently the D line of the sodium spectrum) passing through 1dm of a solution of 100 g in 100 ml; and (4) solubility.

Physical constants of the L isomer at 25°C:
pK_1 (COOH): 2.34; pK_2 (NH_3^+): 9.60
Isoelectric point: 5.97
Solubility (g/100 ml H_2O): 24.99

Glycine has many important functions, including the following:

1. It is incorporated intact into purines.
2. The α-carbon and nitrogen atoms are incorporated into the pyrrole rings of porphyrin.
3. It accepts an amidine group from arginine and a methyl group from methionine to form creatine.
4. It is a constituent of the tripeptide eoenzyme glutathionine (γ-glutamylcysteinylglycine).
5. It can accept formaldehyde from hydroxymethyltetrahydrofolic acid to become serine. This reaction is reversible.

The quantitatively most important biosynthetic pathway for glycine is from serine, which transfers its hydroxymethyl group to tetrahydrofolic acid. Smaller amounts arise by the transamination of glyoxylic acid, which can be formed by cleavage of isocitric acid. Threonine may also be cleaved to glycine and acetaldehyde. *See* SERINE; THERONINE.

During metabolic degradation glycine is deaminated to glyoxylic acid, which is oxidized to formate and carbon dioxide. Under some conditions glyoxylate can be oxidized to oxalic acid. *See* AMINO ACIDS.

[EDWARD A. ADELBERG]

Glycogen

The primary reserve polysaccharide of the animal world. It is found in the muscles and livers of all higher animals, as well as in the cells of lower animals. Because of its close relationship to starch, it is often called animal starch, although glycogen is found in some lower plants, fungi, yeast, and bacteria. A polysaccharide similar to glycogen was isolated in one case from a higher plant, Golden Bantam sweet corn (*Zea mays*). *See* STARCH.

Properties. Glycogen is a nonreducing, white, amorphous polysaccharide which dissolves readily in cold water, forming an opalescent, colloidal solution. It gives a reddish brown color with iodine, is precipitated by alcohol, and has a specific rotation $[\alpha]_D^{20}$ of approximately +200°. It is very resistant to the action of alkalies and may be prepared by boiling liver or muscle tissue in 30% potassium hydroxide to destroy the proteins, and precipitating the glycogen with ethyl alcohol.

The molecular weight of glycogen is usually very high, and it varies with the source and the method of preparation; molecular weights of the order of $1-20 \times 10^6$ have been reported.

In its biochemical reactions, glycogen is similar to starch. It is attacked by the same plant amylas-

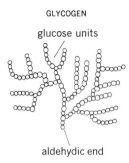

GLYCOGEN

glucose units

aldehydic end

Diagram of branched
structure of glycogen.
(*After K. H. Meyer*)

es that attack starch, and like starch, it is degraded to maltose and dextrins. Both glycogen and starch are broken down by animal or plant phosphorylase enzyme in the presence of inorganic phosphate with the production of α-D-glucose-1-phosphate. *See* CARBOHYDRATE METABOLISM.

Molecular structure. Chemical studies, based on methylation and periodate oxidation procedures, show glycogen to possess a branched structure similar to the amylopectin starch fraction. The molecules of both these polysaccharides consist of chains of D-glucose residues joined by α-1,4 linkages, having similar chains attached through α-1,6 linkages at the branch points (see illustration). Depending on the source, the average chain length of a branch (which is the average length in glucose units of the outer and inner branches) in a glycogen molecule is 11–18 D-glucopyranose units. In amylopectin the average chain length of a branch is 22–27.

Synthesis. About 1940 C. F. Cori and G. T. Cori first showed that glycogen could be synthesized in the test tube and that two enzymes, muscle phosphorylase and a branching enzyme which is present in animal tissues, are required for the formation of this important polysaccharide. The muscle phosphorylase catalyzes a stepwise transfer of α-D-glucosyl units from α-D-glucose 1-phosphate to a nonreducing end of a "primer" (acceptor substrate). Synthesis of polysaccharide from α-D-glucose 1-phosphate does not occur unless a small amount of starch, glycogen, or dextrin is present as a priming agent. In the presence of the primer, the enzyme adds D-glucose units to a preexisting polysaccharide chain, forming long linear chains joined through α-1,4 linkages. The reaction can be written as Eq. (1).

$$x\,\alpha\text{-}D\text{-Glucose 1-phosphate} + (D\text{-glucose})_n \rightleftharpoons$$
$$\text{Acceptor}$$
$$(\alpha\text{-1,4-}D\text{-glucose})_{n+x} + x\,\text{phosphate} \quad (1)$$
$$\text{Glycogen chain}$$

The second enzyme (branching factor) has the ability to unite such chains through α-1,6 linkages, resulting in the formation of a highly branched glycogen structure. It was believed that the combined action of the two enzymes was responsible for the synthesis of glycogen in the animal body.

In 1957 L. F. Leloir and his coworkers obtained an enzymic preparation from liver and other animal tissues that catalyzed the transfer of D-glucose from uridine diphosphate D-glucose to an acceptor (glycogen) according to reaction (2).

$$x\,\text{Uridine diphosphate } D\text{-glucose}$$
$$+ (\alpha\text{-1,4-}D\text{-glucose})_n \rightarrow (\alpha\text{-1,4-}D\text{-glucose})_{n+x}$$
$$\text{Acceptor} \qquad \text{Glycogen chain}$$
$$+ x\,\text{uridine diphosphate} \quad (2)$$

This reaction resembles that of the phosphorylase enzyme, but its equilibrium starting with uridine diphosphate D-glucose is more favorable for synthesis of glycogen than that starting with α-D-glucose 1-phosphate. Since the product obtained is branched, the enzyme preparations must contain another enzyme (6-glucosyltransferase), which transfers α-1,4-glucosyl chains produced by the first enzyme (glycogen glucosyltransferase) to

form a branched molecule. The existence of two mechanisms of glycogen formation raises the question of which of the two mechanisms operates in the animal body. Evidence indicates that synthesis of glycogen in the body occurs through a transfer of D-glucose units from uridine diphosphate D-glucose by an enzyme, glycogen glycosyltransferase, whose function is entirely synthetic. When the chains become about 10 units long, portions are transferred to other chains forming α-1,6-glycosyl linkages by a branching enzyme. The function of phosphorylase is considered to be concerned chiefly with degradation of glycogen.

Metabolic pathways. The metabolic formation of glycogen from glucose in the liver is frequently termed glycogenesis. In fasted animals, glycogen formation can be induced by the feeding, not only of materials that can be hydrolyzed to glucose and other monosaccharides, such as fructose, but also of various other materials. A number of L-amino acids, such as alanine, serine, and glutamic acid, upon deamination in the liver give rise to substances, such as pyruvic acid and α-ketoglutaric acid, that can be converted in the liver to glucose units which are subsequently converted to glycogen. Furthermore, substances such as glycerol derived from fats, dihydroxyacetone, or lactic acid can all be utilized for glycogen synthesis in the liver. Such noncarbohydrate precursors are termed glycogenic compounds. The process of glycogen formation from these precursors is known as gluconeogenesis. The term glycogenolysis is used to connote glycogen breakdown. *See* POLYSACCHARIDE.   [WILLIAM Z. HASSID]

Bibliography: D. M. Greenberg (ed.), *Metabolic Pathways*, vol. 1, 3d ed., 1967; A. White, P. Handler, and E. L. Smith, *Principles of Biochemistry*, 4th ed., 1968.

Gooseberry

Any of several species of the genus *Ribes* belonging to the Saxifragaceae family and occurring in the temperate and cold regions of the world.

The two major species of horticultural impor-

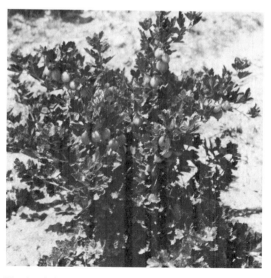

Fig. 1. A 2-year-old Columbus gooseberry plant. (*New York State Agriculture Experiment Station*)

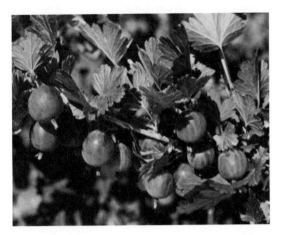

Fig. 2. Poorman, a productive good-quality red-fruited gooseberry. (*New York State Agricultural Experiment Station*)

tance are the English or European gooseberry *(R. grossularia)* and the American gooseberry *(R. hirtellum)*. The term "English gooseberry" is more frequently used than "European gooseberry," because the English gardeners contributed most of the domestication and cultivation of this fruit. English gooseberries are characterized by very large fruit of good quality and high susceptibility to mildew. The American gooseberries are not as susceptible to mildew, but are small-fruited and poor in quality.

Distribution of gooseberry and currants (also of the genus *Ribes*) was restricted in 1932 by law to protect white pines from damage by white pine blister rust, since these fruits serve as alternate host plants for this disease organism. Today, regulations still govern the distribution of gooseberries. Because of these growing restrictions and the low cost of imported fruit, it has not been commercially feasible to produce fruit in the United States. Only a limited acreage is grown, primarily in Oregon, Washington, and Michigan. However, gooseberries are recommended for home gardens throughout the United States, except in the far South and Southwest.

Gooseberry plants are small spreading shrubs (Fig. 1) cultivated for edible fruit or as ornamentals, seldom exceeding 1 m in height. They are spiny or unarmed, deciduous or evergreen. Most of the thornless varieties are unproductive, with small fruit, while the thorny types are more productive, with larger fruit.

Gooseberries are generally propagated from hardwood cuttings made in the fall or by layering. Layers are slower to root, often requiring 2 years. A fertile, well-drained soil with adequate organic matter is best. Currants can tolerate a wetter soil than gooseberries. Perennial weeds should be eliminated before a planting is made. Gooseberries are among the earliest fruits to bloom, so planting in frost pockets should be avoided. Plants are spaced 1 m apart in rows 2½ m apart. Plants should be fertilized regularly, but fertilizers with muriate of potash should be avoided. Plants are pruned like regular shrubs, with removal of old sprawling canes and gradual replacement with young vigorous canes.

The fruits are very acid and contain many soft seeds. The English varieties, when fully ripe, are suitable for eating fresh. The color of gooseberry fruits ranges from dark and light red through various shades of green to near white. The fruits may be canned or frozen for use in pies or as preserves.

The major disease problems are leaf spot and mildew. Leaf spot is relatively easy to control, but if not controlled, complete defoliation may occur in early summer, greatly reducing plant vigor, productivity, and winter hardiness. Mildew is best controlled by good aeration and the growing of more resistant varieties. Aphids and crown borers are serious insect pests. Crown borers can easily destroy a planting.

English gooseberry varieties are seldom sold by United States nurseries. Some of the recommended English varieties include Leveller, Howards Lancer, Whitesmith, Glenton Green, and Scotch Red. Varieties occasionally sold by American nurseries include Columbus, Poorman (Fig. 2), Chautauqua, Downing, Welcome, Oregon Champion, and Pixwell. Columbus and Poorman are the two best varieties. Pixwell is productive although poor in quality, but is the most widely propagated. All of the above varieties have some English gooseberry parentage except Pixwell, which more closely resembles the American types. *See* CURRANT; FRUIT GROWING, SMALL.   [DONALD K. OURECKY]

Grafting of plants

Vegetative propagation by joining a scion (a short section of the stem) to an understock in such manner that the two grow together and continue development as a single plant without change in stock or scion. Success depends upon the scion being nearly dormant, as in spring or early summer, plus genetic compatibility of scion and stock, firm union of their cambia or callus, and protection from desiccation. The various kinds of grafts may be included under either topworking or repair grafting.

Topworking is employed to propagate seedless varieties and hybrids, to change the variety of fruits, to correct pollination problems, or to change the framework of a desirable variety which is subject to trunk or crotch injury. Topworking is done

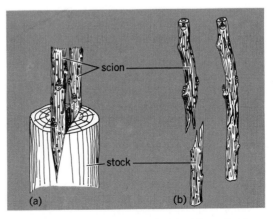

Two types of graft. (a) Cleft graft. (b) Whip graft. (*From H. J. Fuller and Z. B. Carothers, The Plant World, 4th ed., copyright © 1963, by Holt, Rinehart, and Winston; adapted by permission*)

by three methods: root grafting, in which a scion 3–6 in. long is grafted on a root; crown grafting, in which a similar scion graft is made at the root crown just below ground level; and top grafting, including top budding, cleft grafting (illustration *a*), and frameworking. Other methods of top grafting are whip (illustration *b*) or tongue, bark saw-kerf, stub or notch, side, and veneer. *See* BUDDING.

Repair grafting is of two kinds: bridge grafting, in which each of several scions is grafted in two positions on the stock, one above and the other below an injury; and inarching, in which two plants growing on their own roots are grafted together and one plant is severed from its roots after the graft union is established. [JAMES E. GUNCKEL]

Grain crops

Crop plants that belong to the grass family (Gramineae), generally grown for their edible starchy seeds. They also are referred to as cereal crops and include wheat, rice, maize (corn), barley, rye, oats, sorghum (jowar), and millet. The grain of all these cereals is used directly for human food and also for livestock, especially maize, barley, oats, and sorghum.

These large seeded grasses were among the first plants domesticated by man. Archeological studies indicate that some of these crops have been cultivated for 12,000–15,000 years. Cereal grains are the cheapest source of calories for human consumption and provide the most important energy source for three-fourths of the world population.

Cultivation. Wheat, barley, rye, and oats are cool season or temperate zone crops and are generally grown in low-rainfall areas (10–30 in.) because they are better adapted to cultivation under these conditions than other domesticated crops. However, they can produce large crops under higher rainfall, irrigation, and fertilizer applications. Rice is primarily a tropical or subtropical cereal, but Japanese plant breeders have developed types that grow at 45° latitude. Sorghum and some millets originally were tropical crops, but the area of adaptation has been greatly expanded since 1920 by breeding new types. Maize also was a subtropical crop but now is most productive in a temperate climate. Successful rice production is dependent on an abundance of water. Upland or dry-land rice is available but limited in production. Some millets produce crops under dry, low-fertility conditions where other cereals often fail.

All cereals respond to fertilizers, especially nitrogen. Under very favorable conditions maize has yielded 17,000 lb (8½ tons) per acre, and rice and wheat about 12,000 lb (6 tons) per acre. New types of wheat and rice have been developed that have short, stiff straw and respond to high applications of fertilizer. These new types have doubled the yields in certain areas and are contributing significantly to feeding the world population.

Storage and production. Another important attribute of these grain crops is the easy manner in which they can be stored. The grain often dries naturally before harvest to a safe moisture content (10–12%), or can easily be dried with modern equipment. Grain placed in adequate storage facilities can then be protected against insect infestations and maintained in sound condition for years.

The production of wheat, rice, maize, and sorghum has increased significantly since 1950, while that of rye and oats has decreased. Modern agricultural technologies assure further increased production of all cereals on an area basis, especially wheat and rice (see table) [E. G. HEYNE]

Bibliography: H. Helbaek, Domestication of food plants in the Old World, *Science*, 130:365–372, 1959; H. D. Hughes and D. Metcalfe, *Crop Production*, 3d ed., 1972; J. H. Martin and W. H. Leonard, *Principles of Field Crop Production*, 2d ed., 1967.

Grape culture

That division of horticulture concerned with grape growing. The broader term, viticulture, includes studies of grape varieties; methods of culture such as trellising, pruning, and training; and insect and disease control.

The genus *Vitis* consists mostly of plants which climb by means of the coiling of cylindrical-tapering tendrils (Fig. 1). The flowers are polygamodioecious—some plants have perfect flowers, others have only staminate flowers with at most rudimentary pistils. The five flower petals are greenish and narrow, and cohere at the top. The fruit is a pulpy berry. In the Old World species, *V. vinifera*, probably a native of western Asia, the skin and pulp of the mature berry cohere; in many North American

World acreages and production of cereals*

Cereal	Hectares, 10⁶			Metric tons, 10⁶		
	1948–1952	1966	1976–1977	1948–1952	1966	1976–1977
Wheat	173	217	231	177	308	412
Rice	102	126	141	167	253	571
Maize	88	102	118	139	239	336
Sorghum and millets	45	112	105	47	84	93
Barley	52	70	85	59	116	176
Oats	53	31	28	62	48	49
Rye	39	34	16	37	31	29

*Data from U.S. Department of Agriculture Foreign Agricultural Service.

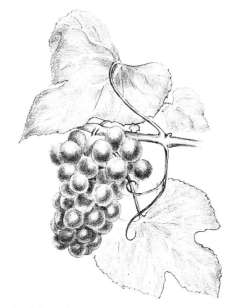

Fig. 1. Foliage, tendrils, fruit, and stem characteristics of the Concord grape (*Vitis labruscana*).

species the skin of mature berries separates freely from the pulp.

Kinds of cultivation. Of the cultivated grapes of the world, more than 90% are clonal varieties of the species *V. vinifera*. In the United States *V. vinifera* is grown on the West Coast. Muscat of Alexandria, Tokay, Emperor, Thompson Seedless or Sultanina, Zinfandel, Carignane, and Grenache are among the leading varieties. Most of the grapes cultivated east of the Rocky Mountains have been derived from American wild vines such as *V. labrusca* and *V. aestivalis*, or from crosses between them and *V. vinifera*. The principal commercial varieties are Concord, Catawba, Delaware, and Niagara. In the southeastern and Gulf states varieties of *V. rotundifolia*, the muscadine grapes (Scuppernong), are grown.

Many *vinifera* varieties are grown with a trunk 1–3 ft high, bearing at the top a ring of short branches which are pruned to produce short spurs each having only a few buds. These trunks are staked in early years but become more woody and self-supporting when older. Other *vinifera* varieties and the American-type grapes are pruned to produce canes bearing 8–15 buds and are supported on a vertical trellis. The muscadine grapes are often grown on overhead arbors.

Production. World grape production probably exceeds that of any other fruit. The largest producers are Italy, France, Spain, the United States, and Turkey. These countries produce about 60% of the world total.

The major area of production in the United States is the West Coast. In the East the Chautauqua-Erie grape belt extends along the southeastern shore of Lake Erie. Another area is about the Finger Lakes of central New York.

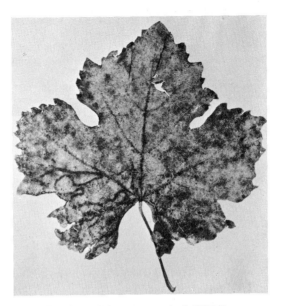

Fig. 3. Powdery mildew on grape leaf. (*USDA*)

The total production in the United States in the period 1972–1974 ranged from 2,569,600 to 4,194,100 tons, averaging 3,652,300 tons (1 ton = 0.9 metric ton). California produced 88, 92, and 90% of the totals in these three years, while the major Concord producers—New York, Washington, Michigan, and Pennsylvania—together produced 10, 6, and 8% of the totals.

About 65% of the total production was crushed for wine, brandy, and juice; the remainder was dried as raisins, canned for use in fruit cocktail, or used as fresh fruit. In California 58% of the production in the 1972–1974 period consisted of raisin varieties, 29% of wine varieties, and 13% of table varieties. The amounts crushed averaged 62% of the total crop. *See* AGRICULTURAL SCIENCE (PLANT).

[JOHN EINSET]

Diseases. Diseases of European bunch grapes (*V. vinifera*), American bunch grapes (*V. labrusca*), and muscadine grapes (*V. rotundifolia*) vary in severity with the varieties planted and the climatic conditions. There are few regions in which grapes can be grown without disease control, and frequently diseases are limiting factors in production. A few fungus diseases are of major importance. *See* PLANT DISEASE CONTROL.

Fungus. Black rot (*Guignardia bidwellii*) is a serious grape disease throughout the world and is the only major disease that attacks muscadines. Symptoms are reddish-brown, circular spots on leaves, black cankers on stems, and on bunch grapes a rot that reduces the berries to shriveled black mummies. On muscadine berries only black scabs and cankers are produced (Fig. 2).

Downy mildew (*Plasmopara viticola*) is serious where the weather is warm and humid. Irregular, yellowed areas covered on the lower surface with a cottony white fungus growth appear on the leaves. Young shoots are shortened, distorted, and covered with the downy growth, as are the young berry clusters. Older grapes turn brown, shrivel slightly, and drop.

Powdery mildew (*Uncinula necator*) occurs even in drier regions where it becomes of greater

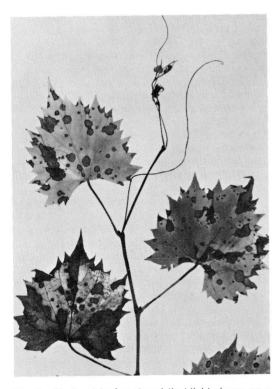

Fig. 2.   Black rot leaf spot and tip blight shown on a portion of a muscadine grape plant.

importance than black rot and downy mildew. Indistinct, mealy, white patches develop on the upper surfaces of leaves (Fig. 3), on succulent stems, and on young berries which drop when infected.

Other fungus diseases include anthracnose (*Elsinoë ampelina*), dead arm (*Cryptosporella viticola*), and bitter rot (*Melanconium fuligineum*).

Bacteria. Blight of the shoots (*Erwinia vitivora*) and crown gall (*Agrobacterium tumefaciens*) cause minor damage.

Viruses. Pierce's disease, caused by the alfalfa dwarf virus, damages vineyards in California and may be responsible for bunch grape failures in the southeastern United States. Leaves scald at the margins and the vines gradually decline and die. Other viruses produce mosaics, leaf-roll, witches' broom, and various growth distortions. *See* PLANT VIRUS.

Control of diseases. Cultural practices helpful in decreasing disease severity include selection of disease-free stock, planting on favorable sites with good air drainage, trellising, pruning, and cultivating to promote air circulation, and vineyard sanitation through removing diseased canes and litter. When fungus diseases threaten the crop, chief reliance must be placed on spraying. Powdered sulfur controls powdery mildew, but at high temperatures it injures the vines. Bordeaux mixture is the most generally effective fungicide for all diseases. Unfortunately, it also causes injury to the vines. Therefore, the organic fungicides, ferbam and zineb, are preferred for control of black rot but are less effective against mildews. *See* FUNGISTAT AND FUNGICIDE; INSECTICIDE.

[E. S. LUTTRELL]

Bibliography: See PLANT DISEASE.

Grapefruit

A citrus fruit, *Citrus paradisi*, including seedy and seedless varieties, with pink, white, or red flesh (see illustration). The trees, evergreen with well-rounded tops, are the largest and most vigorous of commercial citrus types. The grapefruit is thought to have originated as a hybrid of another species, *C. grandis*, which includes the pummelos. Grapefruit from Barbados were first described by Griffith

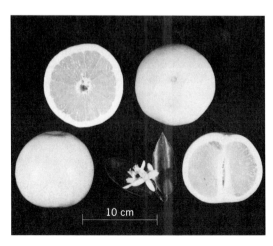

Whole and sectional views of grapefruit. Flowers and foliage are shown below.

Hughes in 1750 under the grouping "Forbidden Fruit." The name "grapefruit" was first used in 1814 in Jamaica. The grapefruit was unknown in Europe and Asia until introduced from the Western Hemisphere. It was first planted in Florida in the early 1800s, with the first commercial shipments in 1885. It was the first citrus to be processed commercially.

The early plantings consisted of white, seedy varieties. The first seedless variety, Marsh, discovered in 1860 and named in 1889, has become the predominant variety because of its seedlessness. Several pink- and red-fleshed varieties have originated as bud-sports from white-fleshed varieties. The Foster, a seedy, pink variety, was discovered in 1907 and replaced by Thompson, a seedless, pink variety discovered in 1924. Redblush, a red-fleshed, seedless variety discovered in 1929, is now the most widely grown because of its deeper flesh color and peel blush. Other pigmented sports have been discovered and named, but none has yet gained prominence.

Most commercial production is limited to areas with high temperatures because high total heat is needed for high-quality fruit. Of the world supply in 1976, almost 75% was produced in the United States. The average yearly sales value of United States crops for the 5-year period ending in 1976 was $130,000,000. Florida is the leading producer, with Arizona, California, and Texas having substantial production. Approximately half of the crop is marketed as fresh fruit, and the rest is processed as canned juice and segments. Other areas producing significant amounts of fruit are Israel, the West Indies, Argentina, and South Africa. *See* FRUIT, TREE.   [R. K. SOOST]

Grass crops

Grasses provide about 53% of the total feed units (forages and grains) consumed by all domestic livestock, in the form of pastures, native range grazing, and harvested forage (hay, green feed, and grass silage). Grasses fill other important roles in the national economy: in conservation of soils, in development and conservation of water resources, in upstream flood control, in wildlife and game management, and in a wide range of outdoor recreation activities. In general, grasses of suitable types, under appropriate methods of management, make effective use of about 1,000,000,000 acres of the national geography that are not adapted because of soil or climate to the production of harvested crops.

Structure. Grass stems have solid joints (nodes) and leaves arranged in two rows, with one leaf at each joint (see illustration). The leaves consist of the sheath, which fits around the stem like a split tube, and the blade, which is commonly long and narrow. Seed heads are made up of minute flowers on tiny branchlets, often several crowded together, but always two-ranked like the leaves. The flowers are generally wind-pollinated. The seeds are enclosed between two bracts, or glumes, which remain on the seed when ripe.

Growth characteristics and distribution. Grass species may be annual or perennial. Some perennial species are perpetuated by creeping stems as well as by seed. Stems that creep underground are termed rhizomes, or rootstocks, whereas surface-creeping stems are called runners, or stolons. Species having creeping stems produce a well-knit sod. These generally tolerate continuous close grazing and are utilized primarily for pastures. Species that do not creep vegetatively tend to grow erect. They make an open or loose sod, and are best suited for hay or silage. In subhumid to semiarid regions, range species are predominantly perennial and are perpetuated mostly by seed. In other areas both annuals and perennials commonly occur. All grasses have a fibrous type of root system that permeates the soil extensively and is effective in preventing soil erosion and restoring soil humus content. Grasses are worldwide in distribution; adapted species are available for nearly all conditions of soil and climate. See separate articles for grasses under their common names.

[HOWARD B. SPRAGUE]

Diseases. Grasses are so commonplace that until recently little heed was paid to agents that killed or injured them. But intensified use on farms and turf areas has made the problem of grass diseases important.

Kinds of pathogens. Grasses are attacked by several hundred kinds of pathogens. No one grass is infected by all, but many grasses are susceptible to 30 or more different disease-causing agents. Fungi cause most of the diseases but bacteria, viruses, and nematodes also attack grasses. The prevalent fungi that attack the leaves of grasses cause the most conspicuous symptoms. They reduce productivity and nutritive value of forage and may result in depletion of stands. Some of the fungi that incite rusts, smuts, and root rots of grasses also attack cereals. Such fungi as those causing stem rust, scolecotrichum brown stripe, and anthracnose of grasses are adapted to a wide range of climatic conditions and can infect numerous species of grass. Such others as stripe rust, stem smuts, and some leafspot fungi are more restricted in host range and distribution.

Some of the viruses that attack grasses also infect cereals and other crop plants. For example, both the barley yellow-dwarf virus and the wheat-streak mosaic virus attack numerous grasses. The virus that causes dwarfing in alfalfa and Pierce's disease in grapevine also occurs in Bermuda grass.

Control measures. The greatest advances in control of grass diseases have been in the identification of disease-resistant varieties and strains of each species; in the breeding of new types that have multiple resistance to several pathogens, combined with high growth potential; and in the multiplication and distribution of seed of superior types. Application of fungicides for control of grass disease is not considered practical except for some lawn and turf grass diseases, and for certain fungi which attack grasses grown for seed production. Consequently, control has been obtained primarily by breeding and selection of resistant varieties or through the use of improved management practices. For example, Sudan grass (*Sorghum vulgare* var. *sudanense*), orchard grass (*Dactylis glomerata*), and Kentucky bluegrass (*Poa pratensis*) can be damaged severely by several foliar diseases. Varieties resistant to some of these diseases have been developed through breeding and selection. Postharvest burning of grass seed fields in western United States is an example of disease control by

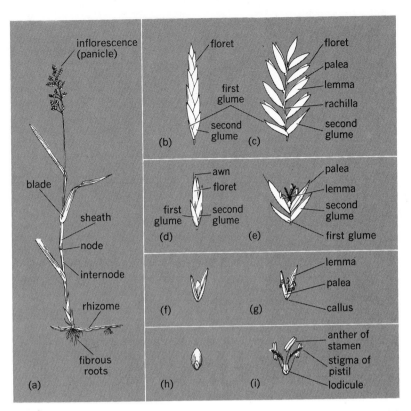

Parts of a typical grass plant. (*a*) Complete plant. (*b*) Many-flowered spikelet. (*c*) Generalized spikelet. (*d*) One-flowered spikelet. (*e*) Spikelet at flowering. (*f*) Floret in fruit. (*g*) Floret in flower. (*h*) A fruit. (*i*) A flower. (*From P. D. Strausbaugh and E. L. Core, Flora of West Virginia, West Va. Univ. Bull., ser. 52, no. 12–2, pt. 1, p. 67, 1952*)

proper management practices. This technique has given practical control of such diseases as blind seed (*Phialea temulenta*) of perennial rye grass and leaf rust (*Puccinia poaesudeticae*) of Kentucky bluegrass. See PLANT DISEASE CONTROL; PLANT VIRUS.   [K. W. KREITLOW]

Bibliography: *Grass,* USDA Yearb. Agr., 1948; H. B. Sprague (ed.), *Grasslands of the United States: Their Economic and Ecological Significance,* 1974.

Growing season

Generally considered to be the period of the year when climatic conditions are favorable for plant growth, common to a place or an area. In middle latitudes, with sufficient moisture, the growing season generally falls between the date of the last freeze in spring and the time of first freeze of autumn. This would apply to most annual plants and crops and to many perennials and biennials. However, some more hardy plants extend their growing season beyond these limits and continue some growth until the soil freezes; but some less hardy plants require minimum temperatures of 40°F, as in the tropics or subtropics.

At the opposite temperature extreme there are areas where high temperatures during the summer (usually also accompanied by lack of rain) retard or prevent plant growth. Such areas commonly have mild winters so that the growing season may extend from the beginning of the autumn rains through the winter to the next dry season.

Some desert areas lack a dependable or well-defined growing season. During occasional but irregular rainy periods plant seeds burst into vigorous growth, covering the desert with a blanket of fast-growing and fast-flowering plants. These quickly produce seeds which then remain dormant until the next rain. Such growing seasons may be only a few days or weeks long and may occur only once in an unpredictable two, three, or several years.

These, however, are special cases. In most usages, the term growing season is of interest in connection with the principal annual food, fiber, and forest crops and, in common climatological practice, is the frost-free season. While the growing season varies from year to year, it is possible to establish an average date for its beginning and ending and its average length for any location or area. Such averages are useful in comparing one location with another in terms of agricultural potential or in deciding the crop varieties suitable for an area. For example, cotton requires a growing season of from 180–200 days, while many corn varieties require only 130–150 days.

In the United States the average length of the growing season ranges from less than 100 days in the higher elevations of the Rockies to practically the whole year in southern Florida. As a rule, the length averages nearly 300 days along the Gulf and South Atlantic coasts and 120 days along the northern border. This is a decrease of about 10 days for every degree of latitude. *See* AGRICULTURAL METEOROLOGY.   [MILTON L. BLANC]

Guava

GUAVA

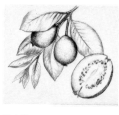

Psidium guajava, showing a branch with leaves and two berries and a berry cut in half.

A plant, *Psidium guajava*, of tropical America that has long been in cultivation. It is a shrub or low tree which belongs to the myrtle family (Myrtaceae). The fruit is a berry, yellow when ripe, and quite variable in size depending on variety and growing conditions, the average being about $2\frac{1}{2}$ in. long (see illustration). The guava is quite aromatic, sweet, and juicy. It is used mostly for jellies and preserves, but also as a fresh fruit.

[PERRY D. STRAUSBAUGH/EARL L. CORE]

Gum

A class of high-molecular-weight molecules, usually with colloidal properties, which in an appropriate solvent or swelling agent are able to produce gels (highly viscous suspensions or solutions) at low dry-substance content. The molecules are either hydrophilic or hydrophobic; that is, they do or do not have an affinity for water. The term gum is applied to a wide variety of substances of gummy characteristics, and therefore cannot be precisely defined.

Various rubbers are considered to be gums, as are many synthetic polymers, high-molecular-weight hydrocarbons, or other petroleum products. Chicle for chewing gum is an example of a hydrophobic polymer which is termed a gum but is not frequently classified among the gums. Quite often listed among the gums are the hydrophobic resinous saps that often exude from plants and are commercially tapped in balsam (gum balsam) and other evergreen trees (gum resin). Incense gums such as myrrh and frankincense are likewise fragrant plant exudates.

Usually, however, the term gum, as technically employed in industry, refers to plant polysaccharides or their derivatives. These are dispersible in either cold or hot water to produce viscous mixtures. Modern usage of the term includes water-soluble derivatives of cellulose and derivatives and modifications of other polysaccharides which in the natural form are insoluble. Usage, therefore, also includes with gums the ill-defined group of plant slimes called mucilages. *See* POLYSACCHARIDE.

Viscosity. Gums are important in that they impart viscosity to aqueous solutions. Their physical properties are manifestations of their chemical structure, the kind and amount of solvent, and the kind and concentration of ions and other substances dissolved in the solvent. Because gums are commonly composed of several different kinds of monomer units with many possible variations in regard to degree of branching, length of branches, and types of linkages, an almost infinite number of structures is possible. Forces act between molecules, between different parts of the same molecule, and between polymer and solvent. These forces include hydrogen bonding, ionic charges, dipole and induced dipole interactions, and van der Waals forces.

All of these forces affect such properties as gel-forming tendency, viscosity, and adhesiveness. The types of linkage due to their effects on chain flexibility are important also in determining physical properties. For example, it is known that linear molecules make more viscous solutions than do long-branch molecules of similar molecular weights, but they have a tendency to precipitate because of association of the chains. If this association is prevented, stability can be achieved without much sacrifice of viscosity. This can be done by introducing groups with ionic charges that repel one another, or by attaching many very short side branches to prevent close approach of the chains. Much work remains to be done in this area. While it is known that solutions of some gums are slimy or mucilaginous, whereas those of other gums are tacky, the reasons for these differences are unknown. Rheological properties of the different gum solutions also differ.

Source and structure. Many plant gums originally used by man still are important items of commerce. Most of these are dried exudates from trees and shrubs, produced with or without artificial stimulation by injury. These gums are collected by hand, usually in the hot, semiarid regions of the world, often from wild plants, but sometimes from cultivated plants. For the most part, these gums have highly branched structures containing two to five different sugar units. They frequently are acidic in that they contain carboxyl groups which are portions of glycuronic acids. Commercial gums often are mixtures of two or more different polysaccharides.

Seed gums, which also have been used for many centuries, likewise are important items of commerce today. The more ancient gums were extracted from quince, psyllium, or flax seeds. The ground endosperm of locust trees grown in the Mediterranean area also has been an item of commerce for many years. It is still important today, along with a similar gum obtained from the endosperm of the guar plant which is native to India and Pakistan but is grown to a small extent in the southwestern United States.

Seaweed gums produced by hot water or alka-

Sources and sugars of important gums

Gum	Source	Sugars present and linkages
Seaweeds		
Agar	Red algae (*Gelidium* sp.)	D-Galactose β-(1 → 4), 3,6-anhydro-L-galactose α-(1 → 3), + sulfate acid ester groups
Algin	Brown algae (*Macrocystis pyrifera*)	D-Mannuronic acid β-(1 → 4), L-guluronic acid β-(1 → 4), Na salt
Carrageenin	Red algae (*Chondrus crispus, Gigartina stellata*)	D-Galactose, 3,6-anhydro-D-galactose + sulfate acid ester groups
Fucoidan	Brown algae (*Fucus* sp., *Laminaria* sp.)	L-Fucose + sulfate acid ester groups
Laminaran	Brown algae (*Laminaria* sp.)	D-Glucose, D-mannitol, β-(1 → 3) chain and β-(1 → 6) branches
Plant exudates		
Gum arabic	*Acacia* sp.	L-Arabinose, D-galactose, L-rhamnose, D-glucuronic acid
Ghatti	*Anogeissus latifolia*	L-Arabinose, D-xylose, D-galactose, D-mannose, D-glucuronic acid
Karaya	*Sterculia urens*	D-Galactose, L-rhamnose, D-galacturonic acid
Tragacanth	*Astragalus* sp.	D-Galactose, D-xylose, D-glucuronic acid
Plant extracts		
Pectin	Cell walls and intracellular spaces of all plants (commercial source, citrus waste)	D-Galacturonic acid α-(1 → 4) partially esterified, L-arabinose α-(1 → 5) and α-(1 → 3) branches, D-galactose β-(1 → 4)
Larch arabino-galactan	Western larch	D-Galactose, L-arabinose
Ti	Tubers of *Cordyline terminalis*	D-Fructose, D-glucose
Plant seeds		
Corn-hull gum	Corn seed coat	D-Xylose, L-arabinose, D-galactose, L-galactose, D-glucuronic acid
Guar	*Camposia teragono-lobus* endosperm	D-Mannose β-(1 → 4), D-galactose α-(1 → 6) branches
Locust bean	Carob tree (*Ceratonia siliqua*) endosperm	D-Mannose β-(1 → 4), D-galactose α-(1 → 6) branches
Quince seed	*Cydonia vulgaris*	L-Arabinose, D-xylose, hexuronic acid, monomethyl hexuronic acid
Psyllium seed	*Plantago* sp.	D-Xylose, L-arabinose, D-galacturonic acid, L-rhamnose, D-galactose
Flax seed	*Linum usitatissimum*	D-Galacturonic acid, D-xylose, L-rhamnose, L-arabinose, L-galactose, D-glucose
Tamarind	*Tamarindus indica*	D-Glucose, D-galactose, D-xylose
Wheat gum	Wheat	D-Xylose β-(1 → 4), L-arabinose branches
Miscellaneous		
Cellulose derivatives	Plant cell walls, wood pulp, and cotton	D-Glucose β-(1 → 4)
Starch Amylose Amylopectin	Cereal grains and tubers	D-Glucose α-(1 → 4), D-glucose α-(1 → 4), α-(1 → 6) at branch points
Dextran	Bacterial action on sucrose	D-Glucose α-(1 → 6) and α-(1 → 3)
Chitin	Exoskeleton of animals of the phylum Arthropoda	*N*-Acetyl-D-glucosamine β-(1 → 4)

line extraction of seaweed are other important industrial raw materials.

Industrially important or potentially useful gums are listed in the accompanying table, together with the plant source, the sugar units, and the most prevalent glycosidic linkage when known.

Use. Gums are used in foods as stabilizers and thickeners. They form viscous solutions which prevent aggregation of the small particles of the dispersed phase. In this way they aid in keeping solids dispersed in chocolate milk, air in whipping cream, and fats in salad dressings. Gum solutions also retard crystal growth in ice cream (ice crystals) and in confections (sugar crystals). Their thickening and stabilizing properties make them useful in water-base paints, printing inks, and drilling muds. Because of these properties they also are used in cosmetics and pharmaceuticals as emulsifiers or bases for ointments, greaseless creams, toothpastes, lotions, demulcents, and emollients. Gums are used to modify texture and increase moisture-holding capacity, for example, as gelling agents in canned meats or fish, marshmallows, jellied candies, and fruit jellies. Their adhesive properties make them useful in the production of cardboard, postage stamps, gummed envelopes, and as pill binders. Other applications include the production of dental impression molds, fibers (alginate rayon), soluble surgery films and gauze, blood anticoagulants, plasma extenders, beverage-clarifying agents, bacteriological culture media, half-cell bridges, and tungsten-wire-drawing lubricants. *See* FOOD MANUFACTURING.

[ROY L. WHISTLER]

Bibliography: American Chemical Society, *Natural Plant Hydrocolloids*, Advan. Chem. Ser. no. 11, 1954; C. L. Mantell, *The Water Soluble Gums*, 1965; W. Pigman and M. L. Wolfrom (eds.), *Advances in Carbohydrate Chemistry*, vol. 13, 1958; R. L. Whistler (ed.), *Industrial Gums: Polysaccharides and Their Derivatives*, vol. 1, rev. ed., 1970; R. L. Whistler and C. L. Smart, *Polysaccharide Chemistry*, 1953.

Heartwater disease

A septicemic, infectious disease of cattle, sheep, and goats in equatorial and southern Africa caused by *Cowdria ruminantium*, a rickettsialike pathogen. It is carried chiefly by the bont tick (*Amblyomma heberaeum*). Man is not susceptible.

Nonapparent infections in certain wild antelope, in addition to range stock, are thought to provide a reservoir in bushveld areas for new generations of young ticks since infection does not pass through tick eggs. Strains of varying virulence cause subacute or acute disease with high mortality. The name is derived from the common lesion of the heart, hydropericarditis. Clumps of organisms are seen in Giemsa-stained cells lining the blood vessels. Young animals are immunized by intentional infection, followed by treatment with sulfonamide or antibiotic drugs.   [CORNELIUS B. PHILIP]

Herbicide

Any chemical used to destroy or inhibit plant growth, especially of weeds or other undesirable vegetation. The concepts of modern herbicide technology began to develop about 1900 and accelerated rapidly with the discovery of dichlorophenoxyacetic acid (2,4-D) as a growth-regulator-type herbicide in 1944–1945. A few other notable events should be mentioned. During 1896–1908, metal salts and mineral acids were introduced as selective sprays for controlling broadleafed weeds in cereals; during 1915–1925 acid arsenical spray, sodium chlorate, and other chemicals were recognized as herbicides; and in 1933–1934, sodium dinitrocresylate became the first organic selective herbicide to be used in culture of cereals, flax, and peas. Since the introduction of 2,4-D, a wide variety of organic herbicides have been developed and have received wide usage in agriculture, forestry, and other industries. Today, the development of highly specific herbicides intended to control specific weed types continues. Modern usage often combines two or more herbicides to provide the desired weed control. Worldwide usage of herbicides continues to increase, making their manufacture and sale a major industry. In 1974, United States sales of herbicides topped $1,000,000,000 for the first time.

The control of weeds by means of herbicides has provided many benefits. Freeing agricultural crops from weed competition has resulted in higher food production, reduced harvesting costs, improved food quality, and lowered processing costs, contributing to the abundant United States supply of low-cost, high-quality food. Not only are billions of dollars saved through increased production and improved quality, but costs of labor and machinery energy necessary for weed control are reduced, livestock is saved from the effects of poisonous weeds, irrigation costs are reduced, and insect and disease control costs are decreased through the removal of host weeds for the undesirable organisms. Still, annual losses of crops due to weeds in the United States are estimated to be $2,500,000,000. Additional benefits due to appropriate herbicide use result as millions of people are relieved of the suffering caused by allergies to pollens and exposure to poisonous plants. Recreational areas, roadsides, forests, and parks have been freed of noxious weeds, and home lawns have been beautified. Herbicides have reduced storage and labor costs and fire hazards for industrial storage yards and warehouse areas. Modern herbicides even benefit the construction industry, where chemicals applied under asphalt prolong pavement life by preventing weed penetration of the surface.

Classification. There are well over a hundred chemicals in common usage as herbicides. Many of these are available in several formulations or under several trade names. The variety of materials are conveniently classified according to the properties of the active ingredient as either selective or nonselective. Further subclassification is by method of application, such as preemergence (soil-applied before plant emergence) or postemergence (applied to plant foliage). Additional terminology sometimes applied to describe the mobility of postemergence herbicides in the treated plant is contact (nonmobile) or translocated (mobile—that is, killing plants by systemic action). Thus, glyphosate is a nonselective, postemergence, translocated herbicide.

Selective herbicides are those that kill some members of a plant population with little or no injury to others. An example is alachlor, which can be used to kill grassy and some broad-leafed weeds in corn, soybeans, and other crops.

Nonselective herbicides are those that kill all vegetation to which they are applied. Examples are bromacil, paraquat, or glyphosate, which can be used to keep roadsides, ditch banks, and rights-of-way open and weed-free. A rapidly expanding use for such chemicals is the destruction of vegetation before seeding in the practice of reduced tillage or no tillage. Some are also used to kill annual grasses in preparation for seeding perennial grasses in pastures. Additional uses are in fire prevention, elimination of highway hazards, destruction of plants that are hosts for insects and plant diseases, and killing of poisonous or allergen-bearing plants.

Preemergence or postemergence application methods derive naturally from the properties of the herbicidal chemical. Some, such as trifluralin, are effective only when applied to the soil and absorbed into the germinating seedling, and therefore are used as preemergence herbicides. Others, such as diquat, exert their herbicidal effect only on contact with plant foliage and are strongly inactivated when placed in contact with soil. These can be applied only as a postemergence herbicide. However, the distinction between pre- and postemergence is not always clear-cut. For example, atrazine can exert its herbicidal action either following root absorption from a preemergence application or after leaf absorption from a postemergence treatment, and thus it can be used with either application method. This may be an advantage in high-rainfall areas where a postemergence treatment can be washed off the leaf onto the soil and nevertheless can provide effective weed control.

Herbicidal action. Many factors influence herbicide performance. A few are discussed below.

Soil type and organic matter content. Soils vary widely in composition and in chemical and physical characteristics. The capacity of a soil to fix or adsorb a preemergence herbicide determines how much will be available to seedling plants. For example, a sandy soil normally is not strongly adsorptive. Lower quantities of most herbicides are needed on a highly adsorptive clay soil. A similar response occurs with the organic portion of soil; higher organic matter content usually indicates that more herbicide is bound and a higher treatment rate necessary. For example, cyanazine is used for weed control in corn at the rate of 1½ lb/acre (1.7 kg/ha) on sandy loam soil of less than 1% organic matter, but 5 lb/acre (5.6 kg/ha) is required on a clay soil of 4% organic matter.

Leaching. This refers to the downward movement of herbicides into the soil. Some preemergence herbicides must be leached into the soil into the immediate vicinity of weed seeds to exert toxic action. However, excessive rainfall may leach these chemicals too deeply into the soil, thereby allowing weeds to germinate and grow close to the surface.

Volatilization. Several herbicides in use today will volatilize from the soil surface. To be effective, these herbicides must be mixed with the soil to a depth of 2 to 4 in. (5–10 cm). This process is termed soil incorporation. Once the herbicide is in contact with soil particles, volatilization loss is minimized. This procedure is commonly employed with thiocarbamate herbicides such as EPTC and dinitroaniline herbicides such as trifluralin.

Leaf properties. Leaf surfaces are highly variable. Some are much more waxy then others; many are corrugated or ridged; and some are covered with small hairs. These variations cause differences in the retention of postemergence spray droplets and thus influence herbicidal effect. Most grass leaves stand in a relatively vertical position, whereas the broad-leafed plants usually have their leaves arranged in a more horizontal position. This causes broad-leaf plants to intercept a larger quantity of a herbicide spray than grass plants.

Location of growing points. Growing points and buds of most cereal plants are located in a crown, at or below the soil surface. Furthermore, they are wrapped within the mature bases of the older leaves. Hence they may be protected from herbicides applied as sprays. Buds of many broad-leafed weeds are located at the tips of shoots and in axils of leaves, and are therefore more exposed to herbicide sprays.

Growth habits. Some perennial crops, such as alfalfa, vines, and trees, have a dormant period in

Important herbicides

Common name*	Chemical name	Major uses†
Acrolein	2-Propenal	Aquatic weed control
Alachlor	2-Chloro-2′,6′-diethyl-N-(methoxymethyl) acetanilide	Sel. PE corn, soybeans, and other crops
Ametryn	2-(Ethylamino)-4-(isopropylamino)-6-(methylthio)-s-triazine	Sel. PE and POE pineapple, sugarcane, bananas
Amitrole	3-Amino-s-triazole	NS weed control in noncrop areas
AMS	Ammonium sulfate	NS POE weed and brush control
Asulam	Methyl sulfanilylcarbamate	Sel. POE sugarcane, range, forests
Atrazine	2-Chloro-4-(ethylamino)-6-(isopropylamino)-s-triazine	Sel. PE or POE corn, sorghum, sugarcane
Barban	4-Chloro-2-butynyl-m-chlorocarbanilate	Sel. POE cereals and other crops
Benefin	N-Butyl-N-ethyl-α,α, α-trifluoro-2,6-dinitro-p-toluidine	Sel. PE legumes, lettuce, tobacco, turf
Bensulide	O,O-Diisopropyl phosphonodithioate S-ester with N-(2-mercaptoethyl)benzene sulfonamide	Sel. PE turf and vegetables
Bentazon	3-Isopropyl-1H-2,1,3-benzothiadiazin-4-(3H)-1-2,2-dioxide	Sel. POE cereals and legume crops
Benzadox	(Benzamidooxy)acetic acid	Sel. POE sugar beet
Bifenox	Methyl 5-(2,4-dichlorophenoxy)-2-nitrobenzoate	Sel. PE soybean, rice, and other crops
Bromacil	5-Bromo-3-sec-butyl-6-methyluracil	NS PE/POE weed and brush control
Bromoxynil	3,5-Dibromo-4-hydroxybenzonitrile	Sel. POE cereals, flax, turf
Butachlor	N-(Butoxymethyl)2-chloro-2′,6′-diethylacetanilide	Sel. PE rice, barley
Buthidazole	3-[5-(1,1-Dimethylethyl)-1, 3, 4-thiadiazol-2-yl]-4-hydroxy-1-methyl-2-imidazolidinone	NS PE/POE weed and brush killer
Butralin	4-(1,1-Dimethyl-ethyl)-N-(1-methyl)-2,6-dinitrobenzeneamine	Sel. PE soybean, cotton
Butylate	S-Ethyl diisobutylthiocarbamate	Sel. PE corn

Important herbicides (cont.)

Common name*	Chemical name	Major uses†
Cacodylic acid	Hydroxydimethylarsine oxide	NS POE general weed control and cotton defoliant
Carbetamide	D-N-Ethyllactamide carbanilate (ester)	Sel. PE or POE alfalfa
CDAA	N,N-Diallyl-2-chloroacetamide	Sel. PE corn and vegetables
CDEC	2-Chloroallyl-diethyldithiocarbamate	Sel. PE vegetables
Chloramben	3-Amino-2,5-dichlorobenzoic acid	Sel. PE soybeans, vegetables
Chlorbromuron	3-(4-Bromo-3-chlorophenyl)-1-methoxy-l-methylurea	Sel. PE soybeans, corn, and potatoes
Chloroxuron	3-[p-(p-Chlorophenoxy) phenyl]-1,1-dimethylurea	Sel. PE/POE soybeans and other crops
Chlorpropham	Isopropyl m-chlorocarbanilate	Sel. PE legume and vegetable crops
Cyanazine	2-[[4-Chloro-6-(ethylamino)-s-triazin-2-yl]amino] 2-2 methylpropionitrile	Sel. PE corn
Cycloate	S-Ethyl N-ethylthiocyclohexanecarbamate	Sel. PE beets, spinach
Cyprazine	2-Chloro-4-cyclopropylamino-6-(isopropylamino)-s-triazine	Sel. POE corn
Dalapon	2,2-Dichloropropionic acid	Sel. PE/POE sugarcane, tree crops, and other crops
Dazomet	Tetrahydro-3,5-dimethyl-2H-1,3,5-thiadiazine-2-thione	Sel. PE turf, tobacco seedbeds, ornamentals
DCPA	Dimethyl tetrachloroterephthalate	Sel. PE turf, ornamentals, vegetables
Desmedipham	Ethyl m-hydroxycarbanilate	Sel. POE sugar beet
Diallate	S-(2,3-Dichloroallyl) diisopropylthiocarbamate	Sel. PE sugar beet, cereals, and other crops
Dicamba	3,6-Dichloro-o-anisic acid	Sel. PE/POE corn, cereals, turf
Dichlorbenil	2,6-Dichlorobenzonitrile	NS PE ornamentals, tree fruits, aquatic weed control
Dichlorprop	2-(2,4-Dichlorophenoxy) propionic acid	NS brush control
Difenzoquat	1,2-Dimethyl-3,5-diphenyl-1H-pyrazolium	Sel. POE cereals
Dinitramine	N^4,N^4-Diethyl-α,α,α-trifluoro-3,5-dinitrotoluene-2,4-diamine	Sel. PE cotton, soybeans, and other crops
Dinoseb	2-sec-Butyl-4,6-dinitrophenol	Sel. PE/POE soybeans, peanuts, and other crops
Diphenamid	N,N-Dimethyl-2,2-diphenylacetamide	Sel. PE turf, peanuts, vegetables, and other crops
Dipropetryn	2,4-Bis(isopropylamino)-6-(ethylthio)-s-triazine	Sel. PE cotton
Diquat	6,7-Dihydrodipyrido[1,2-a:2',1'-c]pyrazinediium ion	NS POE noncrop land and aquatic weed control
Diuron	3-(3,4-Dichlorophenyl)-1,1-dimethylurea	Sel. PE/POE cotton, sugarcane, cereals, tree crops; NS PE/POE general weed killer
DSMA	Disodium methanearsonate	Sel. POE cotton, turf; NS POE general weed killer
Endothall	7-Oxabicyclo[2.2.1]heptane 2,3-dicarboxylic acid	Sel. PE sugar beets; aquatic weed killer; cotton defoliant
EPTC	S-Ethyl dipropylthiocarbamate	Sel. PE corn, potatoes, and other crops
Erbon	2-(2,4,5-Trichlorophenoxy)ethyl-2,2-dichloropropionate	NS PE/POE general weed killer
Ethalfluralin	N-Ethyl-N-(2-methyl-2-propenyl)-2,6-dinitro-4-(trifluoromethyl)benzeneamine	Sel. PE cotton, beans
Fenac	(2,3,6-Trichlorophenyl)acetic acid	Sel. PE/POE sugarcane; general weed killer
Fenuron	1,1-Dimethyl-3-phenylurea	NS PE/POE general weed and brush killer
Fluchloralin	N-(2-Chloroethyl)-2,6-dinitro-N-propyl-4-(trifluoromethyl)aniline	Sel. PE cotton, soybeans
Fluometuron	1,1-Dimethyl-3-(α,α,α-trifluoro-m-tolyl)urea	Sel. PE/POE cotton, sugarcane
Glyphosate	N-(Phosphonomethyl)-glycine	NS POE general weed killer
Ioxynil	4-Hydroxy-3,5-diiodobenzonitrile	Sel. POE cereals
Isopropalin	2,6-Dinitro-N,N-dipropylcumidine	Sel. PE tobacco
Linuron	3-(3,4-Dichlorophenyl)-1-methoxy-1-methylurea	Sel. PE soybean, potatoes, and other crops
MCPA	[(4-Chloro-o-tolyl)oxy]acetic acid	Sel. POE cereals, legumes, flax
MCPB	4-[(4-Chloro-o-tolyl)oxy]butyric acid	Sel. POE legumes
Mecoprop	2-[(4-Chloro-o-tolyl)oxy]propionic acid	Sel. POE turf
Metham	Sodium methyldithiocarbamate	Sel. PE tobacco, turf
Methazole	2-(3,4-Dichlorophenyl)-4-methyl-1,2,4-oxadiazolidine-3,5-dione	Sel. PE cotton
Metolachlor	2-Chloro-N-(2-ethyl-6-methylphenyl)-N-(2-methoxy-1-methylethyl)acetamide	Sel. PE corn
Metribuzin	4-Amino-6-tert-butyl-3-(methylthio)-as-triazin-5(4H)-one	Sel. PE soybeans, potatoes, sugarcane

Important herbicides (cont.)

Common name*	Chemical name	Major uses†
Molinate	S-Ethyl hexahydro-1H-azepine 1-carbothioate	Sel. PE/POE rice
Monuron	3-(p-Chlorophenyl)-1, 1-dimethylurea	NS PE/POE general weed killer
MSMA	Monosodium methanearsonate	Sel. POE cotton, turf; NS POE general weed killer
Napropamide	2-(α-Naphthoxy)N,N-diethylpropionamide	Sel. PE tomatoes, tree fruits
Naptalam	N-1-Napthylphthalamic acid	Sel. PE soybean, peanut, and vegetables
Nitrofen	2,4-Dichlorophenyl-p-nitrophenyl ether	Sel. PE/POE vegetables
Norflurazon	4-Chloro-5-(methylamino)-2-(α,α,α-trifluoro-m-tolyl)-3(2H)-pyridazinone	Sel. PE cranberries
Oryzalin	3,5-Dinitro-N⁴,N⁴-dipropylsulfanilamide	Sel. PE cotton, soybeans
Paraquat	1,1'-Dimethyl-4,4'-bipyridinium ion	NS POE general weed killer
Pebulate	S-Propyl butylethylthiocarbamate	Sel. PE sugar beets, tobacco
Pendimethalin	N-(1-Ethyl)-3,4-dimethyl-2,6-dinitrobenzeneamine	Sel. PE corn, cotton, soybeans
Perfluidone	1,1,1-Trifluoro-N-[2-methyl-4-(phenylsulfonyl)phenyl] methanesulfonamide	Sel. PE cotton
Phenmedipham	Methyl m-hydroxycarbanilate m-methylcarbanilate	Sel. POE beets
Picloram	4-Amino-3,5,6-trichloropicolinic acid	NS PE/POE general weed and brush killer
Procyazine	2-[[4-Chloro-6-(cyclopropylamino)-1,3,5-triazine-2-yl]amino]-2-methylpropanenitrile	Sel. PE/POE corn
Profluralin	N-(Cyclopropylmethyl)-α,α,α-trifluoro-2,6-dinitro-N-propyl-p-toluidine	Sel. PE legumes, cotton, and other crops
Prometryn	2,4-Bis(isopropylamino)-6-(methylthio)-s-triazine	Sel. PE/POE cotton, celery
Pronamide	3,5-Dichloro(N-1,1-dimethyl-2-propynyl)benzamide	Sel. PE/POE legumes, turf, lettuce
Propachlor	2-Chloro-N-isopropylacetanilide	Sel. PE corn, milo, soybeans
Propanil	3',4'-Dichloropropionanilide	Sel. POE rice
Propazine	2-Chloro-4,6-bis-(isopropylamino)-s-triazine	Sel. PE milo
Propham	Isopropyl carbanilate	Sel. PE forages, lettuce, and other crops
Pyrazon	5-Amino-4-chloro-2-phenyl-3(2H)-pyridazinone	Sel. PE beets
Siduron	1-(2-Methylcyclohexyl)-3-phenylurea	Sel. PE turf
Silvex	2-(2,4-5-Trichlorophenoxy)propionic acid	Sel. POE turf; NS POE general and aquatic weed control
Simazine	2-Chloro-4,6-bis-(ethylamino)-s-triazine	Sel. PE corn, forages, and other crops; aquatic weed control
TCA	Trichloroacetic acid	Sel. PE/POE sugar beets, sugarcane, cotton, soybeans
Tebuthiuron	N-[5-(1,1-Dimethyl)-1,3,4-thiadiazol-2-yl]-N,N'-dimethylurea	NS PE/POE general weed killer
Terbacil	3-tert-Butyl-5-chloro-6-methyluracil	Sel. PE sugarcane, tree fruits, and other crops
Terbutryn	2-(tert-Butylamino)-4-(ethylamino)-6-(methylthio)-s-triazine	Sel. PE/POE cereals, milo
Triallate	S-(2,3,3-Trichloroallyl)diisopropylthiocarbamate	Sel. PE cereals
Trifluralin	α,α,α-Trifluoro-2,6-dinitro-N,N-dipropyl-p-toluidine	Sel. PE legumes, cotton, and other crops
2,3,6-TBA	2,3,6-Trichlorobenzoic acid	NS PE/POE general weed control
2,4-D	(2,4-Dichlorophenoxy)acetic acid	Sel. POE cereals, milo, corn, and other crops; aquatic and general weed control
2,4-DB	4-(2,4-Dichlorophenoxy)butyric acid	Sel. POE legume crops
2,4,5-T	(2,4,5-Trichlorophenoxy)acetic acid	Sel. POE rice, forage grasses; general weed and brush control
Vernolate	S-Propyl dipropylthiocarbamate	Sel. PE peanuts, soybeans

*Major trade names can be found in *Farm Chemicals Handbook*, Meister Publishing Co., Willoughby. OH, 1977.

†Sel. = selective herbicide; NS = nonselective herbicide; PE = preemergence; POE = postemergence.

winter. At that time a general-contact weed killer may be safely used to get rid of weeds that later would compete with the crop for water and plant nutrients.

Application methods. By arranging spray nozzles to spray low-growing weeds but not the leaves of a taller crop plant, it is possible to provide weed control with a herbicide normally phytotoxic to the crop. This directed spray technique is used to kill young grass in cotton with MSMA or broad-leafed weeds in soybeans with chloroxuron in an oil emulsion. A recent modification of this technique is an arrangement of nozzles spraying horizontally into a catch basin over the top of the crop in such a manner that weeds taller than the crop pass through the spray streams but the crop does not. Use of a nonselective translocated herbicide in this recirculating sprayer system will then selectively remove the weeds from the crop. Glyphosate is being used experimentally in this system to remove johnson grass from cotton.

Protoplasmic selectivity. Just as some people are immune to the effects of certain diseases while others succumb, so some weed species resist the toxic effects of herbicides whereas others are injured or killed. This results from inherent properties of the protoplasm of the respective species. One example is the use of 2,4-DB or MCPB (the butyric acid analogs of 2,4-D and MCPA) on weeds having β-oxidizing enzymes that are growing in crops (certain legumes) which lack such enzymes. The weeds are killed because the butyric acid compounds are broken down to 2,4-D or MCPA. Another example is the control of a wide variety of weeds in corn by atrazine. Corn contains a compound that removes the chlorine from the atrazine atom, rendering it nontoxic; most weeds lack this compound. A third important example of protoplasmic selectivity is shown by trifluralin, planavin, and a number of other herbicides applied through the soil which inhibit secondary root growth. Used in large seeded crops having vigorous taproots, they kill shallow-rooted weed seedlings; the roots of the crops extend below the shallow layer of topsoil containing the herbicides and the seedlings survive and grow to produce a crop.

Properties. Several factors of the commercial herbicide influence selectivity to crops.

Molecular configuration. Subtle changes in the chemical structure can cause dramatic shifts in herbicide performance. For example, trifluralin and benefin are very similar dinitroaniline herbicides differing only in the location of one methylene group. However, this small difference allows benefin to be used for grass control in lettuce, whereas trifluralin will severely injure lettuce at the rates required for weed control.

Herbicide concentration. The action of herbicides on plants is rate-responsive. That is, small quantities of a herbicide applied to a plant may cause no toxicity, or even a slight growth stimulation, whereas larger amounts may result in the death of the plants. It has long been known that 2,4-D applied at low rates causes an increase in respiration rate and cell division, resulting in an apparent growth stimulation. At high application rates, 2,4-D causes more severe changes and the eventual death of the plant.

Formulation. The active herbicidal chemical itself is seldom applied directly to the soil or plants. Because of the nature of the chemicals, it is usually necessary that the commercial product be formulated to facilitate handling and dilution to the appropriate concentration. Two common formulations are emulsifiable concentrates and wettable powders. Emulsifiable concentrates are solutions of the chemical in an organic solvent with emulsifiers added which permit mixing and spraying with water. Wettable powders are a mixture of a finely divided powder, active chemical, and emulsifiers which allow the powder to suspend in water and to be sprayed. An additional ingredient called an adjuvant is sometimes added to the formulation or to the spray tank when the spray solution is mixed. These adjuvants are normally surface-active agents (surfactants) which improve the uniformity of spray coverage on plants and the plant penetration of the herbicide. An example is the addition of surfactant to paraquat spray solutions to improve its nonselective postemergence action on weeds. Another material sometimes added to spray solutions is a nonphytotoxic oil. These oils may be used to improve postemergence action of herbicides such as diuron which normally have limited foliar absorption.

Available herbicides. In the table, some of the important herbicides used in United States are list-

ed alphabetically by the common name approved by the Weed Science Society of America. The chemical name and some major uses of each herbicide are included.

Many of the chemicals listed in the table are used in proprietary mixtures. These normally combine two or more herbicides in a single formulation and are marketed under brand names. Such mixtures are not included in the table.

[RODNEY O. RADKE]

Bibliography: A. S. Crafts, *Modern Weed Control*, 1975; *Farm Chemicals Handbook*, 1977; *Herbicide Handbook of the Weed Science Society of America*, 3d ed., 1974; G. C. Klingman and F. M. Ashton, *Weed Sciences: Principles and Practices*, 1975.

Histidine

An amino acid widely distributed in proteins. Histidine, like other compounds containing an imidazole ring, may be detected by the Pauly reaction, in which the imidazole ring is coupled to diazotized sulfanilic acid in an alkaline solution to give a red color.

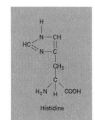

Physical constants of the L isomer at 25°C:
pK$_1$ (COOH): 1.82; pK$_2$ (imidazole): 6.00; pK$_3$ (NH$_3^+$): 9.17
Isoelectric point: 7.59
Optical rotation: [α]$_D$(H$_2$O): −38.5; [α]$_D$ (5 N HCl): +11.8
Solubility (g/100 ml H$_2$O): 4.29

Histidine is present in relatively large amounts in hemoglobin. Histidine derivatives include the dipeptides carnosine (β-alanyl-L-histidine) and anserine (β-alanyl-l-methyl-L-histidine), which are

The major degradative pathway of histidine.

abundant in muscle, and ergothioneine, the trimethylbetaine of thiolhistidine, which is abundant in erythrocytes and seminal fluid; however, the function of these compounds is unknown.

Decarboxylation of histidine results in histamine, which is a vasodilator mediating many of the inflammatory responses of animal tissue. Histidine participates in transamination; however, its keto acid analog, imidazole pyruvic acid, is not an intermediate in the only known histidine biosynthetic pathway. The major degradative pathway of histidine is shown in the illustration. Formiminoglutamic acid is further degraded to glutamic acid, ammonia, and formate or carbon dioxide by reactions that vary according to species. In mammalian tissue the degradation requires folic acid, and individuals deficient in this vitamin excrete formiminoglutamic acid and urocanic acid. Histidinemia is an asymptomatic human metabolic disorder in which the enzyme histidinase is lacking and histidine and its deamination product, imidazole pyruvic acid, are present in abnormal quantities in the blood and urine. *See* AMINO ACIDS.

[DAVID W. E. SMITH]

Honey Dew melon

A long-keeping variety of muskmelon, *Cucumis melo*, of the plant order Violales. The fruit is large (5–7 lb), oval, smooth, creamy yellow to ivory when ripe, and without surface markings. The flesh is thick (1¾ to 2 in.), light green, juicy, sweet, with very mild aroma and flavor; it contains 10% sugar when well ripened, and is rich in vitamin C but not nearly so rich in vitamin A as the orange-fleshed cantaloupes.

Honey Dew is an American name for the variety White Antibes, grown in France and Algeria long before its introduction into the United States about 1900. The Honey Dew melon requires a warm season of about 125 days. It is very susceptible to diseases, which are intensified by rain or high humidity. Except under irrigation in California, Texas, and Arizona, it is little grown in the United States.

Since 1950 the area harvested commercially each year has varied from about 9000 to 11,000 acres. Annual production is about 60,000–70,000 tons. *See* MELON GROWING; MUSKMELON.

[VICTOR R. BOSWELL]

Hop

A dioecious liana (*Humulus lupulus*), belonging to the plant order Urticales. Each season numerous herbaceous vines are produced from a perennial crown. The vines twine in a clockwise direction, grow to a length of 15–25 ft in a season, and die following maturity. *See* STEM (BOTANY).

The inflorescences of the female plants constitute the hops of commerce (see illustration). These inflorescences are catkins (strobiles) with papery bracts and bracteoles. Numerous sticky, yellowish lupulin granules (glands) are produced on the bracts, seeds, and bracteoles. These granules contain resins and essential oils which are of value in the brewing of beer and ale.

Hops are adapted to the temperate regions of the world. In the United States the major areas of production are Washington, Oregon, Idaho, and California. Hops are produced primarily under irrigation on fertile, well-drained soil. Rhizomes from the female plants are planted to produce 680–1030

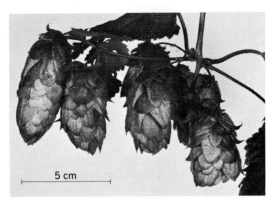

Hop, female inflorescences. (*USDA*)

hills per acre, space 6.5–8 ft apart. The vines are trained to climb strings suspended from an overhead wire trellis and anchored at the hills (bases of plants). The hops are harvested by specialized equipment, dried in forced-air kilns, and baled for market. Net exports amount to about 30% of the annual crop. Production in the United States has been regulated by a Federal marketing order since 1966. Hops have been used by brewers for at least 1200 years. When added to the wort (fermenting material), either whole or in extract form, hops impart a characteristic flavor and aroma to the finished beverage and aid in preservation, head (foam) retention, and protein coagulation.

[STANLEY N. BROOKS]

Horseradish

A hardy perennial crucifer, *Armoracia rusticana*, of eastern European origin belonging to the plant order Capparales. Horseradish is grown for its pungent roots, which are generally grated, mixed with vinegar and salt, and used as a condiment or relish. Propagation is by root cuttings, and the crop is grown like an annual. The individual roots or sets are uncovered by hand usually twice during the summer and stripped of all side roots (see illustration). Maliner Kren is a common variety. Harvesting of the roots occurs in the fall, usually 3½ to 4 months after planting. Production in the United States is limited to northern areas; Illinois, Wisconsin, and Missouri are important producing states. *See* VEGETABLE GROWING.   [JOHN CAREW]

Horticultural crops

Food-producing plants such as tree fruits, small fruits including cane fruits, bush fruits and low-growing berry plants, melons, edible nuts, grapes or vine crops, and vegetables cultivated for their leaves, flowers, fruits, stems, or roots. These plants vary widely in their tolerance to soils, moisture, and temperature, which affects their distribution and adaptation to various localities.

Insects and diseases also greatly influence the survival or the profitable culture of many horitcultural plants. Protection may be provided by chemical spraying, selection of tolerant plants or varieties, or development of resistant types through breeding. Modern research is developing new techniques in biological control of insects as well as more efficient chemicals for the control of insects, diseases, and weeds. Other organic chemical sprays have been developed to improve fruit size

HORSERADISH

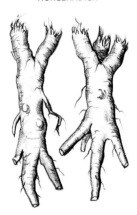

Roots of horseradish stripped of side roots.

and color, advance maturity, initiate flower buds, increase fruit set, and alter growth characteristics for specific purposes. *See* BREEDING (PLANT); PLANT DISEASE; PLANT VIRUS.

Continued progress in developing mechanical harvesting of vegetable crops, strawberries, and cane fruits has initiated breeding research in development of plants or fruits or both better adapted to machine harvest. Tree fruits are being made more adaptable to mechanical harvest by modified tree shape through special pruning, use of dwarf-type trees, changes in planting patterns by using hedgerow systems, and varied methods of tree spacing. The trend in apple and pear orchards is toward higher densities of trees per acre propagated on dwarfing rootstocks.

Many fruit crops are propagated asexually by stem or root cuttings, whereas most vegetable crops are propagated sexually by seed. In propagation of some tree fruits and grapes, certain varieties may be grafted onto more hardy or resistant root stocks, thus better adapting them to adverse soil or weather conditions, or pests. The trend toward dwarf trees of apple and pear has encouraged selection and development of dwarfing stocks. *See* GRAFTING OF PLANTS.

For most horticultural crops, pollination is essential for fruit set. Therefore, varieties in commercial fruit plantings are arranged to ensure maximum cross pollination because some varieties are naturally self-unfruitful, or because the times of blossoming of desirable pollinating varieties may not coincide. Pollination is not known to affect fruit color directly, but in certain species it does affect size, shape, and seed characters of pollinated fruit. *See* FRUIT, TREE; FRUIT GROWING, SMALL; GRAPE CULTURE; MELON GROWING; NUT CROP CULTURE; VEGETABLE GROWING.

[ALBERT F. VIERHELLER]

Bibliography: *See* AGRICULTURAL SCIENCE (PLANT).

Hydroxyproline

An amino acid occurring in certain proteins. Hydroxyproline, the 4-hydroxy analog of proline, shares many of the chemical and biological features of proline. Unlike proline, hydroxyproline is not found generally in proteins but is essentially

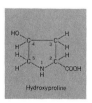

Physical constants of the L-diastereomers at 25°:

Hydroxy-L-proline

pK$_1$ (COOH): 1.82; pK$_2$ (NH$_3$+): 9.68
Optical rotation: [α]$_D$(H$_2$O): −76.0°; [α]$_D$ (5 N HCl): −50.5°
Very soluble in H$_2$O

Allohydroxy-L-proline

pK$_1$ (COOH): 1.98; pK$_2$ (NH$_3$+): 9.60
Optical rotation: [α]$_D$(H$_2$O): −59.5°; [α]$_D$ (5 N HCl): −18.8°
Very soluble in H$_2$O, slightly soluble in ethanol

limited to structural proteins of the collagen type of animals, and to a similar protein in the cell walls of higher plants. It constitutes about 10% of most collagen in vertebrates, but is present in higher content in certain invertebrate collagens (earthworm cuticle and *Hydra* nematocysts). *See* PROTEIN.

4-Hydroxy-L-proline (the major isomer in nature) was first obtained from gelatin in 1902 by E. Fischer; it was first synthesized chemically in 1905 by H. Leuchs.

Isomers. Because it contains two asymmetric carbons (carbon 2 and 4), hydroxyproline can exist as any of four optical isomers; the form with L configuration at both carbon 2 and 4 (trans-relation of the hydroxyl and carboxyl group) is that found in collagen. Other isomers have singular or limited natural occurrence, for example, allohydroxy-L-proline in tissues of the sandalwood tree, and allohydroxy-D-proline in the antibiotic etamycin. In addition, small amounts (about 1%) of the position isomer, 3-hydroxy-L-proline, also occur in many collagens.

Chemistry and metabolic activity. Chemical features of hydroxyproline shared with proline are the yellow color given with ninhydrin and the resistance to nitrous acid deamination. Like proline, hydroxyproline is not a substrate for known pyridoxal-phosphate enzymes.

A number of mammalian tissues contain enzymes that rapidly degrade free hydroxy-L-proline to yield 4-hydroxy-L-glutamic acid, a reaction analogous to the oxidation of L-proline to form L-glutamic acid. 4-Hydroxyglutamic acid can be further decomposed by enzymes to yield pyruvic acid and glyoxylic acid. It is probable that significant amounts of free hydroxyproline are formed in animals from early peptide precursors of collagen, in which prolines are already hydroxylated. These may break down readily to yield hydroxproline both in the form of small peptides and as the free amino acid.

Another path of breakdown of free hydroxy-L-proline has been described in extracts of soil bacteria, which can use hydroxyproline as the entire source of carbon and nitrogen for growth. These reactions convert hydroxy-L-proline to α-ketoglutaric acid through several intermediate compounds; the enzymes for these steps are induced by exposure of the bacterial cells to hydroxyproline.

Medical significance. In humans hydroxyproline is excreted in the urine, predominantly in small peptides. Hydroxyproline excretion in urine is increased during increased breakdown of collagen, and occurs in certain disorders of bone growth or bone destruction and in some metabolic disorders, for example, hyperthyroidism or hyperparathyroidism. A single instance is known in man of the hereditary absence of one of the enzymes degrading hydroxyproline; the subject had abnormally high levels of free hydroxyproline in blood and urine and was mentally retarded. *See* AMINO ACIDS; METABOLIC DISORDERS; PROLINE.

[ELIJAH ADAMS]

Bibliography: J. P. Greenstein and M. Winitz, *Chemistry of the Amino Acids*, vols. 1–3, 1961; A. Meister, *Biochemistry of the Amino Acids*, vols. 1 and 2, 2d ed., 1965.

Ice cream

A commercial dairy food made by freezing while stirring a pasteurized mix of suitable ingredients. They may include but are not limited to milk fat, nonfat milk solids, or milk-derived ingredients; and sugars, corn syrup, water, flavoring, sometimes egg products, stabilizers, and emulsifiers. Air incorporated during the freezing process is also an important component.

The structure of ice cream is complex. It consists of a solid, gaseous, and liquid phase: ice crystals and air cells are dispersed throughout the liquid phase, which also contains fat globules, milk proteins, and other materials.

Composition. In the United States ice cream composition is regulated by Federal Frozen Dessert Standards of Identity, and proposed standards set forth minimum composition requirements. Ice cream must contain not less than 10% milk fat nor less than 2.7% protein, must have not less than 1.6 lb (0.72 kg) food solids per gallon (3.8 liters), and must weigh not less than 4.5 lb (2 kg) to the gallon. In the case of bulky flavors the fat may not be less than 8%, nor can the protein content be less than 2.2% in the finished food. The protein to meet minimum requirements is to be provided by milk solids—nonfat or milk-derived ingredients. Ingredient and nutritional requirements labeling are included in the standards.

The composition of ice cream may vary depending on whether it is an economy brand satisfying minimum requirements, a trade brand of average composition, or a premium brand of superior composition. The components by weight of an average-composition ice cream are 12% fat, 11% milk solids not fat, 15% sugar, and 0.3% vegetable gum stabilizer.

An average serving, $1/6$ qt (155 ml) or 100 g, of vanilla ice cream provides about 200 calories (838 joules), 12 g fat, 3.7 g protein, 18.6 g carbohydrate, 0.122 g calcium, 0.105 g phosphorus, 492 international units of vitamin A, 0.38 mg thiamine and 0.236 mg riboflavin.

Frozen dairy desserts. Products classed as frozen dairy desserts include French ice cream, frozen custard, ice milk, sherbet, water ice, frozen dairy confection, dietary frozen dairy dessert, and mellorine or imitation ice cream.

French ice cream may contain a relatively high fat content, have a deeper color, and contain egg yolk solids. French custard is similar to French ice cream but must contain not less than 1.4% egg yolk solids for plain flavor and not less than 1.12% for bulky flavors. It is usually sold as a soft-serve product but may be sold either as a prepackaged hardened or soft product.

Ice milk meets the provisions for ice cream except that it must contain more than 2% but not more than 7% milk fat, not less than 2.7% protein, and not less than 1.3 lb (0.58 kg) food solids per gallon.

Sherbet has a small amount of milk products but is produced like ice cream. It must weigh not less than 6 lb (2.7 kg) per gallon. It contains not less than 1% nor more than 2% fat, and total milk solids of not less than 2% or more than 5% by weight of the finished food. Sherbet must also contain 0.35% edible citric or natural fruit acid.

Water ice is similar to sherbet but contains no milk solids.

Dietary frozen dessert is a low-calorie product. It must contain less than 2% milk fat and not less than 7% by weight of total milk solids, must weigh not less than 4.5 lb (2.9 kg) per gallon, and must contain 1.1–1.45 lb (0.5–0.65 kg) food solids per gallon.

Mellorine is manufactured in a manner similar to ice cream, but is not limited to milk-derived nonfat solids and may be composed of animal or vegetable fat or both, only part of which may be milk fat. It contains not less than 6% fat nor less than 2.7% protein by weight.

Frozen dairy confections are produced in the form of individual servings and commonly referred to as novelties—including bars, stick items, and sandwiches. These constitute an important segment of the industry.

Soft frozen dairy products have had good sales. The soft frozen product is usually drawn from the freezer at 18 to 20°F (−8 to −7°C) and is served directly to the consumer. Ice milk accounts for about three-fourths of the soft-serve gallonage. Products in the market vary from 2 to 7% fat, 11 to 14% milk solids not fat, 13 to 18% sugar, and about 0.4% stabilizer. Frozen custard and ice cream are also important soft-serve products.

Commercial manufacture. In ice cream manufacture the basic ingredients are blended together (see illustration). The process ranges from small-batch operations, in which the ingredients are weighed or measured by hand, to large automated operations, where the ingredients are metered into the mix-making equipment. The liquid materials, including milk, cream, condensed milk, liquid sugar, and water, are mixed. The dry solids, such as nonfat dry milk, dried egg yolk, stabilizer, and emulsifier, are blended with the liquid ingredients. This liquid blend is called the mix. Then the mix is pasteurized, homogenized, cooled, and aged.

The mix may be pasteurized by the batch method by heating to 160°F (71°C) for 30 min or by a continuous method by heating to 175°F (80°C) for 25 sec. The pasteurization process destroys all harmful bacteria and improves the storage properties of the ice cream.

The hot mix is pumped from the pasteurizer through a homogenizer which reduces the fat globules to less than 2 micrometers in size. Homogenization is accomplished by forcing the mix through the homogenization valves under 1500–3000 psi (103–207 kilopascals). It results in a uniform, smooth product and ensures that the fat will not churn during the freezing process.

The mix is cooled immediately to a temperature of 32–40°F (0–4°C). The mix is then aged for 4–12 hr to improve the body and texture in the finished ice cream due to the favorable hydration and particle orientation effects which develop.

The flavoring materials are usually added to the mix just before the freezing process, but fruits, nuts, and candies are not added until the ice cream is discharged from the freezer. Common flavors of ice cream include vanilla, chocolate, strawberry, butter pecan, peach, and coffee, but there are numerous others.

Ice cream is frozen in batch or continuous freezers. The continuous freezing process is more effective, as it freezes more rapidly and produces a product with finer texture. Continuous freezers vary in capacity from 85 gal (323 liters) to more than 2000 gal (7600 liters) per hour.

During the freezing, air is incorporated into the mix, resulting in increased volume. This increase in volume is called overrun. The drawing temperature of the ice cream from the freezer is about 21°F (−6°C). The ice cream is packaged at this temperature and further cooled to about 20°F (−29°C) in a hardening room, where it is stored until marketed.

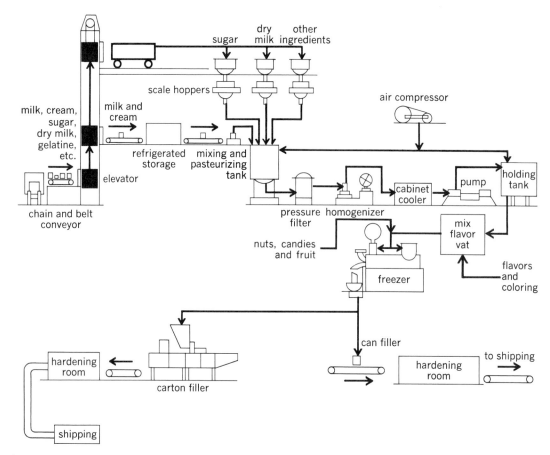

Ice cream manufacture. (*Adapted from S. C. Prescott and B. E. Proctor, Food Technology, McGraw-Hill, 1937*)

The United States ice cream industry has been described as a high-volume, highly automated, progressive, very competitive industry composed of large and small factories. It has developed on the basis of abundant and economical supply of ingredients and has been influenced by such factors as achievement of good-quality products; favorable consumer response; excellent transportation, refrigeration, and distribution; improved merchandising approach; advanced packaging; and adequate home refrigeration.

The annual per capita production is about 15 qt (14 liters) of ice cream or nearly 23 qt (22 liters) of combined production of ice cream and related products. This amounts to more than 7.7×10^7 gal (2.93×10^8 liters) of ice cream and 1.2×10^9 gal (4.56×10^9 liters) of ice cream and related products.   [WENDELL S. ARBUCKLE]

Sources of microorganisms. The cream, condensed- and dry-milk products, egg products, sugar, stabilizers, flavoring and coloring materials, and fruits and nuts used as ingredients in ice cream may be contaminated with microorganisms. Therefore the ice cream mix must be pasteurized before freezing because a low temperature in itself is not sufficient to kill microorganisms. Other possible sources of microorganisms are equipment and utensils used in manufacture, scoops and dippers, vendors, employees, and air. Stringent regulations must be established for all manipulations of ice cream from producer to consumer in order to avoid recontamination, especially with regard to pathogens. Once incorporated, microorganisms

survive a long time in ice cream. This can be seen from the abridged data in Table 1. *See* FOOD MANUFACTURING; PASTEURIZATION.

Kinds of microorganisms. A wide variety of microorganisms may be found, including streptococci, micrococci, coliform bacteria, sporeformers, yeasts, and molds. No selection of species by freezing takes place. Since no growth and only slow destruction of microorganisms in the final product occur, the flora of ice cream consists of organisms surviving pasteurization or incorporated by contamination. With well-controlled sanitation during production, plate counts may be as low as a few thousand; with careless methods they may be in the millions. Normally a slight increase of the

Table 1. Persistence of Salmonella typhosa (Bacterium typhosum) in ice cream*

Time after freezing, days	Typhoid bacteria, $\times 10^3$ per milliliter
Freshly frozen	51,000
5	10,000
20	2,200
104	900
165	640
260	57
342	51
544	13
730	6

*M. J. Prucha and J. M. Brannon, Viability of *Bacterium typhosum* in ice cream, *J. Bacteriol.*, 11:27–29, 1926.

Table 2. Effect of various steps in manufacture on standard plate count of ice cream*

Stage of manufacture	Unsupervised preparation (12 mixes)	Supervised preparation (11 mixes)
Before pasteurization	10,758,566	4,617,535
Before homogenization	105,748	11,850
After homogenization	200,745	18,643
Before aging	289,341	31,381
After aging	354,300	33,227
After freezing	458,325	58,136
After hardening	390,225	39,127

*N. E. Olson and A. C. Fay, The bacterial content of ice cream: A report of experiments in bacterial control in six commercial plants, *J. Dairy Sci.*, 8:415, 1925.

bacterial count takes place during manufacture, especially after homogenization and freezing, due to the breaking up of clumps of bacteria (Table 2). A plate count not greater than 50,000–100,000 per gram is regarded as acceptable from a sanitary point of view in most states.

Hygienic measures. These include proper pasteurization of the mix and adequate sanitizing of equipment. Pasteurization must be more intensive with the mix than with milk because increased milk solids protect microorganisms to some degree. At least 68.4°C for 30 min or 79.5°C for 25 sec are applied to obtain a sufficient margin of safety. In this way all pathogens are killed and total bacterial counts of 10,000 or less per gram are usually reached. Higher counts after pasteurization are due to thermoduric organisms. The source of these organisms is inadequately cleaned farm or plant equipment. Sanitizing of equipment is achieved by cleaning and sterilizing operations with heat or chemicals. *See* DAIRY MACHINERY; STERILIZATION.

Bacteriological control. For determining the hygienic quality of ice cream, the laboratory tests used are similar to those employed for milk. Of these, the standard plate count and the test for coliform bacteria have found widespread application. *See* MILK.   [WILLIAM C. WINDER]

Bibliography: W. S. Arbuckle, *Ice Cream*, 2d ed., 1972; E. M. Foster et al., *Dairy Microbiology*, 1957.

Industrial microbiology

The study, utilization, and manipulation of those microorganisms (in the broad sense including bacteria, yeasts and other fungi, and some algae) capable of economically producing desirable substances, or changes in substances, and controlling unwanted microorganisms.

Industrial fermentation criteria. To be industrially important, microorganisms should be easily cultivable in large quantities; grow rapidly on cheap, available substrates; and carry out the required transformations under comparatively simple and workable modifications of environmental conditions. They should maintain physiological constancy under these conditions and produce economically adequate yields. Above all, the microbiological method must be the cheapest method of producing the desired material or change. The marketing of wastes or other by-products of a

process often serves to keep the process competitive. Lack of current demand for a product may be of little concern, for a market can often be created when the price of the product is low.

The potential uses of microorganisms for the good of man were not appreciated until World War I, when microorganisms were used to produce acetone, butanol, and certain enzymes. The discovery of the usefulness of penicillin during World War II caused an enormous development of the fermentation industry and a fuller realization of the value of microbiological activities. Some of the problems of space travel, pollution, and waste disposal are being solved by the use of microorganisms. *See* FERMENTATION.

Products. Since earliest times microorganisms have been used, intentionally or otherwise, as means of preserving foods or of making them more palatable, as in the making of such products as wine, cheese, butter, vinegar, and silage. They have also been used for such procedures as flax retting, removing mucilage from freshly harvested coffee beans, and copper leaching. *See* BUTTER; CHEESE; FLAX; FOOD MANUFACTURING; FOOD PRESERVATION; WINE.

Microorganisms are used to produce chemical substances, which are then extracted from the culture mixture and purified. Included are (1) solvents such as ethanol, acetone, butanol, 2,3-butylene glycol, and other alcohols, such as glycerol, mannitol, erythritol, and polyhydric alcohols; (2) organic acids such as acetic, lactic, citric, gluconic, fumaric, propionic, itaconic, kojic, and gallic; (3) carbohydrates such as sorbose, fructose, dextrans, and other polysaccharides; (4) vitamins such as B_{12}, thiamine, and riboflavin; (5) amino acids such as lysine, arginine, and glutamic acid; (6) antibiotics such as penicillin, streptomycin, tetracycline, and chloramphenicol; (7) enzymes such as amylases, proteases, and glucose oxidases; and (8) nucleosides. *See* RIBOFLAVIN; THIAMINE; VINEGAR; VITAMIN B_{12}.

Microorganisms are used to produce desired changes in certain types of compounds or materials, such as in the microbiological transformations of steroids by dehydrogenation, hydrogenation, hydroxylation, oxidative cleavage, or reductive rearrangement of the steroid molecules. More ancient are the uses of microorganisms in the textile industry with cotton, wool, and flax. More modern are the applications of bacteriological processes to the generation of electric power in fuel cells and to studies of human wastes as nutrients in closed space ecologies.

As with all life functions, the activities of microorganisms can be reduced to a consideration of enzymes acting on a substrate. The industrial microbiologist is concerned more with the final product or change—the sum total of the activities of a series of enzymes—than with the action of each individual enzyme as such.

Some of the uses already mentioned overlap those where the product is not extracted and purified but is used in the culture mixture. In many cases the product need not be extracted, for the whole culture mixture can be used as in fodder yeast, feed supplement production, upgrading of forages, and nitrogen-fixing organism production.

The field of animal-feed supplementation,

whether with extracted chemicals, whole culture mixtures, or wastes from fermentation, is of great importance and yields large financial return. The production of growth stimulators, growth inhibitors, fungicides, and insecticides is of increasing importance. Because of the vast markets available, the production of materials for use in the agricultural industry, both animal and plant, is receiving increased attention and will probably equal or surpass production for human consumption and therapy, as well as production of industrial chemicals. *See* ANIMAL-FEED COMPOSITION.

Food technology. The leavening of bread and other bakery products; the lactic acid fermentation of pickles, olives, sauerkraut, and other products; the manufacture of cheese, butter, and certain beverages; and the manufacture of shoyu, tempeh, miso, and other Oriental foods involve the activities of one or more microorganisms. In some cases these activities provide a more palatable product, in others they provide a measure of preservation, and in still others they achieve both.

Protein is a necessary basic material for synthetic foodstuffs, not only as nutrient but also as emulsifiers and viscosity extenders, and for color adhesion and improvement of shelf life. Single-cell protein may be obtained from fermentation of agricultural and industrial wastes of many kinds. Protein enrichment by fermentation of starchy materials (such as the dry fermentation of cassava, bananas, and potatoes) is of increasing importance.

Enzymes find use in the degradation of biological polymers (especially renewable resources such as cellulose and lignin) and in the production of single-cell protein.

The control or eradication of unwanted microorganisms is of great importance to prevent spoilage, loss of nutritive value and flavor, and the formation of poisonous substances such as botulins and aflatoxins. *See* FOOD ENGINEERING; FOOD MICROBIOLOGY; FOOD TECHNOLOGY.

Waste and surplus disposal. It may be said that there are no pollution problems—only disposal problems. Microbiological activity may be used merely to dispose of some wastes, such as sewage; with other wastes it may be used to produce material of value. Such wastes may be from other microbiological processes, as in the fermentation of corn-steep liquor, distillers' solubles, and cheese wheys; or they may be from nonmicrobiological processes, such as sugarbeet and sugarcane molasses, waste-sulfite liquor, fish solubles, or cannery wastes. The need to dispose of various agricultural surpluses, such as potatoes and cereal grains, may make feasible their use as fermentation substrates for the production of animal-feed ingredients including single-cell protein. To facilitate disposal, biodegradable detergents have been developed. The reduction of the biological oxygen demand of waste-sulfite liquor prior to disposal, by the production of alcohol or food yeast from it, promises to lessen some pollution.

Bioassay. Microbiological assay procedures for vitamins, amino acids, and antibiotics are in common use because of their relative simplicity, their specificity, and the speed with which they may be carried out. *See* VITAMIN.

Types of fermentations. Fermentations may be of the single organism–one product type, or of the type in which two or more organisms, grown together or in sequence, may be used. Fungi may be used aerobically to saccharify starch, the resulting sugar then being dissimilated by anaerobic bacterial activity to produce desired products. In a patented method of producing *l*-lysine, the precursor diaminopimelic acid is produced by one organism and then decarboxylated by a second organism to give excellent yields of the desired lysine. Organisms producing desired materials, when grown together in one way or another, may be induced to produce new and even more desirable substances.

While many fermentations are still done by the batch process, long-used continuous culture methods have been refined and are finding increased application, as in continuous beer fermentation and in tower fermentors. Computer control and dynamic optimization of fermentation processes are becoming primary bases for increased production. Microbiological modifications of hydrocarbons are more recent entries into the field, as are those organisms which utilize jet fuel and the many which influence the quality of petroleum products. *See* DISTILLED SPIRITS.

[R. H. HASKINS]

Bibliography: C. W. Hessetine, A millennium of fungi, food and fermentation, *Mycologia*, 57:149–197, 1965; D. J. D. Hockenhull (ed.), *Progress in Industrial Microbiology*, vol. 1 et seq.; N. N. Potter, *Food Fermentations in Food Science*, 1973; Protein-Calorie Advisory Group of United Nations System, *PAG Bulletins*, 1976; G. Reed (ed.), *Enzymes in Food Processing*, 1975; Society for Industrial Microbiology, *Developments in Industrial Microbiology*, vol. 1 et seq., AIBS; G. Terui (ed.), *Fermentation Technology Today*, Society of Fermentation Technology, Japan, 1972.

Insect control, biological

The term biological control was proposed in 1919 to apply to the use or role of natural enemies in insect population regulation. The enemies involved are termed parasites (parasitoids), predators, or pathogens. This remains preferred usage, although other biological methods of insect control have been proposed or developed, such as the release of mass-produced sterile males to mate with wild females in the field, thereby greatly reducing or suppressing the pests' production of progeny. Classical biological control is an ecological phenomenon which occurs everywhere in nature without aid from, or sometimes even understanding by, man. However, man has utilized the ecological principles involved to develop the field of applied biological control of insects, and the great majority of practical applications have been achieved with insect pests. Additionally, such diverse types of pest organisms as weeds, mites, and certain mammals have been successfully controlled by use of natural enemies.

History. Man observed the action of predacious insects early in his agricultural history, and a few crude attempts to utilize predators have been carried on for centuries. However, the necessary understanding of biological and ecological principles, especially those of population dynamics, did not begin to emerge until the 19th century. The first great applied success in biological control of an insect pest occurred 2 years after the importation into California from Australia in 1888–1889 of the predatory vedalia lady beetle. This insect feeds on the cottony-cushion scale, a notorious citrus pest that was destroying orange trees at that time, and the vedalia was credited with saving the citrus industry. This successful control firmly established the field or discipline of applied biological control as it is known today.

Ecological principles. Natural enemy populations have a feedback relationship to prey populations, termed density-dependence, which results in the increasing or decreasing of one group in response to changes in the density of the other group. Such reciprocal interaction prevents indefinite increase or decrease and thus results in the achievement of a typical average density or "balance." However, this balance may be either at high or low levels, depending on the inherent abilities of the natural enemies. If the natural enemy is highly density-dependent, it can regulate the prey population density at very low levels. An effective enemy achieves regulation by rapidly responding to any increase in the prey population in two different ways: killing more prey by increased feeding or parasitism, and producing more progeny for the next generation. The net effect is a more rapid increase in prey mortality as prey population tends to increase, so that first the trend is stopped and then it becomes reversed, lowering the prey population. This results in relaxing the pressure caused by the enemy so that ultimately the prey population is enabled to increase again, and the cycle is repeated over and over.

Applications of classical method. Since the vedalia beetle controlled the cottony-cushion scale some 80 years ago, many projects in applied biological control have been undertaken and a large number of successes achieved. There are about 300 recorded cases of applied biological control of insects in 70 countries. Of these recorded cases over 85 have been so completely successful that insecticides are no longer required. In the other cases the need for chemical treatment has been more or less greatly reduced. Also, there are about 47 cases of biological control of weeds by insect natural enemies. In California alone it is estimated that the agricultural industry has been saved $272,000,000 during the past 52 years because of reduction in insect pest-caused crop losses and diminished need for chemical control. A few of the many outstanding successes include the biological control of Florida red scale in Israel and subsequently in Mexico, Lebanon, South Africa, Brazil, Peru, Texas, and Florida; Oriental fruit fly in Hawaii; green vegetable bug in Australia; citrus blackfly and purple scale in Mexico; dictyospermum scale and purple scale in Greece; and olive scale in California.

All the cases of applied biological control mentioned above involved foreign exploration and importation and colonization of new exotic natural enemies of the insect pest in question. In the majority of cases the pest was an invader, being native to another country, and its natural enemies had been left behind. By searching the native habitat for effective enemies and sending them to the new home of the invader pest, the biological balance was reconstituted. This method is considered to be classical biological control, and its scientific application has been responsible for most of the outstanding results obtained. There are, however,

two other major phases of biological control which are categorized under the headings of conservation and augmentation.

Conservation. This phase involves manipulation of the environment to favor survival and reproduction of natural enemies already established in the habitat, whether they be indigenous or exotic. In other words, adverse environmental factors are modified or eliminated, and requisites which are lacking such as food or nesting sites may be provided. Even though potentially effective natural enemies are present in a habitat, adverse factors may so affect them as to preclude attainment of satisfactory biological control. Insecticides commonly produce such adverse effects, causing so-called upsets in balance or pest population explosions.

Augmentation. This phase concerns direct manipulation of established enemies themselves. Potentially effective enemies may be periodically decimated by environmental extremes or other adverse factors which are not subject to man's control. For example, low winter temperatures may seriously decrease certain enemy populations each year. The major means of solving such problems has involved laboratory mass culture of enemies and their periodic colonization in the field, generally after the adverse period has passed. This practice is gaining rapidly in application. *Trichogramma* sp., common egg parasites of lepidopterous pests, have been utilized in this manner with reportedly good results in many countries, and various microorganisms likewise have been successfully used.

Advantages over chemical control. Although research and development costs are modest for biological control projects, they are high for new insecticides. Biological control application costs are minimal and nonrecurring, except where periodic colonization is utilized, whereas insecticide costs are high annually. There are no environmental pollution problems connected with biological control, whereas insecticides cause severe problems related to toxicity to man, wildlife, birds, and fish, as well as causing adverse effects in soil and water. Biological control causes no upsets in the natural balance of organisms, but these upsets are common with chemical control; biological control is permanent, chemical control is temporary, usually one to many annual applications being necessary. Additionally, pests more and more frequently are developing resistance or immunity to insecticides, but this is not a problem with pests and their enemies. Both biological and chemical control have restrictions as far as general applicability to the control of all pest insect species is concerned, although the application of biological control remains greatly underdeveloped compared to chemical control. *See* INSECTICIDE.

[PAUL DE BACH]

Bibliography: R. R. Askew, *Parasite Insects*, 1971; K. F. Baker and R. J. Cook, *Biological Control of Plant Pathogens*, 1974; C. P. Clausen, *Entomophagous Insects*, 1962; P. DeBach (ed.), *Biological Control of Insect Pests and Weeds*, 1964; P. DeBach, *Biological Control by Natural Enemies*, 1974; C. B. Huffaker (ed.), *Biological Control*, 1971; W. W. Kilgore and R. L. Doutt, *Pest Control: Biological, Physical and Selected Chemical Methods*, 1967; E. A. Steinhaus (ed.), *Insect*

Pathology, 1963; L. A. Swan, *Beneficial Insects*, 1964; R. van den Bosch and P. S. Messenger, *Biological Control*, 1973.

Insecticide

A material used to kill insects and related animals by disruption of vital processes through chemical action. Chemically, insecticides may be of inorganic or organic origin. The principal source is from chemical manufacturing, although a few are derived from plants. Insecticides are classified according to type of action, as stomach poisons, contact poisons, residual poisons, systemic poisons, fumigants, repellents, or attractants. Many act in more than one way. Stomach poisons are applied to plants so that they will be ingested as insects chew the leaves. Contact poisons are applied directly to insects and are used principally to control species which obtain food by piercing leaf surfaces and withdrawing liquids. Residual insecticides are applied to surfaces so that insects touching them will pick up lethal dosages. Systemic insecticides are applied to plants or animals and are absorbed and translocated to all parts of the organisms, so that insects feeding upon them will obtain lethal doses. Fumigants are applied as gases, or in a form which will vaporize to a gas, to be inhaled by insects. Repellents prevent insects from coming in contact with their hosts. Attractants induce insects to come to specific locations in preference to normal food sources.

In the United States, about 500 species of insects are of primary economic importance, and losses caused by insects range from $4,000,000,000 to $8,000,000,000 annually.

Inorganic insecticides. Prior to 1945, large volumes of lead arsenate, calcium arsenate, paris green (copper acetoarsenite), sodium fluoride, and cryolite (sodium fluoaluminate) were used. The potency of arsenicals is a direct function of the percentage of metallic arsenic contained. Lead arsenate was first used in 1892 and proved effective as a stomach poison against many chewing insects. Calcium arsenate was widely used for the control of cotton pests. Paris green was one of the first stomach poisons and had its greatest utility against the Colorado potato beetle. The amount of available water-soluble arsenic governs the utility of arsenates on growing plants, because this fraction will cause foliage burn. Lead arsenate is safest in this respect, calcium arsenate is intermediate, and paris green is the most harmful. Care must be exercised in the application of these materials to food and feed crops because they are poisonous to man and animals as well as to insects.

Sodium fluoride has been used to control chewing lice on animals and poultry, but its principal application has been for the control of household insects, especially roaches. It cannot be used on plants because of its extreme phytotoxicity. Cryolite has found some utility in the control of the Mexican bean beetle and flea beetles on vegetable crops because of its low water solubility and lack of phytotoxicity.

Organic insecticides. These began to supplant the arsenicals when DDT [2,2-bis(p-chlorophenyl)-1,1,1-trichloroethane] became available in 1945. During World War II, the insecticidal properties of γ-benzenehexachloride (γ-1,2,3,4,5,6-hexachloro-

cyclohexane of γ-BHC) were discovered in England and France. The two largest-volume insecticides are DDT and γ-BHC. Certain insects cannot be controlled with either, and there are situations and crops where they cannot be used. For these reasons, other chlorinated hydrocarbon insecticides have been discovered and marketed successfully. These include TDE [2,2-bis(p-chlorophenyl)-1,1-dichloroethane], methoxychlor [2,2-bis(p-methoxyphenyl)-1,1,1-trichloroethane], Dilan [mixture of 1,1-bis(p-chlorophenyl)-2-nitropropane and 1,1-bis(p-chlorophenyl)-2-nitrobutane], chlordane (2,3,4,5,6,7,8-8-octachloro-2,3,3a,4,7,7a-hexahydro-4,7-methanoindene), heptachlor (1,4,5,6,7,8,8-heptachloro-3a,4,7,7a-tetrahydro-4,7-methanoindene), aldrin (1,2,3,4,10,10-hexachloro-1,4,4a,5,8,8a-hexahydro-1,4-endo, exo-5,8-dimethanonaphthalene), dieldrin (1,2,3,4,10,10-hexachloro-6,7-epoxy-1,4,4a,-5,6,7,8,8a-octahydro-1,4-endo,exo-5,8-dimethanonaphthalene), endrin (1,2,3,4,10,10-hexachloro-6,7-epoxy-1,4,4a,5,6,7,8,8a-octahydro-1,4-endo, endo-5,8-dimethanonaphthalene), toxaphene (camphene plus 67–69% chlorine), and endosulfan (6,7,8,9,10,10-hexachloro-1,5,5a,6,9,9a-hexahydro-6,9-methano-2,4,3-benzodioxathiepin-3-oxide). TDE is considerably less toxic than DDT but in general is also less effective. It has given outstanding results in the control of larvae of several moths, however. Methoxychlor is even less toxic than TDE and has found considerable use in the control of houseflies and also of the Mexican bean beetle which is not susceptible to DDT. Restrictions have been placed on its use on dairy cattle for the control of flies, and its consumption is declining. Dilan has found some use in the control of the Mexican bean beetle, as well as of some thrips and aphids. Chlordane was the first cyclopentadiene insecticide to reach commercial status. It has been the most effective chemical available for the control of roaches. In addition to lengthy residual properties, chlordane also possesses fumigant action. Related chemicals include heptachlor, aldrin, dieldrin, and endrin. They are effective against grasshoppers and are especially useful for the control of insects inhabiting soil. Registrations for uses of aldrin and dieldrin were reduced in 1966, following extensive investigations of their metabolism and persistence in animal tissues. Toxaphene is used principally for the control of the cotton boll weevil and other insect pests of cotton. Endosulfan, in addition to showing promise for the control of numerous insects, also shows promise of controlling a number of species of phytophagous (plant-feeding) mites that are not generally susceptible to chlorinated hydrocarbon insecticides.

Insect resistance. The resistance of insects to DDT was first observed in 1947 in the housefly. By the end of 1967, 91 species of insects had been proved to be resistant to DDT, 135 to cyclodienes, 54 to organophosphates, and 20 to other types of insecticides, including the carbamates. Among the chlorinated hydrocarbon insecticides, two types of resistance occur. One applies to DDT and its analogs, such as TDE, methoxychlor, and Dilan, and the other to the cyclodiene compounds, such as chlordane, heptachlor, aldrin, dieldrin, endrin, and also γ-BHC and toxaphene. Insecticides are not mutagenic, indicating that resistance preexists in a small part of the natural population even before exposure.

Nearly every country in the world, except mainland China, has reported the presence of resistant strains of the housefly. In many heavily populated urban areas of the United States, it is difficult to obtain control of roaches with chlordane. During 1957 and 1958, many growers of cotton in the southern states changed from toxaphene and γ-BHC to organic phosphorus chemicals because of the resistance of the cotton boll weevil to chlorinated hydrocarbon insecticides. By 1967, resistant strains of the cotton bollworm and the tobacco budworm had developed and proliferated to the extent that in numerous areas the use of chlorinated hydrocarbon insecticides was of doubtful value. The onion maggot has developed widely spread strains resistant to aldrin, dieldrin, and heptachlor, especially in the northeastern United States and in Ontario, Canada. Three species of corn rootworms also are resistant to these insecticides, principally in the corn-growing regions west of the Mississippi River. The development of chlorinated hydrocarbon resistance among several species of disease-transmitting mosquitoes continues to pose a threat to world health. The control of typhus in the Far East could be at stake because strains of vector lice are resistant to DDT. Evidence for insect resistance to the plant-derived insecticides pyrethrum and rotenone has only recently been established.

Organic phosphorus insecticides. The development of this type of insecticide paralleled that of the chlorinated hydrocarbons. Since 1947, more than 50,000 organic phosphorus compounds have been synthesized in academic and industrial laboratories throughout the world for evaluation as potential insecticides. Parathion [O,O-diethyl O-(p-nitrophenyl) phosphorothioate] and methyl parathion [O,O-dimethyl O-(p-nitrophenyl) phosphorothioate] are estimated to have had a world production of 70,000,000 lb during 1966.

A great diversity of activity is found among organophosphorus insecticides. Many are extremely toxic to man and other warm-blooded animals, but a few show a very low toxicity. The more important include tetraethylpyrophosphate, dicapthon [O,O-dimethyl O-(3-chloro-4-nitrophenyl) phosphorothioate], malathion [O,O-dimethyl S-(1,2-dicarbethoxyethyl) phosphorodithioate], dichloro- [O,O-dimethyl O-(2,2-dichlorovinyl) phosphate], diazinon {O,O-diethyl O-[2-isopropyl-4-methylpyrimidyl (6)] phosphorothioate}, dioxathion [2,3-p-dioxanedithiol S,S-bis (O,O-diethylphosphorodithioate)], azinphosmethyl [O,O-dimethyl S-4-oxo-1,2,3-benzotriazin-3-(4H)-yl-methylphosphorodithioate], carbophenothion [S-(p-chlorophenylthiomethyl) O,O-diethylphosphorodithioate], ethion {bis[S-(diethoxyphosphinothioyl) mercapto] methane}, EPN [O-ethyl O-(p-nitrophenyl) phenylphosphonothionate], trichlorfon [O,O-dimethyl (2,2,2,-trichloro-1-hydroxyethyl) phosphonate], dimethoate [O,O-dimethyl S-(methylcarbamoylmethyl) phosphorodithioate], and fenthion {O,O-dimethyl-O-[4-(methylthio)-m-tolyl] phosphorothioate}.

Schradan [bis(dimethylamino) phosphoric anhydride] was unique among organic insecticides in that it showed systemic properties when applied to plants. By direct contact, it has a relatively low order of activity. When sprayed on plants, it is absorbed from areas receiving treatment, is translocated throughout the entire plant, and is metabolized to yield a product highly toxic to such sucking pests as aphids and phytophagous mites. It is selective in that it affects only aphids ingesting juices from treated plants and does not kill predators which destroy aphids. With schradan, it is possible to protect the growing parts of plants without resorting to frequent spraying, because the insecticide is translocated to these growing parts, whereas with most stomach poison or residual insecticides plants outgrow the protection. Several chemicals showing systemic properties have reached commercial or near commercial status. These include demeton [O,O-diethyl O (and S)-(2-ethylthio) ethylphosphorothioates], disulfoton [O,O-diethyl S-(2-ethylthio) ethylphosphorodithioate], phorate [O,O-diethyl S-(ethylthiomethyl)-phosphorodithioate], and mevinphos [2-methoxycarbonyl-1-methyl vinyl dimethyl phosphate].

The use of organic phosphorus chemicals for the systemic control of animal parasites is another facet of interest. During 1958, semicommercial application began of coumaphos [O-(3-chloro-4-methyl-2-oxo-2-H-1-benzopyran-7-yl) O,O-diethyl-phosphorothioate] and ronnel [O,O-dimethyl O-(2,4,5-trichlorophenyl) phosphorothioate] for the control of grubs in cattle. Coumaphos is applied externally as a spray and is absorbed and translocated to kill the cattle grubs. Ronnel is most effective when administered internally. Dimethoate, fenthion, famphur [O-p-(dimethyl-sulfamoyl)phenyl O,O-dimethylphosphorothioate], and menazon [S-(4,6-diamino-s-triazin-2-ylmethyl) O,O-dimethylphosphorodithioate] also show activity for this type of application.

Activity of organic phosphate insecticides results from the inhibition of the enzyme cholinesterase, which performs a vital function in the transmission of impulses in the nervous system. Inhibition of some phenyl esterases occurs also. Inhibition results from direct coupling of phosphate with the enzyme. Phosphorothionates are moderately active but become exceedingly potent upon oxidation to phosphates.

Other types of insecticides. Synthetic carbamate insecticides are attracting increased interest. These include dimetan (5,5-dimethyldihydroresorcinol dimethylcarbamate), Pyrolan (3-methyl-1-phenyl-5-pyrazolyl dimethylcarbamate), Isolan (1-isopropyl-3-methyl-5-pyrazolyl dimethylcarbamate), pyramat [2-n-propyl-4-methylpyrimidyl-(6)-dimethylcarbamate], carbaryl (1-naphthyl-N-methylcarbamate), Bagon, (o-isopropoxyphenyl methylcarbamate), Zectran (4-dimethylamino-3,5-xylyl methylcarbamate), TRANID [5-chloro-6-oxo-2-norbornanecarbonitrile O-(methylcarbamoyl)-oxime], dimetilan [1-(dimethylcarbamoyl)-5-methyl-3-pyrazolyl dimethylcarbamate], Furadan (2,3-dihydro-2,2-dimethyl-7-benzofuranyl methyl-carbamate), and Temik [2-methyl-2-(methylthio) propionaldehyde O-(methylcarbamoyl) oxime]. They are also cholinergic.

Insecticides obtained from plants include nicotine [L-1-methyl-2-(3'-pyridyl)-pyrrolidine], rotenone, the pyrethrins, sabadilla, and ryanodine, some of which are the oldest-known insecticides. Nicotine was used as a crude extract of tobacco as early as 1763. The alkaloid is obtained from the leaves and stems of *Nicotiana tabacum* and *N. rustica*. It has been used as a contact insecticide, fumigant, and stomach poison and is especially effective against aphids and other soft-bodied insects.

Rotenone is the most active of six related alkaloids found in a number of plants, including *Derris elliptica*, *D. malaccensis*, *Lonchocarpus utilis*, and *L. urucu*. *Derris* is a native of East Asia, and *Lonchocarpus* occurs in South America. The highest concentrations are found in the roots. Rotenone is active against a number of plant-feeding pests and has found its greatest utility where toxic residues are to be avoided. Rotenone is known also as derris or cubé.

The principal sources of pyrethrum are *Chrysanthemum cinerariaefolium* and *C. coccineum*. Pyrethrins, which are purified extracts prepared from flower petals, contain four chemically different active ingredients. Allethrin is a synthetic pyrethroid. The pyrethrins find their greatest use in fly sprays, household insecticides, and grain protectants because they are the safest insecticidal materials available.

Synergists. These materials have little or no insecticidal activity but increase the activity of chemicals with which they are mixed, especially that of the pyrethrins. Piperonyl butoxide {α-[2-(2-butoxyethoxy)-ethoxy]-4,5-methylenedioxy-2-propyltoluene}, sulfoxide {1,2,methylenedioxy-4-[2-octyl-(sulfinyl),propyl] benzene}, and N-(2-ethylhexyl)-5-norbornene-2,3-dicarboximide are commercially available. Sesamex [acetaldehyde 2-(2-ethoxyethoxy)ethyl 3,4-methylenedioxyphenyl acetal] and Tropital {piperonal bis[2-(2-butoxyethoxy)-ethyl]- acetal} are active but not fully developed synergists. These synergists have their greatest utility in mixtures with the pyrethrins. Some have been shown to enhance the activity of carbamate insecticides as well.

Formulation and application. Formulation of insecticides is extremely important in obtaining satisfactory control. Common formulations include dusts, water suspensions, emulsions, and solutions. Accessory agents, including dust carriers, solvents, emulsifiers, wetting and dispersing agents, stickers, deodorants or masking agents, synergists, and antioxidants, may be required to obtain a satisfactory product. Insecticidal dusts are formulated for application as powders. Toxicant concentration is usually quite low. Water suspensions are usually prepared from wettable powders, which are formulated in a manner similar to dusts except that the insecticide is incorporated at a high concentration and wetting and dispersing agents are included. Emulsifiable concentrates are usually prepared by solution of the chemical in a satisfactory solvent to which an emulsifier is added. They are diluted with water prior to application. Granular formulations are an effective means of applying insecticides to the soil to control insects which feed on the subterranean parts of plants. Proper timing of insecticide applications is important in obtaining satisfactory control. Dusts are more easily and rapidly applied than are sprays. However, results may be more erratic and much greater attention must be paid to weather conditions than is required for sprays. Coverage of plants and insects is generally less satisfactory with dusts than with sprays. It is best to make dust applications early in the day, while the plants are covered with dew, so that greater amounts of dust will adhere. If prevailing winds are too strong, a considerable proportion of dust will be lost. Spray operations will usually require the use of heavier equipment, however. Application of insecticides should be properly correlated with the occurrence of the most susceptible stage in the life cycle of the pest involved.

During the past decade, attention has focused sharply on the impact of the highly active synthetic insecticides upon the total environment—man, domestic and wild animals and fowl, soil-inhabiting microflora and microfauna, and all forms of aquatic life. Effects of these materials upon populations of beneficial insects, particularly parasites and predators of the economic species, are being critically assessed. The study of insect control by biological means has expanded. The concepts and practices of integrated pest control and pest management are expanding rapidly. Among problems associated with insect control which must receive major emphasis during the coming years are the development of strains of insects resistant to insecticides; the assessment of the significance of small, widely distributed insecticide residues in and upon the environment; the development of better and more reliable methods for forecasting insect outbreaks; and the evolvement of control programs integrating all methods—physical, physiological, chemical, biological, and cultural—for which practicality may have been demonstrated. *See* FUMIGANT; INSECT CONTROL, BIOLOGICAL; MITICIDE; PESTICIDE.

[GEORGE F. LUDVIK]

Bibliography: A. B. Borkovec, *Insect Chemosterilants*, 1966; D. E. H. Frear, *Pesticide Handbook: Entoma*, 1966; D. E. H. Frear, *Pesticide Index*, 4th ed., 1969; M. Jacobson, *Insect Sex Attractants*, 1965; E. E. Kenega, Commerical and experimental organic insecticides, *Bull. Entomol. Soc. Amer.*, 12(2):161–217, 1966; W. W. Kilgore and R. L. Doutt, *Pest Control: Biological, Physical and Selected Chemical Methods*, 1967; H. Martin, *Insecticide and Fungicide Handbook*, 1965; C. L. Metcalf, W. P. Flint, and R. L. Metcalf, *Destructive and Useful Insects*, 1962; R. D. O'Brien, *Insecticides: Action and Metabolism*, 1967; U.S. Department of Agriculture, *Agr. Handb. no. 331*, Agricultural Research Service and Forest Service, 1967.

Irrigation of crops

The artificial application of water to the soil to produce plant growth. Irrigation also cools the soil and atmosphere, making the environment favorable for plant growth. The use of some form of irrigation is well documented throughout the history of humankind. Over 50,000,000 acres (202,300 km²) are irrigated in the United States.

Use of water by plants. Growing plants use water almost continuously. Growth of crops under irrigation is stimulated by optimum moisture, but retarded by excessive or deficient amounts. Factors influencing the rate of water use by plants include the type of plant and stage of growth, temperature, wind velocity, humidity, sunlight duration and intensity, and available water supply. Plants use the least amount of water upon emergence from the soil and near the end of the growing period. Irrigation and other management practices should be coordinated with the various stages of growth. A vast amount of research has been done on the use of water by plants, and results are available for crops under varying conditions. *See* PLANT, WATER RELATIONS OF; PLANT GROWTH.

Consumptive use. In planning new or rehabilitating old irrigation projects, consumptive use is the most important factor in determining the amount of water required. It is also used to determine water rights.

Consumptive use, or evapotranspiration, is defined as water entering plant roots to build plant tissues, water retained by the plant, water transpired by leaves into the atmosphere, and water evaporated from plant leaves and from adjacent soil surfaces. Consumptive use of water by various crops under varying conditions has been determined by soil-moisture studies and computed by other well-established methods for many regions of the United States and other countries. Factors which have been shown to influence consumptive use are precipitation, air temperature, humidity, wind movement, the growing season, and latitude, which influences hours of daylight. Table 1 shows how consumptive use varies at one location during the growing season. When consumptive-use data are computed for an extensive area, such as an irrigation project, the results will be given in acre-feet per acre for each month of the growing season and the entire irrigation period. Peak-use months determine system capacity needs. An acre-foot is the amount of water required to cover 1 acre 1 ft deep (approx. 1214 m² of water).

Soil, plant, and water relationships. Soil of root-zone depth is the storage reservoir from which plants obtain moisture to sustain growth. Plants take from the soil not only water, but dissolved minerals necessary to build plant cells. How often this reservoir must be filled by irrigation is determined by the storage capacity of the soil, depth of the root zone, water use by the crop, and the amount of depletion allowed before a reduction in yield or quality occurs. Table 2 shows the approximate amounts of water held by soils of various textures.

Water enters coarse, sandy soils quite readily, but in heavy-textured soils the entry rate is slower. Compaction and surface conditions also affect the rate of entry.

Soil conditions, position of the water table, length of growing season, irrigation frequency, and other factors exert strong influence on root-zone depth. Table 3 shows typical root-zone depths in well-drained, uniform soils under irrigation. The depth of rooting of annual crops increases during the entire growing period, given a favorable, unrestricted root zone. Plants in deep, uniform soils usually consume water more slowly from the lower root-zone area than from the upper. Thus, the upper portion is the first to be exhausted of moisture. For most crops, the entire root zone should be supplied with moisture when needed.

Maximum production can usually be obtained with most irrigated crops if not more than 50% of the available water in the root zone is exhausted

during the critical stages of growth. Many factors influence this safe-removal percentage, including the type of crop grown and the rate at which water is being removed. Application of irrigation water should not be delayed until plants signal a need for moisture; wilting in the hot parts of the day may reduce crop yields considerably. Determination of the amount of water in the root zone can be done by laboratory methods, which are slow and costly. However, in modern irrigation practice, soil-moisture-sensing devices are used to make rapid determinations directly with enough accuracy for practical use. These devices, placed in selected field locations, permit an operator to schedule periods of water application for best results. Evaporation pans and weather records can be used to estimate plant-water use. Computerizing these data also helps farmers schedule their irrigations. The irrigation system should be designed to supply sufficient water to care for periods of most rapid evapotranspiration. The rate of evapotranspiration may vary from 0 to 0.4 in. per day (10 mm per day) or more.

Water quality. All natural irrigation waters contain salts, but only occasionally are waters too saline for crop production when used properly. When more salt is applied through water and fertilizer than is removed by leaching, a salt buildup can occur. If the salts are mainly calcium and magnesium, the soils become saline, but if salts predominately are sodium, a sodic condition is possible. These soils are usually found in arid areas, especially in those areas where drainage is

Table 1. Example of consumption of water by various crops, in inches (1 in. = 25.4 mm)

Crop	April	May	June	July	Aug.	Sept.	Oct.	Seasonal total
Alfalfa	3.3	6.7	5.4	7.8	4.2	5.6	4.4	37.4
Beets		1.9	3.3	5.3	6.9	5.8	1.1	24.3
Cotton	1.1	2.0	4.1	5.8	8.6	6.7	2.7	31.0
Peaches	1.0	3.4	6.7	8.4	6.4	3.1	1.1	30.0
Potatoes			0.7	3.4	5.8	4.4		14.0

Table 2. Approximate amounts of water in soils available to plants

Soil texture	Water capacity, in inches for each foot of depth
Coarse sandy soil	0.5–0.75
Sandy loam	1.25–1.75
Silt loam	1.75–2.50
Heavy clay	1.75–2.0 or more

Table 3. Approximate effective root-zone depths for various crops

Crop	Root-zone depth, ft (1 ft = 0.3 m)
Alfalfa	6
Corn	3
Cotton	4
Potatoes	2
Grasses	2

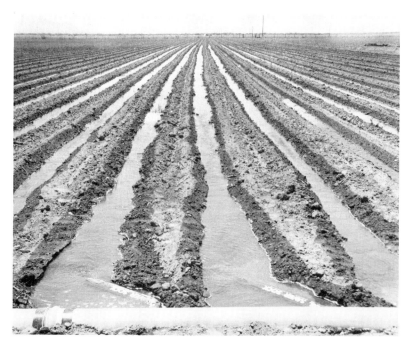

Fig. 1. Furrow method of irrigation. Water is supplied by pipes with individual outlets, or by ditches and siphon tubes.

poor. Rainfall in humid areas usually carries salts downward to the groundwater and eventually to the sea.

Saline soils may reduce yields and can be especially harmful during germination. Some salts are toxic to certain crops, especially when applied by sprinkling and allowed to accumulate on the plants. Salt levels in the soil can be controlled by drainage, by overirrigation, or by maintaining a high moisture level which keeps the salts diluted.

Sodic soils make tillage and water penetration difficult. Drainage, addition of gypsum or sulfur, and overirrigation usually increase productivity.

Ponding or sprinkling can be used to leach salts. Intermittent application is usually better and, when careful soil-moisture management is practiced, only small amounts of excess irrigation are needed to maintain healthy salt levels.

Diagnoses of both water and soil are necessary for making management decisions. Commercial laboratories and many state universities test both water and soil, and make recommendations.

Methods of application. Water is applied to crops by surface, subsurface, sprinkler, and drip irrigation. Surface irrigation includes furrow and flood methods.

Furrow method. This method is used for row crops (Fig. 1). Corrugations or rills are small furrows used on close-growing crops. The flow, carried in furrows, percolates into the soil. Flow to the furrow is usually supplied by siphon tubes, spiles, gated pipe, or valves from buried pipe. Length of furrows and size of stream depend on slope, soil type, and crop; infiltration and erosion must be considered.

Flood method. Controlled flooding is done with border strips, contour or bench borders, and basins. Border strip irrigation is accomplished by advancing a sheet of water down a long, narrow area between low ridges called borders. Moisture enters the soil as the sheet advances. Strips vary from about 20 to 100 ft (6 to 30 m) in width, depending mainly on slope (both down and across), and amount of water available. The border must be well leveled and the grade uniform; best results are obtained on slopes of 0.5% or less. The flood method is sometimes used on steeper slopes, but maldistribution and erosion make it less effective.

Bench-border irrigation is sometimes used on moderately gentle, uniform slopes. The border strips, instead of running down the slope, are constructed across it. Since each strip must be level in width, considerable earth moving may be necessary.

Basin irrigation is well adapted to flatlands. It is done by flooding a diked area to a predetermined depth and allowing the water to enter the soil throughout the root zone. Basin irrigation may be utilized for all types of crops, including orchards where soil and topographic conditions permit.

Subirrigation. This type of irrigation is accomplished by raising the water table to the root zone of the crop or by carrying moisture to the root zone by perforated undergound pipe. Either method requires special soil conditions for successful operation.

Sprinkler systems. A sprinkler system consists of pipelines which carry water under pressure from a pump or elevated source to lateral lines along which sprinkler heads are spaced at appropriate intervals. Laterals are moved from one location to another by hand or tractor, or they are moved automatically. The side-roll wheel system, which utilizes the lateral as an axle (Fig. 2), is very popular as a labor-saving method. The center-pivot sprinkler system (Fig. 3) consists of a lateral carrying the sprinkler heads, and is moved by electrical or hydraulic power in a circular course irrigating an area containing up to 135–145 acres (546,200–586,700 m²).

Extra equipment can be attached in order to irrigate the corners, or solid sets can be used. Solid-set systems are systems with sufficient laterals and sprinklers to irrigate the entire field without being moved. These systems are quite popular for irrigating vegetable crops or other crops requiring light, frequent irrigations and, in orchards, where it is difficult to move the laterals.

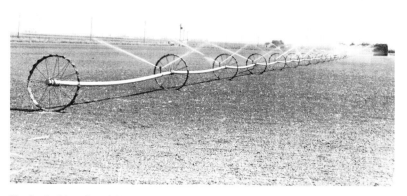

Fig. 2. A side-roll sprinkler system which uses the main supply line (often more than 1000 ft, or 300 m, long) to carry the sprinkler heads and as the axle for wheels.

Sprinkler irrigation has the advantage of being adaptable to soils too porous for other systems. It can be used on land where soil or topographic conditions are unsuitable for surface methods. It can be used on steep slopes and operates efficiently with a small water supply.

Drip irrigation. This is a method of providing water to plants almost continuously through small-diameter tubes and emitters. It has the advantage of maintaining high moisture levels at relatively low capital costs. It can be used on very steep, sandy, and rocky areas and can utilize saline waters better than most other systems. Clean water, usually filtered, is necessary to prevent blockage of tubes and emitters. The system has been most popular in orchards and vineyards, but is also used for vegetables, ornamentals, and for landscape plantings.

Automated systems. Automation is being used with solid-set and continuous-move types of systems, such as the center-pivot and lateral-move. Surface-irrigated systems are automated with check dams, operated by time clocks or volume meters, which open or close to divert water to other areas. Sprinkler systems, pumps, and check dams can all be activated by radio signals or low-voltage wired systems, which, in turn, can be triggered by soil-moisture-sensing devices or water levels in evaporation pans.

Automatically operated pumpback systems, consisting of a collecting pond and pump, are being used on surface-irrigated farms to better utilize water and prevent silt-laden waters from returning to natural streams.

Multiple uses. With well-designed and managed irrigation systems, it is possible to apply chemicals and, for short periods of time, to moderate climate. Chemicals which are being used include fertilizers, herbicides, and some fungicides. Effectiveness depends on uniformity of mixing and distribution and on application at the proper times. Chemicals must be registered to be used in this manner.

Solid-set systems are frequently used to prevent frost damage to plants and trees, since, as water freezes, it releases some heat. A continuous supply of water is needed during the protecting period. However, large volumes of water are required, and ice loads may cause limb breakage. Sequencing of sprinklers for cooling is being practiced for bloom delay in the spring and for reduction of heat damage in the summer.

Humid and arid regions. The percentage of increase in irrigated land is greater in humid areas than in arid and semiarid areas, although irrigation programs are often more satisfactory where the farmer does not depend on rainfall for crop growth. Good yields are obtained by well-timed irrigation, maintenance of high fertility, keeping the land well cultivated, and using superior crop varieties.

There is little difference in the principles of crop production under irrigation in humid and arid regions. The programming of water application is more difficult in humid areas because natural precipitation cannot be accurately predicted. Most humid areas utilize the sprinkler method.

To be successful, any irrigation system in any location must have careful planning with regard to soil conditions, topography, climate, cropping practices, water quality and supply, as well as en-

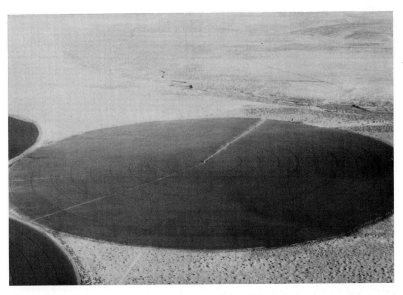

Fig. 3. Center-pivot systems are very popular in new irrigation developments.

gineering requirements.

Outlook. As mentioned, there are over 50,-000,000 acres of land irrigated in the United States. Studies of land that can be developed for irrigation are becoming obsolete with the improvements in irrigation systems. Limitations of water supplies and economics will prevent future developments — not land resources. The limit of simple diversions of natural rivers and streams has been reached, with few exceptions. Future development of large acreages of irrigated land must come through extensive storage; high-lift pumping projects, characteristic of Federal programs and large corporations; transportation of supply water sources to water-poor areas; and better conservation of water supplies.

Since the most economical irrigation projects have already been developed, future development will be more costly, depending upon many factors. Major diversions of stream flow to regions outside the watershed will involve many complicated interstate problems and compacts. As the population increases, there will be greater competition for water by industry, municipalities, power generators, recreational facilities, and wildlife reserves. Some underground water supplies are being depleted and must, at some time, be replenished by transported water if the irrigated area is to remain under cultivation.

Better water conservation could assist in expanding the irrigated acreage. It is estimated that phreatophites (water-loving plants) along streams and irrigation canals transpire 25,000,000 acre-feet of water to the atmosphere. Evaporation from reservoirs accounts for the loss of millions of additional acre-feet. Other losses include seepage from canals and water lost through the soil when more water is applied than the plants can use. *See* AGRICULTURE, SOIL AND CROP PRACTICES IN; LAND DRAINAGE (AGRICULTURE); TERRACING (AGRICULTURE).

[MEL A. HAGOOD]

Bibliography: R. M. Hagan, H. R. Haise, and T. W. Edminster, *Irrigation of Agricultural Lands*, 1967; C. H. Pair, *Sprinkler Irrigation*, 4th ed., 1975.

Isoleucine

An amino acid considered essential for normal growth of animals. The amino acids are characterized physically by the following: (1) the pK_1, or the dissociation constant of the various titratable groups; (2) the isoelectric point, or pH at which a

Physical constants of the L isomer at 25°C:
pK_1 (COOH): 2.36; pK_2 (NH_3^+): 9.68
Isoelectric point: 6.02
Optical rotation: $[\alpha]_D(H_2O)$: +12.4; $[\alpha]_D$(5 N HCl): +39.5
Solubility (g/100 ml H_2O): 4.12

Isoleucine

dipolar ion does not migrate in an electric field; (3) the optical rotation, or the rotation imparted to a beam of plane-polarized light (frequently the D line of the sodium spectrum) passing through 1 dm of a solution of 100 g in 100 ml; and (4) solubility.

The biosynthesis of isoleucine occurs when pyruvate and α-ketobutyrate react to form α-aceto-α-hydroxybutyrate, which undergoes rearrangement and reduction to α,β-dihydroxy-β-methylvalerate. Dehydration to the α-keto acid and transamination complete the biosynthesis. Most or all of the enzymes concerned also catalyze the analogous reac-

$$CH_3-CH_2-CH-C-S-CoA$$
$$|\qquad \|$$
$$CH_3 \quad O$$
α-Methylbutyryl-CoA

↓ −2H

$$CH_3-CH=C-C-S-CoA$$
$$|\qquad \|$$
$$CH_3 \quad O$$
Tiglyl-CoA

↓ H_2O

$$CH_3-CH-CH-C-S-CoA$$
$$|\quad |\qquad \|$$
$$OH \quad CH_3 \quad O$$
α-Methyl-β-hydroxybutyryl-CoA

↓ DPN

$$CH_3-C-CH-C-S-CoA$$
$$\|\quad |\qquad \|$$
$$O \quad CH_3 \quad O$$
α-Methylacetoacetyl-CoA

↓ CoA

$$CH_3-C-S-CoA + CH_3-CH_2-C-S-CoA$$
$$\|\qquad\qquad\qquad \|$$
$$O \qquad\qquad\qquad O$$
Acetyl-CoA   Propionyl-CoA

Pathway for the metabolic degradation of isoleucine after its conversion to α-methylbutyryl-coenzyme A.

tions in valine biosynthesis. See AMINO ACIDS; VALINE.

During metabolic degradation the first steps are deamination and oxidative decarboxylation, forming α-methylbutyryl-coenzyme A (see illustration).

[EDWARD A. ADELBERG]

Jojoba

A unique, wild plant species (*Simmondsia chinensis*) widely distributed in the semiarid regions of Arizona, California, and Baja California over an area of 10^5 mi² (2.6×10^8 km²) between latitudes 25 and 31°N. Jojoba has recently attracted worldwide attention because it is an extremely drought-resistant species; its seeds contain a liquid wax which, in addition to several other uses, can serve as a replacement for sperm whale oil, a product derived from an endangered species; and it can grow in areas of marginal soil fertility, high atmospheric temperatures, high salinity, and low humidity.

Classification, distribution, and botany. Jojoba has 21 pairs of chromosomes. Its unique botanical characteristics have caused taxonomists to place it in the monotypic genus *Simmondsia*; some consider it as the only member of a monotypic family, the Simmondsiaceae, and others include it in the Buxaceae. Obviously, further study of the systematic relationships of the genus *Simmondsia* and the family Buxaceae is required to resolve the above differences of opinion.

Jojoba has a wide adaptation from hot desert environments with about 3 in. (75 mm) of rainfall, such as the Joshua Tree National Park in California, to cool, humid, coastal environments, such as the Ensenada area of Baja California, with up to 15 in. (375 mm) of rainfall. It is usually restricted to coarse, deep, and well-drained soils such as the sandy alluviums and to coarse, attrital mixtures of gravels and clays. It is often found on slopes and along washes from sea level to about 4500 ft (1400 m) elevation.

Jojoba is a dioecious, perennial, evergreen, woody shrub. In inland areas it has a branching, upright growth habit and a spherical or oval outline, 2–15 ft (0.60–4.5 m) in height and in diameter. Ecotypes with a prostrate, creeping growth habit are common along the Pacific coastline from Del Mar, CA, to the tip of Baja California. The mature seed is brown and weighs from 0.2–1.5 g. Its wax content ranges from 44 to 58%.

Jojoba wax can be extracted from the seed with the same equipment and techniques used for other oil seeds such as soybeans and cotton. The wax is not a "fat" or triglyceride but a "liquid wax," or wax ester of high molecular weight. A wax molecule consists of one molecule of a long-chain alcohol esterified with one molecule of a long-chain fatty acid. Jojoba wax consists primarily of two such esters: one with 40 carbon atoms (30%) and one with 42 carbon atoms (50%).

The meal of jojoba contains about 30% protein; it also contains a monoglucoside, called simmondsin, which acts as an appetite depressant when the meal is fed to animals. Simmondsin may find in the future significant uses in the pharmaceuticals industry; at present, however, it constitutes a problem as it makes the meal unsuitable as feed. Research is underway to develop methods of neutralizing simmondsin.

Jojoba flowers usually appear in late summer, in leaf axils at every other node. They remain small, inconspicuous, and dormant until late fall or early winter, at which time the female flowers swell and become receptive and the male flowers release pollen. Bees are often seen visiting male flowers during anthesis, but they rarely land on female flowers; thus, pollination is carried out entirely by wind. After pollination, female flowers continue to enlarge and develop into fruit, reaching maturity in mid or late summer. At that time, the outer tissues of the fruit, the hulls, turn from green to brown, shrivel, and separate, releasing the seed which drops to the ground. Each fruit produces one to three seeds. Harvesting data indicate that shrubs in natural populations produce up to about 10 lb (4 kg) of clean dry seed per plant. A few plants, 40–50 years old, growing in botanical gardens have exceeded 30 lb (13.5 kg) of clean dry seed per plant. The ratio of male to female plants varies in different areas and is either close to 1:1 or males outnumber females. The lifespan of jojoba has not been determined, but all indications are that it lives over 100 years and possibly 200 or more.

Domestication. A major effort to domesticate jojoba was undertaken in California, Arizona, Israel, and Mexico in the early 1970s. Seed harvested from high-yielding wild plants was planted in pilot plantations to study the development and yielding ability of this plant under cultivation, and to develop information on cultural aspects. Present trends are to grow jojoba in rows spaced 10–20 ft (3–7 m) apart, with plants separated by 3–5 ft (1–1.5 m).

Plant propagation can be done from seed, from cuttings, or through tissue culture. With asexual propagation the sex ratio of the seedlings is known in advance, and a plantation can be laid out in accordance with a preplanned pattern and frequency of male and female plants. When seed is used for planting, the sex of seedlings cannot be determined until 2–3 years after planting when flowers appear. To circumvent the problem of sex identification, four or five seeds are planted per hill. After blooming, the desired number and arrangement of male and female plants is maintained in the field while the extra plants are rogued out.

Field plantings of jojoba should be made preferably on light permeable soils and when temperatures are mild. Seedlings should be irrigated during the first 6 months of growth until they establish their root system. Jojoba produces a tap root which at 80°F (27°C) grows to a depth of 12 in. (30 cm) in 1 week, and to 36 in. (90 cm) in about 6 weeks. It responds favorably to fertilization and irrigation; exact requirements, however, have not yet been determined. It appears that 1 acre-foot (1.2 m) of water is sufficient. The greatest need for water occurs during the late winter and spring. Thus, when grown under irrigation jojoba does not compete with other irrigated crops, most of which have their peak requirements for water during the summer.

Jojoba withstands heavy pruning and can easily be trained to grow in desired shapes. Male branches may be grafted onto female ones, and vice versa. A number of herbicides may be used for weed control. No major pests or diseases have been observed as yet. Temperatures of up to 120°F (49°C) do not seem to have adverse effects on plant growth or seed production. Flowers are damaged, however, at 22 to 24°F (−4 to −5°C), and seedling damage may be severe at temperatures below 20°F (−6°C). Dry seed may be stored for over 20 years without any deterioration of the wax it contains.

Jojoba has also attracted interest as a landscape and soil conservation plant. Since it is a perennial, evergreen, nonpoisonous, drought-resistant, low-maintenance, long-lived, and low–fire hazard plant with a deep root system, it can be used in highway and roadside plantings and hedges. Also, it can be used as a soil stabilizer in green belts around desert cities suffering from particulate air pollution.

Harvesting. Seed may be harvested by hand or may be vacuumed or swept and picked from the ground with equipment and techniques comparable to those available for almonds or walnuts. It can also be caught in plastic nets placed under the bushes as is done with macadamia nuts.

Economics. The establishment of a jojoba plantation should not cost any more than that of an almond grove. With lower expenditures for irrigation and fertilization, the maintenance of a producing plantation should be lower than that of most tree crops. Although jojoba starts producing seed in the second or third year, with currently available strains it appears that commercial harvest of seed might not be profitable or even practical until the fifth year after planting. This disadvantage is more than offset, however, by the long life-span of the plant.

Since there are no producing commercial plantations of jojoba available, no detailed data on production and returns are available. Jojoba is not thought of as a crop which will compete for acreage with traditional ones, but as one which will fit in regions where traditional crops cannot be grown profitably, due to various limiting environmental factors. Thus, capital investments for land and expenditures for equipment and energy should be lower than for most tree crops. Extrapolating from data obtained from the harvest of wild plants and from limited information from research plots, it appears that seed yields of 8 years or older plantations might range from 1 to 2 tons (0.9 to 1.8 metric tons) of dry, clean seed per acre (0.4 ha). Development of higher-yielding strains and better cultural techniques should lead to higher yields and lower costs of production per acre.

Current expectations are that the small quantities of wax that will be available initially from cultivated plantations will be absorbed by the more lucrative markets such as cosmetics, waxes, and possibly pharmaceuticals, at price levels of $1–2/lb ($2–4/kg) of wax. The real challenge for jojoba will be to penetrate the larger but less lucrative market of lubricants. This may not be too difficult, however, because with the disappearance of fossil oils, cheap sources of lubricants will also be lost. Lubricants will be needed in the near future as badly as fuels, and none of the new sources of energy now contemplated (solar, atomic, or geothermic) have lubricants as by-products.

Properties and uses of jojoba wax. Jojoba wax has the following properties: melting point, 6.8–7.0°C; boiling point, 398°C; smoke point,

195°C; flash point, 295°C; fire point, 338°; refractive index, 1.4650; specific gravity, .863; iodine value, 82; saponification value, 92; and molecular weight of wax esters, 606.

Jojoba wax is a superior lubricant for high-speed high-temperature machinery, as a cutting, grinding, and transformer oil, and a substitute for sperm whale oil. It has potential use in the cosmetics industry as hair oil, shampoo, soap, face creams, lipstick, tanning lotions, and insect repellents. In the pharmaceuticals industry, it may be of value as a carrier or coating for medicinal preparations, an antifoaming agent, a stabilizer of penicillin products, and as a potential treatment for skin ailments. Other potential applications include linoleum manufacture, printing ink, varnishes, chewing gum, polishing waxes for automobiles, floors, furniture, and vinyl, and a solvent of polyethylene.   [D. M. YERMANOS]

Bibliography: H. S. Gentry, *Econ. Bot.*, 12(3): 261–295, 1958; T. K. Miwa, *Cosmet. Perfum.*, 88: 39–41, 1973; National Academy of Sciences, *Products from Jojoba: A Promising New Crop for Arid Lands*, 1975; D. M. Yermanos, *Econ. Bot.*, 28: 160–174, 1975; D. M. Yermanos and C. Duncan, *J. Amer. Oil Chem. Soc.*, 53:700–704, 1976.

Kale

Either of two cool-season biennial crucifers, *Brassica oleracea* var. *acephala* and *B. fimbriata*, of Mediterranean origin and belonging to the plant order Capparales. Kale is grown for its nutritious green curled leaves which are cooked as a vegetable (see illustration). Distinct varieties (cultivars) are pro-

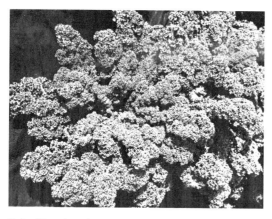

Kale (*Brassica oleracea* var. *acephala*), cultivar Vates. (*Joseph Harris Co., Rochester, N.Y.*)

duced in Europe for stock feed. Kale and collards differ only in the form of their leaves; both are minor vegetables in the United States. Cultural practices are similar to those used for cabbage, but kale is more sensitive to high temperatures. Strains of the Scotch and Siberian varieties are most popular. Kale is moderately tolerant of acid soils. Monthly mean temperatures below 70°F favor best growth. Harvesting is generally 2–3 months after planting. Virginia is an important producing state. The total annual farm value in the United States from approximately 1200 acres is $600,000. *See* CABBAGE; COLLARD; KOHLRABI; VEGETABLE GROWING.

[H. JOHN CAREW]

Kohlrabi

A cool-season biennial crucifer, *Brassica caulorapa* and *B. oleracea* var. *caulo-rapa*, of northern European origin belonging to the plant order Capparales. Kohlrabi is grown for its turniplike enlarged stem, which is usually eaten as a cooked vegetable (see illustration). Kohlrabi is a German

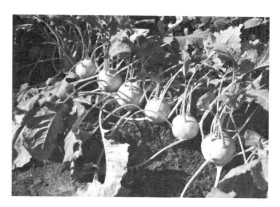

Kohlrabi (*Brassica caulorapa*), cultivar Early White Vienna. (*Joseph Harris Co., Rochester, N.Y.*)

word meaning cabbage-turnip and reflects a similarity in taste and appearance to both vegetables. Cultural practices for kohlrabi are similar to those used for turnips. White Vienna and Purple Vienna are popular varieties (cultivars). Harvesting, when the enlarged stems are 2–3 in. in diameter, is usually 2 months after planting. A common cooked vegetable in Europe, especially Germany, kohlrabi is of minor importance in the United States. *See* CABBAGE; KALE; TURNIP; VEGETABLE GROWING.

[H. JOHN CAREW]

Kudzu

A perennial vine legume, capable of rapid growth in a warm temperate, humid subtropical climate. The name Kudzu has a Japanese origin. Kudzu (*Pueraria thunbergiana*) was introduced into the United States in 1876 and used as a shade plant until 1906, when a few enthusiastic growers in the southeastern United States began to use it as a forage crop, a practice that continued for 30 years. It was then promoted as a soil-conserving plant. However, much prejudice has developed against its use because of its spread into forest borders, drainage ditches, and other areas.

Kudzu is not adapted to tropical or arid climates or to alkaline soils, and probably requires winter cold for growth rejuvenation. The technique for growing kudzu successfully is to set out a few well-developed plants, use enough commercial fertilizer or equivalent for good growth, and protect the plants from weeds, insects, and grazing animals. The vines will spread over the area to be covered, producing roots at the nodes, which, unless killed by severe winter freezing, become independent plants. Thus, a few plants produce many in 2 or 3 years if adequately protected. *See* FERTILIZING.

Kudzu produces moderate yields of forage, but it must be grazed with care to prevent loss of stand. Since the viney stems are difficult to harvest for hay, adapted grasses and clovers are preferred as forage crops.

A simple, economical method is needed for keeping kudzu from spreading into areas where it is not wanted. It may be stopped by a permanent pasture at the border of a kudzu field, or by repeated cultivation or harrowing the borders of cropland. No acceptable method of spread prevention has been developed for uncultivated or non-pastured areas.

Tropical kudzu (*P. phaseolides*) is one of the most important and widely planted cover and green manure crops of the tropics. It makes rapid vigorous growth, providing quick ground cover and suppressing most other vegetative growth. It is increasingly used as a forage crop although careful management is required to prevent complete domination of mixtures with grasses and other species. Its habit of growth is similar to kudzu of subtropical areas. *See* LEGUME FORAGES;

[PAUL TABOR]

Kumquat

Shrubs or small trees that are members of the genus *Fortunella*, which is one of the six genera in the group of true citrus fruits. Kumquats are believed to have originated in China and the Malay Peninsula, but are now widely grown in all citrus areas of the world. Of the several species the most common are *F. margarita*, which has oval-shaped fruit (see illustration), and *F. japonica*, which has round fruit.

The kumquat's stems, leaves, flowers, and fruits resemble those of *Citrus*. Kumquats bear numerous flame- to orange-colored fruits of small size, often less than 1 in. in diameter, having three to five locules filled with an acid pulp and a sweet, edible pulpy rind. The trees are among the most cold-hardy of the citrus fruits; they stay dormant even during protracted warm spells in the winter months, which enables them to withstand low temperatures.

Kumquats, with their brilliant orange-colored fruits and dense green foliage, are highly ornamental and are most frequently grown for this reason. Sprays of foliage and fruit are commonly used for decoration, particularly in gift packages of ordinary citrus fruits. Kumquat fruits can be eaten whole without peeling; they are also used in marmalades and preserves and as candied fruits. *See* FRUIT, TREE.

[FRANK E. GARDNER]

Kwashiorkor disease

A nutritional deficiency disease in infants and young children, caused primarily by diet in which protein is of poor quality or inadequate quantity, or both, and carbohydrate intake is normal or high. The disease has frequently been referred to as protein-calorie malnutrition or deficiency. Kwashiorkor occurs throughout the world, but especially among the underdeveloped areas. According to the World Health Organization, it is the most widespread and important dietary disease in the world today. It is estimated that between 100- and 270,000,000 children, commonly in the 6-month to 3-year age group, are afflicted, many of whom die. Clinical features consist of poor growth and development, edema, dyspigmentation of skin and hair, and psychological changes characterized by apathy and irritability. Pathological changes consist of enlarged fatty liver; atrophy of pancreas, salivary glands, and intestinal glands; and wasting of muscles. Because of its worldwide importance, investigators have studied experimental models of kwashiorkor in animals to understand better the mechanisms involved in the metabolism of dietary constituents, especially protein and its amino acids. This article concerns itself with research with experimental kwashiorkor-like syndromes induced in laboratory animals.

Experimental conditions. It has been frequently demonstrated that the feeding of an amino acid–deficient or imbalanced protein diet to an experimental animal invariably leads to reduced food consumption when the animal is allowed to eat as much as it desires. Under these conditions it has not been possible to demonstrate pathologic changes simulating those found in humans with kwashiorkor. Consequently, investigators have adopted the force-feeding technique on rats and monkeys to assure an adequate intake of a diet deficient in amino acid or protein. With this technique a kwashiorkor-like syndrome has been induced in animals within days or weeks. The chief morphologic alterations consist of an enlarged fatty liver, increased liver glycogen, and atrophy of the pancreas, salivary glands, gastrointestinal glands, thymus, and spleen.

Conclusions. Based on a number of these experimental studies, the conclusion is that a variety of factors are important in the induction of pathologic changes resembling kwashiorkor in animals: Animals must ingest a sufficient amount of food in order to develop the condition; progressive emaciation or marasmus, which is quite different from kwashiorkor, develops if the food intake is decreased; the caloric intake derived mainly from carbohydrates must be quantitatively adequate; adrenal-cortical hormone stimulation is not important, since adrenalectomized animals maintained on low doses of corticosteroids still develop the condition; and finally, single deficiencies of all essential amino acids except arginine and leucine, as well as poor-quality proteins, can produce most of the features of the kwashiorkor-like experimental model.

Among biochemical changes in the livers of these experimental animals were increases in lipid, glycogen, and ribonucleic acid. The results of experiments in which young rats were force-fed an essential amino acid–devoid diet for 3–7 days indicated that protein synthesis is enhanced in the liver but diminished in skeletal muscle of the experimental animals. This has been demonstrated by measuring the incorporation of leucine-C^{14} into proteins of these organs, or of cell-free preparations from these organs. The increased protein synthesis in the liver is related predominantly to enhanced activity of ribosomes, and the aggregates of liver ribosomes (polyribosomes) as measured in a sucrose gradient indicated a shift from lighter toward heavier polyribosomes with a decrease in monomers. Ultrastructural changes in the hepatic cells of experimental animals revealed nucleolar enlargement; increased amounts of lipid and glycogen; increased number of lysosomes, many of which contained glycogen; and an increased amount of free (unbound) polyribosomes. *See* METABOLIC DISORDERS.   [HERSCHEL SIDRANSKY]

Bibliography: H. N. Munro and J. B. Allison, *Mammalian Protein Metabolism*, vol. 2, 1964.

KUMQUAT

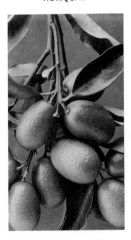

Fruit cluster and foliage of Nagami kumquat (*Fortunella margarita*). (*The McFarland Co.*)

Lactose

Milk sugar or 4-O-β-D-galactopyranosyl-D-glucose. This reducing disaccharide is obtained as the α-D anomer (see formula below, where the asterisk indicates a reducing group); the melting point (mp) is 202°C and the optical activity is $[\alpha]_D^{20} + 85.0 \rightarrow +52.6°$. Crystallization at higher temperatures

(above 93.5°C) gives the β-D anomer; mp 252°C, and $[\alpha]_D^{20} + 35 \rightarrow +55.4°$. Lactose is found in the milk of mammals to the extent of approximately 2–8%. It is usually prepared from whey, which is obtained as a by-product in the manufacture of cheese. Upon concentration of the whey, crystalline lactose is deposited. Lactose is not fermentable by ordinary baker's yeast. In the souring of milk, *Lactobacillus acidophilus* and certain other microorganisms bring about lactic acid fermentation by transforming the lactose of the milk into lactic acid. $CH_3CHOHCOOH$. *See* CHEESE; MILK.

Chemical evidence shows that the glycosidic linkage involves the carbon atom 1 of D-galactose and carbon 4 of D-glucose. Enzymatic studies indicate that the galactosidic linkage has the β-configuration. *See* OLIGOSACCHARIDE.

The mammary glands of lactating animals, and their milk, contain an enzyme, lactose synthetase, capable of transferring the D-galactose unit from uridine diphosphate D-galactose to D-glucose, forming lactose according to the scheme: Uridine diphosphate D-galactose + D-Glucose → Lactose + Uridine diphosphate.

The lactose synthetase can be resolved into two protein components, A and B, which individually do not exhibit any catalytic activity. Recombination of these fractions, however, restores full lactose synthetase activity. The B fraction was identified as α-lactalbumin. [WILLIAM Z. HASSID]

Bibliography: D. M. Greenberg (ed.), *Metabolic Pathways*, vol. 1, 3d ed., 1967; W. W. Pigman (ed.), *The Carbohydrates*, 2d ed., 1957.

Land drainage (agriculture)

The removal of water from land to improve the soil as a medium for plant growth and a surface for crop management operations. Water in excess of that needed by the plants may inhibit growth or the production of the economically important portion of the plant. High water content also lubricates the soil particles and frequently leads to unstable conditions unsuitable to machine and other crop operations. Drainage needs, or the amount of excess water, therefore, varies depending upon the soil, the demands of the crop, and the stability needs of the management practices. If the crops are water-tolerant and only light equipment is needed to manage the crop, the water excess may be small, but for an identical location where either the crop is not tolerant or the management practices place heavy loads on the soil, the water excess may be great.

Excess water creates problems in agricultural production over vast areas. Estimates of the acreage in need of drainage in the United States vary widely. G. D. Schwab stated that 22% of the total cropland, or 94,000,000 acres, has a dominant drainage problem, and Q. C. Ayres indicated that reclamation by drainage would be a benefit on about 216,000,000, or about 24% of all potential agricultural land in the United States. Ayres also indicated that about 33,000,000 acres have already been drained in the humid regions, and about 17,000,000 acres at least partly drained in the irrigated lands of the arid western states. Similar drainage problems exist in other countries.

Water source and disposal. The excess water may be due to rainfall overflow from streams, swamps, or other bodies of water; seepage or runoff from higher areas; or irrigation. The source of water should be identified before a solution is proposed. In general, the solution must fit the soil, the topography, the source of water, the crops being grown, and the management scheme used, including machinery, and must be economically feasible. Obviously, no one ideal solution exists, but a range of solutions may be proposed which

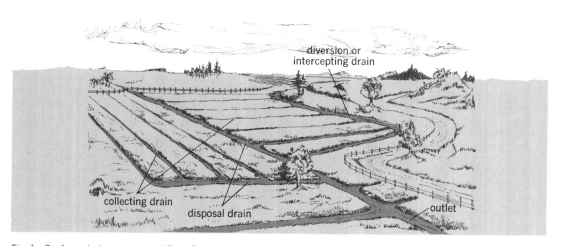

Fig. 1.   Surface-drainage system. (*From Engineering Handbook for Work Unit Staffs, USDA Soil Conservation Serv., 1964*)

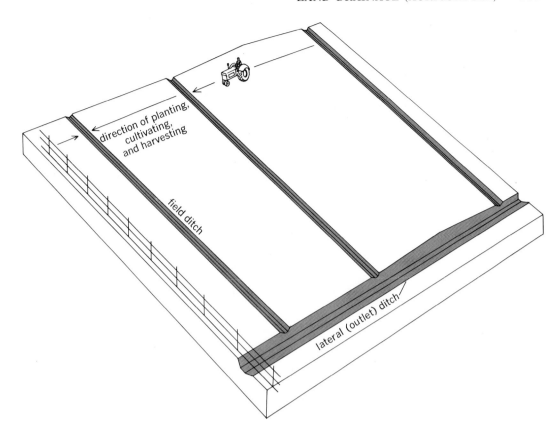

typical cross section of ground surface that has some general slope
in one direction and is covered with many small depressions and pockets

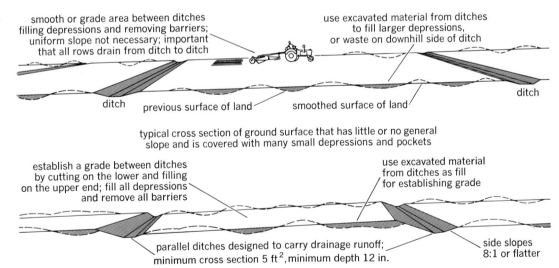

typical cross section of ground surface that has little or no general
slope and is covered with many small depressions and pockets

Fig. 2. Shallow-ditch system for surface drainage. Field ditches should be about parallel but not necessarily equidistant; and the outlet should be about 1 ft deeper than field ditches. It is necessary to clean ditches after each farming operation.

vary in advantage with the individual situation.

Before discussing drainage systems, water disposal must be considered. All drainage systems must have an outlet for disposal of the water collected (Fig. 1); the outlet places restrictions on the type of system that may be used. A good outlet is low enough to permit water removal from the lowest area needing drainage; is stable, neither eroding nor filling rapidly; and is capable of accepting all design flows. Such an outlet is not always easily found; frequently deficiencies in the outlet must be corrected before a drainage system may be designed. In general, drainage outlets may be either natural or artificial, and the water may flow naturally by gravity or be moved by pumps; again, many combinations are possible.

Methods. There are two basic methods of draining land, and these may be combined to form a third. The first method, surface drainage, attempts to remove excess water before it enters the soil;

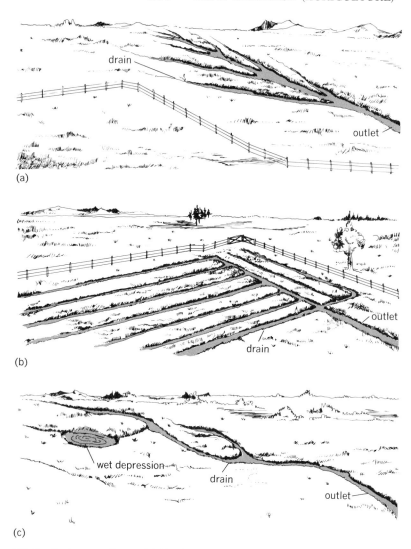

(a)

(b)

(c)

Fig. 3. Drainage patterns. (a) Herringbone. (b) Parallel. (c) Random. (*From Engineering Handbook for Work Unit Staffs, USDA Soil Conservation Service, 1964*)

the second, subsurface drainage, attempts to remove it after it is within the soil. When both are used, the system is called combined drainage. In practice, surface drainage is difficult to isolate from subsurface flow or vice versa, but separation is useful for a discussion of principles.

Surface drainage. This is usually accomplished by using shallow (less than 2 ft deep) open ditches to collect the surface water; the land surface, either between or along the ditches, is either graded or smoothed, or both, to promote movement of water into the ditches (Fig. 2). The ditches are constructed so that they slope toward a collector ditch or the outlet, and water flows naturally down the slope. Surface systems are usually less costly than subsurface or combined systems, and because the ditches are shallow, an adequate outlet is easier to find. Heavy soils that are slow to absorb rainfall, soils that are shallow over impermeable layers, or drainage problems due to surface flow are ideally suited to surface drainage.

Subsurface drainage. This is usually accomplished by burying conduits within the soil. They are buried so that they slope toward a collector or the outlet, and flow is the result of gravity. Outlets

for subsurface systems must be lower in elevation than outlets for surface systems and thus are more difficult to locate. Conduits must be buried at least 2 ft below the soil surface to prevent damage by machines traveling over the surface. They must also be buried deep enough to promote water movement toward the drains at a rapid enough rate to prevent damage to crops and stabilize the soil for machinery operation. The water movement within the soil toward a drainage conduit is primarily by gravity; thus, unless the ability of the soil to conduct water is restricted as depth increases, a deeper drain will provide more rapid drainage over a wider area than will a shallower drain. Soils which are deep and permit rapid movement of water into and through the soil can be said to be ideally suited to subsurface drainage.

Practical applications. Ideal conditions suited exclusively to either surface or subsurface drainage are rare. Most systems operate, by either design or nature, as combined drainage systems. Ditches, even shallow ones, promote some subsurface drainage, and water in excess of that which may infiltrate the soil frequently flows over the surface to some outlet.

Drainage-system patterns. Patterns for drainage systems are of two general types. Where the drainage problem is general over an area, drainage channels may be provided at regular intervals (Fig. 3a and b); where the problem exists in isolated areas within a larger area, channels may be provided at random to include only those areas which need drainage (Fig. 3c). Random systems are usually less expensive to install, and a high proportion of drainage problems first appear as isolatable areas within a larger block. As time passes, however, the second-wettest areas become the limiting factor, and random systems are extended until they look like regularly spaced systems. If expansion at a future date is considered in the initial design, the first cost is increased, but the final system is adequate. Conversely, if expansion is not considered, the initial cost may be much lower, but much of the system may have to be replaced or avoided in order to improve it in the future.

The quantity of water which must be removed by a drainage system is variable and based primarily upon experience. Most drainage system designs permit temporary flooding and require that the system dispose of a quantity of water expressed in inches of depth over the area to be drained in a period of 24 hr (called drainage coefficient). Increased protection is provided in design by increasing the drainage coefficient.

Systems construction. Most drainage systems are constructed with power equipment. Scrapers, graders, bulldozers, draglines, backhoes, plows, and special trenching machines are used to dig open ditches, and the land surface may be shaped and smoothed with some of the same equipment. There are also special machines, land levelers, for smoothing the land. Surface drainage channels are designed with gentle side slopes to permit machines and equipment to cross easily. The earth removed from the channels is deposited where it will not interfere with drainage. Soil from the channels and high spots in the field is used to fill holes or depressions, or it may be used to raise the level of the ground surface to create increased slope into the channel (Fig. 2).

Subsurface drains are of two types. The most common type consists of buried pipes. Special pipes, made of ceramic materials, concrete, plastic, bituminuous impregnated paper, or zinc-coated steel, are constructed for subsurface drainage. Openings are provided into the pipes by holes and slots cut through the pipe walls or by space left between pipe sections and, in rare cases, by permeable wall materials. A machine digs a trench to the required depth with the bottom sloping toward the outlet. The pipes are then placed into the trench and the earth returned over the pipe. In particular soils, special materials may be placed immediately over or around the pipes to prevent soil particles from entering the opening or to promote more rapid drainage. Gravel, sand, fiber glass sheets, and organic materials such as corncobs, hay, grass, or sawdust are used for this purpose. These materials are more open than the surrounding soil but present smaller openings than those present in the pipes. They also contact a larger area of soil than the openings in the pipe and thus promote better drainage.

In some soils, subsurface channels may be provided by pulling a solid object through the soil at the proper slope and depth. This type of drain is called a mole drain and the object used is called a mole. The mole is usually a steel cylinder formed to a wedge-shaped point on one end and attached to a chain or metal plate. The mole is placed in the outlet and then pulled through the soil. The mole is shaped so that it will stay in the ground at a fixed depth; therefore, the land surface must have the desired slope. If the soil has sufficient clay for a binder and enough silt, sand or stones for stability, the channel created will stay open for several years and forms an inexpensive method of subdrainage.

Systems maintenance. All drainage systems require care in design, construction, and maintenance. Erosion or silting may occur in open ditches. Vegetation such as grass may be used along or within the ditch to stabilize the soil against either erosion or siltation, but the grass must be mowed, fertilized, and occasionally replaced. Outlets from subsurface drains may erode, removing support from around the outlets and permitting the pipe to break away, causing further erosion. Animals must be prevented from entering the pipes, and occasionally pipe sections break or collapse and require replacement. Surface entrances into buried conduits may become plugged and need cleaning; roots of perennial plants, for instance, may enter and clog a pipe.

A surface drainage system should last at least 10 years without major improvement if yearly maintenance is provided. Subsurface drainage systems should last 50 years or more if the pipe material is durable. Adequate agricultural drainage, however, is not static. As crops, management, and machines change, different demands are placed upon drainage systems and changes must be made. The soils, crops, water, and technology involved in drainage are dynamic, and the assistance of specialists is needed in devising well-designed drainage systems. The investment in drainage systems is frequently as great or greater than the original price

of agricultural land. Such designs should, therefore, receive careful attention. *See* AGRICULTURE, SOIL AND CROP PRACTICES IN; IRRIGATION OF CROPS; TERRACING (AGRICULTURE).

[RICHARD D. BLACK]

Bibliography: J. N. Luthin, *Drainage Engineering*, rev. ed., 1973; J. N. Luthin, *Drainage of Agricultural Lands*, 1957; G. O. Schwab et al., *Soil and Water Conservation Engineering*, 1966.

Legume

A dry, dehiscent fruit derived from a single, simple pistil. When mature, it splits along both dorsal and ventral sutures into two valves. The term also designates any plant of the order Rosales that bears this type of fruit.

The family Leguminosae characteristically contains a single row of seeds attached along the lower or ventral suture of the fruit. The seeds are highly nutritious and several species of legumes furnish a large amount of food for both man and animals. Nitrogen-fixing bacteria living symbiotically in the roots of legumes accumulate nitrogenous materials and are beneficial for the soil.

Some more common and important legumes are alfalfa, beans, clovers, kudzu, lespedeza, locust, peas, peanuts, soybeans, and vetch. See articles on these individual legumes.

[PERRY D. STRAUSBAUGH/EARL L. CORE]

Legume forages

Plants of the legume family used for livestock feed, grazing, hay, or silage. Legume forages are usually richer in protein, calcium, and phosphorus than other kinds of forages, such as grass. The production, preservation, and use of forage legumes require special skills on most soils. One important requirement is a supply of the needed symbiotic nitrogen-fixing bacteria if these are not already in the soil; commercial cultures for various strains of these bacteria can be purchased and applied to the legume seed just before planting. Additional lime and commercial fertilizers may be needed on all except fertile soils. Protection from weeds, injurious insects, diseases, and other harmful influences is often required. *See* LEGUME; NITROGEN FIXATION (BIOLOGY).

Legume forages may be preserved for future use as dry hay or silage. To obtain high quality, most legume hay crops must be harvested before the mature stage and thoroughly cured without the loss of leaves; high-moisture hay spoils in warm weather. Legumes are more difficult to preserve as silage than grasses due to their high protein content. However, the addition of a high-carbohydrate material, such as molasses, or, as is usually preferred, the mixing of grass and legume are helpful measures. Legume silage often has an objectionable odor if fermentation is not sufficiently rapid to prevent breakdown of the proteins.

Much of the legume forage is grazed. Some crops can be grazed continuously without injury while others require intermittent grazing with rest periods to permit recovery or frequent very light use. A lush growth of a palatable legume crop, such as white clover or alfalfa, often causes bloat in grazing animals, but this may be prevented by restricting intake. The use of drenches in order to prevent or break up foaming in the stomachs of the animals acts as a temporary cure.

Alfalfa is the most important legume forage crop in the United States; it is used mainly for hay but is often grazed. White clover and the annual lespedezas are the most extensively grown legumes for grazing particularly in the southeastern United States. Red clover was an important crop prior to 1930 but is minor now. About a dozen other species of legumes are used for cultivated forage in the United States and a large number for range grazing. *See* ALFALFA; CLOVER; COVER CROPS; COWPEA; KUDZU; LESPEDEZA; LUPINE.

[PAUL TABOR]

Lemon

The fruit *Citrus limon*, commercially the most important of the acid citrus fruits. It most probably originated in the eastern Himalayan region of India or adjoining areas. It was introduced into Europe by the Arabs, probably by the 12th century, and has spread to commercial citrus areas throughout the world. Most varieties are vigorous, upright-spreading, and open in growth habit, attaining large size if not controlled by pruning. New shoot growth is purple-tinted, but mature leaves are a light green in contrast to the dark green of oranges. The large, purple-tinted flowers are produced throughout the year. The yellow fruits are medium-sized and elongate with a prominent nipple (see illustration). The lemon is more sensitive to cold than other major citrus fruits, and thus its commercial culture is restricted to areas with mild winter temperatures. In regions with mild winters and cool summers, marketable fruit is available throughout the year.

The lemon is grown primarily for its acid flavor. For the fresh-fruit market, lemons are picked relatively immature and stored to provide a constant supply of high-quality fruit. Tree-ripe fruits are processed because of their short storage life. Lemon juice, very high in vitamin C, is used in beverages and to garnish meats and fish. It has many culinary uses, especially in pies, cakes, ices, candies, jellies, and marmalades. It is also used widely in proprietary soft drinks. The principal by-products are citric acid from the juice and lemon oil from the peel. *See* ASCORBIC ACID.

Commercial lemon production developed first in Italy, mainly in Sicily. Italy is the largest producer,

followed by California. Spain, Greece, and Argentina are also significant producers, with some commercial production in most Mediterranean countries and also in Australia and South Africa. The average yearly United States production for 1971–1976 was approximately 861,000 metric tons. *See* FRUIT, TREE.

[R. K. SOOST]

Lentil

A semiviny annual legume with slender tufted and branched stems 18–22 in. long (Fig. 1). The lentil plant (*Lens esculenta*) was one of the first plants brought under cultivation. They have been found in the Bronze Age ruins of the ancient lake dwellings of St. Peter's Island, Lake of Bienne, Switzerland. Lentils have been discovered in Poland dating back to the Iron Age. In the Bible the "red pottage" for which Esau gave up his birthright to his brother, Jacob, was probably lentil soup. Large-seeded lentils originated in the Mediterranean region; medium-sized lentils originated in the inner mountains of Asia Minor; and Afghanistan was the original home of the smallest-seeded lentils. *See* LEGUME.

Production. The world's lentil production is centered in Asia, with nearly two-thirds of the production from India, Pakistan, Turkey, and Syria. Whitman and Spokane counties in Washington, and Latah, Benewah, and Nez Perce counties in Idaho grow about 95% of the lentils produced in the United States.

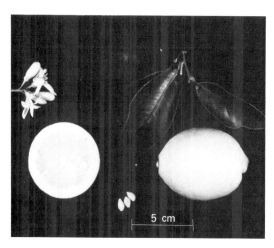

Flowers, foliage, fruit, and seeds of *Citrus limon*.

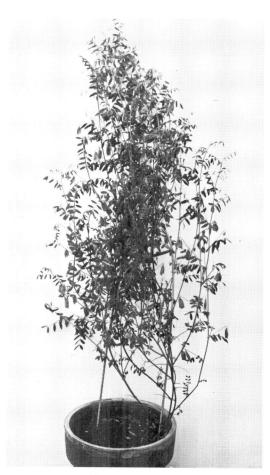

Fig. 1. Lentil plant showing growth habit.

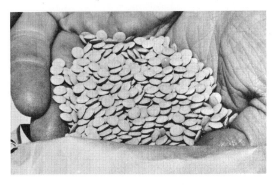

Fig. 2. Lens-shaped lentil seeds.

Description. Lentil leaves are pinnately compound and generally resemble vetch. The plant has tendrils similar to those of pea plants.

The seeds grow in short broad pods, each pod producing two or three thin lens-shaped seeds (Fig. 2). Seed color varies from yellow to brown and may be mottled, although mottled seed are not desirable for marketing. The lentil flowers, ranging in color from white to light purple, are small and delicate and occur at many different locations on the stems.

Lentil seed is used primarily for soups but also in salads and casseroles. Lentils are more digestible than meat and are used as a meat substitute in many countries.

Culture. Lentils require a cool growing season; they are injured by severe heat. Therefore, they are planted in April, when soil moisture is adequate and temperatures are cool. A fine firm seedbed is required; the land is usually plowed in the fall and firmed by cultivation in the spring before seeding. Lentils are usually planted in rotation with winter wheat. Seeds are planted in 7–12 in. rows at depths of $\frac{1}{2}$ to 1 in., on an average of 60–75 lb/acre. Applications of sulfur, molybdenum, and phosphorus are used to increase yields.

Wild oats often infest lentil fields, but chemicals are available to aid weed control. Cowpea and black-bean aphids are the two most important insect pests on lentils. Predators such as ladybird beetles and syrphid-fly larvae usually keep these insects under control. However, when populations of predators are too low to control the aphids, chemical insecticides are used.

Harvesting. Lentils are mowed or swathed when the vines are green and the pods have a golden color. About 10 days later, lentils are ready to combine harvest using the same combines that are used for wheat, oats, and barley. A pick-up attachment picks up the material from the windrows. The combines must be operated at a maximum speed of $1\frac{1}{2}$ mph to prevent loss of, and damage to, the lentil seed. Average yields are about 900 lb/acre. *See* AGRICULTURE, MACHINERY IN; AGRICULTURE, SOIL AND CROP PRACTICES IN.

[KENNETH J. MORRISON]

Bibliography: F. M. Entenmann, K. J. Morrison, and V. E. Youngman, *Growing Lentils in Washington*, Wash. State Univ. Ext. Bull. no. 590, 1968; E. T. Field and G. E. Marousek, *Lentil Production and Marketing in the U.S.A.: A Description and Trends*, Idaho Agr. Res. Progr. Rep. no. 128, 1968; V. E. Youngman, Lentils: A pulse of the Palouse, *Econ. Bot.*, 22:135–139, 1968.

Leren

Calathea allouia is a little-known tuberous rooted crop of the Caribbean region that has special potential as an hors d'oeuvre. Formerly leren was available only in winter months, but the season can now be extended by planting techniques to make this delicacy available for at least half of the year and perhaps as much as 9 months.

Distribution, taxonomy, description. Leren was apparently domesticated in the New World long before the time of Columbus. Fragmentary reports throughout the literature suggest that it is native to Hispaniola and Puerto Rico, some of the Lesser Antilles, the Guianas to Brazil, Venezuela, Columbia, Ecuador, and Peru. At present leren has been recorded as introduced to India, Sri Lanka, Malaysia, Indonesia, and the Philippines.

Leren merits further introduction and trial in the tropics. A member of the family Marantaceae, it belongs to the genus *Calathea*, which consists of more than a hundred species found chiefly in tropical America. Plants are rhizomatous, and the rhizome can be tuberous. Growth requirements are fairly uniform for all species: warm temperatures, high humidities, plenty of water, good drainage, open, organically rich soils, and at least partial shade. Several species produce edible rhizomes or tubers.

Mature leren plants occur in dense clumps formed by mats of upright rhizomes and pseudostems with elongated leaves (Fig. 1). The rhizomes continually branch through the formation of lateral buds. The flowering stock arises from the pseudostem of very old plants and is subtended by a leaf. The flowers are irregular, green and yellowish, or white. The tuberous roots arise normally near the ends of fibrous roots. They are spherical to elongate and measure from 2 to 4 cm in diameter and from 2 to 8 cm in length. The tuber surface is cov-

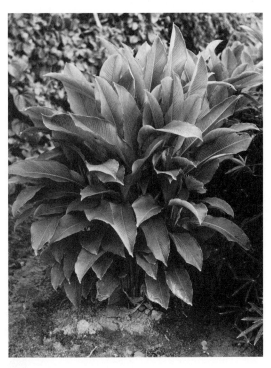

Fig. 1. A mature leren plant.

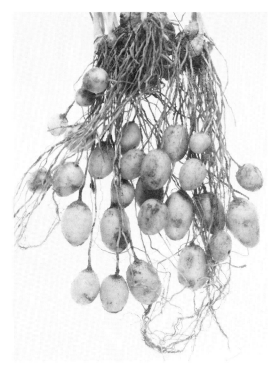

Fig. 2. Tuberous roots of leren.

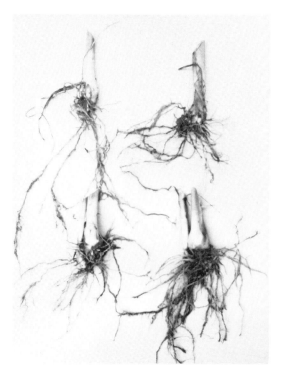

Fig. 3. Rhizome sections from a leren plant.

ered with a fine bark and fine fibrous roots (Fig. 2).

Culture. Leren is adapted to a monsoon climate of alternating dry and wet seasons, with the dry season occurring during the winter, the short-day season. It is planted near the beginning of the rainy season.

The seed material for planting consists of a short section of the rhizome and its upright terminal bud (Fig. 3). These rhizome sections are obtained by breaking up the clump of rhizomes from an old plant. The rhizomes may be left in the ground until spring planting, or may be harvested for their tubers and stored in a cool area. With the beginning of spring rains the plants begin to germinate. Before this time mother plants should be divided into offsets. A single rhizome can produce 50 or more new plants in one season.

The appropriate soil appears to be a loose loam or clay that holds nutrients but permits good drainage. Organic material added to the soil is particularly necessary. Water relationships are also important in the production of leren, and therefore the preparation of the soil should reflect water availability. In areas with heavy, regular rainfall, leren can be planted on ridges. If rainfall is limited, leren should be planted on the flat, or in pits to which organic material is added. Shade or partial shade is often considered necessary for good growth of leren. The best growth is obtained in full sunlight when moisture, nutrients, and drainage are not limited. Leren is planted at distances of from 40 to 80 cm between sets.

Leren rhizomes begin to germinate in March or April after the first rains occur. The plants rapidly develop a large number of leaves or short stalks, and if mature enough, the plants flower briefly. Once established, plantings need very little attention. They are resistant to most insects, although

the rhizomes are sometimes infested by grubs of various beetles. Rhizomes that suffer excessive flooding, especially after planting, may rot.

Vegetative growth continues at a fast pace through the rainy season until October or November. During this time, numerous new side shoots are developed by the rhizome. Tuberization begins in October or November and continues through December if water supply is adequate. The onset of dieback depends on the termination of the rainy season. Leren is harvested beginning in late December. It can be removed from very soft soils by pulling up the plants, but the usual technique is to dig it up with a spading fork. The small tubers are tied together in bunches by the stringlike portions of the roots and are marketed fresh.

Improved techniques. Yield of leren can be maximized by premature harvest of the entire plant, division into offshoots, and replanting under optimum conditions of fertilizer and moisture. Replanting avoids the completion between densely clumped offshoots. The actual amount of tuberization per retransplanted offset is sometimes far higher than that of the whole undisturbed plants.

Mid-November appears to be the most appropriate time for division of the clump. After dormancy has begun, offshoots can germinate but do not tuberize. Because the tuberous roots produced by transplanted offshoots tend to develop later than those of nontransplanted plants, excellent tubers are obtained until at least June.

Uses and food value. Leren tubers can be cooked fresh or stored at room temperature (never in the refrigerator) for up to 3 months. They are used as a snack, but seldom as a principal dish. Tubers are prepared by boiling for 15–20 min, usually without removing the skin. The flesh is uniform white with a translucent core. The texture of the tuber is crisp, which is very agreeable. The flavor resembles that of sweet corn. The thin skin can be peeled away after cooking or can be discarded from the mouth after chewing the entire tuber. Cooked leren may be served by itself, with salt, or with a flavored sauce. The protein content of leren is 1–2% (fresh weight basis), and the starch content is 13–15%.

Future. Although leren is a welcome fresh vegetable, its unique crispness and flavor suggest a specialized role as an hors d'oeuvre. The prices that such a product could command might justify its production and canning by modern techniques. The recently developed technique to increase yields and lengthen season by transplanting makes a commercial breakthrough possible.

[FRANKLIN W. MARTIN]
Bibliography: F. W. Martin and E. Cabanillas, *Econ. Bot.*, 30:249–256, 1976.

Lespedeza

A warm-season legume with trifoliate leaves, small purple pea-shaped blossoms, and one seed per pod. There are 15 American and more than 100 Asiatic species; two annual species, *Lespedeza striata* and *L. stipulacea*, and a perennial, *L. cuneata*, from Asia are grown as field crops in the United States. The American species are small shrubby perennials (see illustration) found in open woods and on idle land, rarely in dense stands; they are harmless weeds. Common lespedeza, once known as Japanese clover, is a small variety of *L. striata*. This variety, unintentionally introduced in the 1840s and used widely until the late 1920s, has been replaced by a larger variety, Kobe. Korean lespedeza (*L. stipulacea*) has been widely grown since the mid-1920s and is preferred in the northern part of the lespedeza belt, from Missouri eastward, while Kobe is preferred in the lower part of the belt (south to the Gulf of Mexico and across northern Florida).

The annual lespedezas can grow on poorer wetter land than most other forage crops. They give a moderate yield of good quality. The plants reseed well and the young seedlings at the two-leaf stage are very tolerant of cold. Most crop damage is from parasitic nematodes and severe drought, especially in the spring.

The perennial lespedeza (*L. cuneata*), commonly known as sericea, is adapted to the same growing conditions as the annuals but persists better on steep slopes and for this reason has been used widely in soil conservation. The young growth from well-established sericea is a moderate-quality forage, but the older growth is poor. The perennial is difficult to establish because the seed does not germinate readily unless scarified or exposed to cold and moisture for several months.

Several large species of lespedeza, such as the widely used *L. bicolor*, are used in plantings for wild life to provide seed and cover. *See* LEGUME FORAGES.   [PAUL TABOR]

Lettuce

A cool-season annual, *Lactuca sativa*, of Asian origin and belonging to the plant order Asterales. Lettuce is grown for its succulent leaves, which are eaten raw as a salad. Four subspecies of this leading salad crop are head lettuce (*L. sativa* var. *capitata*) (see illustration), leaf or curled lettuce (*L. sativa* var. *crispa*), cos or romaine lettuce (*L. sativa* var. *longifolia*), and stem or asparagus lettuce (*L. sativa* var. *asparagina*). There are two types of head lettuce, butterhead, and crisphead or iceberg.

Propagation. The outdoor crop is propagated by seed usually planted directly in the field, but also occasionally planted in greenhouses for later transplanting. Field spacing varies, but usually plants are grown 10–16 in. apart in 14–20-in. rows. Greenhouse lettuce, predominantly leaf and butterhead varieties, is transplanted to ground beds with plants placed 7–12 in. apart.

Uniformly cool weather promotes maximum yields of high-quality lettuce; 55–65°F is optimum. Heading varieties (cultivars) are particularly sensitive to adverse environment. High temperatures prevent heading, encourage seed-stalk development, and result in bitter flavor and tip-burned leaves. However, varieties vary considerably in their resistance to these high-temperature effects and to diseases. Commercial production of lettuce is extensive in several California and Arizona valleys where mild winter and cool summer climates prevail.

Crisphead or iceberg lettuce is the most widely grown type; strains of the Great Lakes and Imperial varieties account for most of the acreage. Popular varieties of other types of head lettuce are butterhead, Bibb, and White Boston. Grand Rapids, cos or romaine, and White Paris are popular types of leaf lettuce.

Harvesting. The harvesting of heading varieties begins when the heads have become firm enough to satisfy market demands, usually 60–80 days after planting. Most western-grown lettuce is field-

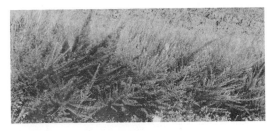

Lespedeza. (*Soil Conservation Service*)

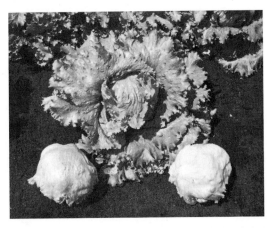

Head lettuce (*Lactuca sativa*), cultivar Fulton, of the plant order Asterales. (*J. Harris Co., Rochester, N.Y.*)

packed in paperboard cartons and chilled by vacuum cooling.

Leaf lettuce and cos lettuce are harvested when full-sized, but before the development of seed stalks or a bitter taste. This varies from 40 to 70 days after planting.

California raises more lettuce than any other state; Arizona and Texas are next in importance. Total annual farm value in the United States from approximately 220,000 acres is about $200,000,000. *See* VEGETABLE GROWING.

[H. JOHN CAREW]

Diseases. Lettuce diseases of greatest importance are caused by fungi and bacteria which disrupt the structure and function of the invaded parts causing malformation, discoloration, and breakdown of tissues. The injuries produced are usually classified as spots, rots, scabs, wilts, or blights.

The most serious fungus diseases and their causal organisms are sclerotinia rot, *Sclerotinia sclerotiorum*; gray mold rot, *Botrytis cinerea*; downy mildew, *Bremia lactucae*; anthracnose, *Marssonina panattoniana*; and bottom rot, *Pellicularia filamentosa*. Several fungi of minor importance cause leaf spots.

The most serious of the bacteria parasitic on lettuce are *Erwinia carotovora* and *Pseudomonas marginalis*, both of which cause soft rots. Soft rots are especially damaging when they follow injuries and diseases, such as spotted wilt and tip burn.

Virus diseases of lettuce are usually transmitted by insects that feed on the plants. Big vein disease, however, is believed to be caused by a soil-inhabiting virus that enters the plant through its root system. Other virus diseases of importance are mosaic, yellows, and spotted wilt.

Tip burn, a physiological disease, is especially damaging to head lettuce. The exact cause of this trouble is not known. *See* PLANT DISEASE; PLANT PHYSIOLOGY; PLANT VIRUS.   [GLEN B. RAMSEY]

Leucine

An amino acid considered essential for normal growth of animals. The amino acids are characterized physically by the following: (1) the pK_1, or the dissociation constant of the various titratable

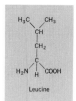

Physical constants of the L isomer at 25°C:
pK_1 (COOH): 2.36; pK_2 (NH_3^+): 9.60
Isoelectric point: 5.98
Optical rotation: $[\alpha]_D(H_2O)$: −11.0; $[\alpha]_D(5\ N\ HCl)$: +16.0
Solubility (g/100 ml H_2O): 2.19

Leucine

groups; (2) the isoelectric point, or pH at which a dipolar ion does not migrate in an electric field; (3) the optical rotation, or the rotation imparted to a beam of plane-polarized light (frequently the D line of the sodium spectrum) passing through 1 dm of a solution of 100 g in 100 ml; and (4) solubility.

In leucine biosynthesis, carboxyl and some carbon atoms of leucine are derived from acetate; the rest of the molecule is furnished by α-ketoisovalerate, which arises in the biosynthesis of valine. A condensation of acetylcoenzyme A (acetyl-CoA) with α-ketoisovalerate, followed by a series of reactions analogous to the tricarboxylic acid cycle, including isomerization, dehydrogenation, and decarboxylation, leads to the formation of α-ketoisocaproic acid. This compound is known to yield leucine by transamination. *See* AMINO ACIDS.

During metabolic degradation the first steps are deamination and oxidative decarboxylation, forming isovalerylcoenzyme A (isovaleryl-CoA). This compound is ultimately converted to acetoacetic acid and acetyl-CoA (see illustration).

[EDWARD A. ADELBERG]

Lime

An acid citrus fruit, *Citrus aurantifolia*, usually grown in tropical or subtropical regions because of its low resistance to cold. The two principal groups of limes are the West Indian or Mexican and the Tahiti or Bearss. The West Indian lime (see illustration) is a medium-sized, spreading tree with numerous, willowly branches densely armed with short, stiff spines. Flowers are small and flowering occurs throughout the year, but mainly in the spring. The fruit is very small (walnut size) and strongly acid, and drops when fully colored. The West Indian lime is more sensitive to cold than the Tahiti lime, which is a more vigorous tree, bearing

Metabolic degradation pathway of leucine.

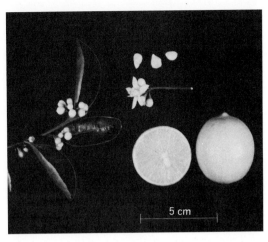

Foliage, seeds, flower, and fruit of the West Indian or Mexican lime.

fruits of lemon size. The Tahiti lime is seedless and its aroma is less pronounced.

The limes are believed to have originated in northeastern India or adjoining portions of Burma or northern Malaysia. It probably was introduced into Europe by the Arabs and was brought to the Americas by the Spanish and Portuguese explorers in the 16th century. It escaped cultivation and became feral in parts of the West Indies, some Caribbean countries, and southern Florida.

Except in the United States, the commercial lime industry is restricted to the West Indian group, which has a high total heat requirement for good-sized fruit. The major producing areas are India, Mexico, Egypt, and the West Indies. Plantings are scattered and production statistics uncertain, but annual world production is over 10,000,000 boxes.

Commercial production of the Tahiti lime is more recent and largely confined to the United States. It is grown mainly in Florida, with some plantings in the warmer areas of southern California. A little over half of the crop is processed, with the remainder utilized fresh. Fruits are harvested before turning yellow because they have maximum aroma and storage life. *See* FRUIT, TREE.

[R. K. SOOST]

Linoleic acid

An 18-carbon straight-chain polyunsaturated fatty acid, chemical name *cis,cis*-9,12-octadecadienoic acid, with two carbon-carbon double bonds of specific geometric configuration at specified locations in the fatty acid chain (see illustration). It is a colorless oil with molecular weight of 280.44, a melting point of $-6.5°C$, and an iodine value of 180.1. It is highly susceptible to oxidation and is a major constituent of semidrying oils, where its oxidation results in formation of an im-

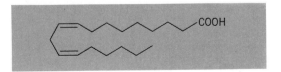

Structure of linoleic acid.

permeable film. Linoleic acid does not appear naturally as a free acid, but is esterified. It appears most commonly as a constituent of triglyceride (triacylglycerol), and is also a constituent of phospholipids, glycolipids, sphingolipids, lipoproteins, and sterol esters. For monogastric animals, the level of linoleate in the depot fats is proportional to the linoleate level in the diet.

Sources. Linoleic acid is the most common polyunsaturated fatty acid and can be synthesized only by plants. Major common sources and their percentages of linoleic acid are soybean (50–55%), cottonseed (40–45%), corn (50–55%), peanut (20–25%), sunflower (50–55%), safflower (70–75%), and sesame (40–45%) oils. In general, good sources of dietary linoleic acid are the natural liquid vegetable oils with the exception of olive oil. Although linoleic acid is a constituent of most solid fats, it is generally at a much lower level than in liquid oils.

EFA function. The stereochemistry of the carbon-carbon double bonds in the carbon chain results in easy susceptibility to oxidation, and is responsible for its function as one of the essential fatty acids (EFAs). Whereas the saturated counterpart of linoleic acid, that is, stearic acid, has a linear carbon chain, the linoleic acid chain is bent back upon itself. This configuration results in a "*cis-cis*-methylene–interrupted," or nonconjugated, double bond. Reactivity of this natural configuration of the polyunsaturation during either oxidation or hydrogenation results in a change in configuration which destroys its EFA character. In addition to its role as an EFA, linoleic acid also serves as a caloric source similar to other fatty acids.

Linoleic acid is essential because there is no evidence that it can be synthesized by animals, at least not in quantities sufficient to prevent EFA-deficiency symptoms. There is, on the other hand, still some doubt that linoleic acid can serve as a sole source of dietary fat, although it is considered the most definitive member of the traditional EFA family of linoleic, linolenic, and arachidonic acids.

EFA deficiency. Because of its ability to alleviate EFA-deficiency symptoms, linoleic acid was originally designated as part of the "vitamin F" group, but since the quantities of EFA required were much greater than that of other known vitamins, the term has been dropped.

The classical symptoms of EFA deficiency in the rat that are alleviated by intake of linoleic acid are: reduced growth rate; dermatitis, skin permeability, or both; susceptibility to infection; reduced hair growth; and infertility. More recently recognized symptoms are decreased prostaglandin biosynthesis, reduced myocardial contractility, and swelling of rat liver mitochrondria.

Physiological function. Linoleic acid is a major constituent of the phospholipids in the body, which in turn are vital components of biomembranes. The function and integrity of biomembranes are apparently dependent on linoleic acid or other EFAs. Membrane dysfunction may be the common denominator of recognized symptoms of EFA deficiency with the exception of decreased prostaglandin biosynthesis. Linoleic acid is converted in the body to dihomo-γ-linoleic acid and arachidonic acids, which in turn are precursor fatty acids of the prostaglandins.

Linoleic acid has been shown to have a hypocholesteremic effect (lowering of blood cholesterol), but it is apparently not unique in this respect since other highly unsaturated fatty acids without EFA activity exhibit the same property.

Minimum requirements. There is at present no consensus as to the recommended minimum requirement for linoleic acid in the diet. The present majority opinion is that the ratio of polyunsaturated fats in the diet should be 1:1 or greater. More sophisticated studies of dose-response curves indicate that in the rat a level of 1–2% linoleate is sufficient to satisfy the biological requirements for EFAs; therefore, some investigators suggest that the range of 3–5% EFA is sufficient for maintenance at maturity. Earlier nutritional literature suggested possible toxic effects due to linoleate intake, but this was later attributed to the by-products of oxidation rather than to the acid itself. *See* LINOLENIC ACID.

[DAVID R. ERICKSON]

Linolenic acid

A polyunsaturated 18-carbon straight-chain fatty acid, chemical name *cis,cis,cis*-9,12,15-octadecatrienoic acid, with three carbon-carbon double bonds located in the 9, 12, and 15 positions, which are in a specific geometric configuration (see illustration). It is a colorless, oily liquid with a melting point of −12.8°C, a molecular weight of 278.42, and an iodine value of 273.5. Linolenic acid is highly susceptible to oxidation and is a constituent of drying oils, where its oxidation results in the formation of an impermeable film. It does not naturally exist as the free fatty acid, but is esterified, most commonly, as a constituent of a triglyceride (triacylglycerol), and is also a constituent of phospholipids, glycolipids, sphingolipids, lipoproteins, and sterol esters. For monogastric animals, the level of linolenate in the depot fats is proportional to the linolenate level in the diet.

Sources. The major industrial source of linolenic acid is linseed oil, where it exists in the triglyceride form at a level of 50–55%. Other industrial sources with the percentage of linolenic are Perilla oil (60–65%) and hempseed oil (20–25%).

Significant sources of linolenic acid in edible oils and their percentages of linolenic are soybean (8–9%), citrus (6–13%), wheat germ (9–10%), rapeseed (7–10%), and walnut (5–6%) oils. Since linolenic acid is highly susceptible to oxidation, it is thought to be principally responsible for "reversion flavors" in food oils, especially soybean oil, and for the characteristic odors of the industrial drying oils. *See* FAT AND OIL, EDIBLE.

EFA function. The stereochemistry of the three carbon-carbon double bonds in the carbon chain makes linolenic acid susceptible to oxidation, and is responsible for its function as one of the essential fatty acids (EFAs). Whereas the saturated counterpart of linolenic acid, that is, stearic acid, has a

linear carbon chain, the linolenic acid chain is bent back upon itself. Ths configuration results in a pair of "*cis-cis*-methylene–interrupted," or nonconjugated, double bonds. Reactivity of this natural configuration of the polyunsaturation during either oxidation or hydrogenation results in a change in configuration which destroys its EFA activity. In addition to its limited role as an EFA, linolenic acid serves as a caloric source similar to other fatty acids.

Soybean oil. The commercial production of soybean oil generally involves the selective hydrogenation of the oil to reduce the linolenic acid to less-unsaturated products, thus resulting in a more flavor-stable and hence acceptable edible oil. Although this processing destroys the EFA of the linolenic acid, it does not affect the remaining EFA (linoleate) and, in turn, the value of the soybean oil as a source of EFA.

Biosynthesis. Biosynthesis of linolenic acid is limited to plants since there is no evidence of synthesis by animals, at least not in sufficient quantities to prevent EFA-deficiency symptoms if it or other EFAs are absent in the diet. Only the natural linolenic acid (all cis) exhibits limited EFA activity. Conversion of the unsaturation to a molecule having one or more trans bonds destroys the EFA activity but apparently does not interfere with the fatty acid serving as a source of calories.

Physiological function. Although linolenic acid is included in the EFA family of linoleic, linolenic, and arachidonic acids, it is not equivalent to either linoleic acid or arachidonic acid, and thus is thought to serve a different function in metabolism and tissue structure. It is more effective than linoleate in stimulating growth and synthesizing fat in rats, but less effective in preventing dermatitis and infertility. This suggests that linolenic acid is less important in biomembranes of mammals than the other essential fatty acids. *See* LINOLEIC ACID.

In fish, however, linolenic acid plays an important role in biomembranes. It has a lower melting point than linoleic acid, and this may be the reason that linolenic acid is the key fatty acid in biomembranes of fish which have a lower body temperature.

Unlike the other EFAs (linoleate and arachidonate), linolenates are apparently not a necessary precursor for prostaglandin synthesis. Linolenic acid has been shown to have a hypocholesteremic effect (lowering of blood cholesterol), but it is not unique in this respect since other highly unsaturated fatty acids without EFA activity also exhibit the same effect.

Nutritional requirements. There is no current agreement as to any recommended minimum requirement for linolenic acid in the diet. To some extent, linolenic acid shows a sparing effect on linoleic acid but this may be temporary. Linoleates apparently cannot serve as the sole fatty acid source in the diet.

Earlier nutritional studies suggested a toxic effect due to linolenic acid, but the effect has since been attributed to its oxidation by-products. This is in agreement with some current thinking that highly unsaturated fatty acids, including linolenic, produce adverse physiological effects due to their oxidation in animals. There is no agreement as to the exact nature or relative importance of this effect in normal diets.   [DAVID R. ERICKSON]

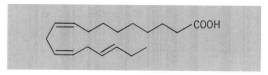

Structure of linolenic acid.

Linseed oil

A product made from the seeds of the flax plant (*Linum usitatissimum*) by crushing and pressing, either with or without heat. After the linseed oil is extracted, it is formulated either raw or boiled, in various grades and with various drying agents, such as litharge, minium, and zinc sulfate. Its most common uses are as the vehicle in oil paints and as a component of oil varnishes; after a longer period of heating (called boiling but actually carried out below the boiling point) and further processing, it is used as a vehicle in printing and lithographic ink, and in the manufacture of oilcloth, linoleum, and some soaps. Oil cake, the residue of the crushed seeds, is a protein- and mineral-rich material used in cattle feed. Most linseed raised for oil comes from plants cultivated for their many seeds rather than for their long fibers in Argentina, the Soviet Union, and India, with lesser quantities from the United States and Canada. It was first used as a drying oil in 12th-century paintings.

[FRANK H. ROCKETT]

Lipid

One of a class of compounds which contains long-chain aliphatic hydrocarbons (cyclic or acyclic) and their derivatives, such as acids (fatty acids), alcohols, amines, amino alcohols, and aldehydes. The presence of the long aliphatic chain as the characteristic component of lipids confers distinct solubility properties on the simpler members of this class of naturally occurring compounds. This led to the traditional definition of lipids as substances which are insoluble in water but soluble in fat solvents such as ether, chloroform, and benzene. However, those lipids (particularly glycolipids and phospholipids) which contain polar components in the molecule may be insoluble in these solvents, and some are even soluble in water. Most of the phosphatides are good emulsifying agents.

Classification. The lipids are generally classified into the following groups:

A. Simple lipids
  1. Triglycerides or fats and oils are fatty acid esters of glycerol. Examples are lard, corn oil, cottonseed oil, and butter.
  2. Waxes are fatty acid esters of long-chain alcohols. Examples are beeswax, spermaceti, and carnauba wax.
  3. Steroids are lipids derived from partially or completely hydrogenated phenanthrene. Examples are cholesterol and ergosterol.
B. Complex lipids
  1. Phosphatides or phospholipids are lipids which contain phosphorus and, in many instances, nitrogen. Examples are lecithin, cephalin, and phosphatidyl inositol.
  2. Glycolipids are lipids which contain carbohydrate residues. Examples are sterol glycosides, cerebrosides, and plant phytoglycolipids.
  3. Sphingolipids are lipids containing the long-chain amino alcohol sphingosine and its derivatives. Examples are sphingomyelins, ceramides, and cerebrosides.

The classification scheme is not rigid since sphingolipids are found which contain phosphorus and carbohydrate, and glycolipids which contain phosphorus. Those lipids not included in the above groupings are of the chemically simpler type and include the fatty acids, alcohols, ethers such as batyl and chimyl alcohols, and hydrocarbons such as the terpenes and carotenes.

The fatty acids found in lipids may be saturated or unsaturated, cyclic or acyclic, and contain substituents such as hydroxyl or keto groups. They are combined in ester or amide linkage.

The alcohols, likewise, may be saturated or unsaturated and are combined in ester or ether linkages; in the case of α-β unsaturated ethers, these are best considered as aldehyde derivatives.

The amino alcohols found in lipids are linked as amides, glycosides, or phosphate esters. Sphingosine is the predominant amino alcohol found in animal tissue lipids, and phytosphingosine is its equivalent in the plant kingdom.

Occurrence. Lipids are present in all living cells, but the proportion varies from tissue to tissue. The triglycerides accumulate in certain areas, such as adipose tissue in the human being and in the seeds of plants, where they represent a form of energy storage. The more complex lipids occur closely linked with protein in the membranes of cells and of subcellular particles. More active tissues generally have a higher complex lipid content; for example, the brain, liver, kidney, lung, and blood contain the highest concentration of phosphatides in the mammal. Fish oils are important sources of vitamins A and D, and seed-germ oils contain quantities of vitamin E. The vitamins K occur chiefly in plants and microorganisms, and carotenoids are widely distributed in both the plant and animal kingdoms. Waxes are found in insects and as protective agents on plant leaves and the cuticles of fruits and vegetables (for instance, the bloom on grapes and plums). Soybeans are used for the commercial preparation of phosphatides.

Extraction. Many of the lipids, particularly glycolipids, phosphatides, and steroid esters, are present in the tissue in association with other cell components, such as protein. The nature of the linkages in these complexes is not fully understood although they are most certainly not covalent. Combinations of lipid and protein, like lipoproteins and proteolipids, have been isolated from sources such as blood serum and egg yolk. For the efficient extraction of lipids from tissues, these complexes must first be disrupted, and this is usually accomplished by dehydration procedures such as freeze-drying or acetone extraction, or by denaturation with alcohol before extracting the tissue with suitable lipid solvents. The use of mixed solvents, such as ethanol and ether, ethanol and benzene, or chloroform and methanol, allows disruption, dehydration, and extraction in one operation. Partial fractionation of lipids may be effected by successive extractions with different solvents.

Separation. Prior to 1948, solvent fractionations or the use of specific complexing agents, such as cadmium chloride for the separation of lecithin, were the only methods available for the separation of lipids, and progress in the chemical identification of individual lipids was slow. Since then, the use of column chromatography (particularly on alumina, silicic acid, and diethylaminoethyl cellulose), thin-layer chromatography, counter-current distribution, and gas-phase chromatography has allowed rapid progress in separation, and many new classes of lipid have been discovered as a result of the application of these techniques. Other methods which allow selective degradation of certain lipids either chemically (for example, the use of dilute alkali to cause preferential hydrolysis of esters) or enzymatically are also being used successfully for the separation of certain lipids.

Identification. Most of the conventional analytical procedures are used in the identification of lipid samples. Physical methods, such as infrared and ultraviolet spectroscopy, optical rotation, proton magnetic resonance, and mass spectrometry, have been used. The advent of gas-phase chromatography allowed a major advance in lipid chemistry by providing a complete analysis of the fatty acid content of lipid mixtures. The high resolving power of thin-layer chromatography has accelerated the routine analysis of the mixture of lipids from many natural sources; qualitative and quantitative methods for the determination of esters, aldehydes, carbohydrates, long-chain bases, and the other important components of lipids such as glycerol, glycerophosphate, ethanolamine, choline, serine, amino sugars, and inositol; and elementary analyses for nitrogen and phosphorus. The nitrogen-to-phosphorus ratio of a phosphatide sample was once used as a criterion of purity because carbon and hydrogen analyses on a single phosphatide species are not highly revealing, owing to the spectrum of fatty acids that may be present. The degree of unsaturation is determined by hydrogenation or iodine number determination, and free hydroxyl groups are expressed by the acetyl value. Lipid samples also may be hydrolyzed under a variety of acid or alkaline conditions and the products investigated by paper chromatography. *See* FAT AND OIL, EDIBLE; LIPID METABOLISM; VITAMIN.   [ROY H. GIGG]

Bibliography: G. B. Ansell and J. N. Hawthorne, *Phospholipids*, 1964; D. Chapman, *Introduction to Lipids*, 1969; H. J. Deuel, *Lipids*, 3 vols., 1951–1957; D. J. Hanahan, *Lipide Chemistry*, 1960; R. T. Holman, W. O. Lundberg, and T. Malkin (eds.), *Progress in the Chemistry of Fats and Other Lipids*, 10 vols., 1952–1969; G. V. Marinetti (ed.), *Lipid Chromatographic Analysis*, 1967; E. J. Masoro, *Physiological Chemistry of Lipids in Mammals*, 1968; R. Paoletti and D. Kritchevsky (eds.), *Advances in Lipid Research*, 5 vols., 1963–1969.

Lipid metabolism

Lipids form a class of compounds composed of neutral fats (triglycerides), phospholipids, glycolipids, sterols, and fat-soluble vitamins (A, D, E, and K). As a group they share the common physical property of insolubility in water. This article describes the assimilation of dietary lipids and the synthesis and degradation of lipids by the mammalian organism.

Fat digestion and absorption. The principal dietary fat is triglyceride, an ester of three fatty acids and glycerol. This substance is not digested in the stomach and passes into the duodenum, where it causes the release of enterogastrone, a hormone which inhibits stomach motility. The amount of fat in the diet, therefore, regulates the rate at which enterogastrone is released into the intestinal tract. Fat, together with other partially digested foodstuffs, causes the release of hormones, secretin, pancreozymin, and cholecystokinin from the wall of the duodenum into the bloodstream.

Secretin causes the secretion of an alkaline pancreatic juice rich in bicarbonate ions, while pancreozymin causes secretion of pancreatic enzymes. One of these enzymes, important in the digestion of fat, is lipase. Cholecystokinin, which is a protein substance chemically inseparable from pancreozymin, stimulates the gallbladder to release bile into the duodenum. Bile is secreted by the liver and concentrated in the gallbladder and contains two bile salts, both derived from cholesterol: taurocholic and glycocholic acids. These act as detergents by emulsifying the triglycerides in the intestinal tract, thus making the fats more susceptible to attack by pancreatic lipase. In this reaction, which works best in the alkaline medium provided by the pancreatic juice, each triglyceride is split into three fatty acid chains, forming monoglycerides. The fatty acids pass across the membranes of the intestinal mucosal (lining) cells. Enzymes in the membranes split monoglyceride to glycerol and fatty acid, but triglycerides are reformed within the mucosal cells from glycerol and those fatty acids with a chain length greater than eight carbons: Short- and medium-chain fatty acids are absorbed directly into the bloodstream once they pass through the intestinal mucosa.

The triglycerides formed in the mucosal cells are associated with proteins and phospholipids and pass into the intestinal lymphatics as the lipoproteins called chylomicrons. The thoracic duct, the main lymphatic channel, carries the chylomicrons to the great veins, where they enter the circulatory system and can be taken up and metabolized by most tissues. *See* DIGESTIVE SYSTEM.

The bile salts are absorbed from the ileum, together with dietary cholesterol. They enter the portal circulation, which carries them to the liver, where they can be reexcreted into the duodenum. The bile also contains pigments which are derived from hemoglobin metabolism.

Abnormalities in the pancreatic secretions, bile secretion, or intestinal wall can lead to either partial or complete blockage of fat absorption and an abnormal excretion of fats in the stool.

Adipose tissue. Accumulations of fat cells in the body are called adipose tissue. This is found beneath the skin, between muscle fibers, around abdominal organs and their supporting structures called mesenteries, and around joints. The fat cell contains a central fat vacuole so large that it fills the cell, pushing the nucleus and cytoplasm to the periphery. The adipose tissue of the body is of considerable magnitude and is quite active metabolically, functioning as a buffer in energy metabolism.

During meals carbohydrates, amino acids, and fats which are absorbed in excess of immediate energy requirements are converted and stored in the fat-cell vacuoles as triglycerides. These fat depots provide an economical storage form for energy requirements and serve as the source of energy between meals and during periods of fasting.

Triglycerides cannot traverse the cell membrane until they are broken down into glycerol and fatty acids. Lipoprotein lipase, an enzyme which catalyzes the hydrolysis of lipoprotein triglycerides, controls entry of triglycerides into the cell; it is induced by feeding and disappears during periods of fasting. The lipase which breaks down triglycerides before they leave the cell is controlled by hormones. Norepinephrine, a hormone released from sympathetic nerve endings, is probably the most important factor controlling fat mobilization. Epinephrine from the adrenal medulla also activates lipase, as do adrenocorticotropic hormone (ACTH) and glucagon. Growth hormone and a separate fat-mobilizing factor released from the pituitary gland of some species also stimulate lipolysis and release of fatty acids from adipose tissue. While the fat-mobilizing factor may activate the same enzyme as the hormones cited above, growth hormone appears to function through a different mechanism, probably requiring protein synthesis.

Obesity is a condition in which excessive fat accumulates in the adipose tissue. One factor responsible for this condition is excessive caloric intake. The metabolic and psychological factors are under investigation. In starvation, uncontrolled diabetes, and many generalized illnesses the opposite occurs and adipose tissue becomes markedly depleted of lipid. *See* METABOLIC DISORDERS.

Blood lipids. Lipids are present in the blood in the form of lipoproteins and as free fatty acids (FFAs), which are bound to albumin. The FFAs originate in adipose tissue and are mobilized for oxidation in other tissues of the body. The lipoproteins are small droplets of lipids complexed with proteins dispersed in the blood. They originate in the liver, with the exception of the small droplets, called chylomicrons, derived from the intestinal tract. The lipoproteins have been divided into arbitrary classes based upon their physical properties. The two methods of classification separate them according to density by ultracentrifugation and according to electrical charge by electrophoresis. The classes of lipoproteins defined by either of these methods differ in their content of triglycerides, cholesterol, and phospholipids. Some disorders of lipid metabolism are manifested in the blood by an abnormality in the pattern of lipoprotein classes.

Fatty acid oxidation. Fatty acids are oxidized to meet the energy requirements of the body by a β-oxidation pathway, that is, the second or β-carbon from the carboxyl group is oxidized. Before oxidation can proceed, the fatty acid must be coupled with coenzyme A (CoA), a compound containing adenosinemonophosphate (AMP), two molecules of phosphate, and the complex nitrogen derivative pantotheine (Fig. 1).

In Eq. (1), showing activation, the fatty acid is as shown in Fig. 2, in which only the terminal 4-carbon atoms are given. The initial activation proceeds in two steps. First, as shown in Eq. (1a), the fatty acid reacts with adenosinetriphosphate (ATP) to form fatty acid adenylate (fatty acid—AMP). This in turn reacts with CoA to form acyl CoA, as shown in Eq. (1b). The enzyme that catalyzes reactions (1a) and (1b) is called the activating enzyme or thiokinase. The fatty acid—CoA cannot penetrate the mitochondrial membrane to gain access to the oxidative enzymes. To traverse the

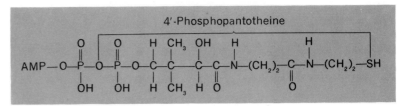

Fig. 1. Structural formula for coenzyme A.

membrane, fatty acid must be esterified with the hydroxyl group of carnitine (Fig. 3), a reaction catalyzed by carnitine acyl transferases. The carnitine–fatty acid ester traverses the membrane, and the fatty acid is again coupled to CoA by a transferase on the other side.

In reaction (2), the first of two oxidation reactions, one hydrogen is removed from the α-carbon and one is removed from the β-carbon, producing an unsaturated fatty acid analogous to crotonic acid. The enzyme is called acyl CoA dehydrogenase, and the cofactor which acts as the oxidizing agent and accepts the hydrogen is flavin adenine dinucleotide (FAD).

In reaction (3), hydration, hydrogen and the hydroxyl group (from water) are introduced at the α- and β-carbons, respectively; a β-hydroxy acid is formed; the enzyme is crotonase.

In (4), the second oxidation, two hydrogens are removed from the α- and β-carbons of the β-hydroxy acid to form a keto acid. The oxidizing agent is diphosphopyridine nucleotide (DPN), also called nicitinamide adenine dinucleotide (NAD).

In reaction (5), showing cleavage, acetyl CoA is split off. Thus a fatty acid two carbons shorter than the original one is formed. Simultaneously, the shortened fatty acid combines with another molecule of CoA at the newly formed carboxyl group to yield a new activated fatty acid. The enzyme is β-ketothidase. The new activated fatty acid undergoes the same series of reactions, and this process is repeated until the entire fatty acid molecule has been reduced completely to acetyl CoA. Oxidation of the higher fatty acids, such as palmitic acid with 16 carbon atoms, yields eight molecules of acetyl CoA. Two fates of acetyl CoA formed in the liver are of immediate interest (Fig. 4): (1) oxidation through the Krebs cycle to carbon dioxide and (2) condensation of two molecules of acetyl CoA with the splitting off of the CoA forming so-called ketone bodies.

LIPID METABOLISM

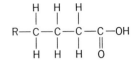

Fig. 2. Structural formula for a fatty acid. R represents chain of up to 14 carbon atoms.

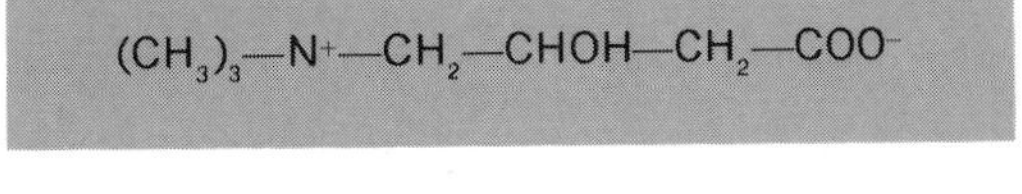

$$(CH_3)_3—N^+—CH_2—CHOH—CH_2—COO^-$$

Fig. 3. Structural formula for carnitine.

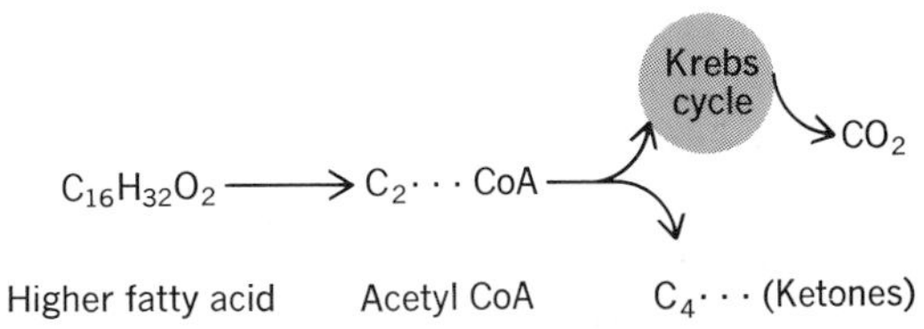

$$C_{16}H_{32}O_2 \longrightarrow C_2 \cdots CoA$$

Krebs cycle $\rightarrow CO_2$

$C_4 \cdots$ (Ketones)

Higher fatty acid   Acetyl CoA

Fig. 4. Fates of acetyl CoA from fatty acid oxidation.

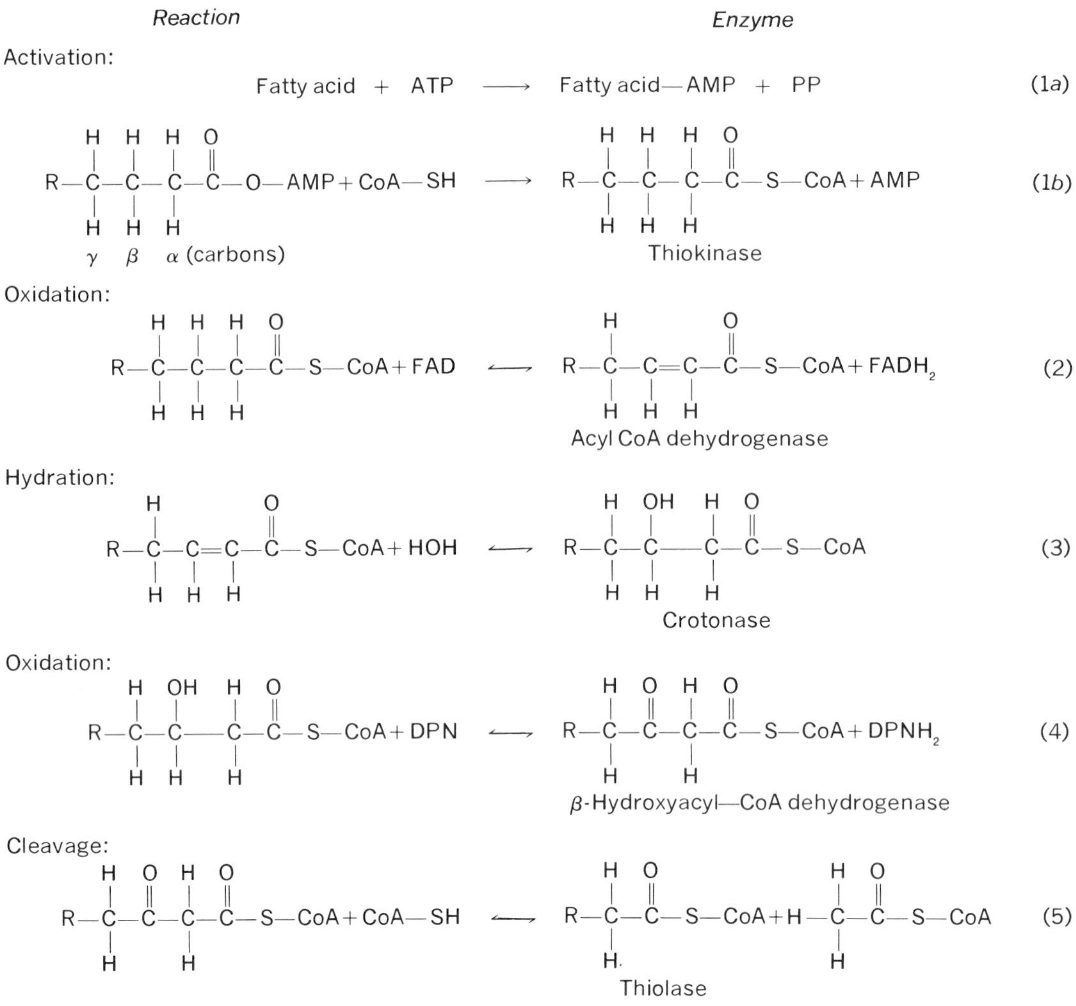

Reaction   *Enzyme*

Activation:

$$\text{Fatty acid } + \text{ ATP} \longrightarrow \text{Fatty acid}-\text{AMP } + \text{ PP} \qquad (1a)$$

Thiokinase   (1*b*)

Oxidation:

Acyl CoA dehydrogenase   (2)

Hydration:

Crotonase   (3)

Oxidation:

β-Hydroxyacyl—CoA dehydrogenase   (4)

Cleavage:

Thiolase   (5)

Ketone body formation. If excessive amounts of fatty acids are mobilized from the depots and metabolized by the liver, as occurs in starvation or diabetes, all the acetyl CoA formed cannot be oxidized. Instead, two molecules of acetyl CoA may form acetoacetic acid, which cannot be further oxidized by the liver but is transformed into β-hydroxybutyric acid or acetone according to reactions (6) and (7). These three compounds, aceto-

Acetoacetic acid

β-Hydroxybutyric acid   (6)

Acetoacetic acid

Acetone   (7)

acetic acid, acetone, and β-hydroxybutyric acid, called the ketone bodies, are formed in excessive amounts in the liver not only because of the excess acetyl CoA present but also because the metabolic disturbances caused by such conditions reduce the capacity of the Krebs cycle for oxidation by diverting oxaloacetate, a key intermediate, to gluconeogenesis (synthesis of glucose from noncarbohydrate precursors).

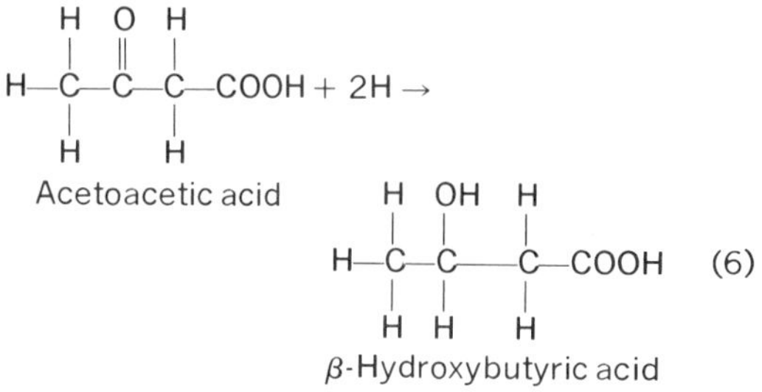

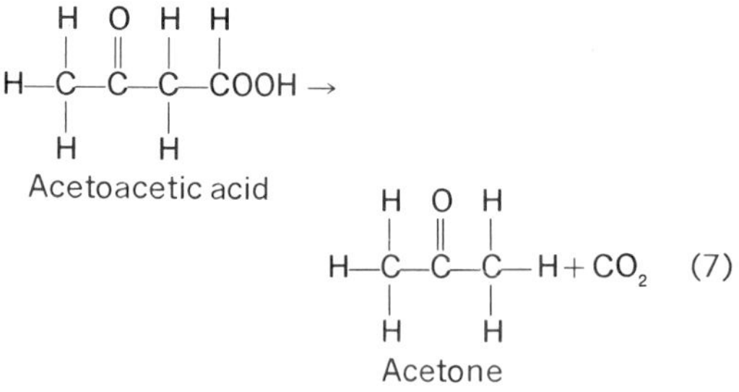

The excessive formation of ketone bodies leads to a high concentration in the blood—a condition called ketonemia. This causes ketone body excretion in the urine, together with water, sodium, and potassium. These losses, along with the excessive acidity of the blood caused by the high concentration of ketone bodies (ketoacidosis), can lead to coma and death if uncorrected. Such fatal acidosis was quite common in diabetics before the advent of insulin. During starvation or diabetic ketosis, muscles are capable of deriving the major portion, if not all, of their energy from oxidizing the ketone bodies. However, in the uncontrolled diabetic subject, the formation of ketone bodies may greatly exceed the utilization of them by the muscle or other tissues, so that ketoacidosis results.

Lipotropic factors. A diet high in fat results in fat accumulation in the liver. This can be prevented by feeding choline, a phosphatide base; the effect has been termed a lipotropic effect. If methionine is present in the diet, it can substitute for

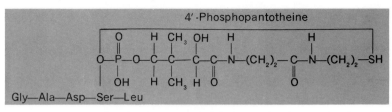

choline, since enzymes are present in the liver which can transfer methyl groups from methionine to ethanolamine to form choline, as shown in Eq. (8).

$$3CH_3^- + H_2NCH_2 \cdot CH_2OH \rightarrow$$
Methyl (from   β-Ethanolamine
methionine)

$$(CH_3)_3 \cdot \overset{+}{N}CH_2 \cdot CH_2OH \quad (8)$$
Choline

Fatty livers can also occur when large amounts of depot fat are mobilized in starvation and diabetes. This type of fatty liver is not affected by choline. Since choline is a constituent of the phospholipid lecithin, it has been suggested that the lipotropic effect of choline is exerted through lecithin. Evidence to support this suggestion has not been forthcoming.

Fatty acid synthesis. Certain carbohydrates, such as glucose and fructose, yield simpler substances, such as lactic acid, pyruvic acid, and acetic acid, as do proteins, which are potential precursors of acetyl CoA. The acetyl CoA molecules thus formed are used to synthesize higher fatty acids.

The initial reaction in fatty acid synthesis is the carboxylation of acetyl CoA to form malonyl CoA. This reaction is catalyzed by acetyl CoA carboxylase, a biotin-containing enzyme (enz-biotin) and probably proceeds in two steps. In the first, reaction (9a), biotin is carboxylated in the 1'-nitrogen position in an ATP-dependent reaction to form 1'-N-carboxamide biotin. In the second step, reaction (9b), the carboxyl group is transferred to acetyl CoA to form malonyl CoA.

For the synthesis to proceed, the malonyl group must be transferred from CoA to a specific carrier protein called the acyl carrier protein (ACP). The compound with which the malonyl group is to be condensed is similarly transferred from CoA to ACP to form an acyl ACP. The acyl group can be acetate or any fatty acid less than 16 carbons in length, depending upon the species. The enzyme catalyzing the transfer from CoA to ACP is specific for each compound and is called a CoA-ACP transacylase. The active group of both CoA

and ACP is 4'-phosphopantetheine (Fig. 5). This group is linked to the protein through the hydroxyl group of serine by a phosphodiester bond. The sulfhydryl group is the functional group of both CoA and ACP linkage occurring through sulfur (thiol ester).

The joining of malonyl ACP with an acyl ACP, as shown in reaction (10), is catalyzed by the acyl-malonyl ACP condensing enzyme. Since carbon dioxide is released in this reaction, the acyl carbon chain is lengthened by two, resulting in a β-keto acid linked to ACP. This compound is converted to a fatty acid by the reverse of reactions (4), (3), and (2). These reactions are catalyzed by a series of enzymes which are associated in a complex protein called fatty acid syntase in yeast and pigeon liver. The individual enzymes have been isolated from bacterial systems and are specific for ACP compounds, in contrast to the specificity of oxidative enzymes for CoA compounds. The reverse reaction (4) is catalyzed by β-keto ACP reductase and the cofactor is triphosphopyridine nucleotide (TPN), also known as nicotinamide adenine dinucleotide phosphate (NADP), rather than NAD. Reverse reaction (3) is catalyzed by enoyl ACP dehydrase and reverse reaction (2) by enoyl ACP reductase.

Repetition of this series of reactions leads to a building up of the fatty acid molecule to a chain containing 16 or 18 carbons. When the fatty acid reaches this length, it is transferred from ACP to CoA. The CoA is split off by an enzyme, deacyclase, yielding the free fatty acid, which in turn

Fig. 5. Active site of acyl carrier protein (ACP). Gly, glycine; Ala, alanine; Asp, aspartic acid; Ser, serine; and Leu, leucine.

$$ATP + CO_2 + Enz\text{-}biotin \longrightarrow Enz\text{-}biotin\text{-}CO_2 + \text{(1'-N-Carboxamide biotin)} + ADP + P_i \quad (9a)$$

$$Enz\text{-}biotin\text{-}CO_2 + CH_3\text{-}\overset{O}{\underset{}{C}}\text{-}SCoA \longrightarrow HO\text{-}\overset{O}{\underset{\underset{O}{||}}{C}}\text{-}CH_2\text{-}\overset{O}{\underset{}{C}}\text{-}SCoA + Enz\text{-}biotin \quad (9b)$$
Acetyl CoA   Malonyl CoA

Acyl ACP + Malonyl ACP ⇌ β-Keto acid—ACP + CO_2 + ACPSH   (10)

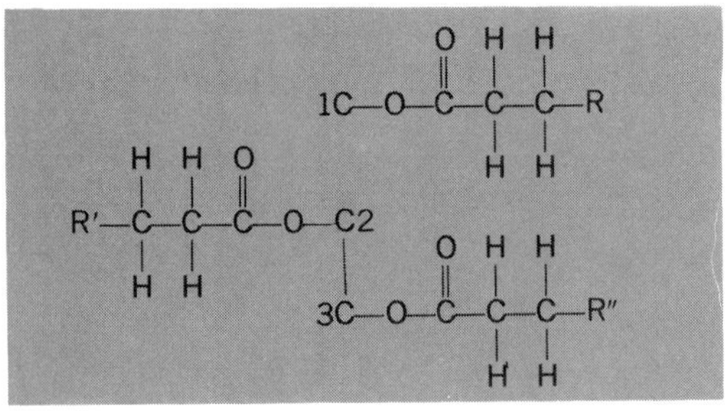

Fig. 6. General structural formula for a triglyceride.

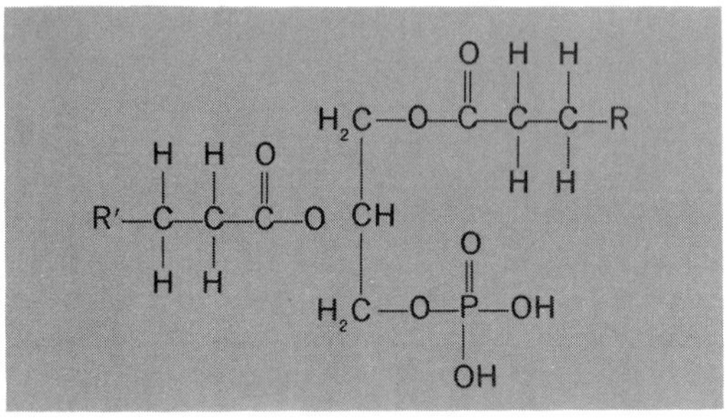

Fig. 7. Structural formula for a phosphatidic acid.

combines with glycerol to form phospholipids and the triglyceride that is stored in depots and circulates in lipoproteins.

Triglyceride synthesis. Triglycerides, which consist of three fatty acids joined to glycerol by ester bonds (Fig. 6), are synthesized in the liver from glycerol phosphate and CoA derivatives of fatty acids. A series of enzymes called transferases catalyze the joining of the first two fatty acids with glycerol phosphate to form a phosphatidic acid (Fig. 7). The phosphate group must be removed to form a 1,2-diglyceride before the third fatty acid can be transferred to form a triglyceride. The removal of phosphate is catalyzed by a specific phosphatase. In the intestinal mucosa, triglycerides can be synthesized from monoglycerides without passing through phosphatidic acid as an intermediate.

Modification of dietary lipids. The fatty acids in the depots of each mammalian species have a characteristic composition. The chain length of ingested fat is either lengthened or shortened by the same pathways used for the synthesis and degradation of fatty acids so that the composition of the depots remains constant. However, when large amounts of a fat of markedly different composition from the animal's depot fat is ingested, the depots slowly change to reflect the characteristics of the ingested fat. The ability to introduce double bonds or reduce them to form an unsaturated or a saturated fatty acid is limited; highly unsaturated fatty acids can only be derived from dietary sources.

Essential fatty acids. Most mammals, including man, probably require arachadonic acid for normal growth and for maintenance of the normal condition of the skin, although the mechanism of these effects has not been elucidated. Linoleic acid, a precursor of arachadonic acid in mammals, is the usual dietary source of unsaturated fatty acid. Highly unsaturated fatty acids cannot be synthe-sized by mammals from either saturated fatty acids or their precursors. Hence, the so-called essential fatty acids must be present in the diet.

Role of phosphatides. The phosphatides are compounds of glycerol, fatty acids, phosphate, and certain bases containing nitrogen, namely, ethanol-amine, serine, and choline, the so-called phosphatide bases. When combined with fatty acids, they tend to make the insoluble fatty acids soluble in water. They are important constituents of both outer cell membranes (plasma membranes) and the network of cytoplasmic membranes (endo-plasmic reticulum).

Phospholipid synthesis. In the liver, phospho-lipid synthesis follows the same pathway as trigly-ceride synthesis to the point of diglyceride forma-tion. The nitrogenous base to be coupled at the 3 position of glycerol must first be phosphorylated by ATP and then reacted with cytidine triphos-phate to form a cytidine diphosphoryl derivative. This derivative can then be coupled with the digly-ceride in a reaction catalyzed by a specific trans-ferase to form a phospholipid. *See* LIPID.

[MARTIN A. RIZACK]

Bibliography: D. S. Fredrickson, R. I. Levy, and R. S. Lees, Fat transport in lipoproteins: Integrat-ed approach to mechanisms and disorders, *New Engl. J. Med.*, 276:34–44, 1967; D. M. Greenberg (ed.), *Metabolic Pathways*, vols. 1–6. 3d ed., 1967–1972; H. A. Krebs, The regulation of the release of ketone bodies by the liver, *Advan. Enzyme Regul.*, 4:339–353, 1966.

Louping ill

A viral disease of sheep, capable of producing cen-tral nervous system manifestations. It occurs chiefly in the British Isles. Infections have been reported, although rarely, among persons working with sheep.

In sheep the disease is usually biphasic with a systemic influenzalike phase, followed by enceph-alitic signs. In man the first phase is usually the extent of illness.

The virus is a member of the Russian tick-borne complex of the group B arboviruses. Characteris-tics, diagnosis, and epidemiology are similar to those of other viruses of this complex.

[JOSEPH L. MELNICK]

Bibliography: F. L. Horsfall, Jr., and I. Tamm (eds.), *Viral and Rickettsial Infections of Man*, 4th ed., 1965.

Lupine

A cool-season legume with an upright stem, leaves divided into several digitate leaflets, and terminal racemes of pea-shaped blossoms. Three species, yellow, blue, and white, each named for the color of its blossoms, are cultivated as field crops (see illustration); several hybrids are grown as orna-mentals; and many species occur as wild plants. The yellow crop varieties are usually the earliest and smallest, the whites latest and largest. Field crop lupines have been grown in Europe since ear-ly Roman times as a soil-improving crop. The older varieties could not be used as forage since the plants contained a bitter, water-soluble, toxic alka-loid. However, since 1912, plant breeders have developed "sweet" varieties with only traces of alkaloid.

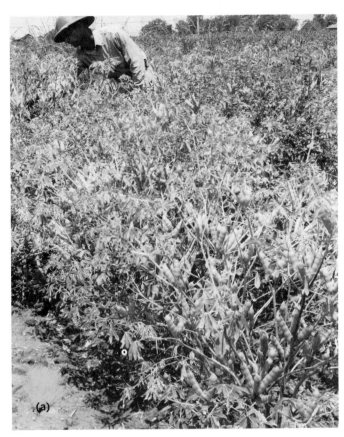

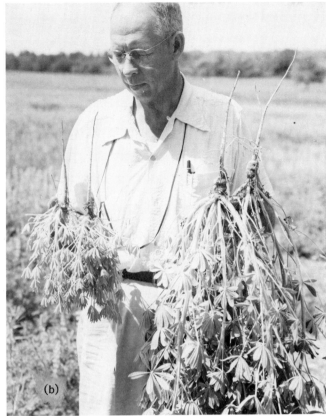

Lupine. (a) A field crop near maturity. (b) Uprooted yellow plants grown without (left) and with (right) needed nitrogen-fixing bacteria. Bacteria grow in the nodules seen on the roots at the right.

Blue lupine was grown extensively as a winter cover crop in the southeastern United States during the 1940s. Since the beginning of the 1950s, however, lupine culture has declined, partly because cheap nitrogen fertilizer competes with the nitrogen-fixing value of the cover crop, and also because diseases and winter killing of lupines have increased. Some progress has been made in developing disease-resistant varieties.

The ornamental lupines are perennials unsuited to areas with hot summers. The many kinds of wild lupines which occur in the western part of the United States vary greatly in length of life, size, and site requirement. In the East a few small perennial wild lupines are found on deep sands. *See* BREEDING (PLANT); COVER CROPS; LEGUME FORAGES.

[PAUL TABOR]

Lychee

The plant *Litchi chinensis*, also called litchi, a member of the soapberry family (Sapindaceae). It is a native of southern China, where it has been cultivated for more than 2000 years. It is now being grown successfully in India, Union of South Africa, Hawaii, Burma, Madagascar, West Indies, Brazil, Honduras, Japan, Australia, and the southern United States.

The fruit is a one-seeded berry. The thin, leathery, rough shell or pericarp of the ripe fruit is bright red in most varieties. Beneath the shell, completely surrounding the seed, is the edible aril or pulp. The fruit may be eaten fresh, canned, or dried. In China the fresh fruit is considered a great delicacy.

[PERRY D. STRAUSBAUGH/EARL L. CORE]

Lysine

An amino acid constituent of proteins that contains a terminal amino group in addition to the usual α-amino group.

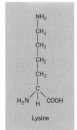

Physical constants of the L isomer at 25°C:
pK$_1$ (COOH): 2.18; pK$_2$ (NH$_3^+$): 8.95; pK$_3$ ($\epsilon \cdot$NH$_3^+$): 10.53
Isoelectric point: 9.74
Optical rotation: [α]$_D$(H$_2$O): +13.5; [α]$_D$(5 N HCl): +26.0
Solubility (g/100 ml H$_2$O): very soluble

Lysine must be supplied in the diet of animals and humans. It is widely distributed in proteins; however, it is absent in some such as zein (a grain protein). It is a precursor of 5-hydroxylysine, an amino acid occurring in only a few proteins such as collagen, and it is found in biocytin (ϵ-N-biotinyl-L-lysine), a complexed form of the vitamin biotin, which is found in yeast.

There are two biosynthetic pathways to lysine. The one which occurs in most bacteria and blue-green algae is characterized by intermediates con-

Major degradative pathway of lysine.

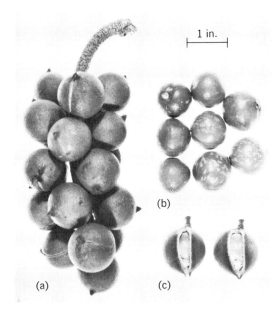

Macadamia integrifolia. (*a*) Mature nuts. (*b*) Nuts without husks. (*c*) Nuts in husk showing method of dehiscence. (*From R. A. Jaynes, ed., Handbook of North American Nut Trees, Humphrey Press, 1969*)

taining seven carbon atoms, including diaminopimelic acid, a constituent of the bacterial cell wall. In most yeast and green algae a pathway of six-carbon intermediates occurs. *See* AMINO ACIDS.

Lysine does not participate in transamination; however, in mammalian tissue and in some microorganisms the major degradative pathway (see illustration) occurs in the irreversible loss of the α-amino group to form α-keto-ϵ-aminocaproic acid. The product of this pathway, glutaric acid, is further metabolized to α-ketoglutaric acid.

In another degradative pathway which occurs in bacteria, lysine is oxidatively decarboxylated and deaminated to form δ-aminovaleric acid, which is metabolized further to glutaric acid.

[DAVID W. E. SMITH]

Macadamia nut

The fruit of a tropical evergreen tree, *Macadamia ternifolia*, native to Queensland and New South Wales and now grown commercially in Australia and Hawaii. The trees grow to 50 ft in height and have dense foliage of glossy, leathery leaves. They bear many small white or pinkish flowers in drooping racemes, each of which may mature from 1 to 20 fruits. These consist of a leathery outer husk (pericarp) which splits along one side at maturity, freeing the very hard-shelled, nearly round seed or nut about an inch in diameter. Two types of nuts are recognized: the most important commercially having a smooth shell and the other having a rough shell and sometimes referred to another species, *M. integrifolia* (see illustration).

Successful culture of the trees as an orchard crop requires a tropical climate, good well-drained soil, abundant rainfall (50 in. or more), and soil management to control competing vegetation. Protection from strong winds is essential. Trees have been grown successfully in Florida and California, but the nuts are commercially important only in Hawaii.

Macadamia nuts ripen over a period of several months: As immature nuts they are of little value; the nuts are allowed to mature on the trees and fall to the ground, where they are picked up by hand, machine-hulled, dried, and stored for processing. After machine-cracking, the kernels are graded by floating in water, where the high-quality kernels float and are skimmed off. They are then roasted, usually in oil, salted, and packed, with glass jars being used for best-grade nuts. The processed nuts are of high quality and find a ready market. *See* NUT CROP CULTURE.

[LAURENCE H. MAC DANIELS]

Malnutrition

A state in which there is a deficiency in one or more of the essential metabolites necessary for maintenance and growth of the intact organism. The deficiency usually arises from a dietary lack, most commonly of protein or vitamins, although deficiencies arising from a lack of essential fatty acids, minerals, and carbohydrates are occasionally seen. The severity and consequences of the malnutritional state will depend not only on the type of deficiency but also on the length of time the deficiency exists. Most malnutritional states, however severe, are easily correctable if accurately diagnosed and treated at an early stage.

Deficiencies may also be the result of increased degradation of essential metabolites or presumably because of antimetabolites which interfere or compete with essential compounds in the cell.

There apparently exists a hierarchy in the degree of importance of various cells in the body. Those that appear to be more essential include the cells controlling the activities of other cells, such as brain cells; those doing constant unexpendable work, as heart cells; certain cells in constant division, such as intestinal cells; and those producing large amounts of necessary extracellular proteins, as the liver and pancreas. These cells may be more susceptible to nutritional deficiencies than supportive cells exemplified by connective tissue cells.

Cell requirements. Most deficiencies resulting in a severe malnutritional state are complex multiple deficiencies and do not result from the loss of a single essential compound. There are seven major constituents of the cell which, in the proper concentrations and proper balance, are necessary in order for the cell to maintain itself. Many of these constituents have a common precursor and their pathways are closely interrelated. It is well known that the labeled carbons of radioactive glucose may eventually appear both in the carbohydrates of the cell and in the proteins, nucleic acids, and fats. The essential constituents of the cell include water, mineral ions, proteins, nucleic acids, carbohydrates, lipids, and porphyrins. Although these substances are usually found in complexes of large molecules within the cell such as the glycolipoproteins, large complex macromolecules are not transported across the cell membrane. Each individual cell is considered to be the site of synthesis of the macromolecular complexes, usually from small precursors which include amino acids, purines, pyrimidines, fatty acids, and glucose.

Essential metabolite deficiencies. When considering a deficiency of the above seven essential cellular constituents, a malnutritional state resulting from protein lack would appear to be not only the most common but the most serious. Proteins make up the large portion of the solid constituents of the cell and serve not only a major structural function but also an important metabolic function, particularly when functioning as enzymes and hormones.

Proteins. Of the 20 amino acids commonly found in man, 8 have been found to be indispensable. Although all 20 are required in the synthesis of most proteins, 12 of these may be manufactured by the cell itself from small carbon fragments, or other amino acids. However, if even 1 of the 8 essential amino acids is missing from the diet, the individual is unable to synthesize any protein and growth ceases. Death does not occur immediately because many proteins are in a constant state of degradation as well as synthesis. Some unessential amino acids become available from protein breakdown for resynthesis of the more essential proteins. The essential amino acids in man are leucine, isoleucine, lysine, phenylalanine, tryptophan, threonine, methionine, and valine. Most malnutritional states do not involve an absolute deficiency of the essential amino acids but rather a relative deficiency when evaluated with the growth and maintenance requirements of the organism or cell. *See* AMINO ACIDS; PROTEIN METABOLISM.

Fats. With regard to the fats, only four fatty acids appear to be essential, again in the sense that only four cannot be synthesized by the cell: arachidonic, γ-linolenic, linolenic, and linoleic. Fats apparently serve a structural function, especially on membranes and interfaces, and usually are combined with proteins as lipoprotein. They also serve as an excellent secondary source of energy when carbohydrates are deficient or unavailable. Malnutritional states involving only fat deficiency are not well recognized. *See* LIPID METABOLISM.

Carbohydrates. The carbohydrates have a somewhat lesser role as structural components within the cell, although their importance as a structural component in the form of extracellular polysaccharide ground substances is well known. Carbohydrates, glucose especially, are considered to be the cell's chief source of energy after degradation, oxidation, and the resultant production of high-energy adenosinetriphosphate (ATP) molecules. *See* CARBOHYDRATE METABOLISM.

Nucleic acids and porphyrins. Nucleic acids are essential to the chromosomal structure and apparently to protein synthesis, but they may usually be synthesized from other smaller substrates. There is no evidence that malnutritional states are due to lack of nucleic acids. Some of the vitamins, however, are essential for nucleic acid synthesis and a vitamin deficiency will decrease new nucleic acid formation. Porphyrins are likewise easily synthesized in the body.

Mineral ions. The mineral ions play a very important role in cellular metabolism. The cations sodium and potassium as well as the anions carbonate, phosphate, sulfate, and chloride are responsible for regulation of the water content of the cell, and a few of them, especially potassium and magnesium, are important as activating ions for many enzymatic reactions. Malnutrition may result in an anemia due to a deficiency in iron, an ion of crucial importance in the synthesis of hemoglobin. Although sodium deficiency, hyponatremia, and potassium deficiency, hypokalemia, are seen in disease states, they are not commonly associated with malnutritional states alone. Iodine deficiency, without other evidence of malnutrition, may result in a colloid goiter of the thyroid gland. Deficiency of the other essential trace elements such as zinc, manganese, cobalt, and copper are apparently present only in severe starvation states.

Generalized malnutrition. The effect of generalized malnutrition, less than 1600 cal per day for a man weighing 70 kg, is usually obvious, resulting in extreme malaise, weakness, lack of growth, anemia, and, in severe cases, edema. The organs shrink in weight as a result of the cells shrinking in size; the fat cells in particular show characteristic changes of shrinkage and the appearance of a clear vacuolar space. Glycogen deposits in the liver and muscle disappear, and the protein structure appears reduced. Generalized malnutrition also results in a lack of resistance to any insult including drastic changes in temperature and infectious agents such as bacteria and viruses. Many of the factors concerned with this resistance are intangible. However, an important factor in resistance is the presence of antibodies. These are specialized proteins formed in response to and combined with antigenic foreign agents such as viruses. Antibody formation and thus resistance to infection is markedly low in malnutritional states.

Kwashiorkor disease. A specific disease associated with malnutrition and more specifically with a lack of dietary protein is called kwashiorkor disease. It is found most commonly in parts of Africa and Asia. The patients, usually children, show severe liver disturbances. There is a reduction of the protein and nucleic acid content of the liver cells, reduction of the serum albumin, which is synthesized in the liver, and increased fat in the liver cells. Analysis of the contents of the small bowel shows markedly decreased intestinal enzyme levels. Other organs commonly affected are the muscle and pancreas, which show markedly altered structure and decreased function. *See* DIGESTIVE SYSTEM; KWASHIORKOR DISEASE.

[DONALD W. KING]

Bibliography: J. S. Fruton and S. Simmonds, *General Biochemistry*, 2d ed., 1958; R. H. S. Thompson and E. J. King (eds.), *Biochemical Disorders in Human Disease*, 3d ed., 1970.

Mandarin

A name used to designate a large group of citrus fruits in the species *Citrus reticulata* and some of its hybrids. This group is variable in the character of trees and fruits since the term is used in a general sense to include many different forms, such as tangerines, King oranges, Temple oranges, tangelos (hybrids between grapefruit and tangerine), Satsuma oranges, and Calamondin, presumably a hybrid between a mandarin and a kumquat. *See* KUMQUAT; ORANGE; TANGERINE.

Many varieties of citrus falling in the mandarin classification are compact trees with willowy twigs and rather small, narrow, pointed leaves. The fruits are usually yellow, orange, or red and have loose skins which peel easily. A distinguishing feature common to the true mandarins and their hybrids is the chlorophyll in the cotyledons (seed leaves), giving them a pistachio-green color.

Although tangerines are the most extensively planted of the mandarin group, others, particularly the Temple orange, the Murcott orange, and the tangelos, of which there are several varieties, are important commercial fruits in the United States. *See* FRUIT, TREE.   [FRANK E. GARDNER]

Mango

The plant *Mangifera indica*, a member of the sumac family (Anacardiaceae) and a native of southern Asia, but now grown in Indomalaysia, Africa,

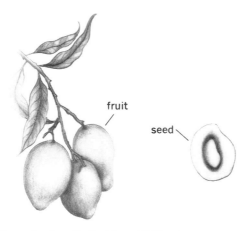

fruit

seed

Mango developed in Florida and California.

tropical America, California, and Florida. The mango has been in cultivation for almost 6000 years. It is an important fruit in tropical countries throughout the world, more important than peaches and apples among temperate climate fruits. It is eaten by at least one-fifth of the world's inhabitants. The fruit is a fleshy drupe, 3–5 in. long, having a thick, yellowish-red skin and a large seed (see illustration). The mango is one of the few tropical fruits which have been improved under cultivation, and over 1000 different varieties are now being grown.

[PERRY D. STRAUSBAUGH/EARL L. CORE]

Manure

Any plant and animal residue that may contain excreta of animals. Manures, classified into animal manure, plant manure, and compost, are added to the soil in various stages of decomposition. In the soil they undergo further degradation through the action of soil microorganisms, raising the soil fertility level and improving soil texture by increasing humus content.

Animal manure includes plant residues like straw, used as litter, as well as solid and liquid excreta. Microorganisms attack the nitrogenous components and the more readily fermentable carbohydrates during storage of the manure. Intense microbial respiration, favored by a loose texture and adequate moisture in the manure, causes a rise in temperature so that thermophilic forms of bacteria, actinomycetes, and fungi grow.

Compost consists of plant and animal residues allowed to rot before being applied to soil. Because they have a lower ratio of nitrogenous to carbohydrate material than animal manure, composts are usually reinforced with inorganic nitrogen and available phosphorus to facilitate microbial action. With moisture and aeration, decomposition proceeds accompanied by a rise in temperature.

Green manure is plant material in the form of a growing crop plowed into the soil. Because the object of manuring is to increase the supply of nitrogen, leguminous crops are grown and then plowed into the soil. Green plants are higher in soluble carbohydrates, nitrogen, and minerals than plant residues used in manures and composts; as a result decomposition sets in more rapidly. Green manures, being low in cellulose and lignin, have little effect on the humus content of soil. *See* SOIL MICROBIOLOGY.

[ALLAN G. LOCHHEAD]

Margarine

An emulsified fatty food product used as a spread and a baking and cooking fat, consisting of an aqueous phase dispersed in the fat as a continuous phase. Hyppolyte Mège-Mouriés invented margarine in 1869 and won the prize offered by Louis Napoleon for the development of an inexpensive butter substitute. Margarine is now considered a food in its own right and is manufactured in forms unknown to butter, such as plastic, soft, or fluid. However, the interrelationship is still acknowledged since margarine is colored, flavored, fortified with vitamins, and otherwise formulated to have the same or similar taste, appearance, and nutritional value as butter. *See* BUTTER.

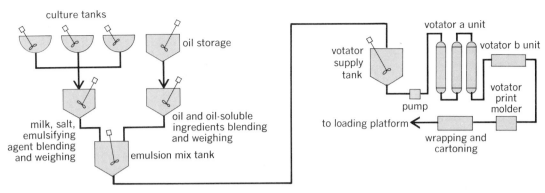

Fig. 1. Flow diagram showing components of a continuous margarine manufacturing process. (*From J. E. Slaughter, Jr., and C. E. Michael, J. Amer. Oil Chem. Soc., 26:623–628, 1949*)

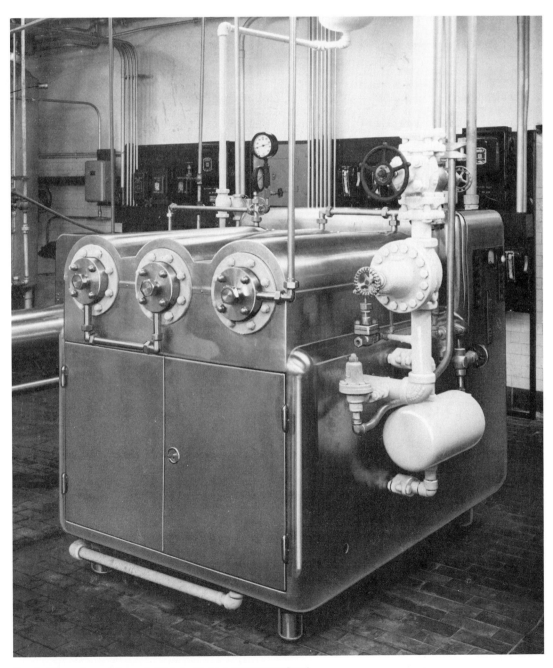

Fig. 2. Margarine votator unit. (*Votator Division, Chemetron Corp.*)

Composition. Margarine is regulated by law in practically every country in which it is manufactured or sold. In 1973 the U.S. Food and Drug Administration revised and broadened its margarine standards to conform to the agreements reached by the Codex Alimentarius Commission, an international body of food and legal authorities charged with the responsibility of unifying foods sold in international trade.

Currently, margarine produced in the United States must contain not less than 80% fat. The fats and oils must be edible but may be from any vegetable or animal carcass source, natural or hydrogenated. The required aqueous phase may be water, milk, or solutions of dairy or vegetable protein, and must be pasteurized. Milk may be cultured after pasteurization. Vitamin A must be added to yield a finished margarine with not less than 15,000 international units per pound (0.45 kg). Optional ingredients include salt or potassium chloride for low-sodium diets, nutritive sweeteners, fatty emulsifiers, antioxidants, preservatives, edible colors, flavors, vitamin D, acids, and alkalies. *See* FAT AND OIL, EDIBLE.

Manufacture. Most margarine is produced in continuous-flow equipment (Fig 1). The oil blend containing the oil-soluble components is held in one supply tank, the aqueous components solution in another. The two components are premixed in appropriate proportions, emulsified, and pumped through an internal chilling machine. The Votator (Fig. 2) is the most frequently selected chilling unit used in the United States. The margarine emulsion is cooled rapidly in the Votator A unit but is still a soupy liquid. It is allowed to rest in the static B unit until it becomes firm enough to be formed into prints for subsequent wrapping. If the margarine is to be filled into 50-lb (22.7 kg) cartons or cans for bakery use or into ½- or 1-lb (0.23 or 0.45 kg) tubs as soft margarine for household use, a working B unit whips the margarine before filling is substituted. Fluid margarines are the latest innovation for both commercial and household use. They differ from solid margarines only in the formulation of the base oils required to give the desired texture and viscosity.

Production. Production of margarine in the United States in 1975 reached almost 2.4×10^9 lb (1.1×10^9 kg). The major oil used was partially hydrogenated soybean oil to the extent of almost 1.6×10^9 lb (7.2×10^8 kg). About 1.9×10^8 lb (8.5×10^8 kg) of corn oil, mostly unhydrogenated, was also used. Other oils in use were cottonseed, palm, and safflower, as well as beef fat and lard. Per capita consumption in the United States approximated 12 lb (5.4 kg) per year during 1970–1976. *See* FOOD ENGINEERING.   [THEODORE J. WEISS]

Bibliography: Federal Register, p. 25671-3, 1973; S. F. Riepma, *The Story of Margarine,* 1970; U.S. Department of Agriculture, *Fats and Oils Situation,* FOS-286, 1977; T. J. Weiss, *Food Oils and Their Uses,* 1970.

Marine fisheries

The harvest of animals and plants from the ocean to provide food and recreation for people, food for animals, and a variety of organic materials for industry. In 1973 the world marine harvest was about 57,100,000 metric tons, plus an undetermined catch by recreational and subsistence fishermen. It is now generally agreed that, with present fishing gear and methods, the world catch is approaching a maximum, which may be less than 100,000,000 metric tons. If methods can be devised to harvest smaller organisms not currently used because they are too costly to catch and process, it has been estimated that the yield could perhaps be increased severalfold. The Soviet Union is said to have succeeded in developing an acceptable human food product from Antarctic krill, an abundant small shrimplike animal which is the principal food of the blue whale. This could lead to a substantial increase in the harvest of the sea. For further information on fishery products and processing *see* FOOD MANUFACTURING.

Harvest of the sea. The world marine commercial fish catch grew more than 6% per year from the end of World War II to 1967. In 1969, however, the catch dropped slightly, and in the period 1970–1973 the average rate of increase was only about 1% per year. Another way of putting it is that in 1960–1967 the world catch increased by nearly 60% (Fig. 1), but in the following 7-year period grew scarcely at all. Much of this decline in rate of growth was caused by the virtual collapse of the Peruvian anchovy fishery, which at its peak accounted for about 20% of the total world catch from the sea.

Whales are not included in these catches because they are recorded by number rather than by weight (Table 1). The 1973 world whale catch yielded about 128,000 tons of whale meat; 38,000 tons of meal; 6000 tons of solubles; 18,000 tons of other products; and 5,600,000 units of vitamin A, in addition to 860,000 barrels of oil.

Most of the world fish catch still comes from the Northern Hemisphere, but the catch in the Southern Hemisphere was growing until the 1970s. In the late 1950s nearly 90% of the world catch came from north of the Equator. By 1967 this had dropped to about 70%, largely through the phenomenal development of the Peruvian anchovy fishery. The decline of this fishery in the 1970s caused the total Southern Hemisphere catch to drop also. By 1975 the Northern Hemisphere produced about 77% of the world total. The Northern Hemisphere includes only about 43% of the total

Table 1. World whale catch in 1973 in numbers of whales*

Whaling area	Fin	Sei and Bryde	Minke	Sperm	Others
Southern Hemisphere					
Antarctic Ocean†	1,288	4,392	7,713	4,927	
Pacific Ocean	11	19		3,227	311
Atlantic Ocean	1	497	650	2,363	
Indian Ocean	41	10	175	3,099	1
Northern Hemisphere					
Pacific Ocean and Bering Sea	460	2,585		8,568	215
Atlantic and Arctic Oceans	342	139	2,445	613	10
Totals	2,143	7,642	10,983	22,797	537

*From *International Whaling Statistics LXXIII* , Bureau of International Whaling Statistics, Oslo, 1974.
†1973–74 season in the Antarctic.

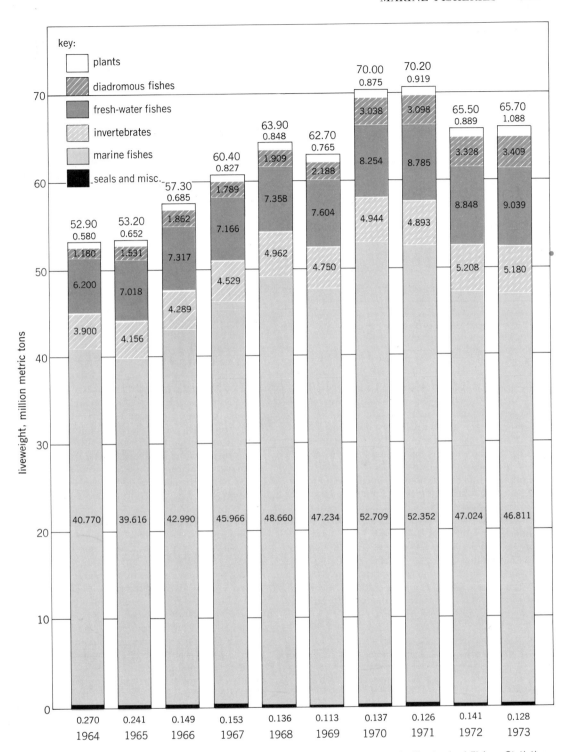

Fig. 1. World catch of fishes and marine invertebrates during the 10-year period from 1964 to 1973. (*From* *L. P. D. Gertenbach, ed., Yearbook of Fishery Statistics 1973, Food and Agriculture Organization, 1974*)

area of ocean, but it contains most of the world's estuaries and continental shelves. It is in these rich and relatively shallow waters that most marine fish and shellfish resources are concentrated.

Sixteen countries landed 1,000,000 metric tons or more of fishery products (live weight) in 1973. These countries accounted for about 84% of the world catch (Table 2). In the late 1950s the United States ranked second in weight of fishery landings;

in 1973 it ranked fifth. This has been cited by many as evidence that the United States is declining as a world fishing power, but like many popular views about fisheries this is a gross oversimplification. Total domestic fishery production has remained about level for many years, while catches by several other nations have been growing. Americans have obtained increasing amounts of fish and shellfish by imports. With less than 7% of the world

Table 2. Leading commercial fishing nations in 1973*

Nation	Weight, 10^6 metric tons†	Percent of world catch
Japan	10,702	18.2
Soviet Union	8,619	14.6
China‡	7,574	12.9
Norway	2,974	5.0
United States	2,670	4.5
Peru	2,299	3.9
India	1,958	3.3
Thailand	1,692	2.9
Republic of Korea	1,655	2.8
Spain	1,570	2.7
Denmark	1,465	2.5
South Africa	1,332	2.3
Indonesia	1,300	2.2
Philippines	1,248	2.1
Canada	1,152	2.0
United Kingdom	1,144	1.9
Totals	49,354	83.8

*From National Marine Fisheries Service, *Fisheries of the United States, 1974*, 1975.

†Live weight; shells of mollusks included.

‡Mainland and Taiwan.

population, the United States consumes more than 12% of world fishery production, and thus is the most attractive fishery market in the world.

The most remarkable fishery development was the climb by Peru from a position of insignificance among fishing nations in the late 1950s to first place by weight landed in the late 1960s. The subsequent decline of this major fishery, based almost entirely on a single species of anchovy, illustrates the inherent instability of most fishery resources. This densely schooling herringlike fish owed its tremendous abundance to the high biological fertility of the Humboldt Current. Fluctuations in anchovy catches are related mainly to fluctuations in the Humboldt Current.

Most marine fisheries are located close to coasts. Only a small part of the world catch is

Table 3. Major kinds of fish and shellfish in the 1973 United States commercial marine fishery catch*

Kinds of fish and shellfish	Landed value, 10^6 dollars†	Weight, 10^3 metric tons‡
Shrimp (less than 10 species)	219.4	168.8
Salmon (5 species)	125.1	96.6
Tuna (5 species)	90.1	155.2
Crab (less than 10 species)	88.1	132.4
Menhaden (2 species)	73.3	857.4
Flounder (about 10 species)	43.9	84.7
Oyster (3 species)	35.2	22.0
Clam (less than 10 species)	34.7	48.2
Cod (9 species)	19.0	63.6
Scallop (4 species)	14.5	3.9
Lobster (3 species)	12.0	5.2
Herring (6 species)	11.0	160.2
Subtotals	766.3	1,798.2
Grand totals of commercial marine catch	907.4	2,146.5

*From B. G. Thompson, *Fisheries of the United States, 1973*, U.S. Department of Commerce, National Marine Fisheries Service, C.F.S. no. 6400, 1974.

†Amount paid to fishermen, not retail value.

‡Weight of shells of mollusks not included.

taken more than 100 mi (160 km) from shore.

No one knows exactly how many different kinds of marine life are used by people. In official statistics many species are lumped together. Several thousand species are included in the world catch, but a surprisingly small number make up the bulk of the catch. For example, most of the domestic catch in the United States, over 83% by weight, is made up of only 12 kinds of fish and shellfish (Table 3). Omitting the considerable part of the world marine fishery catch which is unsorted and unidentified (9,900,000 metric tons), 20 kinds of fish, shellfish, and plants make up about 99% by weight of the world catch. The 10 most important in order of weight landed in 1973 were herring, cod, ocean perch and redfish, mackerel, jack, salmon, tuna, flounder, squid, and shrimp. They made up 74% of the total marine commerical harvest, or about 90% of the harvest exclusive of unsorted and unidentified species.

Changing patterns. Before World War II few fishermen ventured very far away from their home shores in search of marine fish. There were some notable exceptions, however. Some European fishermen had been lured years before to the rich banks of Newfoundland, Nova Scotia, and New England; whaling had begun in the productive waters surrounding Antarctica; the Japanese had started their march across the ocean in search of salmon, tuna, and other species; and the United States tuna fleet was already developing its fishery off Central and South America. But these developments were halted during the war. After the war the need for animal protein stimulated several countries to develop distant water fisheries. In the forefront were Japan and the Soviet Union. These two countries have developed modern, self-sufficient fleets of factory ships, catcher boats, and supply vessels which can and do operate anywhere in the world ocean. Japan more than tripled its catch from 1938 to 1973, from about 3,500,000 to 10,700,000 metric tons. In the same period the Soviet Union more than quintupled its catch, from about 1,600,000 to 8,600,000 metric tons. Almost 99% of the Japanese catch and about 93% of the Soviet catch come from the ocean. Both countries are net exporters of fishery products.

In contrast, the United States fish catch has remained almost static for many years. It rose slightly after the war, reaching an all-time high of about 3,000,000 metric tons (live weight) in 1962. Since 1962 the total catch has dropped about 12%. About $4\frac{1}{2}$% of the United States commercial catch comes from fresh water. The United States is a net importer of fishery products. In 1974 it imported about 2,226,000 metric tons (live weight) and exported less than 4% of that amount.

United States fishing industry. The reasons why the United States supplies most of its demand for fishery products by importing, whereas other major fishing nations produce more than they consume are complicated, and only a brief outline can be given in a short article. First, it must be understood that, although there are a few large fishing companies in the United States, most commercial fishing is conducted by a large number of small, independent operators. Most of them are in competition with each other, either to make the catch or to purchase the raw material from the fishermen. These segments of the industry can be classified in various ways, but the important distinction is between the fisherman and the processing-distributing segment of industry.

Problems of fishermen. Almost all United States fishermen are independent operators. Some are prosperous, but many are struggling to make a living. In many fisheries there are more fishermen and units of gear than are necessary to make the catch. They are hemmed in by laws and regulations, many enacted in the name of conservation, but most merely increasing the cost of catching fish. The living resources fluctuate widely in abundance from natural causes, and their migration patterns change from time to time. Most fishermen in the United States lack the flexibility to shift from one fishery to another in response to these changes. They pay more for boats and gear than do their foreign competitors. Foreign fishermen are liberally subsidized in various ways by their governments, and substantial quantities of this subsidized catch are offered in the United States at prices lower than American fishermen are willing to accept. Foreign fishermen, with their highly organized and efficient fleets, are crowding the independent United States fisherman off traditional fishing grounds, or making incidental catches of resources which support traditional American fisheries. Many of the oldest fishery resources in the United States are fully utilized. Others have been overfished, and attempts to rehabilitate them are being made. These obstacles are almost overwhelming to many fishermen in the United States.

Most Americans believe that elimination of foreign fishing off their shores would solve all the major problems of the domestic fisheries. It is probable that Congress will draft legislation declaring domestic jurisdiction over a coastal zone extending 200 mi (320 km) seaward from the shores. This will remove one source of difficulty for domestic fisheries, but it has not been clearly recognized that it will create other problems. Extended jurisdiction, whether it is accomplished by unilateral action or by international agreement, will focus attention on the remaining domestic fishery management problems. Preoccupation with foreign fishing has caused some exceedingly difficult domestic problems to go almost unnoticed. Many of these problems are long-standing, and have resisted solution. The pertinent states may find that they can no longer afford virtually to ignore fishery management responsibilities.

The United States tuna and shrimp industries generally, and some other segments of the American fishing industry, have been able to avoid most of these problems. One reason is that tuna and shrimp are highly popular seafoods in the United States, and this demand has helped these industries to meet their competition. But as the harvest reaches equilibrium these once prosperous segments of the American fishing industry are having problems. Japan, the Soviet Union, and other nations that fish in distant waters have been able to expand because their flexibility and self-sufficiency allow them to move toward new resources as the catch on older fishing grounds declines. With few exceptions the American fisherman does not have this flexibility.

Problems of processor and distributor. These segments of the United States fishing industry do not usually have the same difficulties as the fishermen. Those who rely upon a single species, as the now defunct California sardine industry did, are at the mercy of a fluctuating supply of raw material and, when the total catch begins to drop, they are likely to encourage fishermen to increase their fishing effort to maintain the total catch at a level that will protect capital investment. Such a policy leads almost inevitably to overfishing and, possibly, destruction of the resource. A reasonable solution is to have alternative resources to turn to as the abundance of a species drops. Unfortunately, however, no two kinds of fish behave exactly alike, and it requires new techniques, and often other types of fishing gear, to catch another kind of fish economically. Thus, while the principal resource is abundant, the industry has no interest in seeking alternate resources, and when the principal resource declines, the capital to develop other fishing methods is hard to find.

Other fish processors in the United States stabilize their supply of raw material by importing partially processed or processed fish in quantity. There has been a growing tendency to merge with large food-processing companies. By diversifying operations and source of supply the processor or distributor of fish can avoid many economic problems.

Sport fisheries. Sport fishing in the ocean is often ignored in discussions of marine fisheries. This is probably because there are not good records of sport fish catches and because the individual sportsman's catch is small. Information on sport catches is gathered by interviews or questionnaires that represent rather small samples of the total number of fishermen. Although these provide estimates rather than precise counts, there is general agreement that sport fishermen in the United States catch large numbers of marine fish and some shellfish. The total catch by weight is at least 11%, and may be as great as 25 to 30%, of the total domestic commercial catch, and it is growing steadily. The catch of some species is as large as, or even larger than, the commercial catch of the same species. Thus, the marine sport fisheries are an important force in determining the condition and the yield of many of the United States coastal fishery resources. Sport fisheries must be considered in any fishery management plan. Marine sport fishing is an important activity in other countries but is probably largest in the United States.

A considerable industry has developed around the marine sport fisheries. The investment in manufacturing and retailing establishments for tackle, boats, motors, bait, fuel, and all the other necessities of the fisherman is large. Operators of marinas, fishing piers, and other establishments in the coastal area may derive all or a considerable part of their income from sport fishing and associated activities.

Fishery management. The aim of modern biological fishery management is maintaining the resource at the level of maximum sustainable yield, which means reaching a balance between the capacity of the resource to renew itself and the harvest that man may safely take. A fishery resource can reach an equilibrium at almost any level of fishing intensity. After fishing begins, the catch increases in proportion to the fishing effort. There is a limit, however, to the total amount that may be caught. If the intensity of fishing increases beyond that point, the total catch will begin to drop because the capacity of the resource to renew itself has been reduced. The catch per fisherman will drop more rapidly than the total catch, for more fishermen will be sharing a smaller catch. Actually, the catch per fisherman will begin to drop before the maximum sustainable yield is reached, for as the fishery grows fishermen begin to compete for the available fish. Many economists believe that the amount of fishing effort should be limited at the point of maximum economic yield, which is reached before the catch reaches a maximum, and which is the point at which the value of the catch over the cost of taking it is at a maximum. From a conservationist's point of view such a restriction would have advantages, for limiting the catch at a level below the maximum biological yield would provide a safety factor against overfishing. A relationship between fishing intensity, total catch, and the numbers or weight of fish in the resource is illustrated in Fig. 2.

Very few marine fisheries are being regulated to maintain the maximum sustainable yield. The classic examples were the Pacific halibut fishery and the fur seal industry on the Pribilof Islands. Both resources had been restored from a condition of overfishing and were producing approximately the maximum sustainable yield. The joint Canadian–United States halibut management program has been affected adversely by incidental catches of foreign trawlers fishing for other species. The North American Pacific halibut catch is now less than half of what it was before intensive foreign fisheries developed in the Gulf of Alaska. In the northwest Atlantic a unique development in the mid-1970s was international agreement on a total catch quota for all species combined, which is less than the sum of the quotas for individual major species and stocks. This approach forces the fishing fleets to make major strategy decisions in advance of the fishing season. The plan was designed to relieve pressure on important species, such as haddock and yellowtail flounder, which have been seriously overfished. Management is made difficult by local traditions, natural fluctuations in abundance, difficulty of surveillance and enforcement of laws, and domestic or international disagreements as to the condition of the resource.

International management. Where fishermen of two or more nations are harvesting stocks of fish jointly, various international arrangements have been developed to deal with mutual problems. The 1958 Geneva Convention on Fishing and Conservation of the Living Resources of the High Seas provides general guidelines for international fishing activities, but developments in the 1970s made that convention obsolete. It was hoped that the round of Law of the Sea Conferences, which convened in Caracas late in 1974, reassembled in Geneva in the spring of 1975, and continued in New York in the fall of 1975, would resolve some major international fishery problems. As already mentioned, however, the United States Congress, impatient at the slow pace of international negotiations, might take matters into its own hands. Unilateral action by the United States and other na-

tions is likely to add complications rather than improve the situation.

The Food and Agriculture Organization of the United Nations, through its Department of Fisheries, has established a number of regional fishery councils and commissions. Several international fishery conventions have been negotiated to deal with single joint-fishery agreements or special fishery problems. Some involve only two nations, such as the International Pacific Salmon Fisheries Convention between Canada and the United States. Others have many members, such as the International Convention for the Regulation of Whaling, which has 15. Often, when special problems develop, as when one nation is fishing off the coast of another, bilateral agreements of relatively short duration are negotiated. Such agreements have been necessary in the continental shelf region between Cape Cod and Cape Hatteras as foreign fishing activities there increased. This region is outside the regulatory area defined by the International Convention for the Northwest Atlantic Fisheries. Although these and other international arrangements for fishery management are far from perfect, they have been considerably more effective in resolving conflicts and promoting rational management than individual nations have been with marine fishery management in their own waters.

[J. L. MC HUGH]

Bibliography: N. G. Benson (ed.), *A Century of Fisheries in North America*, 1970; J. A. Gulland, *The Management of Marine Fisheries*, 1974; National Marine Fisheries Service, *Fisheries of the United States, 1974*, 1975; G. Pontecorvo (ed.), *Fisheries Conflicts in the North Atlantic: Problems of Management and Jurisdiction*, 1974; B. Rothschild (ed.), *World Fisheries Policy: Multidisciplinary Views*, 1972; J. C. Stevenson (ed.), *FAO Technical Conference on Fishery Management and Development*, 1974.

Melon growing

The production of edible muskmelons and watermelons, species of the cultivated gourd family, Cucurbitaceae; they have many ecological requirements in common.

Climate and soil requirements. For successful production a warm, frost-free period of 110 to 140 days is essential. Melons are not adapted to resist even light frost. In some areas, plant protectors (hot caps) are used early in the season. Melons are subject to certain diseases which may attack the above ground parts if there is excessive rainfall or periods of high humidity.

Melons can be grown on almost any fertile, well-drained soil. For early maturity, the lighter soils, such as sandy loams or silt loams, which warm up rapidly in the spring are preferred. Melons require warm soils for successful seed germination; optimum soil temperatures are 75 to 85°F (24 to 29°C). Below 70°F (21°C) germination is slow and poor. Melons are sensitive to acid soils. They thrive best on neutral or slightly alkaline soil. The soil should be free from nematodes, wilt disease, and toxic amounts of alkali. Melons grow best on soil well supplied with organic matter, which can be provided by animal manures. Excellent crops, however, can be produced with commercial fertilizers alone.

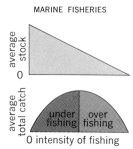

Fig. 2. Relations among fishing intensity, stock size, and average sustainable total catch from a fish population (not to scale).

Cultural requirements. Melons may be planted several ways: by direct field-seeding in rows; by seeding in hills; or by starting the plants in bands or pots in hotbeds or greenhouses and then transplanting them into the field. Melons require thinning regardless of the planting method. The stand should be reduced to two or three plants per hill. Distances between hills may vary according to local practices but, in general, the spacing is 2–4 ft (0.6–1.2 m) for muskmelon and 8–10 ft (2.4–3 m) for watermelon. If seeded in rows, the final stand should consist of single plants 12 in. (0.3 m) apart for muskmelons and 3 ft (0.9 m) apart for watermelons. Muskmelons are generally grown in rows 5–7 ft (1.5–2.1 m) apart, and watermelon in rows 8–10 ft apart.

Melons are insect-pollinated. The domestic honeybee is the only known effective pollinator of melon flowers. Two honeybee colonies per acre (4047 m²) are recommended for adequate pollination.

Harvesting. Nature has provided an excellent means of gaging the stage of maturity of most cultivars of muskmelons (cantaloupes). As the fruit approaches maturity, a light abscission crack develops at the joint where the fruit is attached to the stem. When this crack completely encircles the joint, the melon is market mature. Fruits of Honey Dew, Persian, and casaba muskmelons do not absciss, or absciss only after the melons are overripe. Slight changes in skin color—usually yellowing of part or all of the skin—are measures of maturity in these muskmelons. Several cues can be used to determine the ripeness of watermelon fruit: withering of the tendril at the point of attachment; the soil spot, that is, the area of fruit which rests on the soil, turning from white to creamy yellow; and upon rapping the melon with the knuckles, a hollow sound indicating immaturity or a dull, heavy sound denoting ripeness. *See* MUSKMELON; WATERMELON.　　　　[FRANK W. ZINK]

Metabolic disorders

Disorders which involve an alteration in the normal metabolism of carbohydrates, lipids, proteins, water, and nucleic acids. Deviations in normal metabolic processes are evidenced by various syndromes and diseases. *See* MALNUTRITION.

PROTEIN METABOLISM

Proteins make up the major portion of the body's solid organic material. They are composed of a series of amino acids bound together in long chains by covalent peptide bonds. The chains are folded in irregular configurations and held to each other by disulfide and hydrogen bonds between the side groups of individual amino acid residues. The great individuality and specificity that is characteristic of cellular proteins results from three major factors. First, each protein contains at least 20 amino acids, each of which may appear in a given protein a varying number of times. Second, the sequence of amino acids may vary. The number of sequence combinations of individual amino acids may be considered to be infinite. Third, the long peptide chains may be folded in a variety of configurations. It is therefore theoretically conceivable that every protein in every individual is different from every other protein. Actually, immu-

nological studies have shown great similarity, although not identity, between proteins, not only in one individual but also between species. This is well illustrated by the protein hormone insulin. The complete structure of this protein, which contains 51 amino acids, has been identified in several species including cows, swine, sheep, horses, and whales. The amino acid sequence in cows and sheep is almost identical; in one small portion the sequence in beef insulin is alanine, serine, and valine, while in the sheep it is alanine, glycine, and valine. Most proteins, like other compounds in the body, are complexed with other molecules. They are linked to lipids in the lipoproteins, carbohydrates in the glycoproteins, and nucleic acids in the nucleoproteins. In addition, it is believed that large macromolecular structures incorporating two, three, or four different classes of compounds are present and necessarily interact in an integrated manner for proper functioning of the cell. *See* PROTEIN.

Synthesis. There have been extensive investigations concerning the mechanism by which proteins are synthesized. All proteins arise from single amino acids in the following manner. Plasma proteins are transported and degraded intracellularly into a free amino acid pool. Each amino acid is then activated by an enzyme—amino acid activating enzyme (a specific enzyme has been isolated for each amino acid)—and linked to a molecule of adenosinetriphosphate (ATP), an indispensable energy-donating nucleotide. The amino acid molecule is linked to a ribonucleic acid molecule (transfer RNA) in the soluble portion of the cytoplasm and then the entire complex is transferred to messenger RNA associated with the ribosomes, organelles of the cytoplasm. Here, the sequence of amino acids in the protein being synthesized is determined by the arrangement of the four purine and pyrimidine bases in the nucleic acid. Another enzyme then links the adjacent amino acids by covalent peptide bonding. The long polypeptide chains are released and later are folded in their specific configurations.

Functions of proteins. The functions of proteins are varied. Proteins are present in the major structural component of the cell commonly called the cytoskeleton. This is represented by the cytoplasmic and nuclear membranes of the cell, the particulate organelles such as mitochondria and lysosomes, and a protein network of cisterna and tubules throughout the cell called the endoplasmic reticulum. By definition, enzymes are also proteins. The difference between structural and metabolic enzymatic protein is not distinct in the cell, and there are probably identical proteins which serve both structural and metabolic functions depending on the cellular environment at any one time. Cellular protein is generally considered to be in dynamic equilibrium, that is, a constant state of synthesis and degradation, with its external environment. It is believed, in addition, that each of the thousand or more proteins in a cell has an individual life-span, and the rate of synthesis and degradation of a particular protein varies over a wide range depending on the site and function of the protein involved.

Large amounts of protein are produced intracellularly for use elsewhere. The liver cells are the sole site of albumin synthesis, and the serum albumin usually measures approximately 4 g/100 ml of plasma. As one of the plasma proteins, albumin serves a major role in regulating the osmotic capacity of the blood, as a transport system for fatty acids and as a source of amino acids for cellular protein. The other major group of plasma proteins are the α-, β-, and γ-globulins. The α- and particularly the β-globulins are associated with lipids, and it is in the latter fraction that the large lipoproteins are found. The γ-globulin fraction contains antibodies. Large quantities of enzymatic protein are produced in the intestinal mucosal cells and in the pancreas for use in the digestion of fats, carbohydrates, and proteins. Other proteins are produced in endocrine glands, particularly the pancreas and pituitary, and function as hormones regulating a multitude of cellular activities. Some of the most important extracellular proteins are antibody proteins which are formed in the reticuloendothelial system. They react with antigens, which are usually proteins but may be proteins combined with polysaccharides or lipids. The antigen-antibody reaction usually results in inactivation of the antigen. One example of an antigen-antibody reaction is the neutralization of a bacterial toxin.

General effects of injury to cell proteins. Cell injury in any form results in a change in cell protein. The initial insult may be caused by bacteria, viruses, trauma, nutritional deficiency, antimetabolites, or a variety of other agents. Regardless of the form of injury, part of the cell's protein usually reacts by becoming denatured; that is, the long peptide chain unfolds. This may result in a lessening of the cell's activities, depending on its innate reserves, its ability to repair the damage, and the particular protein affected. If the injury is slight, the process may be reversible and the cell function will return to normal very quickly. Cloudy swelling is a term applied to cells believed to be in a reversible state of injury. Microscopically, such cells appear swollen and exhibit accentuated cytoplasmic granularity. Some investigators believe that this initial reaction represents swollen mitochondria which have changed their shape from the normal rod to a spherical form. If a more severe injury occurs, the denatured protein may coagulate and protein normally in solution may precipitate. This is considered an irreversible state. Associated with these changes in the protein of the cell may be a release of nucleic acid and other proteins into the extracellular fluid. Microscopically, the membrane becomes irregular, various blebs appear on the surface, and discrete water vacuoles form in the cell. These changes are referred to as hydropic degeneration. The denaturation and disruption of the cell's protein network results in a loss of enzymatic activity which culminates in a lack of synthesis of ATP. The subsequent lack of energy makes it impossible for the cell to maintain its ionic equilibrium. There is a reversal of the normally high potassium/sodium ratio. The cell first swells and then shrinks to a nondescript mass of coagulated protoplasm. The changes in the nuclear proteins may proceed at a different rate from those in the cytoplasmic protein. Several terms have been applied to changes in the nucleus alone: karyolysis, a swelling of the nucleus; karyorrhexis, a fragmentation of the basophilic chromosomal

components of the nucleus; and pyknosis, the polymerization and contraction of the nuclear chromosomal components. The mass of denatured coagulated protein, representing the dead cell, is either phagocytized in place by wandering histocytes or partially dissolved in the extracellular fluid and transported via the lymphatics into the bloodstream. Most such particles are removed by the phagocytic activity of the reticuloendothelial cells in the spleen.

Specific effects of injury to cell proteins. While the changes described above may take place very rapidly in experimental situations, various intermediate stages of cell death can be seen in disease states. Lipid or glycogen accumulation, the apprearance of hyaline bodies and vacuoles, and changes in denatured protein are some of the stages commonly seen. Large lipid accumulations occur in degenerating cells of several organs including the heart, liver, and kidney. In some instances these deposits appear to arise through transfer of lipids from the serum; in other instances they are apparently being newly synthesized. Severely damaged cells lose all their glycogen; some slightly injured cells show large accumulations of glycogen, while others merely show vacuolizations which contain water or mucin. In the damage of liver cells associated with nutritional deficiencies, especially when associated with cirrhosis (scarring), the cells may contain large, acidophilic, refractile skeins or discrete bodies near the nucleus which probably represent altered protein. These structures have been called Mallory bodies for diagnostic purposes. In acute hepatitis, another form of liver injury, the entire cytoplasm within the membrane may become acidophilic, homogeneous, and refractile and may eventually be extruded into the liver sinusoids. These bodies in the cytoplasm are known as Councilman's bodies and are useful in differentiating injury by different etiological agents. Whenever cellular or extracellular protein becomes completely and irreversibly denatured and degenerated, it becomes eosinophilic and assumes a homogeneous glassy appearance which is often referred to as hyaline change. It represents an end stage of protein degradation and is found in irreversibly injured cells, inanimate collagen fibrils, and other amorphous extracellular protein deposits. Another change, more commonly seen with extracellular than intracellular protein, is the so-called fibrinoid change. Histologically, this change resembles one of the plasma proteins, fibrin, in many ways. It may be injured protein with fibrin deposited on the outer surface, or it may represent a primary change in the protein which imitates the staining characteristics of fibrin. This condition is most commonly seen in diseases concerned with changes in collagen such as rheumatic fever, rheumatoid arthritis, and lupus erythematosus.

Disorders. The disease associated with abnormal protein metabolism have been classified as follows: (1) diseases associated with increased production of proteins, (2) those associated with decreased production of proteins, (3) diseases associated with the production of abnormal proteins, and (4) diseases associated with the excretion of unusual amounts of amino acids.

Most diseases cause changes in protein metabolism and to a greater or lesser extent result in the cellular changes described above. When a cell is injured slightly, the normal reserve components of the cell plus the ability to resynthesize necessary constituents usually result in a quick return to normal cell function and an inability to recognize any changes morphologically. Damage to a few cells in an organ as large as the kidney, which contains millions of cells, is of little importance in relation to total kidney function and presumably is a common occurrence.

Hyperproteinemia. This is an increase of protein, usually one type of plasma protein. When it occurs, more β- or γ-globulins are produced while fewer total proteins, including α-globulins and albumins, are synthesized. The diseases usually associated with hyperglobulinemia are multiple myeloma, kala-azar, Hodgkin's disease, lymphogranuloma inguinale, sarcoidosis, liver cirrhosis, and amyloid. The mechanisms which stimulate the production of proteins, particularly of one type, are not known, but the plasma cell has been implicated. This may be a compensatory phenomenon because of the deficiency of an essential protein whose pathway has been blocked, or it may be an actual loss of control of the mechanisms which normally regulate the amount and type of protein to be synthesized.

Hypoproteinemia. A decreased amount of protein, hypoproteinemia, may be the result of a lack of essential amino acids for protein synthesis, a metabolic block, or other interference with the normal synthesis mechanism. Increased excretion of protein, particularly in chronic renal disease with a loss of albumin in the urine (albuminuria), is another common cause of hypoproteinemia. Kwashiorkor is the best example of hypoproteinemia resulting from dietary deficiency. Since albumin is synthesized in the liver, severe liver inflammation (hepatitis) or scarring (cirrhosis) will result in decreased synthesis and hypoalbuminemia or decreased levels of albumin in the bloodstream. Since albumin makes up two-thirds of the total protein in serum, this will result in hypoproteinemia. Two recently discovered diseases, hypogammaglobulinemia and agammaglobulinemia, may be classified under hypoproteinemia. In these the total serum albumin and globulin are not markedly depressed but the γ-globulins may fall from a normal of 15–20% of the total protein to levels of 0.4%. As previously mentioned, antibodies are normally part of this fraction, and the patients are unable to synthesize immune antibodies against antigens. In addition to this deficiency there is usually an intractable diarrhea in infants, and in adults, arthritis and bronchiectasis (dilatation of the terminal bronchioles). Although γ-globulins are produced in the reticuloendothelial systems, the lymph nodes show no disarrangement in the endothelial cells, the main supportive cells of the lymph node. There has been noted, however, a lack of plasma cells. These cells have been most commonly associated with the presence of antibodies.

Formation of abnormal proteins. It is impossible to say whether so-called abnormal proteins represent normal intermediates which are in sufficiently small amounts to remain undetected, or whether the proteins really are separate and distinct from any known natural proteins. The primary defect may reside somewhere in the nuclear protein synthesizing system of the cytoplasm, the endoplasmic reticulum, or it may be a result of disturbance in the genic component, desoxyribonucleic acid, of the nucleus.

Myeloma. Multiple myeloma, a neoplastic growth of plasma cells particularly in bone marrow and lymph nodes, is representative of a disease in which an abnormal protein is believed to be produced. The extraordinarily large amounts of γ-globulin present in the serum in this disease may represent only increased, rather than abnormal, synthesis. Many of its physical characteristics are identical with those of normal γ-globulin; however, the Bence-Jones protein found in the urine of multiple myeloma patients differs markedly from any protein found normally in the serum or urine. Its molecular weight is approximately 40,000, one-fourth that of normal γ-globulin (160,000). The use of radioactive glycine has shown that this protein in the urine becomes labeled with radioactive carbon before the plasma globulins do, indicating that it is not merely a degradation product of the plasma protein but is either an entirely new protein or a protein formed as an intermediate on the normal pathway of the larger plasma proteins.

Hemoglobins. Another group of abnormal proteins have been associated with the hemoglobins. Hemoglobin is a protein with a molecular weight of approximately 68,000 containing four porphyrin groups linked to an iron molecule. It functions in the transport of oxygen and carbon dioxide in the blood. Several different hemoglobins in red blood cells in mammals have been described, one of which produces the disease called sickle-cell anemia. The nine different forms of hemoglobin discovered thus far are distinguished by changes in physical characteristics and are named A for adult, F for fetal, S for sickle cell, C, D, E, G, H, and I. The differences between these hemoglobins apparently reside in the arrangement of the amino acids and the folding of polypeptide chains. The sickle-cell hemoglobin, for instance, has a replacement of the glutamyl amino acid residue by a valyl residue.

Amyloid. This material takes on a homogeneous, eosinophilic color when stained with hemotoxylin and eosin. It was originally thought to be starch and later chrondroitin sulfuric acid. In contrast to the two abnormal proteins described above (Bence-Jones proteins of multiple myeloma and the abnormal globin in sickle-cell anemia), amyloid probably represents not a defect in synthesis but an abnormal degradation product of protein. It has also been suggested that it is an abnormal combination of proteins, perhaps an antigen-antibody complex. Its exact composition is unknown but it is believed to contain carbohydrates and to be a glycoprotein. The theory that it is an antigen-antibody complex, formed in response to an autogenous stimulation from dying cells, stems from its being commonly found in diseases where degenerating cells are present. Deposits of amyloid were formerly classified as primary or secondary, depending on the sites of deposits and whether there was a chronic inflammatory reaction present elsewhere in the body. Thus secondary amyloid was usually associated with deposits of amyloid material in the spleen, liver, and kidney, and primary amyloid was associated with deposits in the tongue, mesenchymal tissues, and upper respiratory organs. It is presently thought that there is considerable overlapping between the types, not only in the sites of deposit but also in their being secondary to a chronic disease. In many organs deposits of amyloid may lie free in the extracellular space. In the kidney the material is usually deposited in the extracellular space between the basement membrane and the endothelial lining of the glomerulus; in the liver it lies between the sinus endothelium and the hepatic cell.

Amino aciduria. This is a group of disorders in which there appears to be an increase in the amount of amino acids excreted in the urine. They are due to abnormal protein metabolism and result either from an overflow mechanism where the concentration of amino acids in the serum surpasses the renal threshold of the glomerular membrane, or from defective absorption of amino acids in the renal tubules. The overflow amino acidurias include phenylketonuria, alkaptonuria, and liver disease.

Phenylketonuria. This is a disease in which large amounts of phenylpyruvic acid, a degradation product of the amino acid phenylalanine, is found in the urine of patients who may also be mentally deficient. The biochemical defect in this disease is an absence, presumably hereditary, of the oxidase enzyme which converts phenylalanine to tyrosine. The accumulation of phenylalanine eventually results in accentuation of alternate pathways of phenylalanine degradation leading to phenylpyruvic acid, phenylactic acid, and phenylacetate. The latter products are present in such excessive quantities in the serum that they are excreted in the urine.

Alkaptonuria. In this similar disease there is again failure of complete breakdown of phenylalanine and tyrosine; an intermediate product, homogentisic acid, accumulates in the tissues and serum and is excreted in the urine. It is likely that the enzyme homogentisase which converts homogentisic acid to fumaryl acetoacetic acid is either not formed in alkaptonuria or is in some way inhibited. The deposits of homogentisic acid in the tissues, especially in the cartilages, tendons, ligaments, and sclerae of the eyes, give a bluish discoloration known as ochronosis.

Liver and kidneys. Since the liver plays such a major role in the deamination of amino acids, gross necrosis or advanced cirrhosis may lead to increased levels of amino acids in the blood and subsequent excretion in the urine.

Other diseases having amino aciduria are believed to be the result of defective kidney function. The defect seems to lie in the inability of the renal tubules to reabsorb amino acids from the glomerular filtrate. Thus, in cystinuria, the failure to reabsorb cystine, lysine, arginine, and ornithine results in their appearance in the urine. A similar situation obtains in Wilson's disease, a degeneration involving the liver and brain, although the amino aciduria is highly variable in this disease. Amino aciduria may also occur in Fanconi's syndrome, galactosemia, scurvy, rickets, and toxic poisoning with lead, cresol, and benzene.

NUCLEIC ACID METABOLISM

Originally defined as the acid constituents of the nucleus, nucleic acids are now known to be present throughout the cell. They are divided into two major categories. Deoxyribonucleic acid (DNA) is found principally in the chromosomes of the nucleus of almost all cells and is closely identified, if not synonymous, with the genic material. Ribonucleic acid (RNA) is found in both the nucleus, especially in the nucleolus, and the cytoplasm, and it is closely associated with the process of protein synthesis. Within these two broad categories there may be several subclassifications according to molecular weight and other physical characteristics.

Structure. Each nucleic acid molecule contains purines and pyrimidines bound to a sugar, either ribose (as in RNA) or deoxyribose (as in DNA), and linked together by phosphate bonds. The purines and pyrimidines are referred to as bases; when linked to the sugar the complex is called a riboside; and when the phosphate is added, a nucleotide. Hundreds of nucleotides make up a molecule of nucleic acid. Both DNA and RNA contain the purines adenine and guanine and the pyrimidine cytosine. For the second pyrimidine, RNA contains uracil while DNA contains thymine. The structure of RNA is usually depicted as shown below.

Base—Ribose—Phosphate
|
Base—Ribose—Phosphate
|
Base—Ribose—Phosphate
|

Diseases. Since nucleic acids are closely associated with chromosomes and the process of cell division as well as with protein synthesis, they are one of the most important of cell constituents. They have been shown to be very susceptible to injury by various agents, and interruption of division is one of the earliest signs of cell damage. A disturbance in nucleic acid metabolism is of extreme importance to many other aspects of cell metabolism. The whole field of virus infection of mammalian cells is undoubtedly largely concerned with a disturbance in nucleic acid or nucleoprotein metabolism.

Gout. Gout is a form of arthritis, associated with extreme pain, especially around the smaller joints. There are usually accumulations of uric acid in the blood (hyperuricemia) and deposits of uric acid (tophi) in the soft tissues surrounding the joints, the cartilage of the ear, the diaphysis of bones, the kidneys, and the heart valves. The pathognomonic tophus of gout is readily identified as a collection of sodium urate crystals surrounded by an inflammatory response. The hyperuricemia must result from increased production or decreased excretion of uric acid or a diminished conversion of uric acid to urea. Increased production of uric acid, a degradation product of purines, has been determined in some cases.

Lupus erythematosus. Lupus erythematosus may be classified under abnormalities of either protein or nucleic acid, since it undoubtedly involves a disturbance in nucleoprotein metabolism. The etiology is unknown but the patients are extremely photosensitive and have hyperglobulinemia. There is usually widespread damage to collagen especially in the heart, vessels, kidneys, and skin, and to the pericardial and pleural surfaces. Histologically the lesion shows a granular, friable exudate of fibrin with increased amounts of amorphous ground substance. In some instances eosinophilic necrotic material resembling fibrin is seen coating the collagen fibrils on their free surfaces. Within the fibrinoid material are dark smudges resembling hematoxylin bodies. There is now a reliable diagnostic test, known as the lupus erythematosus phenomenon, available for this disease. When serum from a lupus erythematosus patient is mixed with white blood cells from a control individual, the neutrophilic white blood cells develop large basophilic inclusions which are believed to be nucleoprotein. The significance of this particular nucleoprotein, its origin, or its function is unknown but it does represent an abnormality in nucleic acid metabolism.

Virus infection. Much of the existing knowledge concerning alterations in cell metabolism when a virus enters a cell comes from the study, not of mammalian viruses, but of viruses called bacteriophages which infect bacterial cells. Viruses are parasites since they are dependent on the host cells' mechanism to synthesize the metabolites necessary for their replication. Although the viruses have small amounts of protein, the nucleic acid component is the material responsible for entering the cell and producing infection. A virus may stimulate cellular activity, including growth, may have no apparent effect on cells, or may cause cytolysis and death of cells. The latter phenomenon usually occurs after the virus has multiplied many times and is being released from the cytoplasm. Tissue culture studies have shown an increase in both RNA and DNA as well as protein when the cell is infected with certain viruses. The continued study of viral infections should show that they produce marked effects on nucleic acid metabolism.

LIPID METABOLISM

The basic unit of lipids is the fatty acid which may contain as few as 3 carbons in propionic acid or as many as 18 carbons in stearic acid. The most common fatty acids found in mammalian tissues are stearic acid, $CH_3(CH_2)_{16}COOH$; palmitic acid, $CH_3(CH_2)_{14}COOH$; and the unsaturated oleic acid, $C_8H_{17}CH{:}CH(CH_2)_7COOH$. Arachadonic, linolenic, γ-linolenic, and linoleic acids are considered to be essential fatty acids in that the organism cannot synthesize them. Fats as they exist in the body are generally classified as free fatty acids, neutral fats, chylomicrons, phospholipids, or cholesterol, although there is considerable overlapping of the subdivisions. Free fatty acids probably do not exist alone but are usually bound to proteins as lipoproteins in the plasma or in the cell. Much of the fat is linked to a serum or cellular protein in the neutral fats, which consist of three molecules of fatty acids bonded to three molecules of glycerol by an ester linkage. Large molecules of neutral fat surrounded by a thin layer of protein form microscopically visible globules called chylomicrons. Lecithin is a phosphatidic acid linked to choline and is a representative of the phospholipids. The steroid cholesterol, although not a true fat, is usually included in the lipid group.

Fatty acids may arise from degradation of fats in the intestinal tract or be synthesized from acetate, a degradation product of glucose. When acetate is linked to coenzyme A, a product acetyl-CoA is

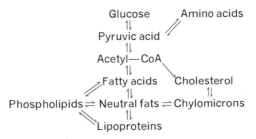

Fig. 1. Interrelationships between lipid compounds.

formed, which is the basic building unit for all fats.

The cell may degrade one class of lipids if synthesis of another group becomes necessary (Fig. 1). Lipids are probably all transported with proteins, either loosely or strongly bound. It has been suggested that a lipoproteinase released by the cells (clearing factor), helped by a coenzyme, heparin, breaks not only the lipoprotein bonding but also the fatty acid glyceral bond of the neutral fat. By this mechanism fatty acids may be transferred from their lipoprotein complex in the serum to the lipoprotein complexes in the cell. Other mechanisms such as pinocytosis, active transport, or diffusion may play a role in the transport of lipid across the cellular membrane. Once in the cell, fats are presumably degraded, oxidized for energy, or used for synthesis of other lipids, carbohydrates, or proteins by alternate metabolic pathways.

Function of lipids. The function of fat is both structural and metabolic. Most of the cell membranes are considered to be lipoprotein complexes. The degradation and oxidation of fats play a role secondary only to carbohydrates in the formation of ATP. Although cholesterol appears in most cells and is present in large amounts in the serum, its function remains unknown.

Obesity, hyperlipemia, lipid tumors. Obesity in general may be attributed to an excess intake of calories and only rarely may glandular deficiencies such as hypopituitarism and hypothyroidism be implicated as its cause. Increased caloric intake results in an increase in the size and number of fat cells distributed throughout normal lipid deposits and many organs of the body.

Hyperlipemia, an excess of lipid in the blood, is usually secondary to uncontrollable diabetes, hypothyroidism, biliary cirrhosis, or lipid nephrosis. A primary type of lipemia is caused by a genic defect. There is marked delay in the clearing of ingested fat so that a milky serum with elevation of all the lipid fractions, especially of the neutral fat, occurs. Severe sclerosis, and occasionally xanthomatosis, is common in this disease in early adulthood. Another primary hyperlipemia, called idiopathic hypercholesteremia, has also been described. Sclerosis of all the vessels is marked, with a high incidence of myocardial infarct.

There are small tumors composed of fat cells called lipomas which are commonly found in the subcutaneous tissue and which occasionally become malignant liposarcomas.

Sources of lipid accumulation. Although readily measurable by chemical methods, fat is not present in sufficient concentration to be seen in normal cells, except for fat cells, under the microscope. In many diseases states, fat appears in cells in excessive amounts and becomes readily visible under the microscope when the cells are examined in the living unstained state. During the fixation and staining of microscopic sections, organic solvents are used which remove the lipids of the cell. Thus in hemotoxylin and eosin stained sections, the space left after the fat has been dissolved presents a well-circumscribed clear vacuolar space. In frozen sections in which the lipid is not removed or in tissues which are not subjected to organic solvents, fat will stain avidly with the Sudan stains. The accumulations of fat in cells have been variously named fat accumulation, fat phanerosis, and fat degeneration. Fat in cells may arise either endogenously from new synthesis or exogenously from the environment surrounding the cell. The origin cannot be determined by examining the tissue alone.

Most cells are capable of synthesizing lipid, and some cells apparently produce excessive amounts under abnormal conditions. This excess lipid may remain in the cell or be released to the extracellular fluid and thence to the bloodstream. Elevated blood lipids and cholesterol may be relatively independent of the diet. The excess lipids present when the dietary lipids are severely restricted must be produced by cells, although not necessarily by the cells in which they ultimately appear. If cells do not manufacture and store lipid within themselves, they must obtain the lipid from extracellular sources, presumably the lipoproteins of the serum.

Lipids and degenerate cells. There are four common major diseases which are associated with accumulations of lipid in and around damaged cells. These are, in order of importance, arteriosclerosis, myocardial infarct, cirrhosis of the liver, and nephrosis.

Arteriosclerosis represents a granuloma of proliferated fibroblasts, chronic inflammatory cells, hyalinized collagen, and large lipid deposits which may ultimately ulcerate or calcify. There has been considerable controversy as to whether the collagen first degenerates and the accumulation of lipid is secondary to the denatured collagen, or whether the lipid accumulation is primary and the fibroblastic proliferation secondary to the presence of lipid. Most of the lipid in arteriosclerotic plaques appears extracellularly. This fact, in addition to the extraordinarily large amounts of lipid which may be present, lends favor to the hypothesis that lipid is being brought in from the serum rather than being newly synthesized in the connective tissue cells of the aorta. However, the fact that the plasma contributes lipid probably means increased synthesis elsewhere in the body. It seems likely too that a change occurs in the collagen or extracellular ground substance which is more conducive to lipid accumulation and precipitation. The primary change remains cellular in nature, and fluctuating serum lipid levels reflect the altered cellular metabolism.

Myocardial infarct results from thrombosis superimposed on severe arteriosclerosis in the coronary vessels. An accumulation of lipid appears intracellularly in the myocardial cells deprived of oxygen, in addition to the lipid in the vessel wall mentioned above. The origin of this intracellular lipid is not known. Since the myocardial cells are not in direct contact with serum and since the large accumulation of lipid does not appear extracellularly, it is conceivable that this lipid arises newly as a result of synthesis from acetate. However, cells in which energy metabolism is altered experimentally with metabolic inhibitors show large accumulations of lipid from extracellular lipoprotein, and ischemic damaged cells probably also incorporate exogenous lipid.

In cirrhosis of the liver, scarring is secondary to liver cell destruction and is commonly associated with nutritional deficiencies. Lipid appears as small and large droplets throughout the damaged liver cells. Again as in arteriosclerosis, there is close physical association with the plasma lipids (the liver cells border the sinusoids containing plasma) which favors an exogenous source of lipid. However, this lipid accumulation is known to be associated with protein deficiencies, and substrates which normally go into protein metabolism may be diverted into lipid synthesis instead. Tissue culture cells in protein deficient media accumulate lipid as a result of synthesis from acetate. The process of lipid accumulation in the liver is reversible when it is produced with protein deficiencies, but not when it is produced with toxic chemicals. Identical results are seen experimentally in tissue culture cells.

The accumulation of lipid in the kidney tubules in lipoid nephrosis, membranous glomerulonephritis, again is representative of a situation in which injured cells are close to the plasma lipids. The arguments for and against exogenous versus endogenous accumulation in the kidney are very similar to those advanced for the toxic damage in the liver.

Lipid storage disease. There is another group of diseases in which lipid accumulates because of a disturbance in lipid metabolism, not dependent as far as is known on external stimuli. These are the so-called lipid storage diseases which are in some ways very similar to the glycogen storage disease. In all of these diseases a large accumulation of lipids appears in many cells, but particularly in the reticuloendothelial cells of the lymph nodes, liver, spleen, and bone marrow. The lipid seems to be distributed throughout the cell and is not well localized. It should be reiterated that in Niemann-Pick and Gaucher's diseases the primary defect is probably in nucleoprotein metabolism which has erred by producing deficient or abnormal enzymatic protein to regulate lipid metabolism and has caused great masses of lipid to be stored in the cells. In Niemann-Pick disease a diaminophosphatide, sphingomyelin, is found to be the principal lipid present. In Gaucher's disease an abnormal glycolipid, cerebroside, is stored.

CARBOHYDRATE METABOLISM

Carbohydrates form a large part of all mammalian diets and play a major role in supplying the necessary caloric requirements for maintenance and growth of the individual organism. The best-known carbohydrate is glucose ($C_6H_{12}O_6$), a monosaccharide which polymerizes to form two important polysaccharides: starch, found in plant tissues, and glycogen, found in animal tissues. In mammals glycolipoproteins, polysaccharides bound to proteins and lipids, are important as macromolecular structural units of membranes and particulate organelles of the cell. Poly-

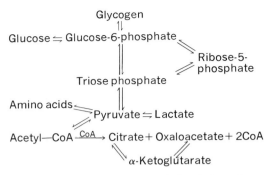

Fig. 2. Pathways for glucose metabolism in the cell.

saccharide-protein complexes are capable of acting as antigens in the stimulation of antibody production; polysaccharides are also a major component of the extracellular ground substance in the body. *See* CARBOHYDRATE.

Although both fat and protein may serve as a source of energy for cellular metabolism, the simple sugar glucose is the major contributor to the energy pool. Each glucose molecule has three major alternative pathways to follow after entering the cell (Fig. 2).

Glucose may polymerize to form glycogen for use as a reserve store of energy, be converted to ribose for use in synthesis of nucleic acid, or be degraded to pyruvic acid. During periods of increased work or oxygen lack, the pyruvate may be converted to lactic acid. Normally, the pyruvate is converted to acetyl-CoA which is used in the synthesis of fatty acids or, after linking with oxalacetic acid, is oxidized to carbon diozide and water. One of the intermediates in the oxidation of carbohydrates is α-ketoglutaric acid which is interconvertible with glutamic acid, an amino acid. Thus the intermediary metabolism and pathway of carbohydrates, fats, and proteins are closely interrelated.

Carbohydrate deficiency. Small molecules in the cell, including sugars such as glucose, fructose, and ribose, cannot be seen with the magnification and resolution powers of the light microscope, although they are readily detected by chemical analyses and chromatographic techniques. The sugar that is seen most easily in the cell is glycogen. This metabolite is particularly prominent in the liver and muscle cells and may appear in a diffuse lace network pattern or as discrete vacuoles, most clearly demonstrated with Best's carmine stain. Other polysaccharides, both intracellular and extracellular, can be seen with special stains. A few of the enzymes concerned with carbohydrate metabolism, notably succinic dehydrogenase, have been identified intracellularly by histochemical methods, but these are, of course, proteins.

A lack of glucose quickly results in a lack of ATP production and a lack of energy for the cells' multitudinous reactions. The cell is unable to maintain its necessary ion concentrations, synthesis ceases, and degenerative changes quickly appear in the protein and nucleic acid structural components. There are undoubtedly many undiagnosed states in which relative deficiencies of energy exist but which are not severe enough to produce clinically recognizable symptoms. Individual cells may die, parts of some organs may

cease functioning, and adaptive alternative metabolic pathways may be utilized in protein and lipid metabolism when energy requirements are not fulfilled by carbohydrates. Most of the diseases ascribed to alterations in carbohydrate metabolism are in reality abnormalities in protein or nucleic acid metabolism. The primary defects are deficient or abnormal enzymes, and the resulting disturbances in carbohydrate metabolism are the effect of this deficiency rather than its cause.

Abnormal carbohydrate metabolism. There are five pathological states which are reasonably well elucidated in terms of deficient mechanisms or in terms of the specific carbohydrate involved: diabetes mellitus, glycogen storage disease (von Gierke's disease), Hurler-Pfaundler's disease, galactosemia, and malignant neoplasm. The end effects of these diseases have been known for many years; the causes still remain obscure.

Diabetes mellitus. Diabetes mellitus is a disease of carbohydrate metabolism in which there is a deficiency of the protein hormone insulin. This deficiency results in an inability of the cells to utilize glucose necessary for energy requirements and hyperglycemia, increased amounts of glucose outside the cell in the bloodstream. To obtain the energy for maintaining the body's activities, the cells oxidize fat with resultant ketonemia, ketone bodies in the blood, and ketonuria, ketone bodies in the urine.

Since insulin is produced by specialized β-cells in the islets of Langerhans, which are scattered throughout the pancreas, logically these cells should be damaged or absent in diabetic states. In some cases of diabetes microscopic examination of the pancreas shows a diminution in the size and number of the islet cells, hydropic vacuolation of the cells, hyaline degeneration (a type of protein denaturation), and replacement fibrosis accompanied by lymphocytic infiltration. However, in 25% of the cases of severe diabetes, the islets appear completely normal. One can only conclude that a functional alteration exists which is not manifested structurally or cannot be demonstrated with existing knowledge of the cell. In a small number of cases, glycogen is found in the convoluted tubules of the kidney and is thought to represent an increased absorption of glucose from the glomerular filtrate.

Glycogen storage disease. Small quantities of glycogen, a polymerization product of glucose, may be found in many cells, where they act as a storage supply for energy when free glucose is unavailable. In glycogen storage disease extraordinarily large amounts of glycogen are deposited in essential organs such as the heart, liver, kidney, and skeletal muscle. The symptoms of the disease arise when the accumulation of glycogen interferes with the normal cells' metabolism. When this occurs in the heart, the muscle fibers appear split by large amounts of glycogen, muscle contractility is impaired, and heart failure and death may eventually result.

The disease has been classified into four general types, although there is considerable crossing over of the classification (Fig. 3).

In classical von Gierke's disease, the major organ involved is the liver. It may contain as much as 16% glycogen wet weight, but the glycogen has a normal structure. The enzyme glucose-6-phospha-

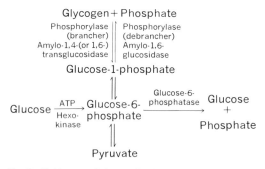

Fig. 3. Pathways of glucose in glycogen synthesis.

tase is deficient so that glucose-6-phosphate is not broken down to free glucose in the blood, and an increased synthesis of glycogen results. The liver is also the site of the second form of the disease, but in this instance the glycogen has an abnormal structure with either short or long outer chains in the frozen molecule. These abnormal structures result from a deficiency of the debranching enzyme, amylo-1,6-glucosidase, and the branching enzyme, amylo-1,4-(or 1-6-) transglucosidase, respectively. The third type of the disease is characterized by generalized glycogen storage throughout several organs of the body. The heart, in particular, shows a lacework appearance of the myocardial fibers. The glycogen is apparently normal and the presumed enzyme defect has not been elucidated. The fourth and rarest type is glycogen disease of skeletal muscle which results in progressive muscle weakness. In a few cases an excess of a low-molecular-weight component of the glycogen has been found.

Hurler-Pfaundler's disease. There is excess storage of a mucopolysaccharide in the spleen, liver, and other tissues in this disease, often called gargoylism. The mucopolysaccharide consists of a family of oligosaccharides, each of which is composed exclusively of D-glucosamine and D-glucuronic acid united in glycosidic linkage. The symptoms, as in glycogen storage disease, result from interference with the cells' function. The enzymatic deficiency in this disease is still unknown.

Galactosemia. This is a disease of the newborn resulting from an inherited deficiency of the enzyme concerned with the conversion of galactose to glucose, phosphogalactose transferase. The principal food of newborns is milk which contains large quantities of lactose. Lactose is usually broken to galactose and glucose, and the glucose is quickly utilized. The galactose, however, must first be converted to glucose. If the galactose is not converted, it accumulates in cells and interferes with their normal functions.

The deficiency of phosphogalactose transference cannot be directly treated at present. If milk is continued in the diet, severe liver damage, cataracts, and mental retardation may result. However, the child with galactosemia can usually be cured if lactose is immediately eliminated from the diet.

Malignant neoplasms. For many years it has been recognized that malignant neoplasms had abnormalities in carbodydrate metabolism. Malignant tissues, to maintain their rapid state of growth and division, require a considerable amount of

glucose as an energy source. There are, however, some tumors in which respiration and aerobic oxidation of glucose are inhibited by excessive amounts of glucose, the Crabtree effect. Normal tissues produce lactic acid from glucose anaerobically; only cancer tissue shows the unusual ability to produce lactic acid from glucose in the presence of oxygen, the Pasteur effect. It has been suggested that the Pasteur phenomenon results from a deficiency of the respiratory enzymes' oxidizing pyruvate to carbon dioxide and water and an acceleration of conversion of glucose to lactic acid by the glycolytic enzymes. No adequate proof for a respiratory deficiency has as yet been presented. Usually the cancer cell is easily distinguished from nonneoplastic cells by its morphology involving characteristics of the chromosomal pattern, size of the nucleus, and irregularity of cell outline. Unfortunately there appears to be no correlation between the abnormal carbohydrate metabolism and the morphological structure of the cell. The carbohydrate abnormalities are believed by many investigators to be secondary to metabolic abnormalities of nucleic acid and protein, including the factors involved in the regulation of the cells' division process.

[DONALD W. KING]

Bibliography: D. H. Brown, Tissue storage of mucopolysaccharides in Hürler-Pfaundler's disease, *Proc. Nat. Acad. Sci.*, 43:783–790, 1957; G. G. Duncan (ed.), *Diseases of Metabolism*, 5th ed., 1964; J. S. Fruton and S. Simmonds, *General Biochemistry*, 2d ed., 1958; H. M. Kalckar, E. P. Anderson, and K. J. Isselbacher, Galactosemia, a congenital defect in a nucleotide transferase: A preliminary report, *Proc. Nat. Acad. Sci.*, 42:49–51, 1956; R. H. S. Thompson and I. D. Wootton, *Biochemical Disorders in Human Disease*, 3d ed., 1970.

Methionine

An amino acid considered essential for normal growth of animals. The amino acids are characterized physically by the following: (1) the pK_1, or the dissociation constant of the various titratable groups; (2) the isoelectric point, or pH at which a

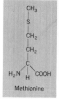

Physical constants of the L isomer at 25°C:
pK_1 (COOH): 2.28; pK_2 (NH_3^+): 9.21
Isoelectric point: 5.74
Optical rotation: $[\alpha]_D(H_2O)$: −10.0; $[\alpha]_D$(5 N HCl): +23.2
Solubility (g/100 ml H_2O): 3.35 (DL)

dipolar ion does not migrate in an electric field; (3) the optical rotation, or the rotation imparted to a beam of plane-polarized light (frequently the D line of the sodium spectrum) passing through 1 dm of a solution of 100 g in 100 ml; and (4) solubility.

A red color is formed when methionine is treated with nitroprusside in alkaline solution and then acidified. Methionine is an important methyl group donor in transmethylation reactions. For this purpose it must first be activated by adenosinetriphosphate (ATP), forming *S*-adenosylmethionine. This compound readily transfers its methyl group to suitable acceptors, leaving *S*-adenosylhomocysteine. Active methyl groups originate during methionine biosynthesis. A hydroxymethyl group is reduced to a methyl group through the mediation either of coenzyme B_{12} or of tetrahydrofolic acid. *See* AMINO ACIDS.

Several metabolic degradation pathways are known:

1. Homoserine may be formed by reversal of the biosynthetic reactions described for microorganisms. Homoserine then can be degraded further by two alternative routes: (*a*) oxidative deamination to α-keto-γ-hydroxybutyrate, followed by cleavage to pyruvate plus formate; and (*b*) nonoxidative deamination to α-ketobutyrate.

2. Homocysteine, arising by demethylation, may be oxidized to homocysteic acid or desulfhydrated to α-ketobutyrate, hydrogen sulfide, and ammonia.

3. Methionine may be deaminated oxidatively to α-keto-γ-methiolbutyric acid, which is further degraded to α-ketobutyrate, methylmercaptan, and ammonia.   [EDWARD A. ADELBERG]

Micrometeorology, crop

Crop micrometeorology deals with the interaction of crops and their immediate physical environment. Especially, it seeks to measure and explain net photosynthesis (photosynthesis minus respiration) and water use (transpiration plus evaporation from the soil) of crops as a function of meteorological, crop, and soil moisture conditions. These studies are complex because the intricate array of leaves, stems, and fruits modifies the local environment and because the processes of energy transfers and conversions are interrelated. As a basic science, crop micrometeorology is related to plant anatomy, plant physiology, meteorology, and hydrology. Expertise in radiation exchange theory, boundary-layer and diffusion processes, and turbulence theory is needed in basic crop micrometeorological studies. A practical goal is to provide improved plant designs and cropping patterns for light interception, for reducing infestations of diseases, pests, and weeds, and for increasing crop water-use efficiency. Shelter belts are modifications that have been used in arid or windy areas to protect crops and seedlings from a harsh environment. *See* AGRICULTURAL METEOROLOGY; AGRICULTURAL SCIENCE (PLANT).

Unifying concepts. Conservation laws for energy and matter are central to crop micrometeorology. Energy fluxes involved are solar wavelength radiation, consisting of photosynthetically active radiation (0.4–0.7 μm) and near-infrared radiation (0.7–3 μm); far-infrared radiation (3–100 μm); convection in the air; molecular heat conduction in and near the plant parts and in the soil; and the latent heat carried by water vapor. The main material substances transported to and from crop and soil surfaces are water vapor and carbon dioxide. However, fluxes of ammonia, sulfur dioxide, pesticides, and other gases or pollutants to or from crop or soil surfaces have been measured. These entities move by molecular diffusion near the leaves and soil, but by convection (usually turbulent) in the airflow. During the daytime generally, and sometimes at night, airflow among and above crops is strongly turbulent. However, often at night a stable air layer forms because of surface cooling caused by emission of far-infrared radiation back to space, and the air flow becomes nonturbulent. Fog or radia-

tion frosts may result. The aerodynamic drag and thermal (heat-absorbing) effects of plants contribute to the pattern of air movement and influence the efficiency of turbulent transfer.

Both field studies and mathematical simulation models have dealt mostly with tall, close-growing crops, such as maize and wheat, which can be treated statistically as composed of infinite horizontal layers. Downward-moving direct-beam solar and diffuse sky radiation are partly absorbed, partly reflected, and partly transmitted by each layer. Less photosynthetically active radiation than near-infrared radiation is transmitted to ground level and reflected from the crop canopy because photosynthetically active radiation is strongly absorbed by the photosynthetic pigments (chlorophyll, carotenoids, and so on) and near-infrared radiation is only weakly absorbed. The plants act as good emitters and absorbers of far-infrared radiation. Transfers of momentum, heat, water vapor, and carbon dioxide can be considered as composed of two parts; a leaf-to-air transfer and a turbulent vertical transfer. As a bare minimum, two mean or representative temperatures are needed for each layer: an average air temperature and a representative plant surface temperature. Because some leaves are in direct sunlight and some are shaded, a representative temperature is difficult to obtain. Under clear conditions, traversing solar radiation sensors show a bimodal frequency distribution of irradiances in most crop communities; that is, most points in space and time are exposed to either high irradiances of direct-beam radiation or low irradiances characteristic of shaded conditions. Models of radiation interception have been developed which predict irradiance on both shaded leaves and on exposed leaves, depending on the leaf inclination angle with respect to the rays. The central concept of both experimental studies and simulation models is that radiant energy fluxes, sensible heat fluxes, and latent heat fluxes are coupled physically and can be expressed mathematically. This interdependence applies to a complex crop system as well as to a single leaf.

Photosynthesis. Studies of photosynthesis of crops using micrometeorological techniques do not consider the submicroscopic physics and chemistry of photosynthesis and respiration, but consider processes on a microscopic and macroscopic scale. The most important factors are the transport and diffusion of carbon dioxide in air to the leaves and through small ports called stomata to the internal air spaces. Thence it diffuses in the liquid phase of cells to chloroplasts, where carboxylation enzymes speed the first step in the conversion of carbon dioxide into organic plant materials. Solar radiation provides the photosynthetically active radiant energy to drive this biochemical conversion of carbon dioxide. Progress has been made in understanding the transport processes in the bulk atmosphere, across the leaf boundary layer, through the stomata, through the cells, and eventually to the sites of carboxylation. Transport resistances have been identified for this catenary process: bulk aerodynamic resistance, boundary-layer resistance, stomatal diffusion resistance, mesophyll resistance, and carboxylation resistance. All these resistances are plant factors which control the rate of carbon dioxide uptake by leaves of a crop; however, boundary-layer resistance and especially bulk aerodynamic resistance are determined also by the external wind flow.

Carbon dioxide concentration and photosynthetically active radiation are two other factors which control the rate of crop photosynthesis. Carbon dioxide concentration does not vary widely from about 315 microliters per liter. Experiments have revealed that it is not practical to enrich the air with carbon dioxide on a field scale because it is rapidly dispersed by turbulence. Therefore carbon dioxide concentration can be dismissed as a practical variable. Solar radiation varies widely in quantity and source distribution (direct-beam or diffuse sky or cloud sources). Many species of crop plants have leaves which can utilize solar radiation having flux densities greater than full sunlight (tropical grasses such as maize, sugar cane, and Burmuda grass, which fix carbon dioxide through the enzyme phosphoenolpyruvate carboxylase). Other species have leaves which may give maximum photosynthesis rates by individual leaves at less than full sunlight (such as soybean, sugarbeet, and wheat, which fix carbon dioxide through the enzyme ribulose 1,5-diphosphate carboxylase). However, in general, most crops show increasing photosynthesis rates with increasing irradiances for two reasons. First, more solar energy would become available to the shaded and partly shaded leaves deep in the crop canopy. Second, many of the well-exposed leaves at the top of a crop canopy are exposed to solar rays at wide angles of inclination so that they do not receive the full solar flux density. These leaves will respond to increasing irradiance also. Furthermore, increased diffuse to direct-beam ratios of irradiance (which could be caused by haze or thin clouds) may increase the irradiance on shaded leaves and hence increase overall crop photosynthesis.

If crop plants lack available soil water, the stomata may close and restrict the rate of carbon dioxide uptake by crops. Stomatal closure will protect plants against excessive dehydration, but will at the same time decrease photosynthesis by restricting the diffusion of carbon dioxide into the leaves. See PHOTOSYNTHESIS.

Transpiration and heat exchange. Transpiration involves the transport of water vapor from inside leaves to the bulk atmosphere. The path of flow of water vapor is from the surfaces of cells inside the leaf through the stomata, through the leaf aerodynamic boundary layer, and from the boundary layer to the bulk atmosphere. Sensible heat is exchanged by convection directly from plant surfaces; therefore there is no stomatal diffusion resistance associated with this exchange. Stomatal diffusion resistance does affect heat exchange from leaves, however, because when stomata are open wide (low resistance) much of the heat exchanged from leaves is in the form of latent heat of evaporation of water involved in transpiration.

Small leaves, such as needles, convect heat much more rapidly than large leaves, such as banana leaves. Engineering boundary-layer theory suggests that boundary-layer resistance should be proportional to the square root of a characteristic dimension of a leaf and inversely proportional to the square root of the airflow rate past a leaf. Experiments support these relationships.

Under high-irradiance conditions, low air humidity, high air temperature, and low stomatal diffusion resistance will favor high transpiration, whereas high air humidity, low air temperature, and high stomatal diffusion resistance will favor sensible heat exchange from leaves. The function of wind is chiefly to enhance the transport rather than determine which form of convected energy will be most prominent. In arid environments, the latent energy of transpiration from crops may exceed the net radiant energy available, because heat from the dry air may actually be conducted to crops which will cause transpiration to increase. In those areas, crop temperature is lower than air temperature.

Flux methods. At least three general methods have been employed to measure flux density of carbon dioxide, water vapor, and heat to and from crop surfaces on a field scale. These methods are restricted to use in the crop boundary layer immediately above the crop surface, and they require a sufficient upwind fetch of a uniform crop surface free of obstructions. Flux densities obtained by these methods will reflect the more detailed interactions of crop and environment, but will not explain them.

The principle of the energy balance methods is to partition the net incoming radiant energy into energy associated with latent heat of transpiration and evaporation, sensible heat, photochemical energy involved in photosynthesis, heat flux into the soil, and heat stored in the crop. Measurement of net input of radiation to drive these processes is obtained from net radiometers, which measure the total incoming minus the total outgoing radiation. The most important components—latent heat, sensible heat, and photochemical energy—are determined by average vertical gradients of water vapor concentration (or vapor pressure), air temperature, and carbon dioxide concentration.

The principle of the bulk aerodynamic methods is to relate the vertical concentration gradients of those transported entities to the vertical gradient of horizontal wind speed. The transports are assumed to be related to the aerodynamic drag (or transport of momentum) of the crop surface. Corrections are required for thermal instability or stability of the air near the crop surface.

The eddy correlation methods are direct methods which correlate the instantaneous vertical components of wind (updrafts or downdrafts) to the instantaneous values of carbon dioxide concentration, water vapor concentration, or air temperature. Under daytime conditions, turbulent eddies, or whorls, transport air from the crop in updrafts, which are slightly depleted in carbon dioxide, and conversely, turbulence transports air to the crop in downdrafts which are representative of the atmospheric content of these entities. More basic and applied research is being done on eddy correlation methods because they measure transports through direct transport processes.

Plant parameters. The stomata are the most important single factor in interactions of plant and environment because they are the gateways for gaseous exchange. Soil-to-air transfers are also very important while crops are in the seedling stage until a large degree of ground cover is attained. Coefficients of absorption, transmission, and reflection by leaves of photosynthetically active, near-infrared, and long-wavelength infrared radiation are not very different among crop species, but the geometric arrangement and stage of growth of plants in a crop may affect radiation exchange greatly. The crop geometry also interacts with radiation-source geometry (diffuse to direct-beam irradiance, solar elevation angle). Crop micrometeorology attempts to show how the plant parameters interact with the environmental factors in crop production and water requirements of crops under field conditions. *See* ECOLOGY, PHYSIOLOGICAL (PLANT); EVAPOTRANSPIRATION.

[L. H. ALLEN, JR.]

Bibliography: Jen-Hu Chang, *Climate and Agriculture*, 1968; J. D. Eastin et al. (eds.), *Physiological Aspects of Crop Yield*, American Society of Agronomy, 1969; E. Lemon, D. W. Stewart, and R. W. Shawcroft, The sun's work in a cornfield, *Science*, 174:371–378, 1971; W. P. Lowry (ed.), *Biometeorology*, 1968; J. L. Monteith (ed.), *Vegetation and the Atmosphere*, vol. 1, 1975, vol. 2, 1976; R. E. Munn, *Descriptive Micrometeorology*, 1966; N. J. Rosenberg, *Microclimate: The Biological Environment*, 1974; W. D. Sellars, *Physical Climatology*, 1965.

Milk

The U.S. Public Health Service defines milk as the lacteal secretion, practically free from colostrum, obtained by the complete milking of one or more healthy cows and containing not less than 8.25% milk solids (not fat) and not less than 3.25% milk fat. Among mammals, man utilizes milk as a source of food. The dairy cow supplies the vast majority of milk for human consumption, particularly in the United States; however, milk from goats, water buffalo, and reindeer is also consumed in other countries. Without qualification, the general term milk refers to cow's milk.

In 1975 the United States ranked nineteenth in world milk production at 542 lb of milk per capita. Statistics show United States consumption of fluid milk at 244 lb (110 kg) per capita and fifteenth on a world basis; butter at 4.7 lb (2 kg) per capita ranked twentieth in the world; while cheese consumption was 14.5 lb (6.5 kg) per capita and fourteenth in the world. *See* BUTTER; CHEESE; ICE CREAM.

Composition. Average composition of milk is 87.2% water, 3.7% fat, 3.5% protein, 4.9% lactose, and 0.7% ash. This average composition varies from cow to cow and breed to breed, as well as during the lactation period and the different seasons of the year, and is dependent upon the feed, nutritional level, age, and health of the animal and mammary gland. *See* CATTLE PRODUCTION, DAIRY.

Nutritionists state that milk is the most nearly perfect food. Although this is true, there are some limitations, particularly in iron and vitamin C. The data in the table compare the daily nutritional requirements of males and females in two age groups with the nutrients supplied by an 8-oz cup of whole milk and skim milk. Whole milk and skim milk are classified as excellent sources of calcium, phosphorus, and riboflavin because 10% of the daily nutritional requirement is supplied by not over 100 kilocalories (kcal). These two beverages are also

classified as good sources of protein and thiamin; and whole milk is a good source of vitamin A. To be classified as good, the source must contribute 10% of a nutrient in not over 200 kcal. Milk is a good source of protein rich in all the essential amino acids. *See* FOOD.

Standards for quality. The U.S. Public Health Service publishes the *Grade A Milk Ordinance*, which is the basic standard for milk sanitation practice for most states and all interstate milk shippers. This ordinance defines milk and each milk product, establishes the requirements for the production of grade A raw milk, gives instructions for the inspection of dairy farms and processing facilities, and gives sanitation requirements for the production of raw and pasteurized milk and milk products. The U.S. Public Health Service certifies the sanitary quality of all raw milk shipped interstate. To accomplish this, the service inspects farms and collection depots.

Grade A raw milk for pasteurization must be cooled immediately and maintained at 50°F or less until processed, cannot exceed 100,000 bacteria/ml per producer, and must have no detectable antibiotic residues. Grade A pasteurized milk and milk products must be cooled immediately and maintained at 45°F or less, contain no more than 20,000 bacteria/ml, contain no more than 10 coliforms/ml, and show a negative phosphatase test. The laws of some states vary from those established by the code. Agriculture Handbook No. 51 (USDA, Agriculture Marketing Service) shows a compilation of all the Federal and state standards for composition of milk products.

Fluid products such as whole milk; 2% milk; 1% milk; coffee, light, whipping, and heavy cream; and half-and-half are all defined by fat or solids contents. Filled (substitution of vegetable fat for milk fat) or imitation (made from nondairy ingredients) products are claiming increased sales. The lower cost of vegetable fat, and therefore lower cost to consumer, and the total lack of standards of identity are two of the significant reasons for the increase.

Nearly all dairy processing equipment in use in the United States has milk contact surfaces made from stainless steel, and these legally must be cleaned and sanitized before use. The fact that stainless steel is used in construction also permits the use of strong cleaning solutions, both alkaline and acid, to properly remove residues on these surfaces. Negligible corrosion or leaching of constituents from stainless steel occurs when these detergents and cleansing compounds are used properly. After being cleaned, the entire milk contact surface is sanitized or essentially sterilized with a chemical usually containing either active chlorine or iodine to render the surface free of pathogenic and most other bacteria. *See* DAIRY MACHINERY.

MILK PROCESSING

Most raw milk collected at farms is pumped from calibrated and refrigerated stainless-steel tanks into tank trucks for delivery to processing plants. The 10-gallon can that was in common use a number of years ago is today found only on a few farms.

Collection and intake. The bulk truck drivers are required to check flavor, temperature, and vol-

Daily nutritional requirements compared with those supplied by fluid whole and skim milk

| Nutrient | National Research Council recommended daily allowances | | | | Nutrients contained in 8-oz cup | |
| | Age 45 | | Age 14 | | | |
	Male	Female	Male	Female	Whole milk	Skim milk
Energy, kcal	3000	2200	3100	2600	165	90
Protein, g	70	58	85	80	9	9
Calcium, g	0.8	0.8	1.4	1.3	0.29	0.30
Phosphorus, g	0.9	0.9	1.2	1.1	0.24	0.25
Iron, mg	10	10	15	15	0.1	0.1
Vitamin A, IU	5000	5000	5000	5000	390	10
Thiamin, mg	1.5	1.1	1.6	1.3	0.08	0.1
Riboflavin, mg	1.8	1.5	2.1	2.0	0.42	0.44
Niacin, mg equiv	20	17	21	17	0.2	0.2
Ascorbic acid, mg	75	70	90	80	2	2
Vitamin D, IU	–	–	400	400	⟨–*⟩	⟨–*⟩

*Most whole milk and skim milk are fortified during processing with 400 IU vitamin D per quart.

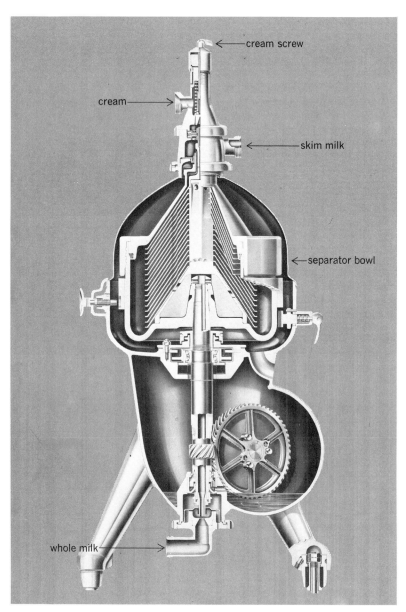

Fig. 1. Cross section of a cream separator. (*De Laval Co.*)

ume of milk in the farm tank and to collect a sample of raw milk for analysis before pumping the milk into the truck. At the receiving area of the processing plant or receiving station, the milk in the farm truck is weighed and pumped into the plant through flexible plastic and stainless steel pipelines.

Separation and clarification. The actual processing of raw milk begins with either separation or clarification. These machines are essentially similar except that in the clarifier the cream and skim milk fractions are not separated. These machines have large high-speed sealed bowls into which whole milk is introduced through ports at the bottom. In the separator, milk passes upward through holes in the closely spaced conical discs. At this point the specific gravity is approximately 1.0. Milk fat (sp gr 0.93 at 20°C) is forced to the center, but skim milk (sp gr 1.037 at 20°C) is forced to the outside. Leukocytes, debris, some bacteria, and sediment carried with the skim milk fraction are deposited in the periphery of the bowl. This single function of a clarifier precludes sediment in homogenized milk. Whole milk or cream and skim milk travel upward to the top of the bowl. A separator contains an upper conical plate without holes to prevent admixing; the clarifier contains no such device.

Separators have two discharge pipes, one for cream and one for skim milk (Fig. 1). Clarifiers have only one pipe for whole milk. Separators have a device called a cream screw by which the fat content in the cream is regulated. This screw allows more or less cream to pass out through the discharge pipe.

Many processers have units called standardizer-clarifiers which separate only a small fraction of the fat from the raw whole milk. Through manipulation of the cream screw, the amount of fat removed can be regulated. This facilitates the production of milk of standard fat content even though that in the raw product may vary. Recent modifications of separators, clarifiers, and standardizer-clarifiers permit the units to be cleaned without disassembly and the bowls to be self-cleaned during operation.

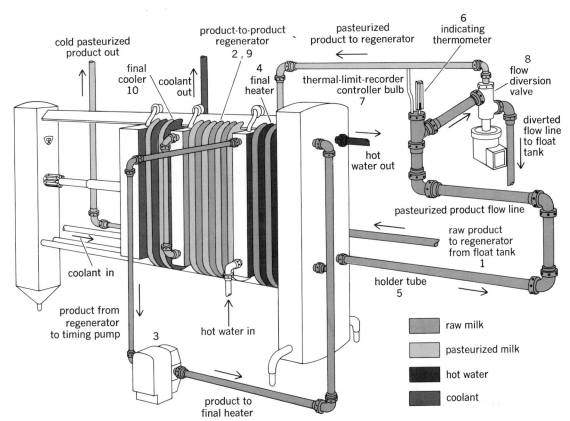

Fig. 2. Typical flow through a high-temperature, short-time plate pasteurizer. (1) Raw product is drawn from float tank into regenerator section by means of product timing pump 3. (2) In regenerator 9 cold raw product is partially heated and hot pressurized product is partially cooled by product-to-product regeneration through stainless steel heat-exchange plates. (3) Product timing pump discharges preheated raw product through tubing to final heater section 4. (4) In holder tube the time required for the product to pass through tube is determined by capacity of pump 3 and length and diameter of the holder tube. (5) Indicating thermometer is at outlet end of holder tube. (6) Bulb from thermal limit recorder controller actuates diversion valve 8. (7) Flow diversion valve diverts product not up to pasteurizing temperature back to raw product float tank. Product up to desired legal temperature is pasteurized product ready for cooling and still under pressure of product timing pump 3. (8) Regenerator 9 receives product into pasteurized product side where it is partially cooled by regeneration with cold incoming product. (9) In final cooler section 10 the cooling medium, usually chilled water, cools product through heat-transfer plates continuously until discharged at the cold pasteurized product outlet. (*CP Division, St. Regis*)

Pasteurization. Milk is rendered free of pathogenic bacteria by pasteurization. This is accomplished in a manner so that every particle of milk is heated to a specified temperature and held at that temperature for a specified time. The U.S. Public Health Service stipulates at least 145°F for 30 min when milk is pasteurized in a vat or at least 161°F for 15 sec when milk is pasteurized continuously. Cream and chocolate milk must be heated to either at least 150°F for 30 min or 166°F for 15 sec. Frozen dessert mixes must be heated to at least 155°F and held at that temperature for 30 min or 175°F for 25 sec. The greater heat treatments for the latter products are required because fat and sugar in greater concentrations than that found in whole milk provide heat resistance to bacteria normally found in milk. Most city and state codes follow these minimum requirements.

Pasteurization requirements were originally established to provide for total destruction of *Mycobacterium tuberculosis* with a safety factor added; this bacterium will not survive 145°F for 6 min or 155°F for 30 sec. Certain spore-forming pathogens will survive pasteurization; however, subsequent refrigeration precludes growth. These organisms, such as *Clostridium botulinum*, become hazardous only after production of toxin and growth. The rickettsia causing Q fever in man can be transmitted through milk, and is not destroyed at 143°F but is at 145°F for 30 min.

Pasteurization on a batch operation requires a jacketed vat where steam or hot water can circulate and heat the milk. This treatment requires the longer times at lower temperatures to accomplish pasteurization (LTLT pasteurizer). If there is a tendency of the particular product to foam, then a space heater is utilized at the top of the vat to ascertain that every particle of product is adequately heat-treated. Modern methods of processing milk and milk products utilize the high-temperature short-time (HTST) pasteurizer. Figure 2 shows a typical pasteurizer and the flows of milk, hot water, and ice water. If milk passing through this pasteurizer is not at a high enough temperature, the flow diversion valve at the end of the holding tube is activated and the milk is diverted back to the

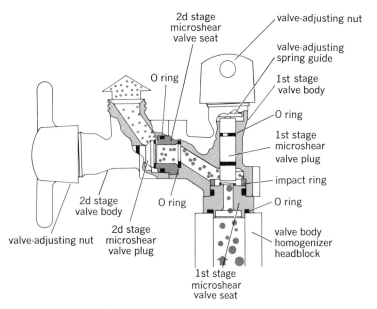

Fig. 3. Flow of the product through a two-stage homogenizer valve assembly. (*CP Division, St. Regis*)

surge or float tank to be reprocessed.

In Europe and to a limited amount in the United States, milk and milk products may be ultra-heat-treated (UHT). This process may use equipment similar to that used for HTST or tubular heating equipment. Aseptic handling is also practiced, in which the equipment is first sterilized by circulating hot water at 295°F for 30 to 45 min, then temperatures are adjusted to allow processing of milk, and packaging is done in sterile containers usually made of paperboard with a foil liner. The UHT processing requires a minimum heat treatment of 280°F for 2 sec. UHT dairy foods have extended shelf-life because all of the bacteria that would survive even HTST pasteurization have been destroyed.

Homogenization. Fat globules in fluid milk products are broken by homogenization into sizes that are 2μ or less and thus are relatively unaffected by gravitational forces. Most fluid milk is homogenized. The flow of product into the homogenizer head is through suction valves, where it is forced by pistons through discharge valves and finally through valves that cause shearing of the fat globules (Fig. 3). These later two valves can be regulated at different pressures, depending on the product being homogenized. Total pressures as high as 3000 psi are used. This reflects 500–700 psi on the second stage and 2300–2500 psi on the first stage. In order to properly homogenize milk, the product must be heated to at least 140°F to liquefy the fat globules and inactivate the enzyme lipase to prevent a rancid flavor. Homogenizers are commonly connected into the HTST pasteurizer where the hot milk comes from the regenerator or heater section (Fig. 2).

There are three theories to explain homogenization or globule fractionation: shearing, shattering, and cavitation. Shearing is the effect produced as whole milk is forced through a minute orifice at high speed. Shattering is the effect that occurs when whole milk under high velocity strikes a flat surface, such as the impact ring. Cavitation is the effect produced as whole milk changes abruptly from an area of high pressure before the valve to an area of somewhat reduced pressure after the valve. All three are evident in a homogenizer.

Efficiency of homogenization can be ascertained by examining the size of the fat globules under an oil immersion lens of a microscope. The U.S. Public Health Service specifies that the fat content of the upper 100 ml of a quart of homogenized milk that has been undisturbed for 48 hr cannot differ by more than 10% from that of the remainder.

Vitamin fortification. Most milk is fortified with 400 international units (IU) of vitamin D per quart, and some skim milk is fortified also with 2000 IU of vitamin A per quart. These vitamins as concentrates are added either by automatic dispensing with a peristaltic pump into a continuous flow of milk prior to pasteurization or as a single quantity in a batch operation. Vitamin concentrates have a potency range of 3000–200,000 IU/ml.

Nonfat dry milk can be enriched with vitamins A and D by adding the vitamin concentrates to the condensed milk just prior to drying or by blending in a dry beadlet form to the dry milk. *See* VITAMIN; VITAMIN A; VITAMIN B_6; VITAMIN B_{12}; VITAMIN D; VITAMIN E; VITAMIN K.

MILK DEFECTS

When milk and milk products are mishandled or good management practices with cows are not followed, some defects can be observed in the flavor and appearance of fluid dairy foods.

Flavor defects. There is an apparent delicate balance between the flavor constituents in milk. These are very subtle flavors, with some well below the threshold concentration where organoleptic detection is impossible. Some of the flavoring materials occurring naturally in milk serve only to potentiate other flavors. Humans vary considerably in their ability to detect flavors. Whereas milk normally has a slight salty character as well as a sweet flavor, the degree to which these background flavors are observed organoleptically varies considerably.

Cooked or heated flavor. Prominent in sterilized milks and baby formulations is a heated flavor. To a much lesser degree this flavor can be detected in fluid milk, cream and ice cream mixes. Conventional pasteurization generally will not cause a noticeable flavor. In fact, a slight cooked flavor is now desired by most consumers. However, when temperatures and holding times greater than the minimums established for pasteurization are used, this defect is discerned.

Heat causes the whey proteins, β-lactoglobulin and euglobulin, to change from the normally helical or springlike structure to random structures. The energy supplied by the heat breaks the chemical bonds that hold these coils together. The result is that numerous sulfhydryl (SH) groups are exposed, which contribute to the flavor.

Prolonged exposure of milk to elevated temperatures will also cause some discoloration or browning. Most of this color change is caused by amino acid–sugar reactions or Maillard-type browning.

Feed flavors. Milk is a good absorbent for flavors whether the flavor itself is in the feed of the animal or in the barn air. Changes from one forage crop to another, feeding of silage within 2 hr of milking, or allowing cows to feed on cabbages, onions, or other highly flavored crops or some weeds will cause objectionable flavors in raw milk. In the southern sections of the United States, deodorization of milk is mandatory to remove objectionable wild-onion flavors. This process involves flashing or injection of a thin stream of milk at pasteurization temperature into a vacuum chamber and can be included in an HTST pasteurizer between the heating chamber and the flow diversion valve.

Oxidized and sunlight flavors. Oxidized flavor is probably the most important single flavor defect in milk and milk products. This flavor is also described by terms such as tallowy, metallic, and cardboard. Lipid material is the source, but the specific flavor compounds differ apparently among milk products. For example, the phospholipids appear to be responsible for the development of oxidized flavor in fluid milk and usually produce the cardboardlike flavor.

Of the factors essential to the development of this flavor, atmospheric oxygen, iron, and copper are important. An adequate heat treatment is a commonly used process to retard the development of this flavor. The chemistry of this oxidation is a complex phenomenon.

When milk is exposed to light for any period of time, another defect can occur. This is sunlight or activated flavor and is attributed to a reaction with the amino acid, methionine, changing to an aldehyde, methional, in the presence of riboflavin (vitamin B_2). Of course, milk in metal or paper containers is resistant to this change because no light can penetrate. Some years ago amber glass bottles were used to prevent this defect in homogenized milk. Glass of this type reduces the amount of energy transmitted but is not totally a preventative.

Rancid flavor. Modern automated methods of handling raw fluid milk promote the onset of this flavor. Each fat globule in milk has a surface coating composed of phospholipids (lecithin and cephalins) and proteins from the serum portion (euglobulin and some casein), among other constituents. Moreover, the enzyme, lipase, is also present in raw whole milk and presumably is associated with casein.

Raw whole milk is stable to the action of lipase until some physical force disrupts the membrane surrounding the fat globules. Forces such as excessive agitation through surging and prolonged pumping in pipelines, mild heat treatment followed by cooling, or freezing can disrupt this membrane. Lipase acts on fat to cause hydrolysis of the triglycerides into glycerol and free fatty acids. Because milk fat contains a significant proportion of short-chain fatty acids which have strong aromas, the defect is easily detected by taste. Lipase, as with most enzymes in milk, is inactivated by proper pasteurization. Moreover, raw whole milk is never homogenized until after pasteurization.

Physical defects. Fluid whole milk is a rather stable product; however, subjection to adverse conditions can cause the appearance of some physical changes.

Destablization. If milk is frozen and then thawed, the fat and protein will aggregate. This can be observed in the thawed fluid product by microscopic flakes of protein and macroscopic fat specks.

Feathering. A defect associated with coffee cream occurs principally because of a salt imbalance in the cream (calcium, magnesium, citrate, or phosphates), too high an acidity, or improper homogenization. Cream is said to feather when a grayish, flaky scum floats to the surface when the cream is added to hot coffee.

Cream plug. Cream and occasionally fluid milk will show some signs of a thick surface. The aggregation of fat that either floats on the surface of fluid milk or forms a thick mass on the surface of cream is caused by churning. Prevention of churning eliminates this, so warming and cooling, freezing, and excessive agitation should be avoided.

TESTING FOR QUALITY

Laboratories associated with dairy processing operations, or private laboratories that analyze milk and milk products, perform many tests to determine compliance with local, state, and Federal regulations; quality control; processing efficiency; and payment to farmers. The test performed in most laboratories for homogenization efficiency is described above in the discussion of homogenization. The subsequent discussion involves other commonly used tests.

Fat determinations. There are several methods used for the determination of fat in milk and its products. The Babcock test developed by S. M. Babcock at the University of Wisconsin in 1890 is classical. This test and the European counterpart, the Gerber test, are volumetric measurements of the quantity of fat in a sample. Sulfuric acid is used to digest the 18-g sample that was added to the special flask. The heat that develops liquefies the fat. Centrifugal force is used to bring the fat into the calibrated neck of the flask. The Babcock test is used as the basis for payment for raw milk received from farms.

Fat can also be determined by extraction from a sample using specific organic solvents and subsequent evaporation of these solvents to obtain a quantity of fatty residue which is weighed. This procedure is outlined in the Mojonnier and Roese-Gottlieb methods. The solvent extraction methods are considered by far the most accurate ever developed; however, they are time-consuming. One skilled operator can complete 30 samples per 8-hr day.

An approved (Association of Official Analytical Chemists) method for fat determination in raw milk involves only the use of the Milko-Tester manufactured by Foss Electric in Denmark. This automated process consists of heating, homogenization to render fat globule size uniform, dilution, and photoelectric sensing of solution opacity. Each analysis requires less than 1 min. Frequent daily calibration of this instrument is required.

Total solids or moisture. Whatever is not lost during analysis for moisture in a food product is considered as total solids. There are several different methods approved by the Association of Official Analytical Chemists as legal for the analysis of milk and milk products. Fundamentally, all involve a heat treatment applied to a sample and then vacuum desiccation or subjection of the sample to treatment in a vacuum oven for a stated period. Other less accurate ways involve the use of specialized hydrometers called lactometers which determine the specific gravity of a fluid sample.

Freezing point. The freezing point of milk is a constant at −0.55°C and consequently can be used for the detection of the addition of water. For this determination a cryoscope is employed which contains a bath to lower the temperature of the sample and a precise thermometer or electrical readout system to determine the temperature at which stable freezing occurs. The sample will be slightly supercooled and when crystallization occurs, the temperature will rise and plateau.

Pasteurization efficiency. To determine whether milk or cream has been pasteurized properly, a test to determine the amount of remaining phosphatase enzyme is employed. The test involves the mixing and incubation of a small sample of milk, buffered solution, and disodiumphenylphosphate. An indicator is added to show colorimetrically the amount of phenol that is liberated. Properly pasteurized milk normally gives a negative test because only 0.1% of the phosphatase remains. However, if this milk were separated and a phosphatase test performed on a sample of the cream, then a positive test would result. This is because this phosphatase enzyme is associated with the fat phase. The phosphatase test is so sensitive that it can determine underpasteurization by 1°F or adulteration with 0.1% raw milk.

Inhibitory and other foreign substances. On occasion raw milk becomes contaminated with antibiotics used in the control of mastitis. Contaminations occur mostly from misuse. Milk containing such foreign substances may not be legally sold.

Detection of antibiotics is mandatory, particularly in cheesemaking and other manufacturing procedures that require bacterial fermentation because approximately 0.2 unit of antibiotic will inactivate most of the fermentating bacteria. Agar which has been inoculated with *Bacillus subtilis* spores is poured into a petri dish and hardened, and filter discs dipped in raw milk are placed on the surface. After incubation, the plates are examined for clear zones around the small disc and a comparison is made with a standard to determine the approximate concentration of antibiotic, if any.

Organochlorine pesticide contamination of milk rarely occurs since these chemicals have been delisted for use. Other organochlorine chemicals, such as polychlorinated biphenyls (PCBs), polybrominated biphenyls (PBBs), and pentachlorophenol (PCP), have accidentally or through misuse contaminated milk products. The route of contamination has been through feed (PCBs and PBB) and licking of preserved wood (PCP). Organophosphorus pesticides and herbicides present no hazard in normal use concentrations since, when contamination occurs, these chemicals are nearly all metabolized to harmless end-products by the dairy cow.

Bacteriological determinations. The microbial content of milk and milk products is an important determination because it relates directly to the sanitary quality and the conditions under which the raw and finished products are handled. Occasionally, dye reduction methods are used to determine the approximate numbers of microorganisms, but usually a direct microscopic technique or an agar plate method is used. These techniques and several others are given in the current edition of *Standard Methods for the Examination of Dairy Products*, published by the American Public Health Association, Washington, D.C.

Milk is an excellent growth medium for microorganisms which, if permitted to grow, will produce changes that render the milk unfit for human use. The U.S Public Health Service Code, which most states and municipalities have adopted, stipulates that pasteurized milk and milk products can contain no more than 20,000 bacterial/ml and no more than 10 coliform bacteria/ml. To ascertain compliance with the law and general product quality, processing plants and regulatory agencies analyze samples of milk and its products for bacterial content. A representative sample of the milk is diluted in sterile buffered water and a quantity of the solution (usually 1 or 0.1 ml) is transferred to a petri dish. Agar is poured into the dish, swirled to distribute the sample, allowed to gel. The dishes are inverted and incubated at 32°C for 48 hr. Colonies of bacteria show as white or pigmented growth on the surface or subsurface. Each is counted as one bacterium times the dilution factor to give total count.

Coliform counts are performed in a similar manner except that a direct sample without dilution is used. Violet-red bile agar is added, swirled, allowed to gel, and overplated with more agar to assure subsurface growth. After the agar has gelled, the plates are inverted to prevent the collection of moisture on the surface of the growth media and the spreading of colonies, and are then incubated 24 hr at 32°C. Coliform bacteria are recognized by their red pigmentation.

One frequent test performed by laboratories associated with processing facilities is to determine the storage stability of the finished product. A container of fluid milk, for example, is stored at 45 or 50°F for 1 week. At the end of this period, a standard plate count would determine the quality of the product. If bacterial analyses show the product to be inferior, then an active program is initiated to correct the problem and protect quality.

The significance of bacteria in milk and milk products depends upon the organism and the product. Because milk is an excellent growth medium, bacteria will be present. Coliform organisms usually are totally destroyed by pasteurization; therefore, the presence of these organisms in the finished product indicates contamination after pasteurization. With present-day facilities for refrigeration, the psychotrophic bacteria, those that multiply at refrigerator temperatures, present problems. These are normally destroyed by pasteurization and are therefore postpasteurization contaminants. Meticulous cleaning and sanitizing in a processing plant is necessary to keep these microorganisms at a minimum in finished products.

Pasteurization practically precludes the presence of pathogens, and those that survive will not survive refrigerated storage and aerobic conditions. Milk and its products also contain thermoduric bacteria, which survive at pasteurization temperatures, and thermophylic bacteria, which have optimal growth at 55°C. Thermoduric organisms are transmitted to milk from poorly cleaned equipment, while thermophylic bacteria are usually contaminants from the farm.

MILK MICROBIOLOGY

Aseptically drawn milk from healthy cows is not sterile. The interior of the udder is open to invasion by bacteria when the opening of the teat comes in contact with the air and fodder. The bacteria present in the udder are distributed internally by their own growth as well as by physical movement. However, only small numbers, averaging about 1000/ml, of a few types are normally found in aseptically drawn milk, although much lower and much higher counts are often reported. During the milking procedure, bacteria are in largest numbers at the beginning and gradually decrease.

Contamination from external sources. There are many sources from which the milk can be contaminated by microorganisms during milking as well as during the subsequent handling of the milk. The most important are given below. However, normal milking practice precludes contamination.

Stable air. This may contain dust in considerable quantities, especially in a dirty stable or when hay is distributed before the milking.

Flies and other insects. A fly may carry as many as 1,000,000 bacteria. Such a fly, falling into a liter of milk, will increase the bacterial count of the milk by 1000/ml, even without bacterial reproduction.

Coat of the animal. Soil, feed, and manure adhere to the cow's coat. During the milking process this material may fall from the coat and a portion of it may get into the milk. Dry manure is a source of heavy contamination. Proper care and preparation of the cow prior to milking precludes most contamination from this external source.

Feed. Hay and silage often contain a great number of spores. Milk may be easily contaminated with portions of the feed.

Milk equipment. Equipment, such as pails, cans, coolers, pipelines, bulk tanks, and milking machines, is the most serious source of bacterial contamination. A dirty can may add several hundred thousands of bacteria to each milliliter of milk. It is very important that utensils be made without seams and sharp corners to facilitate cleaning.

Milking personnel. If the milking personnel are not in good health or have infections on their hands, pathogenic bacteria may be added to the milk. Milk may serve as a carrier of human pathogens from one person to another, and hence the need for pasteurization.

Kinds of microorganisms. The saprophytic and pathogenic microorganisms in milk are discussed in this section.

Saprophytes. Saprophytic microorganisms live on dead or decaying organic matter. The important ones found in milk and dairy products are presented by taxonomic family.

1. Lactobacillaceae. Species of this family found in milk convert milk sugar into lactic acid and other by-products. These bacteria are cocci as well as rods, and belong to such genera as *Streptococcus*, *Leuconostoc*, *Lactobacillus*, and others.

Important species are *S. lactis*, the cause of spontaneous souring of milk and widely used for the making of cheese; *S. thermophilus*, found in fermented milks like yogurt; *Leuconostoc citrovorum*, responsible for the butter aroma; and *Lactobacillus casei*, present in cheese.

2. Enterobacteriaceae. These are gram-negative asporogenous (non-spore-forming) rod-shaped bacteria, commonly occurring in the large intestine of animals. Best known are the species *Escherichia coli* and *Aerobacter aerogenes*. Their presence in pasteurized milk serves as a sensitive index of fecal contamination, after pasteurization.

3. Pseudomonadaceae. These are typical bacteria of surface water and are often motile. The genus *Pseudomonas* is well known for causing spoilage, frequently with pronounced biochemical activity, especially on proteins and fats.

4. Bacillaceae. These are rod-shaped, spore-forming bacteria. The genus *Bacillus* contains aerobic bacilli, like *B. subtilis* and *B. cereus*. Because their spores can survive pasteurizing and sometimes even the sterilizing treatment of milk, members of the Bacillaceae can be important in causing spoilage of pasteurized and sterilized milk. Some species of the anaerobic genus *Clostridium* attack proteins (*C. sporogenes*) and some produce gas (*C. butyricum*). They are well known for causing defects in cheese.

5. Yeasts sometimes ferment carbohydrates and produce gas, and sometimes are lipolytic (hydrolyze fats). They occur as contamination in sour milk products and butter and on cheese rinds. *See* YEAST.

6. Molds which actively dissimilate carbohydrates, fats, and commonly proteins often spoil milk and dairy products, but some are useful. For example, *Penicillium roqueforti* is used in making blue-veined cheese (Blue, Bleu, Roquefort, Stilton, and Gorgonzola cheese). *See* CHEESE.

Pathogens. The milk of diseased animals may contain living germs or pathogenic microbes, and the consumption of such milk (without heat treatment) by other animals and humans may then cause the disease to be transmitted. Tuberculosis, brucellosis (undulant fever in humans), Q fever (caused by *Coxiella burneti*), foot-and-mouth disease, and causative agents of mastitis all may be so propagated. *See* BRUCELLOSIS; FOOT-AND-MOUTH DISEASE.

In addition, milk of healthy animals may become contaminated with pathogens of other origin. Milk has been known to transmit in this manner typhoid and paratyphoid fevers, septic sore throat, diphtheria, and scarlet fever.

Some pathogens do not thrive well in milk but remain alive a fairly long time. They are easily destroyed by pasteurization.

CULTURED PRODUCTS

Many fermented or cultured products are produced from milk. These fermentations require the use of bacteria that ferment lactose or milk sugar. These bacteria are of two general categories: homofermentative, those that produce only lactic acid from lactose; and heterofermentative, those that produce acetic acid, ethyl alcohol, and carbon dioxide in addition to lactic acid from lactose and a flavor precursor, acetoin, from citric acid.

Mother or starter cultures. Bacteria such as *Streptococcus lactis*, *S. cremoris*, *S. diacetilactis*,

S. thermophilus, *Leuconostoc citrovorum*, *Leuconostoc dextranicum*, and *Lactobacillus bulgaricus* are among the common organisms used in cultures. Cultures of these organisms can be purchased from commercial supply houses. Selection of the proper culture to use depends upon the talent and judgement of a trained technologist. Larger quantities of milk are inoculated and ripened to develop the appropriate acidity which is directly related to the populations in the culture, and then large vats of milk are inoculated to produce different fermented products.

Among the problems associated with fermentations, contamination of a culture with bacteriophage is probably the most devastating. Bacteriophage are viral agents that attack and destroy specific bacteria. To preclude this, manufacturers use special media for control of phage growth. Furthermore, rotation of the strains of the particular organisms used in a culture program is advantageous. Moreover, antibiotics and improper manipulations of cultures can be of serious consequence.

Cultured buttermilk. Skim milk or low-fat milk is pasteurized at 180°F for 30 min, cooled to 72°F, and inoculated with an active starter culture containing *S. lactis* and *Leuconostoc citrovorum*. The mixture is incubated at 21°C and cooled when acidity is developed to approximately 0.8%. This viscous product is then agitated, packaged, and cooled. The desired flavor is created by volatile acids and diacetyl, the latter is produced by *L. citrovorum*.

So that the modern product will resemble the classical buttermilk, resulting from the churning of cream to butter, manufacturers often spray or otherwise introduce tiny droplets of milk fat into the product during agitation.

Cultured sour cream. Cream containing 18–20% milk fat is processed and inoculated similar to the milk used in the manufacture of buttermilk. One additional procedure involves homogenization of the hot, pasteurized cream prior to cooling to inoculation temperature to control the consistency. Because of its high viscosity sour cream is often ripened in the package to an acidity of 0.6%.

Yogurt. One of the oldest fermented milks known is yogurt. Historically the people of the Middle East relied on yogurt as an important food item. Later, consumption increased rapidly in Europe because of the suspected correlation with longevity.

Yogurt is prepared using whole or low-fat milk with added nonfat milk solids. The milk is heated to approximately 180°F for 30 min, homogenized, cooled to 115°F, inoculated with an active culture, and packaged. Yogurt cultures are mixtures of *S. thermophilus* and *Lactobacillus bulgaricus* in a 1:1 ratio (Fig. 4). Balance of these organisms in the culture is important for production of a quality product. The product after inoculation is incubated until approximately 0.9% acidity has developed and then cooled.

In the United States, greater sales are realized in yogurts that contain added fruit than in the unflavored product. Three types are marketed: fruit mixed throughout, fruit on top, and fruit on bottom. Current manufacturing procedures and costs demand an automated process where the product is continuously handled. Swiss-style yogurt is prepared, so that after the proper acidity is developed during quiescent incubation, the product is agitated, and fruit is added, cooled to prevent further acid development, and finally pumped to a packaging machine to be filled mostly into 8-fl-oz (0.24 liter) cups. Other styles are ripened in cups. Fortified milk is inoculated, then packaged in cups with a fruit preparation added. These filled cups are placed in a warm room at 100–106°F (38–41° C) until the acidity develops to approximately 0.9%. At this time the cups are transferred to a cold room, where chilling terminates acid development. If the cup is inverted during acid development, fruit will be on the top; otherwise it remains on the bottom.

Yogurt is a custardlike food and is generally eaten with a spoon. The scientific literature contains considerable information relative to the nutritional and therapeutic benefits of eating yogurt, particularly that made with the bacterium *Lactobacillus acidophilus*.

Other fermented milks. A few other types of fermented milks produced in other parts of the world are relatively obscure to people in the United States. Bulgarian buttermilk is made by the inoculation of whole milk with a culture of *Lactobacillus bulgaricus*. It is incubated until approximately 0.9% acidity develops, and then packaged. This product is similar to yogurt except that it is fluid.

Kefir is a fermented milk native to the Caucasus Mountain area of southeastern Europe. Little is produced in the United States. During the

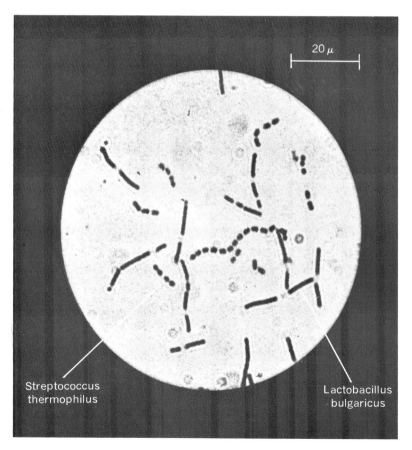

20 μ

Streptococcus thermophilus

Lactobacillus bulgaricus

Fig. 4.   Photomicrograph of yogurt culture.

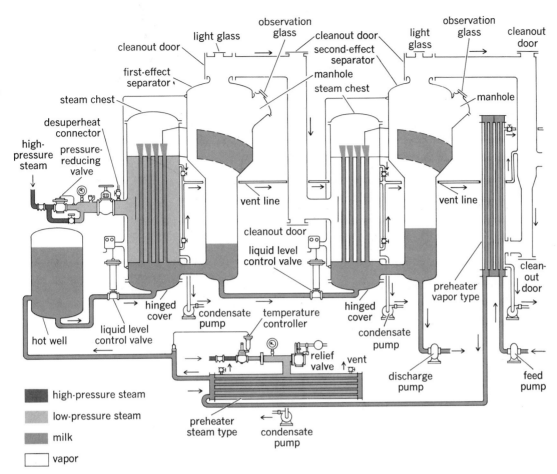

Fig. 5. A double-effect vacuum evaporator. (*Blaw-Knox*)

high-pressure steam

low-pressure steam

milk

vapor

fermentation process, lactic acid is produced by *Streptococcus* and *Lactobacillus* organisms, and alcohol (approximately 1%) is produced by lactose-fermenting yeasts. The latter collect in grains that are about the size of wheat and float on the surface.

Kumiss is another milk beverage in which both acid and alcohol are developed. Commonly, milk from mares is used, and the finished product resembles kefir except that no visible grains float on the surface. Kumiss is a mildly acid milk product with relatively little alcohol (0.5–1.5%) and is native to southern Russia.

CONCENTRATED AND DRIED MILK PRODUCTS

To reduce costs of transportation and handling, either part or all of the water is removed from milk. Moreover, the partly dehydrated milk can either be sterilized or dried to permit unrefrigerated storage for prolonged periods. Many different milk products are produced for these specific reasons. The composition of some of these is controlled by standards of identity and some by request of the commercial buyer.

In the United States nonfat dry milk is defined by Public Law 244, Mar. 2, 1944, as amended by Public Law 646, July 2, 1956. Such milk is the product resulting from the removal of fat and water. In the dry form, nonfat dry milk can contain no more than 5% water and not over 1.5% fat.

Dry whole milk is the result of removing water from whole milk until the dry product contains no more than 4% water and not less than 26% fat.

Dry buttermilk results from the removal of moisture from fluid buttermilk drained from the churn during the manufacture of butter. It contains no more than 5% water and not less than 4.5% fat.

Evaporated milk is the product that results from removing moisture from whole milk so that the final product contains no less than 7.9% fat or 25.9% total milk solids. Emulsifying salts, to reduce the effect of heat on the protein during sterilization and vitamin D, are optional additives and cannot exceed 0.1% and 400 IU (reconstituted), respectively.

Baby formulations are produced to give a product, when reconstituted, that has the same composition as mother's milk. These formulations contain nonfat milk solids, salts, sugars, and vegetable fat. Baby formulations are marketed in either dry or condensed sterilized liquid form.

Sweetened condensed whole or skim milks are prepared to contain not less then 8.5% fat and 28% total milk solids or 24% total milk solids, respectively. Enough sugar is added to prevent spoilage, usually 42–45%.

Condensed milks and buttermilk are the result of removing some water from the fresh fluid product. The concentration of milk solids is generally requested by the food manufacturer; however, if the concentration of skim milk exceeds 36% and this product is stored, lactose will crystallize.

Condensing or evaporating. Water is removed from the exposed milk product by condensing or evaporating. Initially the fluid product is given a heat treatment to destroy bacteria and enzymes and to impart different properties to the finished product. For example, ice cream manufacturers want a low-heat product, whereas bakers need a high-heat product to give loaf volume and crust color to bread. Heat treatments vary from 150 to 210°F, for a few seconds to as much as 60 min. The preheated product is drawn into the vacuum pan from the hot well or surge tank and is boiled at reduced pressure. To increase the efficiency of this operation, two, three, or four stages or effects are connected together. The vapor energy from one pan is used to cause boiling in the next. The vacuum applied to each effect is increased as the final effect is reached. The diagram in Fig. 5 shows a typical double-effect vacuum operation.

Sterilization. Evaporated milk is standardized to meet Federal specifications, canned, sealed, and sterilized. Temperatures and times of 238–245°F for 15–17 min are used. To prevent coagulation of the protein during sterilization, the salt balance of the milk must be examined. If the salt balance or concentration of calcium and magnesium is not in proportion to the phosphates and citrates content, then the defect occurs. However, coagulation can be prevented by the addition of phosphate or citrate salts not to exceed 0.1% in the finished product.

Spray drying. Most of the condensed milks, baby formulations, cheese whey, and buttermilk are dried. The condensed fluid product is pumped directly while still hot from the vacuum pan into a surge tank and then to the spray drier. This piece of equipment can either be in the form of a horizontal stainless steel box or a vertical cylinder that is cone-shaped on the bottom (Fig. 6). The fluid product is atomized to facilitate drying. Atom-

ization is accomplished either by centrifugal force where the product is discharged from a rapidly turning horizontal disc, or by forcing the product through a nozzle with a minute orifice. Drying occurs almost instantaneously in the heated atmosphere in the drier.

The dried product is collected from the drier by several means. One method (Fig. 6) involves the use of a cyclone, where the dried particles are removed by centrifugal force from a swirling air stream. Other methods used in horizontal driers involve mechanical sweeps to push the dried powder across the bottom of the drier to an auger for discharge and a series of cloth filter bags in a separate housing.

The U.S. Department of Agriculture has assigned grades to spray-dried nonfat dry milk on the basis of results from flavor, physical, and laboratory examinations. These are U.S. Extra, U.S. Standard, and U.S. Grade Not Assignable. A product in the latter classification is used as animal feed. Further grading is assigned to denote heat treatments that the product receives during preparation. These are U.S. Low Heat, U.S. High Heat, and U.S. Medium Heat, and these reflect the amount of whey protein change or denaturation.

Roller drying. Little milk for human use is roller-dried. The process involves feeding the concentrated milk between two heated and narrowly spaced stainless steel rollers. A thin film of milk adheres and is dried as these rollers turn. A scraper or doctor blade removes the dried product. The chief disadvantage to this process is the excess exposure to heat incurred by the product. Consequently, the finished product has both a characteristic flavor and limited reconstituting characteristics.

Instantizing. To render spray-dried nonfat dry milk more easily reconstituted, the product is exposed to another heat treatment. Unfortunately, the process decreases the solubility of milk pro-

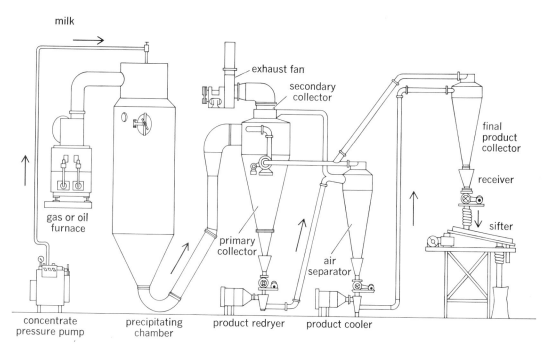

Fig. 6. Flow of product through spray drier. *(Mojonnier Bros. Co.)*

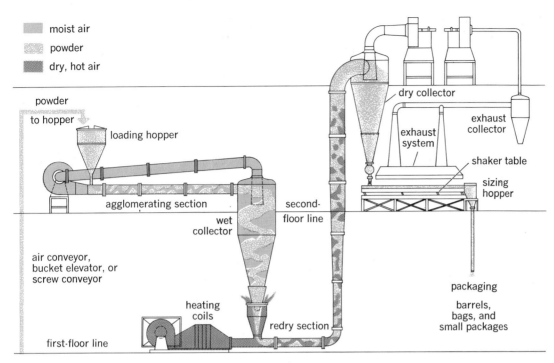

moist air
powder
dry, hot air

Fig. 7. Flow of product through an instantizer. (Cherry-Burrell Corp.)

teins. Instantizing creates an agglomerated powder; therefore, the particles are heavier and sink and wet faster than a noninstantized powder. Nonfat dry milk directly from the spray drier is fed into a hopper and metered into a steam current to cause the product to lump together or agglomerate. This wet (10–15% water) product is redried, and the agglomerates are sieved to the required size. In some commercial operations, sizing rollers are used. Any fine particles are recirculated to the inlet hopper. The diagram in Fig. 7 shows an example of one instantizing process. Most of the nonfat dry milk for fluid consumption is sold in this form.   [ROBERT L. BRADLEY, JR.]

Bibliography: A. W. Farrell, *Engineering for Dairy and Food Products*, 1974; E. M. Foster et al., *Dairy Microbiology*, 1957; C. W. Hall and T. I. Hedrick, *Drying of Milk and Milk Products*, 2d ed., 1971; C. W. Hall and G. M. Trout, *Milk Pasteurization*, 1968; W. J. Harper and C. W. Hall, *Dairy Technology and Engineering*, 1976; J. L. Henderson, *The Fluid Milk Industry*, 3d ed., 1971; L. L. Lampert, *Modern Dairy Products*, 3d ed., 1975; *Official Methods of Analysis of the Association of Official Analytical Chemists*, 12th ed., 1975; U.S. Department of Health, Education and Welfare, *Grade A Pasteurized Milk Ordinance*, Pub. Health Serv. Publ. no. 229, 1965; B. H. Webb, A. H. Johnson, and J. A. Alford, *Fundamentals of Dairy Chemistry*, 2d ed., 1974; B. H. Webb and E. O. Whittier, *Byproducts from Milk*, 2d ed., 1970.

Millet

A common name applied to at least five related members of the grass family grown for their edible seeds: foxtail millet (*Setaria italica*), proso millet (*Panicum miliaceum*), pearl or cat-tail millet (*Pennisetum typhoideum*; formerly *P. glaucum*), Japanese barnyard millet (*Echinochloa frumentacea*), raggee or finger millet (*Eleusine coracana*), and koda millet (*Paspalum scrobiculatum*). Millets have been used since prehistoric times as food crops, primarily in regions where the warm growing season is short (60 to 120 days), or in dry regions where rainfall periodicity provides a short period when soil moisture permits growth and ripening of a short-season crop. Under these climatic conditions, one or more of the millet species are grown in such diverse geographic regions as the Soviet Union, China, India, Africa, and Latin America.

Use. As a crop for human food, pearl millet is grown widely in the tropics and subtropics in regions of limited rainfall where there is a growing season of 90 to 120 days. In Africa and Asia some 20×10^6 metric tons of grain are produced yearly in

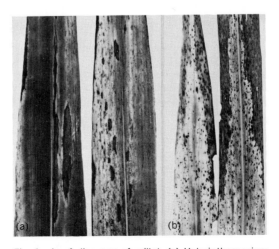

Fig. 1. Leaf diseases of millet. (a) Helminthosporium leaf spot of pearl millet (*Helminothosporium stenospilum* or *H. sacchari*). (b) Cercospora leaf spot of pearl millet (*Cercospora penniseti*). (From E. S. Luttrell et al., *Diseases of pearl millet in Georgia, Plant Dis. Rep.*, 38(7):508,1954)

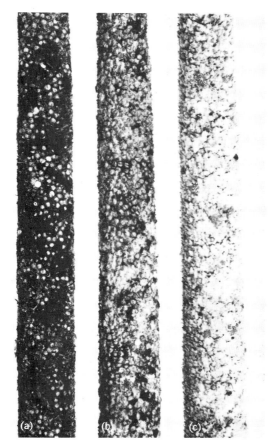

Fig. 2. Head molds of pearl millet. (a) Black mold, which is caused by *Helminthosporium* and *Curvularia*; (b) orange mold, which is caused by *Fusarium*; and (c) white mold, which is caused by *Oidium*.

40 different countries. This millet is grown where the limited rainfall or length of growing season is inadequate for grain sorghum or maize. Pearl millet grain yields average 600 to 700 kg per hectare, but much higher yields are possible with favorable rainfall and soil fertility. The naked seeds are yellowish to whitish in color and about the size of wheat grain. The dried grain is usually pulverized to make a meal or flour and then cooked in soups, in porridge, or as cakes.

In some Asian countries, finger millet is grown as a short-season food grain crop and is used in similar manner as pearl millet. The other millets also are grown as food grains in dry regions, mostly in subtemperate zones or where there is a very short growing season of 45 to 90 days.

Millet grains are high in starchy components— 55 to 65%—and thus serve as energy foods. The protein content and quality vary greatly among the various types, but they are generally low in lysine amino acid and must be used along with animal products or fish to balance the protein diet. Where widely grown, the millets are major food crops.

In North America millets are used to some extent for forage (foxtail millet in northern regions and pearl millet in warm regions). Proso millet is grown for grain, mostly for livestock feed, in the northern Plains region. The feeding value is about equivalent to corn. There is also an increasing demand for proso and foxtail millet for use as birdseed. *See* GRASS CROPS.   [HOWARD B. SPRAGUE]

Diseases. In the United States four general types of disease occur on the millets. These are foliage diseases, head mold, smut, and seedling and root diseases.

Foliage diseases such as Helminthosporium and Cercospora leaf spot diseases of pearl millet usually occur late in the season and, as a rule, damage is slight. Lesions caused by *Helminthosporium* vary in size from brown flecks to large oval or rectangular spots (Fig. 1a), in contrast to the small dark brown, gray, or tan-centered spots caused by *Cercospora* (Fig. 1b). Head molds caused by several fungi may seriously affect seed production, particularly in moist weather (Fig. 2). Individual seeds or entire heads may be covered with wooly mycelial mats which are black, orange, or white, depending on the specific fungi present. Smut diseases, common in other countries, also affect the seed in the heads of foxtail and proso millet in the United States. These smuts may be controlled by seed treatment. Seedling blights and root rots, caused by a number of soil-inhabiting fungi, may reduce stands under unusually moist conditions. *See* PLANT DISEASE.

[HERMAN A. RODENHISER]

Miticide

A chemical useful for killing phytophagous and parasitic members of the order Acarina of the class Arachnida. Although these animals are not insects, their control has become a part of economic entomology. A major difference between the mites and ticks and insects is that mites and ticks have eight legs, whereas insects have only six. The most apparent difference between mites and ticks is that the former are usually very small in size, whereas the latter are quite large and range up to 1/2 in. or more in length. All economically important species of ticks are parasitic. Several species of mites are parasitic, but a considerable number are economically important as plant pests. Chlorinated hydrocarbon insecticides, particularly DDT, benzene hexachloride (γ-isomer), and toxaphene, have proved useful for the control of parasitic ticks and mites, but have little or no value in the control of phytophagous mites.

Miticides are chemicals used specifically for the control of plant-feeding mites. Among the more effective chemicals available are: di-(p-chlorophenyl) methylcarbinol, Kelthane [2,2-bis-(p-chlorophenyl)-2-hydroxyl-1,1,1,-trichloroethane], Chlorobenzilate [ethyl p,p′-dichlorobenzilate], Neotran [bis(p-chlorophenoxy) methane], Ovex (p-chlorophenyl p-chlorobenzene sulfonate), Tedion (2,4,4′,-5-tetrachlorodiphenyl sulfone), Chloroparacide (p-chlorophenyl p-chlorobenzyl sulfide), Sulfenone (p-chlorophenyl phenyl sulfone), and Aramite [2-(p-*tert*-butylphenoxy)-isopropyl 2-chloroethyl sulfite]. All are specific miticides and have little or no insecticidal activity. Many organic phosphorus insecticides, however, are also quite effective as miticides.

The evolution of strains of mites resistant to numerous miticides increased rapidly during the 1960s. Citrus and other fruit growers, particularly in the Pacific Coast states, have experienced difficulty in adequately protecting their crops. This situation is a major factor in stimulating the development of concepts and practices for integrated pest control operations. *See* AGRICULTURAL CHEM-

ISTRY; AGRICULTURE; INSECTICIDE; PESTICIDE.
[GEORGE F. LUDVIK]

Bibliography: D. E. H. Frear, *Pesticide Handbook: Entoma*, 1966; E. E. Kenega, Commercial and experimental organic insecticides, *Bull. Entomol. Soc. Amer.*, 12(2):161–217, 1966; W. W. Kilgore and R. L. Doutt, *Pest Control: Biological, Physical and Selected Chemical Methods*, 1967; C. L. Metcalf, W. P. Flint, and R. L. Metcalf, *Destructive and Useful Insects*, 4th ed., 1962; U.S. Department of Agriculture, *Suggested Guide for the Use of Insecticides*, Agr. Handb. no. 331, 1967.

Monosaccharide

A class of simple sugars containing a chain of 3–10 carbon atoms in the molecule, known as polyhydroxy aldehydes (aldoses) or ketones (ketoses). They are very soluble in water, sparingly soluble in ethanol, and insoluble in ether. The number of monosaccharides known is approximately 70, of which about 20 occur in nature. The remainder are synthetic. The existence of such a large number of compounds is due to the presence of asymmetric carbon atoms in the molecules. Aldohexoses, for example, which include the important sugar glucose, contain no less than four asymmetric atoms, each of which may be present in either D or L configuration. The number of stereoisomers rapidly increases with each additional asymmetric carbon atom. *See* CARBOHYDRATE.

A list of the best-known monosaccharides is given below:

Trioses: $CH_2OH \cdot CHOH \cdot CHO$, glycerose (glyceric aldehyde)
$CH_2OH \cdot CO \cdot CH_2OH$, dihydroxy acetone
Tetroses: $CH_2OH \cdot (CHOH)_2 \cdot CHO$, erythrose
$CH_2OH \cdot CHOH \cdot CO \cdot CHO$, erythrulose
Pentoses: $CH_2OH \cdot (CHOH)_3 \cdot CHO$, xylose, arabinose, ribose
$CH_2OH \cdot (CHOH)_2 \cdot CO \cdot CH_2OH$, xylulose, ribulose
Methyl pentoses (6-deoxyhexoses):
$CH_3(CHOH)_4CHO$, rhamnose, fucose
Hexoses: $CH_2OH \cdot (CHOH)_4 \cdot CHO$, glucose, mannose, galactose
$CH_2OH \cdot (CHOH)_3 \cdot CO \cdot CHOH$, fructose, sorbose
Heptoses: $CH_2OH \cdot (CHOH)_5 \cdot CHO$, glucoheptose, galamannoheptose
$CH_2OH \cdot (CHOH)_4 \cdot CO \cdot CH_2OH$, sedoheptulose, mannoheptulose

Aldose monosaccharides having 8, 9, and 10 carbon atoms in their chains have been synthesized.

Reactions. As polyhydroxy aldehydes or ketones, the monosaccharides undergo numerous reactions.

Reduction and oxidation. On reduction, the aldoses take up two atoms of hydrogen and are converted to the corresponding sugar alcohols. A pentitol or pentahydric alcohol is obtained from a pentose, and a hexitol or hexahydric alcohol is obtained from a hexose. On oxidation, the monosaccharides yield carboxylic acids. Mild oxidation converts aldoses first into the corresponding monocarboxylic acids with the same number of carbon atoms; thus, aldopentoses are transformed into pentonic acids, $CH_2OH \cdot (CHOH)_3 \cdot COOH$, and aldohexoses into hexonic acids, $CH_2OH \cdot (CHOH)_4$

$\cdot COOH$. With stronger oxidizing agents, the process may proceed further, and hexoses, for example, may be oxidized to the corresponding isomeric, saccharic, or tetrahydroxyadipic acids, $COOH \cdot (CHOH)_4 \cdot COOH$. The ketoses, on oxidation, yield acids containing a smaller number of carbon atoms. The reducing properties of the monosaccharides are shown by their behavior with ammoniacal silver nitrate solution, from which metallic silver is precipitated, and particularly with Fehling's solution, from which, on warming, a brick-red precipitate of cuprous oxide is formed. This behavior is characteristic of aldoses as well as ketoses.

Phenylhydrazine. Emil Fischer's introduction in 1884 of phenylhydrazine, $C_6H_5NHNH_2$, as a reagent in sugar chemistry has proved of the greatest value in the separation and identification of the various monosaccharides. When 1 mole of phenlhydrazine reacts with 1 mole of an aldose or ketose sugar, the first product is a hydrazone, as shown in Eq. (1).

$$CH_2OH - (CHOH)_4 - CHO + H_2NNHC_6H_5 \rightarrow$$
$$\text{Glucose}$$

$$CH_2OH - (CHOH)_4 - CH = NHC_6H_5 + H_2O \quad (1)$$
$$\text{Glucose phenylhydrazone}$$

On warming with excess of phenylhydrazine, the hydrazone first formed is oxidized in such a way that the CHOH group adjacent to the original aldehydic or ketonic group is converted into a CO group. The latter then combines with another mole of phenylhydrazine to give a dihydrazone containing group (2). These compounds are termed osazones (Fig. 1).

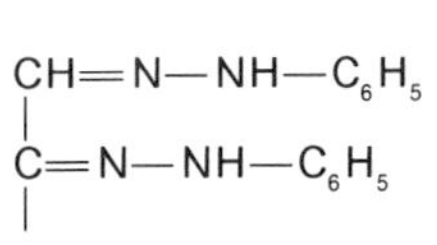

$$\begin{array}{l} CH = N - NH - C_6H_5 \\ | \\ C = N - NH - C_6H_5 \\ | \end{array} \quad (2)$$

The osazones are colored compounds which are difficult to purify. For this reason, their melting points and specific rotations cannot be relied upon. However, since the osazones produced by various sugars possess characteristic crystalline forms, they are frequently used for cursory identification of the parent sugar by examining the crystals under the microscope. The osotriazoles (Fig. 2) obtained by oxidation of the osazones with copper sulfate are to be preferred, because they are colorless crystalline compounds and have more definite melting points and higher specific rotations than the osazones.

Osazones, like all hydrazones, are hydrolyzed when heated with hydrochloric acid, resulting in regeneration of phenylhydrazine. The original sugar, however, is not recovered, because in the process of regeneration of the sugar, group (3) is

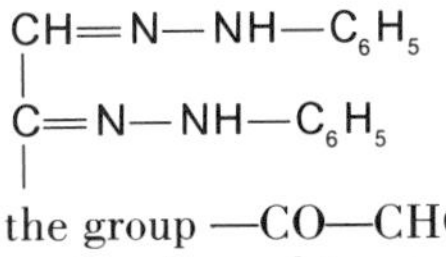

$$\begin{array}{l} CH = N - NH - C_6H_5 \\ | \\ C = N - NH - C_6H_5 \\ | \end{array} \quad (3)$$

converted into the group —CO—CHO. The highly reactive compound so formed is an oxidation product of the original sugar and is termed osone. In the example quoted above, the osazone of glucose yields glucosone, $CH_2OH \cdot (CHOH)_2 \cdot CO \cdot CHO$.

The phenylhydrazine residues from sugar osazones may also be removed with a competing aldehyde, such as benzaldehyde or acetaldehyde, re-

MONOSACCHARIDE

$$\begin{array}{l} CH = N - NH - C_6H_5 \\ | \\ C = N - NH - C_6H_5 \\ | \\ (CHOH)_3 \\ | \\ CH_2OH \end{array}$$

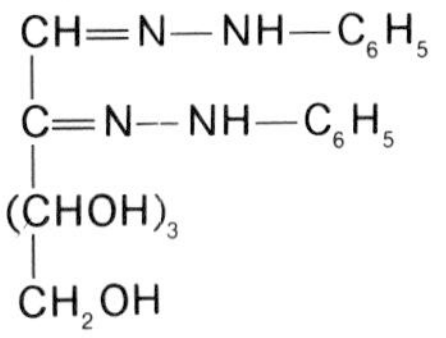

Fig. 1. Structural formula for hexosazone.

MONOSACCHARIDE

$$\begin{array}{l} HC = N \\ \quad\quad\quad NC_6H_5 \\ C = N \\ | \\ (CHOH)_3 \\ | \\ CH_2OH \end{array}$$

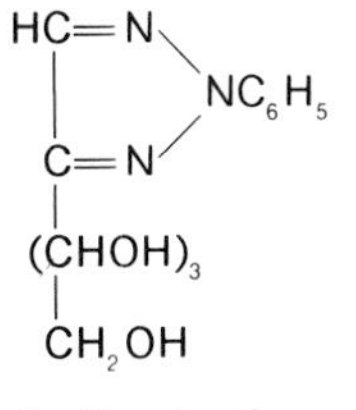

Fig. 2. Structural formula for hexosotriazole.

sulting in osone formation. On mild reduction of this compound with zinc dust and dilute acetic acid, the aldehydic group alone is attacked and converted into an alcoholic group, the keto group remaining unchanged. In the case of glucosazone, the sugar finally obtained is fructose, $CH_2OH \cdot (CHOH)_3 \cdot CO \cdot CH_2OH$, in place of the glucose used as starting material. These reactions may be used as a general method of transforming an aldose into a ketose, according to scheme (4).

$$\text{Aldose} \xrightarrow{\text{Phenylhydrazine}} \text{Osazone} \xrightarrow{\text{Hydrolysis}}$$

$$\text{Osone} \xrightarrow{\text{Reduction}} \text{Ketose} \quad (4)$$

Cyanohydrin synthesis. Monosaccharides, such as aldehydes and ketones, react with hydrogen cyanide to form cyanohydrins. By the use of this reaction, which is due to H. Kiliani, the synthesis of a higher from a lower aldose can be effected. The cyanohydrins are first hydrolyzed to hydroxy acids, which are readily converted into lactones. The latter are then reduced to aldoses by means of sodium amalgam. Thus glucose, under these conditions, results in a new seven-carbon sugar, glucoheptose. This is shown in reaction sequence (5).

$$CH_2OH-(CHOH)_4-CH=O + HCN \rightarrow$$
$$\text{Glucose}$$

$$CH_2OH-(CHOH)_4-CHOH-CN \xrightarrow{\text{Hydrolysis}}$$
$$\text{Glucose cyanohydrin}$$

$$CH_2OH-CHOH-CHOH-CHOH-CHOH-CHOH-COOH \xrightarrow{-H_2O}$$
$$\text{Glucose carboxylic acid}$$

$$CH_2OH-CHOH-CHOH-CH-CHOH-CHOH-CO \xrightarrow{2H}$$
$$\overline{O}$$

$$CH_2OH-CHOH-CHOH-CHOH-CHOH-CHOH-CH=O \quad (5)$$
$$\text{Glucoheptose}$$

Similarly, by using the glucoheptose and continuing with the process of cyanohydrin synthesis, an octose can be obtained. The synthesis has been carried as far as glucodecose.

Since cyanohydrin synthesis introduces a new asymmetric carbon atom, two products are obtained from a single monosaccharide. As an example, both L-gluconic and L-mannonic acids are produced from L-arabinose by this process.

Hydroxylamine. Monosaccharides react with hydroxylamine to yield oximes, the aldehydic or ketonic oxygen being replaced by the group $=N-OH$. Using these compounds, A. Wohl devised a method for effecting degradation of an aldose to one of lower carbon content. Thus, when the aldoxime of D-glucose, $CH_2OH-(CHOH)_4-CH=NOH$, is heated with acetic anhydride, it is converted into the acetyl derivative of the nitrile. $CH_2OAc \cdot (CHOAc)_4 \cdot CN$. On treatment with ammoniacal silver nitrate, this compound is deacetylated and the cyanide is released, leaving the corresponding aldopentose, D-arabinose, as the free sugar, as shown in Eq. (6).

$$CH_2OH-(CHOH)_3-CHOH-CN \rightarrow$$
$$\text{D-Arabinose cyanohydrin}$$

$$HCN + CH_2OH-(CHOH)_3-CH=O \quad (6)$$
$$\text{D-Arabinose}$$

It is also possible to reduce the number of carbon atoms in an aldose carbon chain by O. Ruff's method, in which the calcium salt of an aldonic acid is oxidized with hydrogen peroxide in the presence of ferric acetate. Thus, from calcium arabinate, erythrose is obtained, as shown in Eq. (7).

$$CH_2OH-(CHOH)_3-COO^{1/2}Ca \xrightarrow[Fe(OAc)_3]{H_2O_2}$$
$$\text{Calcium arabinate}$$

$$CH_2OH-CHOH-CHOH \cdot CH=O \quad (7)$$
$$\text{Erythrose}$$

Epimerization. When two sugars or their derivatives, such as sugar acids, differ only in the configuration of the substituents on the carbon atom adjacent to the reducing group, they are called epimers. The aldonic acids are noteworthy for the ease with which they undergo epimerization or partial inversion of the asymmetry at carbon atom 2 upon heating with a weak base, such as pyridine or quinoline, to produce a mixture of the two epimers.

An aldose is first oxidized to the corresponding monocarboxylic acid, which is then heated with aqueous quinoline or pyridine, to yield a mixture of the epimeric aldohexonic acids. The latter may be separated by fractional crystallization of their lactones. Reduction of the lactone yields the corresponding aldose. This process may be illustrated by the transformation of D-glucose to D-mannose, as shown by notation (8).

$$(8)$$

Enolization. Treatment of an aldose sugar with dilute alkali results in a mixture of an epimeric pair and 2-ketohexose. For example, when either D-glucose, D-mannose, or D-fructose is used, a mixture of these three sugars is obtained. The reaction, known as the Lobry de Bruyn-Ekenstein transformation, which is of general application, is due to the production of enolic forms in the presence of hydroxyl ions, followed by a rearrangement.

The transformation serves to show the close relationship between glucose, fructose, and mannose, as in notation (9). The structural representations of these three sugars are identical below the dotted line of the formula.

In a similar manner, the D-galactose series yields a mixture containing D-galactose, its epimer D-talose, and the ketose D-tagatose. When either

$$
\begin{array}{ccc}
\text{CHO} & \text{CHOH} & \text{CHO} \\
\text{HCOH} & \text{COH} & \text{HOCH} \\
\hline
\text{HOCH} & \text{HOCH} & \text{HOCH} \\
\text{HCOH} & \text{HCOH} & \text{HCOH} \\
\text{HCOH} & \text{HCOH} & \text{HCOH} \\
\text{CH}_2\text{OH} & \text{CH}_2\text{OH} & \text{CH}_2\text{OH} \\
\text{D-Glucose} & \text{Enediol} & \text{D-Mannose}
\end{array} \quad (9)
$$

$$
\begin{array}{c}
\text{CH}_2\text{OH} \\
\text{CO} \\
\hline
\text{HOCH} \\
\text{HCOH} \\
\text{HCOH} \\
\text{CH}_2\text{OH} \\
\text{D-Fructose}
\end{array}
$$

D-xylose, D-lyxose, or D-xylulose is used, a mixture of the three sugars is obtained.

Derivatives. Derivatives of the monosaccharides are discussed in this section.

Sugar mercaptals. Reducing sugars, except ketoses, react with mercaptans in the presence of concentrated hydrochloric acid to form mercaptals. The reaction with glucose and ethyl mercaptan is given as an illustration in Eq. (10).

$$
\begin{array}{ccc}
\text{HC}=\text{O} & & \overset{\displaystyle \text{SC}_2\text{H}_5}{\text{HC}} \\
\text{(CHOH)}_4 + \overset{\text{HSC}_2\text{H}_5}{\underset{\text{HSC}_2\text{H}_5}{}} \rightarrow & & \text{SC}_2\text{H}_5 + \text{H}_2\text{O} \quad (10) \\
\text{CH}_2\text{OH} & & \text{(CHOH)}_4 \\
& & \text{CH}_2\text{OH} \\
\text{Glucose} \quad \text{Ethyl} & & \text{Glucose di-} \\
\text{mercaptan} & & \text{ethyl mercaptal}
\end{array}
$$

The mercaptals of the sugars are well-defined crystalline compounds. They are of special interest because they are open-chain compounds and have been found useful for the preparation of other derivatives that have this structure.

Acetone sugars. The reducing sugars yield condensation products with aldehydes and ketones. Those with acetone have played an important role in solving problems of sugar structure. The acetone glucoses such as those shown in Fig. 3 are obtained by treating glucose in acetone with a condensing reagent such as zinc chloride or sulfuric acid.

Acetylated sugars. Acetylation of all free hydroxyls resulting in the formation of an ester may be accomplished by heating the monosaccharide with acetic anhydride in the presence of a catalyst such as anhydrous sodium acetate or zinc chloride, or

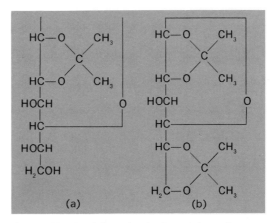

Fig. 3. Structural formulas for two acetone glucoses. Both are furanose derivatives. (*a*) 1,2-Monoacetone-D-glucofuranose. (*b*) 1,2-5,6-Diacetone-D-glucofuranose.

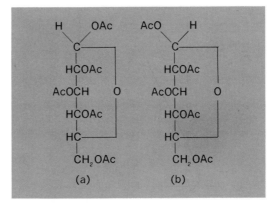

Fig. 4. Structural formulas for two isomers produced from acetylated D-glucose. (*a*) α-D-Glucose pentaacetate. (*b*) β-D-Glucose pentaacetate.

by treating the sugar with acetic anhydride in a pyridine solution. When the hydroxyl at carbon 1 of an aldose is acetylated, two isomers (α,β) may be produced (Fig. 4). The directive influence of the catalyst used in the reaction is important. Glucose acetylated with acetic anhydride in the presence of zinc chloride gives the α-pentaacetate, whereas with a sodium acetate catalyst the β form is produced. Furthermore, the β form, on heating with zinc chloride, is converted into the α isomer.

The free sugar may be recovered by deacetylation with dilute sodium hydroxide, or by catalytic deacetylation with barium or sodium methoxide.

Methylated sugars. Treatment of sugars with methyl iodide and silver oxide or with dimethyl sulfate and sodium hydroxide results in the formation of methylated derivatives (ethers) according to Eqs. (11). Reaction (11*a*) is reversible; thus, in or-

$$
\text{ROH} + \text{ICH}_3 \rightleftharpoons \text{ROCH}_3 + \text{HI(Ag}_2\text{O)} \quad (11a)
$$

$$
\text{ROH} + \text{(CH}_3)_2\text{SO}_4 \xrightarrow{\text{NaOH}} \text{ROCH}_3 + \text{CH}_3 - \text{HSO}_4 \quad (11b)
$$

der to drive it to completion, the acid end product is removed by the addition of silver oxide.

The methyl ethers are the most common derivatives of this type and can be exemplified by fully

MONOSACCHARIDE

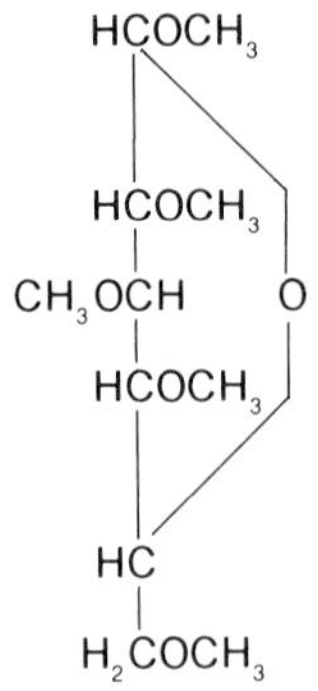

HCOCH₃
HCOCH₃
CH₃OCH   O
HCOCH₃
HC
H₂COCH₃

Fig. 5. Structural formula for methyltetra-O-methyl-α-D-glucose, a methylated ether.

methylated D-glucose, in which the hydrogens of all five free hydroxyls, including that of the glucosidic hydroxyl, are substituted by CH_3 groups (Fig. 5).

The glucosidic methoxyl group of the acetal is easily hydrolyzed with acid; however, the other methoxyls, which are true ethers, are resistant to acid as well as to alkali hydrolysis. The stability of the methoxyl group in these reagents makes the methylated sugars extremely useful in structural investigations. It is possible by appropriate methods to methylate selectively the hydroxyl groups in a monosaccharide. These partially methylated derivatives are utilized as reference compounds in the investigation of the constitution of oligosaccharides and polysaccharides.

Sugar phosphates. The naturally occurring phosphorylated sugars (D-fructose-1,6-diphosphate, D-fructose-6-phosphate, D-glucose-6-phosphate, α-D-glucose-1-phosphate, D-glyceraldehyde-3-phosphate, and a number of others) are of great metabolic importance. They function as intermediates in the processes of glycolysis, fermentation, and photosynthesis, and in most oxidative biological processes. Pentose phosphate esters occur as constituents of nucleic acids and a variety of coenzymes. *See* FERMENTATION; PHOTOSYNTHESIS.

Structurally the phosphorylated sugars are esters. The mono- and diesters of sugars are strongly acidic substances usually isolated as barium, calcium, lead, sodium, cyclohexylammonium, or alkaloid salts. D-Glucose-6-phosphate may be prepared by treating the 1,2,3,4-tetra-O-acetyl-β-D-glucose with diphenylchlorophosphonate. The phenyl groups are removed from the resulting tetra-O-acetyl-D-glucose-6-diphenylphosphate by catalytic hydrogenolysis employing a platinum catalyst, and the product deacetylated by acid hydrolysis. Other phosphorylated sugars may be similarly prepared from the proper acetylated derivatives.

Aldose-1-phosphates may be prepared by reacting the poly-O-acetylglycosyl bromide with trisilver phosphate or silver diphenylphosphate. The resulting phosphate triester is simultaneously deacetylated and hydrolyzed under controlled conditions to give the aldose-1-phosphate. By this procedure, α-D-glucose-1-phosphate, α-D-galactose-1-phosphate, α-D-mannose-1-phosphate, and α-D-xylose-1-phosphate have been prepared. The β anomers may be prepared by reacting the poly-O-acetylglycosyl bromide with silver dibenzylphosphate, followed by catalytic hydrogenation to remove the benzyl groups and saponification of the acetyl groups. They also can be synthesized by coupling the poly-O-acetylglycosyl bromide with monosilver phosphate as the phosphorylating agent.

Sugar alcohols. These are acyclic linear polyhydric alcohols. They may be considered sugars in which the aldehydic group of the first carbon atom is reduced to a primary alcohol group. They are classified according to the number of the hydroxyl groups in the molecule. Thus, erythritol with four hydroxyls is considered to be a tetritol; arabitol with five hydroxyls is a pentitol.

Sorbitol (D-glucitol, sorbite) is one of the most widespread of all the naturally occurring sugar alcohols (Fig. 6a). It is found in higher plants, especially in berries and also in algae (seaweeds). Mannitol (Fig. 6b), like sorbitol, is

MONOSACCHARIDE

CH₂OH   CH₂OH
HCOH   HOCH
HOCH   HOCH
HCOH   HCOH
HCOH   HCOH
CH₂OH   CH₂OH
(a)   (b)

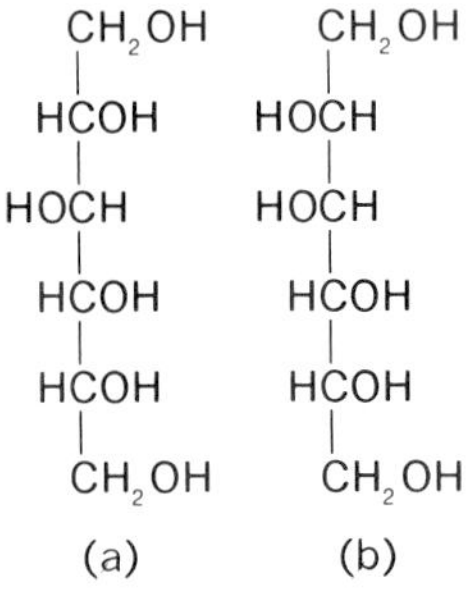

Fig. 6. Structural formulas for two common hexitols. (a) Sorbitol. (b) D-Mannitol.

widespread among plants. However, unlike sorbitol, it is frequently found in exudates of plants.

As a group, the sugar alcohols are crystalline substances, having low specific rotations, and ranging in taste from faintly sweet to very sweet. Their distribution in nature is limited exclusively to plants.   [WILLIAM Z. HASSID]

Bibliography: M. Florkin and E. H. Stotz (eds.), *Comprehensive Biochemistry,* vol. 30, 1972; W. W. Pigman, *The Carbohydrates,* 2d ed., 1972; J. Staněk et al., *The Monosaccharides,* 1963.

Monosodium glutamate

The single sodium salt of glutamic acid used in foods to accentuate flavors. It is also known as MSG. Molecular structure is represented below.

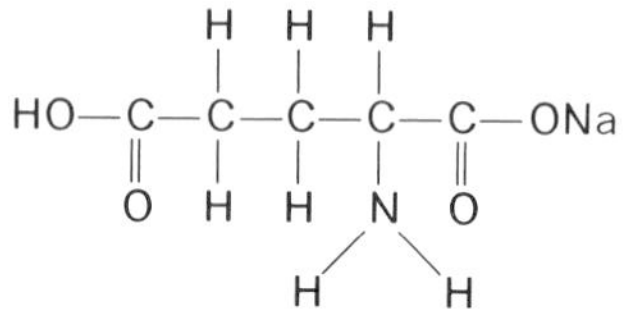

$$HO-\underset{\underset{H}{\overset{\|}{O}}}{C}-\underset{H}{\overset{H}{C}}-\underset{H}{\overset{H}{C}}-\underset{\underset{\underset{H}{N}}{H}}{\overset{H}{C}}-\underset{O}{\overset{\|}{C}}-ONa$$

The crystal form available in commerce is the monohydrate, with structure as represented plus one molecule of water of hydration.

Glutamic acid is one of the more common of the amino acids. Its structural formula is the same as the monosodium salt excepting that the —COONa group on the right is replaced by a —COOH group, making the right end similar to the left.

The formulas for glutamic acid and its salts show an asymmetric carbon atom. This is the fourth carbon atom from the left. It is attached to four entirely different groups. Therefore, the acid itself and each of its salts exist in three forms, the two isomers, L and D, and the racemic of D,L. The L form is the so-called natural or active isomer, and its monosodium salt has the power of bringing out or emphasizing flavors, as distinguished from tastes, of certain foods, notably fish, fowl, meat, and vegetables. It is not a flavoring agent but, like salt, aids in developing the savor of foods. As a major constituent of all proteins, glutamic acid participates in many of the metabolic processes.

Source. Originally produced from seaweed in the Orient, it is now made principally from cereal glutens, such as those of wheat, corn, and soybeans, from solutions evolved in the manufacture of beet sugar, and by microbiological fermentation of carbohydrates. To be commercially feasible as sources, the proteins from cereals must be concentrated and cheap. The two raw materials used for the greater proportion of commercial production are wheat gluten and desugared beet-sugar molasses. The world's largest single producer is a Japanese firm, principally using wheat gluten. In the United States, a number of factories exist; two use wheat gluten, one processes corn gluten, and several work solutions from beet-sugar molasses. The largest United States manufacturer uses a fermentation process and also what is commonly termed concentrated Steffen filtrate (CSF). This results from the multiple effect concentration at the sugar factories of the dilute waste liquor produced in recovering sugar from beet molasses by the Steffen process. Another factory uses liquor that is obtained from both the Steffen and the barium (Deguide) process of sugar recovery.

Glutamic acid appears in the sugar beet as glutamine. During the sugar process, the glutamine changes to the internal anhydride of glutamic acid, pyrrolidone carboxylic acid. The latter is readily hydrolyzed by heating with either acid or alkali, and since it is not a protein, the glutamic acid which results is in the desired L form.

Although basically simple, all of the processes used are somewhat complex because of the many organic substances present in the raw materials. However, commercial production attains a high degree of purity of product, over 99.9% monosodium glutamate.

Glutamic acid produced by the microbiological method using a carbohydrate as raw material is manufactured by a United States pharmaceutical manufacturer and a Japanese firm.

Synthesis. A number of methods for synthesizing glutamic acid from several raw materials have been published in the scientific literature. Synthesis, however, invariably results in the racemized or D,L form. Methods for the resolution of this are known, but the few which have been made public are complex and costly. It has been stated that commercially feasible methods of synthesis and resolution have been developed by two United States chemical manufacturers, one of which is already a large producer of monosodium glutamate. Details have not so far been published.

Uses. United States production includes glutamic acids, its hydrochloride, the mono- salts of sodium, potassium, ammonium, and calcium glutamates, all in the L forms. These find uses in medicine. By far the greatest proportion of glutamic acid production is used as raw material in making monosodium glutamate for the food industry. It is used both in the processing of foods and in the institutional and domestic fields. The Food and Drug Administration has approved it as an additive, and since in itself it is not a flavoring agent, its label designation in use is as a constituent and not as an artificial flavor. Originally, the latter was required because the product made then had a meatlike flavor due to impurities.

Monosodium glutamate is recognized as a standard of identity ingredient in several food preparations now being marketed.

Its principal use is in the preparation of canned and dried soups, but it also enters into the production of some meat, vegetable, fowl, and fish products. It is the "secret" ingredient used by many of the famous restaurant and hotel chefs.

Monosodium glutamate has been and is of great importance in the Oriental diet. In the Orient, it has even been used as a medium of exchange and is often diluted with lactose or salt in order that it may be sold at a price within reach of the poor. *See* FOOD ENGINEERING.

[PAUL D. V. MANNING]

Bibliography: Armed Forces Quartermaster Food and Container Institute, *Proceedings of Monosodium Glutamate Symposium*, 1948; W. L. Faith et al., *Industrial Chemicals*, 3d ed., 1965; L. R. Hac, M. L. Long, and M. J. Blish, The occurrence of free L-glutamic acid in various foods, *Food Technol.*, 3(10):351–354, 1949; International Minerals and Chemical Corp., *The Present Nutritional Status of Glutamic Acid*, 1950; P. D. Manning, M.S.G.:

Savoring agent made in special chemical plant, *Food Ind.*, 20:510–515, 1948; J. Merory, *Food Flavorings: Composition, Manufacture and Use*, 1960.

Multiple cropping

A farming technique for growing several food crops on the same field in one year, thus producing more food. In the temperate regions of the United States and Central Europe, farmers produce, in an average season, enough food to feed their large populations. However, in large areas of the world—in Asia, Africa, and South and Central America, for example—people do not produce enough food to feed even their own families. In such countries more efficient food production techniques are needed. The technique known as multiple cropping shows much promise for meeting these needs, especially in tropical regions with long, warm growing seasons.

Multiple cropping is most widely used in the tropical regions of South and Central America, Africa, and Asia. The advantages of multiple cropping in the densely populated sections of these regions are obvious. It enables farmers to produce on their own small farms the food needed to feed their families. Often four or five different food crops can be grown in succession on the same land in one calendar year. Such practices make it possible to support very dense populations.

Several types of multiple-cropping systems are in widespread use in the densely populated areas of the humid tropics. At the International Rice Research Institute, in the Philippines, multiple-cropping systems produced consistently as much as 13 tons of food per acre (about 28 metric tons per hectare) per year.

Many rotations in the humid tropics start with rice, which is the preferred food of the people. Most farmers in the area propagate their rice crop by transplanting seedlings 6–8 in. (15–20 cm) tall 2–3 in. (5–7.5 cm) deep in mud. Weeds are controlled by cultivation or by herbicides. When the rice plants are 2–3 ft (0.6–0.9 m) tall, they bloom and form long panicles, each often containing 100 or more grains. When ripe the plants turn yellow, and the heads are harvested and threshed. If properly dried, the rice grains can be stored in a dry place for several months, or even a few years. *See* RICE.

Often other crops are planted in the rice, even before it is harvested. For example, research workers in the Philippines grew a five-crop rotation of rice, sweet potatoes, soybeans, sweet corn, grain sorghum, and several vegetables on the same plot of land in one year. This rotation produced on 1 acre (4046 m²) enough food to supply 29 people each 2600 calories and 55 grams of protein per day the year around. In addition, it produced up to 10 tons (9 metric tons) of green forage for cattle feed. *See* AGRICULTURE.

[RICHARD BRADFIELD]

Muskmelon

The edible fruit of *Cucumis melo*, belonging to the gourd family, Cucurbitaceae, as do other vine crops such as cucumber, watermelons, pumpkin, and squash. The muskmelon appears to be indigenous to Africa. There are secondary centers of origin in India, Persia, southern Russia, and China. The muskmelon was a latecomer to the list of domesticated crops. It then exploded into numerous cultivars which were rapidly dispersed throughout Europe and, at an early date, into the Americas. American cultivars encompass the netted, salmon-fleshed cantaloupes; the smooth-skinned, green-fleshed Honey Dew; the green-skinned, bright-orange-fleshed Persian; the delicate-flavored, light-salmon-fleshed Crenshaw; and the wrinkle-skinned, white-fleshed Golden Beauty casaba. Other forms with very different plant and fruit characters are used in the Orient for pickling and in India for cooking. All these melons differ only in varietal characters and all intercross freely. *See* CANTALOUPE; HONEY DEW MELON; PERSIAN MELON.

The plants are annual, trailing vines, with three to five runners that may attain a length of 10 to 12 ft (3 to 3.6 m). The branching vines have coarse, somewhat heartshaped leaves, with almost entire slight-angled, rounded, wavy margins. The runners produce short fruiting branches, which bear the perfect flowers and later the fruits. Most American varieties are andromonoecious, bearing male and perfect flowers (combined male and female). The pollen is heavy and slightly sticky, and therefore insects are required for fertilization. The domestic honeybee is the only known effective pollinator of muskmelon flowers.

Muskmelons maturing on the vine without becoming overripe are superior in quality to those harvested immature. The sugar content, flavor, and texture of the fresh flesh improves very rapidly as the fruit approaches maturity. When mature, the melon is sweet, averages 6 to 8% sugar, and has a slight to distinctly musky odor and flavor, depending upon cultivar and environment. The flesh is rich in potassium, in vitamin C and, when deep orange, also in vitamin A.

Cultivation and culture. Muskmelon plants during all stages of development are easily killed by frost. They require fairly warm weather and are favored by bright sunshine, low humidity, and absence of rain, which tends to prevent certain diseases that often defoliate the plants in humid areas.

Muskmelons can be grown on several types of soil but not on muck. Peat, heavy clay, or adobe soil are not recommended. Soil should be fairly fertile and free from nematodes, wilt disease, and toxic amounts of alkali. Muskmelons are sensitive to acid soils. They thrive best on neutral or slightly alkaline soil.

Light-textured soils that warm up quickly in the spring favor early maturity. Maturity is also hastened by using glassine paper hot caps to increase soil and air temperature around the plants. In some locations the frost-free period may be too short to grow muskmelons from seed planted directly in the field. Muskmelons can be grown at such locations if the plants are started in greenhouses or hotbeds and transplanted to the field when the danger of frost has passed. Muskmelons are generally grown in rows 5–7 ft (1.5–2.1 m) apart, with a single plant 1 ft (0.3 m) apart in the row, or in hills of two or three plants 2 ft (0.6 m) apart. Under irrigation, the rows are on wide ridges with furrows for irrigation water between them. In

the arid West, 2–3 acre-feet (2470–3700 m³) of water per acre is commonly required to grow a crop of muskmelons.

Harvesting. The time from planting to harvest is 85–125 days, depending upon variety and weather. Cantaloupes are harvested at the "full-slip" stage of maturity. At this stage a thin abscission crack encircles the stem where it is attached to the fruit, and the melon separates easily from the stem. Harvest maturity of Persian melons is determined primarily by skin color changes, because in this variety the abscission layer does not develop or is delayed until the fruit is overripe. The ground spot (area resting on soil) of Persian melons develops a pinkish color when the fruits are mature. Honey Dew melons have achieved harvest maturity when the skin color is white and no waxy skin coating is evident. The surface may feel prickly or hairy. With the casaba varieties, Golden Beauty, Crenshaw, and Santa Claus, maturity can be determined by applying firm pressure with the thumb to the blossom end. A slight yielding or softness indicates maturity.

California, Arizona, and Texas account for about 80% of the acreage and 85% of the production of muskmelons in the United States. *See* MELON GROWING.   [FRANK W. ZINK]

Mustard

Any one of a number of annual crucifer species of Asiatic origin belonging to the plant order Capparales (see illustration). Mustards eaten as greens are *Brassica juncea*, *B. juncea* var. *crispifolia*, and *B. hirta*. Table mustard and oils are obtained from *B. nigra*. Cultural practices are similar to those used for spinach. Southern Giant Curled and Ostrich Plume are popular varieties for greens. Long days and high temperatures favor undesirable seed-stalk development. Harvesting is usually 1½–2 months after planting. Important production centers for mustard greens are in the South, where the crop is popular. Montana and the West Coast states are important sources of mustard seed. *See* SPINACH; VEGETABLE GROWING.

[H. JOHN CAREW]

Nitrogen cycle

The continuous cyclic exchange between combined nitrogen in the soil and molecular nitrogen in the atmosphere. It includes all the transformations concerned in the mineralization of nitrogenous organic substances and in the loss or gain of nitrogen by the soil.

Soil nitrogen occurs naturally in organic and inorganic forms as a result of plant, animal, and microbial growth. Nitrogen is stored in soil primarily in organic combinations not utilizable by higher plants, but made available as ammonia through the activities of soil microorganisms. The ammonia may be used by both higher plants and microorganisms either directly or after oxidation to nitrate-nitrogen. Both ammonia and nitrate may be lost from soil by leaching or through microbial action. Soil gains nitrogen chiefly through the addition of fertilizers and through microbial fixation of atmospheric nitrogen. The nitrogen cycle comprises the process of ammonification, nitrification, denitrification, and nitrogen fixation (Fig. 1).

Some authorities further subdivide ammonifi-

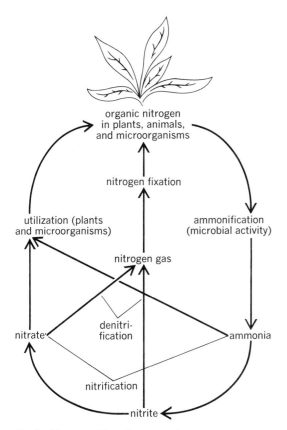

Fig. 1. Diagram of the nitrogen cycle.

cation into proteolysis (protein degradation to amino acids) and ammonification, and nitrification into nitritation (formation of nitrite from ammonia) and nitratation (formation of nitrate from nitrite).

Ammonification. Ammonification refers to the release of nitrogen as ammonia from organic compounds in plant, animal, and microbial residues. This is accomplished chiefly under aerobic conditions through the participation of bacteria, fungi, actinomycetes, and other microscopic forms of life. The first step in the process involves the hydrolytic cleavage of proteins, nucleic acids, and related compounds to amino acids and other simple nitrogenous substances. These are then broken down to ammonia. Uric acid and urea, the excretory products of animals, are rapidly mineralized. The ammonia-nitrogen liberated through microbial action is in excess of the requirements of these organisms for growth. Consequently when a substance that is high in nitrogen, such as protein, is added to a soil, considerable ammonia is liberated, whereas a substance relatively low in nitrogen, such as straw, yields comparatively little, if any, ammonia. Furthermore, if an excessive amount of nonnitrogenous carbonaceous material, for example, carbohydrate, is added to a soil, much available nitrogen, such as nitrate or ammonia, will be used by the rapidly developing microbial population, thus decreasing the available supply for higher plants. Not all organic nitrogen is ammonified, however; a certain portion is retained in slowly decomposable complexes and becomes an integral part of the residual soil organic matter or humus.

Nitrification. Nitrification is the bacterial oxidation of ammonia to nitrate, the chief source of readily available nitrogen for higher plants. It consists of two steps: first, ammonia is oxidized to nitrite by organisms of the genera *Nitrosomonas* and *Nitrosococcus*, and second, the resulting nitrite is oxidized to nitrate by *Nitrobacter*. These highly specialized, autotrophic bacteria obtain their energy from these oxidations and their carbon from the carbon dioxide of the atmosphere. Generally the process of nitrite oxidation is faster than that of nitrite production, so that the level of nitrite in soil is too low to induce toxic effects. The few types of microbes known to be involved in nitrification require a much more restricted set of conditions for optimal activity than do the many types engaged in ammonification. A well-aerated, fertile, neutral to slightly alkaline soil provides optimum conditions for nitrification. The nitrate so formed is utilized by plants and microorganisms, or may be lost from the soil by leaching. Under anaerobic conditions, nitrate may be reduced by the soil microflora.

Denitrification. In denitrification nitrate-nitrogen is reduced to nitrite, nitrous oxide, ammonia, and principally molecular nitrogen. Under conditions of low oxygen tension a variety of soil microorganisms utilize nitrate as a source of oxygen and reduce it to forms which may be lost by leaching or which may escape as gas into the atmosphere. The absence of oxygen, as in waterlogged soil, and the presence of an abundant supply of soluble organic matter provide favorable conditions for this process. Normal agricultural soil is well-aerated, not too moist, and contains moderate amounts of organic matter or nitrate. Here, denitrification is of little economic importance.

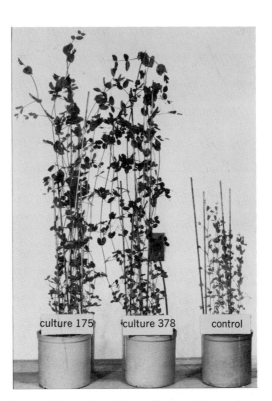

Fig. 2. Effect of inoculation with two strains (cultures 175 and 378) of the nitrogen-fixing *Rhizobium leguminosarum* on the development of peas.

Nitrogen fixation. Molecular atmospheric nitrogen is returned to the soil primarily by man through chemical fixation, and by soil microorganisms through biological fixation. Biological nitrogen fixation is accomplished by symbiotic and nonsymbiotic microorganisms. The symbiotic organisms are bacteria living in the modules of leguminous plants and belong to the genus *Rhizobium*. The nonsymbiotic organisms are free-living bacteria which function either aerobically, as *Azotobacter*, or anaerobically, as *Clostridium*. Certain blue-green algae such as *Nostoc*, *Anabaena*, and *Calothrix* species can fix atmospheric nitrogen. Several other groups of bacteria, including photosynthetic types, and fungi possess this characteristic to a limited degree, as has been demonstrated with isotopic nitrogen. The most important of the nitrogen-fixing bacteria are those that produce nodules on the roots of legumes such as peas, beans, alfalfa, and clover. In this mutualistic association they may add well over 100 lb of atmospheric nitrogen to an acre of soil annually; soils are usually inoculated with active preparations of these organisms wherever legumes are grown. Figure 2 shows the effect of inoculating cultures of symbiotic nitrogen-fixing bacteria on the development of peas. The nonsymbiotic forms, such as *Azotobacter* and *Clostridium*, fix much less nitrogen, with a fair average in fertile soils being about 10 lb/acre annually. Under certain conditions in the tropics, blue-green algae contribute significant amounts to the soil. *See* SOIL MICROBIOLOGY; SOIL MICROORGANISMS; SOIL MINERALS, MICROBIAL UTILIZATION OF.

[HARRY KATZNELSON/R. E. KALLIO]

Nitrogen fixation (biology)

Molecular nitrogen (N_2, dinitrogen) is the major component (approximately 80%) of the Earth's atmosphere. The element nitrogen (N) is an essential component of many chemical compounds, such as proteins and nucleic acids, which are the basis of all life-forms. However, N_2 cannot be utilized directly by biological systems for synthesis of the chemicals required for growth and reproduction. Prior to its incorporation into a living system, it must be altered by combination with the element hydrogen. This process of reduction of N_2, commonly referred to as nitrogen fixation, may be accomplished chemically or biologically.

Nitrogen is the nutrient element most frequently found limiting the growth of green plants. This results from the loss of nitrogen from the reserve of combined or fixed nitrogen which is present in soil and available for uptake and growth by plants. This nitrogen is continually depleted by such processes as microbial denitrification, erosion, leaching, chemical volatilization, and perhaps most important, removal of nitrogen-containing crop residues from the land. The nitrogen reserve of agricultural soils must therefore be replenished periodically in order to maintain an adequate (nongrowth-limiting) level for crop production. This replacement of soil nitrogen is generally accomplished by addition of chemically fixed nitrogen in the form of commercial inorganic fertilizers or by the activity of biological nitrogen-fixing (BNF) systems. The significance of BNF as a major mechanism for recycling of nitrogen from the unavailable atmospheric form to available forms in the biosphere cannot be overemphasized (see table). The reduction of N_2, whether chemical or biological, requires a large input of energy. The chemical process utilizes vast amounts of fossil fuels as an energy source. These materials are nonreplaceable and, ultimately, exhaustible. On the other hand, the process of BNF derives its required energy from the oxidation of carbohydrates which have been generated by the photosynthetic activity of green plants. The energy for photosynthesis is derived from sunlight. The indirect source of energy for BNF is obtained from a universally available and inexhaustible source; the direct source of energy (carbohydrate) is therefore potentially available wherever conditions permit the growth of photosynthetic organisms.

Atmospheric nitrogen (N_2) is a molecule composed of two atoms of nitrogen linked by a very strong triple bond. Large amounts of energy are required to break this bond, and the molecule is therefore quite chemically unreactive. The general chemical reaction for the fixation of N_2 is identical

Nitrogen fixation in the biosphere*

Use		10^6 ha		kg N_2 fixed per hectare per year	10^6 metric tons per year
Agricultural			4,400		
Arable undercrop		1,400			
Legumes		250		140	35
Pulses	63				
Soybeans	34				
Groundnuts	18				
Other	135				
Nonlegumes		1,150			
Rice	135			30	4
Other	1,015			5	5
Permanent meadows, grasslands		3,000		15	45
Forest and woodland			4,100	10	40
Unused			4,900	2	10
Ice-covered			1,500	0	0
Total land			14,900		139
Sea			36,100	1	36
TOTAL			51,000		175

*From R. C. Burns and R. W. F. Hardy, *Nitrogen Fixation in Bacteria and Higher Plants*, Springer-Verlag, 1975.

for both chemical and biological processes: the triple bond of N_2 must be broken and three atoms of hydrogen must be added to each of the nitrogen atoms. In the process of BNF, electrons and hydrogen atoms derived from the oxidation of carbohydrates are transferred sequentially from one specific "carrier" molecule to another, in stepwise fashion. Each carrier molecule is therefore alternately reduced and oxidized as the hydrogen atoms and electrons are transferred. Energy released by these sequential reactions is used to add inorganic phosphate to adenosinediphosphate (ADP), resulting in the formation of adenosinetriphosphate (ATP). This addition forms an energy-rich phosphate bond which essentially traps or stores energy. Other reactions, which break this bond, release the stored energy for use in various other energy-requiring reactions, such as breaking the triple bond of N_2.

The ability of a biological system to fix N_2 is dependent on the presence of a particular enzyme system known as nitrogenase which catalyzes the conversion of N_2 into a reduced form (ammonia combined with certain organic compounds), which can then be assimilated and utilized for growth by microorganisms and higher life-forms. The nitrogenase system consists of two different protein components (enzymes). One of the enzymes (azoferredoxin) is an iron-containing protein composed of two subunits. The second enzyme (molybdoferredoxin) contains both iron and molybdenum and is composed of four subunits. The nitrogenase system is dependent on an energy source (ATP), magnesium ions, and an electron donor in order to function. The two components combine and function together as a single system. The molybdoferredoxin enzyme is extremely sensitive to inhibition by oxygen. Components of the nitrogenase system for different organisms have been combined to form an active "hybrid" nitrogenase system, indicating an apparent general similarity in systems derived from diverse sources. Nitrogenase has so far been detected only in certain prokaryotic microorganisms.

The reduction of N_2, as catalyzed by the nitrogenase system, is a two-step reaction involving (1) electron activation and (2) substrate reduction. Electron activation involves the coupling of ATP hydrolysis (energy release) with electron transfer to the nitrogenase system. This is the rate-limiting step of the nitrogenase reaction and accounts for the observed high-energy requirement of the overall reaction. It is estimated that 15–20 ATP molecules are hydrolyzed per molecule of N_2 fixed.

A number of different organic acids (pyruvate, malate, and formate) and flavoproteins have been identified as electron donors functioning in nitrogenase systems from various sources.

Isotope studies using $^{15}N_2$ have revealed no enzyme-free intermediates between N_2 and ammonia. The ammonia resulting from fixation is rapidly incorporated into certain amino acids, such as glutamine or alanine. The amino nitrogen may then be transferred to other amino acids and N-containing compounds by a variety of commonly occurring amino transfer reactions.

The nitrogenase system is not absolutely specific for N_2 as a substrate. It will catalyze the reduction of several different small nitrogen, oxygen, or carbon triple-bonded substrates, such as acetylene, hydrogen cyanide, isocyanide, and nitrite. The ability of nitrogenase to reduce acetylene to ethylene is the basis for a highly sensitive assay for measurement of nitrogenase activity. The method involves the detection of minute amounts of ethylene by the use of gas chromatography.

Other methods of measurement or detection of nitrogen fixation are less sensitive but may be useful in certain situations. Historically, nitrogen-fixing activity has been detected qualitatively by demonstrating the ability of an organism to grow and reproduce during continued transfer on a nitrogen-free artificial growth medium. A quantitative estimate of N_2 fixed is possible by analyzing for total nitrogen present in the system (Kjeldahl procedure) after an appropriate period of time. A frequently used and more sensitive method using mass spectrometry involves quantitative measurement of the reduction of the stable isotope $^{15}N_2$ by a particular system.

The synthesis and functioning of the nitrogenase system are subject to a number of controlling factors. Ammonia and oxygen will independently inhibit the synthesis of nitrogenase enzymes and will, in addition, inhibit the activity of the enzyme system if it is already present. Such factors as supply of organic substrate, ADP levels, pesticide residues, or micronutrient deficiencies may also severely reduce the activity of the system.

It is estimated that BNF on a global scale may attain a value of 1.75×10^8 metric tons of nitrogen fixed per year. The amount of nitrogen fixed in any restricted situation would depend upon the prevailing environmental conditions and the nature of the biological system(s) present which are capable of nitrogen fixation. For particular situations, nitrogen fixation rates may vary from barely detectable to several hundred kilograms of nitrogen per hectare per year. The significance of the contribution of any system to the nitrogen economy in any situation is a function of the nitrogen supply and demand of the biological community.

BNF is known to occur to a varying degree in numerous diverse environments, including soils; fresh and marine waters and sediments; on or within the roots, stems, and leaves of certain higher plants; and within the digestive tracts of some animals. The potential for nitrogen fixation may be assumed for any environment capable of supporting a diverse microbial population.

Biological systems which are capable of fixing N_2 are historically classified as nonsymbiotic (by free-living microorganisms) or symbiotic (by microorganisms living in association with another organism).

Nonsymbiotic nitrogen fixation by free-living microorganisms is now recognized in approximately 20 genera of bacteria and 15 genera of cyanobacteria (blue-green algae). The amounts of nitrogen fixed by free-living bacteria in the soil, such as *Azotobacter*, *Beijerinckia*, and *Clostridium*, may achieve an approximate maximum of 15 kg N/ha/yr. This relatively low estimated contribution is the result of limited availability of suitable organic substrates and low bacterial populations in the soil environment. Nitrogen fixation is characteristically higher in environments (tropical soils) where such factors as substrate availability, temperature, and moisture are more favorable to the maintenance and activity of a high bacterial population. Anaerobic bacteria *(Clostridium)* predominate in grassland and waterlogged soils and soil aggregates, where oxygen supply to the microenvironment of the bacteria is severely restricted. Amendment of soil with a readily available organic substrate generally results in some increase in nitrogen fixation. Attempts to increase fixation in unamended soil by addition of large populations of bacteria (soil inoculation) are generally unsuccessful. The indigenous microbial population is in equilibrium with the soil environment. The increased population resulting from inoculation is therefore transitory and will rapidly die back to the original equilibrium in an unamended soil, where no provision has been made to create environmental changes supportive of a higher microbial population.

Very little information is available concerning the possible contribution of cyanobacteria to the nitrogen economy of soils, but maximum gains of 50 kg N/ha/yr have been reported. Nitrogen-fixing activity of these aerobic, photosynthetic organisms is strongly dependent on prevailing availability of favorable moisture conditions and adequate sunlight.

Living plant roots release a wide variety of simple organic compounds which may be used as a carbon and energy source by free-living soil bacteria. This continuous supply of substrate supports a higher microbial population in the volume of soil immediately surrounding the plant root (rhizosphere). Evidence indicates that indigenous nitrogen-fixing bacteria are frequent components of this heterogeneous population and that they may fix significant amounts of nitrogen in such associations. This effect may be proportional to the degree of intimacy of the association. Substrate released from the roots would be available in greater concentration to those microorganisms more closely associated spatially with the root. This phenomenon appears most striking in certain combinations of bacteria with some tropical grasses which have a high photosynthetic efficiency and grow under environmental conditions favoring high photosynthetic activity. The roots of such plants therefore supply the nitrogen-fixing microorganisms with a relatively high and sustained supply of substrate (photosynthate) which is more limiting in the rhizosphere associations of most plants. The significant contribution of photosynthetic (cyanobacteria) and nonphotosynthetic *(Clostridium)* microorganisms to nitrogen fixation in the rhizosphere of rice is well recognized.

In addition, nitrogenase activity has been detected in the soil surrounding the mycorrhizal roots of several conifers and in the rhizospheres of marine *(Thalassia)* and freshwater *(Glyceria)* angiosperms. The leaf surface (phyllosphere) of certain plants in warm, humid tropical regions may provide an additional favorable environment for the growth and nitrogen-fixing activity of such free-living bacteria as *Azotobacter, Beijerinckia,* and *Klebsiella.*

Under appropriate environmental conditions, cyanobacteria may contribute significantly to nitrogen gains in freshwater environments, and *Clos-*

tridium may play a similar important role in freshwater sediments. Most of the nitrogen fixation in marine environments (about 20% of the total amount of annual biological fixation) is attributed to the cyanobacteria, but numerous representatives of facultative, heterotrophic and anaerobic, photosynthetic nitrogen-fixers have been isolated from marine environments.

Free-living nitrogen-fixing anaerobic bacteria are present and fix nitrogen in the intestinal contents of a variety of animals (herbivores) and also in humans. Nitrogenase activity is generally quite low, and its significance in terms of satisfying nutritional requirements of the host appears doubtful.

The most significant contribution to BNF comes from the symbiotic association of certain microorganisms with the roots of higher plants. This is classically exemplified by bacteria *(Rhizobium)* which characteristically infect the roots of most plants of the Leguminosae with a high degree of host specificity. On the roots small nodules are formed which become filled with a morphologically and physiologically altered form of the bacteria (bacteroids) which may fix appreciable amounts of nitrogen. This symbiosis alone accounts for 20% of global biological nitrogen fixed annually. The legumes represent a major direct source of food for humans and of forage for livestock, and therefore represent a critical contribution to world food production. It is significant that agricultural scientists have learned to manipulate this symbiotic relationship in agronomic practice, employing selected combinations of bacteria and legumes in specific situations to obtain maximum crop production on land which is low in fertility and frequently unsuitable for growth of nonlegume crops. Nitrogen fixation rates from 75 to 300 kg N/ha/yr are common in various systems.

Numerous genera of nonleguminous angiosperms, such as *Alnus, Casuarina, Ceanothus, Coriaria,* and *Myrica,* form root nodules in response to infection by actinomycetelike organisms. These associations may achieve fixation rates as high as 100 kg N/ha/yr and may occur as climax vegetation or as pioneer species in adverse soil environments. Some gymnosperms, such as *Cycas, Macrozamia,* and *Podocarpus,* are capable of forming similar nitrogen-fixing root nodule associations. A variety of additional plant-microbe symbiotic nitrogen-fixing associations have been reported. Examples include the bacterium *Klebsiella* in leaf nodules of *Psychotria,* and associations of cyanobacteria with fungi (lichens), liverworts *(Blasia),* angiosperms *(Gunnera),* gymnosperms *(Encephalartos),* and the water fern *Azolla.*

Increasing information concerning the genetic information *(nif* gene) in various microorganisms which confers nitrogen-fixing ability now makes the creation of new and perhaps more efficient nitrogen-fixing organisms and symbiotic associations more than a theoretical possibility.

[DAVID H. HUBBELL]

Bibliography: P. S. Nutman (ed.), *Symbiotic Nitrogen Fixation in Plants,* 1976; A. Quispel (ed.), *The Biology of Nitrogen Fixation,* 1974; W. D. P. Stewart (ed.), *Nitrogen Fixation by Free-Living Micro-organisms,* 1975.

Nut crop culture

The cultivation of plants which produce nuts. This term is defined loosely to include a great variety of fruits or seeds (estimated at about 80), which regardless of their morphological structure have at maturity a hard, dry shell enclosing a kernel consisting of cotyledons or endosperm. The botanical term nut is defined as an indehiscent, one-celled, one-seeded, hard fruit derived from a single, simple or compound ovary. The peanut is a notable exception because the plant is a herbaceous legume which is grown as an annual field crop. The so-called nuts are analogous to peapods but mature under the soil surface. The roasted kernels are used in the same way as other nuts. Nut kernels are rich in fat and protein and furnish concentrated, digestible food important in local and world commerce. Coconuts and palm nuts supply large quantities of industrial oil.

Plants producing nut crops are very diverse in their botanical classification, type, and climatic and cultural requirements. Pine nuts are the seeds of conifers, coconuts are from a palm, brazil nuts from a tropical evergreen, and pecans and walnuts from large deciduous trees of the temperate zone. Many nut crops are produced from wild trees which receive little care, for example, pine nuts, brazil nuts, and black walnuts. However, with the destruction of native sources, the increased demand, and particularly the invention of mechanical devices for harvesting and processing, the trend is toward more intensive culture in which sophisticated machines are used at all stages of culture and processing. Cultural methods differ according to the nature of the plant, its soil requirements, the climate, available labor, and other factors.

Nuts important in world commerce

Common name	Scientific name	Plant type	Origin	Climatic zone adaptation	Est. annual production, metric tons in shell*	Principal uses and producing areas
Almond	Prunus amygdalus	Small deciduous tree	Asia Minor	Temperate, subtropical; planted	325,000	Food; Mediterranean countries, California
Brazil nut	Bertholletia excelsa	Very large evergreen tree	Amazon Basin	Tropical; wild	50,000	Food; Brazil, Bolivia
Black walnut	Juglans nigra	Large deciduous tree	Central and eastern United States	Temperate; mostly wild	20,000	Food, lumber, ground-up shells
Cashew	Anacardium occidentale	Evergreen tree to 40 ft	Tropical America	Tropical; wild and planted	160,000	Food, shell oil; India, East Africa
Chestnut	Castanea sp.	Large, spreading, deciduous trees	Eastern United States, Europe, Asia	Temperate; wild and planted	7,000	Food, lumber; Europe, China, Japan
Coconut	Cocos nucifera	Large palm	Probably Polynesia	Tropical; wild and planted	3,689,000 copra	Food, edible and industrial oil, fiber; Philippines, tropics of Pacific
Cola nut	Cola acuminata	Evergreen tree to 40 ft	West Africa	Tropical; wild and planted	100	Stimulant; West Africa
English or Persian walnut	Juglans regia	Large deciduous tree	Eastern Europe, Asia	Temperate; wild and planted	185,000	Food, oil, lumber; Mediterranean basin, California, China
Filbert	Corylus avellana	Deciduous shrub or small tree	Eastern Europe, Asia Minor	Temperate; wild and planted	310,000	Food; Turkey, Italy, Spain, northwestern United States
Macadamia nut	Macadamia ternifolia	Evergreen tree to 60 ft	Queensland, New South Wales	Tropical and subtropical; planted	4,325	Food; Australia, Hawaii
Palm nut	Elaeis guineensis	Large palm	West and Central Africa	Tropical; wild and planted	1,050,000	Edible and industrial oil; West Africa, Indonesia, Brazil
Peanut	Arachis hypogaea	Annual crop plant	Brazil	Tropical, subtropical, warm temperate; planted	18,000,000	Food, edible oil; India, Africa, United States
Pecan	Carya pecan	Large, deciduous tree	Southern and central United States	Warm temperate; wild and planted	120,000	Food; Central and southern United States
Pine nuts	Pinus sp.	Evergreen conifers	Europe, Asia, southwestern North America	Temperate; wild	30,000	Food; Southern Europe, Asia, North America
Pistachio nut	Pistacia vera	Small, spreading, deciduous tree	Asia Minor	Warm temperate; wild and planted	14,700	Food; Iran, Turkey, Syria, Italy
Tung nut	Aleurites fordii	Small tree to 20 ft	Central Asia	Warm temperate, or subtropical; planted	150,000 oil	Industrial oil, paints; China, southern United States

*Figures reflect relative world production for both domestic and commercial use rather than trade statistics for any one year.

As with other orchard crops, pest and disease control is important wherever concentrated plantings are made. Effective control measures are related to the life history of the particular pest or disease, since each may require a different approach in cultural practice or spray program. *See* PLANT DISEASE; PLANT DISEASE CONTROL.

On a world basis, nut-bearing plants have been particularly important in supplying food for native populations and wildlife. Thus the disappearance of the native chestnut in the eastern United States is related to the scarcity of wild turkeys, and the encroachment of civilization on the supply of "mast" (beechnuts and acorns) contributed to the extinction of the passenger pigeon.

With the increasing population pressure on world food resources and the loss of agricultural lands by soil erosion and urbanization, some attention is being given to growing nut crops along with other food-producing trees for erosion control and increasing the overall world food supply. In general, the demand for and world commerce in nut crops have been increasing with the increase in population. Estimate of world commerce in edible (shelled) tree nuts is given as nearly 500,000 short tons (450,000 metric tons) in 1973. Information on the commercially important nut crops is given in the table. *See* ALMOND; BRAZIL NUT; CASHEW; COCONUT; COLA; FILBERT; MACADAMIA NUT; PEANUT; PECAN; PINE NUT; PISTACHIO; WALNUT.

[LAURENCE H. MAC DANIELS]

Nutmeg

A delicately flavored spice obtained from the nutmeg tree (*Myristica fragrans*), a native of the Moluccas, or Spice Islands. The tree is a dark-leafed evergreen 30–60 ft high, and is a member of the

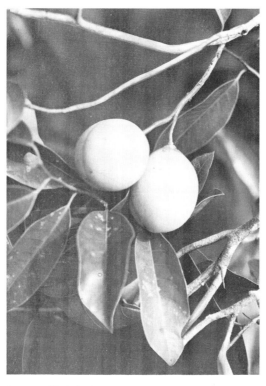

Nutmeg (*Myristica fragrans*), mature fruits. (*USDA*)

nutmeg family (Myristicaceae). The golden-yellow, mature fruits resemble apricots (see illustration). They gradually lose moisture and when completely ripe, the husk (pericarp) splits open, exposing the shiny brown seed covered with a red, fibrous, aromatic aril which is the mace. The kernel inside the seed coat is the nutmeg of commerce. Fruits are produced throughout the year and are picked when the husks split open. The mace is removed from the husks, flattened, and dried. It is used in making pickles, ketchup, and sauces. When the seeds are thoroughly dried, the shells are cracked off, the kernels are removed and sorted, and often treated with lime to prevent damage by insects. Grated nutmeg is used in custards, puddings, and other sweet dishes, also in various beverages. Nutmeg oil is used in medicine, perfumery, and dentifrices, and in the tobacco industry. *See* SPICE AND FLAVORING.

[PERRY D. STRAUSBAUGH/EARL L. CORE]

Nutrition

The science of nourishment, including the study of the nutrients that each organism must obtain from its environment in order to maintain life and reproduce. Although each kind of organism has its distinctive needs which can be studied separately, a far-reaching biochemical unity in nature has been discovered which gives vastly more coherence to the whole subject. Many nutrients, such as amino acids, minerals, and vitamins, needed by higher organisms may also be needed by the lowest forms of life – single-celled bacteria and protozoa. The recognition of this fact has made possible highly important developments in biochemistry.

Mammals need for their nutrition (aside from water and oxygen) a highly complex mixture of chemical substances, including amino acids; carbohydrates; certain lipids; a great variety of minerals, including several which are required only in minute amounts, commonly referred to as trace elements; and vitamins, organic substances of diverse structure which are treated as a group only because as nutrients they are required in relatively small amounts. *See* AMINO ACIDS; CARBOHYDRATE METABOLISM; LIPID METABOLISM; PROTEIN METABOLISM; VITAMIN.

Most nutrients were recognized in the 19th century, but the vitamins and some trace minerals did not become known as fundamental cogs in the machinery of all living things until the early 20th century. The discovery of vitamins, and some of the trace elements, originally came about through the recognition of deficiency diseases, such as beriberi, scurvy, pellagra, and rickets, which arise because of specific nutritional lacks and can be cured or prevented by supplying the needed nutrients. *See* BERIBERI; PELLAGRA; RICKETS; SCURVY.

Different species of mammals have distinctive nutritional needs. Guinea pigs, monkeys, and human beings, for example, require an exogenous supply of ascorbic acid (vitamin C) to maintain life and health, whereas many experimental animals, including rats, do not. It is significant, however, that ascorbic acid is an essential part of the metabolic machinery of animals that do not need an exogenous supply. Rat tissues, for example, are relatively rich in ascorbic acid; unlike guinea pigs these animals are genetically endowed with biochemical mechanisms for producing ascorbic acid from carbohydrate. *See* ASCORBIC ACID.

One of the bases for current and continued interest in nutrition is the fact that individuals who have differing genetic backgrounds have differing nutritional needs, considered quantitatively; for this reason various human ills may arise because the individuals concerned do not get all of the nutrients in amounts compatible with their own distinctive requirements.

Every cell and tissue in the entire body requires continued adequate nutrition in order to perform its functions adequately. Since a multitude of functions, involving the production of specific chemical substances (hormones, for example) and the regulation of numerous processes, are performed by cells and tissues, it is clear that improper nutrition may produce or contribute to almost every conceivable type of illness. *See* MALNUTRITION; METABOLIC DISORDERS.

[ROGER J. WILLIAMS]

Bibliography: G. H. Beaton and E. W. McHenry, *Nutrition: A Comprehensive Treatise*, 3 vols., 1964–1966; R. L. Pike and M. L. Brown, *Nutrition: An Integrated Approach*, 1967; R. J. Williams, *Nutrition in a Nutshell*, 1962.

Oats

An agricultural crop grown for its grain and straw in most countries of the temperate zones of the world. In the major oat-growing states of the midwestern United States (Iowa, North Dakota, South Dakota, Minnesota, and Wisconsin) the crop is raised for grain, whereas in the Southern states (Texas, Oklahoma, and Georgia) it is used for pasture or a combination of pasture and grain. About 90% of the annual oat grain production is used for animal feeds, and about 10% is processed into food for humans, for example, oatmeal and other cereal products.

Among the cereal grains grown in the United States, oats is exceeded in importance only by corn, wheat, and sorghum. Total United States production in 1973 was 664,000,000 bu. harvested from approximately 14,000,000 acres. *See* CORN; SORGHUM; WHEAT.

In general, oats is a cool-season crop which requires a moist climate. It grows well on both light and heavy soils if sufficient moisture and fertility nutrients are available. In the Central and Northern states, oats is spring-sown; but in the Southern states it is fall-sown. In the Corn Belt it is grown in crop rotation with corn, soybeans, and forages.

Origin and description. Oats probably became an agricultural crop about 2000 years ago, most likely starting in the Mediterranean area. The 15 species of oats in the genus *Avena* are divided into three groups on the basis of chromosome number: 14, 28, or 42. Of the seven species that make up the 14-chromosome group, only *A. strigosa* is grown commercially on small agricultural acreage in Portugal and Brazil. The two 42-chromosome species, *A. fatua* and *A. sterilis*, grow in natural stands in the eastern Mediterranean area and provide wild pastures for sheep and goats. Seeds of both wild species shatter at maturity to ensure annual reseeding.

Crosses among the 28-chromosome species and among the 42-chromosome species are easy to make and the hybrids are fully fertile, but only certain 14-chromosome species can be intercrossed. Crosses among species with different chromosome numbers can be made also, but usually the hybrids are sterile or only partly fertile. *See* BREEDING (PLANT).

Within the 42-chromosome cultivated species there is wide variation among varieties for all plant traits. Oats belong to the Graminae (grass) family; thus the oat plant forms a crown at the soil surface from which a fibrous root system penetrates the soil. Most of the roots are concentrated in the upper foot of soil, but some grow to a depth of 5 ft. Under thick seeding only one or two culms develop, but when plants are spaced, 10–30 culms may develop. Culms usually grow 2–5 ft tall, and they are terminated with inflorescences called panicles. Each panicle usually bears 10–75 spikelets on its numerous branches (Fig. 1). A spikelet is enclosed by two papery glumes and bears two or three florets, each with an ovary, two stigmas, and three anthers enclosed in a lemma and palea (Fig. 2). The flowers are normally self-pollinated but 1–2% outcrossing may occur. The stem has 7–9 nodes, and a leaf grows at each node. Internodes of the stems are hollow. *See* GRASS CROPS.

In most varieties the lemma and palea adhere to the oat seed after threshing. A trait used to determine market grade of oats is the color of the lemma, which may be white, yellow, gray, brown, red, or black. The major trait that distinguishes wild from cultivated oats is seed shattering. In cultivated species the seed attachment is persistent, and it can be separated from the panicle only by threshing.

Varieties. The world collection of oats, maintained by the U.S. Department of Agriculture, contains more than 14,000 lines of 42-chromosome types. These represent lines from wild species and from varieties produced at breeding stations. The collection represents a vast range of genetic types that can be used for varietal improvement. Since 1960 breeders have put special emphasis on improving lodging and disease resistance, grain quality, and yield of new oat varieties (see table). These varieties have been developed by crossing strains from the world collection to obtain better combinations of genetic traits. A variety called "multiline" has been developed to control rusts. While each

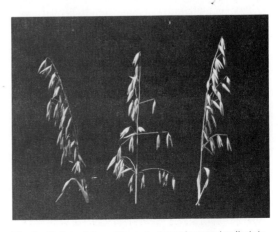

Fig. 1. Oat panicles with many branches and spikelets.

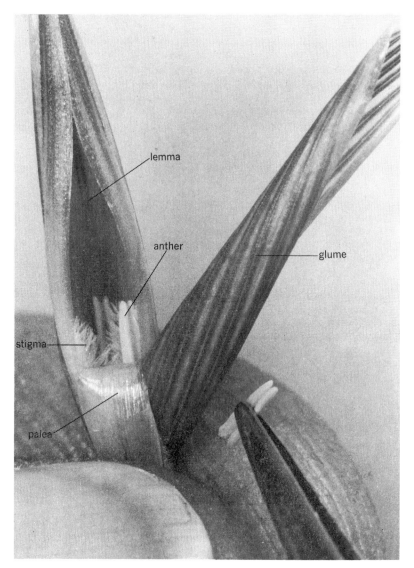

Fig. 2. An oat flower; two oat grains are shown at the lower right.

seeded in March or April at a rate of 2–3 bu/acre on disked or plowed land. Winter oats are sown in October or November. Mature oats are harvested with a combine, either direct or after being windrowed to dry (Fig. 3). For safe storage oat grain should contain no more than 13% moisture. Straw of harvested oats is either worked into the soil for humus or baled and stored for use as bedding for livestock. *See* AGRICULTURE, SOIL AND CROP PRACTICES IN; LEGUME FORAGES.

Uses. Oat grain usually contains 10–16% protein, which makes it especially good for rations for young livestock and for human food. Some strains of *A. sterilis* have up to 30% protein. Dehulled oat seeds are used extensively for making breakfast cereals, such as porridge made from rolled oats. In general, oat grain contains adequate quantities of minerals and B vitamins for normal diet. The fat content is low. Oat hulls are used to make furfural, an important chemical in nylon manufacturing.

[KENNETH J. FREY]

Diseases. Like virtually all agricultural crops, oats are plagued with various diseases, major and minor. Stem rust caused by *Puccinia graminis* var. *avenae*, crown rust caused by *P. coronata* var. *avenae*, two smuts caused by *Ustilago avenae* and *U. kolleri*, and at times root rots are of major importance, and half a dozen leaf, stem, and kernel blights and several virus infections exact their toll in varying degree, depending on weather and soil conditions.

The rusts are the most devastating of all and in seasons particularly favorable to their development may reduce the yield to one-half or even one-fourth of normal. Both rusts are caused by specific fungus parasites that invade tissues of the oat plants, where they grow and absorb nutrients from their host. After about 10 days after infection the fungus bursts through the epidermis of the oat plant in countless places to produce hundreds of thousands of microscopic spores, the fungus "seeds," which invade other oat plants and produce more spores. These rusts can live through the winter in the Northern states and start new epidemics in the spring, provided they have appropriate alternate hosts on which to get started (barberry, *Berberis* sp., for stem rust and buckthorn, *Rhamnus* sp., for crown rust). The most devastating epidemics, however, start in the Southern states, where the rusts can continue to propagate all through the winter on oats alone. In years when abundant rains and dews coincide with the growing seasons over wide areas of the country and when temperatures are favorable, this southern-propagated rust is likely to advance northward over the oat fields as the crop develops. Such waves of destruction may progress from Mexico 2000 mi northward into Canada. Fortunately, the precise combination of circumstances that favor such epidemics occur only occasionally; the last epidemics were in 1953 and 1954. In other years rust may develop to only a moderate degree or not at all.

The loose and covered smuts caused by *Ustilago avenae* and *U. kolleri* likewise are fungus parasites. However, these invade the oat plants only through the sprout of the germinating seed and only while it is below ground. Once inside its host, the parasitic strands of the smut fungus develop gently and

multiline variety is uniform for all agronomic traits, it contains several genes for resistance to a single disease.

Cultural practices. In the Corn Belt, oats usually follow corn or soybeans in crop rotation. It is used as a companion crop for forage seedings; that is, alfalfa and oats are planted simultaneously, and the oats are harvested for grain in the first year and alfalfa for hay in subsequent years. Spring oats are

Average performance of oat varieties from different years

Variety	Years	Yield, bu/acre	Lodging score	Weight, lb/bu
Richland	1930	87	3.8	29.9
Bonham	1945–1950	94	3.1	33.4
Cherokee		95	3.1	33.0
Burnett	1956–1958	99	3.0	33.8
Newton		101	2.4	32.2
Dodge	1960–1964	100	1.9	34.0
Nodaway		99	2.1	34.6
Tonka		97	1.9	36.0

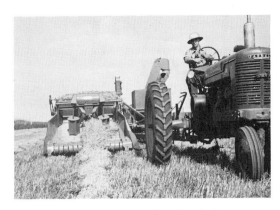

Fig. 3. Combining an oat crop from the windrow.

unseen, keeping pace with the growth of the oat plant until it heads. Then the smut appropriates the host-plant nutrients which are intended to produce grain and changes the young kernels into a mass of black powder (spores), the reproductive bodies of the fungus. These spores contaminate the surface of the grain of nearby healthy plants and there wait to be planted with the seed and infect the next crop.

Red leaf of oats, caused by the barley yellow-dwarf virus, causes frequent crop losses and was particularly destructive in 1949, 1953, and 1959. The virus multiplies in numerous grasses, including barley, wheat, and oats. Aphids acquire the virus by feeding on red-leaf plants and readily transmit it by subsequent feeding on healthy plants. In the South the aphids actively feed and propagate throughout the winter. Occasionally in the spring they are blown northward in great numbers from Texas and Oklahoma into Iowa, Minnesota, and Wisconsin, where they effectively inoculate seedling oats with the virus. *See* PLANT VIRUS.

Most of the various leaf, stem, and grain spots and root rots are caused by other parasitic fungi and bacteria. Red leaf, blue dwarf, and mosaic are caused by viruses. Other disorders may be due to nutrient deficiencies, to soil or climatic factors, or to insects. *See* PLANT, MINERALS ESSENTIAL TO; PLANT DISEASE.

Disease control. Since oats yield a relatively small return per acre, only inexpensive disease-control practices are economical. The least expensive control is the use of resistant varieties produced by plant breeders and pathologists at various state and Federal experiment stations and by some private breeders. Although most commercial varieties of oats have some degree of resistance to one or several diseases, none is resistant to all. In many pathogens—notably the rust fungi—variants arise through hybridization or mutation, and these attack previously resistant varieties. It is then necessary to breed different varieties. For some diseases a second line of defense may be employed, such as chemical seed treatments that control smuts and seedling blights. *See* FUNGISTAT AND FUNGICIDE.

Rotation and maintenance of balanced soil fertility are important controls of root rots and some stem and leaf blights. *See* FERTILIZING; PLANT DISEASE CONTROL.   [M. B. MOORE]

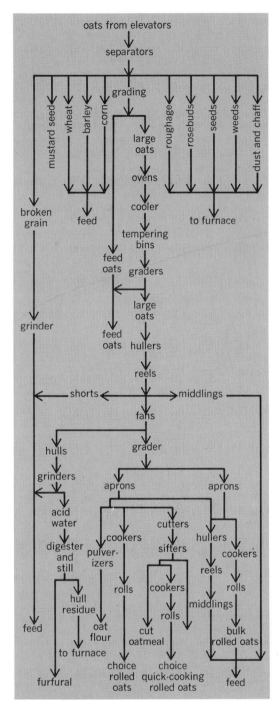

Fig. 4. An oat-mill process flow diagram. (*From M. E. Parker, E. H. Harvey, and E. S. Stateler, Elements of Food Engineering, vol. 1, Reinhold, 1952*)

Processing. The oat kernel has a fibrous hull inedible by humans. The goal in milling oats is to obtain the maximum yield of clean, uniform, sound, whole oat kernels which are free from hulls, floury material, extraneous matter, and undesirable flavors. Oat kernels with the hulls removed are called groats. The percentage of hulls can vary from 21 to 43% but averages about 25%. An oat-mill process flow diagram is shown in Fig. 4.

Separating and grading. Oats, at the start of processing, are called green oats and may contain other grains, foreign materials, and varying quantities of oats not satisfactory for milling. To obtain milling oats, all of these undesirable materials must be removed. This is done by a series of separations and gradings according to length, width, and density. Length graders consist of shaker screens with various-sized openings. Corn, sticks, and trash are separated from oats on the large-hole shaker screens; small seeds, through small-hole screens. Disk separators, which consist of indented plates revolving on a horizontal shaft, are the main type of indent machine. Small indents in the rotating plates lift out seeds and broken material. The oat kernel, being long, falls out of the indents on the plate. Width graders consist of slotted cylindrical-screen machines which separate thin oats through narrow slots and milling oats through wider slots. Materials such as wheat, double oats, barley, and corn pass through the cylindrical screen. Air currents are used to separate light from heavy grain by passing air through the grain as it falls.

Drying. Milling oats are subjected to drying or roasting. The usual type of drier consists of large, open steel pans 10–12 ft in diameter and placed one above another in stacks of 7 to 14. The bottom of each pan is steam-jacketed. Oats are fed to the center edge by sweeps as long as the diameter of the pan. The sweeps, as they ride about on the surface of the pan, mix the grain and prevent any oats from remaining too long in contact with the heating surface. When the oats reach the edge of one pan, they fall into chutes which carry them back to the center of the next pan below; then the process is repeated. It requires 1–1½ hr for the grain to pass through the drier. The moisture of the grain is reduced to between 8½ and 7%. It then passes to a cooler where air circulation further reduces the moisture content about another 1%.

The roasting process serves several purposes, such as developing flavor, improving keeping quality, and facilitating the breaking away of the groats from the hull during milling.

Hulling. The conventional type of huller used to produce oat groats consists of two horizontal circular carborundum or emery-stone disks, one above the other. The lower stone is stationary; the upper one revolves rapidly. Dry oats are fed by gravity through an opening in the center of the upper stone and pass between the stones to the outer edge. The distance between the stones is adjusted to regulate the space so that the hulls may be removed without crushing the groats. To accomplish this, oats are graded for size, including both length and thickness.

A further development in hulling is the use of impact hullers. The oats are fed to the center of a high-speed rotor which has a horizontal plate with fins that throw the oats by centrifugal force against a liner. The liner may have a covering of special-composition rubber. The hulls are loosened from the oat groats by impact. One advantage of this type of huller is that the grading is not quite so important as in the rotating stone system, which requires that the space between the stones be adjusted for different sizes of oats.

The following products are obtained from the hullers: hulls, groats, broken groats and meal, flour, unhulled oats, and a small amount of barley. These materials are separated by air aspiration and screening. The choicest, plumpest groats are used to make package-grade rolled oats, while the less choice groats make either bulk or feed rolled oats. The broken material becomes feed meal.

Products. From milled oats, the following products are produced: steel-cut oats, rolled oats, oatmeal, and oat flour. From oat hulls, furfural is manufactured.

Steel-cutting is done with rotary granulators. The purpose of cutting is to convert groats to uniform granules. The granules are flaked between rolls to produce a quick-cooking breakfast cereal.

Rolled oats are made by treating the groats with live steam just before rolling. After rolling, the flakes are passed through separators to remove all fine material. Rolled oats are used in breakfast foods, cookies, and bread.

Oat flour can be made by several means such as hammer mills, attrition mills, or pulverizers. Oat flours have uses as antioxidants, constituents of baby food, and in soaps and cosmetic preparations.

Oat hulls form the starting material for the manufacture of furfural. It is made by the destructive distillation of oat hulls in the presence of acid and steam under controlled conditions which change the pentosans in the hulls to pentoses. These are then dehydrated to furfural. Furfural is used as a solvent and in the manufacture of plastics and nylon.

[JOHN A. SHELLENBERGER]

Bibliography: F. N. Briggs and P. F. Knowles, *Introduction to Plant Breeding*, 1967; H. J. Brounlee and F. L. Genderson, Oats and oat products: Culture, botany, seed structure, milling, composition, and uses, *Cereal Chem.*, 15:257–272, 1938; F. A. Coffman, *Oats and Oat Improvement*, 1961; M. B. Jacobs, *The Chemistry and Technology of Food and Food Products*, 1951; M. A. Joslyn and J. L. Heid, *Food Processing Operations*, vol. 3, 1964; W. H. Leonard and J. H. Martin, *Cereal Crops*, 1963.

Obesity

Obesity is a major health problem in the United States. The U.S. Public Health Service has reported that between 25 and 45% of all Americans over the age of 30 are more than 20% overweight. The epidemic of obesity relates significantly to the great number of associated diseases that increase morbidity and mortality. Obesity is commonly associated with hypertension, mature-onset diabetes, cardiovascular disease, impaired respiratory function, gallbladder disease, renal disease, and cirrhosis of the liver. There is little doubt that obesity impairs the health of people, reduces their quality of living, and hastens their death.

Causes. As more is learned about obesity, it is increasingly evident that obesity is a complex problem associated with cultural patterns, lifestyle, psychological factors and, in the United States, a tremendous availability of all kinds of foods. Obesity may also be related to familial factors, and adult weight has been strongly correlated with infant weight, parental weight, and educational level. Obesity is seen more often in the lower socioeconomic groups. Very rarely is it due to an identifiable organic cause, such as endocrine imbalance or "glandular difficulty," or specific damage to the appetite and feeding control centers in the central nervous system. No matter what the etiology of obesity, it invariably reflects a caloric intake exceeding caloric expenditure. *See* CALORIE.

Some have postulated that the increased use of bottle feeding for infants, instead of breast feeding, has influenced their caloric intake at the discretion of the mother, rather than having the infant's own physiological control mechanisms tell it to stop feeding at the breast. Obese children have approximately an 80% chance of being obese as adults. Obesity initiated in early childhood not only results in an increased size of fat cells, but also an increase in their number. Normal cellular obesity, in which the adipocytes are increased in size but not in number, generally begins during adulthood. Feeding patterns have been implicated in excessive weight gains wherein large nutrient loads consumed at decreased frequency may lead to increased fat synthesis. Also, glucose intolerance, coupled with high blood levels of insulin, may be a primary cause of obesity. More often, however, it is a secondary effect enhancing the continuation of obesity. It has been said that obesity is impossible in the absence of adequate tissue concentrations of insulin. Insulin is, in fact, a basic requirement for the transfer of glucose from the serum to the cells, where the glucose is further metabolized.

Regardless of the numerous theories that have been proposed as the cause of obesity, the inevitable conclusion is that an excessive accumulation of fat follows the intake of excessive calories, particularly when caloric expenditure is less than caloric intake on an extended basis.

Overeating. The great majority of individuals maintain a normal, if not ideal, weight over a period of many years, which indicates that there must be some mechanism in the normal individual which relates food intake to caloric needs. This "appestat" appears to react primarily to an intake of food, and various mechanisms have been proposed—chemical, nervous, and thermal—to explain why the appestat cuts off food intake at the proper time to prevent obesity. The appestat mechanism is so effective that for most adults caloric intake matches caloric output and the body weight remains constant. In children the balance is so well set that there are enough surplus calories to determine optimal growth without the deposition of excessive fat.

Factors affecting food intake. Genetics seems to have an influence on food intake. The chances of a child being overweight are 75% if both parents are overweight, but only 9% if neither of them is overweight. It is of course difficult to distinguish whether this result is due to the heavy eating patterns which the child observes in the obese adults and copies, or whether this is indeed an inherited characteristic.

As indicated above, there is very little evidence that obese individuals have a significant endocrine disorder. The percentage of obese individuals affected by glandular dysfunction, and particularly thyroid or pituitary gland deficiency, is so small that this cannot be given serious consideration, although it should not be ruled out in the evalua-

tion and treatment of the obese person.

Exercise, or energy expenditure, is an important factor in dealing with obesity. Unfortunately, people who lead sedentary lives do not always reduce their caloric intake in proportion to their low caloric requirements and, as a result, become progressively overweight.

Psychological factors are most commonly given as the cause for overweight. Emotional trauma and a host of daily living stresses, anxieties, frustrations, and insecurities are compensated for by excessive eating. It is also true that many individuals eat a great deal simply because they love food. This is probably the simplest explanation for obesity. Some have thought that individuals overeat and become obese because they gain a sense of security and a feeling of largeness, which may be a compensation for a feeling of inferiority.

The question has been raised as to whether or not there is a specific satiety factor for particular foods or types of foods and whether this factor may be important in determining the appropriate choices of foods for nutritional needs. One of the most common problems associated with food choices is the "sweet tooth" of many individuals who have an inordinate desire for anything sweet, leading to excessive caloric consumption between meals.

One important factor in considering excessive caloric consumption is the caloric density of the American diet, which is very high in fat with approximately 45% of the calories contributed by fat in most diets. It is therefore possible to consume a large number of calories by eating only a small amount of food. In cultures in which the fat content of the diet is much lower, particularly in the Orient, the traditional fat content may be only 15% of the total calories and obesity is far less common. It must be remembered, too, that alcohol contributes seven calories (29 joules) per gram, and the individual consuming two or three drinks per day is encouraging the development of obesity.

Treatment or management. The management or treatment of obesity is difficult, poorly understood, and usually ineffective. Doctors do not as yet have a totally effective way of treating obese people. Even individuals who have reduced may be considered thin "fat people" with their adipocytes continually asking to be refilled. The number of obese individuals who have reduced and stayed so is disappointingly small, particularly over a long period of time. Fortunately, the study of obesity is receiving much interest in the research area and new concepts are developing, offering promise for effective management of the obese individual.

Starvation is undoubtedly a way of losing weight. This method is potentially hazardous and should not be followed unless it is medically supervised. It is true that individuals have fasted for long periods of time without adverse effects, but this does not imply that fasting can be utilized by all individuals in various stages of health.

Numerous research reports indicate that the management of obesity involves three major approaches. The first approach is through nutritional management, after a careful medical evaluation of the individual. The obese person may have many metabolic and health problems, such as mature-onset diabetes with elevations of fasting blood sugar, hypertension, and elevations of blood triglycerides and cholesterol. These factors must be identified and carefully managed to eliminate them as risk factors during the weight reduction program. The second major approach to weight reduction is exercise programming. Energy expenditure must be controlled and carefully supervised, and the exercise activity prescribed for the person should be individualized. The cardiovascular status of the individual should be carefully evaluated prior to any exercise program. The third approach is behavioral modification, or alteration of life-style. This appears to offer the greatest benefit in obesity management, but doubts must be expressed concerning its continued effectiveness in the absence of proper medical evaluation and nutritional management.

A new approach to obesity management is the protein-sparing modified fast. Protein hydrolysates or mixtures of amino acids providing the total amino acid needs of the individual are provided as the exclusive source of calories over reasonably long periods of time. The loss in weight comes first from the temporary water loss and then the continued catabolism and loss of fat tissue. Body protein reserves and physical strength are maintained. With this approach, fat metabolism is emphasized and ketone bodies appear, which tend to minimize sensation of hunger, and the physiological status of the individual remains in a reasonably stable condition.

[WILLARD A. KREHL]

Okra

A warm-season annual, *Hibiscus esculentus*, of Ethiopian origin. Okra, also called gumbo, is grown for its immature pods (see illustration), which are generally used for preparing soups but are also eaten as a freshly cooked vegetable. It is a member of the order Malvales and is related to cotton. Propagation is by seed. Popular varieties are Clemson Spineless and Green Velvet. Okra is

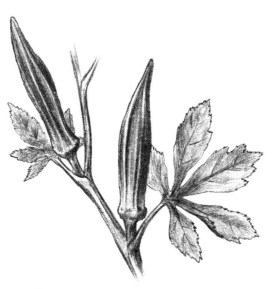

Okra (*Hibiscus esculentus*); branch with pods.

sensitive to low temperatures; commercial production in the United States is primarily in the South. Harvesting begins when the pods are 3–4 in. long, usually 50–60 days after planting. Georgia, Florida, and Louisiana are important producing states. *See* VEGETABLE GROWING.

[H. JOHN CAREW]

Oligosaccharide

A sugar composed of 2 or more monosaccharide units. Those sugars containing up to 6 units, many of which occur in nature, have been isolated as crystalline compounds. Fragments, obtained by controlled hydrolysis of various polysaccharides with acid and consisting of monosaccharides up to 10 units, are also termed oligosaccharides. *See* MONOSACCHARIDE.

Composition. The oligosaccharides may be considered as glycosides in which a hydroxyl (OH) group of one monosaccharide is condensed with the reducing group of another, with the loss of $n-1$ molecules of water (n = number of monosaccharide residues). This condensation process is shown in the following equations.

$$C_6H_{12}O_6 + C_6H_{12}O_6 - H_2O$$
$$= C_{12}H_{22}O_{11} \quad \text{Disaccharide}$$

$$3C_6H_{12}O_6 - 2H_2O = C_{18}H_{32}O_{16} \quad \text{Trisaccharide}$$

If two sugar units are joined in this manner, a disaccharide results; a linear array of three monosaccharides thus joined by glycosidic bonds is a trisaccharide, and so forth. On the basis of the number of constituent monosaccharide units, the oligosaccharides are classified as disaccharides, trisaccharides, tetrasaccharides, and so on. No sharp distinction can be drawn between the oligosaccharides and polysaccharides; it is chiefly a matter of the latter's possessing higher molecular weights. *See* POLYSACCHARIDE.

The oligosaccharides may be considered as glycosidic condensation products of the simple sugars, in which the second sugar unit serves as the aglycone group; that is, the glycosidic hydroxyl of one of the constituent sugars is substituted in the same manner as in glucose in the α- and β-methylglucosides. If the union occurs in such a way that the reducing group of one of the sugars is left free, the complex sugar which is formed is reducing. It will mutarotate, form an osazone, and give the other carbonyl reactions of reducing monosaccharides. If, on the other hand, the union between the sugars involves the glycosidic hydroxyl groups of all the component sugars, the oligosaccharide is nonreducing and will not give any of the reactions characteristic of a sugar with a free carbonyl group. The disaccharides cellobiose and trehalose, which contain two D-glucopyranose residues, are examples of these two types of oligosaccharide. In Fig. 1 the asterisk denotes the reducing group.

Most common disaccharides are dihexoses, although a few naturally occurring members of this group, such as primeverose, are known in which a pentose and a hexose are united together. The monosaccharide units of an oligosaccharide may be alike, as in maltose, which on hydrolysis gives two molecules of D-glucose, or different, as in su-

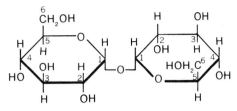

Fig. 1. Cellobiose (α form), a reducing disaccharide.

Fig. 2. Trehalose, a nonreducing disaccharide.

crose or raffinose. Sucrose consists of D-glucose and D-fructose, and raffinose consists of D-glucose, D-fructose, and D-galactose residues.

With the exception of D-fructose, the various monosaccharide residues composing the naturally occurring oligosaccharides have the pyranose structure, or a six-membered ring. When D-fructose serves as the glycosidic component in an oligosaccharide, it always occurs in the furanose form.

Besides the many known naturally occurring free oligosaccharides, a great variety of this class of compounds can be obtained by enzymatic degradation or by controlled hydrolysis of a polysaccharide with acid. For example, the treatment of starch with amylases produces maltose. Under certain conditions of acid hydrolysis, cellobiose can be obtained from cellulose.

Nomenclature. Most of the naturally occurring oligosaccharides have well established trivial names, such as sucrose, lactose, melizitose, raffinose, and stachyose, which were assigned before their complete structures were known. Rational names which indicate the chemical constitution of these and the other known oligosaccharides have been established jointly by the American and British committees on carbohydrate nomenclature. This nomenclature is universally used.

A reducing disaccharide (Fig. 1) is named as a glycosyl aldose (or glycosyl ketose) and a nonreducing disaccharide (Fig. 2) as a glycosyl aldoside (or glycosyl ketoside) from its componet parts. Thus the reducing disaccharide α-lactose, consisting of D-galactopyranose united by a β-glycosyl linkage to C-4 of D-glucopyranose, is designated as 4-O-β-D-galactopyranosyl-α-D-glucopyranose. A nonreducing disaccharide, such as sucrose, which is composed of D-glucopyranose and D-fructofuranose united by α- and β-glycosyl linkages, is named α-D-glucopyranosyl-β-D-fructofuranoside, or β-D-fructofuranosyl-α-D-glucopyranoside. A glycoside of a reducing disaccharide, for example, methyl-α-lactoside, is designated as methyl-4-O-β-D-galactopyranosyl-α-D-glucopyranoside. *See* LACTOSE.

For naming oligosaccharides containing more than two units, the respective positions involved in the glycosidic linkages are indicated by two numbers and an arrow in parentheses. Thus the reducing trisaccharide, maltotriose, is defined as O-α-D-glucopyranosyl-(1 → 4)-O-α-D-glucopyranosyl-(1 → 4)-α-D-glucopyranose.

Properties. Oligosaccharides have the same properties as their constituent monosaccharides, except as those properties may be modified by linking the units together. As an example, disaccharides show alcoholic reactions just like the monosaccharides, but the number of reactive alcohol groups is smaller by 2 than the sum of the alcoholic groups of the two monosaccharides. This is because one hydroxyl position from each monosaccharide unit is involved in the linkage between the two units that constitute the disaccharide and is not reactive until after hydrolysis. A hexose molecule can form a pentaacetate by replacement of 5 hydroxyl groups, but if 2 hexoses are joined to form a 12-carbon disaccharide, 2 hydroxyl positions disappear by union, and only 8 of the original 10 are available for replacement; consequently, the fully acetylated disaccharide is an octaacetate. Similarly, methylation takes place to the extent of introducing 8 methyl groups in a 12-carbon disaccharide molecule.   [WILLIAM Z. HASSID]

Bibliography: *Chem. Eng. News*, 31:1776, 1953; M. Florkin and E. Stotz (eds.), *Comprehensive Biochemistry*, vol. 5, 1965; *J. Chem. Soc.* (London), pp. 5108–5121, 1952; J. Stanek, M. Cerny, and J. Pacak, *The Oligosaccharides*, 1965.

Olive

The evergreen olive (*Olea europeae*) is among the most important of the subtropical fruit crops of the Mediterranean region. It is grown commercially in the United States only in California, where the annual production has a value of $10,000,000. A considerable number of the small white flowers (illustration *a*) borne in the spring frequently contain pollen only, and hence are unable to produce fruit. Pollination is by wind. The fruit (illustration *b*) is a drupe of high oil content (40–65%) which is expressed by mechanical means. A bitter ingredient must be removed by soaking in lye before the fruit is edible. Many varieties are grown for oil or

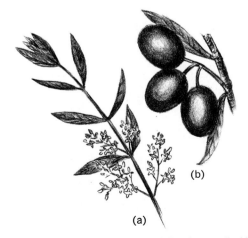

(b)

(a)

Olive (*Olea europeae*) branches. (*a*) Bearing small white flowers. (*b*) Bearing drupes, or fruit.

processing or both. The name Queen refers to the large fruits of any variety used for food when processed either green or black (ripe). *See* FAT AND OIL, EDIBLE; FRUIT, TREE.

[CHARLES A. SCHROEDER]

Onion

A cool-season biennial, *Allium cepa*, of Asiatic origin and belonging to the plant order Liliales. The onion is grown for its edible bulbs (see illustration).

Related species are leek (*A. porrum*), garlic (*A. sativum*), Welsh onion (*A. fistulosum*), shallot (*A. ascalonicum*), and chive (*A. schoenoprasum*).

Propagation. The common onion is grown as an annual and is propagated most frequently by seed sown directly in the field. Onions may also be grown from transplants started in greenhouses or outdoor seedbeds or from small bulbs, called sets, grown the previous year. Field spacing varies; plants are generally grown 1–4 in. apart in 14–18-in. rows. The Egyptian tree or top onion (*A. cepa* var. *vivaparum*) produces little bulbs or topsets in the flower cluster, and the multiplier or potato onion (*A. cepa* var. *aggregatum*) multiplies by branching at the base.

Varieties. Onion varieties (cultivars) are classified mainly according to pungency (mild or pungent) and use (dry bulbs or green bunching). Bulbs may be white, red, or yellow. Varieties differ markedly in their keeping quality and in their response to length of day. Hybrid varieties, produced with male-sterile breeding lines, and with increased disease resistance, longer storage life, and improved quality, are rapidly displacing older varieties. *See* PHOTOPERIODISM IN PLANTS.

Harvesting. The harvesting of dry-bulb varieties usually starts after the leaves begin to turn yellow and fall over, generally 3–4 months after planting. Bulbs to be stored are cured by exposure to warm dry air. Bunching onions are ordinarily harvested when the bulbs are 1/4 in. or larger in diameter.

Texas, New York, and California are important

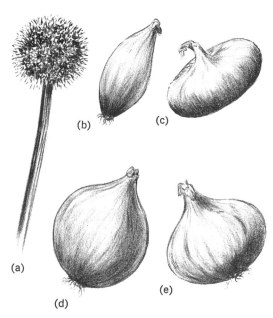

The onion flower and bulbs. (a) Flower head or cluster. (b) Oblong. (c) Flat. (d) Globe. (e) Oblate.

producing states. The total annual farm value in the United States from approximately 100,000 acres is $80,000,000. *See* VEGETABLE GROWING.

[H. JOHN CAREW]

Diseases. The most serious onion diseases are caused by bacteria and fungi. Diseases in the field and in the channels of marketing cause losses amounting to many thousands of dollars each year. All regions that grow onions commerically have diseases of some importance. The weather often determines the kind and amount of disease present in any given year. Wet weather at harvest time, which prevents the proper curing of the bulbs, favors the development of serious diseases, especially during transit, storage, and marketing.

Neck rot, incited by *Botrytis allii* and other species, usually causes greater loss than any other disease. It is reponsible for considerable decay in storage onions that have not been properly cured. Sometimes as much as 50% of the crop is lost.

Bacterial soft rot is probably the second most serious disease of onions. Although it occurs in the field, it causes most damage after harvest. This disease is caused by *Erwinia carotovora* and *Pseudomonas allicola*, bacteria that are common in soil and water. The organisms invade the moist neck of the onion at harvest time and also enter through wounds, particularly under warm, humid conditions.

Where cool, moist weather prevails, downy mildew caused by the fungus *Peronospora destructor* is a very destructive disease. The seedlings and leaves of the growing plants are affected.

Black mold, caused by *Aspergillus niger*, is common on onion bulbs grown in the South. It seldom causes decay. The disease is readily identified by observation of black, powdery spores on the scales at the neck and between the outer scales of the bulb.

Smudge is serious only on white varieties of onions. The causal fungus, *Collectotrichum circinans*, invades the outer scales of the bulbs and causes unsightly dark blotches. However, little damage results to the fleshy part of the bulb.

Smut, a fungus disease caused by *Urocystis cepulae*, occurs in northern-grown onions. It affects seedlings and young green onions, causing black blisters on the leaves and young bulbs.

A bulb rot caused by *Fusarium oxysporum*, a soil-borne organism, frequently causes serious damage to onions late in the season. Infections not apparent at harvest time continue to develop and cause extensive decay during storage and marketing.

Other diseases, usually of minor importance, are caused by viruses, nematodes, and physiological disorders. *See* PLANT DISEASE; PLANT VIRUS.

[GLEN B. RAMSEY]

Orange

The sweet orange (*Citrus sinensis*) is the most widely used species of citrus fruit and commercially is the most important. The sour or bitter oranges, of lesser importance, are distinct from sweet oranges and are classified as a separate species, *C. aurantium*. Citrus belonging to other species are also sometimes called oranges. This article deals only with the sweet orange.

The sweet orange probably is native to north-

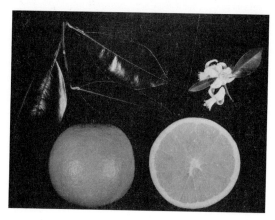
Leaves, flowers, and fruit of *Citrus sinensis*.

extensive worldwide losses of trees on sour orange rootstock. Root rot caused by soil-inhabiting fungi is also widespread, attacking many types of rootstocks. Large-scale selection and breeding programs have developed rootstocks that are tolerant to tristeza and root rot. *See* FRUIT, TREE; FRUIT (TREE) DISEASES.

[R. K. SOOST]

Bibliography: J. Janick and J. N. Moore (eds.), *Advances in Fruit Breeding*, 1975; W. Reuther, L. D. Batchelor, and H. J. Webber (eds.), *The Citrus Industry*, vol. 1, University of California Division of Agricultural Science, 1967.

Paprika

A type of pepper, *Capsicum annuum*, with nonpungent flesh, grown for its long red fruit. A member of the plant order Polemoniales (formerly of the order Tubiflorales) and of American origin, it is most popular in Hungary and adjacent countries. Seeds are removed from the mature fruit, and the flesh is dried and ground to prepare the dry condiment commonly referred to as paprika. Production in the United States is limited, with California the only important producing state. *See* PEPPER; VEGETABLE GROWING.

[H. JOHN CAREW]

Parsley

A biennial, *Petroselinum crispum*, of European origin belonging to the plant order Umbellales. Parsley is grown for its foliage and is used to garnish and flavor foods. It contains large quantities of vitamins A and C and has been grown for 2000 years or more. Two types, plain-leafed and curled, are grown for their foliage; Hamburg parsley (*P. crispum* var. *tuberosum*), also called turnip-rooted parsley, is grown for its edible parsniplike root. Propagation is by seed. Harvesting begins 70–80 days after planting for foliage varieties, and 90 days after planting for Hamburg parsley. *See* VEGETABLE GROWING.

[H. JOHN CAREW]

Parsnip

A hardy biennial, *Pastinaca sativa*, of Mediterranean origin belonging to the plant order Umbellales. The parsnip is grown for its thickened taproot and is used primarily as a cooked vegetable. Propagation is by seed; cultural practices are similar to those used for carrot, except that a longer growing season is required. Parsnip seed retains its viability only 1–2 years. Harvesting begins in late fall or early winter, usually 100–125 days after planting. Exposure of mature roots to low temperatures, not necessarily freezing, improves the quality of the root by favoring the conversion of starch to sugar. *See* CARROT; VEGETABLE GROWING.

[H. JOHN CAREW]

Pasteurization

The application of mild heat for a specified time to a liquid food or beverage to enhance its keeping properties and to destroy any harmful microorganisms present. For milk, the times and temperatures employed are based upon the thermal tolerance of *Mycobacterium tuberculosis*, one of the most heat-resistant of non-spore-forming pathogens. A temperature of either 143°F (61.7°C) for 30

eastern India and southern China, but has spread to other tropical and subtropical regions of the world. The introduction of this delicious fruit into the Mediterranean region in the 15th century aroused much interest in citrus. The orange was first introduced into the Western Hemisphere by Columbus, and has become a major crop in Florida and California and in Brazil. The United States is the largest producer of oranges, followed by Spain, Italy, and Brazil. It is also a major crop in several other countries.

Sweet orange fruit is consumed fresh or as frozen or canned juice. A large portion of the crop, particularly in the United States, is used as frozen concentrate. After the juice is extracted, the peel and pulp are used for cattle feed. Peel oil is used in perfumes and flavoring, and citrus molasses is used as a livestock feed.

The sweet orange tree is a moderately vigorous evergreen with a rounded, densely foliated top. The fruits are round (see illustration) or somewhat elongate and usually orange-colored when ripe. They can be placed in four groups: the common oranges, acidless oranges, pigmented oranges, and navel oranges. They may also be distinguished on the basis of early, midseason, and late maturity. The common oranges are orange-colored and have varying numbers of seeds. Several, such as the Valencia, are important commercial cultivars throughout the world. The acidless oranges are prized in some countries because of their very low acidity, but generally are not major cultivars. The pigmented or "blood" oranges develop varying amounts of pink or red in the flesh and peel and have a distinctive aroma and flavor. Most originated in the Mediterranean area and are popular there, but are little grown in the United States. Navel oranges are so named because of the structure at the blossom end. Because they are usually seedless, some have become important cultivars for the fresh-fruit market. Many, if not all, of the cultivars appear to have been selected as bud sports, with the original type being small, seedy, and nonpigmented.

Sweet oranges are propagated by budding or grafting on rootstocks in order to obtain uniform, high-yielding plantings. Many citrus species and relatives have been used as rootstocks. Diseases have severely restricted the use of some major rootstocks. Tristeza, a virus disease, has caused

min or of 161°F (71.7°C) for 15 sec is employed. Vegetative cells of most bacteria are killed by the heat treatment, but endospores are unaffected. *See* MILK; WINE.

Pasteurization originated with Louis Pasteur in the 1860s, who demonstrated that spoilage of wine and beer could be prevented by heating these beverages to approximately 135°F (57.2°C) for a few minutes.   [CHARLES F. NIVEN, JR.]

Pea

The pea is one of the oldest cultivated crops. It is a native to western Asia from the Mediterranean Sea to the Himalaya Mountains. It appears to have been carried to Europe as early as the time of the lake dwellers of prehistoric times. Peas were introduced into China from Persia about A.D. 400; they were introduced into the United States in very early Colonial days.

Description. Garden peas (*Pisum sativum*) have wrinkled seed coats at maturity when dry; field peas (*P. arvense*) have a smooth seed coat. Both types are annual leafy plants with stems 1–5 ft long. Each leaf bears three pairs of leaflets and ends in a slender tendril (see illustration). The blossoms are reddish-purple, pink, or white, with two or three on each flower stalk. Five to nine round seeds are enclosed in a pod about 3 in. long. Seed color varies from white to cream, green, yellow, or brown. Smooth-seeded varieties may be harvested fresh for freezing or canning, or harvested dry as edible peas. Dry peas may be split or ground and prepared in various ways, such as for split-pea soup.

Culture. Peas require a cool growing season. They should be sown in early spring as soon as a fine, firm seedbed can be prepared. Early-seeded peas develop before the heat of early summer can harm them and usually produce higher yields. Peas are seeded 2–3 in. deep. Then the fields are usually rolled immediately to firm the seedbed and aid germination. In the Palouse area of Washington and Idaho, peas are usually planted in early April, while elsewhere irrigated fields are often seeded in March. Garden peas may be seeded as early as February in home gardens in the southern half of the United States.

Applications of lime, sulfur, molybdenum, phosphorus, and potassium are commonly made for pea production.

Harvesting. The peas are mowed and windrowed with a swather. Self-propelled viners, which have replaced stationary viners, pick up the windrowed crop and separate the fresh green peas from the vines and pods. To maintain high quality, this must be done within 2 hr after the peas have been mowed. *See* AGRICULTURE, SOIL AND CROP PRACTICES IN.

A tenderometer is used to determine when green peas for processing should be harvested. Dry peas are harvested with a regular grain combine when the moisture content in the seed drops below 14%. Adjustments are made to minimize damage to the pea seed.

The Grain Division of the Agricultural Marketing Service, U.S. Department of Agriculture, has set standards and issues a grade certificate to define the relative market value of different-quality dry peas.

[KENNETH J. MORRISON]

Production. Wisconsin, Washington, Minnesota, Oregon, Illinois, New York, Pennsylvania, Utah, and Idaho lead in the production of peas harvested green. In dry- and seed-pea production the leading states are Washington, Idaho, Oregon, California, Colorado, Montana, North Dakota, Wyoming, and Minnesota. Seed for all garden varieties is grown primarily in the same areas that grow the dry commercial peas. Washington and Idaho produce more than 84% of the total seed and dry commercial pea crop. The two main export markets for dry peas are Europe and Latin America. The European market is somewhat sporadic, depending on the total production of Europe's usually large acreage of peas. *See* LEGUME; VEGETABLE GROWING.

[WILLIAM A. BEACHELL]

Diseases. The pea plant is subject to numerous diseases caused by bacteria, fungi, nematodes, and viruses. Some of these diseases can be controlled by seed treatments and planting of resistant varieties; for many, however, no control measures are available.

Root diseases. Root rots in the northern pea canning areas of the United States are caused by *Aphanomyces euteiches*, *Fusarium solani* f. *pisi*, *Pythium* sp., *Ascochyta pinodella*, and *Rhizoctonia solani*; in the Southern states root rots are caused by *Sclerotium rolfsii* and *Phymatotricum omnivorum*. These fungi probably live permanently in the soil and attack many crops other than peas; the root rots therefore constitute a major problem in pea production, control being almost impossible. *Aphanomyces euteiches*, the most prevalent and severe of the root rots, can survive in field soils for 10–20 years. Present control measures are limited to keeping field infestation to a minimum by cultural practices and to using a special land-selection program to avoid fields already infested.

Two wilt diseases affect peas, common wilt caused by *Fusarium oxysporum* f. *pisi* race 1, and near-wilt caused by *F. oxysporum* f. *pisi* race 2. In both diseases, the organism becomes established in the soil and infects the roots of the pea plant. The organism grows through the water-conducting vessels up into the stem, thus interfering with the passage of water through the stems and into leaves. Affected plants wilt, the lower leaves turn yellow, and the plant dies either in the early stage of development or soon after flowering. Wilt diseases are best controlled by the use of resistant varieties. Both market-garden and canning varieties of peas resistant to common wilt are available, but only a few canning varieties are resistant to near-wilt.

The root knot nematode (*Heterodera marioni*) attacks the roots of peas, causing a reduction in growth and yield and often killing the plants. The disease is most prevalent in the southern and southwestern United States.

Foliage diseases. Bacterial blight caused by *Pseudomonas pisi*, anthracnose caused by *Colletotrichum pisi*, Septoria blotch caused by *Septoria pisi*, Mycosphaerella blight caused by *Mycosphaerella pinodes*, and Ascochyta leaf and pod spot caused by *Ascochyta pisi* are some of the more important foliage diseases other than the mildews and viruses. Most of these pathogens are known to live from one season to the next in and on seed and in the plant refuse left in the field from the pre-

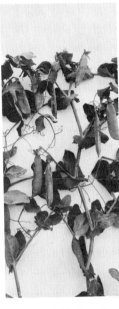

Typical wrinkled-seed type of pea, showing fruit (pod) containing seeds (peas). (*Dumas Seed Co., Inc.*)

vious crop. Partial control is obtained through the use of clean, treated seed, crop rotation, and sanitary practices to reduce the plant refuse.

Downy mildew caused by *Peronospora pisi* and powdery mildew caused by *Erysiphe polygoni* seldom become severe outside the pea-growing areas of the Northwest. There are no effective control measures for downy mildew, but fungicides are sometimes used for powdery mildew control.

The virus diseases of peas may cause severe damage in some seasons. They are generally widespread, the mosaic types being the most prevalent. Varieties resistant to some of the viruses are available. See PLANT DISEASE; PLANT VIRUS.

[THOMAS H. KING]

Bibliography: R. Delorit and H. L. Ahlgren, *Crop Production*, 4th ed., 1973; H. D. Hughes and D. Metcalfe, *Crop Production*, 3d ed., 1972; H. M. Reisenauer et al., *Dry Pea Production*, Wash. State Univ. Ext. Bull. no. 582, 1965; W. W. Rufener, *Production and Marketing of Dry Peas in the Palouse Area*, Agr. Exp. Sta. Bull. no. 391, Washington State University, 1940; J. C. Walker, *Plant Pathology*, 3d ed., 1968.

Peach

The fruit *Prunus persica*. It originated in the temperate region of China (see illustration) and has been cultivated as long as there has been knowledge of domesticated plants. It was carried from Europe to America in the 16th century. The seeds were quickly disseminated by the Indians, and strains of the so-called Indian peaches still persist in the wild in parts of the southern United States. Various varieties of peaches are grown in nearly all parts of the United States, in Canada around the Great Lakes, and in both North and South Temperate zones throughout the world.

Peach trees are generally short-lived—8 to 10 years in the warmer areas of cultivation and up to 30 years in the most favorable areas. They usually bear a small crop 3 years after planting, and healthy trees continue to increase in production for 6 to 12 years. The trees are often killed when the temperature drops below −26°C. Conversely, the trees need a certain number of days of sustained temperatures below 10°C in order to leaf out and bloom in the spring. Varieties (cultivars) vary as to their cold requirements, and good commercial cultivars are now available for United States areas as far south as northern Florida. Choosing the most suitable cultivar for a given area is important to successful production.

Propagation and cultivation. Peach trees are propagated by budding onto 1-year-old peach seedlings to maintain varietal characteristics of the top part of the tree. Budding is generally done in June, and the young trees are set in the orchard the following winter or spring. Peaches do best on sites with good air and water drainage—sandy or sand loam soils with a clay subsoil are best. Trees are usually planted 10 to 20 ft (3 to 6 m) apart in rows 20 to 24 ft (6 to 7 m) apart. Peach trees should not be set on land that has been previously planted to peaches since such trees tend to die earlier in spite of the best known methods of cultivation and disease control. Rye or another grain crop should precede peaches on the land, and preparation should include liming and subsoiling. Peaches are generally clean-cultivated, that is, cultivated dur-

ing the growing season to keep the land reasonably free of weeds. Certain chemical weed killers can be used satisfactorily to replace or supplement mechanical cultivation. Deep cultivation is detrimental to the shallow-feeding roots.

Proper fertilization, pruning, and fruit thinning are important. Bearing trees require a complete fertilizer in the spring and nitrogen alone in summer. Early spring is the best time to prune. Peach trees are pruned to three to five scaffold limbs between 16 to 30 in. (40 to 75 cm) from the ground and shaped to an open vase form. Mechanical shearing with machines is partially replacing annual hand pruning. Thinning by hand is aided by chemical thinners.

Harvesting. Ripe peaches are removed from the tree by hand for local markets. Successful mechanical harvesters are available for cannery peaches and for "hard ripe" peaches for shipment. Machines sort the fruit by size. Defective fruits are removed by hand as they move on the conveyors. The fuzz on the fruit is removed with mechanical brushes. The fruit is then precooled, waxed, packed in suitable containers, and iced. *See* FRUIT, TREE.   [FRANCIS E. JOHNSTONE, JR.]

Diseases. Brown rot, caused by *Monilinia fructicola* and *M. laxa*, is a destructive fungus disease of the peach throughout the world. Blossoms, twigs, and fruit are infected. Major loss is from the decay of the fruit, which is converted into a soggy mass unfit for human consumption. Control is achieved by spraying or dusting the trees at regular intervals with powdered sulfur or with captan, an organic fungicide. For best results it is essential also to control the plum curculio, a common fruit insect, whose punctures facilitate entrance of the fungus into the fruit. *See* FUNGISTAT AND FUNGICIDE.

In contrast to brown rot, which requires strenuous efforts for its control, peach scab (*Cladosporium carpophilum*), although universally present, is readily controlled by one or two sprays of sulfur shortly after the blossom petals drop. Leaf curl caused by *Taphrina deformans*, a leaf-distorting fungus, can be prevented by one spray of lime sulfur, bordeaux mixture, or ferbam applied before the buds begin to swell.

Bacterial spot, caused by *Xanthomonas pruni*, is a serious disease of peaches in the United States, China, Japan, and New Zealand. The bacteria kill small groups of cells in the leaves, twigs, and fruit. Infected leaves drop prematurely and this devitalizes the trees mainly through reduced photosynthesis, the most serious long-time effect of the disease. Diseased fruit is edible, but its appearance is marred and its market value reduced. The bacteria survive the winter in small cankers formed on the twigs. Control is difficult because of the prolonged infection period. A mixture of zinc sulfate and hydrated lime, applied as a spray at intervals of 10–14 days, reduces the severity of the infection in most years.

Other fungus diseases affecting peaches are rust caused by *Tranzschelia discolor*, peach blight caused by *Coryneum beijerinckii*, and mildew caused by *Sphaerotheca pannosa*. These diseases cause serious losses in various parts of the world. *Rhizopus nigricans*, occurring throughout the world, causes rapid decay of harvested and stored peaches.

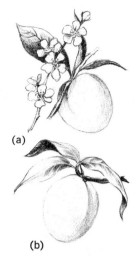

PEACH

Peaches. (*a*) Chinese peach grown from seed of wild trees in China. (*b*) Elberta peach.

Among the more than 20 virus diseases known to affect peaches in the United States, yellows, rosette, phony peach, and mosaic are the most serious. The first two kill the trees in a few years, whereas phony peach and mosaic reduce both quality and quantity of fruit, and the trees eventually become worthless. *See* PLANT VIRUS.

Peaches are also injuriously affected by nutrient deficiencies in the soil, the symptoms of which often resemble those resulting from disease organisms. Fluctuations in temperature during the winter, particularly in the Southern states, frequently kill many peach trees. *See* FRUIT (TREE) DISEASES; PLANT, MINERALS ESSENTIAL TO; PLANT DISEASE CONTROL.

[JOHN C. DUNEGAN]

Peanut

A self-pollinated, one- to six-seeded legume which is cultivated throughout the tropical and temperate climates of the world. The oil, expressed from the seed, is of high quality, and a large percentage of the 20,000,000-ton annual world production is used for this purpose. In the United States some 65% goes into the cleaned and shelled trade, the end products of which are roasted or salted peanuts, peanut butter, and confections. *See* LEGUME.

Origin and description. Peanuts originated in Bolivia and northeastern Argentina where a large number of wild forms are found. The cultivated species, *Arachis hypogaea*, was grown extensively by Indians in pre-Columbian times. Merchant ships carried seed to many continents during the early part of the 16th century. Although grown in Mexico before the discovery of America, the peanut was introduced to the United States from Africa.

Botanically, peanuts may be divided into three main types, Virginia, Spanish, and Valencia, based on branching order and pattern and the number of seeds per pod. The USDA Marketing Standards includes an additional type, Runner, which refers to the small-seeded Virginia type produced in Georgia and Alabama.

The peanut's most distinguishing characteristic is the yellow flower, which resembles a butterfly (papilionaceous) and is borne above ground. Following fertilization the flower wilts and, after a period of 5–7 days, a positively geotropic (curving earthward) peg or ovary emerges. Penetrating the soil 2–7 cm, the peg assumes a horizontal position and the pod begins to form (Fig. 1).

The pod, a one-loculed legume, splits under pressure along a longitudinal ventral suture. Pod size varies from 1 by 0.5 cm to 2 by 8 cm, and seed weight varies from 1/5 to 5 g. The number of seeds per pod usually is two in the Virginia type, two or three in the Spanish, and three to six in the Valencia.

The plant may be upright, prostrate, or intermediate between these forms. The main stem is usually upright and may be very short in some varieties. The leaves are even-pinnate with four obovate to elliptic leaflets. Leaves occur alternately and have a 2:5 phyllotaxy (arrangement on stems).

Harvesting and value. Peanuts are harvested by running a special wing-type plow under the plants. After wilting they are either stacked or allowed to cure in windrows before picking. *See* AGRICULTURE, MACHINERY IN; AGRICULTURE,

PEANUT

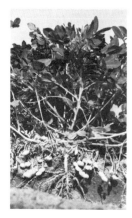

Fig. 1. A typical Virginia-type peanut.

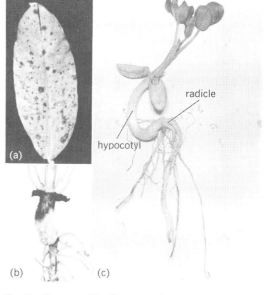

Fig. 2. Nonparasitic diseases of peanut. (*a*) Necrotic areas caused by manganese deficiency. (*b*) Heat canker. (*c*) Primary roots and curled hypocotyl of a seedling with an injured radicle. (*Photograph by L. W. Boyle*)

SOIL AND CROP PRACTICES IN.

The main production areas in the United States extend southward from Virginia and westward to Oklahoma and Texas. Peanuts are under strict acreage controls. In 1975, Georgia had the largest acreage with 520,000 acres, followed by Texas, 309,000; Alabama, 204,000; North Carolina, 168,000; Oklahoma, 121,000; and Virginia, 104,000. Total annual value of the crop amounts to about $700,000,000. *See* AGRICULTURAL SCIENCE (PLANT).   [ASTOR PERRY]

Diseases. Yields of peanut hay and fruit may be reduced by at least one-fourth because of nonparasitic, insect, bacterial, fungous, nematode, and virus-caused disorders.

Nonparasitic. Calcium deficiency may initiate fruit decay. A deficiency of manganese causes chlorosis and necrotic spots on peanut leaves (Fig. 2). Mechanical injury to the seed radicle causes a curvature of the hypocotyl and retards foliar growth (Fig. 2). Radiant energy from the Sun causes heat canker on young seedlings. *See* PLANT, MINERALS ESSENTIAL TO.

Insects. The southern corn rootworm (*Diabrotica undecimpunctata howardii*) acts as an inoculating agent for the fungi and bacteria that cause fruit rot. The potato leafhopper (*Empoasca fabae*) secretes a toxic substance on the leaves and causes a disorder known as hopperburn. The tobacco thrip (*Frankliniella fusca*) causes puckered leaflets and retards the growth of seedlings. *See* INSECTA.

Bacteria. Bacterial wilt, caused by *Pseudomonas solanacearum*, occurs in all peanut growing areas and occasionally causes significant losses. Several peanut varieties that are resistant to bacterial wilt have been developed in Java.

Fungi. Species of *Aspergillus, Rhizopus, Mucor, Diplodia, Fusarium, Pythium, Rhizoctonia, Sclerotium, Botrytis*, and *Phymatotrichum* either cause, or play an important role in, the development of rots of planted seed, rots of root, pegs, and fruit, a collar rot of the hypocotyl and lower stem, concealed damage of the cotyledon interfaces, and blue damage discoloration of the seed coat and cotyledon of harvested fruit (Fig. 3). Rust of the foliar parts, caused by *Puccinia arachidis*, occasionally causes serious plant damage in South America, the West Indies, and southern Texas. The leaf-spot disease, caused by *Cercospora arachidicola* and *C. personata*, results in premature leaf fall and is the most common and one of the most destructive diseases wherever the crop is grown. Southern blight, caused by *Sclerotium rolfsii*, occurs in all peanut-growing areas, and occasionally causes severe losses. *S. rolfsii* is a soil-borne fungus which kills the succulent tissues of the hypocotyl, stem, branches, peg, and fruit.

Nematodes. The northern rootknot nematode (*Meloidogyne hapla*) is a common pest of the peanut. It feeds inside the root, peg, and fruit and causes small galls on these parts (Fig. 4). The peanut rootknot nematode (*Meloidogyne arenaria*) causes large galls to form on all underground parts. It is known to occur in the United States and Africa and is far more injurious than the northern rootknot nematode. The sting nematode (*Belonolaimus gracilis*) and an unidentified species of *Belonolaimus* are very destructive; however, they are known to occur only in the lighter soils of the United States. Sting nematodes feed on the outside of the peanut root, peg, and fruit and cause a reduced root system and smaller fruit. The smooth-headed meadow nematode (*Pratylenchus brachyurus*) feeds inside the peanut root, peg, and fruit and causes necrotic lesions on these parts.

Viruses. Viruses causing chlorotic rosette, green rosette, bunchy plant, mosaic, mottle, marginal chlorosis, ringspot, rugose leaf curl, stunt, and spotted wilt have been reported from all the principal peanut-producing areas. The rosette viruses of Africa, spotted wilt of Australia, and peanut stunt of the United States are known to cause severe losses. *See* PLANT DISEASE; PLANT DISEASE CONTROL; PLANT VIRUS.

[LAWRENCE I. MILLER]

Processing. Peanut processing begins in the fields where the peanuts are removed from vines by portable, mechanical pickers. The freshly dug peanut plants are windrowed in the field, and the peanuts, with a moisture content of 25–30%, are picked from the vines within 3 days.

The Spanish-type peanut has led others in the United States since 1940; however, Runner-type is increasing and the Valencia is grown only in limited quantities in the Southwest. Spanish is the prodominant type used in candy, Runner leads in peanut butter, and practically all peanuts retailed in shell are Virginia.

Cleaning. Peanuts from the pickers are delivered to warehouses for cleaning. This consists of removing sticks, stems, small rocks, and faulty nuts by a series of screens and blowers. The operation reduces the bulkiness of the nuts by 10–20%.

Storing. Cleaned peanuts are stored unshelled in silos or warehouses for continuous shelling and delivery to end users; shelled, they are stored in refrigerated warehouses at 32–36°F with 65% relative humidity (RH). Refrigeration ensures protection against insects and rancidity.

Shelling. This consists of breaking the shells by passing the nuts between series of rollers. The

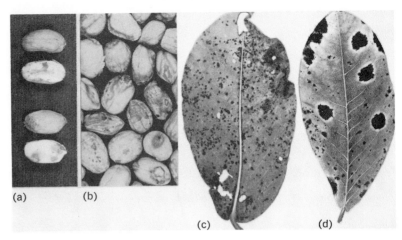

Fig. 3. Fungus diseases of peanut. (*a*) Concealed damage of cotyledon interfaces. (*b*) Blue damage of seed coat and cotyledon (*photograph by D. C. Norton*). (*c*) Rust of leaf caused by *Puccinia arachidis* (*photograph by B. B. Higgins*). (*d*) Leaf spot caused by *Cercospora arachidiacola* (*photograph by M. McB. Miller*).

shells and small, immature pegs are separated by screens and blowers, and the discolored kernels are removed by hand and by electric eye. Shelling reduces the weight of peanuts 30–60%, the space occupied 60–70%, and the shelf life 60–75%, depending upon the variety.

Blanching. This consists of removing the skins (seed coats) and usually the hearts of peanuts prior to use in peanut butter, bakery products, confections, and salted nuts. Blanching may be done with heat or with water. Heat blanching consists of embrittling the skins by exposure to 126–145°C heat for 5–20 min, followed by rubbing the kernels between soft surfaces and removing the skins by blowers and the hearts by screens.

In water blanching, kernels are wet with steam and arranged longitudinally in troughs and passed beneath spring fingers with blades which slit the skins from end to end. Skins are removed as a spiral conveyor carries the kernels through a 1-min bath of scalding water. An improved and more

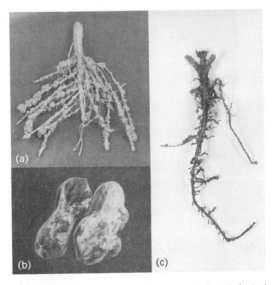

Fig. 4. Nematode diseases of peanut. (*a*) Root infected by the peanut rootknot nematode. (*b*) Fruit infected by the peanut rootknot nematode. (*c*) Root injury caused by the feeding of the sting nematode.

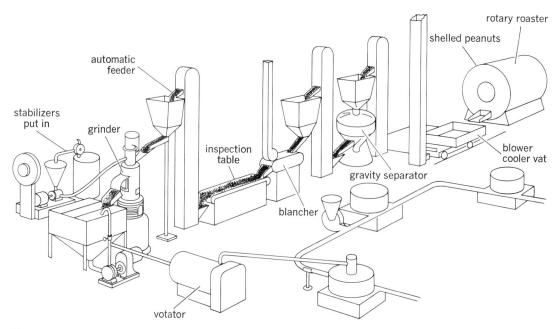

Fig. 5. Apparatus for the manufacture of peanut butter. (*From Food Processing*)

rapid method is to wet the nuts with 60°C water and remove the skins by rapidly revolving spindles. The kernels are dried to 7% moisture prior to storage or conversion into peanut products.

Dry roasting. Peanuts for use in peanut butter, confections, or bakery products are dry-roasted to develop desirable color, texture, and flavor. Unblanched peanuts are heated to 204°C for 20–30 min, after which they are cooled and blanched.

Shelled, ground, and parched peanuts were first prepared about 1890 as food for infants and invalids. From a kitchen operation this has become a major industry, with individual plants manufacturing 20,000,000 lb of peanut butter annually (Fig. 5). The product consists of blanched, dry-roasted peanuts, ground to a size to pass through a 200-mesh screen. Additives to improve smoothness, spreadability, and flavor include 1.5% salt, 0.125% hydrogenated vegetable oil, 2% dextrose, and 2–4% corn syrup or honey. Additives to improve nutritive qualities include 185 ml/100 g ascorbic acid and yeast.

Shelled peanuts are dry-roasted in a gas-fired rotary roaster at 204°C. When cooking is complete, as indicated by photometer, the peanuts are automatically dumped into a blower-cooler vat where they are brought to 30°C. The cool peanuts pass through a gravity separator which removes foreign material, then to a blancher which removes the hearts by a shaker screen and the skins by a blower. After passing over the inspection table the nuts pass through an automatic feeder and into a grinder. Stabilizers are metered into the mill simultaneously with the peanuts and are thoroughly dispersed in the butter. The stabilized peanut butter is cooled in a votator (rotating refrigerated cylinder), automatically packed, labeled, and stored.

Peanut butter contains 50–52% fat, 28–29% protein, 2–5% carbohydrate, and 1–2% moisture. *See* ASCORBIC ACID; YEAST.

Oil roasting. Peanuts for salting are roasted in coconut oil or partly hydrogenated vegetable oil at 148.9°C for 15–18 min. The end point is based on change of color and is controlled electrically or manually.

Salting. Peanuts either blanched or unblanched are roasted in oil and salted. Finely ground salt (2–3%) and an oil-base binder are mixed with freshly cooked nuts, which are then placed in flexible bags or canned under vacuum.

Salting in the shell. Peanuts may be salted in the shell. This involves soaking in a surface-active agent at 60°C for 15 min, rinsing, submerging in saturated brine, and subjecting nuts to 20 in. vacuum two or three times for 5-min periods, rinsing, and drying.

Extraction of oil. The recovery of oil from peanuts is by one of three methods—hydraulic pressing, expeller pressing, or solvent extraction. Hydraulic pressing is essentially the same as used for oil recovery from cottonseed. The peanuts are broken between rollers, and the shells are removed by blowers. The meats are crushed and heated under 25 lb steam pressure for 10 min, stabilized at 7% moisture, and pressed at 137.8°C. The yield of oil by hydraulic pressing is 41–47%, and the press cake contains 42–45% protein, 5–6% moisture, and 7–8% oil.

Solvent extraction of oil from ground peanuts is similar to that from soybeans. The direct-solvent process was introduced in the late 1940s, and was followed in 1950 by the prepress-solvent process, which in turn was followed in 1954 by the high-speed screw press. The yield of oil by solvent extraction is 48–50%, and the meal contains 50–52% protein, 1–2% oil, and 1–2% moisture. In 1965 a method was developed for hydraulically pressing out up to 80% of the oil of whole moistened peanuts. The nuts are dried for storage, subsequently reshaped by moistening, and finally oil-roasted for salting. *See* FOOD ENGINEERING; SOYBEAN.   [JASPER G. WOODROOF]

Bibliography: M. A. Watson, Virus diseases, in *Pest Control in Groundnuts*, Pans Manual no. 2,

Ministry of Overseas Development, London, 1967; J. G. Woodroof, *Peanuts: Production, Processing, Products*, 1973.

Pear

A fruit native to western Asia or nearby Europe and of very old culture, having been known nearly 1000 years B.C. (see illustration). It spread across Europe and was extremely popular in Belgium and France during the 18th and 19th centuries.

Early settlers throughout North America made extensive efforts to grow pears, but it does best in an equable, dry climate with sufficient summer heat to develop good quality. Trees require winter cold to break the dormant period but are injured by temperatures below −10 to −15°F (−23 to −26°C). Over 95% of United States commercial production is in the interior valleys of California, Oregon, and Washington where these climatic conditions are found.

Commercial types and varieties. Nearly all United States pear production is of the European pear *(Pyrus communis)* which includes the varieties Bartlett (known as Williams in Europe), d'Anjou, Bosc, and Comice. Other major types are *P. serotina*, the Oriental sand pear, with roundish shape and gritty flesh; hybrids between *P. communis* and *P. serotina*, represented by Kieffer and Leconte; and *P. nivalis*, the snow pear, grown in Europe for cider or perry (a fermented liquor).

Propagation and cultivation. The pear is usually propagated by budding onto seedlings grown from seeds of Bartlett or the wild French pear. Vegetatively propagated rootstocks of Old Home and Old Home X Farmingdale are coming into wider use. The pear may be dwarfed by propagating onto roots of quince *(Cydonia oblonga)*. Oriental rootstocks are seldom used because of their sensitivity to a "pear decline" desease. Orchard care and culture are similar to the apple. *See* APPLE; QUINCE.

Disease. Most commercial pear varieties are extremely susceptible to fireblight, a bacterial disease caused by *Erwinia amylovora* which spreads from blossoms and new shoot tips throughout the branches of a tree. Properly timed sprays of copper or streptomycin provide partial control, but removal of infected branches is always necessary in blighted orchards. The disease is most severe in warm, humid areas, which accounts for the restricted pear production in many regions of the United States. Pear psylla *(Psylla pyricola)*, the major insect pest of pears, is becoming an increasing problem because of inadequate chemical or biological control procedures.

Harvesting, handling, and production. For best quality, pears are picked early and ripened off the tree. They are first held in cold storage at 30 to 32°F (−1 to 0°C) and thereafter ripened for several days at 60 to 70°F (15 to 21°C), with 80 to 85% relative humidity. Winter pears, such as d'Anjou, may be held in cold storage for many months before ripening.

Average annual commercial production in the United States for the 5-year period 1972–1976 was 733,000 tons (659,700 metric tons), of which California produced 320,000 (288,000), Washington 203,000 (182,700) and Oregon 167,000 (150,300). The Bartlett variety made up 69% of the United States total; 42% of the average 5-year crop was marketed fresh, 57.7% canned, and 0.3% dried. *See* FRUIT, TREE; FRUIT (TREE) DISEASES.

[R. PAUL LARSEN]

Pecan

A large tree *(Carya illinoensis)* of the family Juglandaceae, and the nut from this tree. Native to valleys of the Mississippi River and tributaries as far north as Iowa, to other streams of Texas, Oklahoma, and northern and central Mexico, this nut tree has become commercially important throughout the southern and southwestern United States and northern Mexico. Limited plantings have been made in other regions, being reported of interest in such diverse areas as California, South Africa, Israel, Brazil, and Peru. The tree's major importance is in areas with a long growing season of over 200 days and midsummer average temperatures of 26°C (79°F) or higher, though a few early-ripening cultivars are grown in slightly cooler regions. There are different cultivars for arid, irrigated regions and humid summer regions. The United States cultivars have an indistinct winter chilling requirement but fruit best where the coldest winter month averages less than 16°C (61°F).

Botany. The tree is deciduous with compound, pinnate leaves. Flowers are unisexual with staminate flowers borne on year-old wood and pistillate flowers formed terminally on new spring growth. The period of pollen shedding of a cultivar usually does not overlap the time of stigma receptivity, so a choice of cultivars is necessary in large plantings to ensure cross pollination. Pollen is windblown for distances up to 1 km, and usually there is enough diversity of bloom habits to ensure fruit set in smaller orchards and home plantings. Because of the bloom habits, pecans are heterozygous and seedlings are highly variable.

Production. Nuts from native seedlings and from named grafted cultivars are marketed in roughly equal amounts. The former are more important in Texas, Oklahoma, and Louisiana while the latter are more important in Georgia, Alabama, other southeastern states and in new producing areas of western Texas, New Mexico, and Arizona. The tree requires good soil fertility and culture, and usually some spraying to give satisfactory production. Total annual production usually exceeds 210,000,000 lb (94,500,000 kg) but varies as much as 20% from year to year because of strong tendencies toward biennial bearing. Heavy production in one season, combined with premature leaf drop from disease, insects, or poor nutrition will result in light cropping the next year. Research studies in almost all southern states attempt to find spray programs and cultural methods to even out and increase total production. Mechanization of harvest has progressed rapidly in recent years. Local extension information, grower meetings, and circulars and magazines are available to growers.

Breeding. As in all agricultural endeavors, the cultivar is the base for success. Old selections like Stuart and Western, dating from the late 19th century, are still grown extensively. Intensive breeding work by U.S. Department of Agriculture workers since 1950 has produced new cultivars (Fig. 1) which come into production early and have 7–8-g nuts with over 60% kernel content. Combined with

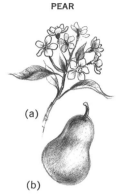

PEAR

Pear *(Pyrus communis)*.
(a) Flower cluster.
(b) Fruit.

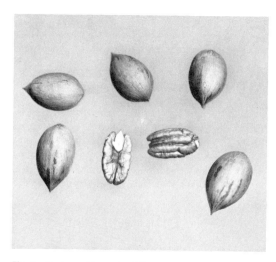

Fig. 1. Nuts and kernels of the relatively new Cherokee pecan cultivar developed by the U.S. Department of Agriculture. (*Pecan Quarterly*)

tree spacings as close as 10 m, these can make orchards profitable sooner and double or triple yields. Converting this large forest-type tree to a smaller, highly productive orchard-type tree is thus becoming reality. See NUT CROP CULTURES.

[RALPH H. SHARPE]

Processing. Pecans constitute about 60% of domestic tree nut production and 10% of United States consumption.

Pecan processing began with the development of mechanical equipment for removing faulty nuts, sizing, cracking, separating meats and shells, grading of meats, drying, and packaging. Utilization has been increased by year-round storage at 34°F or lower, with 65% relative humidity, in an

odor-free atmosphere. Pecans may be stored at 25°F or lower for 2 years or more.

Pecans are palatable, nutritious, very high in energy (700 cal/100 g), and almost completely digestible. They contain 55–75% fat, 9–9.5% protein, 10–15% carbohydrates, 2.2% fiber, and 1.6% ash; they are a good source of vitamin A, thiamin, riboflavin, and phosphorus.

Shelling reduces the weight about 60%, the volume 50%, and the storage life 25%. Shelled nuts are more susceptible to insects, mold, staleness, and rancidity. However, nut meats are preferred because of added convenience, eye appeal, and ease of packaging. The distribution and uses of pecans and pecan meats are approximately as shown in Fig. 2.

Faulty nuts are removed by passing field-run pecans on a perforated conveyor belt under a vacuum hood to remove the light nuts. The pecans are then air-dried at 100°F or lower to a moisture content of 4% for storage or further processing.

To prevent shattering of the meats during cracking, the nuts are conditioned by raising the moisture to 9%. This is accomplished by immersing the pecans in water containing 1000 ppm of chlorine with a wetting agent and allowing them to equalize for 12 hr.

The nuts are cracked as they pass through a hopper in the processing machine. They are momentarily positioned, then struck by a plunger which crushes them to about 75% of their length. Crackers arranged in series have a capacity of about 800 lb of nuts per day.

Shells are removed by series of shaker screens, which also separate the meats into mammoth, jumbo, large, medium, small, midget, and granule pieces. While moving on conveyor belts, the meats are further graded by electric eye and by hand.

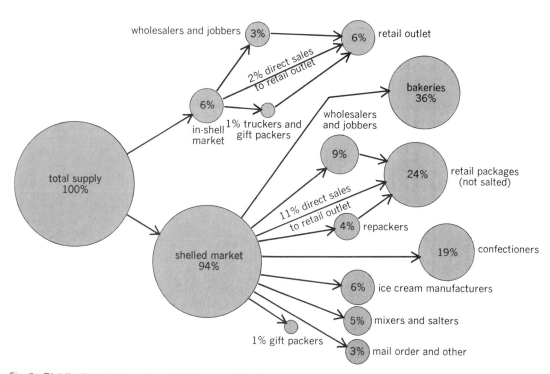

Fig. 2. Distribution of pecans since 1960, by products. (*Courtesy of U.S. Department of Agriculture*)

They are then dried to a moisture content of $3\frac{1}{2}-4\%$ for further processing or storage.

Pecans have a very desirable flavor, aroma, texture, and appearance, and they are used to impart these qualities to such foods as baked goods, dairy products, confections, salads, desserts, fowl stuffings, puddings, soufflés, meat combinations, cereals, and vegetable dishes. The flavor of pecans is compatible with that of most foods, so that they may be used natural, sweetened, salted, or spiced. The texture is such that they may be used as halves or pieces of any desired size. They may be eaten raw or toasted. There are more than 1200 formulas for using pecans in prepared dishes.

[JASPER G. WOODROOF]

Bibliography: J. G. Woodroof, *Tree Nuts: Production, Processing, Products*, 2d ed., 1973.

Pellagra

A disease resulting from severe deficiency of the vitamin B complex. Niacin deficiency is the principal dietary defect in pellagra; the low tryptophan content of some foods also plays a role in this disease. Skin, gastrointestinal, and neurologic symptoms may occur. Wheat, milk, or egg proteins afford ample dietary requirements, but corn protein may be deficient. This accounts for the regional, or endemic, form of pellagra in areas of restricted diet. *See* NIACIN.

Redness, scaling, and brownish discoloration of the skin, particularly in areas exposed to sunlight, are common lesions. Marked enlargement of the tongue and drooling are prominent symptoms. The mucous membranes of the mouth, eyes, urethra, and vagina may show swelling and have a bright red, smooth appearance. Gastrointestinal symptoms may be vague or may take the form of severe nausea, vomiting, and bloody diarrhea. Early nervous system involvement is displayed by the neurasthenic syndrome characterized by restlessness, anxiety, and insomnia. Organic psychoses may follow continued deficiency and are marked by memory loss, confusion, and a variable pattern of affective behavior, such as depression or paranoia. Actual delirium, limb rigidity, and certain uncontrolled reflexes mark the severe case.

Diagnosis may be difficult because of incompletely developed symptoms. In addition, pellagra is almost always accompanied by other vitamin B deficiencies of some degree. Education and preventive medicine have largely eliminated pellagra from areas in the United States where it was prevalent. *See* VITAMIN.

[EDWARD G. STUART/N. KARLE MOTTET]

Pepper

The garden pepper, *Capsicum annuum* (family Solanaceae), is a warm-season crop originally domesticated in Mexico. It is usually grown as an annual, although in warm climates it may be perennial. This species includes all peppers grown in the United States except for the "Tabasco" pepper (*C. frutescens*), grown in Louisiana. Other cultivated species, *C. chinense*, *C. baccatum*, and *C. pubescens*, are grown primarily in South America. Some 10–12 strictly wild species also occur in South America. Peppers are grown worldwide, especially in the more tropical areas, where the pepper is an important condiment. *Piper nigrum*, the black pepper, a tropical climbing vine, is botanically unrelated to the common pepper. *See* PEPPER, BLACK.

Sweet (nonpungent) peppers, harvested fully developed but still green, are widely used in salads or cooked with other foods. Popular varieties (cultivars) are California Wonder and Yolo Wonder. Perfection pimento, harvested red ripe, is used for canning. Paprika is made from ripe red pods, dried and ground, of several distinct varieties. *See* PAPRIKA; PIMENTO.

Hot (pungent) peppers may be picked before ripening for fresh use, pickles, or canning. "Wax" peppers are yellow instead of green before ripening. Ripe pods dried and ground are used to make red pepper powder or mixed with spices to make chili powder. Cayenne and Anaheim Chili, respectively, are the major varieties for grinding. Hot sauce is made from the fresh fruit of the Tabasco pepper ground with vinegar. Pungency is due to the compound capsaicin, located in fragile glands on the internal partitions or "ribs" of the fruit. Seed and wall tissue are not pungent.

The ripe color of most varieties is red, a few varieties are orange-yellow, and in Latin America brown-fruited varieties are common. Nutritionally, the mature pepper fruit has three to four times the vitamin C content of an orange, and is an excellent source of vitamin A. *See* ASCORBIC ACID; VITAMIN A.

Propagation is by planting seed directly in the field or by plants started in greenhouses or hotbeds and transplanted to the field after 6–10 weeks. Field spacing varies: plants 12–24 in. (30–60 cm) apart in 30–36 rows are common. Long warm, but not hot, seasons favor yield and quality.

Green peppers are harvested when fully developed but before appearance of red or yellow color, about 60–80 days after transplanting. Hot peppers, picked red ripe, require about 70–90 days. Florida, California, North Carolina, and New Jersey, in that order, are the most important growing areas. *See* VEGETABLE GROWING.

[PAUL G. SMITH]

Pepper, black

One of the oldest and most important of the spices. It is the dried, unripe fruit of a weak climbing vine, *Piper nigrum*, a member of the pepper family (Piperaceae), and a native of India or Indomalaysia (see illustration). The fruits are small one-seeded berries which, in ripening, undergo a color change from green to red to yellow. When in the red stage, they are picked, sorted, and dried. The dry, wrinkled berries (peppercorns) are ground to make the familiar black pepper of commerce. White pepper is obtained by grinding the seed separately from the surrounding pulp. *See* SPICE AND FLAVORING.

[PERRY D. STRAUSBAUGH/EARL L. CORE]

Peppermint

The mint species *Mentha piperita* (family Lamiaceae), a sterile interspecific hybrid believed to have occurred in nature from the hybridization of fertile *M. aquatica* with fertile *M. spicata*. Peppermint grows in wet, marshy soil along streams in Europe at latitudes of 40–55°. Overwintering sto-

PEPPER, BLACK

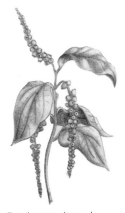

Berries on a branch of *Piper nigrum*.

lons, the leafless underground stems, produce new plants, giving the species a perennial habit.

Strains. Numerous clonal strains brought by pioneers for medicinal use in colds and stomach disorders or as flavoring herbs have persisted in North America in wet areas for more than 100 years. These and a few strains cultivated prior to 1890 are frequently called American peppermint to distinguish them from the single clonal strain called Black Mitcham peppermint, obtained from Mitcham, England, near London. Due to its excellent flavor and aroma, Black Mitcham, with a red anthocyanin stem color, became the exclusive cultivar source of United States peppermint oil from 1910 to 1972. A similar, green-stemmed strain called White Mitcham proved less winterhardy and is no longer cultivated. Irradiation breeding during 1955–1972 at A. M. Todd Company produced two *Verticillium*-resistant varieties registered as Todd's Mitcham (1972) and Murray Mitcham (1977). These were vegetatively propagated and distributed to farmers by certified seed-producing agencies at the state universities of the mint-producing states. Mitcham peppermint is also grown in Bulgaria, Italy, and the Soviet Union and to a limited extent in other countries but is restricted by its long-day–short-night photoperiod to an area north of 40° latitude that is not subject to severe mid-June freezes.

Cultivation and harvesting. In mint farming the dormant stolons are scattered by hand in 10–12-in.-deep (25–30 cm) furrows and covered with soil in rows 36–38 in. (90–95 cm) apart that can be cultivated for weed control with a maize cultivator. In the United States machine planting and preemergence application of terbicil herbicides (such as Sinbar) for weed control are standard practice to minimize labor costs. Peppermint has rather high water requirements, hence supplementary overhead or sprinkler irrigation may be used on the organic soils of the Midwest area (southern Michigan, northern Indiana, Wisconsin) and must be used on alluvial soils of the Willamette Valley of western Oregon and the Madras area of central Oregon. In all these areas the first-year crop is row mint, and all subsequent crops are meadow mint in a solid stand, whereas rill or ditch irrigation necessitating row culture has generally been used on the volcanic soil of eastern Washington and in part on alluvial soils of the Snake River Valley of Idaho.

The crop is mown and windrowed, as hay, about the time that peak vegetative growth is attained or flower buds are beginning to form (July 15–September 10). The windrowed, partially dried hay is picked up by a loader that chops the hay and blows it into a mobile metal distillation tank mounted on four wheels or on a dump truck chassis.

Peppermint oil. The oil of commerce is obtained by steam distillation from the partially dried hay. Steam under pressure traverses the chopped hay in the mobile tank, removing the oil, and is then cooled in a condenser. The oil floats on the water in a receiving receptacle and is removed to metal drums for storage and sale. Stills are expensive since automatic valves and stainless steel construction are needed. The oil is complex, having 3 major constituents and over 80 minor ones

that are necessary to the flavor and aroma. Oil yields in pounds per acre are generally 40–65 (45–73 kg/hectare) in the Midwest, 65–85 (73–96 kg/hectare) in the Willamette Valley and Idaho, and 85–110 (96–125 kg/hectare) in eastern Washington. The United States produces 50,000–80,000 acres (202–324 km²) of peppermint. The main uses of peppermint oil are to flavor chewing gum, confectionary products, toothpaste, mouthwashes, medicines, and as a carminative in certain medical preparations for the alleviation of digestive disturbances. *See* SPICE AND FLAVORING.

Diseases. Principal diseases are Verticillium wilt, which occurs everywhere, and Puccinia rust in the western United States. In the Willamette Valley, where rust is severe, fields are flamed with a propane burner to interrupt the rust cycle in early spring as plants are emerging. Genetic control of Verticillium wilt is through use of the new varieties.

[MERRITT J. MURRAY]

Peptide

A compound that is made up of two or more amino acids joined by covalent bonds which are formed by the elimination of a molecule of H_2O from the amino group of one amino acid and the carboxyl group of the next amino acid. Peptides larger than about 50 amino acid residues are usually classified as proteins.

In the reaction shown, the α-linkage between

L-Glutamic acid   D-Alanine

L-Glutamyl-D-alanine

the α-amino group of alanine and the α-carboxyl group of glutamic acid is by far the most common type of linkage found in peptides. However, there are a few cases of γ-linkage in which the side-chain carboxyl group of one amino acid is linked to an α-amino group of the next amino acid, as in glutathione and in part of the structure of the bacterial cell wall. Linear peptides are named by starting with the amino acid residue that bears the free α-amino group and proceeding toward the other end of the molecule. Sometimes the configuration of the asymmetric carbon atom of each residue is included in the name, as shown in the reaction. A three-letter notation is convenient to use, for example, L-Glu-D-Ala.

Occurrence. Peptides of varying composition and length are abundant in nature. Glutathione, whose structure is γ-L-glutamyl-L-cysteinyl-glycine, is the most abundant peptide in mammalian tissue. Hormones such as oxytocin (8), vasopressin (8), glucagon (29), and adrenocorticotropic hormone (39) are peptides whose structures have been deduced; in parentheses are the numbers of amino acid residues for each peptide. Some of the hormone regulatory factors which are secreted by the hypothalamus are peptides that govern the release of hormones by other endocrine glands. In the peptides indigenous to mammalian tissues all of the amino acid residues are of the L-configuration.

Many of the antimicrobial agents produced by microorganisms are peptides that can contain both D- and L-amino acid residues. Penicillin contains a cyclic peptide as part of its structure. Other peptide antibiotics include the gramicidins, the tyrocidines, the polymyxins, the subtilins, and the bacitracins. See ANTIBIOTIC.

Synthesis. For each step in the biological synthesis of a peptide or protein there is a specific enzyme or enzyme complex that catalyzes each reaction in an ordered fashion along the biosynthetic route. However, it is noteworthy that, although the biological synthesis of proteins is directed by messenger RNA on cellular structures called ribosomes, the biological synthesis of peptides does not require either messenger RNA or ribosomes.

In the methods most commonly used in the laboratory for the chemical synthesis of peptides, the α-carboxyl group of the amino acid that is to be added to the free α-amino group of another amino acid or peptide is usually activated as an anhydride, an azide, an acyl halide, or an ester, or with a carbodiimide. To prevent addition of the activated amino acids to one another, it is essential that the α-amino group of the carboxyl-activated amino acid be blocked by some chemical group (benzyl oxycarbonyl-, t-butyloxycarbonyl-, trifluoroacetyl-) that is stable to the conditions of the coupling reaction; such blocking groups can be removed easily under other conditions to regenerate the free α-amino group of the newly added residues for the next coupling step. In order to ensure that all the new peptide bonds possess the α-linkage, the reactive side chains of amino acid residues are usually blocked during the entire synthesis by fairly stable chemical groups that can be removed after the synthesis. For a successful synthesis of a peptide or protein, all of the coupling steps should be complete, and none of the treatments during the progress of the synthesis should lead either to racemization or to alteration of any of the side chains of the amino acids. In the earlier techniques for the chemical synthesis of peptides the reactions were carried out in the appropriate solvents, and the products at each step were purified if necessary by crystallization ("solution method"). An innovation devised by R. B. Merrifield uses a "solid phase" of polystyrene beads for the synthesis. The peptide, which is attached to the resin beads, grows by the sequential addition of each amino acid. The product can be washed by simple filtration at each step of the synthesis. See AMINO ACIDS; PROTEIN.   [JAMES M. MANNING]

Persian melon

A long-keeping variety of muskmelon, *Cucumis melo*, of the plant order Violales. The fruit weighs 6–8 lb and is globular and without sutures; it has dark-green skin and thin, abundant netting; and the flesh is firm, thick, orange, and sweet, with mild but distinctive flavor. Persian melons require a long warm season, and are highly susceptible to diseases, which are intensified by rain or high humidity.

In the United States the Persian melon is a very minor crop with significant commercial acreage only in the great central valley of California. It is a luxury product for which demand declined during the 1960s. The average annual production of 7600 tons during 1961–1965 declined to 3000 tons in 1974, and harvested acres declined from 1280 to 500. The average annual farm value declined from some $1,000,000 during the 1950s and $800,000 during 1961–1965 to $700,000 in 1974. See MUSK-MELON.   [VICTOR R. BOSWELL]

Pesticide

A material useful for the mitigation, control, or elimination of plants or animals detrimental to human health or economy. Algaecides, defoliants, desiccants, herbicides, plant growth regulators, and fungicides are used to regulate populations of undesirable plants which compete with or parasitize crop or ornamental plants. Attractants, insecticides, miticides, acaricides, molluscicides, nematocides, repellants, and rodenticides are used principally to reduce parasitism and disease transmission in domestic animals, the loss of crop plants, the destruction of processed food, textile, and wood products, and parasitism and disease transmission in man. These ravages frequently stem from the feeding activities of the pests. Birds, mice, rabbits, rats, insects, mites, ticks, eel worms, slugs, and snails are recognized as pests.

Materials used to control or alleviate disease conditions produced in man and animals by plants or by animal pests are usually designated as drugs. For example, herbicides are used to control the ragweed plant, while drugs are used to alleviate the symptoms of hay fever produced in man by ragweed pollen. Similarly, insecticides are used to control malaria mosquitoes, while drugs are used to control the malaria parasites—single-celled animals of the genus *Plasmodium*—transmitted to man by the mosquito.

Some pesticides are obtained from plants and minerals. Examples include the insecticides cryolite, a mineral, and nicotine, rotenone, and the pyrethrins which are extracted from plants. A few pesticides are obtained by the mass culture of microorganisms. Examples are the toxin produced by *Bacillus thuringiensis*, which is active against moth and butterfly larvae, and the so-called milky disease of the Japanese beetle produced by the spores of *B. popilliae*. Most pesticides, however, are products of chemical manufacture. Two outstanding examples are the insecticide DDT and the herbicide 2,4-D.

The development of new pesticides is time-consuming. The period between initial discovery and introduction is frequently cited as being about 5 years. Numerous scientific skills and disciplines are required to obtain the data necessary to establish the utility of a new pesticide. Effectiveness under a wide variety of climatic and other environmental conditions must be determined, and minimum rates of application established. Insight must be gained as to the possible side effects on other animals and plants in the environment. Toxicity to laboratory animals must be measured and be related to the hazard which might possibly exist for users and to consumers. Persistence of residues in the environment must be determined. Legal tolerances in processed commodities must be set and directions for use clearly stated. Methods for analysis and detection must be devised. Economical methods of manufacture must be developed. Manufacturing facilities must be built. Sales and education programs must be prepared. See AGRICULTURAL CHEMISTRY; AGRICULTURE; FUMIGANT; FUNGISTAT AND FUNGICIDE; HERBICIDE; INSECTICIDE; MITICIDE.   [GEORGE F. LUDVIK]

Bibliography: B. P. Beirne, *Pest Management*, 1966; D. E. H. Frear, *Pesticide Index*, 4th ed., 1969; W. W. Kilgore and R. L. Doutt, *Pest Control: Biological, Physical and Selected Chemical Methods*, 1967.

Phenylalanine

An amino acid considered essential for normal growth of animals. The amino acids are characterized physically by the following: (1) the pK_1, or the dissociation constant of the various titratable groups; (2) the isoelectric point, or pH at which a

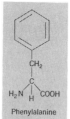

Physical constants of the L isomer at 25°C:
pK_1 (COOH): 1.83; pK_2 (NH_3^+): 9.13
Isoelectric point: 5.48
Optical rotation: $[\alpha]_D(H_2O)$: −34.5; $[\alpha]_D$(5 N HCl): −4.5
Solubility (g/100 ml H_2O): 2.97
Absorption spectrum: peak at 260 mμ (ultraviolet)

Phenylalanine

dipolar ion does not migrate in an electric field; (3) the optical rotation or the rotation imparted to a beam of plane-polarized light (frequently the D line of the sodium spectrum) passing through 1 dm of a solution of 100 g in 100 ml; (4) solubility; and (5) absorption spectrum or the wavelength at which maximum absorption occurs.

Dietary phenylalanine is the source of tyrosine in animal tissues. Phenylalanine originates biosynthetically from phosphoenolpyruvic acid and D-erythrose-4-phosphate by way of shikimic acid and prephenic acid. See AMINO ACIDS.

During metabolic degradation the major pathway in mammals is by oxidation to tyrosine, which is then degraded to fumarate and acetoacetate. Phenylalanine also can be deaminated to phenylpyruvic acid, of which three metabolic products are known: benzoic acid, phenylacetic acid, and phenyllactic acid. See TYROSINE.

[EDWARD A. ADELBERG]

Phenylpyruvic oligophrenia

A type of mental deficiency caused by an inherited defect in the metabolism of the amino acid phenylalanine. Postmortem examination of affected individuals discloses absence of the liver enzyme responsible for the metabolism of phenylalanine. The condition, also known as phenylketonuria, is rare with an incidence of 1 in 25,000 in the general population and 3 in 2300 mental deficients. The concentration of unmetabolized phenylalanine is associated with diminution of activity in the higher mental centers and in permanent intellectual retardation. However, research has opened the possibility of preventing some types of mental deficiency caused by mutant genes through medical identification of genetic factors in the parents. See PHENYLALANINE.

Phenylpyruvic mental deficiency is diagnosed by the presence of phenylpyruvic acid in the urine. This is accomplished by the addition of a 5% solution of ferric chloride, which causes a characteristic deep-green color in the presence of the acid. The generally accepted Guthrie test is a simple serological technique in which a drop of blood, taken from the baby's foot prior to its release from the hospital, is tested for elevated phenylalanine levels. With greater awareness of the condition, the development of improved techniques of identification, and the recognition of the beneficial effects of dietary regimen, many states in the United States have adopted statutes which permit or require appropriate tests on all infants.

It is possible to alter the levels of such abnormal metabolites in the body by changing the diet; phenylalanine-free diets have been developed. There are many indications that if diet control can be applied in early infancy, damage to the nervous system can be halted and more normal maturation anticipated.

The mental defective of this type is usually blond and has blue eyes and fair skin, with signs of eczema; the urine is characterized by a musty odor. These individuals generally show severe mental retardation, although occasionally they may be classified as moderate. Bizarre behavior reactions, including withdrawal, fright reaction, negativism, and posturing, are observed in some cases. They rarely benefit from special education.

From the genetic standpoint the condition is due to a single mutant gene which follows the recessive pattern of inheritance. It is estimated that the recessive gene exists in a 1:173 ratio in the general population. The parents are apparently normal heterozygotes with no overt clinical evidence of the disease, and the child is a homozygote with marked signs of the abnormal metabolite in the urine. Studies of the heterozygous parents have demonstrated abnormal phenylalanine tolerance curves. By using this finding, it may be possible to predict the existence of the recessive gene and therefore the probable occurrence of a homozygote offspring. Such a technique may provide a concrete basis for genetic counseling of the parents, thus reducing the incidence of the condition in the population.

[MAURICE G. KOTT]

Photoperiodism in plants

The growth, development, or other response of the organism (plant) to the length of night or day or both. Since this implies an ability to measure time, there must exist in living organisms a biological clock.

DEFINITION OF PARAMETERS

The study of photoperiodism in plants has largely been directed toward an understanding of the initiation of flowers. If a plant flowers in response to a given day or night length, it will flower at some specific time during the year. Response to short nights causes flowering in midsummer, while response to longer nights allows flowering in late summer or fall. Detection of seasonal time by measurement of length of day or night is highly dependable, much more so than response to factors such as temperature. The photoperiodic response is also a function of latitude. For example, if very long days (very short nights) are required, the species will only be able to flower in the far north. This is clearly important in the distribution of plants, and there are important applications in agriculture. Day length may restrict crop distribution in addition to restrictions of temperature, moisture, or other factors. Some varieties of soybeans, for example, can be grown successfully only in a belt of latitude about 50 mi wide. Plant breeders may control the flowering of several species, and in ornamental horticulture flowering of some plants (for example, chrysanthemums, poinsettias, and orchids) is controlled on a commercial scale in greenhouses by controlling the length of day and night. To extend the day, lights are hung above the greenhouse benches, while black curtains are placed on racks over the plants to shorten the day.

There are many aspects of photoperiodism in plants besides the formation of flowers in higher plants. These include development of reproductive structures in lower plants (mosses); stem elongation in many herbaceous species, as well as evergreen and deciduous trees; formation of winter dormant buds; development of frost hardiness; formation of many underground storage organs such as bulbs (onion), tubers (potato), and storage roots (radish); runner development in strawberries (a long-day response—flowering is a short-day response in many varieties); balance of male to female flowers or flower parts (cucumbers); and certain less well-known responses, such as the formation of foliar plantlets and the fixation of carbon dioxide in the dark (both with *Bryophyllum*).

There are also many responses to photoperiod in animals such as control of several stages in the life cycle of insects (diapause), and the long-day promotion in birds of molting, development of gonads, deposition of body fat, and migratory behavior. Even feather color may be influenced by photoperiod (as in the ptarmigan). In certain mammals the induction of estrus and spermatogenic activity may be influenced by photoperiod, as is fur color in

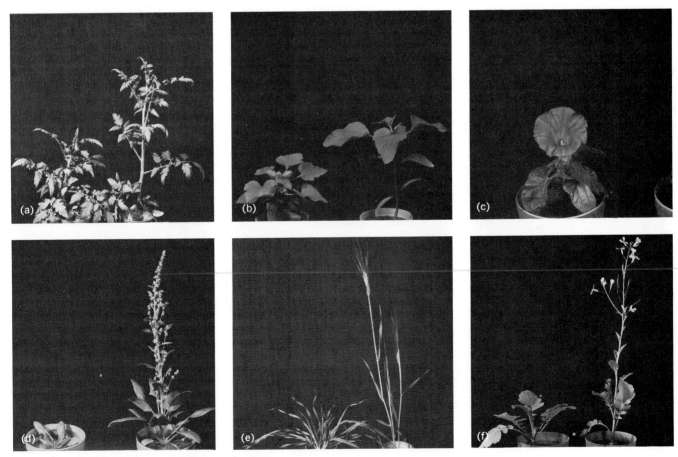

Fig. 1. Plant responses to photoperiodism. Short-day responses on left and long-day on right for each plant. (*a*) Tomato, a day-neutral plant (110 days). (*b*) Cocklebur (60 days). (*c*) Japanese morning glory (35 days). (*d*) Spinach, a long-day plant (35 days). (*e*) Barley (35 days). (*f*) Radish (54 days). (*From F. B. Salisbury, The Flowering Process, Pergamon Press, 1963*)

certain species (for example, snowshoe rabbit).

Many descriptive facts have been discovered about photoperiodism. Often there is little theory to help understand these phenomena. Furthermore, the topic is becoming almost unbelievably complex as investigators continue to document individual differences in response among various species. This article reviews the discovery of photoperiodism, outlines some of the descriptive facts about the phenomenon, and considers certain lines of modern research. The discussion concerns flowering exclusively, since little information is available about other plant responses.

Discovery. It is interesting that the importance of day length was essentially overlooked until rather recently. Georg Klebs obtained data before 1918 which might have allowed him to discover photoperiodism. Certain plants flowered in his greenhouses in the wintertime, providing they were kept under electric lamps. Klebs interpreted these results and others, however, in terms of a nutrition theory of flowering. The real discovery was published in 1920 by Whiteman Wells Garner and Harry Ardell Allard, who observed among other things that Maryland Mammoth tobacco flowered in their greenhouses in the winter but not during the summer in the fields. All of the environmental factors which might differ between the summer

fields and the winter greenhouses were investigated. One of these was day length. Maryland Mammoth tobacco plants bloomed profusely when subjected to days shorter than about 12 hr, but remained vegetative if days were longer. Since these plants responded to shortening days, Garner and Allard referred to them as short-day plants; plants which responded to lengthening day were called long-day plants. Some plants seemed to show no flowering response to day length; these were called day-neutral plants (Fig. 1).

There is a qualitative difference between the long-day and short-day responses. As illustrated in Fig. 2, short-day plants flower as the days become shorter, while long-day plants flower as the days become longer. The actual day length allowing flowering may overlap considerably in the two response types. Both henbane and cocklebur flower when days are 12–15 hr long, for example, although their response types are quite opposite.

Complications. Many species do not seem to require a given day length to flower (sooner or later they flower anyway), but they may be promoted in their flowering by some specific day length. At proper temperatures, for example, tomato is slightly promoted in its flowering by short days (Fig. 2). Plants requiring a given day length are said to be qualitative or absolute short- or long-day plants, while those only promoted by proper day length are said to be quantitative or facultative in response. Several species exist which require short days followed by long days (short-long-day plants) or long days followed by short days (long-short-day plants). Furthermore, certain species (for example, sugarcane) seem to require an intermediate day length; they remain vegetative if days are either too short or too long.

Often there is a strong interaction between temperature and day length, and various combinations are known. Some species (for example, Japanese morning glory) have an absolute short-day requirement at high temperatures but are day-neutral at lower temperatures, for example, close to freezing. Furthermore, many plants have an absolute requirement for low temperatures given over a period of days to weeks if they are to flower. Typically this requirement is followed by a long-day requirement (vernalization).

The complexity of response may be surprisingly intricate as detailed researches yield more facts. *Silena armeria* requires long days at 20°C to flower, but it is completely day-neutral at 5° or 32°C. It can also be made to flower at any temperature by treatment with GA$_7$ (one of the gibberellic acids). Complications such as these make it difficult to assess the significance of photoperiodism and vernalization for plant distribution. *See* GIBBERELLIN.

Species also differ in sensitivity to photoperiod. *Chenopodium rubrum* responds as a minute seedling in a petri dish. The cotyledons (seed leaves already present in the embryo) of Japanese morning glory are highly sensitive. In cocklebur the cotyledons are not sensitive, but the first true leaf becomes highly sensitive when it is half expanded (plants about 30 days old). Certain trees do not flower until they are 5–40 years old, although it is not known whether they are actually responding to photoperiod.

Plants also vary in the number of photoperiodic

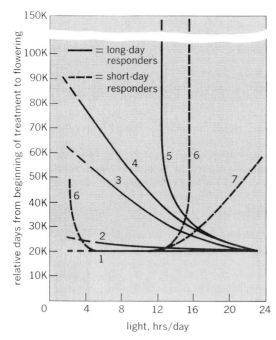

Fig. 2. Schematic indicating flowering response to various day lengths. K varies for each plant; each line represents a different hypothetical plant. Low parts of the curves indicate that flowering occurs in relatively few days and hence is promoted by the indicated day length. (1) Truly day-neutral plant. (2) Plant slightly, but probably insignificantly, promoted in its flowering by long days. (3 and 4) Both plants are quantitatively promoted by long days (to different degrees), even though they flower on any day length. (5) Qualitative long-day plant such as henbane (flowers only when days are longer than about 12.5 hr). (6) Qualitative short-day plant such as cocklebur (flowers only when days are shorter than 15.6 and longer than about 3 or 4 hr). (7) Quantitative short-day plant flowers on any day length but sooner under short days. (*From F. B. Salisbury, The Flowering Process, Pergamon Press, 1963*)

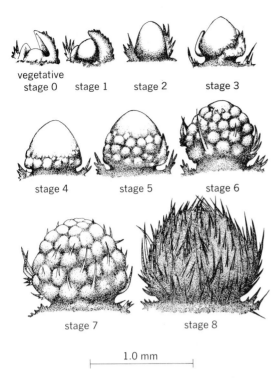

vegetative
stage 0   stage 1   stage 2   stage 3

stage 4   stage 5   stage 6

stage 7   stage 8

|— 1.0 mm —|

Fig. 3.   Appearance of tip of cocklebur stem as its growing point develops from vegetative condition (stage 0)
into small flower primordium (stage 8). Plants exhibit
stages when examined microscopically at intervals after
one long dark period. (*From F. B. Salisbury, The dual role
of auxin in flowering, Plant Physiol., 30:327–334, 1955*)

cycles required for induction. Cocklebur, Japanese morning glory, and other species respond to a
single cycle. Biloxi soybean requires at least three
cycles, while chrysanthemums and many other
plants require several more. The cocklebur becomes induced by exposure to a single cycle; that
is, flowering continues even though short days are
no longer being given. Conversely, in chrysanthemums when short days are replaced by long days,
the developing flower buds abort.

MECHANISMS

Many techniques have been devised to investigate photoperiodism. One of the most important
concerns the quantitative measurement of
flowering. To measure flowering, one counts the
number of flowers or flowering nodes produced by
a given treatment, the number of days until flowers
first appear, the height of the flowering stem, or
other indicators. It is also possible to observe the
development of the floral bud under a dissecting
microscope a few days after floral induction. A series of numerical stages can be arbitrarily assigned
to the steps in the development of this bud (Fig. 3).
In cocklebur, for example, buds can be examined 9
days after plants have been exposed to a single
long night, and effectiveness of the long night is
proportional to the stage of the flower buds when
they were examined.

Seeing light and dark. K. Hamner and J. Bonner
in 1938 asked whether day or night was most important in photoperiodism. They combined constant day length with various intervals of darkness
and constant dark periods with various intervals of
light. They found that cocklebur plants would

flower when the dark period exceeded about 8.5 hr
and that this response was essentially independent
of the length of the day, at least for the light periods used.

The 8.5-hr dark period essential to achieve the
first perceptible signs of flowering in cocklebur is
referred to as the critical night. The critical day
would be the minimum or maximum day lengths
required to induce flowering. On a 24-hr cycle if
the critical night is 8.5 hr, then the critical day
would be 15.5 hr.

Hamner and Bonner also interrupted the day
with a short period of darkness and the night with
a brief interval of light. Darkness during the day
had essentially no effect, but plants completely
failed to flower when the long dark period was interrupted by light. Other workers found that long-
day plants were promoted in their flowering by a
night interruption (Fig. 4). It was concluded that
day length was of secondary importance to night
length, and that short-day plants might more properly be called long-night plants. The importance of
the dark period opened up an unexplored area of
research in photoperiodism.

Light interruption of dark period. The light interruption of the dark period was studied to determine when the interruption is most effective, how
much light is required, and which colors work
best.

The effective time of light interruption can be

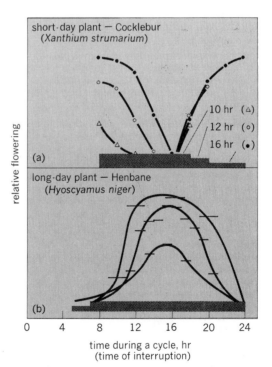

Fig. 4.   Effects of a brief interruption of light given to
plants during long dark periods, as indicated by dark-
gray bars. (a) Plant inhibited in flowering by light interruptions (most effectively about 8 hr after beginning of
dark period). Inhibition begins sooner with shorter dark
periods (*from F. B. Salisbury and C. W. Ross, Plant Physiology, Wadsworth, 1969*). (b) Plant flowering promoted by
a light interruption (1 or 2 hr long as indicated by length
of horizontal bars). Maximum promotion near middle of
dark period (*from H. Claes and A. Long, Die Blütenbildung
von Hyoscyamus niger in 48 stündigen Licht-Dunkel-Zyk-
len und in Zyklen mit aufgeteilten Lichtphasen, Z. Natur-
forschung, 26:56–63, 1947*).

measured by exposing a large number of plants to a suitable dark period and then illuminating a few of these for short intervals at various times. Flowering several days later is plotted as a function of time of illumination (Fig. 4). Obviously some times of illumination (8 hr after the beginning of the dark period for cocklebur) are much more effective than others.

The intensity of an inhibitory light interruption (short-day plants) depends upon the duration of illumination. Higher intensities required shorter exposure times in a manner analogous to the rules of exposure in photography. With cocklebur 2–6 sec of light from four photoflood lamps held about 2 ft away are sufficient to saturate the inhibitory process. If light is applied all night, only 0.02 footcandles of incandescent illumination inhibits flowering.

To investigate the most effective wavelengths (colors), a large spectrograph is used in which an intense beam from a carbon arc passes through a prism, forming a spectrum which can be projected in a band several inches high and 6–10 ft across. Leaves can be illuminated in this spectrum in the middle of the night to determine which wavelengths are most effective in inhibiting or promoting flowering. The orange-red wavelengths are by far the most active. If response (in this case, inhibition of flowering in cocklebur) is plotted as a function of wavelengths, an action spectrum is obtained as in Fig. 5. The action spectra for inhibition of flowering in short-day plants and for promotion of flowering in long-day plants were similar to each other and to spectra for several other responses, such as the germination of lettuce seeds, formation of pigments in apple skins and other plant parts, inhibition of elongation of stems of pea and other

species grown in the dark, opening of the hook on seedlings of such dark-grown species, expansion of leaves on such seedlings, and several other sometimes relatively obscure responses. These are not photoperiodism responses, but other photoperiodism reactions in plants besides flowering do exhibit the same action spectrum. These responses indicate that plants contain some substance, by definition a pigment, capable of absorbing orange-red light, leading to several often unrelated plant responses.

Role of phytochrome. In 1952 it was discovered that the responses could be reversed if, immediately following exposure to red light, plants were illuminated with light of somewhat longer wavelengths, called far-red (Fig. 5). This was a highly significant discovery which opened up a number of areas for research in plant physiology. Investigators suggested that a pigment (subsequently called phytochrome) existed in plants, and that this pigment could be converted from one form to another by absorbing red light, and from the second form back to the original by absorbing far-red. Plants respond as though they are exposed to a preponderance of red light during the days. (The red-absorbing form is most active so that even if there is a mixture of red and far-red, the plant responds as though it is being illuminated with red.) Yet after they have been in the dark a short time, red light is most effective in inhibiting flowering. Hence some kind of shift must occur in the dark; that is, plants must have a preponderance of far-red absorbing pigment when they go into the dark, but in a short time the pigment must be primarily in the red-absorbing form. There must be a conversion from one form to the other, or alternatively (as recent evidence indicates) the far-red absorbing form may be destroyed in the dark while the red-absorbing form is synthesized. The far-red absorbing form (Pfr, sometimes expressed as P_{fr}) which is produced by red light is active in cocklebur or soybean for about 30 min, after which its inhibitory act is apparently complete; that is, the effects of a red interruption can be reversed by a subsequent far-red interruption, but only when the far-red is within about 30 min of the initial red interruption. This is how a plant "sees": When Pfr is present in abundance, the plant is in the light; Pr indicates to the plant's biochemistry that it is in the dark.

In 1959 a group of researchers extracted phytochrome from dark-grown corn seedlings using an intricate piece of equipment capable of detecting the shift between the two forms of phytochrome. Phytochrome is present in plants in such dilute quantities that no color can be observed in dark-grown plants which contain no chlorophyll. After suitable laboratory concentration of the pigment, its blue color becomes apparent. A slight shift (bluish-green to greenish-blue) can be observed with the naked eye upon illumination of the extracted pigment with red or far-red light.

Time measurement. The flowering process can be divided into a series of component steps or partial processes: The dark period must be preceded by light; phytochrome is shifted from one form to the other at the beginning of the dark period; time is measured (the critical night); flowering is then initiated, probably by synthesis of a flowering hormone; the hormone is translocated out of the

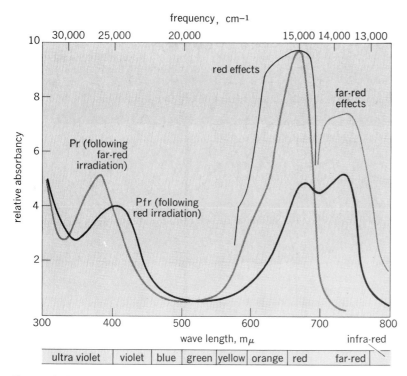

Fig. 5. Action spectra (curves labeled red effects and far-red effects) of plant response and absorption spectra (curves labeled Pr and Pfr) for two forms of phytochrome. (*From F. B. Salisbury, The Flowering Process, Pergamon, 1963*)

leaf; and finally it acts at the bud to initiate a flower. From the synthesis of the hormone on, the investigator is dealing more with the physiology of flowering than with photoperiodism itself, but time measurement is the very essence of photoperiodism.

With the discovery of the reversible nature of phytochrome, it was suggested that time measurement might simply be the time required for pigment shift. Most experiments to test the proposal had negative results. For example, time measurement was shown to be relatively temperature-independent, but conversion of pigment would be expected to be strongly influenced by temperature. Other experiments seem to imply that phytochrome shift is complete in an interval considerably less than the critical night.

There is another important example of time measurement in living organisms: the circadian rhythms. It was shown in the late 1920s that the movement of the leaves of a bean plant (from a horizontal position at noon to a vertical position at midnight) would continue uninterruptedly even when the plants were placed in total darkness and at constant temperature, and that the period between given points on the cycle was not exactly equal to 24 hr but varied as much as 2 or 3 hr either way. Bean plants apparently have an internal clock which oscillates from one position to another and back to the original position in about 24 hr. Many other cycles have been found with similar characteristics in virtually all groups of plants and animals.

Properties of the circadian rhythms have been extensively studied. Their period lengths, for example, are remarkably temperature independent, but they exhibit a high degree of sensitivity to light, which may shift the cycle. Often there is either an advance or delay in the rhythm, depending upon when the light interruption is given during the cycle.

Could time measurement in photoperiodism utilize the circadian clock? Hamner and coworkers have shown that photoperiodism in soybeans and Japanese morning glory exhibits several of the features of circadian rhythms (Fig. 6). For example, there is both an optimum day and an optimum night. Furthermore, if extended periods of darkness are given to short-day plants, such as soybean, and interruptions are given at various times during this long dark period, peaks of promotion occur at about 24-hr intervals, as do troughs of inhibition.

Frank B. Salisbury performed a number of experiments on the light period. Cocklebur (or Japanese morning glory) plants are given a phasing dark period of 7–8 hr, too short to induce flowering, followed by an intervening light period which varies in several ways, and a final test dark period of perhaps 12 hr (long enough normally to induce flowering). The intervening light period has to be at least 5 hr (cocklebur) when the test dark period equals 12 hr. As the intervening light period increases beyond this length, flowering is strongly promoted. This is the typical long-day response exhibited by a classical short-day plant. Five hours may not seem like a long day, but the important point is that flowering is promoted by increasing day length. Low intensities of light are found to be

quite effective during the intervening light period, and red light is by far the most effective, with far-red the least (or inhibitory). Hence in cocklebur red light (Pfr) is highly inhibitory during one phase of the inductive cycle but highly promotive during the other. This is a feature often observed in circadian rhythms.

Herbert Papenfuss, working with Salisbury, further studied time measurement in cocklebur. It was found that the clock could be delayed slightly when light interruptions came close to the beginning of an inductive dark period, but that it was completely rephased (in a sense advanced) when the interruption came 5 or 6 hr after the beginning of the dark period. These responses are also typical of the circadian rhythms.

It would appear then that photoperiodism is a time measurement with a biological clock similar to, or identical with, the one used in control of the circadian rhythms. This clock is apparently coupled to the environment, in some yet to be discovered manner, by the phytochrome system. The

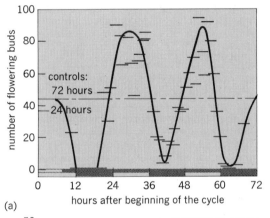

(a)

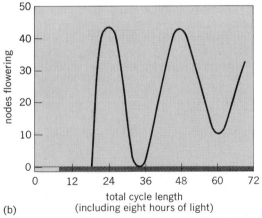

(b)

Fig. 6. Examples of a rhythmic response in the flowering process. (a) Plants given seven cycles, including 8 hr of light and 64 hr of darkness (top bar on abscissa). When the long dark period was interrupted with 4 hr of light (horizontal bars), flowering was greatly inhibited at some times (12–20 hr, 39 hr, and 64 hr) but promoted at other times (24–36 hr and 48–55 hr). If the plant goes through cycles during which light is promotive at one time and inhibitory at another (bottom bar on abscissa), results would be expected. (b) Flowering response to 8 hr of light plus periods of darkness. Flowering is promoted at total cycles of 24 and 48 hr; inhibition occurs at about 34 and 60 hr. (From F. B. Salisbury, The Flowering Process, Pergamon Press, 1963)

mode of action of the biological clock remains the frontier for research in photoperiodism.

Flowering hormone. The site of the photoperiodic response is the plant leaf. Exposing the stem or the bud to the inductive daylength typically has no effect. Thus it was suggested that some substance must be synthesized in the leaf and translocated to the bud, where flowers are initiated. Such a substance if not a nutrient and if effective in small quantities would be called a hormone (florigen). The likelihood of such a material was further demonstrated by grafting experiments in which plants which had been exposed to suitable day lengths were grafted to plants which had not been so exposed, causing the receptors to flower. Furthermore, a flowering short-day plant grafted to a long-day plant might cause it to flower when kept under short days and vice versa. Translocation of this hypothetical hormone can be studied by removing the leaves of cocklebur or Japanese morning glory at various times following exposure to a single dark period. When leaves are removed immediately, plants remain vegetative as though the hormone had not had time to be translocated from the leaf. After several hours, however, the leaves can be removed and the plants flower nearly as well as when the leaves were left on indefinitely.

These experiments led to several attempts to extract florigen, but most have so far failed. Tentative successes have been reported with extracts applied to vegetative plants. They cause only a minimal level of flowering, however, and so this remains another frontier of research in this field.

There are also evidences for a negative-acting inhibitor of flowering produced by photoperiodism. For example, if the tip of a cocklebur leaf is darkened with folded black paper while the base remains in long day (light of low intensity), flowering is completely inhibited. If the leaf tissue between the veins at the base of the leaf is removed, then flowering occurs, showing that the tip is quite capable of producing florigen. Apparently this tissue produces an inhibitor when it is maintained under long-day conditions. This and other evidence for inhibitors indicate that flowering apparently results from the interaction of promoters and inhibitors and that several of both may be involved.

The metabolism of flowering has been studied by the application of chemicals. Plant-growth regulators such as the auxins may inhibit flowering, for example. Gibberellic acid completely replaces the requirement for a long day (or for low temperatures) in many (but not all) species. It has little effect on short-day plants. Abscisic acid induces flowering in black currants but inhibits flowering in *Lolium temulentum*. Cobaltous ion seems to inhibit the running of the biological clock, and various herbicides stop development of the floral bud. Unfortunately, this tells little about the biochemistry of flowering, since little is known about the action of these materials. *See* ABSCISIC ACID; AUXIN.

Certain metabolic inhibitors or antimetabolites have been used, and somewhat more is known about their mode of action. Dinitrophenol and other compounds inhibit the production of respiratory energy, and they inhibit the synthesis of florigen, as though this depends upon such energy. A few antiamino acids, known to inhibit the synthesis of protein, inhibit flowering, although many do not. Several antinucleic acids inhibit flowering, and it is quite likely that the synthesis of nucleic acids, both deoxyribonucleic acid (DNA) and ribonucleic acid (RNA), is an essential part of floral initiation. Often simultaneous application of suitable amino acids or nucleic acid precursors overcomes the effects of the inhibitors. Certain antisteroids are highly effective in inhibiting flowering, but their effects cannot be overcome by application of appropriate steroids or precursors, nor can changes in natural steroids be correlated with flowering.

Florigen action. It appears likely that the arrival of the hormones at the bud results in a shift in the active genes in the cells of the bud. The result of this derepression of genetic material is the initiation of new metabolic steps in these cells which lead to the growth and development of the flower. The process can be described in these general terms, but the details of how such a change in metabolism could result in the formation of a new kind of organ are completely unknown. *See* PLANT GROWTH; PLANT HORMONES.

[FRANK B. SALISBURY]

Bibliography: L. T. Evans, *Induction of Flowering: Some Case Histories*, 1969; A. Lang, in W. Ruhland (ed.), *Encyclopedia of Plant Physiology*, vol. 15, pp. 1381–1536, 1965; F. B. Salisbury, *The Biology of Flowering*, 1969; F. B. Salisbury and C. W. Ross, *Plant Physiology*, 1969; N. E. Searle, Physiology of flowering, *Annu. Rev. Plant Physiol.*, 16:97–118, 1965.

Photorespiration

All respiratory activity in which CO_2 is released and O_2 is taken up by illuminated green plants. The respiration of plants in sunlight is quite different from "dark" respiration, although for many years most scientists tacitly assumed that they were identical. In the late 1950s J. P. Decker, the pioneering investigator of photorespiration, questioned this assumption and performed experiments based on the rationale that an illuminated leaf, when suddenly placed in darkness, might exhibit a momentarily perturbed dark respiration if light and dark respiration were different. The rationale proved to be correct for certain plants, as shown in Fig. 1 with *Panicum bisculatum* leaves. As the light is extinguished, photosynthesis ceases almost immediately, but the leaf rapidly releases a burst of CO_2 for about a minute before gradually returning to the normal, steady dark rate of respiration. The complex shape of this postillumination CO_2 curve is not fully explainable, but clearly light has a large momentary effect on the subsequent dark respiration, and it is assumed that light respiration also is affected.

As these types of measurements were extended to other plants, it was discovered that, in certain species, postillumination CO_2 metabolism simply returns to the normal dark respiration rate, as in Fig. 1 with crabgrass. Thus, in certain species, leaf photorespiration is not easily detectable. It was quickly recognized that most major crop plants in the world had photorespiration, whereas in many other plants photorespiration could not be detected. Simultaneously it was recognized that plants with easily detectable photorespiration assimilated

CO_2 photosynthetically via the pentose phosphate cycle (C_3), whereas with plants in which photorespiration could not be detected, CO_2 was assimilated via the C_4-dicarboxylic acid cycle (C_4) of photosynthesis.

Photorespiration apparently is a wasteful process energetically in that no useful form of energy, such as adenosinetriphosphate (ATP), is derived from the oxidation reactions and CO_2 is lost, although two amino acids, glycine and serine, are produced (Fig. 2). Hence much research is aimed at discovering methods for controlling photorespiration either chemically, genetically, or environmentally. Several chemicals have been discovered which influence laboratory culture assays of photorespiration, but none are effective on whole plants. Genotypes with various levels of photorespiration have been detected, but the genetics of photorespiration are unknown. Plant species with levels of photorespiration intermediate between C_3 and C_4 plants also have been discovered by R. H. Brown, including *P. milioides* and *P. hians*. Environmentally, photorespiration can be reduced in whole plants by raising the CO_2 level above atmospheric (0.03%) or by lowering the oxygen level below 21%.

Since photorespiration involves CO_2 and O_2, the problem of accurately measuring photorespiration comes into focus because the most dominant biochemical process occurring in green plant tissues is photosynthesis. Photosynthesis in full sunlight results in a net uptake of CO_2 and evolution of O_2 which may exceed the rate of normal "dark" respiration some 10 to 30 times, depending upon the plant species. Obviously, photorespiration and photosynthesis both involve the same gases, so that there simultaneously occurs opposite processes of gas uptake and release in an illuminated leaf. Seemingly all gas measurements to determine absolute rates of photosynthesis or photorespiration in intact tissues are somewhat in error due to this intractable problem of CO_2 and O_2 equilibration inside the tissue. *See* PHOTOSYNTHESIS.

Due to the inherent problems of quantitatively measuring photorespiration, early research was not readily accepted. However, other types of information have been discovered, and the older findings have been reevaluated, so that photorespiration now can be described in biochemical terms with reasonable confidence. The major carbon substrate for photorespiration is glycolic acid. The enzymes involved in glycolic acid metabolism in leaves have been studied, and a new leaf organelle, the peroxisome, which contains some of the enzymes of the glycolic acid pathway, has been isolated and partially characterized. The contribution of normal mitochondrial respiration to photorespiration is unknown. Although primary consideration will be given to peroxisomal respiration, mitochondrial respiration is involved in the entire process of photorespiration.

Methods of estimation. All measurements of photorespiration with intact tissues employ indirect methods, each of which includes at least one limiting assumption. The following methods have been employed to estimate photorespiration. The postillumination CO_2 burst discussed above and shown in Fig. 1 is a method in which it is assumed that a remnant of light respiration can be measured in the dark. A second method is to measure

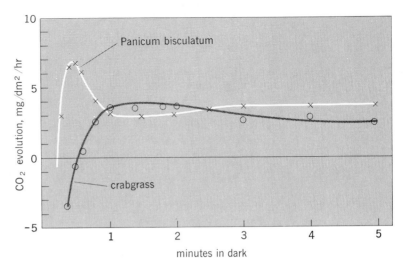

Fig. 1. Leaf postillumination CO_2 metabolism of *Panicum bisculatum*, a pentose-cycle plant, and of crabgrass, a C_4-cycle plant. The respective rates of leaf photosynthesis prior to extinguishing the lights were 34 and 45 mg of CO_2 taken up per square decimeter per hour. (*Data courtesy of R. H. Brown*)

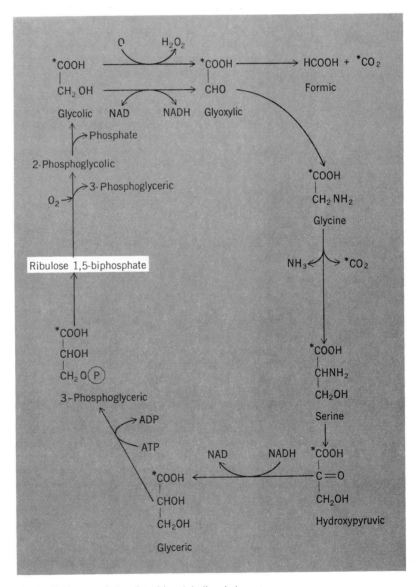

Fig. 2. Pathways of glycolic acid metabolism in leaves.

the release of CO_2 by an illuminated leaf into CO_2-free air. Unfortunately, this method is confounded because in photosynthesis CO_2 is required and glycolate production is a function of the CO_2 concentration. A common method to detect photorespiration is to place a plant in an illuminated sealed chamber and to allow the plant to reduce the CO_2 concentration to a point where CO_2 output equals CO_2 uptake, which is defined as the photosynthetic CO_2 compensation concentration. Perhaps the best method is to measure the rate of net leaf photosynthesis in low O_2 (1 or 2% approximately) and in 21% O_2 since photorespiration is dependent upon O_2 concentration, whereas photosynthesis and respiration generally are not. The decrease in rate of net photosynthesis in 21% O_2 compared to the lower O_2 level is a reasonably quantitative measurement of photorespiration in C_3 plants.

Environmental factors. Photorespiration is favored by high-intensity illumination, high temperature, high O_2 concentration, and low CO_2 concentration.

Light. The magnitude of photorespiration is correlated with light intensity in that photorespiration increases as the light intensity increases in a fashion similar to a light intensity response curve for C_3 photosynthesis. The action spectrum for photorespiration indicates that chlorophyll is the light-absorbing pigment. Photosynthetic electron transport inhibitors also inhibit photorespiration in intact tissues.

Temperature. Temperature has a pronounced effect on photorespiration. Although a reliable Q_{10} has not been reported, photorespiration increases severalfold as the temperature rises from 15 to 35°C. The temperature optimum for photorespiration is near 35°C.

Oxygen. Photorespiration in leaves increases linearly as the concentration of O_2 is varied from 1 to 100%. Dark respiration usually is saturated near 1 to 2% O_2, which clearly distinguishes photorespiration from dark respiration. It has been shown that O_2 competes with CO_2 on the enzyme ribulose 1,5-bisphosphate carboxylase during photosynthesis.

Carbon dioxide. Changing the CO_2 concentration between 0 to 300 ppm (parts per million) probably affects photorespiration indirectly in that photosynthesis is proportional to these CO_2 concentrations; thus the production of glycolate is affected. At CO_2 concentrations much higher (1000 to 5000 ppm CO_2) than physiological (300 ppm CO_2), the synthesis of glycolate is markedly inhibited. Therefore at CO_2 concentrations above atmospheric the metabolic contribution of photorespiration is minimal.

Substrate. It has been discovered that, during photosynthesis in certain algae and in leaves, a sizable amount of carbon can pass through the glycolate pathway intermediates, glycine and serine (Fig. 2). Indeed, in some instances as much as 50% of the photosynthetic carbon has been estimated to pass through the glycolate pathway. Some likely pathways of glycolic acid metabolism are outlined as a guide for the path of photorespiration carbon flow, and the sites of O_2 uptake and CO_2 evolution during photorespiration are indicated in Fig. 2.

Glycolic acid is the major source of carbon for the CO_2 evolved during photorespiration. Using glycolate labeled in carbon positions 1 or 2, it has been shown that CO_2 evolved in the light can arise from the carboxyl carbon of glycolate. In Fig. 2 the asterisk denotes a labeled carbon atom. In another type of experiment, glycolate oxidase, which catalyzes the oxidative conversion of glycolic to glyoxylic acid, can be inhibited fairly specifically by adding an α-hydroxysulfonate. With tobacco leaf disks at 35°C, addition of the inhibitor stimulated photosynthetic CO_2 uptake an average of about 3.8-fold. Furthermore, the inhibitor caused glycolate to accumulate since glycolate oxidation was blocked.

Synthesis of glycolic acid. In the early 1950s it was discovered that glycolate is a very early labeled product of photosynthesis in $^{14}CO_2$. Now, G. Bowes has demonstrated that ribulose 1,5-bisphosphate (RuDP) carboxylase not only carboxylates CO_2, Eq. (1), but that it also is an oxygenase, Eq. (2). Thus this ubiquitous and key photosynthetic protein has two catalytic functions. During oxygenase activity, RuDP is cleaved between the second and third carbon atoms to form 3-phosphoglyceric acid and 2-phosphoglycolic acid, Eq. (2). The site

$$RuDP + CO_2 \xrightarrow[\text{carboxylase}]{RuDP}$$

$$\text{3-phosphoglyceric acid} + \text{3-phosphoglyceric acid} \quad (1)$$

$$RuDP + O_2 \xrightarrow[\text{oxygenase}]{RuDP}$$

$$\text{3-phosphoglyceric acid} + \text{2-phosphoglycolic acid} \quad (2)$$

of glycolate production is the chloroplast. Plant chloroplasts contain an enzyme, phosphoglycolate phosphatase, which irreversibly removes the phosphate.

Glycolic acid oxidation enzymes. Two enzymes in higher plants may oxidize glycolic to the corresponding keto acid, glyoxylic. Glycolic acid oxidase irreversibly catalyzes the oxidation, using O_2 as the electron acceptor, with the production of hydrogen peroxide. Glycolic acid oxidase is localized in the peroxisome. Glyoxylate reductase reversibly catalyzes the oxidation, using a pyridine nucleotide as an electron acceptor. The equilibrium for this reaction, however, strongly favors glycolic acid formation. Glyoxylate reductase is localized in the chloroplasts and may act in a shuttle system with glycolic acid oxidase in the peroxisomes, having a net action of oxidizing reduced pyridine nucleotides in the chloroplasts.

Catalase also is present in the peroxisomes in large quantities and efficiently removes the H_2O_2 produced by glycolic acid oxidase. It has been suggested that the glyoxylic acid is nonenzymatically decarboxylated by H_2O_2 to produce formic acid and the CO_2 of photorespiration (Fig. 2). However, this appears very unlikely, since catalase is over a thousand times more active than any other glycolate pathway enzyme in the peroxisomes. In addition, the isolated peroxisome does not produce CO_2 when fed glycolate.

Glyoxylic acid is converted to glycine through the action of an aminotransferase. Both glutamate–glyoxylate aminotransferase and serine–glyoxylate aminotransferase are present in the peroxisome and catalyze this essentially irreversible glycine production.

Two molecules of glycine then are converted to serine, with the release of NH_3 and the CO_2 of photorespiration. Serine hydroxymethyl transferase is the enzyme which catalyzes this conversion. The peroxisome, however, does not contain this transferase; rather it is localized in the mitochondrion. Hence the CO_2-releasing reaction of photorespiration is in the same organelle which also releases the CO_2 of dark mitochondrial respiration. Again, further proof of the site of CO_2 release is the discovery that isolated peroxisomes, when fed glycolate, do not evolve CO_2.

The fate of both glycine and serine is uncertain since they could be used in many processes, such as protein synthesis. However, by feeding labeled serine to illuminated leaves, it is known that serine is converted primarily to carbohydrates. In the peroxisomes, serine–pyruvate aminotransferase converts the serine to hydroxypyruvic acid, and hydroxypyruvate reductase converts the hydroxypyruvic acid to glyceric acid by utilizing reduced pyridine nucleotides. Chloroplasts contain a glyceric acid kinase which phosphorylates glyceric acid with ATP to form 3-phosphoglyceric acid, the well-known intermediate of the photosynthetic C_3 cycle.

Leaf organelles. About 1965 researchers described a leaf particle of unknown function bounded by a single membrane. Mostly through the efforts of N. E. Tolbert, this leaf particle was isolated and partially characterized. The leaf particle has been termed a peroxisome since it somewhat resembles the peroxisome found in animal tissues. Morphologically, peroxisomes are characterized by a single limiting membrane and a granular matrix, and frequently exhibit a dense or crystalline inclusion. Peroxisomes have a buoyant density of 1.24–1.26 g/cm³ in sucrose, which is utilized in isolating peroxisomes by gradient centrifugation. Leaf peroxisomes tend to be globular and to vary in diameter from about 0.2 to 1.5 μm.

Figure 3 is an electron micrograph of a leaf cross section demonstrating the general appearance of a leaf peroxisome in comparison to a mitochondrion and a chloroplast. Frequently in electron microscopy studies with leaves, these three organelles are found in close proximity. The peroxisomes frequency in leaves relative to mitochondria and chloroplasts varies with species and even in adjacent cells within leaves of plants with the C_4 cycle of photosynthesis, such as crabgrass. In the C_3 plants spinach and sunflower, peroxisomes are quite frequent and represent 1 to 1.5% of the total soluble leaf protein.

Isolated leaf peroxisomes are characterized by a specific enzyme content: glycolic acid oxidase, catalase, glutamate–glyoxylate aminotransferase, serine–glyoxylate aminotransferase, serine–pyruvate aminotransferase, and hydroxypyruvic reductase. Several other enzymes are present, but their role in photorespiration is uncertain. Therefore the glycolate pathway outlined in Fig. 2 is only partially localized in the peroxisome.

Peroxisome respiration does not involve phosphate or phosphate esters. Thus, in contrast to

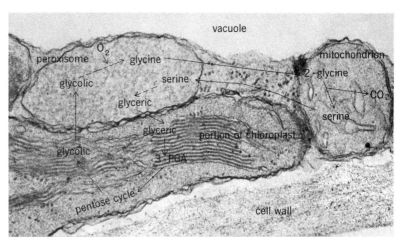

Fig. 3. Electron micrograph of a section from a *Sedum* leaf mesophyll cell. The glycolic acid pathway is inserted in outline, where broken lines indicate that other components of the pathway have been omitted. (*Courtesy of H. H. Mollenhauer*)

mitochondrial respiration, the oxidation reactions are not linked to energy-conserving reactions such as ATP synthesis. Rather the peroxisome is characterized by the production of H_2O_2 and the loss of energy as heat through the destruction of H_2O_2 by catalase.

The complete process of photorespiration involves three cellular organelles. As depicted in Fig. 3, glycolate is synthesized in the chloroplast and moves to the peroxisome, where it is converted to glycine. The glycine moves to the mitochondrion, where CO_2 is released and serine is formed. The serine moves back to the peroxisome, where glycerate is formed, which then moves to the chloroplast and enters the C_3 cycle as 3-phosphoglyceric acid.

In the cyclic pathway in Fig. 2, the ratio of O_2 uptake to CO_2 evolution is 1.5:0.5, since the hydrogen peroxide is split to form $H_2O + 1/2\ O_2$ and two molecules of glycine are required to produce a molecule of CO_2 and serine.

Apparent absence of photorespiration. Most methods of measuring leaf photorespiration fail to detect CO_2 from photorespiration in specific plant species, such as crabgrass, corn, sugarcane, and pigweed; note that all of these plants fix CO_2 photosynthetically via the C_4 cycle. However, leaves of these plants do contain peroxisomes, RuDP oxygenase, and enzymes of the glycolate pathway. It has been speculated that the lack of detectable leaf photorespiration in such plants is due to an internal leaf gas equilibration and recycling of the CO_2 released during photorespiration.

In relation to internal leaf CO_2 recycling, in fully developed leaves of C_4-cycle plants two distinct cell types are present in intact tissues. These cell types, bundle sheath and mesophyll, have been isolated from C_4 plant leaves. The glycolate pathway enzymes are present in both cell types, but the specific activities of most enzymes are about fourfold higher in bundle sheath cell extracts than in mesophyll cell extracts, and in electron micrographs the number of peroxisome profiles are about threefold higher. Each layer of bundle sheath cells is surrounded by one layer of mesophyll cells which are low in peroxisome content and enzyme activity; thus most of the CO_2 released would have to pass through or between the mesophyll cell layer before escaping to the atmosphere. The trapping of CO_2 by the active C_4 cycle in the mesophyll cells before it can escape would greatly decrease the amount of CO_2 which eventually reaches the outside of the leaf. This situation is quite different from that in C_3 plant leaves, such as spinach, which have loosely packed mesophyll cells containing many peroxisomes and very poorly defined bundle sheath cells. Thus, because C_4 plant leaves have an unusual leaf anatomy combined with a spatial distribution of enzymes and organelles, they do not exhibit photorespiration, although the process is present in the intact leaf.

In algae the photorespiration process is somewhat different from higher plants in that spatial specialization may not occur and other environmental factors such as media pH are involved. However, the enzymes of glycolate metabolism are present and glycolate is produced. Indeed, in culture some algae excrete large quantities of glycolate, but until additional data are available few conclusions can be reached about photorespiration in algae.

Function. Photorespiration is an accepted physiological process in plant leaf metabolism. Certainly many unanswered questions remain, but the foundation for future research has been laid in that a substrate (glycolate) and its biosynthesis have been identified, the enzymes to operate the glycolate pathway are present in leaves, and a spatial separation of function into organelles and cell types has been demonstrated. Clear data are not available on the rate-limiting step or steps, nor on the rate of photorespiration. The ratio of CO_2 release to O_2 uptake in the most controlled experiments is about 0.25, which is lower than the theoretical ratio of 0.33 This raises questions regarding substrate oxidations external to the glycolate pathway. The control of photorespiration is a complex process, since intermediates of other metabolic pathways are involved, plus three cellular organelles, the cytoplasm, and specific cell types. Future research holds the possibility of uncovering means for controlling photorespiration, which could result in phenomenal increases in the production of food, fiber, and shelter crops.

[CLANTON C. BLACK, JR.]

Bibliography: G. Bowes, W. L. Ogren, and R. H. Hageman, *Biochem. Biophys. Res. Comm.*, 45: 716–722, 1971; R. H. Brown and W. V. Brown, *Crop Sci.*, 15:681–685, 1975; R. H. Burris and C. C. Black (eds.), *CO_2 Metabolism and Productivity of Plants*, 1976; W. A. Jackson and R. J. Volk, *Annu. Rev. Plant Physiol.*, 21:385–432, 1970; N. E. Tolbert, *Annu. Rev. Plant Physiol.*, 22:45–74, 1971.

Photosynthesis

The manufacture of organic compounds from inorganic materials, with liberation of oxygen, by chlorophyll-containing plant cells in light. Photosynthesis ranks as the most significant process of the biological world. Although it is important in several aspects, the fundamental importance is in the conversion of radiant energy of the Sun to chemically bound energy in the form of sugar and related compounds. This sugar or glucose is sometimes called the primary food of the biological world, since it is from glucose that other energy-containing molecules such as starches, fats and oils, and protein can be directly or indirectly traced. Units of glucose can also be linked together in long chains, forming molecules of cellulose. Cellulose is a main constituent of plant cell walls and makes up a large part of the woody portion of trees. It is the most abundant organic molecule on Earth. Although cellulose cannot be used as a food by most organisms, it does contain a great deal of chemical energy, which can be liberated by the direct burning of wood. Wood and other plant materials produced thousands of years ago, which have since been subjected to pressures below the surface of the Earth, form the origins of fossil fuels such as coal, oil, and natural gas. Thus energy derived from these fossil fuels can likewise be traced back to the photosynthetic process.

Oxygen, another product of photosynthesis, is also of great importance to the biological world. When the Earth was first formed, it is thought that little or no oxygen gas existed in the atmosphere. The atmosphere at present contains over 20% oxygen, most of which can be traced to the photosynthesis of plants over many thousands of years. Ironically, the fossil fuels mentioned above would be of little value if there were no oxygen in which to burn them. Of perhaps more basic importance is the requirement of oxygen for the aerobic respiration process of most plants and animals. Respiration involves the controlled oxidation of foods within the cells of living organisms. Again, both the fuel (food) and the oxygen required in aerobic respiration can be traced back to photosynthesis.

BASIC PROCESS

Early studies of the photosynthetic process date back to about 1800. By about 1815 investigators such as J. Ingen-Housz, J. Priestley, and N. T. de Sarssure had determined that CO_2 gas was used in the process and that O_2 gas was a product when green plants were illuminated. By about 1900 the basic photosynthetic process was known in its summary form. This process is shown in Eq. (1).

$$6CO_2 + 6H_2O \xrightarrow[\text{Green plant}]{\text{Light energy}} C_6H_{12}O_6 + 6O_2 \quad (1)$$

Blackman reaction. In the next few years F. Blackman, working in England, did experimentation which began to indicate that photosynthesis involved more than one kind of reaction. In studying plants under conditions of low light intensities which limited the rate of photosynthesis, he was able to demonstrate that changes in temperature did not change the rate of reaction. Under full light, however, increasing the temperature caused an increase in the rate of the process. It is known that reactions which are purely photochemical do not change in rate with temperature, whereas reactions which are chemical and require enzymes are greatly affected by changes in temperature. Thus it could be inferred that under full sunlight one or more enzymatic reactions limited the rate of reaction, whereas in low light intensities a photochemical process seemed to be limiting the rate of reaction. The name "Blackman reaction" was applied to that portion of photosynthesis which is under enzymatic control. The true significance of the light reactions versus enzymatic reactions of photosynthesis was not completely understood at that time, however.

Hill reaction. In 1937 R. Hill showed that when the chlorophyll-containing organelles (chloroplasts) were extracted from leaves and placed in an illuminated test tube, oxygen gas was produced. The production of oxygen gas occurred only if an additional compound capable of reacting with (accepting) hydrogen was also put in the reaction mixture. It appeared in this reaction that water was being split, with the oxygen escaping as a gas and the hydrogen combining with a hydrogen acceptor. This splitting of water was called photolysis, and the entire reaction was named the Hill reaction. The Hill reaction did not involve a consumption of CO_2 and did not produce sugar. This was the first strong evidence that photosynthesis might involve a light-mediated water-splitting phase which was somewhat independent of the direct production of sugar.

In the Hill reaction, the compound used to accept the hydrogen portion of the water molecule is said to be chemically reduced. (Any molecule which gains either a hydrogen atom or a hydrogen electron becomes reduced.) As a molecule gains

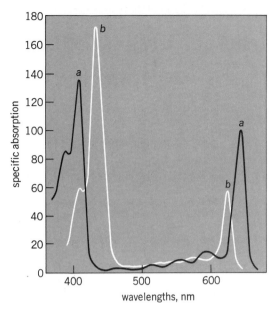

Fig. 2. Absorption spectra of chlorophylls *a* and *b* in ether solution. (*After P. P. Zscheile and C. L. Comar, Bot. Gaz., 102:463–481, 1941*)

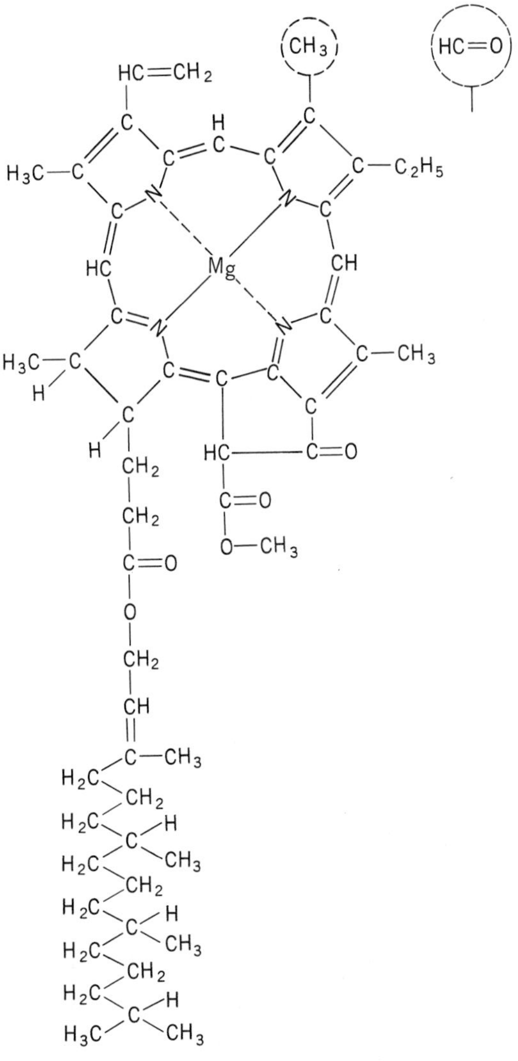

hydrogen, it also gains chemical energy. It had long been recognized that photosynthesis involved a chemical reduction. The carbon of carbon dioxide on the left side of photosynthesis equation (1) has no hydrogen associated with it. However, the carbon of glucose ($C_6H_{12}O_6$) on the right side has considerable hydrogen associated with it. It can therefore be stated that carbon is reduced during the photosynthetic process. Since glucose is a more reduced compound than CO_2, it is not surprising that glucose has considerably more chemically bound energy than carbon dioxide.

One question remaining in understanding the photosynthetic process was how the hydrogen originally split from water was able to become attached to the carbon of CO_2 in the formation of $C_6H_{12}O_6$. A direct reaction of the two did not seem likely. Many years elapsed before the natural hydrogen acceptor in leaf chloroplasts was determined. This compound was found to be nicotinamide adenine dinucleotide phosphate (NADP). When the Hill reaction is run using NADP as the hydrogen acceptor, the process is referred to as the light phase of photosynthesis. This phase is now known to be a fundamental stage in the overall photosynthetic process as it occurs in green plant tissue.

LIGHT PHASE

In the years since the early 1960s, the rather complex nature of the light phase has begun to be unraveled. A portion of these studies have centered on the main pigment involved in this process, chlorophyll (Fig. 1).

Absorption of light. As photons of light reach a leaf, some light passes directly through the leaf (transmitted light) and some bounces off of the leaf surface (reflected light). Neither of these forms of light affect chlorophyll in any way. Only light which is absorbed by a chlorophyll molecule can be effective in the photosynthetic process. Chloro-

Fig. 1. Structural formula for chlorophyll *a*. Substituting the group shown in the broken circle will indicate chlorophyll *b*. (*From B. S. Meyer et al., Introduction to Plant Physiology, Van Nostrand, 1973*)

phyll does not absorb all wavelengths of light equally well (Fig. 2). Although the absorption spectra for chlorophyll *a* and chlorophyll *b* are not identical, both show absorption peaks at the blue end of the spectrum (about 400–450 nm) and the red end of the spectrum (about 640–690 nm). The shorter a wavelength, the greater the energy associated with a photon. Thus, for example, a photon of blue light is much more energetic than a photon of red light. Certain leaf pigments other than chlorophyll, such as the carotenes, can absorb light in ranges of the spectrum where chlorophyll absorption is poor. Energy absorbed by such accessory pigments is thought to be transferable, at least in part, to chlorophyll molecules, and as a result this energy can ultimately be used in the photosynthetic process.

Dissipation of energy. As a photon of light is absorbed by a chlorophyll molecule, an electron of this molecule absorbs the energy of the photon. This electron is in an "excited state." The excited electron jumps to a more external orbit, creating a rather unstable condition. As this excited electron drops back to its original orbit (ground state), a pulse of energy must be dissipated. The dissipation of energy can take several forms: The energy can be completely dissipated as heat. Such energy is "wasted" in terms of involvement in the photosynthetic process. A second means of dissipating the energy as the electron falls back to the ground state is through fluorescence, the production of a photon of red light which is reemitted from the chlorophyll molecule. Energy lost from a leaf by fluorescence cannot be involved in the photosynthetic process. Fluorescence can easily be observed in chlorophyll when an acetone extract of ground leaf material is placed in a strong beam of light. Light striking such an extract produces a steady stream of photons of reemitted red light which makes the solution glow with a blood red color. (This reemitted light should not be confused with reflected light discussed earlier.)

Photosystem I. The two means of dissipation of the energy of an excited chlorophyll electron thus far discussed play no role in the photosynthetic process. There are two other ways that an excited chlorophyll molecule can achieve the ground state.

Both are important in the light phase of photosynthesis. The first of these processes is called resonance transfer. In this process, the energy of an excited electron is passed to an adjacent chlorophyll molecule, and an electron of the second molecule then reaches the excited state. This energy of the second molecule can then be passed to a third molecule in the same manner, and so on. It is thought that chlorophyll molecules exist in groups of about 200. Each group is referred to as a photosynthetic unit. These 200 molecules can be thought of as a network of closely packed molecules. As a photon excites any one of these molecules, energy can travel by resonance transfer from molecule to molecule throughout the network. The energy lost by any one molecule in going from the excited to the ground state is about equal to the energy required to raise the next molecule from the ground to the excited state, provided the molecules are identical. However, for every photosynthetic unit of 200 "normal" chlorophyll molecuels which have an absorption maximum for light with a wavelength of about 685 nm, there is a single modified chlorophyll molecule which has an absorption maximum of about 700 nm. This unusual form is called P_{700}. The P_{700} chlorophyll molecule is thought to be complexed with a protein molecule. As energy from an adjacent normal chlorophyll travels to P_{700} by resonance transfer, there is more than enough energy to excite the P_{700} molecule. However, because the excited electron of P_{700} is slightly less energetic than that of the normal chlorophyll, this energy cannot be transferred back to any of the normal molecules. Thus the energy is trapped in the P_{700} molecule. A photosynthetic unit can therefore be conceived of as a network of molecules which absorbs light energy and funnels it specifically to the P_{700} molecule (Fig. 3).

The energy trapped in P_{700} is dissipated in yet another way. The excited electron leaves the P_{700} molecule and combines with a molecule known to exist, but as yet not identified, which has temporarily been given the name "X." This electron is then rapidly passed sequentially to the compound ferridoxin, and then to NADP. This last reaction can be seen more completely in reaction (2), which

$$H^+ + NADP + e^- \rightarrow NADPH \qquad (2)$$

shows the reduction of NADP to NADPH. Through this sequence of events the energy from a photon of light eventually resides in the high-energy compound NADPH, a fairly stable molecule. This series of events is the most important sequence in the biological world, since it bridges the gap between radiant energy (a photon) and chemical energy (NADPH).

The P_{700} which loses its excited electron to compound X then receives an unexcited electron from a compound called plastocyanin (Fig. 3). Once the P_{700} is reconstituted, its electron can again become excited through resonance transfer from another excited chlorophyll molecule. With 200 chlorophyll molecules funneling energy to P_{700}, it is believed that the rapidity by which P_{700} can be repeatedly excited by resonance transfer is manyfold greater than if it were to directly receive photons of radiant energy.

Photosystem II. The portion of the light phase thus far discussed is generally referred to as photo-

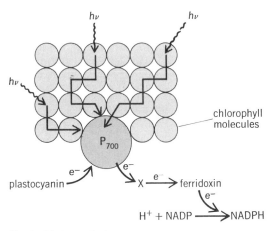

Fig. 3. Photosynthetic unit shown in diagrammatic form indicating the trapping of light energy and subsequent conversion of this energy to chemical energy in the form of NADPH.

system I (PS I). A second type of photosynthetic unit similar to the one already described, photosystem II (PS II), is also known to be involved in the light phase of photosynthesis. The composition of the pigments involved in PS II is slightly different, however. Although both photosystems contain chlorophyll a, the content of chlorophyll b and other accessory pigments appears to be in somewhat different proportions in PS II than in PS I. PS II is thought to be more closely associated with the photolysis of water than PS I.

Summary of light phase. The complete light phase of photosynthesis is now thought to require two photons of light, acting in sequence on PS II and PS I (Fig. 4). In PS II an excited electron is transferred to a yet unidentified compound temporarily named "Q." From Q the electron is sequentially transferred to a number of compounds, including plastoquinone, cytochrome f, and plastocyanin. The electron energy level decreases with each transfer in this sequence (Fig. 4). As the energy level of the electron falls, part of this dissipated electron energy is recaptured in the formation of the high-energy compound adenosinetriphosphate (ATP) from the compound adenosinediphosphate (ADP) plus inorganic phosphate (P_i). ATP plays an important role in other photosynthetic reactions to be discussed later.

In PS I (which follows PS II), a second photon is required to transfer an excited electron to compound X, as discussed earlier. Although the electron of reduced compound X is generally thought to be indirectly transferred to NADP, it should be pointed out that an alternate pathway occurs under certain conditions. This alternate system involves the return of the electron from X back to P_{700}, from which it had originally come. As the electron returns to P_{700}, an ATP is generated from ADP and P_i. Because this phosphorylation of ADP involves an electron which completes a circuit back to P_{700}, this process is called cyclic photophosphorylation (Fig. 4).

In summary, the entire light phase of photosynthesis involves the absorption of at least two photons of light energy by chlorophyll; the photolysis of water; and the generation of two important high-energy compounds, ATP and NADPH. As will be seen in later discussion, these high-energy compounds are used in the conversion of CO_2 to glucose.

CHLOROPLAST STRUCTURE

The photosynthetic process occurs within the organelle known as the chloroplast. The number of chloroplasts per cell can vary with the type of plant: some algae have one large chloroplast per cell, while most photosynthetic cells of higher plants have from 20 to 50 chloroplasts per cell. A typical chloroplast is an ovate structure which is about 2 to 4 μm in length and is surrounded by a double lipid-protein membrane. Within the chloroplast there are areas of dense, compact membranes interspersed with less dense matrixlike areas. The stacks of dense membranes (Fig. 5), referred to as the grana, are composed of flattened saclike subunits called thylakoids. Each thylakoid is so compressed that its saclike nature is not evident in the chloroplast cross section seen in Fig. 5. Each consecutive pair of membranes making up

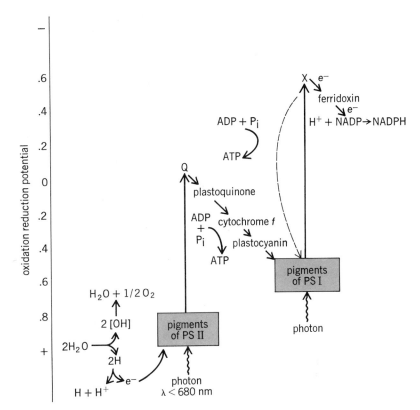

Fig. 4.   Diagram representing the reactions associated with the light phase of photosynthesis. Cyclic photophosphorylation is represented by the broken arrow.

the granum actually represents the top and bottom membrane of a flattened thylakoid sac. The surface view of the inner side of such a membrane, when seen under very high magnification, reveals tiny cubelike units known as quantosomes (Fig. 6). Each quantosome may be the visual equivalent of the photosynthetic unit discussed earlier, although this theory has not yet been completely confirmed. The chlorophyll molecules are known to be associated with the grana membranes. Thus it is fairly well established that the light phase of photosyn-

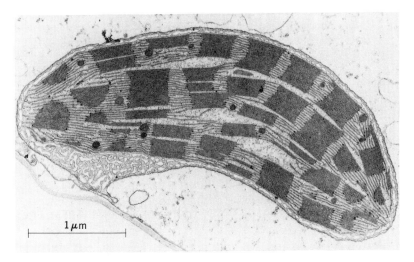

Fig. 5.   Chloroplast of corn shown in section, revealing areas of denser membranes (grana) and gray matrix (stroma). (*From W. A. Jensen and R. B. Park, Cell Ultrastructure, Wadsworth, 1967*)

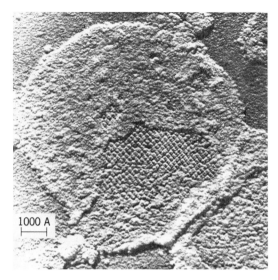

1000 A

Fig. 6. Surface view of a granum membrane showing tiny cubelike units (quantosomes) arranged in an orderly fashion on a portion of this membrane. (After R. B. Park, Science, 144:3621, copyright 1964 by the American Association for the Advancement of Science)

thesis occurs in this membrane system.

The less dense matrixlike area of the chloroplast is known as the stroma. This area contains the many enzymes required in the non-light-requiring phase of photosynthesis.

NON-LIGHT-REQUIRING PHASE

The word "photosynthesis" implies two processes: a "photo" or light phase and a "synthesis" phase. "Synthesis" in this case refers to the making of sugar or glucose. From summary equation (1), logic might suggest that six CO_2 molecules directly combine with one another to produce the 6-carbon sugar glucose ($C_6H_{12}O_6$). Indeed, early investigators studied the problem from this point of view. It was not until about the early 1950s that scientists began to realize that the six CO_2 molecules entering the reaction do not react with one another at all. Instead, sugar is synthesized by a rather complex and somewhat circuitous sequence of reactions. Insight into this sequence was first gained through the work of M. Calvin and coworkers, who used radioactive carbon in CO_2 to trace the pathway of carbon in photosynthesis. The reactions involved in the non-light-requiring phase of photosynthesis are now generally referred to as the Calvin cycle.

Calvin cycle. With short durations of light, the first product of photosynthesis was not found to be glucose, but phosphoglyceric acid (PGA), a 3-carbon compound. The steps leading to the production of PGA involve a 5-carbon sugar, ribulose diphosphate, which must already be present in a chloroplast before the non-light-requiring phase of photosynthesis can proceed. Each CO_2 which enters reacts with this 5-carbon sugar to form a very unstable 6-carbon molecule which immediately cleaves in half, ultimately forming two PGA molecules. Actually, six CO_2 molecules enter the reaction, so six ribulose diphosphate molecules must be present, and the total yield is twelve PGA molecules. Each of the PGA molecules then proceeds

through a sequence of reactions which structurally modifies these 3-carbon units. More importantly, these units are phosphorylated by a high-energy phosphate donated by an ATP molecule which had been generated earlier in the light phase. In addition, each 3-carbon unit becomes further reduced by accepting a hydrogen from NADPH, which likewise had been generated in the light phase. Since twelve 3-carbon units are involved in the total process, twelve ATP and twelve NADPH molecules are used at this point. The NADP and ADP which remain after these reactions are completed are then recycled to the light phase where they can again be converted to NADPH and ATP. These high-energy carriers can be thought of as molecules which shuttle back and forth between the light and non-light-requiring phases of photosynthesis in a cyclic manner. They deliver energy from the light phase to the 3-carbon units of the non-light-requiring phase in the form of a high-energy phosphate from ATP and reducing power (hydrogen) from NADPH. The result of this input of energy causes the 3-carbon units to become very reactive.

As shown in Fig. 7, two of the reactive 3-carbon units (now called trioses) combine in a sequence of reactions leading to the production of one glucose molecule. This glucose molecule represents the net gain resulting from the input of the original six CO_2 molecules. The other ten triose molecules (which can be thought of as a 30-carbon pool) react with each other in a complex sequence of intercoversions which results in the ultimate production of six 5-carbon ribulose monophosphate molecules. Each of the six ribulose monophosphate molecules gains an additional high-energy phosphate by reacting with ATP. The six ATP molecules required in this reaction come from the light phase. The production of these six ribulose diphosphate molecules thus completes the Calvin cycle. The six ribulose diphosphate molecules which are regenerated can then react with six more CO_2 molecules, and the cycle begins again. Notice that although six ribulose diphosphate molecules are used in the process, six are also regenerated, so there is no net consumption or production of these molecules. In summary, the production of one glucose molecule requires six molecules of CO_2, twelve of NADPH, and eighteen of ATP.

Hatch-Slack pathway. In the last few years, plants such as corn and sugarcane have been found to be much more efficient in fixing CO_2 into sugar than most other plants. A study of these plants has shown that they do not use CO_2 directly from the air during the non-light-requiring phase, as do most other plants. Instead, CO_2 in air first reacts with the 3-carbon compound phosphoenolpyruvic acid (PEP) to form the 4-carbon compound oxalacetate. Oxalacetate is then converted to malic acid, another 4-carbon compound. Plants which produce these 4-carbon compounds in this manner are referred to as C4 plants. This reaction sequence is called the Hatch-Slack pathway, named after the scientists who elucidated these reactions.

In most plants, leaf mesophyll cells carry on the complete photosynthetic reaction. In C4 plants, however, mesophyll cells can carry on the Hatch-Slack reactions outlined above, but they appear to lack at least some of the enzymes required to complete the Calvin cycle. However, around each vascular bundle (vein) there is a layer of cells called bundle sheath cells which have very dense chloroplasts and can carry on the entire photosynthetic process. Vascular bundle sheath cells are in contact with vascular tissue on one side, but are in contact with mesophyll cells on the other. Studies with the electron microscope have revealed that at points where mesophyll cells are in contact with bundle sheath cells, there are many channels (plasmodesmata) which interconnect the cytoplasm of adjacent cells. It is likely that malic acid produced in the mesophyll cells travels through these plasmodesmata to the bundle sheath cells. Once inside the bundle sheath cell, the malic acid loses a molecule of CO_2 and is converted to the 3-carbon compound pyruvic acid. Pyruvic acid is then thought to pass back through the plasmodesmata to the mesophyll cell. The pyruvic acid is subsequently converted to PEP, and thus the cycle is completed (Fig. 8).

The significant aspect of this entire cycle is that malic acid "delivers" a relatively large quantity of CO_2 to the bundle sheath cells. It is believed that the concentration of CO_2 which could build up in bundle sheath cells via the malic acid route is many times greater than the concentration of CO_2 which could enter these cells by simple diffusion from the air. Since bundle sheath cells contain all the enzymes required to complete photosynthesis, the normal Calvin cycle process can utilize the CO_2 present to form glucose. Because of the high concentration of CO_2 in these cells, the rate of sugar production is quite rapid. It is likely that the high photosynthetic efficiency of C4 plants is related, at least in part, to the relatively high concentration of CO_2 which exists in the photosynthesizing cells. Other factors relating to this higher efficiency will be discussed later.

C3 and C4 plants. Since the discovery of the Hatch-Slack pathway, those plants which lack this system and use CO_2 from air in the Calvin cycle are now called C3 plants (PGA and the trioses are 3-carbon compounds). However, the use of the terms C3 and C4 has caused a certain amount of confusion. A common misconception is that C4 plants produce sugar through a different pathway than C3 plants. Actually, both C3 and C4 plants produce sugar through the Calvin cycle but differ in their mechanism of obtaining CO_2. C3 plants obtain CO_2 directly from the air, whereas C4 plants utilize CO_2 derived from organic compounds such as malic acid. It is mainly the steps preceding the Calvin cycle that differ. Perhaps it would be less confusing and more representative of the facts if C4 plants were called C4/C3 plants, with other plants simply called C3 plants.

Enzymes. Although the concentrating of CO_2 in photosynthesizing cells of C4 plants has been mentioned as a factor in their greater photosynthetic efficiency, at least two other factors should also be noted. In recent enzyme studies it has been found that the enzyme which catalyzes the reaction combining CO_2 with PEP is very efficient. This reaction can proceed relatively rapidly even when CO_2 concentrations in air are very low. The subsequent malic acid formation, as well as liberation of CO_2 to bundle sheath cells, can occur at a relatively

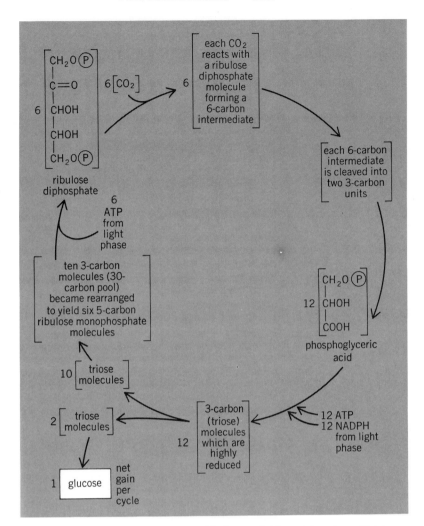

Fig. 7. Metabolic pathway associated with the non-light-requiring phase (Calvin cycle) of photosynthesis.

rapid rate. Thus CO_2 can be maintained at a relatively high concentration in bundle sheath cells and photosynthesis can continue at a moderately fast rate, even though the air surrounding the plant has a low CO_2 concentration.

Studies of the enzyme which catalyzes the reaction between CO_2 and ribulose diphosphate in the Calvin cycle have shown that this enzyme is relatively inefficient, even when CO_2 in the air is at a relatively high concentration. Under low CO_2 concentration, the incorporation of CO_2 through this reaction is very marginal. For C3 plants, the ribu-

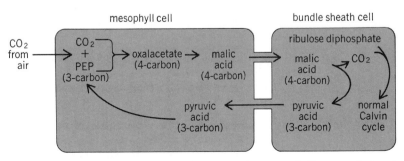

Fig. 8. Reactions of the Hatch-Slack pathway as they occur in the mesophyll and bundle sheath cells of some C4 plants.

lose diphosphate pathway is the only means of incorporating CO_2. Thus CO_2 fixation is relatively poor in C3 plants under conditions of low CO_2 concentration.

Another factor of possibly great significance has also recently been discovered relative to the enzyme which catalyzes the reaction between CO_2 and ribulose diphosphate. It has been found that this same enzyme also catalyzes a reaction between ribulose diphosphate and O_2. This reaction with O_2 leads to oxidative steps in a sequence called photorespiration. Photorespiration can waste as much as 30% of the carbon which was previously fixed in photosynthesis. It appears to be a totally detrimental process. *See* PHOTORESPIRATION.

It is quite unusual for a single enzyme to catalyze two completely different reactions. The fixation of CO_2 in the Calvin cycle by this enzyme probably ranks as one of the most important reactions in biology. It seems ironic and very unfortunate that this same enzyme should catalyze a competing reaction that can waste nearly a third of this photosynthetic output.

C3 versus C4 productivity. Equation (3) indicates that CO_2 and O_2 compete as substrates in the reac-

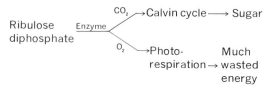

(3)

tion. Changing the relative concentrations of these gases can change the relative rates of the two processes. For example, one way to slow or prevent photorespiration is to decrease the concentration of O_2. Another method of accomplishing the same result is to increase the concentration of CO_2. This is done commercially in systems where CO_2 is pumped into greenhouses to increase crop yields. However, C4 plants have developed a natural means of concentrating CO_2 in photosynthetic cells, as discussed above. Tests on C4 plants indicate that practically no photorespiration occurs in their cells. There is little doubt that this factor is involved in the higher photosynthetic efficiency of C4 plants as compared with C3 plants.

In years to come, as food production becomes critical, scientists will certainly need to study ways to circumvent photorespiration in crop plants. Corn, sugarcane, and some of the few other C4 crop plants may become more dominant crops in future years. At present there are about 15 families of plants which are known to have one or more species capable of carrying out C4 metabolism. Geneticists will need to try to cross present C3 crop plants with known C4 noncrop plants in an attempt to introduce the C4 gene complement into crop plants. This accomplishment could have immense ramifications on worldwide food production.   [DOUGLAS G. FRATIANNE]

Bibliography: R. K. Clayton, *Molecular Physics in Photosynthesis*, 1965; H. Gaffron, Energy storage in photosynthesis, in *Plant Physiology: A Treatise*, vol. 1B, 1960; M. D. Kamen, *Primary Process in Photosynthesis*, 1963; B. Kok and A. T. Jagendorf (eds.), *Photosynthetic Mechanisms of Green Plants*, 1963; J. M. Olson (ed.), *Energy Conversion by the Photosynthetic Apparatus*, 1966; E. I. Rabinowitch, *Photosynthesis and Related Processes*, 3 vols., 1945–1956; E. I. Rabinowitch and Govindjee, *Photosynthesis*, 1969; J. B. Thomas and J. H. C. Goedheer (eds.), *Currents in Photosynthesis*, 1966; L. P. Vernon and G. R. Seely (eds.), *The Chlorophylls: Physical, Chemical and Biological Properties*, 1966.

Pimento

A type of pepper, *Capsicum annuum*, grown for its thick, sweet-fleshed red fruit. A member of the plant order Polemoniales, pimento is of American origin, and gets its name from the Spanish word designating all sweet peppers. In the United States, however, the term pimento generally refers to the heart-shaped varieties (cultivars) grown in the South for canning and used for stuffing olives and flavoring foods. Perfection is a popular variety. Harvesting begins when the fruits are fully red, usually $2\frac{1}{2}$–3 months after planting. Georgia is the only important pimento-producing state. *See* PEPPER; VEGETABLE GROWING.

[H. JOHN CAREW]

Pine nut

The edible seed of more than a dozen species of evergreen cone-bearing trees in the genus *Pinus*, native to the temperate zone of the Northern Hemisphere. The important nut-producing species are the stone pine (*P. pinea*) of southern Europe; the Swiss stone pine (*P. cembra*), native to the Swiss Alps and eastward through Siberia to Mongolia;

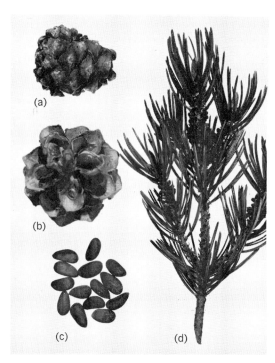

Piñon pine, *Pinus cembroides* var. *edulis*. (a) Unopened cone. (b) Opened cone. (c) Nuts in shell. (d) Branch with needles and old staminate cones.

and the piñon pine (*P. cembroides* var. *edulis*) of the arid regions of the southwestern United States. The seeds or nuts, variable in size according to species, are borne in cones which take 3–4 years to develop.

The cones of the stone pine are 4–6 in. long, each containing a hundred or more nuts $\frac{5}{8}-\frac{3}{4}$ in. in length. Cones are picked from the trees before the cone scales separate and later dried in the sun to free the nuts. The nuts are removed from the cone by hand and cracked mechanically to free the kernels which are cleaned and packed for export. Imports to the United States, coming mostly from Italy and Spain, average approximately 250 tons per year.

The piñon pine (see illustration) of Colorado, New Mexico, Arizona, and northern Mexico grows in forests of scattered trees on arid land with only 12–14 in. annual rainfall. The trees are dwarf and grow slowly. The relatively small cones open on the trees, freeing the nuts, which are picked up, mostly by local Indians, and are either used as food or for commerce. The harvest varies greatly from year to year but is of the order of 3,000,000–5,000,000 lb annually.

Pine nuts are an important staple food over large areas of the Northern Hemisphere. Only a small part of the nuts produced reaches local or world markets. The raw nuts of some species have a strong turpentine flavor which disappears when they are roasted.

[LAURENCE H. MAC DANIELS]

Pineapple

A low-growing perennial plant, indigenous to the Americas. The cultivated varieties (cultivars) belong to the species *Ananas sativus* of the plant order Bromeliales.

The edible portion of the pineapple develops from a mass of ovaries on a fleshy flower stock having persistent bracts (see illustration). On the cultivated types, the flowers are usually abortive. The leaves are long and swordlike, usually rough-edged, and grow to a height of 2–4 ft. Commercial plantings bear fruit at the age of 12–20 months, and may continue to be productive for as much as 8–10 years. Propagation is by suckers or offsets which may be rooted in sand, but are usually set directly in the field where they are to produce. The leafy crowns may also be used as cuttings, but because they are harvested with the fruit, other methods of propagation are more satisfactory.

The pineapple, a warm-climate plant, is injured by temperatures below 32°F. It does best in a dry atmosphere and relatively poor soil, but responds well to fertilizers. The major producing area is Hawaii, where special methods of culture and harvesting have been developed. A paper mulch is used in the production of much of the Hawaiian pineapple crop. The paper is laid in long strips by a special machine which pulls soil over the edges of the strips to hold them in place. The mulch aids in weed control and decreases moisture evaporation from the soil. Because of the tendency to iron chlorosis of plants growing on these soils, spraying with an iron salt is frequently a part of the fertilization program. Careful control of the nitrogen sup-

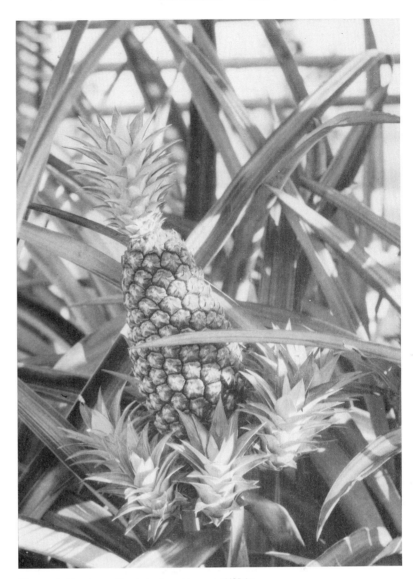

Pineapple (*Ananas sativus*), fruit and leaves. (*USDA*)

ply in relation to the hours of sunshine, together with the use of hormone sprays under certain conditions, has made possible considerable control over the time of ripening, an important consideration in obtaining maximum year-round use of processing facilities. Pineapples are also grown in the West Indies and other tropical areas, and to a limited extent in southern Florida.

Pineapples are consumed fresh in considerable quantity, but because of distance from markets and the problems of transporting fresh fruit, most of the crop is canned as sliced pineapple or as juice. In Hawaii, the average annual value of the processed crop is about $91,000,000. *See* FRUIT GROWING, SMALL.

[J. HAROLD CLARKE]

Pistachio

A small (15–30 ft) spreading evergreen tree, *Pistacia vera*, native to the dry parts of Asia and Asia Minor and now grown in the Mediterranean region, Turkey, Iran, and Afghanistan as a nut crop. Although pistachio nuts can be grown in California and other parts of the arid Southwest, no commercial industry has developed in the United States. The green or reddish oval fruits, 3/4 to 1 in. long, are borne in clusters along the smaller branches. Classified botanically as a drupe, the fruit consists of an outer fleshy husk within which is a thin tough shell enclosing the usually green kernel which is covered with brown seed coats. The husk splits at maturity and is separated easily from the shell.

Most of the commercial production of pistachio nuts comes from wild seedling trees which cover large areas of dry wastelands. However, because of increased demand for the nuts, attention has been given to selecting improved types and varieties which are propagated by budding on seedling stocks. The trees are dioecious so that pollen-bearing trees must be planted along with nut-bearing trees.

In harvesting, the clusters of nuts are picked, or beaten from the trees and caught on cloths spread on the ground. The nuts are then hand-pulled from the clusters and either husked immediately and dried in the sun or dried with the husks on, stored, and later husked after soaking in water.

Processing the husked nuts consists of floating out the empty nuts and sorting out those with split shells. These are roasted and salted. Many are colored with a pink dye before packaging. The nuts that do not split naturally are cracked and the kernels are sold to the baking, ice cream, and confectionery trade. Most of the United States imports, estimated at about 10,000,000 lb, come as nuts in shell and are processed by the importers.

Pistachio nuts are an important food in central Asia, where much of the crop is used locally. *See* NUT CROP CULTURE.

[LAURENCE H. MAC DANIELS]

Plant, mineral nutrition of

Beginning in the early 1800s, botanists became interested in determining the mineral requirements of plants. To determine the essential elements and the amounts required, scientists resorted to artificial culture techniques: Plants were grown in water, sand, or some other inert medium to which a nutrient solution of known chemical composition could be added.

When all elements believed to be required, except one, were supplied, it was possible to determine whether the omitted element was required—that is, essential. These experiments showed that most higher green plants required the elements carbon, hydrogen, oxygen, nitrogen, potassium, phosphorus, sulfur, calcium, iron, magnesium, boron, manganese, zinc, copper, chlorine, and molybdenum.

Artificial culture techniques, or hydroponics, proved useful and in fact mandatory for determining which elements were essential. This approach is still used to discover whether additional elements are also required. The technique has been adopted on a limited scale for the commercial production of plants. In some areas where there is no true soil or in those where the soil contains toxic constituents or pathogenic organisms, hydroponics has proved commercially practical. It has also been used for specialty crops in green-

houses when its advantages have justified the extra cost.

When plants are grown hydroponically, provision must be made for the basic growth requirements: light, nutrient salts, water, aeration for the roots, and anchorage or support for the plants. Plant growth and yields are essentially the same whether plants are grown in water culture or sand culture, or in a soil which has adequate nutrients, water, and aeration.

Essential elements. Plants require various amounts of the essential elements. A nutrient solution or a good soil solution may have as much as 100 parts per million (ppm) each of potassium and calcium. On the other hand, boron or manganese need be present only to the extent of 1/2 ppm and molybdenum, 1 or 2 parts per billion. For micronutrient elements, such as copper, boron, molybdenum, manganese, and zinc, the range of tolerance is quite narrow. Whereas 1/2 ppm of boron is adequate for most higher, green plants, as little as 2 ppm may prove lethal for certain species. *See* PLANT, MINERALS ESSENTIAL TO.

Fortunately, the concentration of most of the essential elements can vary over a considerable range without greatly altering plant growth and yield, so long as the concentration of an essential element is neither low enough to cause a deficiency nor high enough to result in toxicity. Plant roots absorb relatively less of an element when it is present in a high concentration, and relatively more when in a low concentration. This is undoubtedly an equalizing factor which explains why plants tend to grow equally well over a wide range of concentrations of the various essential elements.

For example, in field corn plants (Table 1) most of the dry weight is composed of carbon (43.6%), oxygen (44.4%), and hydrogen (6.2%). Carbon and oxygen, in the form of carbon dioxide, enter the plant through pores in the leaves called stomata. The carbon of carbon dioxide is built into carbohydrates, fats, proteins, and all the other organic

Table 1. Elements in corn plants*

Element	Total dry weight of roots, stems, leaves, cobs, and grain, %
Oxygen	44.4
Carbon	43.6
Hydrogen	6.2
Nitrogen	1.5
Phosphorus	0.2
Potassium	0.9
Calcium	0.2
Magnesium	0.2
Sulfur	0.2
Iron	0.1
Silicon	1.2
Aluminum	0.1
Chlorine	0.1
Manganese	0.05
Undetermined elements	0.9

*Adapted from W. L. Latshaw and E. C. Miller, Elemental composition of the corn plant, *J. Agr. Res.*, 27:845–860, 1924.

(carbon-containing) compounds of the plant. (Amazingly, the plant obtains its vast amount of carbon from the air, in which there are only 3 parts of carbon dioxide per 10,000 parts of air.) Oxygen involved in these organic compounds comes from carbon dioxide, the atmosphere, soil "air," and water absorbed by the roots.

Hydrogen is derived from the water absorbed by the roots. The rest of the essential elements are absorbed from the soil, and they are usually present in lower concentrations in plants than are carbon, oxygen, and hydrogen.

Salt-absorption processes. Elements may enter roots by any one or a combination of four processes. Three of these—diffusion, Donnan equilibrium, and ionic or adsorption exchange—are purely physical processes. The fourth, active absorption or active transport, is a vital process which is dependent on the metabolism of living cells. In each process the first step is adsorption of ions on the surface of the roots.

Diffusion. Diffusion is a physical process in which ions enter the cells of the root only when the ions exist in a higher concentration outside the cells than inside. A given ion continues to enter the cell until the internal and external concentrations are equal. The cell plays no active role in the process, and ions enter by kinetic energy; that is, the ions are in motion. This process cannot account for the concentration of ions within cells, and there is no selection of the types of ions which enter; nonessential and even toxic ions can enter.

Donnan equilibrium. This special type of diffusion occurs when positively charged cations or negatively charged anions inside the cells are unable to pass through the membrane. It has been demonstrated by nonliving, physical systems that this situation can lead to a higher concentration of diffusible ions inside the root cells than in the external environment. Although root cells characteristically have higher concentrations of certain ions inside rather than outside the cells, the Donnan process is not regarded as important for the accumulation of ions by cells.

Ionic exchange. Ionic exchange, or adsorption exchange, is also a physical process by which ions can enter root cells. This process may best be visualized by thinking of the root as a sponge, with the air pockets representing the vacuoles (cell sap) of cells and the solid portions the cytoplasm and cell walls. The adsorbed ions remain outside the vacuoles and are free to exchange position with ions in the external medium or in neighboring cells. The cytoplasm and cell walls (solid parts of the sponge) are a continuum extending throughout the plant; therefore the ions are free to move throughout the plant or to return to the external environment of the root. The ions are said to be in the "outer space" of the cells; that is, the ions have not moved into the cell sap or vacuoles as they do in active absorption.

In this physical process, as in diffusion, the plant plays no active role, and there is no selectivity with regard to what ions enter. As in diffusion, ionic exchange permits the concentration of ions to become only as high internally as externally. For reasons that will become apparent when active absorption is discussed, ionic exchange is regarded as the most important of the entry processes.

Active absorption. The fourth process by which ions may enter roots is active absorption, or active transport, that is, transport across the vacuolar membrane of the cell. The term active indicates that the cells play a role in the process; only living, metabolizing cells are capable of this type of salt absorption; that is, cells must be carrying on respiration, the energy-liberating process. Furthermore only aerobic respiration, involving oxygen, sustains active absorption.

If cells are deprived of oxygen and are therefore forced to carry on anaerobic respiration (in which oxygen is not involved and only one-twenty-fifth as much energy is released), not only will cells fail to accumulate additional salts but they will lose to the external environment the ions of an element whose concentration is higher internally than externally. It is by aerobic respiration that active absorption can occur, resulting in a concentration of ions within cells. This process is more important than Donnan equilibrium, which can result also in the concentration of ions within cells.

In active absorption the absorbed ions enter the vacuole or cell sap and, for the most part, tend to remain there; that is, their movement into the vacuole is largely a one-way, irreversible step. In the vacuole, therefore, the concentration of various ions may be many times their concentration in the external solution. The cells must have a source of energy and must "work" to accumulate and retain ions against such a concentration gradient.

Since the ions which enter by active absorption pass irreversibly into the vacuoles, they are not free to move to the top of the plant where nutrient ions are also required. For this reason, active salt absorption is not regarded as the important process for ionic transportation within plants. Active absorption is, however, the only salt-absorption process in which there is selectivity of the ions which enter the cell. Thus this type of entry alone explains why different species of plants may have different internal concentrations of various ions. Some type of "carrier" compound is thought to be involved in this selective activity.

Carriers. The unique feature of active transport is that special compounds called carriers are thought to be involved. They are believed to be in the differentially permeable membranes of cells and to regulate the entry of cations and anions. One theory proposes that the transport of anions is mediated through cytochrome oxidase and that cytochromes may be anion carriers; consequently anions would be absorbed actively and the cations passively. Cytochromes would not account for the observed selectivity in the absorption of ions.

Another theory suggests that a phospholipid, lecithin, may be involved in the entry of cations and anions into cells. The synthesis of at least one of the components of the proposed "phosphatide cycle" requires adenosinetriphosphate (ATP). While this theory accounts for the active absorption of cations and anions, it gives no indication as to how selectivity in absorption is controlled. Although the chemical nature of the carriers is unknown, they act somewhat like the specialized, proteinaceous, organic catalysts called enzymes.

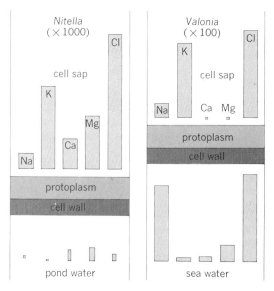

Fig. 1. Diagrammatic representation of the differences in absorption of ions by plants growing in low-salt and high-salt environments. (*From P. J. Kramer, Plant and Soil Water Relationships, McGraw-Hill, 1949*)

In fact, the kinetics of carrier action in salt uptake may be studied in the same manner as that of enzyme systems. It is postulated that carriers make a temporary union with an ion that results in an unstable carrier-ion complex and by a second reaction the complex releases the ion on the other side of the membrane.

Carriers are produced by the metabolism of

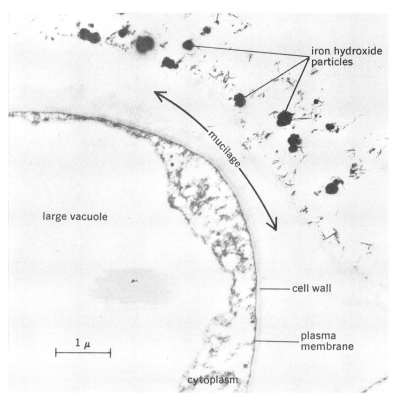

Fig. 2. The root-soil boundary, as revealed in an electron micrograph. (*From H. Jenny and K. Grossenbacher, Root-soil boundary zones as seen by the electron microscope, Calif. Agr., 16(10):7, 1962*)

cells, and they appear to have a high degree of specificity with regard to the ions whose entries they regulate. For example, one carrier has been shown to be involved in the entry of potassium, rubidium, and cesium. Any one of these ions competes with the others for the cation-carrying site on this carrier. A different carrier appears to be involved in the entry of sodium. The possibility that different carriers regulate the entry of potassium and sodium might explain why two species of plants differ widely in their absorption of potassium and sodium from a common external environment. In other words, the two species of plants may contain widely different concentrations of sodium- and potassium-carrying carriers; therefore, differences in the permeability of roots to two kinds of ions may depend on the relative concentrations of the carriers that transport these ions. There are also specific carriers for lithium; calcium, barium, and strontium; magnesium; sulfate and selenate; chloride and bromide; nitrate; phosphate ($H_2PO_4^-$), arsenate, and hydroxyl (OH^-); and phosphate (HPO_4^{--}) and hydroxyl (OH^-).

Under certain conditions or with time during the life cycle of a plant, there are changes in the absorption rates of various ions. Since carriers are formed by the metabolism of cells and since carriers break down in time, the relative rates of production of the different carriers may be altered by changes in cell metabolism. Therefore, not only would carriers explain the different rates of absorption of various ions by different species, but changes in the relative concentrations of carriers would explain the observed changes in cell permeability with time.

The involvement of carriers in the irreversible movement of ions into vacuoles would explain the differences in the inorganic composition of roots, stems, and leaves of various species. From a common environment, one species might move considerable quantities of potassium and comparatively little sodium into the vacuoles; another species might do just the opposite. Though both species may have the same concentrations of potassium and sodium in the cytoplasm and cell walls, or "outer space," by virtue of ionic or adsorption exchange, the differences in movement of ions into the vacuoles could explain the compositional differences of two species growing in a common environment.

Growing in dissimilar external solutions, two species of plants may show striking differences in their abilities to concentrate or exclude certain ions. In Fig. 1 all ions shown reach a higher concentration in the sap of *Nitella* (a fresh-water plant) than in the external solution. In *Valonia* (a seawater plant) the cell sap contains primarily potassium and chloride, whereas the sea water contains chiefly sodium and chloride.

In view of the characteristics of ionic exchange and of active absorption, it seems that the ions which are free to move to the tops of plants are those which escaped absorption (into the vacuoles) by the root cells. It is for this reason that ionic exchange is generally regarded as the most important of the four types of salt absorption from the standpoint of plant nutrition. Differences in the inorganic composition of species, on the other hand, may result from active absorption, that is, the extent to which different ions accumulate in the vacuoles of cells in roots, stems, and leaves.

Ion absorption from soil. Nutritive elements are contained in soil in two ways: dissolved in water, or loosely adsorbed on the surfaces of minute (less than 0.2 μ in diameter) soil particles called colloids. There are two types of colloids: mineral or clay and organic. The latter arise from the decomposition of organic matter. Whereas elements which are in solution may be washed or leached from the root zone by rain, those which are adsorbed on colloidal surfaces are resistant to leaching. Per unit of surface area, organic colloids have a greater capacity than clay colloids to adsorb and retain ions such as potassium, calcium, and magnesium.

Colloids on the surfaces of roots are in intimate contact with soil colloidal particles (Fig. 2), from which the plant may take an adsorbed ion directly, that is, without the ion's passing into solution. Nutrients which enter the cell in this manner are said to do so by contact feeding or contact absorption. This is not, however, another type of salt absorption; it refers to the external location of the ion, that is, whether it is in the soil solution or on the surface of a colloid. The first step in absorption from a colloid also involves adsorption of the ion onto the root surface. In contact feeding the colloidal surfaces of the root and of the soil colloid are in such intimate contact, each with adsorbed ions, that an ion associated with the surface of the colloid may readily exchange with one associated with the root surface.

Whether an ion is absorbed from the soil solution or the surface of a colloid, the plant must exchange an ion for the one it absorbs (Fig. 3). Because the roots in carrying on respiration produce carbon dioxide, the plant has a source from which to yield ions for ions it absorbs. Carbon dioxide dissolves in the water of the root cell to form carbonic acid, which in turn dissociates into positively charged hydrogen (H^+) ions and negatively charged bicarbonate (HCO_3^-) ions. When a plant absorbs a cation, such as potassium, the root usually yields a hydrogen ion to the external medium.

As more hydrogen ions are introduced into the soil in exchange for ions such as potassium and calcium which are absorbed by the plant, the soil tends to become acidic and requires liming. When the plant absorbs an anion, such as nitrate or phosphate, it generally yields a bicarbonate anion to the external medium (Fig. 4). The hydroxyl (OH^-) anion may also be involved. It is interesting to note that the ions which the plant uses in "swapping" for essential nutrients are hydrogen and bicarbonate ions produced as a result of respiration.

The most active part of the root for salt absorption is about 1/8 in. from the tip; for water absorption it is about 1/2 in. from the tip, where root hairs (extensions of epidermal cells) are most numerous. Since these two regions tend to mature with time and lose their ability for absorption, it is important that the roots continue to grow. Otherwise the root matures almost to the tip, the root hairs in the root-hair zone die, and the root tips are no longer effective for either salt or water absorption.

Foliar nutrition of plants. A plant may receive nutrients through the leaves as well as through the roots. Any essential element can be supplied, at least in part, by application to the foliage. In fact, there may exist in the soil some condition which makes a certain element more or less unavailable to the roots. Iron and manganese, for example, may be rendered largely unavailable by the alkalinity of the soil, and the tops of the plants may show extreme iron or manganese deficiencies or both.

A foliar application of missing ions is a very practical way—indeed the only way—to supply the missing essential elements. Often foliar nutrients are added to sprays that are applied for the control of fungi, bacteria, or insects.

Foliar nutrition is particularly useful during periods when the soil is waterlogged, and the roots are relatively ineffective in the absorption of nutrients. Similarly, early in the spring, when the soil is cold, nitrification is proceeding slowly, and plant roots are relatively ineffective in absorbing nutrients, the application of nutrients (particularly nitrogen) to the tops may be most beneficial. These conditions are particularly likely to occur with turf grasses, such as on golf courses, where foliar nutrition is widely practiced. Foliar nutrition is also widely used to supply nitrogen, usually in the form of urea, to apple and citrus trees.

Translocation. Water and mineral salts absorbed by the roots generally move upward through the plant in the woody portion of the stem in a tissue called xylem. Organic substances, such as sugars, are made in the leaves and move downward to the roots through the bark of the stem in a tissue called phloem. However, sugars also use the phloem when they move upward from the mature leaves of the plant to the growing point of the stem. Apparently all substances which come from the leaves move through the plant by way of the phloem.

A mystery of transport or translocation which has long been studied is that some substances, such as sugars, move in one direction in the phloem at the same time that other organic substances, such as amino acids, move in the opposite direction. Evidence indicates that some vertical strands of phloem cells carry materials in one

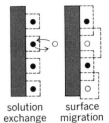

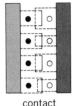

solution   surface
exchange   migration

contact
exchange

Fig. 3. Diagram of various modes of ionic migration, especially ionic or contact exchange. (*From E. Truog, ed., Mineral Nutrition of Plants, University of Wisconsin Press, 1951*)

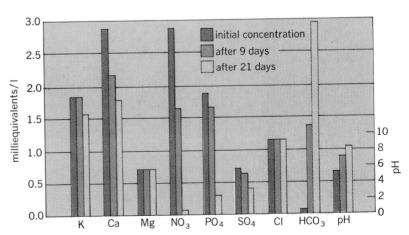

Fig. 4. The levels of the principal ions initially in solution and then after 9 days and 21 days of a mass culture of the alga *Scenedesmus*. (*From R. W. Krauss, Inorganic nutrition of algae, in J. S. Burlew, ed., Algal Culture from Laboratory to Pilot Plant, Carnegie Inst. Wash. Publ., 600:85–102, 1953*)

direction while other strands of phloem carry materials in the opposite direction; that is, an entire bundle or ring of phloem does not act in unison.

There is no generally recognized explanation for the rapidity with which substances move in the phloem or for the amounts of substances which move through a cross-sectional area of phloem in a given time. It is obvious that simple diffusion cannot account for the rapid rates of movement. Similarly, simple diffusion does not explain the vast quantities of sugars, for example, which have been shown to move through a given cross-sectional area of phloem to a rapidly developing fruit, such as pumpkin, squash, or watermelon.

The Münch mass-flow hypothesis, which can account for movement of solution en masse in only one direction in the phloem, is not in accord with numerous reports of simultaneous, bidirectional movements in the phloem. Activated diffusion — movement of substances in or over interfaces — could account for rapid, massive movement of substances in the same or in opposite directions. Activated diffusion is dependent solely on the relative concentration of substances in two regions of the plant. Concentrations of substances tend to equalize in the interfaces (such as planes of contact of cell wall with cytoplasm, or of portions of protoplasm with different densities of protoplasm), and this equilization process involves rapid movement of materials. If a given substance, such as sugar, is added at one point, it spreads rapidly throughout the interfaces toward regions with a lower sugar concentration. Since the withdrawal of a substance from the interfaces may be continuous, such as the removal of sugar by root cells, there tends to be a continual flow of sugar from the leaves, where an excess is produced, to the roots.

Although activated diffusion is a purely physical process, active metabolism of living phloem cells is somehow required for the translocation of the organic substances in the phloem. It seems likely that a unique organization of protoplasm must be maintained in order for this physical process to occur, and cellular metabolism is undoubtedly required to maintain the unique physical structure of protoplasm.

It is generally recognized that the aboveground portions of the plant are dependent on the roots for water and mineral salts. Less generally recognized, however, is the dependence of the roots on the substances, particularly sugar, produced in the tops. In perennial plants, renewed growth in the spring may be largely or entirely dependent on food reserves stored in the roots. For many plants whose tops die at the end of the growing season, renewed growth is entirely dependent on the roots, for example, even trees, whose trunks store some material for growth. This is shown strikingly when a complete ring of bark (in which the phloem is located) is removed from a tree by field mice. The tree shows few or no effects during the first season after the damage, but it may fail to grow the following spring because destruction of the phloem stops translocation of food reserves to the roots. A tree can often be saved by bridge grafting across such a break in the bark. See GRAFTING OF PLANTS.

Relation of nutrition to yield. The ultimate goal of commerical production of plants is yield—either of the vegetative plant, as in the case of hay, or of

Table 2. Raw materials used by corn plants producing 100 bu/acre*

Substance	Approximate amount, lb/acre	Approximate equivalent
Water, H_2O	4,300,000 – 5,500,000	19–24 in. rain
Oxygen, O_2	6800	Air is 20% O_2
Carbon, C	5200 C, 19,000 CO_2	Amount of C in 4 tons of coal
Nitrogen, N	160	Eight 100-lb bags of 20% fertilizer
Potassium, K	125	Three 100-lb bags of muriate of potash
Phosphorus, P	40	Four 100-lb bags of 20% superphosphate
Sulfur, S	75	78 lb of yellow sulfur
Magnesium, Mg	50	170 lb of epsom salt
Calcium, Ca	50	80 lb of limestone
Iron, Fe	2	2 lb of nails
Manganese, Mn	0.3	1 lb of potassium permanganate
Boron, B	0.06	1/4 lb borax
Chlorine, Cl	Trace	Amount in rainfall
Zinc, Zn	Trace	Shell of one dry-cell battery
Copper, Cu	Trace	25 ft no. 9 copper wire
Molybdenum, Mo	Trace	2–3 oz ammonium molybdate

*From G. Hambidge (ed.), *Hunger Signs in Crops: A Symposium*, American Society of Agronomy and the National Fertilizer Association, 2d ed., 1950.

the fruit. Thus the most practical and fundamental question about the mineral nutrition of plants is how to produce the greatest yield. Consequently man is interested in what chemical elements and how much of each a plant requires (Table 2).

Once it is known that all plants require potassium, for example, then the problem is the determination of how much potassium a particular crop needs for maximal production. If there is insufficient potassium, the plant may show potassium deficiency symptoms: stunted growth and little or no fruit. A certain concentration of potassium in the plant is required for maximal yield. With increasing amounts of potassium above the deficiency level, increasing growth occurs. Obviously, beyond some given concentration of potassium in the plant, there is no further increase in yield commensurate with increase of the element. The sufficiency values or levels for certain essential elements have been determined in some plants. Information on the essential elements is needed for all crop plants if maximal production is to be attained.

If a crop is to produce maximal yield, all factors, including the essential elements, must be at sufficiency concentrations or levels. If all the essential elements are present in sufficiency except one, growth and yield of the plants are limited to the extent that this essential element is lacking. Around 1840 the German scientist Justus von Liebig proposed this concept in the law of limiting factors, according to which, growth is dictated by the element which has the most insufficient concentration. From this law it follows that, if the crop is only slightly deficient in phosphorus but extremely deficient in potassium, an increase in phosphorus will be essentially without effect on growth and yield since potassium is the pacesetter. On the other hand, if potassium is added to bring the concentration of the element to sufficiency, growth of the plants will be increased only to the extent that the next most limiting factor, phosphorus, permits.

Sometimes it appears obvious that a certain crop is not growing as it should, although the plants do not indicate any particular deficiency. Upon the addition of a fertilizer containing nitrogen, phosphorus, and potassium, the plants may suddenly exhibit some clear-cut deficiency, for instance, manganese. This may be explained on the basis that the plants were originally deficient, to varying degrees, in nitrogen, phosphorus, potassium, and manganese. When sufficient amounts of the first three were added, clear-cut and striking manganese deficiency symptoms developed.

Relation of inorganic to organic nutrients. The inorganic nutrition of the plant cannot be evaluated without consideration of its organic nutrition. Proteins, for example, contain carbon, hydrogen, oxygen, nitrogen, and sometimes phosphorus and sulfur. Protein formation depends on carbohydrates, which are formed by photosynthesis. Therefore, even though a plant might be tested and found to contain less nitrogen that is known to be associated with maximal yield, the addition of nitrogen would be without beneficial effect if the plant was deficient in sugars because of prolonged cloudly weather or for some other reason.

Soil moisture. Soil moisture is another factor in the mineral nitrition of plants. Absorption of nutrients by roots is related to the growth of roots. When soil moisture is inadequate, new root growth is limited or ceases, and salt absorption is accordingly decreased. From a practical point of view there is no benefit in adding a known deficient nutrient, such as nitrogen, if the roots are not prepared to absorb it. Nutrient salts cannot substitute for water, and water cannot substitute for nutrients. The interdependence or interrelationships between water, nutrients, sugars, and so on are often overlooked. Successful agricultural experts in crop production have to take all these factors into consideration. It is important economically to know what factor is limiting plant growth, even if man has no control over it, such as sunshine. There would be no economic advantage in adding a fertilizer if sunshine was the limiting factor. On the other hand, if some essential element was found to be the limiting factor, its addition might more than pay for the cost of the added fertilizer. *See* FERTILIZER.

The most frequent limiting factor in crop production is undoubtedly the amount of soil moisture. Only in recent years has this become generally recognized, resulting in the installation of facilities for supplemental irrigation even in relatively humid regions of the United States, such as the Eastern states. In many cases the installation of an irrigation system has paid for itself in a single year, when because of a prolonged drought the yield of the crop would otherwise have been a total failure. *See* SOIL.

Excessive salt concentration. In the semiarid or arid regions of the West, where irrigation is widely practiced, the low rainfall and the salt content of the irrigation waters combine to cause undesirably high concentrations of salts in many soils. The low rainfall is insufficient to leach accumulated salts from the soil, and the irrigation waters naturally contain appreciably more salt than does rainwater. For example, the water of the Colorado River, which is widely used in irrigation, contains about 700 ppm of salt. About 27,000,000 acres of land in the Midwest and Far West are under irrigation. Even in areas which are not already clearly "salinity" areas, there is always a potential danger of the development of salinity. In some of these soils the salts which accumulate are alkaline in reaction, and the soils are called alkali soils. When the accumulated salts are essentially neutral in reaction, such as sodium chloride or sodium sulfate, the soils are properly called saline soils. Salinity is regarded as a problem when the concentration of salts reaches 0.2% of the dry weight of a loam soil; most species of plants die when the concentration is around 2%.

Salinity conditions are often unsuspected because there are no plants of the same species growing on nonsaline soil in the same area. Therefore, actual reductions in growth and yield may go undetected if salinity conditions are not too pronounced. With higher levels of salinity it becomes obvious that plant growth is restricted, and the plants may show "burning" or "firing" of the leaves, particularly the oldest, lower leaves which have accumulated toxic concentrations of salts.

In contrast with deficiency symptoms, the predominance of a toxic salt in the soil does not usually produce symptoms indicative of the type of salt which is present. On the basis of symptoms, it cannot ordinarily be determined whether there is a high concentration of sodium chloride or of sodium sulfate in the soil. In either case the symptoms are very much the same—stunting and firing of the leaves, particularly at the tips or margins or both.

A toxic concentration of boron in the soil solution induces specific symptoms, particularly on the oldest leaves, which trained scientists can usually identify.

Soil analyses of course may be used to determine the nature of the accumulated salts in saline or alkali soils. Often this information is useful in prescribing a remedy for the removal of salts. If the soil is permeable enough to water and if sufficient irrigation water (preferably of low salt content) is available, the toxic salts may be leached out of the root zone and carried away in the drainage water.

When sodium salts accumulate, they usually impart undesirable physical characteristics to the soil, such as reduced permeability to water and reduced aeration. If the sodium concentration is not too high and if the value of the land is sufficient to warrant it, this condition can often be overcome by the application of a calcium-containing salt, such as gypsum, to the soil. Calcium replaces the sodium on the clay and organic colloids, and the sodium may then be leached from the root zone. With the substitution of calcium for sodium, the permeability of the soil to water usually improves with time so that it becomes increasingly easier to wash the sodium salts from the root zone. Along with this change the overall physical characteristics of the soil, including tilth and aeration, become more conducive to plant growth.

[HUGH G. GAUCH]

Bibliography: A. S. Crafts, *Translocation in Plants*, 1961; R. M. Devlin, *Plant Physiology*, 2d ed., 1969; A. W. Galston, *The Life of the Green Plant*, 1961; H. G. Gauch, Mineral nutrition of plants, *Ann. Rev. Plant Physiol.*, 8:31–64, 1957;

B. S. Meyer, D. B. Anderson, and R. Bohning, *An Introduction to Plant Physiology*, 2d ed., 1973; L. A. Richards (ed.), *Diagnosis and Improvement of Saline and Alkali Soils*, USDA Handb. no. 60, 1954; F. C. Steward (ed.), *Plant Physiology*, vols. 1A–6C, 1959–1972.

Plant, minerals essential to

Beginning in the middle of the 19th century, botanists sought to determine the chemical elements required for the growth of plants. Elements such as nitrogen, phosphorus, and potassium, required in relatively large amounts, were among the first shown to be essential. The essentiality of certain elements, such as copper and molybdenum, was not established until chemical compounds of greater purity were produced. Earlier, many of the elements were present in sufficient amounts as impurities in a nutrient solution to preclude their detection as essential elements when they were "omitted" from the solution. Elements which are required in small amounts, such as copper, molybdenum, manganese, zinc, boron, iron, and chlorine, are sometimes called trace elements. They have also been called minor elements, but this term erroneously implies that these elements play only a minor role in plant nutrition. The term micronutrients is generally favored, since it implies that small amounts are required and that they perform a nutritive role.

Most plant scientists agree that the following elements are essential for higher plants: carbon, hydrogen, oxygen, phosphorus, potassium, nitrogen, sulfur, calcium, magnesium, iron, boron, manganese, zinc, copper, chlorine, and molybdenum. The last seven are micronutrients. Nitrogen, phosphorus, and potassium are the three most important and are the components of a 5-10-5 fertilizer (5% nitrogen, 10% phosphorus, calculated as phosphorus pentoxide, and 5% potassium, calculated as potassium oxide). Certain algae require vanadium, sodium, and cobalt. Additional elements may possibly be added to the present list of essential elements for plants.

Criteria of essentiality. In order to be considered essential, an element must meet the following criteria: (1) Absence of the element results in abnormal growth, injury, or death of the plant; (2) the plant is unable to complete its life cycle without the element; (3) the element is required for plants in general; and (4) no other element can serve as a complete substitute. Most scientists prefer to add a fifth criterion, namely, that the element have a specific and direct role in the nutrition of the plant. This last criterion is difficult to determine since known, direct roles for potassium and calcium, for example, are not as yet agreed upon; their essentiality, however, is unquestioned. Without exception, when the essential elements were experimentally removed from the external environment, drastically reduced growth ensued. The direct, specific roles of the elements were then pursued, most of which have been elucidated.

Roles of essential elements. The following paragraphs discuss the roles in plants of carbon, hydrogen, oxygen, phosphorus, nitrogen, sulfur, potassium, calcium, magnesium, iron, manganese, copper, zinc, molybdenum, boron, and chlorine.

Carbon. Carbon may constitute as much as 44% of the dry weight of a typical plant such as corn. It is a component of all organic compounds, such as sugars, starch, proteins, and fats, in plants (and animals). One of its main roles, is as a constituent of a vast array of compounds which in turn are synthesized from sugar. Carbon may indeed be said to be involved in all the roles played by all the carbon-containing compounds. This would include such compounds as the plant hormones, which regulate plant growth, flowering, and reproduction. *See* CARBOHYDRATE; PLANT HORMONES; PROTEIN; STARCH.

Hydrogen. This element is also a constituent of all organic compounds, and what applies to carbon similarly applies to hydrogen. Hydrogen constitutes about 6% of the dry weight of a plant.

Oxygen. This element is a constituent of all carbohydrates, fats, and proteins and, in fact, of most organic compounds. Some organic compounds, such as carotene, which gives rise to vitamin A, are composed only of carbon and hydrogen. Since oxygen is a constituent of most organic compounds, it is involved in whatever functions those compounds perform. Oxygen constitutes about 43% of the dry weight of a plant.

Carbon, hydrogen, and oxygen are constituents of the bicarbonate ion (HCO_3^-), which is believed to be one of the chief anions (along with hydroxyl, OH^-) exchanged by the plant for anions absorbed from the soil. Because of this role, these three elements are involved in the process of salt absorption by roots.

In the process of oxidation (aerobic respiration) of foods by the cell, oxygen is the final acceptor of hydrogen. When a food, such as sugar, is respired by the removal of hydrogen and carbon dioxide, the latter and water appear as end products. Water is formed in the terminal step in these oxidation reactions when oxygen and hydrogen unite.

Phosphorus. Certain special proteins in all cells, the nucleoproteins, contain phosphorus. Nucleoproteins are in the nucleus of the cell and hence in the chromosomes which carry the hereditary units, the genes. Since phosphorus is a constituent of the nucleoproteins, cell division is dependent on phosphorus. The transmission of hereditary characteristics also depends on this element.

Cellular membranes are believed to consist, in part, of special phosphorus-containing fats or lipids called phospholipids. These, along with hydrated protein molecules, are very likely the chief components of cellular membranes. Differentially permeable membranes regulate the entry and exit of materials from the cells; phosphorus therefore plays a role in the permeability of cells to various substances and in the retention of substances by cells.

Phosphorus is a constituent of the special compounds diphosphopyridine nucleotide (DPN) and triphosphopyridine nucleotide (TPN). DPN and TPN are commonly called NAD (nicotinamide, adenine dinucleotide) and NADP (nicotinamide adenine dinucleotide phosphate), respectively. These compounds are involved in the transfer of hydrogen in aerobic respiration, and life itself depends on this important energy-liberating process.

The early stages in the combustion or utilization of sugar by cells involve the addition of phosphorus to the sugar molecule. Only after phosphorus is added to both ends of the sugar molecule is it cleaved and prepared for further transformations which release the chemical energy stored in the sugar molecule.

Also, phosphorus is a constituent of adenosinediphosphate (ADP) and adenosinetriphosphate (ATP). In ADP one of the two phosphate bonds is a high-energy bond, and in ATP two of the three phosphate bonds are high-energy bonds. This unique concentration of energy in these special phosphorus bonds is one of the ways in which potential energy is stored within the cell. The bond is important not only because it represents a form of stored energy, but also when it is broken the released energy can accomplish "work." Many synthetic reactions, such as the syntheses of sucrose and starch from glucose, require energy which the high-energy phosphate bond delivers.

The reduced forms of diphosphorpyridine nucleotide ($DPNH_2$) and triphosphopyridine nucleotide ($TPNH_2$) constitute the other major form of energy storage in cells. This chemically stored energy is also available for work—driving certain chemical reactions that would otherwise proceed at imperceptibly low rates.

Nitrogen. Along with carbon, hydrogen, and oxygen, nitrogen is a constituent of all amino acids: the building blocks of proteins. Protoplasm usually has a high percentage of water, but the substance portion is primarily proteinaceous. Thus nitrogen and certain other elements such as carbon, hydrogen, and oxygen are a part of the living substance, protoplasm.

All enzymes thus far isolated are protein in nature. Therefore nitrogen is a constituent of these remarkable organic catalysts, which accomplish at room temperature, or below, chemical reactions that man can perform only with high temperature, pressure, or other special conditions.

As a constituent of chlorophyll (four nitrogen atoms in each molecule), nitrogen is required in photosynthesis, the food-manufacturing process which only plants can accomplish.

Sulfur. Certain amino acids, such as cystine, cysteine, and methionine, contain sulfur and are often components of plant proteins. Sulfur is also a constituent of the tripeptide, glutathione, which may function as a hydrogen carrier in the respiration of plants and animals. Biotin, thiamine, and coenzyme A are examples of still other sulfur-containing compounds in plants. *See* CYSTEINE; CYSTINE; METHIONINE.

Potassium. Although potassium was one of the first elements shown to be essential and often accounts for 1% or more of the dry weight, there is no known potassium-containing compound in plants. Despite numerous researches, it still is not known why plants require potassium in such seemingly large amounts. Although it functions as a cofactor for certain enzyme systems, the need for such high concentrations is not known. Virtually all the potassium in plants appears to be water-soluble, emphasizing further that it is not a constituent of any compound and certainly not of the larger, relatively insoluble and immobile compounds.

Calcium. Although calcium may typically be present in plants to the extent of 0.2% of the dry matter, it also is not clear why plants require so much calcium. Many workers consider the cementing substance between cells, the middle lamella, to be composed of calcium pectate. No other calcium-containing compounds of biological

significance have been reported for plants, and yet they contain far more calcium than would be required for its postulated role in the middle lamella. Excesses of oxalic and other organic acids may appear in the cell as crystalline calcium salts of low solubilities. These salts, however, are considered waste products and serve no vital function. Their removal from solution by calcium may prevent a toxicity that would otherwise result from such acids.

Magnesium. Magnesium is a constituent of chlorophyll molecule, each molecule containing one atom of magnesium in the center. Although other metallic ions may be made to replace the magnesium, chlorophyll functions in photosynthesis only when it contains a magnesium atom. Despite much speculation, it has not yet been determined why only magnesium is effective in chlorophyll and in photosynthesis.

In addition to the unique role which magnesium plays in chlorophyll and photosynthesis, it is also required for the action of a host of enzymes. It may have two roles in protein synthesis: as an activator of some enzymes involved in the synthesis of nucleic acids, or as an important binding agent in microsomal particles where protein synthesis occurs. It is also apparently required for an enzyme concerned with oil formation in plants, since oil droplets are not formed in the alga *Vaucheria* in the absence of magnesium. The seeds of plants, which contain large amounts of oil, are consistently high in magnesium.

Iron. Iron is required for the formation of chlorophyll but is not a constituent of the molecule. In plant leaves about 80% of the iron is associated with chloroplasts, the chlorophyll-containing plastids. Iron is a constituent of cytochrome *f*, which may have a role in photosynthesis.

Iron is a constituent of the enzymes cytochrome oxidase, peroxidase, and catalase. Cytochrome oxidase is involved in respiration, and catalase catalyzes the breakdown of any hydrogen peroxide that forms in cells as a result of certain metabolic

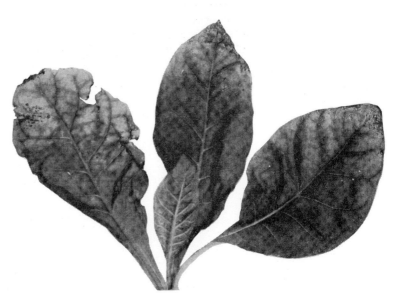

Fig. 1. Young tobacco seedling showing potassium-deficiency symptoms consisting of interveinal chlorosis and marginal and apical scorch of older leaves. (*From G. Hambidge, ed., Hunger Signs in Crops: A Symposium, American Society of Agronomy and National Fertilizer Association, 2d ed., 1950*)

reactions. Why plants require so much iron is not known, since a smaller quantity would appear sufficient for its known roles. Iron is also a component of ferredoxin.

Manganese. There are no known compounds in plants of which manganese is a constituent. There is considerable evidence that the element may be a cofactor or an activator in certain enzyme systems. For example, manganese may be involved in nitrate reduction and hence in nitrogen metabolism. Manganese is known to be needed for photosynthesis, particularly by algae growing in an inorganic medium. *See* PHOTOSYNTHESIS.

Copper. Copper is a constituent of laccase, ascorbic acid oxidase, plastocyanin, and tyrosinase (polyphenoloxidase). The last enzyme is believed to be involved in most plants with the terminal step in aerobic respiration, the transfer of hydrogen to oxygen to form water. This action thus links copper with energy release in plant cells.

Zinc. Although the enzyme has not been isolated, it has been shown that the enzyme which synthesizes the amino acid tryptophan requires zinc. Tryptophan in turn is the precursor from which the plant hormone indoleacetic acid is made. Zinc then is directly necessary for the formation of tryptophan and indirectly necessary for the production of indoleacetic acid. *See* TRYPTOPHAN.

Two zinc-containing enzymes have been isolated from plants, namely, carbonic anhydrase and alcohol dehydrogenase.

Molybdenum. Molybdenum is required in the external solution to the extent of 1 or 2 parts per billion. In the dry matter of the plant it may be present only to the extent of about 10 parts per billion. It has been calculated that the number of molybdenum atoms required per cell of *Scenedesmus obliquus* and *Azotobacter* is 3000 and 10,000, respectively.

Molybdenum is the metal component of xanthine oxidase and of the enzyme nitrate reductase, which effects reduction of nitrate nitrogen to the reduced form of nitrogen that is incorporated into amino acids and then into proteins. Molybdenum-deficient tomato plants may accumulate nitrate to the extent of 12% of the dry weight of the plant. If such plants are given a few parts per billion of molybdenum in the external medium, the nitrate content will drop to around 1% within 2 days. *Aspergillus niger*, *Scenedesmus obliquus*, and *Chlorella pyrenoidosa* also require molybdenum for the reduction of nitrate nitrogen. Fixation of atmospheric nitrogen by one of the free-living, nitrogen-fixing bacteria, *Azotobacter*, and by a blue-green alga, *Anabaena cylindrica*, requires molybdenum. The element is therefore intimately associated with nitrogen metabolism and synthesis of protein and hence, synthesis of protoplasm. *See* NITROGEN FIXATION (BIOLOGY).

Certain species of plants appear to require molybdenum for one or more unidentified roles other than nitrate reduction or nitrogen fixation. For example, cauliflower plants grown on urea and ammonium, as reduced nitrogen sources, nevertheless develop characteristic molybdenum-deficiency symptoms known as whip tail when molybdenum is withheld.

Boron. The essentiality of this element was established around 1910. Approximately 1/2 part per million (ppm) in the external solution suffices for growth of most plants. Garden and sugarbeets, as well as alfalfa, have a somewhat higher boron requirement, 5–10 ppm being optimal.

There are no known compounds in plants of which boron is a constituent, and no enzyme system has been shown to require boron. In most plants boron is immobile, suggesting that it is combined with large, immobile molecules, and plants therefore have to receive boron continually throughout the life cycle.

Numerous functions have been proposed for boron, including roles in carbohydrate and protein metabolism. One theory states that boron is required for the translocation of sugar from the leaves (where sugar is made) to the flowers, fruits, and the growing points of stems and roots. In the absence of boron, stem and root tips die, and flowering and fruiting are drastically reduced or altogether curtailed. A certain degree of deficiency of boron, for example, that which results in almost complete failure to set seeds in alfalfa, may not materially reduce the size of the plants. This well-established phenomenon signifies its unique role

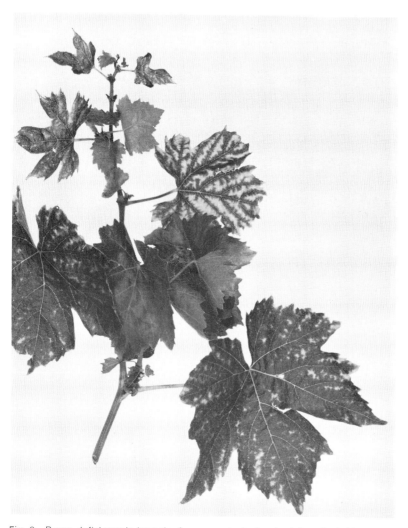

Fig. 2. Boron deficiency in branch of a grape plant, showing interveinal chlorosis of terminal leaves and necrotic terminal growing point. (*From J. A. Cook et al., Light fruit set and leaf injury from boron deficiency in vineyards readily corrected when identified, Calif. Agr., 15(3):3–4, 1961*)

in flowering and fruiting. Successful germination of pollen grains and the production of the pollen tubes require boron.

Boron-deficient plants lose the normal response to gravity, indicating that boron is involved in the production, movement, or action of the natural plant hormones that cause the stem of a horizontally placed plant to turn up and the roots to turn down.

Chlorine. In the tomato plant, chlorine deficiency results in wilting of the leaf tips and chlorosis (yellowing), bronzing, and necrosis (death) of the leaves. If chlorine is added early enough, as little as 3 ppm banishes the symptoms and normal growth proceeds. Tomato plants show deficiency when they contain about 200 ppm of chlorine (dry-weight basis), whereas they show molybdenum deficiency when the concentration is about 0.1 ppm. Therefore, the tomato plant requires several thousand times more chlorine than molybdenum.

It should be made clear that plants cannot tolerate more than a few parts per million of chlorine in the molecular, gaseous state. Ordinarily plants absorb chlorine in the ionic form as chloride. Most plants tolerate 500 ppm or more of chloride without much effect upon growth, and certain halophytes (salt plants) can grow vigorously in high concentrations of chloride slats.

Other elements. Vanadium is required for the growth of *Scenedesmus obliquus*, and it plays a role in photosynthesis in *Chlorella*. There is no evidence of its essentiality for plants other than the green algae. Silicon is required for diatoms.

Sodium is an essential element for certain blue-green algae but is not required for green algae or higher plants.

Cobalt is required only for certain blue-green algae and the nitrogen-fixing bacteria in nodules of leguminous plants.

Deficiency symptoms. A deficiency of any one of the 16 essential elements results in stunted growth and reduced yield.

Deficiency symptoms are best identified by specially trained persons, since a deficiency of a particular element has different symptoms on different plants, for example, corn and beans. Furthermore, the application of nutrients to correct deficiencies, particularly of boron, copper, manganese, zinc, and molybdenum, requires specialists in plant nutrition.

The elements which are most likely to have a limiting effect on growth are nitrogen, phosphorus, and potassium; these are present in a typical, commercially available fertilizer, such as 5-10-5. Some generalizations can be made about the deficiency symptoms of these three main elements. When nitrogen moves out of the older, hence lower, leaves of a plant, the deficiency is generally characterized by yellowing of these leaves. Phosphorus deficiency is often characterized by a purpling of the stem, leaf, or veins on the underside of the leaves.

In corn, phosphorus deficiency causes purpling of the stem and sometimes of the leaf blades. Potash (potassium) deficiency results in burn or scorch of the margins of the leaves, particularly the older, lower leaves (Fig. 1). Recognition of the deficiency symptoms of these three elements can

be corrected by the application of readily available commercial fertilizer.

Chemical tests (tissue tests) can often be made of key plant tissues to determine whether a particular element is lacking. These tissue tests can detect a near-deficiency state before the symptoms become manifest. In general, these tests should be made by trained persons.

The best approach for the average homeowner or farmer, however, is to have the soil tested if there is any question as to its productive capacity. Commercial laboratories and state agricultural experiment stations provide this service. A soil test can predict in advance of planting what nutrients are lacking. By the time deficiencies appear, plant growth and yield are usually irretrievably retarded. If they are used early enough, tissue tests can detect an incipient deficiency in time for correction.

In addition to the widespread need for nitrogen, phosphorus, and potassium, it is often necessary to add other elements. The following elements have been found to be deficient in one or more areas of the United States: boron (Fig. 2), magnesium, copper, manganese, zinc, iron, calcium, sulfur, and molybdenum. A deficiency of chlorine has not been observed under field conditions. In one soil or another, a deficiency of every essential element except chlorine has been found. Considering the number of years that some soils have been under cultivation and the amounts of essential elements which have been removed by crops, it is not surprising that agricultural soils are becoming deficient in certain essential elements. When plants are unusually low in calcium or phosphorus, for example, people and particularly grazing animals may develop certain deficiency diseases. Thus there is a very intimate relationship between plant and animal nutrition that is receiving considerable attention. *See* PLANT, MINERAL NUTRITION OF.

[HUGH G. GAUCH]

Bibliography: J. Bonner and J. E. Varner (eds.), *Plant Biochemistry*, 1965; R. M. Devlin, *Plant Physiology*, 1966; C. A. Lamp, O. G. Bentley, and J. M. Beattie (eds.), *Trace Elements*, 1958; W. D. McElroy, *Cell Physiology and Biochemistry*, 3d ed., 1967; H. B. Sprague (ed.), *Hunger Signs in Crops: A Symposium*, American Society of Agronomy and National Fertilizer Association, 3d ed., 1964; F. C. Steward (ed.), *Plant Physiology*, vols. 1A–6C, 1959–1972.

Plant, water relations of

Water is the most abundant constituent of all physiologically active plant cells. Leaves, for example, have water contents which lie mostly within a range of 55–85% of their fresh weight. Other relatively succulent parts of plants contain approximately the same proportion of water, and even such largely nonliving tissues as wood may be 30–60% water on a fresh-weight basis. The smallest water contents in living parts of plants occur mostly in dormant structures, such as mature seeds and spores. The great bulk of the water in any plant constitutes a unit system. This water is not in a static condition. Rather it is part of a hydrodynamic system, which in terrestrial plants involves absorption of water from the soil, its translocation throughout the plant, and its loss to the environment, principally in the process known as transpiration.

Cellular water relations. The typical mature, vacuolate plant cell constitutes a tiny osmotic system, and this idea is central to any concept of cellular water dynamics. Although the cell walls of most living plant cells are quite freely permeable to water and solutes, the cytoplasmic layer that lines the cell wall is more permeable to some substances than to others. This property of differential permeability appears to reside principally in the layer of cytoplasm adjacent to the cell wall (plasma membrane, or plasmalemma) and in the layer in contact with the vacuole (vacuolar membrane, or tonoplast). This cytoplasmic system of membranes is usually relatively permeable to water, to dissolved gases, and to certain dissolved organic components. It is often much less permeable to sugars and mineral salts. The permeability of the cytoplasmic membranes is quite variable, however, and under certain metabolic conditions solutes that ordinarily penetrate through these membranes slowly or not at all may pass into or out of cells rapidly.

Osmotic and turgor pressures. If a plant cell in a flaccid condition—one in which the cell sap exerts no pressure against the encompassing cytoplasm and cell wall—is immersed in pure water, inward osmosis of water into the cell sap ensues. Osmosis may be defined as the movement of solvent molecules, which in living organisms are always water, across a membrane that is more permeable to the solvent than to the solutes dissolved in it. The driving force in osmosis is the difference in free energies of the water on the two sides of the membrane. Pure water, as a result of its intrinsic properties, possesses free energy. Since there is no certain way of measuring the free energy of water, it is arbitrarily given a value of zero when exposed only to atmospheric pressure. The free energy of water is influenced by temperature, but this discussion will be restricted to isothermal systems. This free energy has been designated water potential and may be expressed in either energy or pressure units. It is more meaningful to use pressure units in considerations of the water potential of plants.

Inward osmosis of water takes place under the conditions specified above because the water potential of the cell sap is less than that of the surrounding pure water by the amount of its osmotic pressure. Introduction of solutes always lowers the potential of water by the amount of the resulting osmotic pressure. If the osmotic pressure of the cell sap is 15 atmospheres (atm), then the water potential of the cell sap is 15 atm less than that of pure water at the same temperature and under the same pressure.

The gain of water by the cell as a result of inward osmosis results in the exertion of a turgor pressure against the protoplasm, which in turn is transmitted to the cell wall. This pressure also prevails throughout the mass of solution within the cell. If the cell wall is elastic, some expansion in the volume of the cell occurs as a result of this pressure, although in many kinds of cells this is relatively small.

Because of the solutes invariably present, the cell sap possesses an osmotic pressure. The osmotic pressures of most plant cell saps lie within a 5- to 40-atm range of magnitudes, although values

as high as 200 atm have been found in some halophytes (plants that can tolerate high-solute media). The osmotic pressures of the cells of a given plant tissue vary considerably with environmental conditions and intrinsic metabolic activities. More or less regular daily or seasonal variations occur in the magnitude of cell sap osmotic pressures in the cells of many tissues. It is the osmotic pressure of the cell sap, coupled with the differential permeability of the cytoplasmic membranes and the relative inelasticity of the cell walls, which permits the development of the more or less turgid condition characteristic of most plant cells.

With continued osmosis of water into the cell, its turgor pressure gradually increases until it is equal to the final osmotic pressure of the sap. Subjection of the water in the cell sap to pressure increases its water potential by the amount of the imposed pressure. In the example given above, disregarding the usually small amount of sap dilution as a result of cell expansion, the water potential of the cell sap is reduced 15 atm because of the presence of solutes (the osmotic pressure is the index of this lowering of water potential) and raised 15 atm as a result of turgor pressure when maximum turgor is reached. Hence, when a dynamic equilibrium is attained, the water potential of the cell sap is zero and thus is equal to that of the surrounding water, a necessary condition if equilibrium is to be achieved.

If the same cell in a flaccid condition is immersed in a solution with an osmotic pressure of 6 atm, inward osmosis of water occurs, but does not continue as long as when the cell is immersed in pure water. Disregarding sap dilution, a dynamic equilibrium will be attained under these circumstances when the turgor pressure of the cell sap has reached 9 atm, because at this point the water potential in the cell sap and the water potential in the surrounding solution will be equal. Since the water potential of the cell sap was originally diminished 15 atm because of the presence of solutes and then raised 9 atm because of turgor pressure, the net value of the water potential in the cell at equilibrium is −6 atm. This is also the value of the water potential in the surrounding solution, as indexed by its osmotic pressure. At dynamic equilibrium the number of water molecules entering the cell and the number leaving per unit of time will be equal.

Water potential. As the examples just given indicate, the effective physical quantity controlling the direction of osmotic movement of water from cell to cell in plants or between a cell and an external solution is the water potential WP of the water. In most plant cells this quantity is equal to the osmotic pressure OP of the water less the turgor pressure TP to which it is subjected. Since the osmotic pressure is the index of the amount by which the water potential of a solution is less than that of pure water under the same conditions, it must be treated as a negative quantity. Turgor pressures usually have a positive value, but if water passes into a state of tension, they are negative. Examples of the occurrence of water under tension in plants will be discussed later in this article. In an unconfined solution the water potential is equal to the osmotic pressure, since there is no turgor pressure. In a fully turgid plant cell the water potential is zero, since the turgor pressure is equal to the osmotic pressure. In a fully flaccid plant cell the turgor pressure is zero and the water potential is equal to the osmotic pressure. The interrelationships among these quantities may be expressed: $WP = (-OP) + TP$.

Since the osmotic pressure must be treated as a negative quantity and since turgor pressures rarely exceed osmotic pressures, the water potentials in plant cells are negative in value. The only well-known exception to this is root pressure, discussed later, during which small positive water potentials can be generated in the water-conductive tissues.

The relationships expressed in the equation are illustrated graphically in Fig. 1, in which allowance has been made for the effect of the volume changes which are characteristic of some kinds of cells with shifts in turgor pressure. The conditions which would prevail in the cell if the cell sap passed into a state of tension (negative pressure) are indicated by the dotted extension of curves to the left.

Cell-to-cell movement of water in plants always occurs from the cell of greater (less negative) water potential to the cell of lesser (more negative) water potential. Such movement of water in plant tissues apparently often occurs along water potential gradients in which the water potential of each cell in a series is less (more negative) than that of the preceding one.

Plasmolysis. If a turgid or partially turgid plant cell is immersed in a solution with a greater osmotic pressure than the cell sap, a gradual shrinkage in the volume of the cell ensues; the amount of shrinkage depends upon the kind of cell and its initial degree of turgidity. When the lower limit of cell wall elasticity is reached and there is continued loss of water from the cell sap, the protoplasmic layer begins to recede from the inner surface of the cell wall. Retreat of the protoplasm from the cell wall often continues until it has shrunk toward the center of the cell, the space between the protoplasm and the cell wall becoming occupied by the bathing solution. This phenomenon is called plasmolysis. If a cell is immersed in a solution with an osmotic pressure which just slightly exceeds that of the cell sap, withdrawal of the protoplasm from the cell wall would be just barely initiated. The stage of plasmolysis shown in Fig. 1 is called incipient plasmolysis, and it is the basis for one of the methods which is commonly used in measuring the osmotic pressure of plant cells.

Imbibition. In some kinds of plant cells movement of water occurs principally by the process of imbibition rather than osmosis. The swelling of dry seeds when immersed in water is a familiar example of this process. Imbibition occurs because of the more negative water potential in the imbibant as compared with the water potential in some contiguous part of the system. An equilibrium is reached only when the water potential in the two parts of the system has attained the same value. The water potential in a dry seed is extremely low, being equal in value, but with a negative sign, to its imbibition pressure. The water potential of pure water is zero; hence movment of water occurs into the seed. Even if the seeds are immersed in a solution of considerable osmotic pressure, which in an unconfined solution is an index of its negative water potential, imbibition occurs. However, if the osmotic pressure of the solution is high enough (of the order of 1000 atm), the seed will not gain water

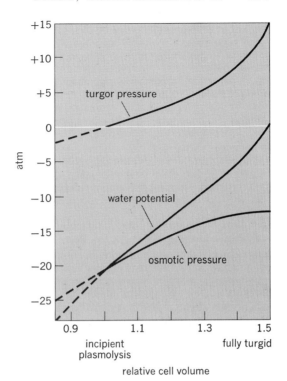

Fig. 1. Curves showing interrelationships among osmotic pressures, turgor pressures, water potentials, and volumes of a plant cell. (*Based on data of K. Höfler, Ber. Deut. Botan. Ges., 38:288–298, 1920*)

from the solution and may even lose a little to the solution. In other words, if the water potential of the solution is negative enough, imbibition does not occur.

However, a more negative water potential in the imbibant, as compared with the surrounding or adjacent medium is not the only condition which must be fulfilled if imbibition is to occur. Many kinds of seeds swell readily if immersed in water but not when immersed in ether or other organic solvents. On the other hand, rubber does not imbibe water but does imbibe measurable quantities of ether and other organic liquids. Certain specific attraction forces between the molecules of the imbibant and the imbibed liquid are therefore also a requisite for the occurrence of imbibition.

In an imbibitional system the imbibition pressure *IP* of the imbibant is the analog of the osmotic pressure in an osmotic system; hence in such a system water potential is related to the imbibition pressure and turgor pressure: $WP = (-IP) + TP$. The imbibition pressure may be regarded as an index of the reduction in water potential in an imbibant insofar as it results from attractions between the molecules of the imbibant and water molecules. For an unconfined imbibant immersed in water, the negative water potential initially equals the imbibition pressure, since there is no turgor pressure. The more nearly saturated such an imbibant becomes, the smaller its imbibition pressure and the less negative its water potentials. A fully saturated imbibant has a zero imbibition pressure and a zero water potential.

Stomatal mechanism. Various gases diffuse into and out of physiologically active plants. Those gases of greatest physiological significance are carbon dioxide, which diffuses into the plant during photosynthesis and is lost from the plant in respiration; oxygen, which diffuses in during respiration and is lost during photosynthesis; and water vapor, which is lost in the process of transpiration. The great bulk of the gaseous exchanges between a plant and its environment occurs through tiny pores in the epidermis called stomates. Although stomates occur on many aerial parts of plants, they are most characteristic of, and occur in greatest abundance in, leaves.

Each stomate or stoma (plural, stomates or stomata) consists of a minute elliptical pore surrounded by two distinctively shaped epidermal cells called guard cells. Stomates are sometimes open and sometimes closed; when closed, all gaseous exchanges between the plant and its environment are greatly retarded. The size of a fully open stomate differs greatly from one species of plant to another. Among the largest known are those of the wandering Jew (*Zebrina pendula*), whose axial dimensions average 31 by 12 microns (μ). In most species the stomates are much smaller, but all of them afford portals of egress or ingress which are enormous relative to the size of the gas molecules that diffuse through them. The number of stomates per square centimeter of leaf surface ranges from a few thousand in some species to over a hundred thousand in others. In many species of plants stomates are present in both the upper and lower epidermises, usually being more abundant in the lower. In many species, especially of woody plants, they are present only in the lower epidermis. In floating-leaved aquatic species stomates occur only in the upper epidermis.

Rates of transpiration (loss of water vapor) from leaves of the expanded type often are 50% or even more of the rate of evaporation from a free water surface of equal area under the same environmental conditions. Loss of water vapor from leaves may occur at such relatively high rates despite the fact that the aggregate area of the fully open stomates is only 1–3% of the leaf area. Much more significant is the fact that the rate of diffusion of carbon dioxide, essential in photosynthesis, into the leaves through the stomates is much greater than through the equivalent area of an efficient carbon dioxide – absorbing surface.

Although some mass flow of gases undoubtedly occurs through the stomates under certain conditions, most movement of gases into or out of a leaf takes place by diffusion through the stomates. Diffusion is the physical process whereby molecules of a gas move from a region of their greater diffusion pressure to the region of their lesser diffusion pressure as a result of their own kinetic activity. Molecules of liquids and solids (to a limited extent), molecules and ions of solutes, and colloidal particles also diffuse whenever the appropriate circumstances prevail.

Diffusion of gases through small pores follows certain principles which account for the high diffusion capacity of the stomates. In the diffusion of a gas through a small pore, an overwhelming proportion of the molecules escape over the rim of the pore relative to those escaping through its center. Hence, diffusion rates through small apertures vary as their perimeter rather than as their area. The less the area of a pore, therefore, the greater is its diffusive capacity relative to its area. Therefore, a gas may diffuse nearly as rapidly through a septum pierced with a number of small orifices, whose aggregate area represents only a small proportion of the septum area, as through an open surface equal in area to the septum. The high diffusive capacity of the stomates can be accounted for in terms of these principles. Since diffusion of gases through stomates is proportional to the perimeter of the pore rather than to its area, the diffusion rate through a partially open stomate is almost as great as that through a fully open stomate.

In general, stomates are open in the daytime and closed at night, although there are many exceptions to this statement. The mechanism whereby stomates open in the light and close in the dark seems to be principally an osmotic one, although other factors are probably involved. Upon the advent of illumination, the hydrogen ion concentration of the guard cells decreases. This favors the action of the enzyme phosphorylase, which in the presence of phosphates causes transformation of insoluble starch into the soluble compound glucose-1-phosphate. The resulting increase in the solute concentration of the guard cells causes an increase in their osmotic pressure, and hence also in the negativity of their water potential. Osmotic movement of water takes place from contiguous epidermal cells, in which there is little daily variation in osmotic pressure, into the guard cells. The resulting increase in turgor pressure of the guard cells causes them to open. With the advent of darkness or of a relatively low light intensity, the reverse train of processes is apparently set into operation, leading ultimately to closure of the stomates.

Light of low intensity is, generally speaking, less effective than stronger illumination in inducing stomatal opening. Hence stomates often do not open as wide on cloudy as on clear days, and often do not remain open for as much of the daylight period. A deficiency of water within the plant also induces partial to complete closure of the stomates. During periods of drought, therefore, stomates remain shut continuously or, at most, are open for only short periods each day, regardless of the light intensity to which the plant is exposed. Opening of the stomates does not occur in most species at temperatures approaching freezing. Hence in cold or even cool weather stomates often remain closed even when other environmental conditions are favorable to their opening. Nocturnal opening occurs at times in some species, but the conditions which induce this pattern of stomatal reaction are not clearly understood.

TRANSPIRATION PROCESS

The term transpiration is used to designate the process whereby water vapor is lost from plants. Although basically an evaporation process, transpiration is complicated by other physical and physiological conditions prevailing in the plant. Whereas loss of water vapor can occur from any part of the plant which is exposed to the atmosphere, the great bulk of all transpiration occurs from the leaves. There are two kinds of foliar transpiration: (1) stomatal transpiration, in which water vapor loss occurs through the stomates, and (2) cuticular transpiration, which occurs directly from the outside surface of epidermal walls through the cuticle. In most species 90% or more of all foliar transpiration is of the stomatal type.

Stomatal transpiration. The dynamics of stomatal transpiration is considerably more complex than that of cuticular transpiration. In the leaves of most kinds of plants the mesophyll cells do not fit together tightly, and the intercellular spaces between them are occupied by air. A veritable labyrinth of air-filled spaces is thus present within a leaf, bounded by the water-saturated walls of the mesophyll cells. Water evaporates readily from these wet cell walls into the intercellular spaces. If the stomates are closed, the only effect of such evaporation is to saturate the intercellular spaces with water vapor. If the stomates are open, however, diffusion of water vapor usually occurs through them into the surrounding atmosphere. Such diffusion always occurs unless the atmosphere has a vapor pressure equal to or greater than that within the intercellular spaces, a situation which seldom prevails during the daylight hours of clear days. The two physical processes of evaporation and diffusion of water vapor are both integral steps in stomatal transpiration. Physiological control of this component of transpiration is exerted through the opening and closing of the stomates, previously described.

Environmental factors. Light is one of the major factors influencing the rate of transpiration because of its controlling effect on the opening and closing of stomates. Since stomatal transpiration is largely restricted to the daylight hours, daytime rates of transpiration are usually many times greater than night rates, which largely or entirely represent cuticular transpiration. Since leaves in direct sunlight usually have temperatures from one to several degrees higher than that of the surrounding atmosphere, light also has a secondary accelerating effect on transpiration through its influence on leaf temperatures. Increase in leaf temperatures results in an increase in the pressure of the water vapor molecules within the leaf.

The rate of diffusion of water vapor through open stomates depends upon the steepness of the vapor pressure gradient between the intercellular spaces and the outside atmosphere. When the vapor pressure in that part of the intercellular spaces just below the stomatal pores is high relative to that of the atmosphere, diffusion of water vapor out of the leaf occurs rapidly; when it is low, water vapor diffusion occurs much more slowly.

Temperature has a marked effect upon rates of transpiration, principally because of its differential effect upon the vapor pressure of the intercellular spaces and atmosphere. Although leaf temperatures do not exactly parallel atmsopheric temperatures, increase in atmospheric temperature in general results in a rise in leaf temperature and vice versa. On a warm, clear day such as would be typified by many summer days in temperate latitudes and with an adequate soil water supply, increase in temperature results in an increase in the vapor pressure of the intercellular spaces. Such a rise in vapor pressure occurs because the vapor pressure corresponding to a saturated condition of an atmsophere increases with rise in temperature, and the extensive evaporating surfaces of the cell walls bounding the intercellular spaces make it possible for the intercellular spaces to be maintained in an approximately saturated condition most of the time. An increase in temperature ordinarily has little or no effect on the vapor pressure

of the atmosphere, and this is especially true of warm, bright days, when transpiration rates are the highest. Hence, as the temperature rises, the vapor pressure of the intercellular spaces increases relative to that of the external atmosphere, the vapor pressure gradient through the stomates is steepened, and the rate of outward diffusion of water vapor increases.

Wind velocity is another factor which influences the rate of transpiration. Generally speaking, a gentle breeze is relatively much more effective in increasing transpiration rates than are winds of greater velocity. In quiet air, localized zones of relatively high atmospheric vapor pressure may build up in the vicinity of transpiring leaves. Such zones retard transpiration unless there is sufficient air movement to prevent the accumulation of water vapor molecules. The bending, twisting, and fluttering of leaf blades and the swaying of stalks and branches in a wind also contribute to increasing the rate of transpiration.

Soil water conditions exert a major influence on the rate of transpiration. Whenever soil conditions are such that the rate of absorption of water is retarded, there is a corresponding diminution in the rate of transpiration.

Daily periodicity of transpiration. The rate of every major plant process, including transpiration, is measurably and often markedly influenced by the environmental conditions to which the plant is exposed. Many of the environmental factors exhibit more or less regular daily periodicities, which vary somewhat, of course, with the prevailing climatic conditions. This is especially true of the factors of light and temperature. Many plant processes, including transpiration, therefore exhibit daily periodicities in rate that are correlated with the daily periodicities of one or more environmental factors.

The daily periodicity of transpiration in alfalfa, as exhibited on three clear, warm days with adequate soil water available, is illustrated in Fig. 2. A similar daily periodicity of transpiration is exhibited under comparable environmental conditions by many other species. During the hours of darkness, the transpiration rate is relatively low, and in most species water vapor loss during this period may be regarded as entirely cuticular or nearly so. The transpiration rate shows a steady rise during the morning hours, culminating in a peak rate which is attained in the early hours of the afternoon. The increase in transpiration rate during the forepart of the day results from gradual opening of the stomates, beginning with the advent of light, followed by a steady increase in the steepness of the vapor pressure gradient through the stomates, which occurs as a result of increasing atmospheric temperature during the morning and earlier afternoon hours.

In most plants, if transpiration is occurring rapidly, the rate of absorption of water does not keep pace with the rate at which water vapor is lost from the leaves. In other words, the plant is gradually being depleted of water during the daylight hours. In time the resulting decrease in the water content of the leaf cells results in a reduced vapor pressure within the intercellular spaces, and a diminution in the rate of transpiration begins. Stomates also start to close as a result of the diminished leaf water content, and their closure is accelerated during the later part of the afternoon by the waning light intensity. By nightfall complete closure of virtually all stomates has taken place, and water vapor loss during the hours of darkness is again restricted largely or entirely to the relatively low rate of cuticular transpiration. It is noteworthy that the peak rate of transpiration occurs during the early afternoon hours, correlating more closely with the daily temperature periodicity than with the daily periodicity of light intensity.

Under environmental conditions differing considerably from those postulated in the preceding discussion, patterns of transpiration periodicity may show a considerable variance from the one described. On cloudy days, for example, stomates generally open less completely than on clear days, and a curve for daily transpiration periodicity presents a greatly flattened appearance as compared with those shown in Fig. 2. A cool temperature, even in a range somewhat above freezing, greatly diminishes and may even cause cessation of stomatal transpiration, resulting in a pronounced modification in the daily march of transpiration periodicity. A deficient soil water supply is probably the most common cause of departures from the pattern of transpiration described above. A reduction in soil water content below the field capacity (optimum water availability) results not only in a general flattening of the transpiration periodicity curve, but frequently also in appearance of the peak of the curve somewhat earlier in the day. Since, even in temperate zone regions, drought periods of greater or less severity are of common occurrence during the summer months and in many habitats are the rule rather than the exception, transpiration periodicity curves of this flattened and skewed-peak type are undoubtedly of frequent occurrence.

Magnitude of transpiration. Transpiration of broad-leaved species of plants growing under temperate zone conditions may range up to about 5 g per square decimeter of leaf area per hour. Sufficient quantities of water are often lost in transpiration by vegetation-covered areas of the Earth's surface to have important effects not only on soil water relations, but also on meteorological conditions. The quantities of water lost per acre by crops, grasslands, or forest are therefore a matter of basic interest. An acre of corn (maize), for example, transpires water equivalent to 15 in. of rainfall during a usual growing season. Transpiration of deciduous, largely oak, forest in the southern Appalachian Mountains has been estimated as equivalent to 17–22 in. of rainfall per year. Marked variations occur in such values from year to year,

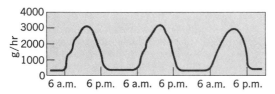

Fig. 2. Daily periodicity of transpiration of alfalfa on three successive clear, warm days with adequate soil water. Rate of transpiration expressed as grams per hour per 6-ft² plot of alfalfa. (*From M. D. Thomas and G. R. Hill, Plant Physiol., 12:285–307, 1937*)

however, depending upon prevailing climatic conditions.

Significance of transpiration. Viewpoints regarding the significance of transpiration have ranged between the two extremes of considering it a process that is an unavoidable evil or a physiological necessity. Neither of these extreme views appears to be tenable. Some of the incidental effects of transpiration appear to be advantageous to the plant, but none of them is indispensable for its survival or even for its adequate physiological operation. Likewise, while some of the incidental effects of transpiration appear to be detrimental to the plant, none of them is so in such a critical fashion that survival of plants, considered in the aggregate, is endangered.

Transpiration is a necessary consequence of the relation of water to the anatomy of the plant, and especially to the anatomy of the leaves. Terrestrial green plants are dependent upon atmospheric carbon dioxide for their survival. In terrestrial vascular plants the principal carbon dioxide–absorbing surfaces are the moist mesophyll cells walls which bound the intercellular spaces in leaves. Ingress of carbon dioxide into these spaces occurs mostly by diffusion through open stomates. When the stomates are open, outward diffusion of water vapor unavoidably occurs, and such stomatal transpiration accounts for most of the water vapor loss from plants. Although transpiration is thus, in effect, an incidental phenomenon, it frequently has marked indirect effects on other physiological processes which occur in the plant because of its effects on the internal water relations of the plant.

WATER TRANSLOCATION

In terrestrial rooted plants practically all of the water which enters a plant is absorbed from the soil by the roots. The water thus absorbed is translocated to all parts of the plant. In the tallest trees (specimens of the coast redwood, *Sequoia sempervirens*) the distance from the tips of the deepest roots to the tips of the topmost branches is nearly 400 ft, and water must be elevated for this distance through such trees. Although few plants are as tall as such redwoods, the same mechanisms of water movement are believed to operate in all vascular species. The mechanism of the "ascent of sap" (all translocated water contains at least traces of solutes) in plants, especially tall trees, was one of the first processes to excite the interest of plant physiologists.

Water-conductive tissues. The upward movement of water in plants occurs in the xylem, which, in the larger roots, trunks, and branches of trees and shrubs, is identical with the wood. In the trunks or larger branches of most kinds of trees, however, sap movement is restricted to a few of the outermost annual layers of wood. This explains why hollow trees, in which the central core of older wood has disintegrated, can remain alive for many years. The xylem of any plant is a unit and continuous system throughout the plant. Small strands of this tissue extend almost to the tip of every root. Other strands, the larger of which constitute important parts of the veins, ramify to all parts of each leaf. In angiosperms most translocation of water occurs through the xylem vessels, which are nonliving, elongated, tubelike structures. The vessels are formed by the end-to-end coalescence of many much smaller cells, death of these cells ensuing at about the same time that coalescence occurs. In trees the diameters of such vessels range from about 20 to 400 μ, and they may extend for many feet with no more interruption than an occasional incomplete cross wall. In gymnosperms no vessels are present, and movement of water occurs solely through spindle-shaped xylem cells called tracheids. Vertically contiguous tracheids always overlap along their tapering portions, resulting in a densely packed type of woody tissue. Individual tracheids may be as much as 5 mm in length. Like the vessels, they are nonliving while functional in the translocation of water. Small, more or less rounded, thin areas occur in the walls of vessels and tracheids that are contiguous with the walls of other tracheids, vessels, or cells. Structurally, three main types of such pits are recognized, but all of these types appear to facilitate the passage of water from one xylem element to another.

Root pressure. The exudation of xylem sap from the stump of a cutoff herbaceous plant is a commonly observed phenomenon. Sap exudation ("bleeding") from the cut ends of stems or from incisions into the wood also occurs in certain woody plants, such as birch, currant, and grape, especially in the spring. A single vigorous grapevine often loses a liter or more of sap per day through the cut ends of stems after spring pruning. This exudation of sap from the xylem tissue results from a pressure originating in the roots, called root pressure. A related phenomenon is that of guttation. This term refers to the exudation of drops of water from the tips or margins of leaves, which occurs in many species of herbaceous plants as well as in some woody species. Like sap exudation from cut stems, this phenomenon is observed most frequently in the spring, and especially during early morning hours. The water exuded in guttation is not pure, but contains traces of sugar and other solutes. Guttation occurs from special structures called hydathodes, which are similar in structure to but larger than stomates. In most species water loss by guttation is negligible in comparison with the water lost as vapor in transpiration. Like xylem sap exudation, guttation results from root pressure.

Root pressure is generally considered to be one of the mechanisms of upward transport of water in plants. While it is undoubtedly true that root pressure does account for some upward movement of water in certain species of plants at some seasons, various considerations indicate that it can be only a secondary mechanism of water transport. Among these considerations are: (1) There are many species in which the phenomenon of root pressure has not been observed. (2) The magnitude of measured root pressures seldom exceeds 2 atm, which could not activate a rise of water for more than about 60 ft, and many trees are much taller than this. (3) Known rates of xylem sap flow under the influence of root pressure are usually inadequate to compensate for known rates of transpiration. (4) Root pressures are usually operative in woody plants only during the early spring; during the summer months, when transpiration rates, and hence rates of xylem sap transport, are greatest, root pressures are negligible or nonexistent.

Water cohesion and ascent of sap. Although invariably in motion, as a result of their kinetic energy, water molecules are also strongly attracted to each other. In masses of liquid water the existence of such intermolecular attractions is not obvious, but when water is confined in long tubes of small diameter, the reality of the mutual attractions among water molecules can be demonstrated. If the water at the top of such a tube be subjected to a pull, the resulting stress will be transmitted, because of the mutual attraction (cohesion) among water molecules, all the way down the column of water. Furthermore, because of the attraction between the water molecules and the wall of the tube (adhesion), subjecting the water column to a stress does not result in pulling it away from the wall.

The observations just mentioned have been made the basis of a widely entertained theory of the mechanism of water transport in plants, first clearly enunciated by H. H. Dixon in 1914. According to this theory, upward translocation of water (actually a very dilute sap) is engendered by an increase in the negativity of water potential in the cells of apical organs of plants. Such increases in the negativity of water potentials occur most commonly in the mesophyll cells of leaves as a result of transpiration.

Evaporation of water from the walls of the mesophyll cells abutting on the intercellular spaces reduces their turgor pressure and hence increases the negativity of the water potential in such cells. Consequent cell-to-cell movements of water cause the water potentials even of those mesophyll cells which are not directly exposed to the intercellular spaces to become more negative. The resulting decrease in the water potential of those cells directly in contact with the xylem elements in the veinlets of the leaf induces movement of water from the vessel or tracheids into those cells. Whenever transpiration is occurring at appreciable rates, water does not enter the lower ends of the xylem conduits in the roots as rapidly as it passes out of the vessels or tracheids into adjacent leaf cells at the upper ends of the water-conductive system; therefore the water in the xylem ducts is stretched into taut threads, that is, it passes into a state of tension. Each column of water behaves like a tiny stretched wire. The tension is transmitted along the entire length of the water columns to their terminations just back of the root tips. Subjection of the water in the xylem ducts to a tension (in effect, a negative pressure) increases the negativity of its water potential. The water potential in the xylem conduits is also subject to some lowering because of the presence of solutes, but xylem sap is usually so dilute that this osmotic effect is rarely more than a minor one. As a result of the increased negativity of the water potential in the xylem elements, movement of water is induced from adjacent root cells into those elements in the absorbing regions of roots.

The tension engendered in the water columns can be sustained by them because of the cohesion between the water molecules, acting in conjunction with the adhesion of the boundary layers of water molecules to the walls of the xylem ducts.

The existence of water under tension in vessels has been verified in a number of species of plants by direct microscopic examination. There is some evidence that, under conditions of marked internal water deficiency, the tensions generated in the water columns are proliferated into the mesophyll cells of leaves and cells in the absorbing regions of roots. Conservative calculations indicate that a cohesion value of 30–50 atm would be adequate to permit translocation of water to the top of the tallest known trees. However, under conditions of internal water deficiency, tensions considerably in excess of 50 atm are probably engendered in the water columns of many plants, especially woody species.

WATER ABSORPTION

This process will be discussed only from the standpoint of terrestrial, rooted plants. Consideration of the absorption of water by plants necessitates an understanding of the physical status of the water in soils as it exists under various conditions.

Soil water conditions. Even in the tightest of soils, the particles never fit together perfectly and a certain amount of space exists among them. This pore space of a soil ranges from about 30% of the soil volume in sandy soils to about 50% of the soil volume in heavy clay soils. In desiccated soils the pore space is occupied entirely by air, in saturated soils it is occupied entirely by water, but in moist, well-drained soils it is usually occupied partly by air and partly by water. In a soil in which a water table is located not too far below the surface, considerable quantities of water may rise into its upper layers by capillarity and become available to plants. In arid regions, however, there ordinarily is no water table. Even in many humid regions the water table is continuously or intermittently too far below the soil surface to be an appreciable source of water for most plants. In all soils lacking a water table or in which the water table is at a considerable depth, the only water available to plants is that which comes as natural precipitation or which is provided by artificial irrigation. If water falls on, or is applied to, a dry soil which is homogeneous to a considerable depth, it will become rapidly distributed to a depth which will depend on the quantity of water supplied per unit area and on the specific properties of that soil. After several days further deepening of the moist layer of soil extending downward from the surface virtually ceases, because within such a time interval capillary movement of water in a downward direction has become extremely slow or nonexistent. The boundary line between the moist layer of soil above and the drier zone below will be a distinct one. In this condition of field equilibrium the water content of the upper moist soil layer is, in homogeneous soils, essentially uniform throughout the layer. *See* Soil.

The water content of a soil in this equilibrium condition is called the field capacity. Field capacities range from about 5% in coarse sandy soils to about 45% of the dry weight in clay soils. The moisture equivalent of a soil, often measured in the laboratory, is usually very close in value to the field capacity of the same soil. It is defined as the water content of a soil which is retained against a force 1000 times gravity as measured in a centrifuge. A soil at its field capacity is relatively moist, but is also well aerated. Soil water contents at or near the field capacity are the most favorable for growth of most kinds of plants.

A considerable proportion of the water in any soil is unavailable in the growth of plants. The permanent wilting percentage is the generally accepted index of this fraction of the soil water. This quantity is measured by allowing a plant to develop with its roots in soil enclosed in a waterproof pot until the plant passes into a state of permanent wilting. The water content of the soil when the plant just passes into this condition is the permanent wilting percentage. The range of permanent wilting percentages is from 2–3%, of the dry weight in coarse sandy soils to about 20% in heavy clay loams. About the same value is obtained for the permanent wilting percentage of a given soil, regardless of the kind of test plant used.

The potential of soil water is always negative and has two major components. One is the osmotic pressure of the soil solution, which in most kinds of soils is only a fraction of 1 atm, although saline and alkali soils are marked exceptions. The other component is the attractive forces between the soil particles and water molecules, which may attain a very considerable magnitude, especially in dry soils. In moist soils, those at the field capacity or higher soil water content, the former of these two components is principally responsible for the negative soil water potential. In drier soils the latter component is almost solely responsible for the negative water potential. In the majority of soils the water potential is only slightly less than zero at saturation, not less than −1 atm at field capacity, and in the vicinity of −15 atm at the permanent wilting percentage. With further reduction in the water content of a soil below its permanent wilting percentage, its water potential increases rapidly in negativity at an accelerating rate. Almost no water can be absorbed by plants from soils with such extremely negative water potentials; for this reason the permanent wilting percentage is the index of soil water unavailable to plant growth (Fig. 3).

Root growth and water absorption. The successively smaller branches of the root system of any plant terminate ultimately in the root tips, of which there may be thousands and often millions on a single plant. As generally employed, the term root tip refers to the region extending back from the apex of the root for a distance of at least several centimeters. The terminal zone of a root tip is the root cap. Just back of this are the regions in which cell division and cell elongation occur and in which all growth in length of roots takes place. Just back of these regions, in the majority of species, is the zone of root hairs. Each root hair is a projection from the epidermal cell of which it is an integral part. A single root tip may bear thousands of root hairs, ranging in length from a few millimeters up to about a centimeter. In most species the root hairs are short-lived structures, but new ones are constantly developing just back of the growing region of the root as it elongates. Most absorption of water occurs in the root tip regions, and especially in the root hair zone. Older portions of most roots become covered with cutinized or suberized layers through which only very limited quantities of water can pass.

Whenever the potential of the water in the root

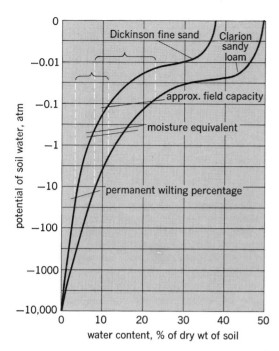

Fig. 3. Relation between soil water potentials and soil water contents of two soils over the entire range of soil water contents. Horizontal braces show the range for each soil over which water is readily available to its plants. Vertical scale is logarithmic. (*Based on data of M. B. Russell, Amer. Soil Sci. Proc., 4:51–54, 1939*)

hairs and other peripheral cells of a root tip is less than that of the soil water, movement of water takes place into the root cells. If the soil water content exceeds the field capacity, water may move by capillarity toward the region of absorption from portions of the soil not immediately contiguous with the root tips, and the supply of readily absorbable water is maintained in this way. Elongation of the roots, although slower in most species in relatively wet soils, also helps maintain contact between the root tips and untapped areas of soil water.

Many plants much of the time grow in soils with a water content in the range between the field capacity and the permanent wilting percentage. In this range of soil water contents, capillary movement of water through the soil is extremely slow or nonexistent, and an adequate supply of water cannot be maintained to rapidly absorbing root tips by this means. In such soils maintenance of contact between the root tips and available soil water is assured only by continued elongation of the roots through the soil. Mature root systems of many plants terminate in millions of root tips, each of which may be visualized as slowly growing through the soil, absorbing water from around or between the soil particles with which it comes in contact. The aggregate increase in the length of the root system of a rye plant averages 3.1 mi/day. Calculations indicate that the daily aggregate root elongation of this plant is adequate to permit absorption of a sufficient quantity of water from soils at the field capacity to compensate for daily transpirational water loss.

Mechanisms of water absorption. As previously indicated, tension, generated in the water col-

umns of a plant, most commonly as an indirect result of transpiration, is transmitted to the ultimate terminations of the xylem ducts in the root tips. The water potential in the water columns is diminished by the amount of the tension generated, which is equivalent to a negative pressure. As soon as the water potential in the water columns becomes less than that in contiguous cells in the root tip, water moves from those cells into the xylem. This activates further cell-to-cell movement of water in a lateral direction across the root and presumably in the establishment of gradients of water potentials, diminishing progressively in magnitude from the epidermal cells, including the root hairs, to the root xylem. Whenever the water potential in the peripheral root cells is less than that of the soil water, movement of water from the soil into the root cells occurs. There is some evidence that, under conditions of marked internal water stress, the tension generated in the xylem ducts will be propagated across the root to the peripheral cells. If this occurs, water potentials of greater negativity could develop in peripheral root cells than would otherwise be possible. The absorption mechanism would operate in fundamentally the same way whether or not the water in the root cells passed into a state of tension. The process just described, often called passive absorption, accounts for most of the absorption of water by terrestrial plants.

The phenomenon of root pressure, previously described as the basis for xylem sap exudation from cuts or wounds and for guttation, represents another mechanism of the absorption of water. This mechanism is localized in the roots and is often called active absorption. Water absorption of this type only occurs when the rate of transpiration is low and the soil is relatively moist. Although the xylem sap is a relatively dilute solution, its osmotic pressure is usually great enough to engender a more negative water potential than usually exists in the soil water when the soil is relatively moist. A gradient of water potentials can thus be established, increasing in negativity across the epidermis, cortex, and other root tissues, along which the water can move laterally from the soil to the xylem. There is evidence, however, that a respiration mechanism, as well as an osmotic one, may be involved in the correlated phenomena of active absorption, root pressure, and guttation.

Environment and absorption. Any factor which influences the rate of transpiration also influences the rate of absorption of water by plants and vice versa. Climatic conditions may therefore indirectly affect rates of water absorption, and soil conditions indirectly affect transpiration. Low soil temperatures, even in a range considerably above freezing, retard the rate of absorption of water by many species. The rate of water absorption by sunflower plants, for example, decreases rapidly as the soil temperature drops below 55°F.

Within limits, the greater the supply of available soil water, the greater is the possible rate of water absorption. High soil water contents, especially those approaching saturation, result in decreased water absorption rates in many species because of the accompanying deficient soil aeration. In the atmosphere of such soils the oxygen concentration is lower and the carbon dioxide concentration is higher than in the atmosphere proper. In general, the deficiency of oxygen in such soils appears to be a more significant factor in causing retarded rates of water absorption than the excess of carbon dioxide. This retarding effect on water absorption rate is correlated with a retarding effect on root respiration rate.

Likewise, if the soil solution attains any considerable concentration of solutes, water absorption by the roots is retarded. In most soils the concentration of the soil solution is so low that it is a negligible factor in affecting rates of water absorption. In saline or alkali soils, however, the concentration of the soil solution may become equivalent to many atmospheres, and only a few species of plants are able to survive when rooted in such soils.

Wilting. Daily variations in the water content of plants, more marked in some organs than in others, are of frequent occurrence. The familiar phenomenon of wilting, exhibited by the leaves and sometimes other organs of plants, particularly herbaceous species, is direct visual evidence of this fact. In hot, bright weather the leaves of many species of plants often wilt during the afternoon, only to regain their turgidity during the night hours, even if no additional water is provided by rainfall or irrigation. This type of wilting reaction is referred to as temporary, or transient, wilting and clearly results from a rate of transpiration in excess of the rate of water absorption during the daylight hours. As a result, the total volume of water in the plant shrinks, although not equally in all organs or tissues. In general, diminution in water content is greatest in the leaf cells, and wilting is induced whenever the turgor pressure of the leaf cells is reduced sufficiently.

Even on days when visible wilting is not discernible, incipient wilting is of frequent occurrence. Incipient wilting corresponds to only a partial loss of turgor by the leaf cells and does not result in visible drooping, folding, or rolling of the leaves. Leaves entering into the condition of transient wilting always pass first through the stage of incipient wilting. Occurrence of this invisible first stage of wilting is almost universal on bright, warm days on which environmental conditions are not severe enough to induce the more advanced stage of transient wilting.

Confirmation of the inferred cause of transient wilting has been furnished by investigations of the comparative daily periodicities of transpiration and absorption of water (Fig. 4). As illustrated in this figure, there is a distinct lag in the rate of absorption of water as compared with the rate of transpiration during the daylight hours. During the

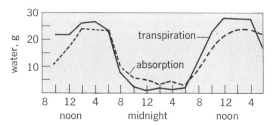

Fig. 4. Comparative daily periodicities of transpiration of water and absorption of water in the loblolly pine (*Pinus taeda* L.). (*From P. J. Kramer, Plant and Soil Water Relationships, McGraw-Hill, 1937*)

night hours, on the contrary, the rate of water absorption is continuously greater than the rate of transpiration. Thus, during the daylight hours the tissues of the plant are being progressively depleted of water, whereas the store of water within the plant is being steadily replenished during the night hours. The lag in the rate of absorption behind the rate of transpiration during the daylight hours appears to result largely from the relatively high resistance of the living root cells to the passage of water across them.

Both incipient and transient wilting should be distinguished from the more drastic stage of permanent wilting. This stage of wilting is attained only when there is an actual deficiency of water in the soil, and a plant will not recover from permanent wilting unless the water content of the soil in which it is rooted increases. In a soil which is gradually drying out, transient wilting slowly grades over into permanent wilting. Each successive night recovery of the plant from temporary wilting takes longer and is less complete, until finally even the slightest recovery fails to take place during the night.

Although the stomates are generally closed during permanent wilting, cuticular transpiration continues. Plants in a state of permanent wilting continue to absorb water, but at a slow rate. Restoration of turgidity is not possible, however, because the rate of transpiration even from a wilted plant exceeds the rate of absorption of water from a soil at the permanent wilting percentage or lower water content. During permanent wilting, therefore, there is a slow but steady diminution in the total volume of water within the plant, and a gradual intensification of the stress in the hydrodynamic system. Tensions in the water columns of permanently wilted plants are relatively high and have been estimated to attain values of 200 atm in some trees, although this is probably an extreme figure.

As previously mentioned, the permanent wilting percentage, an important index of soil water conditions, is defined as the soil water content when a plant just enters the condition of permanent wilting. The sunflower is the most commonly used test plant in making determinations of the permanent wilting percentage of a soil. Permanent wilting of the basal pair of leaves, judged to have occurred when they fail to recover if placed in a saturated atmosphere overnight, is taken as the critical point in the measurement. The range of soil water contents between the first permanent wilting of the basal leaves of sunflower plants and the permanent wilting of all the leaves is called the wilting range. The water content of the soil at the time all the sunflower leaves have become wilted is termed the ultimate wilting point. In general, the wilting range is narrower in coarse-textured soils than in fine-textured soils, and may be 10–30% of the soil water content between the field capacity and the ultimate wilting point. Although plants cannot grow while the soil in which they are rooted is in the wilting range, many kinds of plants can survive for considerable periods under such conditions. This is especially true of many shrubby species indigenous to semidesert areas.

Internal redistributions of water. For convenience, the processes of transpiration, translocation of water, and absorption of water are often dis-

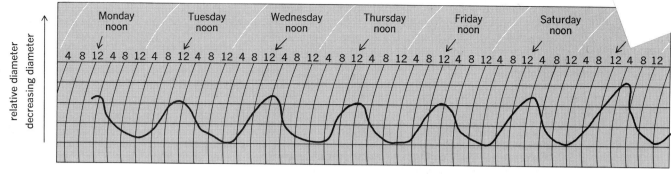

Fig. 5. Daily variations in diameter of lemons. (*From E. T. Bartholomew, Amer. J. Botany, 13:102–117, 1926*)

cussed separately, although there is a close inter-relationship among these three processes. The hydrodynamic system of a plant is essentially a unit in its operation, and changes in the status of the water in one part of a plant are bound to have effects on its status in other parts of the plant.

Whenever a plant is saturated, or nearly so, with water, differences in water potential from one organ or tissue to another are minimal. But whenever the rate of absorption of water lags behind the rate of transpiration, an internal water deficit develops in the hydrodynamic system of the plant, which in turn favors the establishment of marked differences in water potential from one part of the plant to another. Under such conditions redistribution of some of the water present from some tissues or organs of a plant to others generally occurs.

Internal movements of water from fruits to leaves and vice versa seem to be of common occurrence. Mature lemon fruits, while still attached to the tree, exhibit a daily cycle of expansion and contraction (Fig. 5). The lemon fruits begin to contract in volume early in the morning and continue to do so until late afternoon. Since transpirational loss from a lemon fruit is negligible, it is obvious that during this part of the day, corresponding to the period of high transpiration rates from the leaves, water is moving out of the fruits into other parts of the tree. Most of this movement probably occurs into the leaves. During the daylight hours, the water potentials of the leaf cells presumably decrease until they soon are lower than those of the fruit cells, thus initiating movement of water from the fruits to the leaves. During the late afternoon and night hours, the volume of the fruits gradually increases, indicating that water is now moving back into the fruits. During this period, transpirational water loss from the leaves is small, leaf water contents increase, and the water potential of the leaf cells becomes less negative. Less of the absorbed water is translocated to the leaves than during the daylight hours, and more can move into the fruits, despite the relatively high water potential of the fruit cells. Marked daily variations take place in the diameters of lemon fruits, even under environmental conditions which result in no observable wilting of the leaves.

In growing cotton bolls, however, as long as enlargement is continuing, increase in diameter continues steadily both day and night and even during periods when the leaves are severely wilted. Movement of water is obviously occurring into the growing bolls without interruption during this period.

Once the bolls cease enlarging, however, reversible daily changes occur in their diameter, similar in pattern to those which take place in mature lemon fruits (Fig. 6). Similarly, it has been shown that in a tomato plant the topmost node, within which growth in length occurs, continues to elongate at approximately the same rate both day and night. The stem below the first node, however, shrinks measurably in length during the daytime and elongates equally at night, undoubtedly as a result of reversible changes in the turgidity of the stem cells. The growing cells in the terminal node of the tomato stem obviously continue to obtain water during the daylight hours while the rest of the stem is losing water, and some of the water utilized in their growth probably comes from the cells of the lower nodes.

In general, as the last two examples illustrate, actively meristematic regions such as growing stems and root tips and enlarging fruits, under conditions of internal water deficiency, apparently develop more negative water potentials than other tissues. Hence water often continues to move toward such regions even when an internal water deficiency of considerable magnitude has developed within the plant. However, under conditions of drastic internal water deficit, approaching or corresponding to a state of permanent wilting, growth of all meristems is greatly retarded or inhibited.

Drought resistance. The term drought refers, in general, to periods during which the soil contains little or no water which is available to plants. In relatively humid climates such periods are infrequent and seldom of long duration except in certain local habitats. The more arid a climate, in

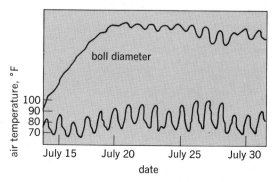

Fig. 6. Daily variations in diameter of a cotton boll (still growing for first 5 days). (*From D. B. Anderson and T. Kerr, Plant Physiol., 18:261–269, 1943*)

general, the more frequent is the occurrence of droughts and the longer their duration. Most species of plants can survive short dry periods without serious injury, but a prolonged period of soil water deficiency is highly injurious or lethal to all except those species of plants with a well-developed capacity for drought resistance.

Most species which grow in semidesert regions, such as those of the southwestern United States and adjacent Mexico, or in locally dry habitats must be drought resistant in one sense of the word or another. Annual species which grow in many arid regions during short rainy spells are exceptions to this statement. Such species complete their brief life cycle from seed to seed during a period when soil water is available and can survive in arid regions because they evade rather than endure drought.

Succulents, such as cacti, are found in most semidesert regions, and are also often indigenous to locally dry habitats such as sand dunes and beaches in humid climate regions. Succulents are able to survive long dry periods because of the relatively large quantities of water which accumulate, in some species in fleshy stems and in other species in fleshy leaves, during the occasional periods when soil water is available. Many succulents can live for months on such stored water.

Those plants which are drought resistant in the truest sense are those whose cells can tolerate a marked reduction in water content for extended periods of time without injury. Many shrubby species of semidesert regions have this property. Certain structural features undoubtedly aid in the survival of such plants for long periods of arid habitats. Many xerophytes (plants that can endure periods of drought) have extensive root systems in proportion to their tops; such a structural characteristic aids in maintaining a supply of water to the aerial portions of the plant longer than would otherwise be possible. Other drought-resistant species are characterized by having diminutive leaves; the transpiring surface of the plant may thus be small relative to the absorptive capacity of the roots. In still other species the leaves abscise (fall) with the advent of the dry season, thus greatly reducing transpiration in the period of greatest internal stress in the hydrodynamic system.

Despite any structural features which may help maintain their internal water supply, shrubby plants of semiarid regions regularly undergo a gradual depletion in the store of water within them and a gradual intensification of the stress prevailing in the internal hydrodynamic system over dry periods often lasting for months. Only drought-resistant species can endure this condition, which is in essence a state of permanent wilting, for long periods of time without injury. A fundamental factor in the drought resistance of plants therefore appears to be a capacity of the cells to endure a substantial reduction in their water content without suffering injury. This capacity probably is based in part on structural features of the cells of such species and in part on the distinctive physiological properties of their protoplasm. See ECOLOGY; PLANT, MINERAL NUTRITION OF.

[BERNARD S. MEYER]

Bibliography: G. E. Briggs, *Movement of Water in Plants*, 1967; A. S. Crafts and C. E. Crisp, *Phloem Transport in Plants*, 1971; T. T. Kozlowski, *Water Metabolism in Plants*, 1964; A. J. Rutter and F. H. Whitehead (eds.), *Water Relations of Plants*, 1963; R. O. Slatyer, *Plant-Water Relationships*, 1967.

Plant disease

A great obstacle to the successful production of cultivated plants, plant disease is also sometimes destructive in natural forests and grasslands. Despite large expenditures for control measures, diseases annually destroy close to 10% of the crop plants in the United States, before and after harvest, resulting in a financial loss of more than $3,000,000,000.

Diseases may destroy plant parts outright by rotting, or may cause stunting or other malformations. Most diseases are caused by parasitic microscopic organisms such as bacteria, fungi, algae, and nematodes or roundworms, although a few are caused by parasitic higher plants, such as dodder and mistletoe. Many are caused by viruses, and some are caused by poor soil conditions, unfavorable weather, or harmful gases in the air.

The living organisms and viruses which cause disease are called pathogens. Most pathogens can multiply extremely rapidly, the bacteria by simple division, the fungi by producing spores which behave as seeds but are much smaller and simpler in structure. Bacteria are about 0.0005 in. long, and fairly large fungus spores about 0.001 in. Virus particles are not visible with ordinary microscopes; they can multiply a millionfold in a short time. Roundworms reproduce by means of eggs.

Most pathogens can be disseminated quickly and widely by wind, water, insects, man, and other animals. They infect plants through wounds or pores (stomata) or by penetrating plant surfaces. Each kind of pathogen can attack only certain kinds of plants or plant parts. Once inside the plant, living pathogens obtain their nourishment from it in various ways, destroying plant tissues or weakening the plant by robbing it of its food substances. The rapidity of growth and reproduction of pathogens and of disease development varies with the kind of pathogen and host and with soil and weather conditions. Some pathogens thrive best in hot weather, others in cool weather. Extensive and destructive epidemics develop when all conditions favor the most rapid development of the pathogen.

Good cultural practices, chemical disinfestation of planting materials, spraying or dusting with appropriate chemicals to protect against airborne infection, and the use of resistant varieties are the principal control measures.

Discussed in the following sections are the economic importance, nature, and causes of plant diseases; the characteristics, growth, and reproduction of pathogens; the infection stage and development of diseases; the dissemination of pathogens; and the diseases to which plants are subject in storage. Discussion of other aspects can be found under separate titles or under the names of plants infected.

Economic importance. All plants and their parts are subject to diseases which may be caused at various stages of their life cycles not only by microorganisms, but also by higher plants, injurious salts in the soil, and harmful gases in the air. Diseases may rot the seed, kill plants, or make them poor and unsightly; they may cause root rots, stem cankers and rots, leaf spots and blights, blossom blights, and fruit scabs, molds, spots, and rots. In transit and storage they cause rots of fleshy fruits and vegetables; mold sickness of wheat, rice, corn, and other grains; and discoloration or rotting of wood and wood products.

When weather favors their development, some diseases become epidemic and ruin vast acreages of economically important plants. The historic potato famine in Ireland in the 1840s, resulting in the death of 1,000,000 people, was due to epidemics of potato late blight. Chestnut blight ruined the chestnut forests of the United States. Stem rust destroyed about 300,000,000 bu of wheat in the United States and Canada in 1916. In the United States it destroyed 60% of the spring wheat in 1935, and 75% of the macaroni wheat and 25% of the spring bread wheat in both 1953 and 1954. Stem rust, only one of more than 3000 kinds of plant rusts, has been similarly destructive in other wheat-growing areas of the world, and it continually menaces wheat, oats, barley, rye, and many grasses. The *Helminthosporium* disease of rice was the principal cause of a famine in which a million or more people died in India in 1943.

Plant diseases are a dangerous threat to man's future subsistence. Much of the world is now underfed, and acute food shortages often occur in many areas. The situation tends to become worse as population increases by many millions each year. Plant diseases, old and new, are a critical limiting factor in food production. The degree to which they can be controlled will help determine whether the world can feed its rapidly growing population.   [E. C. STAKMAN]

Nature of diseases. In the broad sense, disease in plants may be considered as any physiological abnormality which produces pathological symptoms, reduces the economic or esthetic value of plant products, or kills the plant or any of its parts. Damage, caused by wind or lightning or predation of insects or other animals, is not usually called disease, although such injury to living plants may result in a physiological disturbance which is truly disease. Decay of storage organs, such as tubers and roots, is disease because such plant parts are living; decay of lumber is disease only by extension of the definition, although the processes may be similar.

Disease in plants is usually evidenced by abnormalities in appearance, called symptoms, or by the presence of a pathogen in or on the plant. Some diseases, however, have no obvious symptoms; potato virus X, for example, reduces the yield of potatoes without apparent changes in the appearance of the plants.

The symptoms of plant diseases may be death (necrosis) of all or any part of the plant, loss of turgor (wilt), overgrowths (hypertrophy and hyperplasia), stunting (hypoplasia), or various other changes in the structure and composition of the plant. Necrosis may affect any part of the plant at any stage of growth. A rapid death of foliage is often called blight (Fig. 1), whereas localized necrosis results in leaf spots and fruit spots. Necrosis of stems or bark results in cankers. Wilting may be

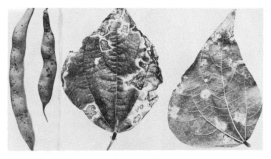

Fig. 1. Common bacterial blight of bean. (*From J. C. Walker, Plant Pathology, 3d ed., McGraw-Hill, 1969*)

slow or rapid, and it is usually more pronounced in dry than in moist soil. Necrosis eventually follows persistent wilting (Fig. 2). Overgrowths composed primarily of undifferentiated cells are called galls (Fig. 3), the term tumor being less commonly used to designate these structures. A bunch of small, abnormal shoots is often referred to as a witches'-broom. Underdevelopment or stunting may affect the entire plant or only certain of its parts.

Chlorosis (lack of chlorophyll in varying degree) is the most common nonstructural evidence of disease. For example, in leaves it may occur in stripes or in irregular spots (mosaic). Various degrees of curling and crinkling of the foliage often accompany chlorosis. Sometimes there is also other abnormal coloration, such as shades of red and brown.

A number of diseases may cause similar symptoms. These may be characteristic enough to permit diagnosis, but often it is necessary to identify the causal organism for exact diagnosis.

Causative agents. Usually two or more causes operate simultaneously to produce plant disease. For example, if a parasite is involved, the weather will influence the growth of the parasite as well as the plant's susceptibility to the parasite. The following subsections describe the influence on plant diseases of animals, plants, and viruses; soil conditions; weather; agricultural practices; industrial by-products; and plant metabolism.

Animals, plants, and viruses. Nematodes and insects are the animals that most commonly cause plant disease (Fig. 4). Although herbivorous animals, including many insects, bite off and swallow plant parts, the parts removed are not diseased and the animals are predators, not pathogens.

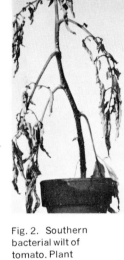

Fig. 2. Southern bacterial wilt of tomato. Plant shows leaf epinasty and wilt. (*After Kelman, from J. C. Walker, Plant Pathology, 3d ed., McGraw-Hill, 1969*)

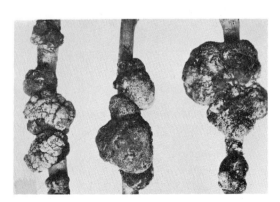

Fig. 3. Crown gall of apple. (*A. J. Riker, from J. C. Walker, Plant Pathology, 3d ed., McGraw-Hill, 1969*)

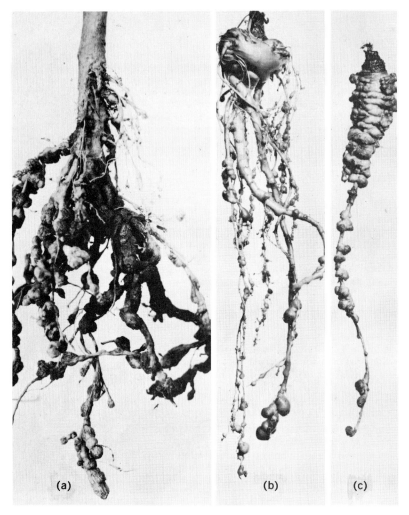

Fig. 4. Nematode galls incited by *Meloidogyne* sp. (*a*) On tomato. (*b, c*) On parsnip. (*After Cox and Jeffers, from J. C. Walker, Plant Pathology, 3d ed., McGraw-Hill, 1969*)

However, the loss of the parts eaten may cause the rest of the plant to become diseased. Conversely, some insects are true pathogens because they remain on or in the plant and cause disease symptoms typically associated with the insects involved. Such symptoms may include yellowing, leaf curl, and overgrowths. Many nematodes are

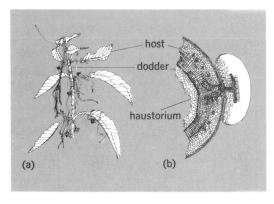

Fig. 5. Dodder (genus *Cuscuta*). (*a*) Plant attached to host. (*b*) Section through host showing haustorium of dodder extending into host. (*From F. W. Emerson, Basic Botany, 2d ed., Blakiston, 1954*)

true parasites, hence pathogens, since they cause rots, overgrowths, and other plant abnormalities.

Certain algae, fungi, and bacteria are plant pathogens that cause disease. Most plant diseases are due to fungi; less than 200 are known to be caused by bacteria, and even fewer are caused by algae and parasitic seed plants, such as dodder and mistletoe (Fig. 5).

Many plant diseases are caused by viruses, which are neither plants nor animals but are similar to living things in many ways and may properly be called pathogens. *See* PLANT VIRUS.

Soil conditions. Deficiencies of mineral nutrients in the soil are a frequent cause of plant disease (Fig. 6). Often the deficiency can be identified by characteristic plant symptoms. For example, yellowing of the leaf tip and midrib of corn indicates nitrogen deficiency; yellowing of the margins, potassium deficiency. However, the symptoms may vary somewhat in different plant species. In addition, deficiency diseases may be difficult to diagnose, since they sometimes resemble those caused by viruses.

Besides nitrogen, potash, and phosphorus, which plants need in relatively large amounts, smaller quantities of sulfur, calcium, and magnesium are required. Boron, iron, copper, manganese, molybdenum, zinc, and other minerals are used in such minute amounts that they are called trace elements. However, if one of the latter is missing, a typical disease may result, such as dry rot of rutabagas, which is due to boron deficiency (Fig. 7). *See* PLANT, MINERALS ESSENTIAL TO.

Frequently deficiencies of minerals cannot be determined by soil analysis alone, because the minerals may be present in chemical combinations that plants cannot use. For example, iron is often unavailable on high-lime soils, even if it is present in the soil in appreciable quantities. *See* PLANT, MINERAL NUTRITION OF.

Besides lime, excess amounts of many other chemicals may be present in the soil and cause plant disease. Excess of soluble salts causes "alkali injury" and aggravates drought damage; too much nitrogen may stimulate abnormal growth; while an excess of boron may cause necrosis and stunting. Unfavorable chemical balance in the soil may also result in excess acidity (low pH) or alkalinity (high pH), either of which may inhibit normal plant growth. *See* PLANT GROWTH.

The soil is the principal source of water, which all plants need in varying amounts, depending upon the species. Too little available water slows growth and, below certain limits, results in wilting. Plants can recover from limited (transient) wilting, but if it is prolonged the affected parts die. *See* PLANT, WATER RELATIONS OF.

Conversely, too much water in the soil results in oxygen deficiency, which causes suffocation of the tissues of roots and other underground parts of most plants. Water-inhabiting plants, such as rice, are exceptions. Excess water in the soil favors certain kinds of fungus and bacterial diseases, and these are often confused with the purely physiologic effects of too much water.

High soil temperature during the growing season may also cause disease, for instance, internal necrosis of potato. Lack of oxygen in storage may result in blackheart of potato tubers, especially at temperatures above 40°F (Fig. 8).

The structure of soil (particle size and organic content) determines its water-holding capacity and hence affects both the conditions mentioned above and the ease with which plant roots penetrate the soil. *See* SOIL.

Weather conditions. Wind, lightning (Fig. 9), and hail may injure plants and cause true diseases such as those resulting from unfavorable temperatures (Fig. 10). Temperature effects range from poor development of plants grown in climates too cold or too warm to actual frost or heat damage. For example, tomatoes grow poorly and drop their blossoms in cool weather; direct sunlight on the fruit may kill the tissue, causing sunscald; and the foliage is severely damaged by even light frosts that would not harm cabbage.

Although high temperatures may literally cook plant tissue, with such results as "heat canker" of young flax and sunscald of tomato fruit, the commonest effect is to increase water loss by transpiration, resulting in drought damage. Wind has the same effect, the degree depending upon its velocity and relative humidity.

In most green plants deficiency of light causes weak, spindly growth and chlorosis, although some species can endure much shade. House plants are frequently affected in this manner, but excess shading by buildings or other plants will produce the same effect outdoors.

Agricultural practices. Mismanagement of soil, including untimely applications of irrigation water and fertilizer, can cause plant disease, but other agricultural practices are frequently injurious. The more common of these injuries result from the improper use of chemicals such as fungicides, insecticides, and herbicides. *See* AGRICULTURE; FUNGISTAT AND FUNGICIDE; HERBICIDE; INSECTICIDE.

Nearly all fungicides are injurious to plants as well as to fungi, although the damage to the plants is usually much less than the potential injury from the diseases controlled by the fungicides. Examples of effects are increased transpiration caused by Bordeaux mixture on tomatoes, russeting of fruits caused by lime sulfur on apples, and yield reductions without visible symptoms caused by other chemicals. Conversely, the fungicide may contain a nutrient such as zinc which, if deficient in the soil, may result in much better growth of the plant.

Chemicals used for seed treatment are frequently toxic, especially to some species of plants. For example, plants of the cabbage family are stunted by copper-containing seed treatment materials. Vegetative organs, such as potato tubers, are very susceptible to chemical injury, and strong poisons, such as mercuric chloride, often do more harm than good. Materials applied to the soil to control fungi, bacteria, and nematodes may injure plants grown in the soil too soon after treatment.

Some crop plants are very sensitive to herbicides, being affected by very minute amounts of such things as 2,4-D (2,4-dichlorophenoxyacetic acid). Tomatoes may be affected from sources far removed. Symptoms of 2,4-D are sometimes confused with those of virus diseases.

Industrial by-products. The fumes from ore smelters frequently cause widespread symptoms

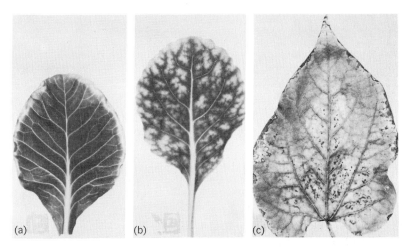

Fig. 6. Mineral deficiencies. (*a*) Potassium-deficiency disease of cabbage. (*b*) Iron-deficiency disease of cabbage. (*c*) Magnesium-deficiency disease of bean. (*From J. C. Walker, Plant Pathology, 3d ed., McGraw-Hill, 1969*)

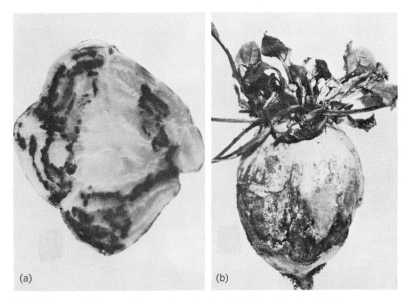

Fig. 7. Boron-deficiency disease of garden beet. (*a*) Internal necrosis of tissue occurs in the secondary cambial rings. (*b*) Leaves become stunted, and dormant buds of the crown are stimulated but form small distorted leaves. Internal necrosis near the exterior of the root leads to collapse of the outer tissue to form cankers. (*From J. C. Walker, Plant Pathology, 3d ed., McGraw-Hill, 1969*)

of plant disease, including stunting, yellowing, and necrosis. Where atmospheric inversion layers prevent their escape, even traffic and domestic fumes may be toxic. *See* ATMOSPHERIC POLLUTION.

Plant metabolism products. Brown areas on stored apples (scald) may be caused by ethylene gas produced by the apples (Fig. 11). This gas occurs in small quantities in many healthy plant tissues but is produced in greater amounts by diseased and aging cells. Ethylene gas may also cause yellowing in plants, and it accelerates ripening in certain fruits such as banana.

PLANT DISEASE PATHOGENS

Most pathogens are grouped primarily on the basis of their structure; but bacteria, being morphologically simple, are classified to a considerable extent by physiological characters. Viruses

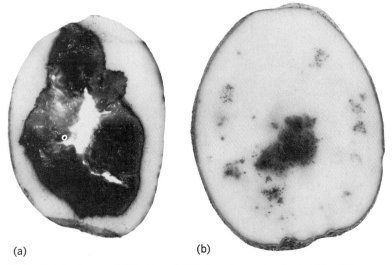

Fig. 8.   Potato disease. (a) Blackheart. (b) Internal necrosis, due to high soil temperature. (*From J. C. Walker, Plant Pathology, 3d ed., McGraw-Hill, 1969*)

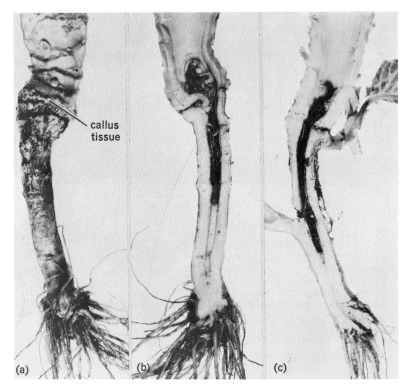

Fig. 9.   Lightning injury of cabbage, seen several weeks after occurrence. (a) Callus tissue on stem at ground level where charge entered plant. (b) Interior of plant. Paths whereby the charge passed through the cortex and the vascular ring are evident. The pith was killed, and as the tissue collapsed, adventitious roots formed in the cavity. (c) Dormant buds stimulated to growth at leaf axes just below entry point of the charge. (*From J. C. Walker, Plant Pathology, 3d ed., McGraw-Hill, 1969*)

represent a special problem, and such considerations as means of transmission and host symptoms are used in classifying and naming them.

Fungi, bacteria, and a few seed plants are heterotrophs; that is, they lack chlorophyll and consequently are dependent, directly or indirectly, upon green plants (autotrophs) for carbohydrates. Animals and some fungi and bacteria are also dependent upon other organisms for nutrients such as amino acids and vitamins. Viruses (Fig. 12) multiply or are replicated by synthesizing virus nucleic acids and proteins from amino acids and other compounds present in the host cell. *See* PHOTO-SYNTHESIS; PLANT VIRUS.

Plant pathogens usually penetrate into the host plant and grow within or between the cells (Fig. 13). Viruses are usually intracellular, and some are confined to the phloem, whereas plant pathogenic bacteria are usually intercellular or occur in the xylem. Fungi are composed of microscopic tubes called hyphae, by means of which plant pathogenic species penetrate into or between the host cells (Fig. 14). The powdery mildew fungi grow principally outside of the plant but send special absorptive organs (haustoria) into the host cells (Fig. 15). Some intercellular species of fungi also produce haustoria. Pathogenic seed plants, such as mistletoe and dodder, usually penetrate the host by means of rootlike absorptive organs. Pathogenic insects and nematodes may be wholly within the plant, or they may remain superficial and penetrate the host with specialized mouthparts.

Most plant pathogens are parasites. Some, such as the rusts and powdery mildews, are obligate parasites, that is, can grow only on a living host plant. Viruses are also in this category, although they are not typical organisms. Fungi and bacteria that can use only nonliving food sources are called saprophytes.

Most fungi and all plant pathogenic bacteria can grow on nonliving organic matter as well as parasitically on living matter; these are called facultative saprophytes. Some organisms live primarily as saprophytes but also have the ability to parasitize weakened plants and are therefore called facultative parasites. Many plant pathogens have both a parasitic (or pathogenic) and a saprophytic phase of development.

Symbiotic relations of organisms. Parasitism is the one of a series of associations characterized by intimate physical union of taxonomically dissimilar organisms. Such relationships are known as symbiosis, and may be neutral, beneficial, or harmful to the symbionts. An association such as that of legumes and nodule bacteria, beneficial to both partners, is called mutualistic symbiosis. Parasitism is antagonistic symbiosis.

There are different degrees of parasitism. In the early stages, the association between rust fungi and their hosts may appear to be almost neutral, harming the plants little. Other fungi, such as those rotting fruit, can become established only in dead tissue, producing enzymes or toxins that kill adjacent living cells which they then inhabit. Some biologists say that such organisms are saprophytes, not parasites, because they never colonize living host tissue. But the term parasitism is generally used to refer to a relationship with the host plant as a whole, because the degree of intimate relationship is often difficult to determine.

Ecologic relations of organisms. Associations of organisms in the same environment without physical union are called ecologic and are often very important in plant disease. As in symbiosis, the effects may be beneficial, neutral, or harmful. Metabiosis occurs when one organism uses a substance for food and produces a by-product that enables another to grow. If the benefits are reciprocal, the relationship is called synergism, as when the fungus *Mucor ramannianus* produces pyrimidine and *Rhodotorula rubra*, a nonsporulating yeast, makes thiazole. These chemicals are components of thiamine, which both organisms need but which neither can produce alone. If deleterious substances (antibiotics) are produced, the relationship is called antibiosis. Usually the term antibiosis refers only to the deleterious effects of one microorganism on another, but similar relationships exist between plants of all kinds.

All of these relationships may be important to the survival of certain plant pathogens, especially some of those which live in the soil part of the time. Metabiotic and synergistic relationships may help them to survive; antagonistic relationships hinder survival. One of the goals of the plant pathologist is to encourage antibiosis that eliminates certain soil-inhabiting pathogens.

Ecologic associations may exist between two or more pathogens inhabiting the same host plant as a common environment. When fire-blight bacteria parasitize apple twigs and permit the entrance of canker and wood-rotting fungi, the relationship between the bacteria and the fungi is metabiotic. The molds *Oospora citri aurantii* and *Penicillium digitatum* can rot fruit more rapidly together than either can alone; this is synergism. Antagonism seems to exist between races of the potato late blight fungus, and one will replace the other when they parasitize a potato plant together.

Even the relationship of host and pathogen may be ecologic at first. For example, *Rhizoctonia solani* in the soil causes visible injury to the roots of soybean before touching them. Accordingly, the fungus is at first toxic to soybean; later it becomes parasitic and pathogenic.   [CARL J. EIDE]

Growth and reproduction. Many plant pathogens, especially among the bacteria, fungi, and viruses, multiply with amazing rapidity under favorable conditions. Viruses, although not generally considered living organisms, may increase a millionfold a few days after introduction into the right place in the right kind of living plant, when temperature and other environmental conditions are favorable to the virus.

Food requirements of bacteria and fungi. Although lack of chlorophyll prevents these organisms from using solar energy to synthesize basic carbohydrates from carbon dioxide and water as green plants do, their basic nutrient requirements are essentially the same as those of higher plants. They require carbon, hydrogen, oxygen, nitrogen, phosphorus, and sulfur as structural elements. In addition, they need the metallic elements potassium, magnesium, iron, zinc, copper, calcium, gallium, manganese, molybdenum, vanadium, and scandium. Potassium and magnesium, needed in relatively large amounts, are designated macroelements; the others, some of which are needed in minute amounts, are often designated microelements. Vitamins are also needed by some species for growth and reproduction.

For experimental purposes, pure cultures of facultative saprophytes are grown in the laboratory on sterilized synthetic media containing sugars or some other source of carbon, salts of the other necessary elements, and essential vitamins and amino acids for those organisms which cannot syn-

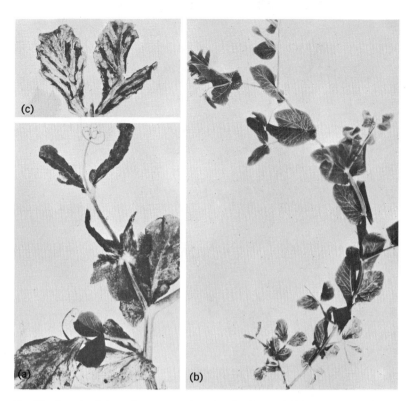

Fig. 10. Freezing injury of pea, several weeks after injury. (*a*) Enlargement of the injured growing point in *b*; in the youngest leaf the stipules and the first pair of leaflets have assumed abnormal shapes, and the second pair of leaflets did not form. (*b*) Following killing of the growing point at the left, a lower dormant bud grew out to form the main stem. (*c*) Necrotic bands in a pair of leaflets which were developing at the time of injury. (*From J. C. Walker, Plant Pathology, 3d ed., McGraw-Hill, 1969*)

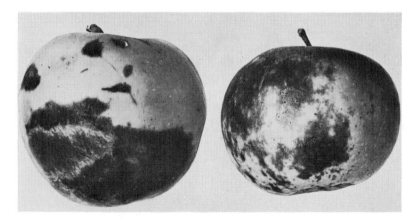

Fig. 11. Apple scald. (*USDA*)

thesize their own. Natural plant products, such as potato broth, steamed cornmeal, or oatmeal, often are used as nutrient bases. Liquid media are used for some purposes; for others, the nutrient solutions are solidified with gelatin or agar. Nutrient requirements for growth and reproduction are best determined by varying the composition of synthetic media. Studies on the effects of temperature, light, and other environmental factors are facilitated when organisms can be grown on culture media. Although all pathogenic organisms have some requirements in common, they differ greatly in special requirements, both on artificial media and on host plants. By growing pathogens artificially,

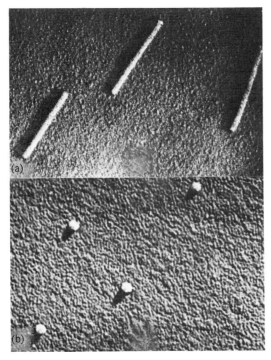

Fig. 12.   Plant viruses. (a) Rod-shaped particles of the tobacco mosaic virus. (b) Polyhedral particles of the squash mosaic virus. Electron micrographs of preparations made by the freeze-drying technique. Magnification approximately 100,000×. (P. Kaesberg, from J. C. Walker, Plant Pathology, 2d ed., McGraw-Hill, 1957)

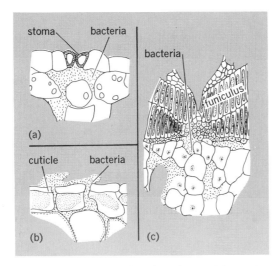

Fig. 13.   Common bacterial blight of bean. (a) Invasion through stomata. (b) Invasion through rift in the cuticle of the cotyledon. (c) Invasion of the seed through the tissue of the funiculus. (After Zaumeyer, from J. C. Walker, Plant Pathology, 3d ed., McGraw-Hill, 1969)

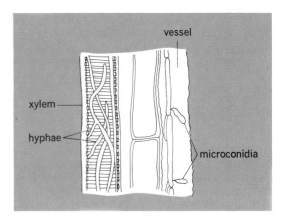

Fig. 14.   The cabbage-yellows organism in tracheae of the cabbage plant. Note formation of microconidia in the vessel. (After Gilman, from J. C. Walker, Plant Pathology, 3d ed., McGraw-Hill, 1969)

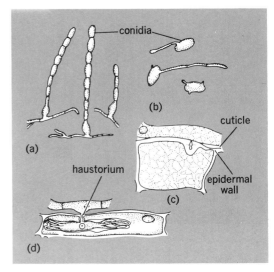

Fig. 15.   Erysiphe graminis. (a) Conidiophores and conidia (spores); (b) germinating conidia (after Reed). (c) Penetration of cuticle and epidermal wall; (d) haustorium. (after G. Smith). (From J. C. Walker, Plant Pathology, 3d ed., McGraw-Hill, 1969)

much is learned about them which enables the development of better control measures.

Host selectivity of bacteria and fungi. Among the approximately 150 species of pathogenic bacteria and the many thousands of fungi, there are wide differences with respect to the kinds of plants and plant parts on which they can grow. Flax rust (*Melampsora lini*) grows only on wild and cultivated flax, asparagus rust (*Puccinia asparagi*) prin-

cipally on asparagus; *Xanthomonas campestris*, the bacterium which causes black rot of cabbage, cauliflower, and related plants, parasitizes members of the mustard family only. On the other hand, the fungus *Rhizoctonia solani* causes root rot of potatoes, alfalfa, clover, and hundreds of other species in many different plant families; the bacterium *Agrobacterium tumefaciens* causes crown gall on grape, raspberry, chrysanthemum, and numerous other plants; the bacterium *Erwinia carotovora* causes soft rot of almost all kinds of fleshy vegetables.

Some pathogens attack only a few plant parts or tissues, others attack many. Some attack roots only, others attack stems, others cause leaf spots, and still others attack fruits. Some attack young tissues, others attack old ones. There are diseases of youth and of age, of herbaceous plants, and of woody plants. Some pathogens parasitize all plant parts of susceptible hosts at all stages of development. To understand and control the numerous diseases of thousands of kinds of plants, it is necessary to learn the conditions under which each pathogen thrives.

Environmental factors. The rate and kind of growth and reproduction of pathogens are affected by nutrition, moisture, temperature (Fig. 16), light, the acidity or alkalinity of the medium, the relative amounts of oxygen and carbon dioxide, and by other microorganisms with which they must compete. Most pathogens require free moisture for germination and infection, although some powdery mildews can germinate in dry air. Soil moisture sometimes is a determining factor in growth and reproduction. Some pathogens that live in the soil thrive best at high moisture content, some at low. Temperature determines the geographical and seasonal occurrence of many diseases, since the cardinal temperatures—the minimum, optimum, and maximum—differ for different pathogens. The peach leaf curl fungus, the potato late blight fungus, and yellow rust of wheat develop best at a relatively low temperature; the peach brown rot fungus, the potato wilt and brown rot bacterium, and stem rust of wheat develop best at a relatively high temperature. Light has less influence than temperature on the growth of pathogens in nature, but it strongly affects reproduction of some fungi. Some soil organisms, such as the potato scab bacterium, like an alkaline (high pH) soil; some, such as the cabbage clubroot fungus, like an acid soil (low pH).

Reproduction of bacteria and fungi. A single bacterium divides into 2, the 2 into 4, and so on. As division may occur every 20 to 30 min, a single bacterium could produce a progeny of 300,000,000,000 within 24 hr. The rate, however, varies with the kind of bacterium, its nutrition, temperature, and other environmental conditions.

Most fungi, however, reproduce both asexually and sexually. In many fungi asexual reproduction results in rapid multiplication (Fig. 17), whereas sexual reproduction results in the production of spores that can survive unfavorable conditions. In general, fungi continue to grow and produce asexual spores while the environment is favorable and nutrients are easily available, but they tend to produce sexual spores when growth is checked. Thus an asexually produced urediospore (summer spore) of wheat stem rust (*Puccinia graminis* var. *tritici*) can cause infection, the resulting mycelium grows for a time and then forms a pustule containing 50 to 400,000 new urediospores. The time required is only about a week at 75°F, but it increases to a month at 50°F and even longer as temperature decreases. Each new spore can cause a new infection, and this process continues at a rate that varies greatly with temperature, moisture, and light, until the wheat starts to ripen or growth is otherwise checked. Then the winter spores (teliospores) are produced; these differ from urediospores in appearance and cannot normally germinate until they have been exposed to winter weather. The apple scab fungus (*Venturia inaequalis*) may produce many successive crops of asexual spores (conidia) on the fruit and leaves during the growing season. But it does not produce sexual spores until the following spring, on infected leaves that have fallen to the ground the previous autumn. Some fungi, such as the ergot

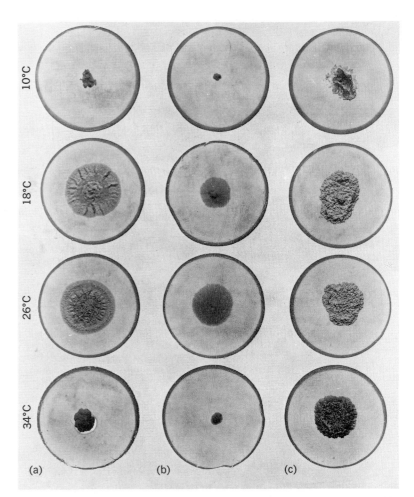

Fig. 16. Effect of temperature on growth rate of mutant lines of corn smut (*Ustilago maydis*). Note difference in ability of lines to grow at extremes. (*a*) Line W. Va. A8-3-1 is intermediate; (*b*) line W. Va. A8-5-4 scarcely grows at extremes; and (*c*) line W. Va. A8-5-2-1 grows fairly well at 10°C. (*Univ. Minn. Agr. Exp. Sta. Tech. Bull. no. 65*)

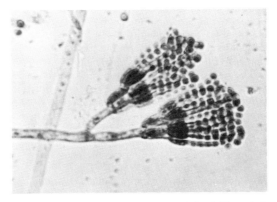

Fig. 17. Spore-producing branches of *Penicillium* similar to the one from which the drug penicillin is obtained. Chains of spores are produced on the ends of branches. (*Univ. Minn. Agr. Exp. Sta.*)

fungus (*Claviceps purpurea*), produce sclerotia, bodies made up of densely interwoven hyphae, which may survive winters or other unfavorable conditions and then produce fruiting structures under appropriate conditions in the spring.

Special stimuli are sometimes necessary to initiate the formation of fruit bodies (Fig. 18); some

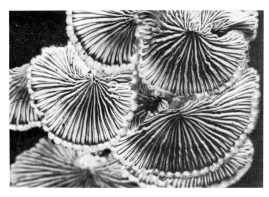

Fig. 18. Fruit bodies of a tree-inhabiting mushroom, *Schizophyllum*. Basidiospores are produced on the sides of the gills. In *Schizophyllum* gills are split lengthwise; in dry weather they curl up to conceal and protect surface on which spores are borne. (*Univ. Minn. Agr. Exp. Sta.*)

fungi require the stimulus of light for fructification, although they grow well in darkness; some require special temperature; others require certain nutrients or vitamins.

How, where, when, and the rate at which fungi grow and reproduce depend on their inheritance and their environment. The inheritance determines the limits within which the behavior of each kind of fungus can vary, and the environment determines its behavior under particular combinations of conditions.

[CARL J. EIDE; E. C. STAKMAN]

INFECTION AND DEVELOPMENT OF DISEASE

Infection of plants by a pathogen terminates a series of events that begins with inoculation, which is the contact of a susceptible part of a plant by the inoculum. Inoculum is any infectious part of the pathogen, such as spores, bacterial cells, and virus particles. Typically, inoculation is followed by entrance into the host, and infection follows entrance. A plant is infected when the pathogen starts taking nourishment from it. However, some pathologists consider penetration part of the infection process.

The time between inoculation and infection is the incubation period. Because it is often difficult to tell when infection occurs, the incubation period is usually counted as the time between inoculation and the appearance of the first symptoms of infection.

The probability that infection will follow inoculation depends upon the susceptibility of the host, the virulence and amount of inoculum in contact with the host, and the duration of favorable environmental conditions. A single unit of inoculum (propagule) of many pathogens can infect a plant; this is probably true of all pathogens when conditions are ideal. Actually only part of the propagules on a plant cause infection, and hence the amount of inoculum on a plant helps to determine how many infections result. This fact has given rise to the concept of inoculum potential, which has been defined as the product of the number of propagules per unit area of the host plant and their physiological vigor. Because of the usually haphazard dissemination of inoculum of plant pathogens, only a small part of that produced actually reaches a sus-

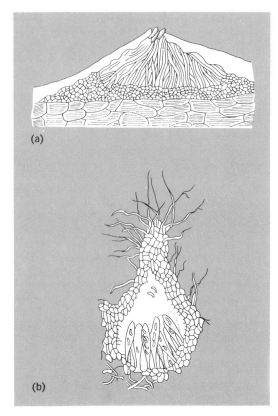

Fig. 19. *Glomerella cingulata*. (*a*) Acervulus on apple fruit. (*b*) Perithecium. (*From J. C. Walker, Plant Pathology, 3d ed., McGraw-Hill, 1969*)

ceptible plant. Consequently, most plant pathogens survive as species and are destructive partly because they produce fantastically large amounts of inoculum.

The inoculum. Inoculum of viruses and bacteria consists of the individual virus particles or bacterial cells, respectively; the inoculum of fungi may be spores, pieces of hyphae, or specialized structures, such as sclerotia. Pathogenic plants such as dodder produce true seed, and nematodes produce eggs, both of which function as inoculum.

Bacteria and viruses produce billions of cells or virus particles in infected plants, and each new unit theoretically can infect another plant. Fungi produce spores on the surface of hyphal growth or in a variety of specialized structures which may be large, as the giant puffball, or almost invisible to the unaided eye (Fig. 19). Some of the spore-producing structures function over a considerable period of time and, like bacteria, produce prodigious amounts of inoculum.

Bacteria and viruses are somewhat restricted as pathogens by having no special means of liberating themselves from the host, although the bacteria may ooze out in sticky droplets. For dissemination or transmission these pathogens depend chiefly upon plant contact, insects, or man, although bacteria may be spattered short distances by rain. Some fungi produce spores in sticky masses, like bacterial ooze, and are disseminated in much the same ways as bacteria. Other fungi have ways to liberate or forcibly eject spores into the air, where they can be carried by the wind. This gives fungus pathogens the potential of much farther and faster spread than the bacteria or viruses, although their arrival on a susceptible plant is much more a matter of chance than if insects carry the inoculum, because insects often seek similar plants for food. (Dissemination is considered in greater detail in a later section of this article.)

Dormant inoculum is one of the most important, but not the only, means by which plant pathogens survive during periods when parasitic life is impossible. If the pathogen is within a perennial host, it is usually quiescent during the rest period of the host. Sclerotia and even the vegetative hyphae of some fungi may survive periods of drought and cold independently of the host. Other pathogens require the protection of the dead host plant, not so much against cold and drought as against antagonistic organisms. This is especially true of plant pathogenic bacteria, few of which survive long if separated from host tissue. Some viruses can live only minutes apart from the living host; others, such as tobacco mosaic virus, remain infective for years in dried leaves.

At the beginning of the growing season, the first inoculum of a pathogen is called primary inoculum; that which is produced later on infected plants, secondary inoculum. The primary inoculum of fungi may be resting spores or the surviving hyphae or sclerotia; often the hyphae or sclerotia produce spores which function as primary inoculum.

Many fungi produce two or more kinds of spores. Those formed late in the growing season (resting spores) usually will not germinate until after a period of dormancy and will survive more cold and drought than spores produced during the growing season. Some, like the spores of the cabbage clubroot fungus and the chlamydospores of the onion smut fungus, stay dormant for several years, thus assuring the species of survival if susceptible hosts are not grown on the land for several seasons. Such diseases are difficult to control by crop rotation.

"Repeating" spores typically are morphologically distinct from the resting spores and are produced in great numbers on diseased plants during the growing season. They usually germinate rapidly whenever environmental conditions are favorable. Before germination, repeating spores can survive for periods ranging from several hours to several weeks, depending upon the species. This determines largely how far and under what conditions a pathogen will spread during the growing season.

Spore germination. Germination, as applied to spores or seeds, means the resumption of vegetative growth leading to the development of a new individual. In fungi this usually means the production of a hypha, called a germ tube (Fig. 20). Cell division of bacteria and the hatching of nematode and insect eggs are comparable processes, so far as their function as pathogens is concerned.

Germination occurs if the spore is not dormant and if environmental conditions are favorable. This usually requires a certain temperature range and liquid water, although a few species of fungi (powdery mildews) germinate in humid air. Certain species also require the presence of food substances, special stimulants associated with the host, absence of inhibitors that may be produced

by the pathogen or associated organisms, or certain degrees of acidity. Such requirements limit germination but may be a benefit to the species. For example, the necessity for a host stimulant prevents wastage of spores in the absence of the host.

When a nondormant spore is placed under favorable conditions, germination may follow in 45 min or only after several days, depending upon the species, age of the spores, and variations in the environment. Since conditions change rapidly, germination is a critical time for a fungus, because if it does not penetrate the host quickly the germ tube may be killed, especially by dryness. It is at this stage that fungi are most easily killed by fungicides.

Establishment in the host. For bacteria and viruses, entering a host is a passive process. Bacteria accidentally get into injuries or are put there by insects or other agencies; they may also be drawn by water into stomata, hydathodes, or nectaries. Viruses often are placed in the host by insects, but many can be transmitted when the sap from infected plants comes in contact with minute wounds in healthy plants.

Spores of fungi may also be carried into plants by various agencies, but many species have active means of penetration, the method usually being characteristic of the species. In some, germ tubes enter stomata by producing a flat structure (appressorium) over the stoma from which a hypha grows through the opening (Fig. 21). Others ignore the stomata; instead the appressorium adheres to the cuticle of the plant and forces a slender infec-

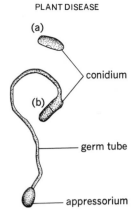

Fig. 20. *Glomerella cingulata.* (a) Conidium (spore). (b) Conidium that has become septate during germination; appressorium at tip of germ tube. (*From J. C. Walker, Plant Pathology, 3d ed., McGraw-Hill, 1969*)

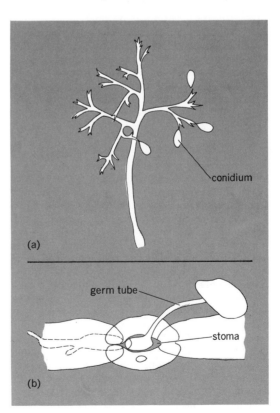

Fig. 21. *Peronospora destructor.* (a) Conidiophore bearing conidia. (b) Conidium germinating by a germ tube, the latter penetrating a stoma. (*From J. C. Walker, Plant Pathology, 3d ed., McGraw-Hill, 1969*)

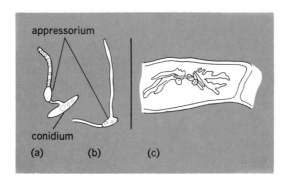

Fig. 22. *Colletotrichum circinans*. (a) Conidium which has germinated and formed an appressorium, which in turn has germinated. (b) A germinating appressorium. (c) Conidia and appressoria on surface of host and sub-cuticular mycelium developing after penetration. (*From J. C. Walker, Plant Pathology, 3d ed., McGraw-Hill, 1969*)

tion peg directly through the protective layer (Fig. 22). This apparently is accomplished entirely by pressure, as no enzyme action has been demonstrated.

Animal pathogens, such as nematodes, have special mouthparts that pierce the plant, and the nematode may remain external or it may actually enter the plant.

Even after penetration, pathogens may fail to invade the plant because of the presence of mechanical barriers, lack of proper nutrients, or the presence of inhibiting toxic substances. These factors depend not only on specific interactions between host and pathogen but also upon the environment. Successful establishment of the pathogen may mean killing the host cells and living upon the dead tissue, with or without the actual penetration of living cells.   [CARL J. EIDE]

Development within the host. After a pathogen has become established in a susceptible host, the rate of disease development under favorable conditions follows a sigmoid (S-shaped) curve with three major aspects: (1) the lag phase or incubation period, when infection is not evident externally; (2) the exponential phase, when the pathogen spreads rapidly in host tissues and symptoms and signs of disease appear; and (3) the senescence phase, when limiting mechanisms of either host or pathogen restrict further extension.

Disease development varies with genetic susceptibility of the host, genetic aggressiveness of the pathogen, and with many environmental factors that influence the host, the pathogen, and the interactions between the two. Environmental factors influence the growth rates and the metabolism of the host and the pathogen; and the interrelations between these activities determine the pattern of disease development. Furthermore, the effects of past environmental conditions on the host may affect disease development, a condition known as predisposition when host susceptibility is increased. The combined effects of these factors on growth and development of healthy crop plants in nature are poorly understood, and the problem becomes increasingly complex when the plants become diseased.

Climate often determines the adaptability of plant species to geographic areas and may also determine the geographic distribution of their diseases. For each disease there are minimum, optimum, and maximum values for each critical environmental factor. The mean measurements of weather, however, are often less important than the exact combinations of weather at critical times. Those environmental factors that deviate most from the optimum limit the development of a disease.

Effect of temperature. Temperature has a major effect on disease development and determines the seasonal and regional incidence of most diseases. For example, a succession of diseases attacks certain creeping bent grasses on golf greens in northern United States: snow mold occurs beneath melting snow in winter; red thread during the moderate temperatures of spring and fall; dollar spot during the warm temperatures of early and late summer; and brown patch during the hot weather of midsummer. The fungi causing these diseases may attack the leaves, grow into the crowns of the plants, and may kill the plants entirely in patches of characteristic size for each disease. These diseases produce similar effects, but temperature determines when each disease is most destructive.

The length of the incubation period of disease is governed by prevailing temperatures. Many diseases, such as rusts, mildews, and leaf spots, cause only small lesions on aboveground plant parts. The damage to the plant depends on the number of lesions, which in turn depends on the number of disease cycles. The elapsed time from infection to spore production—the length of the incubation period—determines the frequency of disease cycles. Thus temperature often determines whether pathogens can produce enough disease cycles for development of an epidemic. Temperature likewise may influence the symptom expression. Thus symptoms of many virus diseases disappear or are masked at high temperatures. Temperature also determines whether certain wheat varieties are susceptible or resistant to certain parasitic races of stem rust. The effect of temperature on disease development may be principally on the pathogen, or it may be on the host. When the cardinal temperatures are the same for growth of the pathogen in culture and for development of the disease, the effect is principally on the pathogen. However, when the optimum temperature for growth of the pathogen in culture differs from that for maximum disease development, the temperature probably predisposes the host plant by weakening it.

Effect of light. Light affects disease development principally by its effect on photosynthesis and the assimilative processes of the host. Obligate parasites, such as rusts and powdery mildews, generally develop best when assimilation is maximal, although the severity of the disease lesion caused by some pathogens on some hosts may be decreased by high light intensities. Low light often weakens plants and thus predisposes them to diseases caused by facultative saprophytes.

Effect of moisture. Moisture is a major factor in germination and entrance of pathogens into the host. The moisture requirements of the established pathogen are supplied by the host, since the osmotic value (water absorption capacity) of the hyphae of the pathogen is always greater than that of the parasitized host cells. Transpiration (water vapor loss) from diseased aboveground plant parts is greater than that of healthy parts. The water economy of the host is disrupted in wilt diseases by the effects of the pathogen on the translocation of water in the xylem and the osmotic permeability of foliage parenchyma, and in root diseases by the destruction of the tissues for water absorption and conduction. The rate of symptom development and death of the plant tissue in wilts and root rots is accelerated by excessively low atmospheric humidities and low soil moisture availability.

Relation of soil. Soil reaction, as regards hydrogen ion concentration, affects the development of many diseases in the soil. Potato scab is less severe in acid soils (below pH 5.2) while cabbage clubroot is not so severe in less acid soils (above pH 5.7). However, the extent to which the soil reaction affects the infectivity of these pathogens and the subsequent development of the diseases has not been determined. As the hydrogen ion concentration of the plant cell is relatively constant despite differences in the range of soil reaction, soil pH probably affects disease development indirectly by its effects on the availability to the host or pathogen of mineral nutritional elements in the soil.

Soil oxygen and carbon dioxide concentrations affect the development of root diseases. The effects on infectivity of the pathogen, predisposition of the host, and disease development have not been distinguished, although the development of the host is more adversely affected by high carbon dioxide and low oxygen tensions in the soil than is the growth of many fungal pathogens.

Effects of nutrients. The effects of nutrients are largely indirect since plants and their pathogens require the same essential mineral elements. However, the available amount of each mineral element and the balance between them affect the structure and physiology of the host and thus may be either favorable or unfavorable to the development of different pathogens. The principal mineral elements in fertilizers (nitrogen, phosphorus, potassium, and calcium) have the most pronounced effects. Diseases caused by obligate parasites such as rusts, powdery mildews, and many viruses develop best in "normal" plants having optimal mineral nutrition; while subnormal plant development due to inadequate or unbalanced mineral nutrition favors the development of many diseases, such as root rots, that are caused by facultative saprophytes. Some vascular pathogens are affected directly by the concentration of nitrogen compounds in the conductive tissues of the host.

[J. B. ROWELL]

Plant disease epidemics. When a disease spreads rapidly in a crop or other plant population, it constitutes an epidemic. Strictly speaking, the increase does not have to be spectacularly rapid to be an epidemic; the essential feature is that the pathogen, and hence the disease, is increasing in a population of host plants.

The population of plants may be small, as a single field of potatoes, or large as the total of all wheat fields from Texas to Canada. Thus epidemics may be local or regional in extent.

The time required for an epidemic to reach a destructive climax and subside may be a few days or weeks or it may go on for years. For example, an epidemic of stem rust (*Puccinia graminis* var. *tritici*) occupied roughly 3 weeks from its beginning until 100% of the plants were infected (Fig. 23). On the other hand, chestnut blight (*Endothia parasitica*) was introduced into the United States in 1904 and continued to spread through the chestnut forests for about 40 years, after which nearly all the chestnut trees were dead.

Typically the progress of an epidemic follows the same course as the growth of a population of any organism. The pathogen (for example, a fungus such as *Phytophthora infestans*, which causes late blight of potatoes) infects the host plants; in a few days the infected spots produce a crop of spores (propagules) which in turn infect new host tissue. As long as there is fresh host tissue to infect and the weather is favorable, this cycle will be repeated every 5 to 7 days. During the period of optimum development the population of the pathogen, and hence the severity of the disease, increases logarithmically, and it is possible to express the rate of increase mathematically.

Some pathogens, such as *Phytopthora infestans* and *Puccinia graminis*, may increase very rapidly, causing true population explosions. These two fungi may, on the average, double in numbers every 2 to 7 days during the logarithmic phase of development (Fig. 23). Disease of perennial plants may increase much more slowly, but still do so logarithmically.

The rate of logarithmic increase of a pathogen is dependent upon the existing population of individuals at any given time, that is, the numbers which are producing reproductive units or propagules. Other factors that affect the rate of increase can be put into three categories: (1) the number of host plants in a given area; (2) the susceptibility of the host plants; and (3) the inanimate environment.

Crops grown in fields of only one kind of plant provide ideal conditions for epidemics, because propagules of the pathogen (for example, fungus spores) can encounter more susceptible plants. Plants growing wild are usually (but not always) mixed with other species, and propagules of a pathogen, disseminated at random, have less chance to encounter susceptible plants. By growing pure stands of crop plants, disease problems are aggravated.

The pathogen itself affects the population of host plants. As an epidemic develops, plants or areas of tissue in plants become diseased and are no longer available for infection. Thus fewer of the propagules that are produced cause new infections, and the rate of increase of the pathogen and the disease slows down (Fig. 23).

Similarly, differences in host resistance influence reproduction of the pathogen. If a variety is immune, of course there is no disease, but such immunity is usually effective against only certain races of the pathogen. Varieties that are not immune may have different degrees of resistance that reduce penetration by the pathogen, increase its incubation time, and reduce the number of propagules produced. This slows down its rate of reproduction.

Environmental factors that affect individual organisms, such as temperature, light, moisture, and

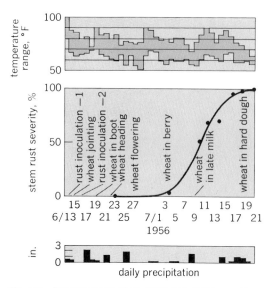

Fig. 23. Development of an epidemic of stem rust on Marquis wheat. (*From J. B. Rowell, Oil inoculation of wheat with spores of Puccinia graminis var. tritici, Phytopathology, 47(11):689–690, 1957*)

soil in which the plant is growing, naturally also affect the increase in the population of the pathogen and hence the rate at which the disease increases. Adverse environment tends to limit both the number of propagules that infect and the rate of development of the pathogen within the host, thus reducing the production of more propagules.

Fungicides applied to host plants reduce epidemics by killing some of the propagules of the pathogen before they can infect. Most fungicides are not completely effective, their essential effect is to reduce reproduction of the pathogen.

Epidemics, then, are characterized by the increase of successive generations of a pathogen in a population of host plants. Host and environmental factors affect the rate of increase, and anything that can be done to manipulate such factors may reduce the increase of the pathogen to relatively harmless proportions.

DISSEMINATION OF PLANT PATHOGENS

Insect and nematode plant pathogens can within limits move about and find plants on which to live: fungi, bacteria, viruses, and seed plants have no such means of locomotion and are dependent upon other agencies for dissemination. Most fungi produce spores that are adapted for transport by the wind, but bacteria and viruses are usually carried from place to place by insects, although bacteria are often spread by water. Occasionally other animals carry plant pathogens, and man, because of his ability to travel fast and far, often becomes the unwitting means of dissemination of destructive plant pathogens.

Dissemination, which means to disperse or spread abroad, is often closely associated with transmission, which refers to the inoculation of a new host plant, as well as to the transport of inoculum. This is often accomplished by insects. However, a pathogen such as *Xanthomonas phaseoli*, which causes common bean blight, usually penetrates the seed of the plant which it has parasit-

ized. When such a seed is planted, the new plant becomes infected. Such a pathogen is said to be seed-transmitted. Therefore this bacterium can be disseminated long distances by transporting infected seed and can also be disseminated from plant to plant in the field by splashing rain or insects.   [CARL J. EIDE]

Dissemination by wind. The plant spore is a form in which many pathogens of plants and animals spread between and within populations. Dispersal by air operates both locally and over great distances. Many viruses and bacteria that attack animals and man can be dispersed in exhaled droplets. Those that infect plants are mostly spread by vectors which range from fungi to nematodes, but the most common are insects, such as aphids or leafhoppers, which are also easily carried by wind. A few viruses can be spread within pollen and spores.

Local dissemination. Fungi are unique in the variety of physical processes they utilize to traverse the boundary layer of relatively still or smooth-flowing air adjacent to the substrates on which they grow. Powdery accumulations of detached spores, such as formed by many rust and smut fungi (or pollen), are removed by the shearing stress of moving air and, at least in the light winds usual among crops, in approximately logarithmically increasing numbers with linear increases in wind speed. Many ascomycetes and basidiomycetes have developed delicately adapted hydrostatic pressure mechanisms for releasing spores. Conidia were long assumed to be released without specialized discharge mechanisms, but some are now known to be released by the rupture of weak points in cell walls forced apart by internal pressures, by hygroscopic twisting, or (as D. S. Meredith showed) by drying mechanisms that produce great tensions in specially strengthened structures that are released when the cohesive force of the cell sap is abruptly overcome, with the formation of a gas phase within the cell. The kinetic energy of falling water drops is also used by some fungi with cup-shaped fructifications, but more often by the collision of raindrops with spore-bearing surfaces. Large transient increases of spore concentration can result from "rain tap and puff" the dual effects of the vibration of impact and the fast radial displacement of air caused by the spreading of raindrops falling on dry surfaces. Once the surfaces are wetted, these processes are replaced by the dispersal of spores in splash droplets. Most splashed spores are in large droplets and are soon deposited, but those released in small droplets that quickly evaporate must become dry, airborne spores.

Weather and airflow factors. As so many fungi form spores on surfaces and need particular weather to liberate them, it is not surprising that the concentration of airborne spores changes dramatically with changing weather. Changes are abrupt, for example, when rain falls or cyclical in time with circadian rhythms. Spores of some pathogenic fungi are liberated only into dry air, others only into damp air, and so some are most abundant by day and others by night. Such properties have important effects on dispersal and establishment. Spores released during rain, although probably soon deposited, are more likely to find congenial conditions for germination than are spores liberated in hot dry weather; but if these can survive, they may be carried much greater distances.

Concentrations of airborne spores are determined both by the rate they are liberated and the rate they are diluted by diffusion when they reach turbulent air. The diffusion processes that meteorologists have described for aerosols show that velocities in eddies often greatly exceed the terminal velocity of spores (ranging from about 0.02 to 5.0 cm/sec for fungus spores and even up to 20 cm/sec for large pollen grains). Deposition by sedimentation is certainly important in sheltered places, but elsewhere it may be a less frequent method than impaction from moving air or washout by rain.

Range of dispersal. It is often necessary to measure the proportions of spores deposited at increasing distances from sources, propose safe isolation distances, explain the development of epidemics, and help forecast diseases. Typically, the intensity of deposition on the ground decreases fast within the first tens of meters from sources and even faster near sources close to the ground than around higher ones. P. H. Gregory drew attention to the paradox that, despite these steep deposition gradients, enough spores must escape local deposition to travel far and to establish disease hundreds or perhaps thousands of miles from their sources. Local deposition is much greater in the calmer air at night than on hot windy days with both thermal and frictional turbulence. As spores are carried higher, their distribution is increasingly determined by vertical temperature lapse rates and atmospheric pressure systems, although sedimentation and diffusion in small eddies continue. Aircraft sampling over the North Sea downwind of the British Isles has revealed the remnants of spore clouds produced over Britain on previous days and nights. Understanding these transport processes better helps to explain disease outbreaks and the dispersal tracks suggested by J. C. Zadoks.

Application of aerobiological information. Advances in aerobiology have given much information on the formation and transport of biological aerosols, but its relevance to disease attacks is often uncertain because too little attention has been paid to the viability of the spores being dispersed. This situation will not be remedied until there are better methods of growing the spores of obligate parasites and of fungi too featureless to be identified except in culture and better ways of relating contemporary spore concentration in the air to deposition on crops.   [J. M. HIRST]

Dissemination by water. Nematodes and certain fungi and bacteria which inhabit the soil may be carried from place to place by surface water. This becomes important when a pathogen such as *Plasmodiophora brassicae*, which causes clubroot of cabbage, is introduced into a field. Spores from a small center of infection can be carried all over the field. Dissemination from field to field in drainage or irrigation ditches occurs, but such dissemination for long distances is much less frequent than by wind or insects.

Splashing rain, especially if accompanied by wind, is often responsible for local spread of pathogens, especially bacteria and those fungi which produce spores in sticky masses.

Dissemination by insects. Bacteria and fungi which produce sticky spores are often disseminated by insects that sometimes are attracted to them by sweet- or putrid-smelling substances. The spores or bacteria stick to the mouthparts or other parts of the insect body and are carried from plant to plant in an apparently incidental manner. Actually this is a more effective way of dissemination than by either wind or water, because through evolutionary adaptation many insects and pathogens have developed an affinity for the same kinds of plants. Consequently a greater proportion of insect-carried spores arrive on plants they can infect than if they were scattered by the wind.

In other instances the relationship between insect and fungus is much more highly specialized. Dutch elm disease is caused by *Ceratocystis ulmi*, the spores of which are introduced into the vascular system of the tree by bark beetles (*Scolytus multistriatus* or *Hylurgopinus rufipes*) when they feed on the small twigs of healthy elm. After feeding, the beetles lay their eggs on weak or dying trees. The larvae feed beneath the bark and then pupate; when the new adults emerge, they are contaminated with the spores of the fungus which are in the pupal chambers. If the beetles did not feed on the young twigs, the fungus probably would not cause such a destructive disease, although it might still be a relatively harmless bark fungus as are similar species found only in weak trees. This is a case of transmission being more important than dissemination, although the beetle is the agent of both.

Many plant viruses are completely dependent upon insects for transmission from one plant to another. In the process the virus is also disseminated. Although a few viruses are transmitted by chewing insects, by far the most important vectors are the sucking insects, including aphids, leafhoppers, thrips, whiteflies and mealy bugs.

The diversity of relationships between viruses, plants, and insects is very great. Some viruses are transmitted by only one species of insect, some by several, and a few by many. Some insects, for example, the peach aphid (*Myzus persicae*), transmit many viruses: some only one. In some instances the insect can transmit the virus immediately after feeding upon a virus-infected plant: in others hours or days elapse before it can do so. Some viruses persist in the insect only a few hours after it has fed on a diseased plant, others persist for the rest of the life of the insect, and in some the virus is transmitted from adult to offspring through the eggs for an indefinite number of generations. In such instances the virus increases in the insect as it does in the plant, and the insect can be considered an alternate host of the virus, not merely a carrier.

The epidemiology of insect-transmitted viruses depends upon the ease and frequency with which an insect transmits the virus, which varies a great deal, and upon the life habits of the insect. If it is active, like leafhoppers, the virus may be spread far and rapidly; if it is sedentary, like mealybugs, spread may be very slow.

Dissemination by other animals. Besides insects, mites and nematodes transmit and disseminate a number of plant viruses. Among higher animals few are important as agents of dissemination of plant pathogens, though occasionally they may be very important. *Endothia parasitica*, the fungus which causes chestnut canker, produces sticky spores which adhere to the feet of birds. These birds carry the spores over considerable distances; in fact, they made it impossible to eradicate the fungus after it had been accidentally introduced into the eastern United States from the Orient.

Dissemination by man. Man is an important disseminator of plant pathogens if they lack other means of transport. Some pathogens are not adapted for widespread dissemination by wind, water, insects, or other natural means. Others have natural means for widespread dissemination, but still may be unable to surmount natural barriers such as oceans, high mountain ranges, or deserts.

Plant pathogens, as other flora and fauna, were usually confined to certain areas of the Earth before man began to alter the terrestrial environment. Frequently in his commercial, agricultural, or recreational activities, man has carried pathogens to new localities where they have caused tremendous damage, even though they were relatively harmless in their native habitat. For example, the chestnut blight fungus (*Endothia parasitica*) is a relatively mild parasite on the chestnut (*Castanea molissima*) in the Orient. When the fungus was brought to the United States about 1904 on imported chestnut trees, it spread to the native American chestnut (*Castanea dentata*), which is much more susceptible. The American chestnut forests were completely destroyed in about 40 years. Such lack of resistance in species of plants which have not evolved in the presence of the pathogen is very common, and it is the principal reason for the great danger involved in carrying pathogens to areas where they have not been before.

Dissemination by man may be hazardous even where natural barriers do not exist. Soil-borne pathogens such as *Plasmodiophora brassicae* and *Fusarium oxysporum* f. *conglutinans*, both of which attack cabbage, have been widely distributed on young cabbage seedlings which were grown in infested soil and sold for transplanting elsewhere. Neither fungus is disseminated by wind or insects, and water ordinarily carries them only to other parts of the field where they have already been introduced on infected transplants.

Plant pathogens disseminated by man are most frequently carried on infected plants. Some pathogens, such as certain cereal smuts (*Ustilago* sp.), bacterial blight (*Xanthomonas phaseoli*), and mosaic virus of bean, are transmitted and disseminated through seeds. However, this is less common and less hazardous than transmission in vegetative propagative parts such as potato seed tubers, flower bulbs, and nursery stock. Plant viruses in particular are more likely to be in the vegetative parts than in the seed.

Pathogens in either seed or planting stock have a good chance to become established in a new area because they have already infected the plant and need only to continue development when the plant starts to grow again. Similar plants and a favorable environment are likely to be present to permit further spread. Spores or bacteria disseminated independently are much less likely to survive or to find a host or favorable conditions for growth. The same may be said of pathogens in seeds, fruits, or vegetables to be used for food or in plant parts, such as lumber, to be used for manufacture.

Control of dissemination by man is attempted by quarantine.   [CARL J. EIDE]

PLANT DISEASES IN STORAGE

Tubers, fruits, and fresh vegetables are subject to spoilage by a variety of pathogenic and nonpathogenic agents during storage and transit, and often this hazard remains acute up to the time of consumption. Seeds such as those of wheat, corn, barley, soybeans, and flax, which often are stored in bulk for months or years, also are subject to deterioration. At times, the losses in transit and storage equal those that occur while the plants are growing. In general, storage diseases are divided into those caused by nonpathogenic factors and those caused by living organisms or pathogens.

Nonpathogenic storage diseases. Fruits and vegetables in storage suffer from a number of serious nonpathogenic or physiological diseases. Typically, these show up as discolored spots or areas on the surface of or within the affected parts, sometimes accompanied by collapse of the tissues, leaving pits on the surface or hollows within. These diseases are caused mainly by an excess of gases, such as certain esters or carbon dioxide, given off by the fruits or vegetables themselves or by chemicals introduced into the storage rooms. These diseases can be controlled by maintaining proper storage conditions, including temperature, humidity, and aeration. Fruits, vegetables, and seeds har-

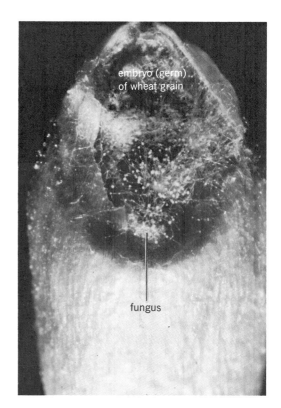

embryo (germ) of wheat grain

fungus

Fig. 24. Damaged grain of wheat, from commercial storage bin, with *Aspergillus* (fungus) growing from germ (embryo). Approximately 250,000 bu in this bin were affected, with a loss of more than $240,000.

bor abundant microflora, and damage beginning from nonpathogenic causes may be increased greatly by subsequent invasion of the tissues by bacteria and fungi able to cause rapid decay.

Pathogenic storage diseases. Common fungi, such as *Botrytis*, *Penicillium*, *Rhizopus*, and *Sclerotinia*, invade and rot many fruits and vegetables. Losses up to 25% of a shipment between harvest and consumption are common in fruits such as oranges, apples, peaches, pears, and plums and in vegetables such as potatoes, sweet potatoes, tomatoes, and peppers. Bacteria, or a combination of fungi and bacteria, often rot stored potatoes and root vegetables. These diseases may be controlled by harvesting only sound, disease-free products, careful handling to prevent bruising, the use of clean containers, maintenance of low (about 40°F) temperatures in transit and storage, and at times the use of fungicides.

Grains stored in bulk are subject to invasion by a number of fungi, principally those in the genus *Aspergillus* (Fig. 24), which have the ability to grow at moisture contents in equilibrium with relative humidities above 70%. These reduce germinability of seeds, which is important in those to be used for malting or planting, and may reduce the quality of the grains or seeds for processing. Some storage fungi produce potent toxins; the resulting deterioration may not be detected until most of the damage has been done. Research is gradually making available to men in the grain trade the facts and principles that will enable them to reduce such losses. *See* PLANT DISEASE CONTROL.

[CLYDE M. CHRISTENSEN]

Bibliography: F. G. Bawden, *Plant Viruses and Virus Diseases*, 4th ed., 1964; W. J. Dowson, *Plant Diseases due to Bacteria*, 2d ed., 1957; P. H. Gregory, *The Microbiology of the Atmosphere*, 2d ed., 1973; W. R. Jenkins and D. P. Taylor, *Plant Nematology*, 1967; E. C. Stakman and J. G. Harrar, *Principles of Plant Pathology*, 1957; J. E. van der Plank; *Plant Diseases: Epidemics and Control*, 1963; J. C. Walker, *Plant Pathology*, 3d ed., 1969; R. K. S. Wood, *Physiological Plant Pathology*, 1967.

Plant disease control

Plant diseases may be controlled by a variety of methods which can be classified as cultural practices, chemicals, resistant plant varieties, eradication of pathogens, and quarantines. Often a combination of methods is most effective.

Cultural practices. Cultural practices help to control disease by eliminating or reducing the effectiveness of the pathogen or by altering the susceptibility of the host plant. *See* AGRICULTURE, SOIL AND CROP PRACTICES IN.

If the primary inoculum is seed-borne, its prevalence may be reduced by getting seed from an area where the disease is absent or is controlled by other means. For example, bean growers in the humid parts of the United States get seed from arid western states to avoid seed-borne *Xanthomonas phaseoli*, which causes bacterial blight. Potato growers buy certified seed which is almost free of viruses that are kept under control through isolation and rogueing, that is, destroying infected plants.

Some pathogens, for example, the bacterium

X. phaseoli, live in infected plant debris so long as the debris remains undecayed. Accordingly, bean growers not only buy western seed but also use a 2–3 year rotation plan, which allows the debris to decay, thereby eliminating the bacteria. Sometimes it is practical to remove or burn crop residue, thus reducing the amount of the pathogen that is returned to the soil. *See* SOIL MICROBIOLOGY.

Bacteria such as *X. phaseoli* that survive only so long as the crop residue is undecayed probably are killed by antagonistic microorganisms in the soil. Attempts have been made to reduce or eliminate some of the more persistent soil-borne plant pathogens by introducing antagonistic species into the soil or by increasing those already present. Most of these efforts have not been successful.

Certain plant pathogens, for example, viruses, infect biennial or perennial weeds which supply primary inoculum. Eradication of the weeds is often an effective means of controlling the disease in crop plants. *See* PLANT VIRUS.

The elimination of primary inoculum usually is not complete by any of the above methods and is less effective as a means of control if the pathogen increases rapidly during the growing season from a few initial infections. Sometimes the rate of spread can be reduced. For example, the spread of viruses which are transmitted by insects can be delayed by controlling the insect. *See* INSECT CONTROL, BIOLOGICAL.

The inherent resistance of plants to disease is usually altered by environmental factors such as temperature, moisture, and available nutrients. Moisture sometimes can be controlled, as in irrigated areas, and soil nutrients can be regulated to some degree by fertilizer practice. For example, apple trees are more susceptible to fire blight, caused by *Erwinia amylovora*, if they are growing rapidly; growth can be reduced by withholding fertilizers, especially nitrogen. *See* FERTILIZING; IRRIGATION OF CROPS; PLANT, MINERALS ESSENTIAL TO.

Since some pathogens enter plants through wounds, avoiding injury often reduces infection. This applies particularly to fleshy vegetables, such as potato tubers, and to fruits which are subject to storage diseases caused by bacteria and fungi. Even seeds, for example, soybean, can be cracked if harvested when too dry and become infected by soil organisms when planted.

[CARL J. EIDE]

Chemical control. Infectious plant diseases are caused by four major classes of agents: fungi (molds), nematodes (minute worms), bacteria, and viruses. These are arranged in the order of importance in chemical control, bacteria and viruses being the most difficult to control by chemicals. Hence the major tonnage of chemicals are fungicides and nematicides. *See* FUNGISTAT AND FUNGICIDE.

The last published list of antidisease chemicals showed 267 trade materials, many of which are duplicate trade names for the same chemicals.

The chemical control of plant disease differs sharply from the chemical control of human disease. Chemicals must be used to protect plants rather than to cure them, by killing the parasites while they are still in the environment and before

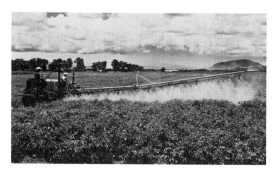

Fig. 1. Chemical control of potato late blight, Toluca Valley, Mexico. (*Rockefeller Foundation*)

they invade the plant.

External protection. Plant diseases attack all parts of the plant: seeds, roots, stems, leaves, and fruits. They attack plants in the field, packing shed, trains and trucks in transit, market, and home. This means that a variety of compounds and methods must be used to control parasitic forms.

Many fungi and a few nematodes attack seeds. If the organism is inside the seed, an organic mercury compound is sometimes effective. If the organism is merely on the surface of the seed, an organic sulfur compound, called a dithiocarbamate, may be used. Seeds are commonly treated by tumbling them with the dry compound in a drum or by mixing them in slurries and then drying.

Nematodes and fungi which attack plant roots must be flushed out of the soil with fumigant gases that can seep into all the crevices and spaces in the soil. A common fumigant is a mixture of methylisothiocyanate and 1,3-dichloropropene. Soil fumigants are commonly inserted several inches deep in the soil through holes in the lower end of special thin "chisels" on a machine pulled with a tractor. Soil and seed may be treated together by spilling the chemical over the seed and adjacent soil as the seed is planted. Nematicides and fungicides for use in the soil are being developed rapidly.

The biggest tonnage of chemicals for plant disease control goes onto foliage and developing fruit for protection from fungi. Foliage fungicides are known as protectants; that is, they must be applied to the plant before an invading fungus arrives. Since the waiting period may be long, serious limitations are imposed on a compound. To work effectively, it must resist erosion by rain and dew, and it must withstand the heat of the summer sun.

Few chemicals have proved to be effective. The first was elemental sulfur, used since about 1803 to control powdery mildew diseases. Although it sublimes somewhat in the heat, it survives sufficiently for effective use. The next was Bordeaux mixture, a copper-containing substance that saved the French wine industry in the 1880s. It is both exceedingly resistant to rain erosion and does not sublime. It was over 60 years before another really good type of chemical was discovered, namely, the dithiocarbamates—organic sulfur compounds which are now used worldwide. Other fungicides were developed in rapid succession, including the imidazolines, dinitrocaprylphenyl crotonate, trichloromethylthioimides, and guanidines.

Foliage and fruit fungicides are generally applied as sprays delivered by powerful machines that move through the crops. In areas where fields are large, farmers use airplanes as flying sprayers. Compounds are seldom effective if applied as dry dusts to foliage and fruit because the dusts do not stick well and consequently do not resist rain action (Fig. 1).

Fruits and vegetables are subject to disease and decay after picking. Much of this postharvest loss is not yet subject to chemical control, but oranges and other citrus fruits are widely treated in the packing shed with such compounds as diphenyl and sodium *o*-phenylphenate.

Chemotherapy. The newest frontier of the science of plant disease control is chemotherapy, the control of disease by internal treatment rather than by external protection (Fig. 2).

Although extensive researches have gone into chemotherapy of plant disease, the biological obstacles to success are great. Effective compounds have been discovered, but to move them inside the plant to the right place at the right time and to keep them there for a long enough time is extremely difficult. Sap in the sap stream passes a given point only once; therefore if the compound cannot cure the infection in one pass, it fails. An even more severe limitation is that plants have nothing even faintly similar to white blood cells. In animals the white cells clean up the few straggler germs left by the drug. Unless the chemical treatment kills every pathogen in a plant, however, the infection flares again and eventually kills the plant. *See* PESTICIDE.   [JAMES G. HORSFALL]

Disease resistance. Plants are surrounded by a vast number of microorganisms that inhabit the air and soil. A few invade plants and injure them by disrupting their normal growth and development (disease). Such microorganisms are called pathogens. It is remarkable that plants are not injured by most microorganisms around them. Many microorganisms actually are essential for the growth and development of plants. The ability of plants to grow in an environment of microorganisms is evidence of how well they resist the harmful effects caused by pathogens (disease resistance). Most pathogens cause disease to only a certain plant, for example, pathogens of corn do not cause disease on wheat or geraniums. In addition, there are cer-

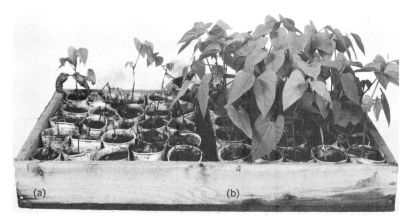

Fig. 2. Control of downy mildew of lima beans with a streptomycin sulfate compound, Agristrep. (*a*) Untreated, 100% infection. (*b*) Sprayed with 100 ppm of streptomycin, excellent control. (*W. J. Zaumeyer, USDA*)

tain varieties of plants that are resistant and others that are susceptible, for example, a pathogen may attack a certain kind of wheat but not another.

What makes a plant resistant to disease? Each plant cell carries the genetic information that can be translated into chemical reactions and structures which determine whether a plant is resistant or susceptible. The mechanisms for disease resistance in plants are highly efficient since susceptibility is the rare exception in nature. Resistance may be due to the inability of the microorganism to penetrate the plant, inability to develop in the plant because the microorganism lacks nutrients or encounters compounds that inhibit its growth or reproduction, or the ability of the plant to resist microbial toxins.

Barriers to penetration. To cause disease, microorganisms must first establish physiological contact with the plant. Plants are covered by a coating of waxlike material called the cuticle, which serves as a nonspecific physical barrier. Plant storage organs also have outer protective tissues commonly referred to as peel. In addition to serving as a physical barrier, the outer coverings of many plants also contain chemical compounds that are toxic to many microorgansims. The peel of the Irish potato tuber contains chlorogenic acid, caffeic acid, α-solanine, and α-chaconine, whereas the outer scales of red onions contain protocatechuic acid and catechol. Natural openings (stomata and lenticels) exist in the barrier layer, and also this outer barrier is often broken by injury. Some pathogens invade plants through the natural openings and others only through wounds, but a few can grow through the barriers by mechanical pressure or by producing enzymes which dissolve parts of the protective barrier. The thickness of cuticle or peel is important in the resistance of certain plants to disease. In general, however, the contribution of cuticle or peel to resistance is thought to be small, except with microorganisms that invade plants only through wounds.

Nutrient factors. The absence of a factor necessary for microbial growth may be part of the disease-resistance mechanism of a plant. Certain bacteria can attack plants only if nutrients are available on the plant surface. Invasion of plum tree bark by *Rhodosticta quercina*, a fungus requiring myoinositol, is related to the myoinositol content of the bark. Susceptible varieties contain more than 10 times the amount of myoinostol found in resistant varieties. Except for microorganisms that can grow only in living plants, the presence or lack of nutrient factors is not considered a major mechanism for disease resistance. Most microorganisms grow on plant extracts or dead plant tissue from healthy susceptible or resistant plants.

Production of inhibitors. Once the microorganism has established physiological contact with the plant, it can influence the chemical reactions (metabolism) in the plant. Often this interaction of plant and microorganism results in the production of compounds (phytoalexins) around sites of penetration which inhibit the growth and reproduction of the microorganism. Phytoalexins include chlorogenic and caffeic acids, ipomeamarone, pisatin, phaseollin, 6-methoxy-mellein, orchinol, gossypol, oxidation products of phloretin, and an inhibitor not yet characterized from soybeans. Ian Cruickshank and coworkers established a relationship between the resistance of pea pods to fungi and the production of the phytoalexin, pisatin. Fungi unable to cause disease in pea pods were found to stimulate production of pisatin in amounts which markedly inhibited their growth, whereas pathogens of peas stimulated production of less pisatin. The amount of phytoalexin produced by the plant, therefore, is not the sole factor in disease resistance. The sensitivity of the microorganism to the amount of phytoalexin produced is also important. This suggests that at least two distinct biochemical mechanisms are involved in determining disease resistance—one controlling biosynthesis of phytoalexin and the other controlling the sensitivity of the microorganism to the inhibitor.

It is not surprising therefore to encounter situations where more of phytoalexin is produced by a plant after inoculation with a pathogen than with a nonpathogen. Some plants produce more than one phytoalexin after infection. Chlorogenic acid and 6-methoxy-mellein are produced by carrot and reach toxic levels around sites of microbial penetration within 24 hr after inoculation with microorganisms that do not cause disease on carrot. Microscopic examination of the inoculated tissue indicates that the inhibition of microbial growth in the carrot coincides with the production of 6-methoxy-mellein and chlorogenic acid at levels toxic to the microorganisms. It has also been demonstrated that the foliage of resistant but not susceptible varieties of soybeans produce a phytoalexin when inoculated with the pathogen *Phytophthora sojae*. Nonpathogens induce the production of the phytoalexin regardless of the susceptibility of the soybean variety of *P. sojae*. The appearance of phloretin in apple leaves following injury or inoculation with the pathogen *Venturia inaequalis* illustrates not the synthesis, but the liberation of a phenol from its nontoxic glycoside.

Phloridzin, the glucoside of phloretin, is found in leaves of apple varieties susceptible or resistant to attack by *V. inaequalis*. There is no correlation between the phloridzin content of leaves and resistance to the pathogen. When the pathogen penetrates the leaf of a highly resistant variety, the plant cells around the point of penetration immediately collapse, phloridzin is hydrolyzed by the enzyme β-glycosidase to yield phloretin and glucose, and phloretin is oxidized by phenol oxidases to yield highly fungitoxic compounds. In susceptible varieties the fungus penetrates the leaves and makes extensive growth beneath the cuticle for 10–14 days without causing collapse of plant cells. Thus phloridzin is not hydrolyzed and the pathogen is not inhibited. After 10–14 days the fungus sporulates on the leaves of susceptible varieties, and the affected tissue collapses. As with the resistance of soybeans to *P. sojae*, the potential for resistance appears to be present in all plants, and resistance may be determined by the ability of the microorganism to trigger synthesis or liberation of an inhibitor in the host. A similar series of reactions involving arbutin and hydroquinone may be important in determining the resistance of pear to the bacterium *Erwinia amylovora* that causes the disease fire blight.

Some compounds that accumulate around sites

of infection or injury, for example, chlorogenic and caffeic acids, are widely distributed throughout the plant kingdom. The synthesis of others appears limited to a narrow host range, for example, 6-methoxy-mellein in carrot, phaseollin in the green bean, pisatin in the garden pea, and ipomea-marone in sweet potato. Apparently the plant has the potential for synthesis of the compound, and the microorganism used for inoculation determines the quantitative response of the plant. Where two or more compounds are produced in response to infection, the microorganism controls the relative concentration of each.

Resistance to toxins. The ability of plants to resist factors arising from plant-microbial interaction, which lead to tissue disintegration or impaired metabolic activity, may also be part of a disease-resistance mechanism. This resistance mechanism may include the presence of resistant structural components and metabolic pathways, mechanisms for detoxication, and the presence of alternate pathways for metabolism in the plant.

The resistance of immature apple fruit to many fungi that cause rots has been related to the resistance of pectic compounds in the cell walls of the green fruit to enzymes produced by the fungi. In mature fruit the microbial enzymes dissolve the cell walls, but the cell walls of immature fruit are not destroyed. During the growing season the amount of water-insoluble, resistant cell-wall material decreases as the apple matures. A major drop in the polyvalent cation content of cell-wall material occurs at about the time the fruit becomes susceptible. Conversely, the potassium content of the cell-wall material is higher in susceptibility than resistant fruit, with a major increase occurring with the onset of susceptibility. It appears that a pectin-protein polyvalent cation complex making up the cell-wall material of resistant fruits is responsible for the resistance of the fruits. The cell walls become susceptible as the polyvalent cations are lost.

Further evidence for the role of polyvalent cations is provided in the resistance of old bean seedlings to the fungus *Rhizoctonia*. Calcium ions accumulate in and immediately around developing lesions caused by the fungus. Barium, calcium, and magnesium ions inhibit tissue maceration by enzymes produced by the fungus, whereas potassium and sodium ions do not significantly influence the process. Bean tissue with lesions is more difficult to macerate with enzymes produced by the fungus than comparable healthy tissue. The cementing material (middle lamella) between plant cells around lesions is more difficult to dissolve than the middle lamella of cells more distant from lesions. The accumulation of polyvalent cations in advance of the fungus makes pectic substances of the tissue resistant to breakdown by the fungus.

In addition to producing enzymes which destroy plant cells, microorganisms have also been reported to produce toxic compounds that injure the plant without dissolving the plant tissue. The toxins that are produced are very specific for the plant in which the microorganism can cause disease. Varieties of the plant that are resistant to the microorganism are also resistant to the action of the toxin. The mechanism by which the plants are able to resist the toxin is not known; however, resistant plants may be able to change the toxin into nontoxic forms, or the toxin may be unable to penetrate into vital parts of the resistant cell. Microorganisms known to produce host-specific toxins include *Alternaria kikuchiana, Helminthosporium victoriae, Periconia circinata,* and *Helminthosporium carbonum.*   [JOSEPH KUC]

Breeding and testing for resistance. The use of disease-resistant varieties that prevent or limit infection is one of the most widely used methods of disease control. Much of man's food and fiber supply depends upon the growth of disease-resistant crops.

In dealing with disease resistance, modern scientists must recognize not only the genetic system of the host plant but also the genetic system of the pathogen. Infectious diseases, in the final analysis, are the end result of gene-controlled chemical processes that are modified to some extent by the environment.

Use. The use of disease-resistant varieties with satisfactory yield and quality characteristics is the best and most economic means of disease control. It is the only feasible means of control for many virus and bacterial diseases, most soil-borne diseases, and many foliage diseases of extensively grown crops. Over 75% of the diseases of field crops and over 50% of the diseases of vegetable crops are controlled by means of host resistance.

The meat supply for human consumption depends on corn and sorghum hybrids resistant to blights, smuts, and other diseases, and the vegetable-processing industry depends on varieties of corn, peas, cucumber, beans, and tomatoes resistant to wilts, viruses, and other diseases. The list can be extended manyfold. Most of these crops are annual plants with which rapid breeding programs are possible. Resistance is less frequently used in crops with a long life-span or in high-value crops possessing special qualities or ornamental characteristics.

Disease tolerance. Tolerance is the ability of a variety to endure disease attack without suffering the same reduction in yield or quality as another variety. Although disease tolerance is a valuable attribute of a plant, tolerant varieties have the disadvantage of allowing pathogen reproduction to take place, thus exposing nearby nontolerant varieties to infection.

Disease escape. Some plant varieties, normally susceptible to disease, escape being inoculated and therefore are less damaged by disease than are other varieties grown in the same area at the same time. For example, early varieties of plants may mature before the pathogen reaches the area in which they are grown. Plants with an upright growth habit may be less frequently infected than plants with a prostrate type of growth. A plant may be resistant or unattractive to an insect that is a carrier for a virus and thereby may escape infection.

Genetics of resistance. The expression of resistance is an inherited character in the plant and can take several forms. The simplest mode of inheritance is a single gene. Gene action may be completely dominant, incompletely dominant, or recessive. When studied in detail, genes for resistance are frequently found to exist in a large number of separate functional forms or alleles. Resistance in a variety may also be due to two or more genes acting individually or through some form of gene interaction. When two or more genes must be present simultaneously in a variety for resistance to occur, gene action is spoken of as complementary. Modifier genes may individually show no effect on disease reaction, but together with another gene for resistance may either enhance or reduce the expression of resistance.

Disease reaction sometimes is under the control of a large number of gene loci. In these situations disease reaction in segregating populations usually grades continuously between, and sometimes beyond, the limits of the susceptible parent reactions. Gene action is largely additive, but sometimes dominant and epistatic effects are seen.

Stability of resistance. Resistance can fail to function because of certain environmental conditions or because of genetic changes in the pathogen which may enable it to overcome the resistance of the host.

Cabbage varieties with multiple-gene resistance to yellows become susceptible at soil temperatures above 24°C, whereas varieties with single-gene resistance do not. Certain cereal varieties are resistant to rust in cool summers but may be susceptible when air temperatures are high. Resistance to root-invading fungi may break down when roots are injured by nematode feeding.

The most common failure of resistance, however, originates from genetic changes in the pathogen. Pathogens are living organisms with systems for the storage and release of genetic variation. Most rust, smut, and powdery mildew fungi occur in the form of races that differ from each other in ability to infect varieties of their host plants. New races that have the ability to attack a currently grown variety can appear in nature. Resistance to the new race must then be found and the breeding program repeated. Experiments indicate that this phenomenon is true for certain forms of resistance but not for others. Thus certain forms of generalized plant resistance give protection even against pathogens that are made up of many races. In other organisms, specialized races with reference to pathogenicity are not known. This is true for many organisms that cause root and culm rots, vascular wilts, and numerous foliage diseases. Resistance to these organisms seems to be lastingly effective.

Testing for disease resistance. In breeding for disease resistance or in selecting among established varieties, a reliable method for determining differences in disease reaction is necessary. Sometimes natural infection must be used; more commonly, however, carefully designed, artifical inoculation procedures are employed in field, greenhouse, or laboratory tests.

The inoculation method must be reliable so that escapes do not occur. Conditions for disease development should not be so severe, however, that different gradations of reaction to disease do not appear. It is desirable that a large number of plants be inoculated and that the method does not interfere with the breeding and selection scheme for the crop.

The inoculum should be a pure culture of the pathogen with an optimal degree of virulence. In many instances pathogenic races must be carefully selected so that plants with the desired type of resistance can be identified.

Environmental control, particularly of temperature and moisture, is needed during the inoculation and testing period. Comparable results from test to test can then be achieved, and different types of resistance can be distinguished.

Sources of resistance. Resistant germ plasm for use in breeding programs has been found in native and exotic varieties and even in wild species. When adapted native varieties are available, breeding objectives are more rapidly achieved. Resistant selections may need only to be identified and put into production. Exotic varieties have been valuable sources of resistance. For example, cottons from India and Africa have provided bacterial blight resistance; wheats from Australia and Kenya have furnished valuable genes for rust resistance; barleys from Ethiopia have provided yellow-dwarf-virus resistance; and sugarcanes from Java and India have provided the resistance to mosaic needed in American varieties of these crops. Noncultivated plant species frequently have more resistance to disease than cultivated species. Sterility, lack of chromosome pairing, and presence of undesirable characters are limitations in the use of wild plants in breeding programs. Nevertheless, wild relatives of tobacco, tomato, potato, sugarcane, wheat, oats, and other crops have contributed valuable genes for disease resistance to cultivated species.

Employment of resistance. Superior genes for disease resistance are usually exploited rapidly by plant breeders, and numerous varieties with similar resistances are put into production. With the recognition of different types of disease resistance, more careful attention is now given to the type of resistance used in the breeding program. Greater attention is directed to the less complete but more generalized types of resistance. Diversity of resistance and combinations of resistant types are also regarded as important. This has been necessary because of the repeated failure of varieties with only specific types of resistance to maintain this resistance in nature.

To maximize the effectiveness of genes for specific resistance, multiline varieties and hybrids are being developed. Multiline varieties are composed of a mechanical mixture of backcross-derived lines; each line contains different genes for resistance, but all are similar in maturity, appearance, and other respects. The components of the mixture can be varied from year to year, depending upon the pathogen races present. In addition, since some plants in the mixture are resistant each year, disease development on susceptible plants is delayed, enabling the plants to mature with light damage.

Breeding methods. Methods of breeding for disease resistance do not differ greatly from those employed for other characters. Selection, varietal hybridization and selection, and backcrossing are the methods most commonly employed. Simple selection procedures have resulted in the isolation of resistant varieties from heterogeneous crops.

Where agricultural technology is more advanced and pure-line varieties of crops are grown, genetic variation must be achieved. Simple or complex crosses are made between sources of disease resistance and varieties possessing other desirable qualities. This is followed by careful selection and testing during the segregating generations so that superior disease-resistant varieties can be identified. As breeding programs have become more advanced, the only improvement needed in a variety may be additional disease resistance. In these situations the backcross breeding method is commonly employed. The method consists of repeatedly crossing each generation of resistant plants with the susceptible variety. After several generations, this is followed by selfing and selection. The breeding procedure allows for the recovery of nearly all the characteristics of the original variety but with resistance added.

Breeding for disease resistance has been a process of challenge and response. As each new disease has threatened the destruction of a crop, resistant varieties have been developed and put into production. Although breeding for resistance has been highly effective, it is expected that further gains in the efficiency and effectiveness of the method will be made. To achieve this, modern research is aimed at the identification of superior forms of disease resistance and a greater understanding of the genetical and biochemical nature of resistance. *See* BREEDING (PLANT).

[ARTHUR L. HOOKER]

Eradication campaigns. These are designed either to eliminate recently introduced pathogens completely or to protect economic plants by destroying alternate, or weed, hosts. Success in eliminating pathogens depends on early detection of the pathogen and on the efficiency of eradication measures.

Attempts made in the United States to eradicate chestnut blight and the Dutch elm disease were unsuccessful. The citrus canker disease, however, was eliminated from Florida by burning infected trees. Flag smut of wheat, which was introduced locally into Mexico, was also successfully burned out. Similarly, persistent eradication of infected plants has helped restrict many diseases. *See* FRUIT (TREE) DISEASES.

Certain rusts can be controlled wholly or partly by eradicating alternate hosts. For example, the destruction of red cedars near apple orchards protects apples against the *Gymnosporangium* rust, because this rust cannot maintain itself on either host alone. To help control stem rust of wheat and other small grains, the growing of barberries, *Berberis* sp., has been prohibited by law in some countries. Denmark began a successful campaign against barberries in 1904, and in the United States about 500,000,000 barberries have been destroyed since 1918, with substantial reduction of the stem-rust menace (Fig. 3). Likewise in the United States white pines and other susceptible species are partly protected from blister rust by eradicating nearby currants and gooseberries, *Ribes* sp.

Like legal public health measures for human beings and for domestic animals, those for plants are essential in keeping many diseases in check.

[E. C. STAKMAN]

Quarantines. Plant disease quarantines are legal measures taken by Federal or state governments to prevent the introduction of foreign plant diseases or pests into an area. Quarantines are based on the philosophy that government has the right and obligation to protect its agricultural resources and industry from the destructive effects of exotic plant diseases and pests.

The transportation of plants and plant parts was long a matter of private concern, with the result that many plant pathogens became widely distributed by international travelers or through unrestricted trade channels. The dangers of this situation became dramatically apparent following the accidental importation of the chestnut-blight fungus into the United States from Asia between 1900 and 1905 and the ultimate destruction of the American chestnut forests.

As a consequence of this and other bitter lessons, the United States government in 1912 passed the national Plant Quarantine Act. Today essentially all nations have enacted protective quarantine regulations. Quarantine laws authorize Federal or state officials to intercept and inspect shipments of plant materials and to release, fumigate, or confiscate the shipment in accordance with legal provisions. Quarantine inspectors are stationed at ports of entry, border stations, and at receiving and distributing points for freight and mail.

Value of quarantines. The value of quarantines has long been disputed. Antagonists claim that man is unable to prevent the movement of microscopic pathogens, that many quarantines are scientifically unsound, and that on occasions quarantines have been used as economic sanctions in restraint of free trade and have caused unnecessary economic losses. Supporters insist that even though not 100% effective, quarantines do prevent the introduction of many pests and diseases and retard the movement of others, giving scientists time to combat them before they become well established; that quarantines annually save the agricultural industry millions of dollars; and that these economic gains are many times greater than any possible business losses resulting from the application of quarantine measures.

Improvements in the practice of quarantining may provide assurance that all quarantines will be established on sound biological bases for maxi-

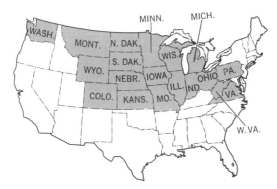

Fig. 3. More than 513,500,000 rust-susceptible barberry bushes were destroyed on 153,000 rural and urban properties in 19 barberry-eradication states. (*USDA*)

mum effectiveness, that they can be lifted with equal facility when it becomes clear that they are no longer necessary, and that, insofar as possible, new quarantine laws would be preceded by international consultation in an attempt to obtain mutual agreement and to ensure minimum disruption of the international exchange of commodities.

International disease protection. Joint efforts are made by nations to protect their agricultural resources and industries without impairment of exchange of commodities. Ideally, available knowledge on plant pests and pathogens is utilized to devise methods to limit their geographic spread and to prevent the outbreak of epidemics. Changes in cropping patterns, trade agreements, and the distribution of pests and pathogens necessitate a continuing program consisting of (1) annual plant disease surveys by the several nations with free exchange of results, (2) rigorous practice of local sanitation and plant protection, (3) prompt distribution of resistant varieties of crop plants, (4) exchange of information in improved control measures, and (5) international consultation with respect to the establishment and enforcement of quarantines.

International plant protection can be successful only when regulatory activities are fortified by scientists investigating the etiology of plant diseases, life cycles of pathogens, host-parasite relationships, and chemical and other control measures. Exchange visits by scientific personnel further strengthen understanding and lead to logical and amicable agreements. Among international organizations active in plant protection are the Food and Agriculture Organization of the United Nations, and the International Commission on Plant Disease Losses.

[J. GEORGE HARRAR]

Bibliography: E. Evans, *Plant Diseases and their Chemical Control*, 1968; R. N. Goodman, Z. Kiraly, and M. Zaitlin, *The Biochemistry and Physiology of Infectious Plant Disease*, 1967; J. B. Harborne (ed.), *Biochemistry of Phenolic Compounds*, 1964; A. L. Hooker, The genetics and expression of resistance in plants to rusts of the genus *Puccinia*, *Annu. Rev. Phytopathol.*, 5:163–182, 1967; T. Johnson et al., The world situation of the cereal rusts, *Annu. Rev. Phytopathol.*, 5:183–200, 1967; J. Kuć, Resistance of plants to infectious agents, *Annu. Rev. Microbiol.*, 20:337–370, 1966; E. E. Leppik, Relation of centers of origin of cultivated plants to sources of disease resistance, *USDA Agr. Res. Serv. Plant Introd., Invest. Pap.*, no. 13, 1968; C. J. Mirocha and I. Uritani (eds.), *The Dynamic Role of Molecular Constituents in Plant-Parasite Interaction*, 1967; K. S. Quisenberry and L. P. Reitz (eds.), *Wheat and Wheat Improvement*, 1967; E. C. Stakman and J. G. Harrar, *Principles of Plant Pathology*, 1957; J. C. Walker, *Plant Pathology*, 3d ed., 1969; W. Williams, *Genetical Principles and Plant Breeding*, 1964; R. K. S. Wood, *Physiological Plant Pathology*, 1967.

Plant fiber, dietary

There is no concise definition of fiber, certainly none that can describe its role in human nutrition. In general, fiber can be defined as a complex of substances of plant origin that appear not to be absorbed or digested by humans. Most, but not all, of these substances are found in the plant cell wall.

Knowledge about fiber has increased due to advances in analysis of this material and easier means of identifying its components. Most nutrition literature provides values for the crude fiber content of foods. These values represent only that portion which is resistant to solvents, acid, and alkali. Current methodology permits scientists to obtain a fractionation of so-called fiber, which may help establish the biological properties of each fraction.

Cell wall fibers. Cellulose is the most widely distributed component of the cell wall. It is an unbranched 1-4β-D-glucose polymer with a molecular weight of about 600,000. Hemicellulose, on the other hand, represents a wide variety of polysaccharide polymers that contain a mixture of pentose and hexoses, many of which are branched. It also contains sugars that have a terminal carboxyl group, uronic acids. The compounds most commonly found in hemicellulose are xylose, arabinose, mannose, galactose, glucose, rhamnose, galacturonic acid, and glucuronic acid. The average hemicellulose molecule contains 150–200 carbohydrate units, in contrast to cellulose which contains about 3000 glucose units. Pectins are present in small amounts in most cell walls (1–5%), but certain plant tissues, such as citrus rinds, may contain up to 30%. The terms "pectic substances," "pectin," "pectinic acid," and "pectic acid" are all used to describe the pectins. The backbone of pectin structure is a polymer of 1-4β-D-galacturonic acid. Other component sugars are galactose, arabinose, xylose, rhamnose, and fucose. There is also an appreciable amount (up to 10%) of methyl substitution on the hydroxyl groups. Pectins have a molecular weight in the region of 60,000–90,000.

The fourth major constituent of cell walls is lignin, the only noncellulosic material among the main components. Lignin is a highly insoluble substance comprising several polymeric hydroxyphenylpropane derivatives. The molecular weight of lignin is about 1000–4500.

Other fibers. Plant gums and mucilages can also be classified as fiber. They are highly branched polymers of glucuronic and galacturonic acids and usually contain xylose, arabinose, and mannose. Algal polysaccharides, such as alginic acid, agar, and carageenan, should also be included as fiber. Agar and carageenan are sulfated galactans, whereas alginic acid is a linear 1,4-β-D-manuronic acid polymer with L-glucuronic acid substitutions. It can form fibrils as cellulose does.

Among fiber-associated substances are phytic acid (inositol hexaphosphate), silica, waxes, cutins (hydroxyacid polymers), tannins, and some proteins.

Relation to disease. Early interest in fiber (or roughage as it was known) was centered mainly on its laxative properties. Current interest was catalyzed by publications which attributed to a low-fiber diet many of the diseases common to the Western world; among these are coronary disease, diabetes, colon cancer, and diverticular disease. Whereas the early theory was that any type of fiber was sufficient dietary protection, it has now become evident that specific components of fiber may play individual metabolic roles.

Cholesterol metabolism. The influence of dietary fiber on cholesterol metabolism in animals and humans has been under intensive study. In humans, an elevated serum cholesterol level is one of several factors that increase the risk of development of coronary disease. A survey of the literature has shown that bran, even in quantities as high as 100 g daily, has no effect on either cholesterol or triglyceride levels. Pectin, on the other hand, has an effect on cholesterol. Studied in nine subjects over a 3-week period at a dosage level of 15 g per day, pectin did not influence serum triglyceride levels but reduced cholesterol by 15%. The treatment did not affect intestinal transit time but did increase fecal dry weight and excretion of cholesterol and its metabolites. Guar gum (36 g per day) lowered cholesterol levels by an average of 16% in seven patients. The assessment of the influence of dietary fiber on actual coronary disease in humans will require careful long-term studies. In cynomolgus monkeys it was found that neither wheat, soya, nor rice bran had any effect on serum lipid levels.

In rats it is possible to examine both serum and liver cholesterol levels. In rats fed 0.5% cholesterol and 7% fiber, pectin lowered serum cholesterol by 21% and liver cholesterol by 64%. Carageenan lowered serum cholesterol to the same extent as pectin but raised liver cholesterol slightly (9%). Agar and cellulose did not change serum cholesterol levels but raised liver cholesterol by 105 and 32%, respectively. Rabbits and vervet monkeys fed atherogenic diets containing wheat straw or alfalfa exhibited less atherosclerosis (arterial fat deposition) than controls who were fed similar diets containing cellulose.

The American Diabetic Association prescribes a 2200-calorie (9.2 kilojoule) diet which contains 43% of its calories as carbohydrate (about half as simple sugar) and 4.7 g of fiber. In one study 13 diabetics were fed a 2200-calorie diet in which 75% of the calories were from carbohydrates (about one-quarter as simple sugar) and which contained 14.2 g of fiber. After 2 weeks, levels of plasma cholesterol, triglycerides, and glucose had fallen by 24, 15, and 26%, respectively, and a number of the subjects were able to discontinue insulin or sulfonylurea therapy.

Colon cancer. To date, data relating to the influence of fiber on colon cancer in humans are epidemiological. That is, there are apparent correlations between incidence of colon cancer and low-fiber diets. Another school of thought attributes the rise in cancer incidence to high meat diets. A recent study, however, shows no increase in incidence of colon cancer in the United States over the past 30 years, despite increasing consumption of meat and decreasing intake of fiber. There are also conflicting epidemiological data since Seventh Day Adventists (a primarily vegetarian group) and Mormons (who eat a mixed diet) both show lower incidence of colon cancer than the standard United States population.

One animal study in which colon cancers were induced chemically in rats fed 20% fat with or without 20% bran showed about 19–39% fewer colon tumors in the rats fed bran. The variation in incidence is due to different schedules of chemical treatment.

Negative properties. Fiber is not without some negative properties. Principal among these is the possibility that dietary fiber may decrease the bioavailibility of certain essential nutrients. Continued ingestion of fiber-rich foods or of individual components of fiber can result in decreased absorption and reduced blood levels of calcium, magnesium, iron, and zinc. Another concomitant of a high-fiber diet is increased flatulence.

There is no evidence that any disease is due directly to lack of dietary fiber. High- and low-fiber diets are manifestations of other differences in lifestyle, social as well as dietary. Both of these types of differences contribute to disease. In addition, many of the diseases prevalent in developed countries are diseases of old age, and observed differences between high- and low-fiber societies may be partly due to differences in life-span.

Outlook. Methodology for fiber analysis must be improved and simplified. It is important to learn the mechanisms by which individual fiber components affect lipid metabolism, heart disease, and cancer. It is also necessary to learn how these components interact when present in food. Finally, the general population should be made aware that the amount of a dietary component that is added is important both for its own value and for the nutritional values of the food being replaced. If a little is good—as in the case of fiber—a lot is not necessarily better.

[DAVID KRITCHEVSKY]

Plant growth

An irreversible increase in cell numbers and cell size in plants. In contrast, animal growth is almost wholly the result of increase in cell numbers. Another important difference in growth between plants and animals is that animals are determinate in growth and reach a final size before they are mature and start to reproduce. Plants have indeterminate growth and as long as they live continue to add new organs and tissues. In animals growth of the different parts of the body is more or less simultaneous; in plants growth is restricted to the growing points or meristems. Therefore, in an animal most body cells attain about the same age and the individual dies as a unit, but in a plant new cells are produced all the time, and some parts, such as leaves and flowers, may die, while the main body of the plant persists and continues to grow. However, the basic process of growth, cell multiplication, is very much the same in plants and animals, and mitosis and cell division will not be considered here in detail.

This article discusses the various phenomena of growth, followed by sections on reproductive growth, dominance and germination, periodicity and abscission, and seasonal thermoperiodicity.

Factors affecting growth. The factors which control plant growth can be separated into three groups. First are the inherent genetic factors, the genes, carried by all cells, which give every cell the potentiality to grow, and which control the limits within which each cell, organ, or plant can develop. These factors can be controlled only by breeding, and once the egg cell has been fertilized, the genetic potentialities of the future plant can no longer be altered.

Second are the internal factors, such as the interactions between cells, the hormonal control system, the internal food distribution, and all correlations in general. These will be discussed in the section on plant hormones.

The third group includes the root and aerial environment.

The balance between the available water in the soil and the water loss through transpiration is a major factor in plant growth. Another major factor is the availability of nutrients. This is a function of the concentration of nutrients in the soil, and also depends on such factors as the soil water and air content, the size of the root system, the presence of a proper soil microflora, the temperature of the soil, and the balance between the nutrients.

For land plants the aerial environment is of paramount importance. The components of this environment are temperature, light, humidity, wind, air composition, and such extreme conditions as frost, excessive heat, rain, extremes of barometric pressure, invisible radiation, periodic changes, and the living plants and animals in the immediate surroundings.

It is important to realize how complex the interrelationship between external and internal environment is. The effects are both direct and indirect, for a change in growth rate or in development influences the subsequent behavior of the plant as well. At present, knowledge about the interrelationship between these factors is only fragmentary. This is partly because of the difficulty of investigating these effects. In studying this relationship it is necessary to control the external environment and to work with genetically uniform plant material. This is being done in so-called phytotrons, in which each of the environmental factors can be controlled separately.

The additional problem of the irregularities and unpredictability of the climate arises in dealing with the effects of climate on plant growth. The growth responses of plants to individual factors will be discussed in this article.

Plant hormones. The cell is the smallest unit of the organism which has all the attributes of life and which can persist as a unit. It has been shown that not only the fertilized egg cell, but also isolated cells from a tissue, can grow and develop into a complete plant. This is already known about certain leaf cells which, upon regeneration, give rise to plantlets on the excised leaf. Therefore, if not all, at least a considerable number of cells in the body of a plant, when isolated, can give rise to a complete plant. However, as long as these cells are in contact with their neighboring cells in the intact plant, they do not exhibit their full potentialities but remain only a part of the whole. This means that there is a controlling mechanism inside the plant which integrates the individual cells, the tissues, and the organs into a complete organism.

It has been proved in a number of cases that the interrelations between the cells which mold them into an organism are brought about by minute amounts of chemicals produced in one part of the plant body which activate or inhibit other parts after the chemical has been transported to them. Such chemicals, produced in small amounts in one part of the body and regulating other parts, are called hormones. In animals most hormones are carried in the bloodstream; in plants they are transported through the living cells or in the transpiration stream.

A cell that is completely self-sufficient, producing all the organic substances it needs for growth and metabolism, cannot be part of an organism. Many unicellular algae grow in this way, although they may develop into irregular masses of cells (colonies) with or without specific shape.

In yeast, a slight modification of this growth pattern exists. These cells can grow provided the concentration of some of the substances they produce themselves, such as biotin and thiamin, is high enough in the liquid in which they grow. Thus, a single cell of yeast will not grow by itself, but is dependent on many other cells in its surroundings. Once enough biotin and thiamin is produced by all the cells, they will start to grow collectively. *See* YEAST.

An organism results when part of the cells have lost the ability to produce certain essential substances which are still produced by other cells of the same organism. This is perhaps best illustrated in the case of root growth.

When a root tip 1 cm long is cut off a tomato plant and placed aseptically in a medium consisting of a 2% sugar solution to which the necessary mineral salts are added, such a root tip will grow only a small amount. But when thiamin in a concentration of 1 part in 100,000,000 is added to the medium, growth is rapid. Tips of the cultured root, when cut off and placed in fresh medium, will also continue to grow. Therefore, this medium contains all that is necessary for continued root growth. In the normal plant the salts are supplied by the soil, the sugar by the photosynthesizing leaves, and the thiamin by the younger leaves. The roots cannot grow faster than the production of sugar and thiamin in the leaves allows and, as a result, balanced growth occurs. *See* PHOTOSYNTHESIS.

In all excised roots investigated, the addition of thiamin is essential for continued growth. In other roots additional substances, such as vitamin B_6 and niacin, are also essential. Thus, thiamin satisfies the definition of a plant hormone, and vitamin B_6 and niacin may also be hormones in such cases as pea roots. *See* VITAMIN.

Many other hormones are involved in the growth of a flowering plant. For example, if the stem tip is cut off, the stem underneath stops growing in length. But when the stem tip is replaced, or when auxin, the stem-growth hormone, is applied instead of the stem tip, growth of the stem is resumed. The amounts of auxin produced by the stem tip and required for normal growth of the stem itself are infinitesimal (about 10^{-6} mg) and this places auxin in the category of hormones. *See* AUXIN.

Growth correlations. A number of the correlations which exist in plants and which are usually influenced by hormones are shown in Fig. 1. Young leaves grow because purines, such as adenine, are supplied to them by mature leaves. Similarly an unknown growth factor, produced by roots, is essential for stem growth. It is not known where gibberellin or kinetin (a plant hormone) fit into this scheme, but it is clear that the growth of the different plant organs is intimately interrelated

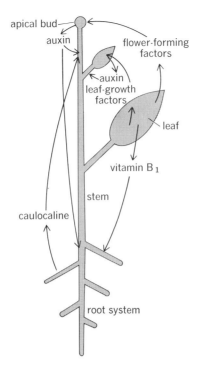

Fig. 1. Schematic drawing of a plant with root system, stem, old and young leaf, and apical bud, showing correlations for some known growth factors. Sugar interrelations not shown. (*From F. R. Moulton, ed., The Cell and Protoplasm, Science Press, 1940*)

through the need of some plant parts for substances produced in other parts of the plant. Often these substances are simple compounds, and may be effective by being prosthetic groups of enzymes, and these enzymes could not function without such groups. *See* GIBBERELLIN.

In an unexpectedly large number of cases, correlations in plants are produced by auxin, a simple substance first discovered as the plant-growth hormone which causes elongation of cells. Another substance has been found, gibberellin, which more spectacularly influences elongation of stems, leaf stalks, and leaves. It is present in plant organs, but its role in normal growth has not been established.

Other correlations affected by auxin are (1) control of lateral bud inhibition by the apical bud; (2) prevention of abscission of leaf petioles or of peduncles of flowers; (3) root formation at the basal end of cuttings; (4) tissue growth and induction of cancerous growth; (5) induction of xylem elements in regenerating vascular bundles; and (6) production of parthenocarpic fruits.

To explain how auxin can take part in so many reactions and can control so many correlations, it has been assumed that auxin controls one master reaction involved in each of the above-mentioned processes. This master reaction has been variously assumed to be a change in cellular permeability, a step in cellular respiration, a synthetic process, or a stimulation of translocation of other substances, but no universal master reaction has been found. Researchers are still looking for the mechanism of each of the above-mentioned processes.

Embryonic growth. After fertilization of the egg cell by one of the sperms produced by the generative nucleus of the pollen tube, the resulting zygote

starts to develop. This occurs either immediately after fertilization, as in most rapidly developing seeds, or after a delay of several months, as in the case of pines. During the first 5–10 cell divisions an undifferentiated mass of more or less globular tissue is produced within the endosperm. In some seeds, such as those of orchids, development does not proceed immediately beyond this point. Even after germination of orchid seeds, the globular cell mass continues to grow evenly in all directions until a body one to several millimeters in diameter is produced, which is called the protocorm. Differentiation of stem and root is delayed until the protocorm has reached this size, which takes several months.

In most plants the undifferentiated cell mass derived from the zygote proceeds directly to differentiate into an embryo consisting of a growing stem tip bearing two or more leaf primordia at one end and a root primordium at the other. Food for the growth and differentiation of the embryo is supplied by the mother plant either directly from the cotyledons, or indirectly by means of the endosperm. It has been found that the fully developed embryo can be excised and cultivated aseptically on a medium containing sugar and mineral salts. However, an immature embryo needs in addition small amounts of organic nutrients, such as vitamins. A still smaller embryo in which only the beginning of the cotyledons is indicated will not grow when excised unless it is supplied with coconut milk, a very rich source of organic nutrients since it is a liquid endosperm itself.

As soon as the embryo inside the seed is fully grown, it passes into a dormant condition which is broken only upon germination. The embryo differs from all other developmental stages of the plant most remarkably in its ability to withstand almost complete dehydration, a conditions which causes death at any other stage in the life of the higher plant.

Vegetative meristematic activity. The stem primordium of the embryo, upon germination of the seed, immediately becomes the growing stem tip which continues to produce more stem cells and leaf primordia. There is a remarkable control of the cell divisions in this growing point and the sequence of leaves follows a perfect order (phyllotaxis) which in its regularity compares with that of the structure of a crystal.

Little is known about control of the cell divisions in the growing point. In general, long days are usually required to keep the cells dividing in this growing point, especially in shrubs and trees of temperate regions. It has not been possible to change the growth pattern of the stem growing point, or apical meristem, with chemicals. Micrurgy, the science of microdissection, has shown that the youngest leaf primordia have an influence on the location of the subsequent primordia. This means that the cells of the growing point, although remarkably autonomous in their growth, are to some extent dependent upon each other. This is perhaps best indicated by the existence of sectorial and periclinal chimeras (mixed organisms). When two different plant species are grafted together, a new plant combining the properties of both occasionally develops on the junction of their tissues. This happens when a new growing point regenerates at the graft union which is made up of cells of both species. If the two halves of the growing point are different, a plant results in which the two species are joined lengthwise. An example of such a sectorial chimera is shown in Fig. 2. Although there is a considerable difference in size and growth rate between the two species composing this sectorial chimera—for example, a nightshade and a tomato—when in direct contact with each other, the cells in the growing point and all along the stem grow and act in unison; that is, they divide and elongate at exactly the same rate.

Perhaps even more remarkable are the periclinal chimeras. They have been studied in greatest detail in the case of nightshade and tomato. Occasionally a bud develops on the graft union of these two species that produces a plant in which the characters of both species are perfectly blended and in which the leaves, flowers, and fruits are intermediate between the two species in size, form, and color. No actual fusion of the nuclei of the two species has occurred; this is shown by the fact that a seed produced by these intermediate forms develops either into a nightshade or a tomato plant. Through chromosome counts and other evidence it was found that in these periclinal chimeras the different layers of tissue, such as the epidermis, the cortex, and the central cylinder (stele), belong to the two different species. Either the epidermis or the epidermis and cortex belong to one species, while either the cortex and central cylinder or the central cylinder alone belong to the other species. This is possible because in the growing point there are three layers of cells: the dermatogen, which gives rise to the epidermis; the periblem, which produces the cortical cells (outside the pericycle); and the plerome, which gives rise to all the cells of the center (stele) of the stem from the pericycle inward. All four possible periclinal chimeras between nightshade and tomato have been obtained in extensive grafting experiments. Such periclinal chimeras are also known combining hawthorne and *Mespilus*, and between *Cytisus* and *Laburnum*, and in each case intermediate forms are produced. This means that all cells and tissues influence each other during their stages of growth so that each partakes of the form and size of the other. In general, the cells produced by the periblem have the greatest effect on the final shape of leaves and flowers.

Similar periclinal chimeras were produced in *Datura* by colchicine treatment of the growing point. This causes formation of tetraploid cells. When only the dermatogen or periblem or plerome cells of the growing point are tetraploid, and the others are normally diploid, periclinal chimeras are formed in which the difference in cell size does not result in distorted plants but gives rise to harmonious structures.

Occasionally a growing point enlarges beyond its normal size. This can be stimulated by auxin treatments. It then gives rise to fasciated (flattened and malformed) stems with abnormal phyllotaxis (leaf arrangement on the stem).

The stem growing point can be cultured in a test tube by placing it on an agar medium containing sugar and salts. It will then develop into a stem with leaves which, upon regeneration of roots, will become a complete plant. Growing points of mono-

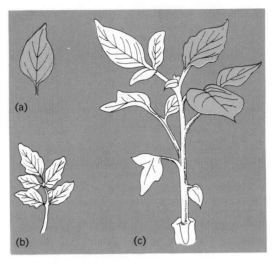

Fig. 2. An example of a sectorial chimera. (a) Leaf of black nightshade (*Solanum nigrum*). (b) Leaf of tomato (*Solanum lycopersicium*). (c) Base shows tomato stem into which a wedge of nightshade tissue was grafted. Following combination of the two tissues, a shoot developed which consisted of nightshade tissue (right) and tomato tissue (left). (*After Winkler*)

cotyledons and ferns (neither of which regenerate easily) are easier to culture than growing points of dicotyledons (which have a much greater capacity for regeneration).

In addition to the apical meristems the plant has lateral meristems called the cambium, the cork cambium and the adventitious growing points. It is known that the activity of the cambium is under the control of the buds and leaves of the plant. In deciduous trees divisions in the cambium, giving rise to phloem and xylem cells, start as soon as the buds become active in spring. During the period of bud opening and young-leaf expansion, the elements of the spring wood are formed. Later the presence of mature leaves causes the cambium to produce summer wood with smaller cells, thicker cell walls, and often fewer vessels. This periodicity in cambial activity gives rise to the annual xylem rings in the wood. This is not an autonomous periodicity, for when the leaves are removed the cambial activity stops. If in the same year more buds and leaves develop, new spring wood is produced, followed by summer wood, and an extra complete annual ring is formed.

Auxin application to a stem can stimulate cambial activity in the same way that growing buds and young leaves do. Therefore, it is likely that the spring wood is formed under the influence of auxin coming from the buds and young leaves. Actually, it has been found that the auxin production of these growing plant parts shows the same cycle as that of cambial activity. Also, in most cases cambial activity starts in the younger branches and is followed by cambial growth in the trunk, with a time lag that approximates the rate of auxin transport from buds through branches to the stem base.

Cambium cells have been grown in a test tube. In most cases, however, they regenerate undifferentiated callus cells, indicating that the stimulus for cambial growth is normally more complex than merely an auxin supply. This is also indicated by the periodic changes in the cells differentiating from the cambium. For example, in a rubber tree, *Hevea*, at intervals of 1–4 months, a layer of latex vessels is produced in the phloem, alternating with layers of sieve tubes and other phloem elements; and in the xylem of members of the plant family Sapotaceae layers of wood parenchyma alternate with layers of vessels and fibers.

REPRODUCTIVE GROWTH

Reproduction in plants can either be sexual or vegetative (asexual). Some reproduction mechanisms in higher plants are discussed here.

In plants such as *Ficaria*, some lilies, or *Hydrocharis*, many axillary buds swell and store food in their bud scales. These buds may then become detached and behave like seeds; that is, when conditions become favorable, these buds start to grow and form new plants. In *Hydrocharis* or *Stratiotes* the buds are formed in autumn, as a response to the shortening of the days, and they "germinate" only after having been subjected to cold during winter. In many bulbous plants, such as tulips, hyacinths, daffodils, and onions, reproduction is mostly vegetative. The bulb consists of a markedly foreshortened stem on which thick scale leaves are implanted, and when completely developed, the stem usually ends in a flower. Toward the end of the season, two or more axillary buds on the foreshortened stem develop into new bulbs. This causes the clustering of bulbs on these plants. When the scale leaves of these bulbs are halved by cutting off the upper half, a large number of adventitious buds may form on the cut surface, each one producing a tiny bulb which can grow into another plant. *See* PHOTOPERIODISM IN PLANTS.

In a number of plants, thickened buds, or bulblets, are formed in place of flowers. Some plants, such as *Polygonum viviparum*, reproduce entirely in this way. In others, such as *Agave*, only occasionally do flowers fail to develop, but the flowers are replaced by such vegetative bulblets. The factors causing this transformation are unknown.

Very peculiar forms of vegetative reproduction exist in the genus *Bryophyllum*. The Madagascarian species *B. tubiflorum* and *B. daigremontianum* produce, under long-day conditions, adventitious buds in the notches of the teeth of their leaves. When they have formed their first two pairs of leaves, these buds drop off, root, and form new plants. In *B. calycinum* these buds are formed in the leaf notches only after the leaf is cut off.

A large number of plants, for example, iris and lotus, form rootstocks which branch and form aboveground shoots at their apices. As the older portion of the rootstock dies, the original plant becomes divided into a number of individual rootstocks and consequently multiplies. When the rhizomes remain aboveground, they are called runners. Strawberries and many grasses multiply this way. Runner formation in the strawberry is strictly a long-day response and occurs at higher temperatures.

In potatoes underground runners enlarge at the end producing tubers. This tuber formation is the result of a stimulus (or perhaps hormone) which comes from the shoot and is produced only at low temperature or in short days. This stimulus can pass through a graft union. The tubers which are formed are dormant, and to sprout require either a chemical treatment with ethylene chlorohydrin or several months of dormancy at room temperature. This ensures vegetative reproduction: the plants survive the cold winter as dormant tubers and new shoots develop the next spring. In many other plants, such as dahlia and sweet potato, roots swell in the same manner as the underground shoot tips of the potato and growing points on these roots develop into new shoots the following season.

Many agricultural crops are reproduced vegetatively. In addition to potatoes, sweet potatoes, and strawberries there is sugarcane, which grows from stem cuttings. A cutting is a piece of stem with one or more nodes, which, when placed under suitable conditions (moist, usually partly buried in soil, sand, or peat), will produce roots and shoots so that a complete plant results. Many other plants, such as Lombardy poplar and many shrubs and trees grown by horticulturists, are propagated by cuttings. The roots which develop on these cuttings either arise from preformed root primordia, present near the node, as in sugarcane, or are new formations, mostly near the basal cut end of the cutting. This root formation is an expression of the tendency of a part of a plant to regenerate lost organs. The hormones necessary for root formation and root growth are formed in the shoots and usually flow downward to the roots. When this downward transport is interrupted by cutting the stem, these hormones accumulate near the cut surface where they stimulate new formation of roots. It was found that in the majority of cases the stimulus for root formation coming from the plant top can be replaced by auxin; thus, auxin application at the base of the cutting is very commonly practiced by horticulturists to ensure good rooting. The auxin in most instances speeds up rooting on a large proportion of the cuttings. In some cases vitamins and amino acids were also found to stimulate root formation. *See* AMINO ACIDS.

In cases in which cuttings will not root, plants may be propagated by layering or budding.

Floral initiation and development. At a certain moment in the development of a vegetative growing point, the regular sequence of vegetative cell divisions is interrupted and the growing point is transformed into a flower primordium. This change is induced by a stimulus received by the leaves and transmitted through the phloem of the stem. When a purely vegetative scion is grafted on a photoperiodically induced stock, the scion will under certain conditions, such as the removal of the larger leaves from scion, start to flower. *See* GRAFTING OF PLANTS.

Morphologically, the first change in the transformed growing point is a broadening. Then, instead of the regular leaf phyllotaxis, the sepals are laid down simultaneously, usually in a whorl. After a time interval of a few days, another whorl of primordia, the petals, is formed. Then the stamens and carpels are produced. In exceptional cases this sequence is partly reversed; for example, in the case of inflorescences the flower primordia are produced acropetally (from the base upward) or basipetally (from the apex downward) on the large meristematic dome.

The initiation of flower primordia is not exclusively under the control of the photoperiod. In many cases, such as beet and peach, flower initiation occurs only after a cold treatment called vernalization. This is an induction phenomenon, but there may be an interval of one or several months between exposure to cold and transformation of the growing point. When the plant is subjected to high temperatures during this induction period, occasionally devernalization occurs with resultant nonflowering. In many plants, such as deciduous trees, coffee, and the dove-orchid (*Dendrobium crumenatum*), the flower buds develop only to a certain size and then become dormant. It takes exposure to relatively low temperatures to break the dormancy of these buds. In peaches, pears, and other deciduous trees the buds need a period of weeks or months below 40°F before they will open. This means that they have to pass through a winter for best flowering. In the dove-orchid a rapid cooling of 80°–65°F will make the dormant flowerbuds enlarge, and exactly 9 days later they open. In coffee the first heavy rain of the season usually triggers the flowerbud development, and 8 days later all trees which have received the rain are festooned with flowers.

Flower biology. The opening and closing of flowers and the process of pollination is a fascinating field of study. Whereas many flowers, such as roses, camellias, snapdragons, and orchids, open only once and then remain open for the rest of their lives, many other flowers, such as tulips, poppies, tobacco, and gazania, open and close several times with a daily rhythm. On clear days the California poppy opens its flowers at 10 A.M., and the petals close again at 4 P.M. Also on clear days, the tobacco plant *Nicotiana affinis* opens its flowers at sunset and closes them the next morning at 9 A.M. The flower movements of the California poppy are induced by the light-dark change of the previous day; they close 21 hr after the previous sunset. The flowers of the night-blooming cactus open 24 hr after darkening on the previous day. Tulips and crocuses open upon a rise in temperature and close again upon cooling; gazania flowers open above 18°C and close below this temperature. These responses to light and temperature are so regular that the time of day or the air temperature can be told fairly accurately by observing which flowers are open or closed. It is actually possible to use flowers as clocks. Carolus Linnaeus, the great Swedish botanist, planted part of his garden as a flower clock.

The life of flowers varies from a fraction of a day to a month or more. There are several factors which control the life span. In many flowers the petals are abscised (dropped), as in poppies and pelargoniums; in others they wilt, as in cacti and orchids. Wilting is the result of loss of vitality of the cells of the petals either because their sugars have been respired, as in *Chrysanthemum*, or because their proteins have decomposed, as in cacti. In others, such as orchids, the auxin released by the pollinia causes wilting. *See* PROTEIN.

Most flowers have mechanisms for cross pollination; many are actually self-sterile. Sterility in flowers may be the result of a large number of factors, such as genetic block (especially in triploids and others where abnormal meiosis occurs), lack of germination of pollen, insufficient growth in length of pollen tubes, as in the long styles of *Oen-*

othera or corn, or lack of chemotropism (attraction of the pollen tubes to the ovules).

Pollination is most commonly effected by flying insects which are attracted to the flowers by color or smell. In many flowers the development of odor is periodic. In the night-blooming jasmine and in tobacco, the flowers open at sunset and at the same time become fragrant; the odor disappears again the following morning at about the time the flowers close. These flowers are pollinated by night-flying moths. Other pollinators are ants, hummingbirds, or bats.

A large group of plants, such as ragweed, grasses, conifers, and trees with male flowers in catkins, is pollinated by the wind; flowers of this group are usually inconspicuous. Their pollen, which is discharged in large amounts, is a major cause of hay fever.

Pollination by mechanical means is sometimes required when the pollen does not readily come out of the anthers, for example, the shaking of the flowers of tomato. Very rare are cases of pollination by water (the male flowers of *Vallisneria* float on the water and thus their open anthers come in contact with the stigmata of the female flowers). In a few cases the pollen is ejected by the snapping open of the flowers, as in *Pilea*.

Most interesting are the honey-excreting nectaries. These are usually found at the base of the flower or in spurs (over 1 ft long in *Angraecum sesquipedale*), or sometimes outside the flower on bracts, as in the plant family Marcgraviaceae or in the genus *Euphorbia*. This honey is excreted by special glandular cells or it is pressed out of the phloem. The pollen in insect-pollinated flowers is usually sticky because it is covered with a waxlike material.

Many flowers show marked movements before opening or after pollination, for example, poppies and *Linaria*. These movements are usually due to differential growth of the two sides of the flower stalk caused by auxin.

Fruit development. Auxin plays a very important role in the growth of the ovary after pollination. The pollen itself provides the auxin, or the auxin is produced in the fertilized ovules. An ovary of a nonpollinated flower usually does not enlarge, but if treated with auxin it may produce parthenocarpic fruits, such as seedless tomatoes or watermelons. In the naturally parthenocarpic fruit of the navel orange, the pulp in the developing fruit provides the auxin necessary for growth. Auxin application will only lead to the formation of parthenocarpic fruit at low temperatures; during the middle of summer it has no effect.

If every flower grew into a fruit, most plants would not be able to support the crop. However, many flowers drop off before fruits start to grow and some of the growing fruits also fall. Auxin sprays are sometimes effective in preventing fruit drop; at present such sprays are generally applied to prevent the preharvest drop of apples.

As a fruit grows its total respiration increases until it is almost ripe, then respiration decreases. In some fruits, for example, the avocado, a so-called climacteric rise in respiration occurs when the carbon dioxide production more than doubles just prior to the fully ripe stage; however, this happens only after the fruit is picked off the tree.

DOMINANCE AND GERMINATION

Every leaf carries a bud in its axil which can grow into a shoot with leaves and buds. Each of these buds in its turn has the potential of growing into a leafy shoot. Should this happen, the plant would soon become an inextricable clump of branches. Although it does not occur naturally, there are certain diseases which cause all the axillary buds to grow. For example, a fungus causes the development of masses of small branches called witches' brooms in trees.

Apical dominance. In a normal plant only a small percentage of the axillary buds grow into shoots. When, for one reason or another, the apical bud ceases growth, a few axillary buds lower down the stem will develop. This suppressing effect of the apical bud on lateral or axillary buds is called apical dominance. For some time it was suspected that the apical bud exerted its influence through the production of a hormonelike substance. After auxin was discovered to be the stem-elongation hormone produced in the stem tip, it was also shown to be the material produced by the apical bud that is responsible for inhibition of axillary bud growth. Removal of the apical bud releases this inhibition, but replacement of the apical bud with an adequate auxin supply restores the lateral bud inhibition. However, only a few hours' interruption of the auxin supply releases the lateral bud inhibition irreversibly.

Apical dominance has many interesting characteristics. For instance, the inhibition increases with distance from the tip and the buds farthest removed from the apical bud are most inhibited, whereas the buds nearest to it have the best chance for development. Upon removal of the apical bud, the uppermost axillary buds start to grow; once they start growing they inhibit buds farther down from the stem tip.

In nature conditions occur in which the basal buds grow more than those nearer the apex. For example, after a warm winter peaches show delayed foliation; that is, the apical buds fail to open in spring and buds lower down the stems are the only ones which grow.

Many hypotheses have been offered to explain the mechanism of auxin action in lateral bud inhibition. The direct-action hypothesis states that this is merely a matter of auxin concentration; at low concentration auxin accelerates stem growth; at high concentration it inhibits growth. However, this does not account for the all-or-none nature of inhibition. Besides, it has been shown that it is not the total amount of auxin, but the relative amounts in bud and stem that control growth. Only when the auxin concentration in the bud exceeds that in the adjacent stem is bud growth possible. In a somewhat different light, the hypotheses of indirect action assume that auxin releases inhibitors, or controls transport of other essential growth factors.

Apical dominance can appear in other ways. In conifers the perpendicular growth of the primary shoot is called orthotropic, whereas all lateral shoots grow more or less horizontally, or plagiotropically. When the apex is removed, or the apical bud is injured, one or more of the higher side-branches will become orthotropic and take over the vertical position and function of the original apical bud. This occurs in pines and firs, but in *Araucaria* the plagiotropic growth of the lateral shoots is not a response to the dominance of the apical bud, for they remain plagiotropic even in the absence of an apical bud.

Bud dormancy. As explained previously, because of the correlative inhibition established by the growth of the apical bud, the majority of buds do not grow. As soon as this correlative inhibition is removed, some of the axillary buds begin to grow, usually within a few days. Many buds, however, do not start to grow when the growing conditions become favorable and when apical dominance is removed. Such buds are dormant. Dormant buds occur on most deciduous plants in winter.

When a lilac, oak, or peach branch is cut off a plant growing outside and brought into a greenhouse, the buds will not develop between October and February. In April, or even in early summer, these plants have nondormant buds, and they start to grow as soon as the branches are removed and the cut ends put in a moist medium. Dormancy of the buds is induced by the short-day light exposure of the branches in autumn. When such deciduous trees are kept throughout the summer under long-day conditions, their buds do not become dormant and they will develop at any time when the temperature is favorable and the correlative inhibition is removed.

Induced bud dormancy can be broken in several ways. In nature it is done by exposure for several months to near-freezing temperatures. Peach or pear trees brought into the greenhouse in late summer or autumn are dormant, and they can remain dormant for more than a year because the buds have not been exposed to cold. The bud itself must be kept cold. On a branch which has been partially cooled, only the buds on the cooled part develop.

In a number of cases chemical treatment can substitute for the cold requirement, and ether or ethylene chlorohydrin vapors as well as nitrophenol and ethylene have been used to break bud dormancy. Chemical treatments have the advantage of requiring only a few days in contrast to the cold exposure which must last weeks or months.

Bulbs and tubers commonly have to go through a dormant period before they can sprout. In some cases this is a question of straight dormancy (gladiolus, potato, and lily-of-the-valley) which cold or ethylene chlorohydrin will break. Other cases will be discussed below in the section on seasonal thermoperiodicity.

Germination. In the section on embryonic growth the formation of the seed was described, and it was stated that upon ripening, the seed passes into a dormant condition from which it emerges upon germination.

The seed represents a stage in the development of a plant which is particularly resistant to cold, heat, and drought. The main function of a seed is to provide for progeny by carrying the plant over unfavorable conditions and facilitating distribution of the species.

In germination three distinct stages can be distinguished. The first stage is the intake of water, and is completed when all cell walls and protoplasts have sufficient water content. Associated with the water uptake is an increase in respiration. The second stage is a curious one. Except for respiration no measurable changes occur; the embryo does not enlarge; and the seed seems to be in a condition of suspended animation. During these first two stages germination is a reversible process; the seeds can be dried and rewetted a number of times without any effect on their future germinability. Large numbers of seeds persist in the soil for years or even decades without reaching the third stage – actual enlargement of the embryo. However, once this third stage has set in, there is no holding back and the embryo either dies or grows to form the seedling.

The second stage, that of suspended animation, is the most critical because it is the period when it is decided whether the seed will germinate or not; it is an all-or-none process. No matter how long or short this second stage of germination is, once the inhibition has been released, growth of the seedling will always be the same.

Some of the mechanisms involved in preventing growth of the embryo and the events occurring during the second stage of germination can now be discussed.

Some seeds contain substances which inhibit germination. When such inhibitors are removed, either by decomposition or by leaching, embryo growth proceeds normally. In at least one seed, *Amaranthus*, and probably in many others, such inhibitors also repress respiration. Thus, *Amaranthus* seeds can be kept for many years in moist soil without germinating or utilizing all their storage food.

In other seeds the seed coats, or certain layers of them, are impermeable either to water or to oxygen. Breaking (scarifying) of such impermeable layers leads to germination.

In many leguminous seeds in which the seed coat is so hard that the embryo cannot break through, scarification suffices for germination.

In the seeds of wild plants, a large number of mechanisms delay germination until the growing conditions for the seedling are favorable. Cultivated plants are not sown until the season is proper for germination and growth; consequently, germination delays are unnecessary and may be unfavorable. The germination behavior of seeds of cultivated and wild plants should be clearly distinguished.

Many seeds fail to develop and ripen under conditions which seem unusually favorable for germination, such as the moist interior of a melon or of a tomato fruit. In such species there are substances in the fruit pulp which inhibit germination. In exceptional cases, however, germinated seeds are found inside the fruit, for example, occasionally in oranges or peaches.

Some seeds of northern crop plants, such as barley and wheat, germinate at low temperatures and can be sown in autumn or early spring. Others, such as corn, sugarbeet, and tobacco, require higher temperatures and are sown much later in spring; or they are sown in greenhouses and the young seedlings are transplanted in the field, for example, tomato and chili pepper. The latter plants originated in warm climates and grow only during the summer.

Seeds of tropical forest trees usually have a short life, and unless they germinate immediately, they decompose in the humus layer.

Many seeds which normally remain dormant during winter need stratification, that is, treatment with low temperatures (near freezing), before they will germinate. This treatment is effective only when the seeds are moist.

Most of the seeds which have inhibitors, hard or impermeable seedcoats, or need stratification before they can germinate, have normal embryos which will start to grow as soon as conditions are favorable. Other seeds have embryos which will not develop even when excised. Such embryos are either immature or have embryo dormancy. In both cases germination can occur after a sufficient period of waiting during which after-ripening (physiological change) takes place.

The seeds of many plants germinate very irregularly, only a few at a time. In this way germination is sometimes spread over a period of many years, with occasional peaks of germination at about yearly intervals.

Seed germination of desert plants has been studied in some detail. These seeds show a number of different mechanisms which prevent premature germination. When rains are few and far between, the chance that a small amount of rain will be augmented by another rain is slight. Under these conditions germination in desert plants would best be delayed until after 1 in. of rain has fallen continuously, and when the soil is sufficiently wetted to ensure normal development of the seedling. Some seeds have four or more mechanisms for delayed germination. Among these belong (1) presence of germination inhibitors which can be removed by leaching, as occurs during a heavy rain; (2) excess mineral salts in the seedcoat or in soil, also removed by heavy rain; (3) remains of fruit covering, which has to be removed before seed can germinate; and (4) hard seedcoat, which may be removed by scarification, usually by rubbing of the seeds with sand or stones; for example, after a heavy rain a slurry of water, sand, and gravel rushes down the wash carrying with it the seeds of smoke tree, palo verde, and other shrubs.

Growing plants have a strong inhibitory effect on seeds present in the soil around them. Germination of many plants does not occur in a closed vegetation. Interesting exceptions are seeds of parasitic or semiparasitic plants, such as *Striga* and *Euphrasia*. These seeds germinate only under the influence of excretions from the roots of their host plants. The reverse phenomenon is found for the guayule rubber plant (*Parthenium argentatum*), whose seedlings are killed by excretions, consisting partly of cinnamic acid, from the roots of the mature plants.

PERIODICITY AND ABSCISSION

There are relatively few plants whose growth is not periodic. Basically, all processes in the growing point are periodic; for example, the laying down of leaf primordia is cyclic and occurs in a definite sequence producing a specific phyllotaxy.

Growth periodicity. Each individual cell and each internode go through a succession of growth rates, the so-called grand period of growth. When

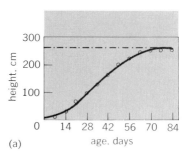

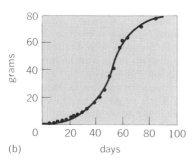

Fig. 3.   Graphs showing growth curves. (a) Growth in height of sunflower stem (*from E. P. Odum, Fundamentals of Ecology, Saunders, 1953*). (b) Growth of entire corn plant as measured by increase in dry weight (*from Gustav Backman after Stefanowska, in D. W. Thompson, On Growth and Form, Cambridge, 1942*).

the length of a cell or of an internode is recorded as a function of time, a sigmoid (S) curve is obtained, showing that after an initial slow start, growth increases to a maximal rate, and then gradually decreases (Fig. 3). This is typical for the individual cell, for a colony of cells, such as a bacterial or yeast culture, and even for a whole organism. Because a growing plant usually has the same number of dividing, growing, and maturing cells in its stem, the growth rate of a whole stem is regular and linear, always maintaining the same proportion of growing cells in its different stages. Thus, the regular growth rate of the whole plant is the integration of thousands of sigmoid growth curves of the individual cells.

As was explained in the section on dormancy, the periodicity of growth of a pear or peach tree is partially induced by the external conditions. But there is an inherent periodicity in growth of a number of plants, often based on the morphology of the plant. In tulips and other bulbous plants the growing point goes through a cycle of forming scale leaves, true leaves, and a flower. Because the flower terminates the growing point, a new axillary bud takes over and a new cycle is started. In the tomato plant the same phenomenon occurs. After forming 8–17 nodes (depending on the variety), the growing point transforms into a terminal flower. Then a lateral bud starts to grow, forms 2–4 nodes, and likewise terminates in a flower. Thus the tomato stem is a sympodium (many-forked), and a definite periodicity in development can be observed. In pines, peaches, and most other trees there is a sequence of formation of nodes bearing leaves and bud scales. Even if there is no cessation of growth when the bud with bud scales is formed, for example, because the bud did not become dormant as a response to short-day treatment, the cycle of scale and leaf formation is repeated several times per year, giving evidence of an internal growth periodicity.

Many cases of periodicity in development are induced by external factors. The daily fluctuation of growth rates of stems, roots, and leaves is due, at least in part, to the daily light-dark cycle, to the periodicity in temperature, or to the change in relative humidity from day to night. However, in the nyctinastic ("sleep") movements of leaves, there is also an autonomous component of growth periodicity which has a 24-hr cycle and becomes synchronized with the 24-hr climatic cycle.

Very curious periodicities are known in the flowering of orchids, coffee trees, and other plants. For example, the dove-orchid (*Dendrobium crumenatum*) flowers in the lowlands of Java once every few months, but all plants in the same locality flower on the same day. This was found to be the result of a sudden drop in temperature accompanying certain heavy rains.

The simultaneous flowering of all bamboo plants of a particular species every 11 or 33 years has tentatively been connected with the 11-year cycle in sunspots. But other plants, such as *Strobilanthes* in Ceylon and Java, flower simultaneously at 4- or 7-year intervals. Such periodicities seem to be of the same type as those of the 13- or 17-year cicada.

Typical yearly periodicities in growth and flowering are often induced by the yearly cycle of temperatures or photoperiods.

Abscission in plants. Because special tissues are produced between stem and leaf stalk, or between stem and fruit stalk, or at the base of petals, each plant does not remain burdened with its dying and dead leaves, flowers, or fruits (Fig. 4). These dead parts drop off (abscise) and are regenerated to carbon dioxide in the carbon cycle of nature, often before the whole plant has died and fallen to the ground. *See* ABSCISSION.

Although not much is known about how or why a leaf abscises, a great deal has been learned about how to stimulate or prevent abscission. The abscission layer at the base of the petiole is formed when the leaf blade is removed, or when the leaf is no longer active, as in autumn. The formation of this abscission layer can be delayed by applying auxin, or other substances with similar physiological activity, on the leaf stalk stump.

The reaction of the ovary and fruit is similar to that of the leaf. When the ovules in the ovary have not been fertilized, no auxin reaches the place of attachment of the fruit stalk to the stem, and the young fruit abscises. The lack of the inhibitory effect associated .with developing seeds can be rectified by auxin application to the ovary. This

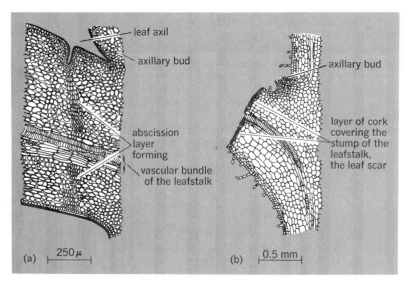

Fig. 4.   Abscission. (a) Longitudinal section through base of leaf of *Prunus*. Divisions of cells from an abscission layer, shown vertically. (b) Vertical section through part of a stem and leafbase of *Coleus* after abscission of leaf. (*From R. D. Gibbs, Botany, An Evolutionary Approach, Blakiston–McGraw-Hill, 1950*)

means that auxin production by the developing seeds has at least a dual function: causing the growth of the ovary, and preventing its abscission, as explained in the preceding section on fruit development.

There are several practical applications of these auxin effects. One is the spraying of ripening apples with auxins to prevent preharvest drop, and also to prevent bruising of the fruit as it falls on the ground. Another is the use of auxin sprays in tomato growing to prevent the flowers on the first clusters from dropping off, and to cause the continued growth of the young fruit.

In a number of flowers, fertilization causes abscission of all the flower parts except the ovary; this presumably is also connected with the auxin production by the developing ovules or by the auxin released by the pollen. The latter is the case in the postfloration phenomena in orchids. Instead of placing the pollinia on the stigma, auxin can be applied and will produce swelling of the ovary and wilting of the petals.

Mechanical cotton pickers work properly only when the cotton plants are leafless. Therefore, methods have been developed to defoliate cotton fields. This can be done either by killing the leaf blades, which will cause abscission of the petiole as though it had been debladed, or by applying abscisin or other antiauxin.

Not only petioles, but also whole branches may be dropped through the formation of an abscission layer. This occurs in *Castilloa* and *Sterculia*, and results in a self-pruning operation in which the older branches, shaded by the higher ones, are abscised.

Tissue culture in plants. Often, under the heading of tissue cultures the problem of organ culture is also considered. The growth of roots in cultures was discussed under the general heading of plant hormones, and the culture of growing points was treated under vegetative meristematic activity. Typical plant tissue cultures were achieved for the first time about 1938. When pieces of stem, root, or other organs are placed aseptically on an agar medium containing sugar and mineral nutrients, they either regenerate buds and roots and grow as a complete plant, or they produce a small mass of undifferentiated tissue called callus, which develops into a globular mass on top of the piece of stem. To make this globular mass of undifferentiated parenchyma cells grow to a larger mass, it is necessary to add auxin to the medium. *See* AUXIN.

Thus callus tissue, transplanted aseptically in a medium containing sugar, mineral salts, and auxin, will grow to a large mass of undifferentiated cells. This mass of callus can be subdivided into smaller pieces, and each piece will continue to grow equally well on this medium. Whereas this is the rule, occasionally a piece of such a callus culture will lose the requirement for auxin in the medium, and will then continue to grow on a medium containing only sugar and salts. This is called habituation, and makes these tissues less dependent upon their environment.

Usually plant tissues are completely dependent for growth upon the surrounding tissues and organs, and such tissues fail to grow when the adjacent parts become mature. An exception exists in the case of crown gall, an abnormal growth which

usually occurs near the root crown on stems. Crown gall is induced by *Bacterium tumefaciens* and it is largely a mass of callus. It is possible to keep the crown gall callus growing even when the bacteria have been eliminated because the callus tissue loses the requirement for auxin in the medium. It will grow in the same sugar-nutrient medium in which habituated cultures develop. Because of its independence of auxin, it has escaped the growth control of the plant. This explains why a crown gall develops.

A number of substances have been isolated and identified which increase growth of callus cells, usually manyfold. Many are present in coconut milk. Among them kinetin, or 6-furfuryl-aminopurine, has been investigated most extensively.

The most interesting development in tissue culture is that it has been found possible, by several different means, to make a single callus cell develop into a large callus mass, and to have this differentiate into a shoot and ultimately into a complete plant. Thus, a single undifferentiated cell has the potentiality of developing into the complete organism, just as the egg cell has.

Usually, no differentiation of tissues and organs occurs in a callus mass. Upon transplanting a piece of differentiated tissue into it, however, a differentiation of callus cells in the immediate vicinity of the transplant will occur.

THERMOPERIODICITY

Temperature influences most physiological processes. The optimal temperature is the temperature at which a process is fastest or most efficient. Above the optimal temperature, the rate of the process decreases, often rapidly, as a result of injury to the protoplasm. There is also a minimum temperature below which the process does not go on at all. In many cases this lowest temperature is 0°C or even slightly below freezing. Because of the osmotic value of the cell contents, cells do not freeze unless cooled to well below 0°C. Above the minimum temperature, the rate of the process increases rapidly, in an exponential manner, much as temperature influences the rate of chemical processes. This means that for every rise in temperature of 10°C, the rate of the process is doubled or tripled. The rate of the process at a given temperature divided by the rate at a temperature 10°C lower is called the temperature coefficient, or Q_{10}.

Seasonal thermoperiodicity. Many plants cannot develop normally in a constant temperature or when the daily temperature range is kept within the same limits. For example, sugarbeet plants kept every day at 23°C and every night at 17°C will continue to grow vegetatively for 3–4 years, after which time the base rots away. A peach tree can be kept for many years under the above-mentioned temperature regime without ever flowering. Tulip and hyacinth bulbs, planted in the even climate of the tropics, even at higher altitudes, will not develop normally, and will die in 1–2 years. All these plants will develop normally when they are subjected to a yearly cycle of low temperatures followed by high temperatures. This requirement is called seasonal thermoperiodicity.

In tulip and other bulbs, the seasonal thermoperiodicity has been investigated in great detail. Each developmental stage of the plant has its own optimal temperature. When the aboveground part of the tulip plant has died, the bulb is completely filled with storage food in the scale leaves, and the growing point has formed only a few leaf primordia. During the next few weeks, more leaf primordia and a flower primordium are produced. This process of morphogenesis has a relatively high temperature optimum of about 25°C. When the bulbs are subsequently kept at that temperature, very little else will happen. Although ultimately a few weak leaves may appear, the flowerstalk never elongates. To make the plant develop normally the temperature must be lowered after the flower primordia have been initiated. By keeping the bulbs at 0°C, they can be stored for 6 months or longer without damage, following which they can be forced to flower, producing tulip flowers at any desired time.

At a somewhat higher temperature, 5–10°C, the bulbs still seem to remain dormant, but when they are brought to 13–17°C, they sprout rapidly. This does not happen in bulbs kept at 0°C. It is evident that pretreatment at 5–10°C for 1–2 months is essential for later growth. Thus 5–10°C is a delayed optimum in which the effect becomes apparent some time after the treatment.

After the 5–10°C treatment, the initial optimal temperature for stem elongation is about 13°C until flower opening, when it shifts to 17°C. In this way the following sequence of optimal temperatures has been found for tulip development, each lasting 1–2 months: 25°, 5–10°, 13°, and 17°C. A period of blooming and photosynthesis follows, after which the same temperature sequence must be repeated.

For hyacinths the optimal temperature sequence is 34°, 25°, 13°, 21°C. In this plant each temperature is also connected with a specific phase of development. Therefore, these bulbs must pass through a sequence of different temperatures to allow the various morphogenetic and physiological processes to take place. In a tropical climate with constant temperature, the bulbs do not pass through such a sequence and hence the plants do not develop normally. In a temperate climate with the proper yearly cycle of temperatures, the bulbs not only develop properly but also become synchronized with the climate.

A large number of plants in temperate climates have to pass through a cycle of high-low-high temperatures within a period of about 1 year before they develop normally. In beets, carrots, and other biennial plants, a low-temperature period is necessary before flower initiation can occur later at higher temperatures. In deciduous trees the lower temperatures are necessary for later flower initiation, and for breaking of bud dormancy.

Daily thermoperiodicity. Practically everywhere in the world the temperature during the day exceeds that during night. Plants grow better when subjected to such a daily temperature fluctuation than when exposed to a constant temperature. From the limited information available, a 6°C temperature differential between day and night seems to be optimal. In desert plants this optimal differential seems to be higher; in some tropical plants it may be lower.

Only part of the explanation of this phenomenon lies in the different processes which predominate in the plant in darkness and in light, each with its own optimal temperature. In the tomato plant, for instance, most growth occurs during the night at an optimal temperature of 17–18°C. During the day the optimal temperature is about 23°C, which coincides with the higher optimum of photosynthesis.

This explanation, however, accounts for only part of the daily thermoperiodicity. In most plants it seems that the autonomous 24-hr cycle is of paramount importance for normal development. If the internal cycle does not coincide with the period of the external cycle, or if there is no external cycle to synchronize the cyclic processes inside the plant, development slows down or becomes abnormal. Thus the daily temperature cycle and the light-dark cycle tend to steer development into normal channels. *See* PLANT PHYSIOLOGY.

[FRITS W. WENT]

Bibliography: W. Crocker, *Growth of Plants*, 1948; W. Crocker and L. V. Barton, *Physiology of Seeds*, 1953; A. C. Leopold, *Plant Growth and Development*, 1964; W. E. Loomis, *Growth and Differentiation in Plants*, 1953; F. W. Went, *Experimental Control of Plant Growth*, 1957; P. R. White, *Cultivation of Animal and Plant Cells*, 2d ed., 1963.

Plant hormones

A plant hormone, or phytohormone, is an organic compound that is synthesized in minute quantities in one part of a plant and translocated to another part, where it influences a specific physiological process. The term hormone is derived from the Greek word *hormaein*, which means "to step up." As the term was first used by both animal and plant scientists, it was intended to convey the idea of the action of a substance at a distance from the site of production. Two modifications have since been included: Hormones are naturally occurring substances, and only small amounts are needed to influence a physiological process. In animals, hormones are produced in the glands of the endocrine system and transported in the body fluid to definite target organs, so that the concept now embodied in the term evolved rather easily. This was not so in plants where definite sites of production and sites of action are more difficult to delineate, and where there is a complexity of interactions between the various regulators to control a physiological process. In plants, moreover, it was relatively easy to synthesize chemicals that would modify growth, so there was a tendency to call these chemicals hormones. However, the term hormone presently means essentially the same for botanists and zoologists, that is, a chemical messenger produced naturally in small amounts with the site of action different from the site of production. Historically, this chemical-messenger idea served both animal and plant experimenters well. In plants, chemical regulators of growth and reproduction have received a great deal of attention.

Physiological classification. Plants contain many chemically and physiologically distinct types of plant-regulatory substances, some of which properly can be called hormones. For example, auxins, gibberellins, cytokinins, and growth inhibitors are classes of plant regulators, some of which satisfy the criterion of being hormonal in nature. Thus only certain natural plant-regulatory substances are hormones, while synthetic chemicals with hormonelike action are not hormones. These natural and synthetic chemicals, which are not hormones, are referred to as plant regulators; or the term may be modified to designate the process affected, for example, plant growth regulator. This does not mean that synthetic or natural chemicals other than hormones cannot act as chemical messengers, but rather that hormones have certain characteristics that are not limited to physiological action.

Other classes of plant regulatory substances, for example, abscisin, dormin, florigen, and vitamins, can also be classified as hormones, and still other classes, for example, components of growth retardants and Vernalin, may prove to be hormonal in nature for some plants. Regulators are grouped primarily by the influence that the substances have on certain physiological processes. This is implied by the names of many of the groups; for example, abscisins regulate abscission; auxins regulate cell elongation; cytokinins influence cytokinesis and hence are involved in the regulation of cell division; dormins are involved in regulating dormancy; and florigen, one or possibly more than one substance since chemical identification has not been established for a member of this group, is involved in floral initiations.

Chemical classification. Since hormones and regulators are classified on the basis of a physiological action, a single chemical, or closely allied group of chemicals, can be classified several ways since they may influence more than one process, depending on various factors including interactions with other regulators. For example, in the isolation and identification of a hormone that was an abscisin and one that was a dormin both proved to be the same chemical. Ethylene, a simple gaseous hydrocarbon that has been known for years to have drastic effects on plants, is a fruit-ripening hormone for certain types of fruits, an abscisin because of its action on abscission, and a growth inhibitor because of its interaction with auxins on growth. To add complexity to classification by action is the observation that certain physiological processes depend on the interaction of several regulators, for example, the correlative development of a plant shoot. The correct intermeshing of a chemical and physiological classification will be forthcoming once the identity of the various chemical regulators and the mode of action are known.

Commercial uses. As the list of natural regulators continues to grow, it is reasonable to assume that it will ultimately be shown that plants contain many chemicals of a hormonal nature which interact to control growth and development. The increase in knowledge of hormones and other regulators will be used by man to modify plants and plant communities for his benefit. For example, some uses presently being made are auxins and growth inhibitors as herbicides; auxins and gibberellins to increase fruit set; gibberellins to stimulate the sprouting of buds; growth inhibitors to check the growth of buds; ethylene to hasten the ripening of fruits and to improve color development; cytokinins to increase the shelf life of vegetables; and growth retardants to dwarf plants. *See* ABSCISIC ACID; AGRICULTURAL SCIENCE (PLANT); AUXIN; CYTOKININ; GIBBERELLIN; HERBICIDE; PLANT GROWTH; PLANT PHYSIOLOGY.

[ROBERT H. BIGGS]

Bibliography: A. W. Galston, Regulatory systems in higher plants, *Amer. Sci.*, 55:144–160, 1967; A. C. Leopold, *Plant Growth and Development*, 1964; G. E. Nelson, G. G. Robinson, and R. A. Boolootian, *Fundamental Concepts of Biology*, 3d ed., 1974; G. Pincus and K. V. Thimann (eds.), *The Hormones*, vol. 4, 1964; J. Van Overbeck, Plant hormones and regulators, *Science*, vol. 152, 1966.

Plant physiology

The branch of botany which comprises knowledge of the processes which occur in plants. It is a fundamental tenet of physiology as a science that the usually complex processes occurring in living organisms can be resolved into the relatively simpler processes of physics and chemistry. The field of plant physiology therefore grades imperceptibly into the fields of plant biochemistry and plant biophysics. Much progress in elucidating the detailed mechanisms of the physiological processes that occur in plants has been achieved by using physical and chemical methods as tools of experimentation. No exception has ever been found in which plant processes do not operate in accordance with the fundamental principles of physics and chemistry.

All processes occurring in plants are subject to the dual control of the genetic factors inherent within a plant and the environmental factors to which it is subjected. The study of the effects of environmental factors upon physiological processes therefore often comes within the purview of plant physiology. In this area of knowledge plant physiology overlaps with the field of plant ecology in a borderline domain of knowledge which is often called physiological ecology.

The effects of genetic factors upon the physiology of plants are under implied consideration whenever the same process is studied comparatively for two different species of plants, or even different varieties of the same species. Differences in physiology between species are as much a reflection of their genetic differences as are their more obvious differences in external morphology. Genetic differences in physiology are often much more subtle than morphological differences; varieties of the same species, indistinguishable morphologically or nearly so, often differ to a marked degree in their physiology.

Investigations of the mechanism whereby specific genetic factors—the genes of the chromosomes—influence physiological processes involves precise probing into the metabolic pathways within cells and into the patterns of enzymatic activity which control such pathways. This subdivision of biology is often called physiological genetics. No sharp boundary can be drawn, however, between this realm of knowledge and the realm of plant physiology.

An intimate relation exists between the cellular structure of a plant and the processes which occur in it. This relationship is a dual one. The organs and tissues of a plant originate as a result of growth, which is itself a complex of coordinated physiological processes. Once materialized, however, the organization of a cell or the cellular structure of a given tissue or organ may have marked effects on the manner in which continuing physiological processes proceed within it. Process and structure are inseparable facets of the phenomenon of growth in plants. *See* PHOTOSYNTHESIS; PLANT, MINERAL NUTRITION OF; PLANT, WATER RELATIONS OF; PLANT GROWTH; PLANT HORMONES; PLANT RESPIRATION.

[BERNARD S. MEYER]

Plant translocation of organic solutes

The transport of organic compounds through plant vascular tissues over a considerable distance. In tree species translocation distances often exceed 100 ft.

The process of organic translocation is necessary for survival in higher land plants in which specialized organs of synthesis and utilization are separated by a considerable distance. In general the movement occurs from a place of supply or production, such as the leaves, to a place of use or storage, such as the shoot apex or roots. Sources of translocated organic material include products of photosynthesis, nitrogenous compounds formed in the roots, and materials moving out of senescing leaves. The ability to move organic materials at a high velocity over a long distance depends on the presence of structurally adapted vascular tissue.

Importance of conductive tissues. The relative importance of phloem and xylem tissues as conducting channels in organic translocation is a function of the nature of the organic compound transported and, more significantly, the site of origin of the compound in the plant. Quantitatively, the most important compounds translocated in plants are sucrose, certain closely related sucrose-galactose oligosaccharides, such as stachyose, and sugar alcohols, such as mannitol and sorbitol. Smaller quantities of amino acids and organic phosphate compounds may be translocated. These compounds are transported predominantly in the phloem both acropetally and basipetally, that is, in the direction of the shoot tips and root tips, respectively. Numerous ringing experiments have been conducted in which the continuity of the phloem is interrupted by removal of a narrow ring of tissue external to the xylem. These experiments demonstrate that xylem tissue plays no significant role in the conduction of sugars. *See* OLIGOSACCHARIDE.

Sugar transport in phloem. The importance of phloem in the translocation of sugars has been established by data from ringing experiments and radiochemical assays and by the analysis of sieve-tube exudate. Chromatographic analyses of sieve-tube exudate collected from an incision in the bark (Fig. 1) or from a severed stylet of phloem-feeding aphids (Fig. 2) have contributed greatly to the knowledge of sugar transport. Although the sieve-tube sap obtained by incision or aphid stylet is probably not identical with the contents of the undisturbed sieve tube, it does give data consistent with radiochemical experiments and gives a valid picture of the compounds in transit. The organic components of sieve-tube sap consist of 10–25% sugar by weight with less than 1% amino acids and possibly traces of sugar phosphates. Although glucose and fructose are frequently abundant throughout the plant, they are much less readily translocated than sucrose. Analysis of sieve-tube sap from many different species of plants reveals a consistent absence of hexose sugars with the occasional presence of the sugar alcohols mannitol or sorbitol. Only the nonreducing oligosaccharides of the raffinose family have been found: sucrose, raffinose, stachyose, and verbascose. These sugars

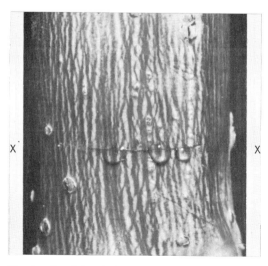

Fig. 1. Droplets of sieve-tube sap exuding from a phloem incision which was made at the level X-X in the bark of a box elder (*Acer negundo*). (*From C. A. Swanson, in F. C. Steward, ed., Plant Physiology: A Treatise, vol. 2, Academic, 1959*)

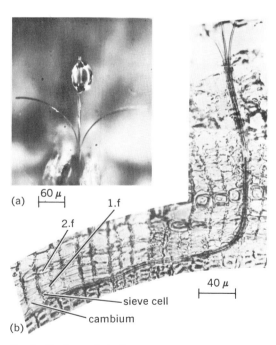

(a) ⊢ 60 μ ⊣
1.f
2.f
40 μ ⊢───┤
— sieve cell
— cambium
(b)

Fig. 2. Findings of studies on a phloem-feeding aphid. (*a*) Droplet of sieve-tube sap exuding from severed proboscis of aphid *Eupressobium juniperi*. (*b*) Cross section through a 2-year-old twig of juniper (*Juniperus communis*) showing the path of penetration of the stylets which terminate in a young sieve cell; 1.f and 2.f are the first and second bands of bast fibers. (*From R. Kollmann and I. Dörr, Z. Pflanzenphysiol., 55(2):131–141, 1966*)

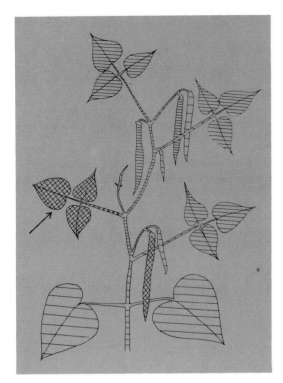

Fig. 3. Distribution of radioactive products of photosynthesis in a bean plant. Arrow indicates leaf supplies with C¹⁴O₂. Density of hatching indicates amount of radioactivity present as determined by autoradiography. (*From H. Wanner and R. Bachofen, Planta, 57:531, 1961*)

form a series consisting of sucrose with one, two, or three galactose residues joined to form a series of di-, tri-, and tetra-, and pentasaccharides. Sucrose is the dominant sugar in the sieve-tube sap of most species analyzed.

Import and export by leaves. The nature and physiological activity of the source region influence the contents of the sieve-tube sap and the pattern of translocation. Early in its development a leaf is dependent on the import of a significant quantity of organic material via the phloem. Not until the leaf is about half expanded does it begin to export the products of photosynthesis. Export starts in the tip region of the leaf and extends baseward until the entire leaf is exporting. Import ceases with the onset of export in a given leaf region. For a time the blade is both importing and exporting organic material. A mature leaf may export nearly half of the carbohydrate produced during photosynthesis; much of the rest will be accumulated as starch which will contribute to translocated materials during darkness. Materials are translocated both upward and downward from a given leaf toward regions which can be characterized physiologically as regions of utilization. Young leaves, root tips, shoot tips, and developing fruits are examples of such sink regions (Fig. 3). The distribution pattern from a leaf also depends on the pattern of vascular connections with other organs (Fig. 4). Carbohydrates from the leaves provide carbon "skeletons" for synthesis of nitrogenous compounds in the roots; these compounds then may ascend to the shoot via the phloem or the xylem. In sugarbeet it has been found that many of

the protein amino acids and amides, particularly glutamic acid and glutamine, are translocated via the phloem to young leaves. Other nitrogen compounds from the roots are distributed more generally to the leaves via the xylem.

Xylem sap. During translocation through the petiole and stem, a considerable quantity of sugar in transit may move into the cortex, phloem parenchyma, or xylem parenchyma cells and be stored as starch available for later mobilization. In spite of the proximity of the phloem and of carbohydrate reserves, only negligible quantities of sugar appear in sap from the xylem elements during most of the growing season. During the dormant season, when the flow of water in the xylem elements practically ceases, sugars often accumulate in readily detectable amounts. Although the average maximal concentration seldom exceeds 0.05%, a concentration as high as 8% has been reported for the sugar maple (*Acer saccharum*). Even in this species, ringing the stem just below the terminal bud results in severe reduction in growth of the emergent shoot, showing that, even when the sugar content of xylem is high, the phloem is still the most important channel for translocation of sugars. *See* PLANT, WATER RELATIONS OF.

Channels for nitrogen compounds. The xylem sap contains amino acids and amides whose concentration remains moderately high throughout the growing season. In apple the amino acid–amide concentration averages about 0.03 *M* glutamine-equivalent in the xylem sap, while in sieve-tube exudate the concentration is of the order of 0.001 *M*. Although the xylem constitutes an important channel of transport of nitrogenous compounds from the roots to the leaves, stem, and fruits, ringing and radioisotope studies suggest that the phloem is also important in this regard at certain times. Redistribution of nitrogenous compounds from the leaves occurs mainly by the phloem. During senescence (yellowing) large

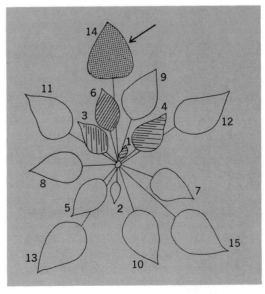

Fig. 4. Distribution of radioactivity in the leaves of a beet plant 1 week after administration of C¹⁴O₂ for 4 hr to a single leaf. Hatching indicates the approximate intensity of radioactivity from autoradiographs of leaves. Numbers increase with leaf ages.

amounts of nitrogen- and phosphorus-containing organic compounds are exported from the leaves and large amounts of these compounds appear in the sieve-tube exudate. *See* PLANT, MINERAL NUTRITION OF.

Plant disease control. A practical application of translocation is in the area of systematic insecticides, fungicides, herbicides, and bactericides. Interest has centered on modifications of molecules which increase their capacity to be translocated and thus be distributed throughout the plant. For example, many herbicidal carbamate compounds are not readily translocated from mature leaves unless the lactic acid group is incorporated. Much work remains to be done on the relationship between molecular structure and translocatability via the phloem. *See* PLANT DISEASE CONTROL.

Requirements for organic nutrients.

The specific requirements of fruits for organic nutrients translocated from other parts of the plant appear to be simple. Excised pollinated ovularies of tomato and gherkin can be cultured in the laboratory and will form fruits on a culture medium containing only sucrose, the usual complement of inorganic ions (nitrate, phosphate, sulfate, calcium, magnesium, and so on), and water. Large quantities of organic solutes, principally sugars, are translocated to fruits. For example, in the course of a growing season, up to 150 kg of organic solutes are translocated to the fruits in a single apple tree under favorable conditions.

Although differences in composition of fruit might be expected when fruits are grafted onto various stocks, the differences in some cases are small. Grafting sour lemon fruits to a sweet lemon stock does not materially change the organic acid content when the fruits are mature; the same is true of the reciprocal grafting experiment. The rootstock, however, does affect the chemical composition and quality of the fruit, sometimes to a significant extent. Consistent differences have

been found, for example, in the bitterness of the juice of the Washington navel orange relatable to the type of rootstock used. Though such changes are sometimes subtle, they are of interest to agriculturalists. *See* GRAFTING OF PLANTS.

Mechanism of translocation.

The mechanism of phloem translocation is not known with certainty. Proposed mechanisms fall into two classes: One stresses the role of the path tissues in generating the moving force, and the other views the region of supply and utilization as the source of this force. In the former group are mechanisms which depend on cytoplasmic streaming and electroosmosis, and activated diffusion in the sieve-tube elements. The second group of theories, which has received the more general acceptance in spite of a number of admitted limitations, includes a variety of massflow mechanisms based on theory developed principally by E. Munch about 1930. In his view, a solution of dissolved materials is carried along as a whole as a result of an osmotically produced pressure gradient generated in the regions of supply and possibly of utilization. Theories of translocation must account for the following important observations: polarity, bidirectional movement, velocity, energy requirement, and turgor pressure.

Polarity. Solutes move from a place of production or mobilization to points of storage or utilization. In addition to a source of translocatable compounds, there is need for a metabolically active region where growth or accumulation is occurring. The direction of translocation is determined more by physiological states of source and accumulation areas than by structural relations, as can be seen by comparing Figs. 4 and 5. Growing regions of a plant, especially rapidly developing fruits, exert a strong mobilizing effect on solutes translocated from source regions. In apple trees it has been shown that the fruits and the supplying leaves can be separated by distances up to 10 ft without loss in size or quality of the fruit.

Bidirectional movement. Translocation in the path may occur in opposite directions. Solutes may move both up and down a stem or petiole simultaneously, even in the same phloem bundle; but it has not been shown that this bidirectional movement can occur within a single sieve tube.

Velocity. Translocation is rapid and conveys large quantities of solutes. Velocity measurements by radioactively labeled compounds and by growth rate studies reveal that the velocity of translocation is about 1–2 cm/min, with velocities of over 20 cm/min reported for a rapid component of translocation. The mass transport rate for sugar beet has been measured at 9 mg sucrose/hr out of a 100-cm² leaf. In the sausage tree (*Kigelia africana*) as much as 32 g/day of organic material must pass through the slender stem to account for the dry weight gain of the cluster of four fruits. These rates are many orders of magnitude greater than could be accounted for by diffusion.

Energy requirement. The high rate of directed mass transfer observed necessitates a considerable expenditure of energy both to move the stream of solutes and to maintain the structural integrity of the conducting tissue. As a consequence, living phloem cells are necessary for translocation of organic solutes, in contrast to xylem transport.

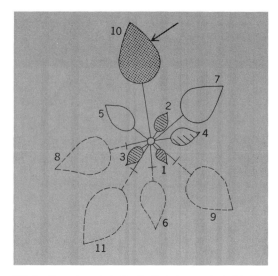

Fig. 5. Experiment similar to that demonstrated in Fig. 4 except for removal of all fully expanded leaves from one side of the stalk. Young leaves on both sides of the plant now receive the translocated C¹⁴. The leaves are numbered to show relative age; 1 is youngest. (*From K. W. Joy, J. Exp. Bot., 15(45):485, 1964*)

Killing the cells in a localized zone of the stem by heating is as effective a barrier to transport of phloem-limited solutes as is ringing. The sieve elements, which are enucleate at maturity, are commonly held to be metabolically inactive as compared to other tissues. In cold-tolerant plants translocation continues at an undiminished rate through a petiole at 0°C for many hours, indicating that energy expenditure in the path tissue is primarily required for maintenance of structure of the phloem rather than for moving the translocate stream. On the other hand, treatments, such as cooling, which lower the metabolism in source or in accumulation regions slow translocation markedly.

Turgor pressure. Sieve-tube contents are under positive turgor pressure. Aphid stylet and bark incision methods for collecting sieve-tube exudate indicate that the pressure, estimated at up to 30 atm in some trees, is the result of an influx which continues for many hours.

Mass-flow theory. Although none of the theories proposed to explain solute translocation are without limitations, the mass-flow theory, as modified by several investigators, has received wide acceptance. According to this theory, companion cells associated with the phloem endings in source regions deliver solutes into the sieve tubes by a process which requires metabolic energy. A square centimeter of leaf may contain 70 cm of these endings. In some plants the walls of the companion cells associated with the minor veins have ingrowths which increase the area of the plasma membrane severalfold. In the phloem endings where sugar concentration in the sieve tubes is high, water enters from surrounding cells and from the xylem in particular; the resulting hydrostatic pressure causes the solutes to flow along under the force of turgor pressure. At points of utilization or storage, solutes are removed from the sieve tubes, probably by a process requiring metabolic activity. The resultant lowering of solute concentration causes a lowering turgor pressure, also aiding translocation stream movement. The functioning of the proposed mass-flow system has been studied by mathematical models. The simulated working of the system corresponds generally to translocation as observed in living plants.

Observations of phloem structure are also important in evaluating theories of phloem translocation. The sieve element itself has a specialized protoplast which is not expected to be a major source of energy involved in longitudinal transport, while the phloem parenchyma cells or companion cells associated with terminal regions of the phloem are large and have dense cytoplasm with numerous mitochondria. These latter cells appear to be well suited to controlling the concentration of solutes in the sieve elements. Studies of these phloem cells by autoradiography and analysis of solute concentration indicate that the minor-vein phloem accumulates solutes to a very high level by a process known as phloem loading. Many objections remain unanswered in the presently proposed theories and much work in evaluating them remains.

Because the bulk of organic translocation takes place via phloem cells, considerable research has been directed toward a better understanding of the mechanism of translocation as well as to the elucidation of factors, both environmental and internal, which influence this process. The technological importance of these studies derives from the fact that many crop management practices are, in their final analysis, efforts to control the rate and direction of translocation of organic compounds from leaves to roots or fruits. *See* AGRICULTURAL SCIENCE (PLANT).

[DONALD GEIGER]

Bibliography: A. S. Crafts and C. E. Crisp, *Phloem Transport in Plants*, 1971; K. Esau, *Plants, Viruses and Insects*, 1961; B. S. Meyer et al., *Introduction to Plant Physiology*, 1973; M. Zimmermann and J. Milburn (eds.), *Encyclopedia of Plant Physiology*, vol. 1, 1975.

Plant virus

A pathogenic (disease-causing) agent, too small to be seen with the optical (light) microscope. Viruses replicate only in living susceptible cells, and they attack all forms of living things from bacteria to man; more than 300 different viruses have been described from plants, including algae (Fig. 1). The first scientific discovery of a virus was made in 1892 by Dimitrii Iwanowski, who showed that the sap of a tobacco plant infected with the mosaic disease was still infectious, after passing through a filter which removed all visible organisms, when rubbed on the leaves of a healthy tobacco plant. From this experiment arose the term "ultramicroscopic filter-passing viruses," now rendered obsolete by improvements in scientific techniques. The symptoms of plant virus diseases are very varied and when the number of plant viruses is taken into consideration, it is not surprising that this multiplicity is reflected in an equally varied response on the part of the host plant.

Plant viruses are more dependent on organisms for their transfer from infected to healthy hosts than any other kind of pathogen. It has been demonstrated that almost all types of organisms feeding upon or parasitizing plants can act as carriers of viruses, or "vectors," as they are called.

No virus was actually seen until the invention of the electron microscope. With this instrument it is possible not only to see the virus but, with the development of special staining methods, to identify the structural components of the virus particle itself. Magnification of 40,000 times and upward

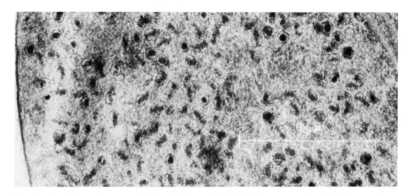

Fig. 1. Electron micrograph of part of a cell of the blue-green alga *Plectonema boryanum* infected with a virus; note most of the virus particles are in the form of a helix, a developmental form. (*Courtesy of K. M. Smith, R. M. Brown, Jr., and P. L. Walne*)

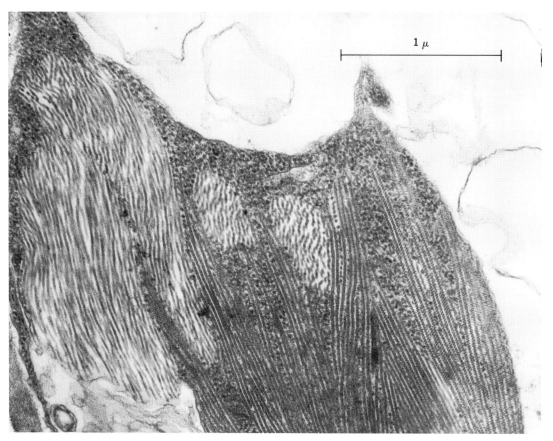

Fig. 2. Electron micrograph of part of *Lantana horrida* cell infected with a mosaic virus; note the long helices on the right side of the figure which may be a developmental stage of the virus. Mature virus rods are at top left. (*Courtesy of H. J. Arnott and K. M. Smith*)

are easily obtainable on an electron microscope.

The development of the ultramicrotome, which uses a glass or diamond knife, allows sections of the infected cell and the virus particles contained therein to be cut 300 mμ in thickness. Thus by using the electron microscope, a study can be made of the relationships of the virus with the plant cell, and some knowledge can be gained of how a virus reproduces itself (Figs. 2 and 3). Such a study forms a substantial part of molecular biology and has contributed much to the knowledge of hereditary mechanisms. It is also possible by this means to visualize certain plant viruses in the cells of the insect which transmits them.

Modern methods of isolation have made it feasible to obtain some plant viruses in a pure state in sufficient quantities to allow for the investigation of their chemical composition.

Symptoms. The most common expression of a virus disease in a plant is known as "mosaic," a term first used by G. E. Mayer because of a resemblance of the leaf mottling to a mosaic pattern. Diseases in this category include tobacco mosaic, cucumber mosaic, and potato mosaic, in which the leaves are mottled with light- and dark-green patches, sometimes interspersed with yellow (Figs. 4–6). Although the most noticeable symptoms occur on the leaves, all parts of the plant, including the roots, may be affected. Changes in the flower color are common; the most familiar is the tulip break, in which the flower of the self-colored tulip is flecked or streaked with yellow. These "broken"

flowers, as they are called, can be very attractive. Other symptoms include stunting of the plant (rice dwarf disease), outgrowths on the leaves, and formation of tumors on roots and stems (wound-tumor disease).

Transmission. Some viruses which are in high concentration in the plant, such as that causing tobacco mosaic, can be transmitted from diseased to healthy plants in the field by mere contact. In addition, all vegetative parts produce a diseased plant if the parent plant is virus-affected. A few viruses are also transmitted through seed. The majority, however, are dependent for their spread upon an intermediary or vector organism. Vectors may be insects and other arthropods, nematode worms, or spores of parasitic fungi.

The greatest number of vectors occurs in the insect order Hemiptera, which includes the sap-sucking insects such as aphids (greenflies), leaf-hoppers, and whiteflies. These insects all feed by means of four fine stylets which come together to form two canals. These stylets are thrust into the tissues of the plant; the plant sap passes up one canal while saliva flows down the other into the plant. If the insect has been feeding previously on a virus-infected plant, virus accompanies the saliva into the plant. Such insects are ideally suited for transmission of plant viruses. Aphids are the most numerous vectors but leafhoppers are also important; some viruses have a close biological relationship and multiply inside these insects. Thus the unusual situation arises of a plant virus

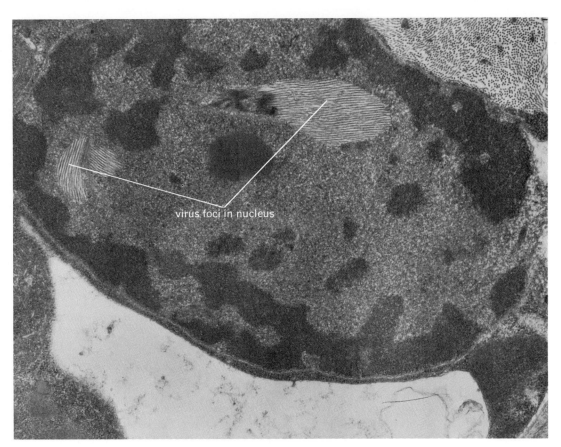

virus foci in nucleus

Fig. 3. Electron micrograph of part of cell of *Lantana horrida* infected with mosaic virus. The nucleus contains two virus foci. At the top right is another concentration of virus, multiplying independently in the cell cytoplasm. (*Courtesy of H. J. Arnott and K. M. Smith*)

which can replicate in an animal. Several plant viruses, notably that of peach mosaic, are transmitted by mites (Eriophyidae), and nematode worms spread a number of plant viruses of economic importance. The spores of the fungus *Olpidium brassicae* transmit two viruses that affect tobacco and lettuce plants.

Morphology. The shapes of plant virus particles fall into two general categories: the anisometric and isometric particles. Among the viruses with anisometric particles, those which are rod-shaped are the most common (Fig. 7) and they vary in appearance from the rigid type to long, flexuous rods (Fig. 2). The small isometric viruses appear at first sight to be spherical when viewed in the electron microscope, but they are actually icosahedrons, possessing 20 sides.

In essence, a plant virus particle consists of a strand of ribonucleic acid (RNA) surrounded by a protein coat, which provides a protective covering for the RNA. The different parts of the virus particle are named as follows: The whole particle is called a virion, the protein coat the capsid, and the individual protein subunits the capsomeres. Essentially all viruses seem to have the outside surfaces composed of regularly arranged protein units with the RNA intertwined among them.

The particle of the tobacco mosaic virus is a rod 300 mμ in length by 150 mμ in diameter; it consists of a helical array of protein subunits containing a single chain of RNA.

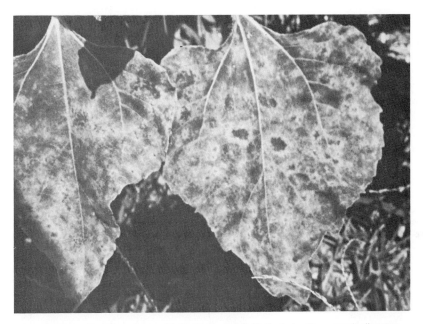

Fig. 4. Leaves of wild sunflower (*Helianthus annuum*) infected with a mosaic disease; note mottling and blotching. (*Courtesy of H. J. Arnott and K. M. Smith*)

The virus of turnip yellow mosaic is a very small icosahedron measuring about 21 mμ in diameter. The protein framework has a surface structure of 32 knobs, known as morphological units, but these

PLANT VIRUS

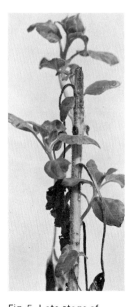

Fig. 5. Late stage of sunflower mosaic; growing point and many leaves are killed; secondary growth of small distorted leaves then develops. (*H. J. Arnott and K. M. Smith*)

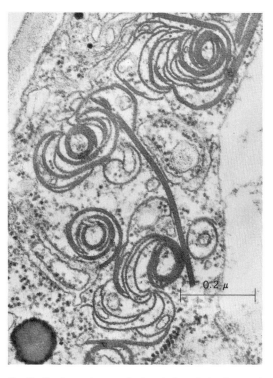

Fig. 6. Electron micrograph of part of a cell of a diseased sunflower. Note peculiar "pinwheel" intracellular inclusions caused by the virus; their exact nature is not known. (*Courtesy of H. J. Arnott and K. M. Smith*)

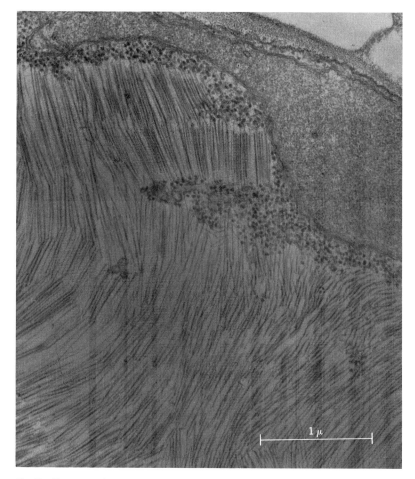

Fig. 7. Electron micrograph of part of a cell of a tomato plant infected with tobacco mosaic virus; note massed array of the virus and its rodlike shape.

are in turn composed of 180 units, called structural units. The actual position of the RNA is not definitely known, but it is thought to be deeply embedded within the protein shell.

Replication. When a virus particle enters a susceptible cell, the first event to occur is the release of the viral nucleic acid by the removal of the protein coat. Not much is known about the exact method of assembly of plant virus particles, and most of the work has been carried out with tobacco mosaic virus. From a great number of experiments, there is much evidence that both the virus protein and the RNA are first formed in the nucleus before the assembly of the virus particle in the cytoplasm.

Electron microscope studies of a virus from the plant *Lantana horrida* show quantities of virus apparently in process of assembly in both cytoplasm and nucleus. Associated with the virus, which is a very long rod, are helices and crystalline material from which the helices appear to be assembled (Fig. 2).

Electron micrographs of thin sections of leaves infected with certain viruses and of the organs of virus-carrying leafhoppers reveal the virus particles in crystalline formation in both plant and insect vectors. This is further evidence that certain plant viruses are capable of replication inside the insect.

Isolation. By using chemical precipitation methods and the ultracentrifuge, it is now possible to isolate some plant viruses in pure form. All the small plant viruses so far isolated consist of protein and RNA only. It has also been shown that the RNA of the tobacco mosaic virus is capable of replication by itself, thereby indicating that the RNA contains the genetic material of the virus. This means that not only can the RNA reproduce itself but also it controls the synthesis of its particular protein. *See* PLANT DISEASE.

[KENNETH M. SMITH]

Bibliography: F. C. Bawden, *Plant Viruses and Virus Diseases*, 4th ed., 1964; K. M. Smith, *Plant Viruses*, 4th ed., 1968; K. M. Smith and M. A. Lauffer (eds.), *Advances in Virus Research*, vols. 1–17, 1953–1972.

Plum

Any of the smooth-skinned stone fruits grown on shrubs or small trees. Plums are widely distributed in all land areas of the North Temperate Zone, where many species and varieties are adapted to different climatic and soil conditions.

Types and varieties. There are four principal groups: (1) Domestica (*Prunus domestica*) of European or Southwest Asian origin, (2) Japanese or Salicina (*P. salicina*) of Chinese origin, (3) Insititia or Damson (*P. insititia*) of Eurasian origin (see illustration), and (4) American (*P. americana* and *P. hortulana*). The Domesticas are large, meaty, prune-type plums, the principal varieties being Agen or French Prune (grown in California) and Italian or Italian hybrids (grown primarily in Oregon, Washington, Idaho, and Michigan).

A prune is a plum which dries without spoiling. Commonly but incorrectly the term "prune" is applied to all Domestica-type plums, whereas the term "plum" is used only for Japanese-type plums. Japanese plums are typically round, reddish or yellow, and juicy, and are represented by such

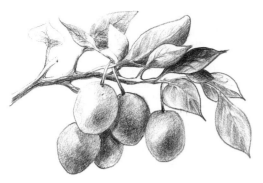

Branch of a Damson plum.

varieties as Beauty, Santa Rosa, Duarte, Burbank, Wickson, and Satsuma. Insititias (Damson), represented by Shropshire, are small, meaty fruits grown sparingly for jam. American plums are small, watery fruits of low quality, represented by De Soto, Pottawattomi, and Golden Beauty, and valued chiefly for cold hardiness of the tree.

Propagation and culture. Plums are propagated by budding on seedlings of the myrobalan plum (*P. cerasifera*) and less commonly on the peach and certain strains of *P. domestica*. *See* GRAFTING OF PLANTS; PEACH.

The Domestica and Insititia plums are slightly hardier than the peach; the Japanese plums have about the same hardiness as the peach; and native American plums are considerably hardier than the other groups.

Trees of the Domestica and Damson types may grow 20–25 ft (1 ft = 0.3 m) high unless kept lower by training and pruning. They are usually planted about 20 ft apart, and are adapted to a wide range of soils, from light to heavy. Trees of the Japanese type are smaller (15–20 ft) and are best adapted to lighter soils. They are normally planted 18–20 ft apart, but in the hands of skilled horticulturists they are adaptable to close spacings and controlled shapes. Most plums require cross-pollination.

Production and economic importance. Average commerical production of the prune-type, Domestica plums in the United States was approximately 509,000 tons (1 short ton = 0.9 metric ton) annually during the 5-year period 1970–1974. California produced 451,000 tons (100% dried as prunes), Oregon 21,800, Washington 14,700, Michigan 14,500, and Idaho 8400. In the states other than California, 52% of the prune-type plums were sold fresh, 40% canned and 8% dried. During 1970–1974 Japanese-type plum production averaged 112,000 tons; nearly all was produced in California, and 98% was sold fresh. The 1974 farm value of plums sold in the five states totaled $114,000,000.

[R. PAUL LARSEN]

Plum and prune diseases. Brown rot, a fungus disease caused by *Monilinia fructicola*, is the limiting factor in production of plums under humid conditions. Infected fruit decays rapidly and is covered with gray masses of fungus spores. Punctures made by the plum curculio, a common fruit insect, increase the risk of fungus infection. Control is difficult and must include measures for control of the plum curculio as well as the fungus. Commercial production of plums and prunes is confined almost entirely to the Pacific Coast states where the plum curculio does not occur and cli-

matic conditions are less favorable for development of the fungus.

Japanese varieties of plums and their hybrids are so susceptible to attacks of the bacterial spot organism (*Xanthomonas pruni*) that their commercial production is likewise confined to the far western states where the organism does not occur.

Other fungus diseases are plum pockets (a form of the leaf curl disease), rust, and scab. These diseases usually cause little damage.

Diamond canker and prune dwarf are two important virus diseases that cause prune trees to become unproductive. Control involves removal of affected trees and use of virus-free nursery stock. *See* FRUIT (TREE) DISEASES; PLANT DISEASE CONTROL; PLANT VIRUS.

[JOHN C. DUNEGAN]

Bibliography: W. H. Chandler, *Deciduous Orchards*, 1957; N. F. Childers, *Modern Fruit Science*, 1973.

Polysaccharide

A class of high-molecular-weight carbohydrates, colloidal complexes, which break down on hydrolysis to monosaccharides containing five or six carbon atoms. The polysaccharides are considered to be polymers in which monosaccharides have been glycosidically joined with the elimination of water. A polysaccharide consisting of hexose monosaccharide units may be represented by the empirical equation below.

$$nC_6H_{12}O_6 \rightarrow (C_6H_{10}O_5)_n + (n-1)H_2O$$

The term polysaccharide is limited to those polymers which contain 10 or more monosaccharide residues. Polysaccharides such as starch, glycogen, and dextran consist of several thousand D-glucose units. Polymers of relatively low molecular weight, consisting of two to nine monosaccharide residues, are referred to as oligosaccharides. *See* GLUCOSE; GLYCOGEN; MONOSACCHARIDE; STARCH.

Polysaccharides are either insoluble in water or, when soluble, form colloidal solutions. They are mostly amorphous substances. However, x-ray analysis indicates that a few of them, such as cellulose and chitin, possess a definite crystalline structure. As a class, polysaccharides are nonfermentable and are nonreducing, except for a trace of reducing power due, presumably, to the free reducing group at the end of a chain. They are optically active but do not exhibit mutarotation, and are relatively stable in alkali.

The polysaccharides serve either as reserve nutrients (glycogen and inulin) or as skeletal materials (cellulose and chitin) from which relatively rigid mechanical structures are built. Some polysaccharides, such as certain galactans and mannans, however, serve both functions. Through the action of acids or certain enzymes, the polysaccharides may be degraded to their constituent monosaccharide units. Some polysaccharides yield only simple sugars on hydrolysis; others yield not only sugars but also various sugar derivatives, such as D-glucuronic acid or galacturonic acid (known generally as uronic acids), hexosamines, and even nonsugar compounds such as acetic acid and sulfuric acid.

The constituent units of the polysaccharide molecule are arranged in the form of a long chain, either unbranched as in cellulose and amylose, or branched as in amylopectin and glycogen. The linkage between the monosaccharide units is generally the 1,4- or 1,6-glycosidic bond with either the α or β configuration, as the case may be. The branched glycogen and amylopectin contain both the 1,4 and 1,6 linkages. However, other types of linkage are known. In plant gum and mucilage polysaccharides, 1,2, 1,3, 1,5, and 1,6 linkages occur more commonly than the 1,4 type.

In an attempt to systematize the carbohydrate nomenclature, the generic name glycan was introduced as synonymous with the term polysaccharide. This term is evolved from the generic word glycose, meaning a simple sugar, and the ending, "an," signifying a sugar polymer. Examples of established usage of the "an" ending are xylan for polymers of xylose, mannan for polymers of mannose, and galactomannan for galactose-mannose copolymers. Cellulose and starch are both glucans or glucoglycans, since they are composed of glucose units.

Polysaccharides are often classified on the basis of the number of monosaccharide types present in the molecule. Polysaccharides, such as cellulose or starch, that produce only one monosaccharide type (D-glucose) on complete hydrolysis are termed homopolysaccharides. On the other hand, polysaccharides, such as hyaluronic acid, which produce on hydrolysis more than one monosaccharide type (N-acetylglucosamine and D-glucuronic acid) are named heteropolysaccharides. *See* CARBOHYDRATE

[WILLIAM Z. HASSID]

Bibliography: R. L. Whistler and C. L. Smart, *Polysaccharide Chemistry*, 1953; A. White, P. Handler, and E. L. Smith, *Principles of Biochemistry*, 5th ed., 1973.

Potato, Irish

The plant *Solanum tuberosum* of the nightshade family, Solanaceae. The origin of the potato was in the South American continent. Many wild tuber-bearing species are found in Central and South America, some at altitudes as high as 4800 m.

Potatoes have been under cultivation for several thousand years in these areas, supplying a large portion of the food for the inhabitants. They were introduced into Europe early in the 16th century and into the United States from Ireland in 1719.

The potato is an annual, herbaceous, dicotyledenous plant. It is sometimes regarded as a potential perennial because of its ability to reproduce vegetatively by means of tubers. Tubers, which are shortened, thickened underground stems, form on the ends of lateral stems (stolons) underground. The principal areas in the mature tubers from the exterior inward are the periderm, cortex, vascular ring, perimedullary zone, and central pith. Lateral buds (eyes) on the mature tuber are the growing points for the new crop when whole tubers or pieces with at least one eye are planted (Fig. 1).

Varieties. There are 75–80 varieties certified for seed propagation in the United States. Six of these, however, account for more than 80% of the commercial acreage planted. These are Russet Burbank, Kennebec, Katahdin, Superior, Norchip, and Norgold Russet.

Production. Potatoes are grown commercially in every state in the United States. The number of farms on which potatoes are grown is decreasing at a rather rapid rate, accompanied by more potato-planted acres per farm. With more efficient methods of growing and harvesting potatoes, higher yields and better methods of storing have resulted.

There has been a remarkable shift in production from the Eastern and Central states to those in the West, particularly the Northwest. Most of the production is concentrated in 15 states, as shown in Table 1. Since 1951 potato acreage in the United States has been within the range 1,250,000–1,540,000 (5058–6230 km²). Yields, however, have increased from an average of 150 hundredweight/acre (16,875 kg/hectare) in the early 1950s to 254 cwt/acre (28,125 kg/hectare) in 1976.

Consumption. Per capita consumption of potatoes in the United States declined from 198 lb (89 kg) early in this century to about 103 lb (46 kg) in 1956. Availability of processed potatoes of various forms reversed this trend, resulting in consumption increase to 121.6 lb (54.7 kg) in 1975. Before World War II, per capita consumption of pro-

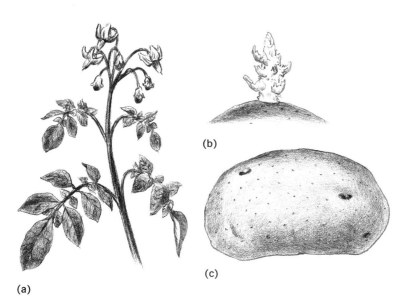

(a)

(b)

(c)

Fig. 1.   Irish potato. (*a*) Flowering stem. (*b*) "Eye" with buds. (*c*) Tuber.

Table 1. Fifteen leading states in potato production, 1975

State	Acres harvested*	Yield/acre, cwt†	Production, 10^3 cwt
Idaho	322,000	233	75,090
Washington	105,000	460	48,300
Maine	122,000	220	26,840
Oregon	52,100	437	22,779
California	59,100	351	20,740
North Dakota	110,000	160	17,600
Wisconsin	49,500	300	14,850
New York	47,300	250	11,818
Minnesota	65,100	181	11,796
Colorado	39,700	264	10,485
Michigan	36,400	222	8,076
Pennsylvania	29,000	235	6,815
Florida	27,500	194	5,344
Nevada	12,500	330	4,125
Texas	14,100	211	2,975
U.S. total	1,257,000	(251, av. yield)	315,647

*1 acre = 0.00405 km².   †cwt = 45.36 kg.

Table 2. United States production and per capita consumption of potatoes, 1960–1975

Year	Production, 10^6 cwt*	Total fresh and processed, lb†	Fresh, lb	Processed‡				
				Total, lb	Canned,§ lb	Frozen, lb	Chips and shoestrings, lb	Dehydrated, lb
1960	257.1	108.4	83.3	24.6	1.5	6.6	11.6	4.9
1961	293.2	109.3	83.8	25.5	1.5	6.8	12.3	4.9
1962	264.8	107.3	78.4	28.9	1.6	9.4	13.1	4.8
1963	271.2	111.4	79.9	31.5	1.7	11.0	13.9	4.9
1964	241.1	111.0	74.6	36.4	1.7	14.6	14.8	5.3
1965	291.1	107.0	68.2	38.8	1.7	14.3	15.8	7.0
1966	307.2	116.8	72.4	44.4	1.7	17.3	16.7	8.7
1967	305.8	108.0	62.0	46.0	1.7	19.0	16.9	8.4
1968	295.4	115.2	65.9	49.3	1.9	21.2	17.1	9.1
1969	312.4	116.8	61.6	55.2	2.0	24.6	17.7	10.9
1970	325.8	117.6	58.4	59.2	2.0	27.7	17.7	11.8
1971	319.4	118.9	57.0	61.9	2.2	30.3	17.3	12.1
1972	296.0	119.2	57.2	62.0	2.1	30.6	17.0	12.3
1973	299.4	116.5	51.6	64.9	2.3	33.2	16.6	12.8
1974	342.1	113.8	47.9	65.9	2.3	33.0	16.1	14.5
1975¶	315.6	121.6	54.5	67.1	2.3	34.7	15.2	14.9

*10^6 cwt = 45,360,000 kg.   †1 lb = 0.454 kg.   ‡Fresh-weight basis.   § = Includes potatoes canned in soups, stews, and other combinations.   ¶Preliminary.

cessed potatoes was about 3 lb (1.4 kg), increasing at a rather remarkable rate to 67 lb (30 kg) in 1975. Per capita consumption of fresh potatoes dropped to 54.5 lb (24.5 kg) in 1975. More than 75% of all potatoes were consumed fresh in 1960, dropping to 42% by 1974 (see Table 2).

Constituents. Chemical composition varies with variety, area of growth, cultural practices, maturity at harvest, subsequent storage history, and other factors. Average composition of potatoes is approximately 78–80% water, 14–18% starch, 2% protein, 1% minerals, 0.1% fat, with some sugars, organic acids, amino acids, and vitamins.

Starch comprises about 65–80% of the dry weight of the potato and, calorically, is the most important nutritional component. The texture of a cooked potato is determined largely by its starch content. The nutritional or biological value of protein in potatoes is rather high. Potato protein contains substantially more of all the essential amino acids, except histidine, than does that of whole wheat. As a world average 226 kg/hectare of potato protein is produced, which is greater than that·in wheat grain or in rice grain. Potatoes provide the world with 6,000,000 metric tons of protein.

Potatoes contain appreciable amounts of the B vitamins: niacin, thiamine, riboflavin, and pyridoxine. Potatoes are an excellent source of vitamin C. One medium-sized baked potato yields 20 mg of vitamin C, or about 33% of the 60 mg which is the recommended allowance per human per day. On a national basis potatoes contribute more vitamin C to the United States food supply than any other one major food. Inorganic constituents or minerals of potatoes are predominately potassium, phosphorus, sulfur, chlorine, magnesium, and calcium. Iron is present in sufficient quantity for potatoes to be a good nutritional source of this mineral. Sodium content is low, rendering potatoes a good food for those individuals requiring a low sodium diet. *See* VEGETABLE GROWING.   [ORA SMITH]

Diseases. The potato is especially subject to disease for three principal reasons: (1) It is propa-

gated vegetatively, which permits transmission of many pathogens from generation to generation. (2) Clonal propagation results in genetically homogeneous populations, which favor epidemic diseases. (3) The product is perishable and subject to storage diseases.

Viruses cause the most economically important diseases. Most common are mild, rugose, and latent mosaics, leaf roll, and spindle tuber. Viruses reduce yield and sometimes lower the quality of the tubers. Because they are tuber-borne, viruses are controlled principally by rogueing out diseased plants and growing seed crops in isolation. Some potato varieties are resistant or immune to certain viruses. *See* PLANT VIRUS.

Several species of bacteria cause potato diseases. *Corynebacterium sepedonicum* (causing ring rot and wilt) is seed-borne, like viruses, and is controlled by the same methods. *Pseudomonas solonacearum* (causing brown rot or southern wilt) is also seed-borne and in the humid South survives in the soil over the winter, making potato culture unprofitable on fields that have become infested. *Erwinia atroseptica* (cause of blackleg) is also seed-borne and is similar to *E. carotovora*, which causes soft rot of tubers in storage. Proper storage of tubers and careful handling of seed pieces at planting reduce incidence of these diseases.

The most destructive fungus disease is late blight, caused by *Phytophthora infestans* (Fig. 2). Primary infection is from infected seed and typical epidemics occur when the weather is mild and wet. Genes for immunity have been bred into new varieties, but the genetic plasticity of the fungus has resulted in failure of such resistance. There are, however, potato varieties with generalized but partial resistance which are useful in reducing the spread of epidemics. Fungicides are still the principal means of control. *See* FUNGISTAT AND FUNGICIDE.

Alternaria dauci f. *solani* causes early blight, and various species of *Rhizoctonia*, *Verticillium*, and *Fusarium* cause stem cankers, wilts, and stor-

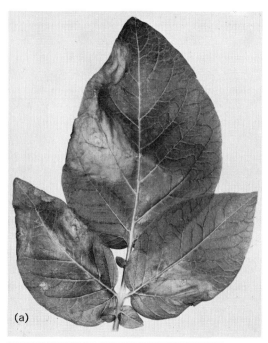

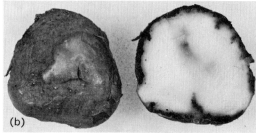

Fig. 2. Late blight (*Phytophthora infestans*) of Irish potato. (*a*) Foliar infection. (*b*) Tuber infection. (*USDA*)

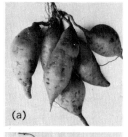

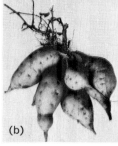

Fig. 1. Sweet potatoes. (*a*) Porto Rico, a yam variety. (*b*) Big-stem Jersey type. (*USDA*)

age rots. Tubers are also subject to diseases that are principally blemishes, such as common scab, caused by *Streptomyces scabies*; silver scurf, caused by *Spondylocladium atrovirens*; and black scurf, caused by *Rhizoctonia*.

In addition to storage diseases caused by organisms, potato tubers are subject to nonparasitic disorders such as black heart, hollow heart, and various kinds of internal necroses and discolorations due to growing or storage conditions.

Nematodes cause root knots and tuber rots. The most destructive is the golden nematode (*Heterodera rostochiensis*). At present it is not widespread, but once introduced into the soil it will persist indefinitely. *See* PLANT DISEASE.

[CARL J. EIDE]

Potato, sweet

The fleshy root of the plant *Ipomoea batatas*. The sweet potato was mentioned as being grown in Virginia as early as 1648. In 1930 the selection of outstanding strains of the Porto Rico variety, which was introduced into Florida in 1908, was begun in Louisiana, and the best strain, Unit I Porto Rico, was released in 1934. The Unit I Porto Rico is now being replaced by the Centennial, a yam type which has three times its vitamin A content. More than 70% of the commercial crop in the United States is of the Centennial variety. Another va-

riety, Nemagold, is used largely in the Virginia area because of its resistance to nematodes. Most varieties released now have multiple disease resistance, particularly resistance to wilt and soil rot.

In 1937 new techniques were developed for inducing the sweet potato to bloom and set seed. This stimulated a surge of research on breeding for higher yield, greater nutritional value, better shape, storage ability, market and canning quality, greater disease resistance, and new food products and industrial uses for the sweet potato throughout the Southern states and from New Jersey to California. In Louisiana, the leading state for commercial production of both the canned and fresh products, the annual value of the crop varies from $15,000,000 to $20,000,000, depending on seasonal conditions and demand.

Types. There are two principal types of sweet potato, the kind erroneously called yam and the Jersey type (Fig. 1). The chief difference between the two is that in cooking or baking the yam, much of the starch is broken down into simple sugars (glucose and fructose) and an intermediate product, dextrin. This gives it a moist, syrupy consistency somewhat sweeter than that of the dry (Jersey) type. On cooking, the sugar in the dry type remains as sucrose.

The yam is produced largely in the Southern states; however, because of the breeding of more widely adapted varieties, it is now being grown farther north. The Jersey sweet potato is grown largely along the eastern shore of Virginia, Maryland, Delaware, and New Jersey, and also in Iowa and Kansas (Fig. 2).

The total consumption of sweet potatoes in the United States, like that of white potatoes, rice, and other high-carbohydrate foods, is now somewhat lower than in former years. Nevertheless, the value of the sweet-potato industry in Louisiana is increasing at the rate of about $500,000 of market value each year. With the development of new varieties, the northern limits of sweet-potato production have been extended to Canada and the northern United States. This has come about by breeding early and better varieties. In Michigan and Iowa a number of baby-food manufacturers are growing this crop for processing.

Breeding. The principal objectives in sweet-potato breeding are higher nutritional values, including higher vitamin and mineral contents; increased yield; greater disease resistance; and wider adaptation. Louisiana, Oklahoma, Georgia, North and South Carolina, and California have initiated breeding programs. The U.S. Department of Agriculture and several states jointly test and evaluate the newer seedlings and varieties (cultivars). For example, each year in Louisiana about 40,000–50,000 seedlings are grown and studied. Men from all parts of the world are being trained in breeding, producing, and handling the crop. The better varieties are sent to practically all the countries in the tropical and subtropical zones and to most of the temperate zone. *See* BREEDING (PLANT).

Processing. In the United States the sweet potato is canned extensively in Louisiana and along the Eastern seaboard. The frozen product has also appeared on the market. The sweet-potato chip is another new product, similar to the Irish-potato

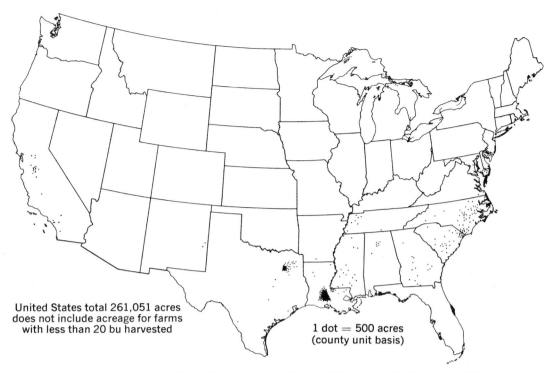

United States total 261,051 acres
does not include acreage for farms
with less than 20 bu harvested

1 dot = 500 acres
(county unit basis)

Fig. 2. Sweet-potato acreage in the United States for 1 year. (*Bureau of the Census, U.S. Department of Commerce*)

chip but higher in vitamins and carbohydrates. Another development is the making of sweet-potato flakes, similar to corn flakes, which can be used as cereal, in pie filling, in doughnuts, and in casserole form. These are being processed in Louisiana, North Carolina, and Virginia, and are being used extensively by the armed forces, the civilian trade, and the school lunch program. In addition, many livestock growers use fresh and dehydrated sweet potatoes for feeding swine, poultry, and dairy cattle.

Use of the sweet potato as feed stimulates milk production and increases the vitamin A content of the milk.

True yam. The true yam (*Dioscorea*) includes both edible and medicinal varieties. The latter are grown primarily for their cortisone, a steroid. Cor-

tisone yams can be grown in the southern United States, particularly in Louisiana. *See* POTATO, IRISH; VEGETABLE GROWING; VITAMIN A.

[JULIAN C. MILLER]

Diseases. Sweet-potato diseases, caused by fungi, nematodes, and viruses, affect both plants growing in the field and edible roots in storage and transit (Fig. 3). Diseases incited by the different fungi are black rot, stem rot, soft rot, soil rot, scurf, circular spot, Java black rot, charcoal rot, foot rot, root rot, mottle necrosis, leaf blight, leaf spot, white rust, and true rust. The primary nematode disease is root knot. Virus diseases, important in sweet-potato production mainly since 1940, are mosaic, feathery mottle, internal cork, mottle leaf, dwarf, and others still unidentified.

Disease control, of any great importance in suc-

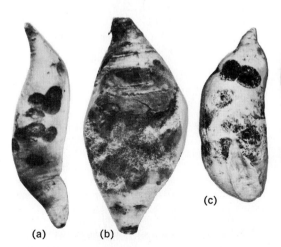
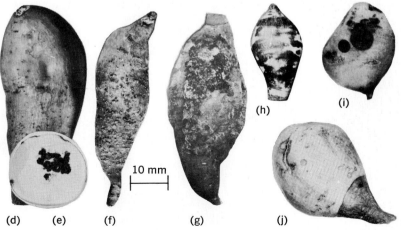

10 mm

(a)   (b)   (c)   (d)   (e)   (f)   (g)   (h)   (i)   (j)

Fig. 3. Some important sweet-potato diseases, caused by fungi, nematodes, or viruses. (*a*) Black rot. (*b*) Soft rot. (*c*) Soil rot. (*d*) Internal cork. (*e*) Section through internal cork-affected root. (*f*) Root knot. (*g*) Java black rot. (*h*) Scurf. (*i*) Circular spot. (*j*) Charcoal rot. (*Louisiana Agricultural Experiment Station*)

cessful production and distribution of sweet potatoes, is difficult because sweet potatoes are propagated vegetatively. Essential control practices are selection of disease-free roots for propagation, chemical treatment of selected roots to destroy unseen traces of fungi, and crop rotation to reduce soil infestation. Soil treatments with fungicides or nematocides sometimes are necessary to rid infested soils of disease-producing organisms. Since 1940 resistant varieties obtained through breeding and selection have aided in control of stem rot, and to some extent soil rot, black rot, and root knot. Worldwide search for disease-resistant strains among the numerous sweet-potato types available, combined with breeding programs, should result in development of more resistant varieties. *See* FUN-GISTAT AND FUNGICIDE; PLANT DISEASE; PLANT VIRUS. [WESTON J. MARTIN]

Poultry production

Poultry production can be divided into two major categories, meat production and egg production. Heavy-breed chickens, turkeys, ducks, and geese are used for meat, while light-breed chickens are used primarily for egg production. The subject of poultry production will be discussed here with particular reference to chickens.

Trends in both broiler and egg production have been toward vertical integration. This means that the various aspects of production and marketing (production of hatching eggs, incubation, feeding, growing, processing, and marketing) are being merged within the framework of a single organization.

Broiler production. The meat or broiler industry has become one of the largest agricultural businesses in the United States. In 1934 broiler production was around 34,000,000 per year. By 1945 production had grown to about 365,000,000 annually, and by 1974, according to the U.S. Department of Agriculture census, 2,992,844,000 broilers were grown for a total value of $2,437,050,000. The leading states in broiler production in 1974 were Arkansas, Georgia, Alabama, and North Carolina. To grow a chick to broiler size, that is, 3–4 lb, required 7–8 weeks in 1974 as compared with 13–14 weeks in the late 1940s. Improvements in diet, breeding, and management have been responsible for this tremendous change.

Egg production. The commercial egg industry in the United States had its start in the early 1900s. According to the Department of Agriculture census, of the eggs laid by chickens raised on farms in 1928, 43% were hatched under hens (of which only

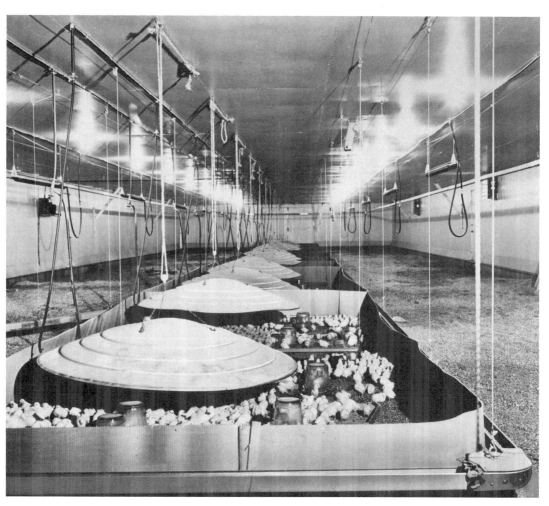

Fig. 1. Chicks in gas-fired brooder to provide supplementary heat. As chicks grow, guard used to keep them close to brooder stove is removed so they can eat from mechanical feeder and have access to total floor area. (*J. C. Snavely and Co.*)

23% were bought as baby chicks) and 57% of the eggs were sold. By 1938, 66% of all baby chicks were bought from commercial breeders and hatcheries and this increased to nearly 100% by 1974. Equally significant was the change in number of eggs laid per hen. Between 1925 and 1937, annual egg production per laying hen in the United States averaged around 120 eggs. By 1974 this rate increased to 231 eggs. However, in 1974 on many of the better commercial egg farms the number of eggs produced ran as high as 265 eggs per layer annually. Gross income from the sale of eggs in 1974 amounted to nearly $2,934,542,000. The leading states in number of eggs produced in 1974 were California, Georgia, Arkansas, and Pennsylvania. Egg consumption per person in the United States increased from about 300 eggs a year prior to 1937 to 403 eggs per person by 1945. Since this maximum was reached the number has declined to about 294 eggs per person.

Incubation. Incubation is a period requiring 21 days during which fertile eggs are converted into baby chicks. In contrast with natural incubation by a hen, baby chicks are now incubated in large machines which can provide precise automatic control of temperature, humidity, and air. The optimum temperature for incubation is 99.75°F. A relative humidity of 60% is satisfactory for the first 18 days of incubation but at hatching it should be raised to 70%. Rate of air exchange is also important to assure adequate supplies of oxygen and for the removal of carbon dioxide and other harmful gases.

With carefully operated incubators, hatchability of 88–92% of all eggs set is not uncommon. Fertility of eggs, a major factor influencing the number of chicks hatched, should exceed 90%; levels of 95–97% are frequently achieved. Other factors influencing the number of chicks hatched are: incubation conditions; diet and age of the breeding stock; length of time the eggs are stored; environmental conditions under which the hatching eggs are stored before being placed in the incubator; and possible bacterial contamination of the egg shell.

Brooding and rearing. The procedures for caring for chicks after they have been removed from the incubator is known as brooding. Some artificial heat is required to keep the chicks comfortable during the first 6–8 weeks of brooding. Rearing refers to the growing period, which lasts about 8–20 weeks.

Chicks need to be placed in an environment having a temperature near the incubation level. This is accomplished by using a brooder stove which provides artificial heat and can be thermostatically controlled (Fig. 1). Weekly adjustments of thermostats are made for temperature control. Temperature is maintained at 90°F during the first week and then is dropped 5°F weekly until the chicks are about 6 weeks old.

Feeding troughs and waterers are also needed during brooding. For the first 5 days feed is placed in cardboard lids from chick boxes and set underneath and around the edges of the brooder stove. After 5 days the cardboard lids are replaced with an adequate number of small troughs. Water may be provided in small glass or tin water fountains placed around the edge of the brooder stove. After

6–8 weeks larger chick feeders and waterers may be installed. In commercial installations, with flocks of 20,000–60,000 broilers, mechanical feeders and automatic waterers are employed by the second or third week after hatching.

Feeding. No feed is required for the first 48 hr after chicks are hatched and removed from the incubator because the yolk of the egg is absorbed into the body cavity of the chick just before hatching and provides the necessary food requirements. This makes it possible to ship baby chicks to all parts of the world as well as to the most remote areas of the United States.

Ordinarily, chicks are fed as soon as they are delivered on the farm where they are to be grown. The diet is determined on the basis of age and the purpose for which the chicken is grown (see table), although chicks grown for egg production or broiler meat have similar nutrient requirements. The growing period for broilers requires a protein level over 20%. For laying chickens and growing pullet chicks from 8 to 20 weeks, when egg production starts, the protein level is reduced to 15–17% because less productive energy per pound of feed is required.

Nutrients are provided from a wide choice of feed ingredients. Among the more common ingredients are yellow corn, wheat or wheat by-products, oats, soybean meal, and alfalfa meal, with animal, fish, and milk by-products as protein supplements. Oyster shell and calcium carbonate are used to provide the calcium needed especially by laying and breeding flocks.

The various ingredients of the diet are mixed together and ground to form mash. This mash is fed to the chicks as soon as they are placed in the brooder house. In addition, chicks are fed a hard, insoluble grit, such as granite, which aids them in grinding feed particles. Sometimes the mash is compressed and fed in pellet form or the pellets may be reground to a crumbly consistency. Chicks are fed as much as they can consume daily. *See* ANIMAL-FEED COMPOSITION.

Suggested levels of certain nutrients in practical rations (total feed basis) for chickens

Nutrient	Starting chicks and broilers	Growing chickens	Laying chickens
Metabolizable energy, cal/lb	1400–1500	1250–1300	1250–1300
Crude protein, %	20–27	14–18	16–18
Calcium, %	1.00	0.80	2.75–3.50
Phosphorus, available,* %	0.40–0.45	0.35–0.40	0.45–0.65
total, %	0.70–0.80	0.50–0.80	0.70
Salt, total, %	0.45	0.45	0.45
Iodine, mg/lb	0.16	0.15	0.15
Manganese, mg/lb	35	35	20
Zinc, mg/lb	25	25	25
Selenium, ppm	0.1	0.1†	0.0
Vitamin A, IU/lb	3000–4000	3000–4000	3500–4000
Vitamin D_3, ICU/lb	300	300	400
Riboflavin, mg/lb	2.0	2.0	2.0
Pantothenic acid, mg/lb	5–7	4–5	4–5
Vitamin B_{12}, μg/lb	5	3–4	2
Choline, mg/lb	700	700	500
Niacin, mg/lb	20	17	15
Folacin, mg/lb	0.25	0.25	0.11
Vitamin K, mg/lb	0.5	0.5	0.5
Vitamin E‡ mb/lb	7.5	5.0	?

*Includes phosphorus from inorganic sources and animal sources and 30% of that from plant sources.
†Feed up to 16 weeks of age only.
‡Spared by antibiotics.

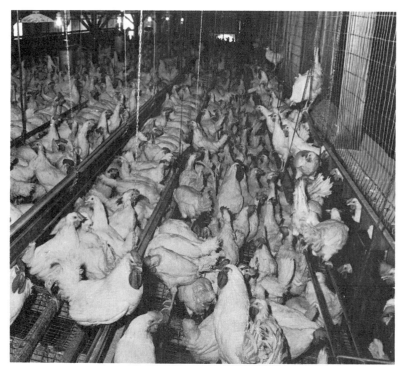

Fig. 2. Sloping wire floor egg production system. The water troughs have mechanical feeder lines on each side, and a double tier of roll-away nests is visible on the right. (*Pennsylvania State University*)

Egg production systems. There are two major systems for commercial egg production, the floor system and the cage system.

Floor system. The earlier method was to place litter, such as shavings, straw, or corn cob, on the floor and to allow $2\frac{1}{2}$–3 ft² of floor space per layer. This is gradually being replaced by housing with high-density floor for laying chickens. With the sloping wire floor system (Fig. 2), layers can be housed successfully at $\frac{2}{3}$ ft² floor space per layer.

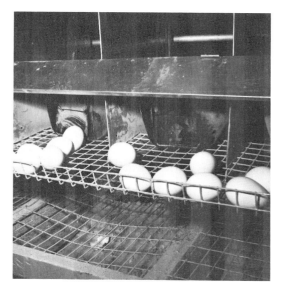

Fig. 3. Roll-away nest (rear view). After hen lays egg in nest, egg rolls through a flexible gate and comes to rest on open tray for rapid cooling to maintain quality. (*Pennsylvania State University*)

No litter is required and the chickens are removed from contact with their own droppings. Flocks of 10,000–20,000 layers in a single group are common and eggs are gathered from roll-away nests (Fig. 3) either mechanically or by hand. Food and water are supplied automatically. A combination of two-thirds wooden-slat floor and one-third litter is another floor system popular for commercial egg and breeder flocks.

Cage system. In the cage system layers are confined in rows of wire cages of various sizes separated by service aisles (Fig. 4). A common method is to confine three or four layers in a cage 12×16 in. Larger cages, 3×4 ft, accommodating about 25 layers, have also been used. Layers in these cages may be fed by a mechanical feeder or by an electric- or gasoline-powered feed cart. Individual water valves in each cage or water trough are used for watering. As in floor operations, eggs can be gathered mechanically or by hand.

Housing. Poultry houses, similar in both types of egg production systems, are designed to protect the chickens and to provide optimum conditions by preventing wide environmental fluctuations. This is accomplished by control of light, temperature, moisture, and air. Many of the poultry houses constructed today are prefabricated and are assembled on the farm site (Fig. 5).

The side walls of the houses are generally insulated with 2-in. fiber-glass batts or their equivalent in the form of styrofoam, urethane, or other types of insulating materials; 4-in. batts are used in the ceiling in northern areas of the United States. In the warmer Southern states, houses may be more open and have side drop curtains to protect flocks from the weather. However, in hot climates there is much interest in the use of totally enclosed and insulated houses for both temperature and light control.

Light stimulates egg production and, until pullets are nearing 20 weeks of age, they should not be exposed to an increase in day length, either by natural or artificial light, for this encourages early maturity. After 20 weeks an increase in day length is desirable to encourage maximum egg production. In short-day winter months, artificial lights controlled by a time clock are used to add to natural day length both at morning and evening. From 14 to $16\frac{1}{2}$ hr of light daily has been found satisfactory for optimum egg production, although much depends on how many hours of light the pullets were exposed to daily while growing.

Housing is designed to avoid extreme temperatures. Temperatures around 65–70°F are ideal for the most efficient broiler meat production, while the ideal temperature range for the most efficient and economical egg production is 55–75°F. Higher temperatures result in reduced egg size, thin shells, and decreased egg production. Between 32 and 55°F laying hens perform well but require more feed per dozen eggs; also, moisture problems in the house become more difficult to control. At temperatures below freezing, hens are uncomfortable, egg production may decrease, and feed requirements per dozen eggs increase significantly. In very cold weather, with house temperatures of 0–10°F, combs on cockerels (males) begin to freeze and fertility is lowered in breeding flocks.

Control of temperature and moisture is achieved

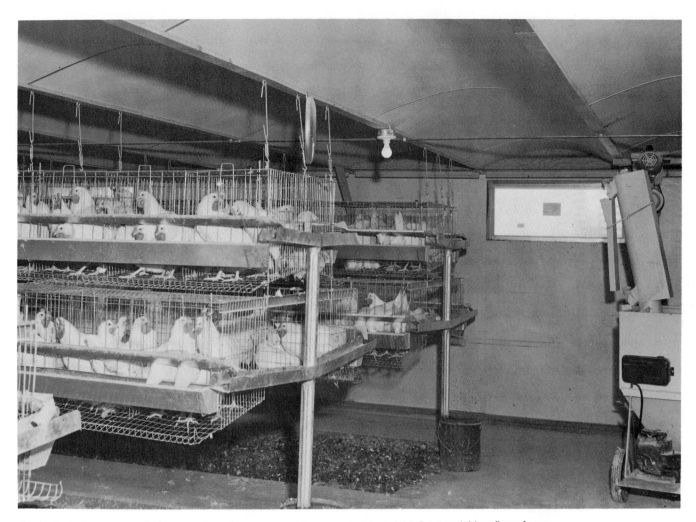

Fig. 4. Typical arrangement of cage system of egg production. Note the feed trough and water trough in front of each cage. Feed is augered into trough by using electric powered cart on right. Eggs are laid on floor of cage and roll to lower outside edge for gathering by hand or mechanically. (*J. C. Snavely and Co.*)

by the ventilation system. Thermostatically controlled fans exchange warm, moisture-laden air for cooler, drier air. Animal heat is the major source of heat in egg producing flocks: a $4\frac{1}{2}$ lb laying hen will produce about 42 Btu of heat per hour, which can be used for warming the poultry house and for moisture evaporation. A flock of 3000 hens produces about the same amount of heat per hour as a furnace in an average family-size house. However, since hens and broilers produce considerable amounts (75–80%) of water through respiration and droppings, this heat supply may not be adequate in cold weather if a house temperature above 55°F is to be maintained. Incoming cold air must be warmed and structural heat losses must be replaced. The balance of heat available may be insufficient to evaporate the amount of water produced, and thus the relative humidity rises, causing the interior walls and ceilings of the house to become damp. In such cases the house temperature may be lowered by reducing the temperature setting on the thermostat to move more fresh air

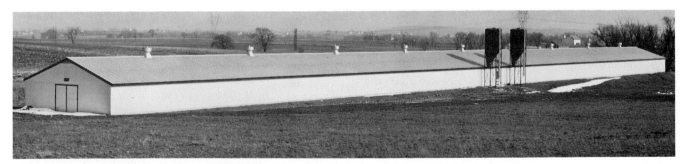

Fig. 5. Modern prefabricated environment-controlled poultry house used for both broiler and egg production. Note the bulk feed bins in center. Feed flows into mechanical feeder as needed. (*J. C. Snavely and Co.*)

through the house. For average weather conditions (32–70°F), 2 ft³ of air exchange per minute per layer is generally adequate.

In broiler production similar ventilating practices are followed. However, ventilation can become very critical. For the first 2 or 3 weeks, when chicks are small, very little ventilation is required. As broilers approach maturity (6–8 weeks), more air exchange is required because the brooder stoves may create dust. This can be a major problem since high levels of dust are not healthy for either the caretaker or the broilers.

Breeding. The application of genetic principles to poultry breeding has resulted in rapid advances in the improvement of growth and feed efficiency in broiler production, in increasing annual egg production, in improving egg quality factors, and in developing strains of chickens resistant to various diseases. Methods of intensive inbreeding of strains, followed by crossing inbred lines, has resulted in sharp increases in egg production. Breeding chickens resistant to avian leukosis offer new hope for reducing or eliminating the tremendous losses resulting annually from this disease. Development of a smaller laying chicken, without impairing production and egg size, can further reduce feed requirements and possibly housing and equipment costs because of lesser space requirements.

Breeding operations are highly specialized. Capital investment and operation costs are high and the results achieved will determine the direction of the poultry industry in the future. *See* BREEDING (ANIMAL).

Health. Poultry health is of paramount importance in the operation of a successful and profitable poultry farm. Improvements in housing and equipment can provide a more healthful atmosphere for poultry; however, death losses from diseases are still heavy in some commercial operations. Emphasis is directed toward the use of disease-resistant stock, vaccination against specific diseases, and the use of antibiotics and drugs in the feed or drinking water.

Pullorum disease has practically been eliminated, and respiratory diseases, such as Newcastle disease, bronchitis, and laryngotracheitis, as well as fowl pox, can be controlled by following a sound vaccination program. Coccidiosis, a protozoan disease attacking both young and adult stock, can be controlled by using various drugs in the feed. Leukosis, a highly complex disease manifesting itself in paralysis or total disability. A very effective vaccine has been developed to control Marek's disease, which is part of the avian leucosis complex.

Economics of production. The poultry industry is an excellent example of the effect of applied science and technology in lowering production costs. In 1932 the cost of producing a dozen eggs was 26 cents; in 1948, 53 cents; and in 1968, about 30 cents. The reduction in costs by almost 50% since World War II was the result of better breeding practices, more efficient use of feed, better diets, improvement of housing, and labor-saving mechanical equipment. However, by 1974 costs had risen to about 42 cents per dozen eggs due to inflation. About 4 lb of feed per dozen eggs were required in 1968–1974 as compared with 6–8 lb in 1946–

1947. Labor efficiency also improved. During the late 1940s, 3000–5000 hens provided adequate income for a family living, while 30,000–40,000 hens were considered a family-size operation in 1974. Environmentally controlled housing reduced housing costs per layer without seriously impairing egg production. The development of mechanical poultry feeders, automatic watering systems, mechanical poultry manure removal devices, and improved ventilation systems cut labor costs sharply. These improvements resulted in a rapid expansion of the egg industry. The egg supply has exceeded demand for a great portion of the time, with the result of a general reduction of egg prices to the producer as well as for the consumer. In broiler production a similar pattern has developed.

Marketing. Production of poultry meat or eggs is closely tied to the marketing of these products. A producer must be assured of a market before investing capital in a production enterprise. Chain-store merchandising has resulted in the negotiation of many types of production-marketing contracts which call for the production of large quantities of poultry products of uniform grade and quality. There are also many individual producers who develop their own market outlets through restaurants, hospitals, and other institutions and through retailing operations. Direct delivery from the farm to the consumer has the advantages of a fresher product reaching the market and also can be profitable for the producer. *See* AGRICULTURAL SCIENCE (ANIMAL); EGG PROCESSING.

[GLENN O. BRESSLER]

Bibliography: G. O. Bressler, T. W. Burr, and H. D. Bartlett, *Sloping Wire Floors in Poultry Houses*, Penn. Agric. Exp. Sta. Bull. no. 795, 1974; L. E. Card and M. C. Nesheim, *Poultry Production*, 10th ed., 1966; E. J. Gardner, *Principles of Genetics*, 5th ed., 1975; M. S. Hofstad et al., *Diseases of Poultry*, 6th ed., 1972; National Research Council, *Nutrient Requirements of Poultry*, 6th ed., 1971; M. L. Scott, M. C. Nesheim, and R. J. Young, *Nutrition of Chickens*, 1969; U.S. Department of Agriculture, *Commerical Broiler Production*, Agr. Handb. no. 320, 1967.

Proline

A common amino acid of proteins occurring in varying amounts in essentially all individual proteins, and in mixtures of proteins at about 4% by weight. It is a major amino acid (10–15%) in the collagen proteins. It was first synthesized in 1900

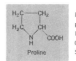

Physical constants of the L isomer at 25°C:
pK₁ (COOH: 1.99; pK₂ (NH₃⁺): 10.96
Isoelectric point: 6.30
Optical rotation: [α]ᴅ(H₂O): −86.2; [α]ᴅ(5 N HCl): −60.4
Solubility (g/100 ml H₂O): very soluble

by R. Willstätter and first isolated from protein in 1901 by E. Fischer. Like hydroxyproline, proline contains the pyrrolidine ring with its secondary amine, conferring unusual properties both chemically and biologically, compared with the primary amino acids common in proteins. Chemically, it gives a yellow instead of blue-purple color reaction with ninhydrin, and it is not deaminated by nitrous

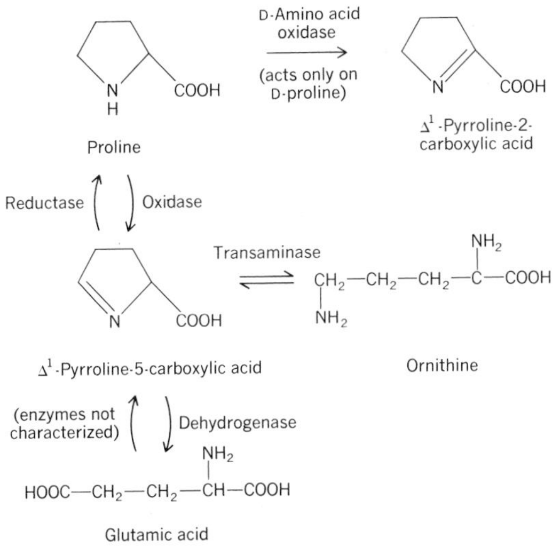

Metabolic reactions of proline.

acid treatment. In peptide linkage, its nitrogen lacks the hydrogen atom retained by amino acids, and the pyrrolidine ring hinders rotation about the bond between the nitrogen and α-carbon atom; in consequence the geometry of the peptide chain of proteins is altered by proline. The structural features of collagen are also greatly influenced by their high content of proline and hydroxyproline as well as glycine. See AMINO ACIDS; HYDROXYPROLINE.

Nutritionally, proline is not required in the diet of man or other mammals, since it is formed freely from glutamic acid, which in turn is derived from products of carbohydrate metabolism. Free L-proline, like many amino acids, occurs at several milligrams percent in human blood and tissues. It occurs at high concentration (up to 600 mg %) in the hemolymph of certain insects. See CARBOHYDRATE METABOLISM; GLUTAMIC ACID.

An apparent consequence of the secondary nitrogen in the amino group of proline (and hydroxyproline) is failure of these compounds to undergo enzymatic reactions involving pyridoxal phosphate as a coenzyme. Thus, direct transamination or decarboxylation of proline is not known, although many primary amino acids undergo such reactions catalyzed by pyridoxal phosphate enzymes. A racemase for proline (interconverting L-proline and D-proline) occurs in certain bacteria, but this enzyme uses a mechanism other than pyridoxal-catalyzed racemization.

In its biological formation and degradation, proline is closely related to two other 5-carbon amino acids, glutamic acid and ornithine. Proline is formed enzymatically from glutamic acid through the intermediate compound, Δ¹-pyrroline-5-carboxylic acid. The enzymes that catalyze this process are not yet fully characterized. A separate set of enzymes present in both animals and bacteria oxidizes proline to glutamic acid through the same intermediate, Δ¹-pyrroline-5-carboxylic acid. The latter reactions account for the manner in which proline can be completely oxidized to carbon dioxide.

In addition, ornithine transaminase, an enzyme that occurs in many cells, can interconvert ornithine and Δ¹-pyrroline-5-carboxylic acid. Since the latter compound is readily formed from or converted to proline, ornithine transaminase provides a route for the interconversion of proline and ornithine. These metabolic transformations are shown in the illustration.

D-Proline is oxidized by the enzyme D-amino acid oxidase (present in tissues of animals) to yield Δ¹-pyrroline-2-carboxylic acid.

A rare hereditary human disease, prolinemia, occurs when one or another of the degradative enzymes converting proline to glutamic acid is absent. Affected persons have a high content of proline in blood and urine and may suffer from mental retardation and renal malfunction.

[ELIJAH ADAMS]

Bibliography: J. P. Greenstein and M. Winitz, *Chemistry of the Amino Acids*, vols. 1–3, 1961; A. Meister, *Biochemistry of the Amino Acids*, vols. 1 and 2, 2d ed., 1965.

Protein

A polymeric compound made up of various amino acids as the monomeric units. Proteins generally contain from 50 to 1000 amino acid residues per polypeptide chain. The amino acids are joined by peptide bonds between the α-carboxyl groups and the α-amino groups of adjacent amino acids in which the α-amino group of the first amino acid residue is usually free, as shown below.

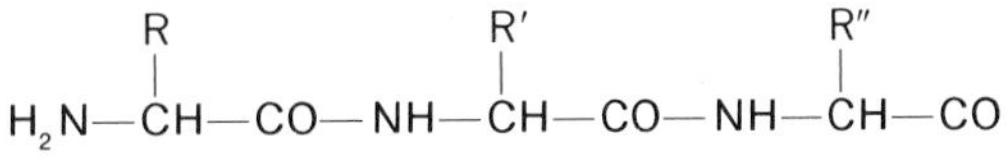

$$H_2N-CH-CO-NH-CH-CO-NH-CH-CO$$

with R, R', R'' substituents on the respective CH groups.

Occurrence. Proteins are of importance in all biological systems, playing a wide variety of structural and functional roles. They form the primary organic basis of structures such as hair, tendons, muscle, skin, and cartilage. All of the enzymes, the catalysts in biochemical transformations, are protein in nature. Many hormones, such as insulin and growth hormone, are proteins. The substances responsible for oxygen and electron transport (hemoglobin and the cytochromes, respectively) are conjugated proteins that contain a metalloporphyrin as the prosthetic group. The chromosomes are highly complex nucleoproteins, that is, proteins conjugated with nucleic acid. The viruses are also nucleoprotein in nature. Thus, proteins play a fundamental role in the processes of life.

Of the more than 200 amino acids that have been discovered either in the free state or in small peptides, only 20 amino acids, or derivatives of these 20, are present in mammalian proteins. They are glycine, alanine, isoleucine, leucine, valine, serine, threonine, aspartic acid, glutamic acid, asparagine, glutamine, arginine, lysine, cysteine, methionine, phenylalanine, tyrosine, tryptophan, histidine, and proline. The amino acids thus far examined in mammalian proteins have the L configuration, but both the D and L isomers of amino acids occur in the free state and in peptides. Commonly occurring derivatives of these 20 amino acids are cystine, hydroxyproline, and hydroxylysine. Cystine results from the oxidation of two cysteine residues to form a disulfide bridge. Hydroxyproline and hydroxylysine are formed by the enzymatic hydroxylation of specific proline and lysine residues, respectively, while the polypeptide chain of collagen is being synthesized on the ribosome. Other examples of biological modification of parent amino acid residues are O-phosphoserine in phosvitin, ^3N-methylhistidine in actin, and ϵ-N-methyllysine in histones. *See* AMINO ACIDS.

Specificity. The linear arrangement of the amino acid residues in a protein is termed its sequence (primary structure). The sequence in which the different amino acids are linked in any given protein is highly specific and characteristic for that particular protein.

This specificity of sequence is one of the most remarkable aspects of protein chemistry. The number of possible permutations of sequence in even so small a protein as insulin, of molecular weight 5732 and with 51 amino acid residues, is astronomic: 10^{51} permutations. Yet it has been established that the pancreatic cell of a given species has only one of these possible sequences. The elucidation of the mechanism conferring such a high degree of specificity on the biosynthetic reactions by which proteins are built up from free amino acids has been one of the key problems of modern biochemistry.

The task of determining the sequences of proteins has been a major preoccupation of a large number of scientists since the mid-1940s. Major innovations in the techniques for the isolation of proteins in the pure state and for the separation and quantitative determination of their constituent amino acids were necessary before substantial progress could be made.

Preparation. The solution to the total structure of a protein begins with its purification to homogeneity from the tissue of origin. The isolation of a protein in the pure state usually requires a combination of several of the techniques described below. If the protein is an enzyme, a hormone, or an antibody that has a biological activity that can be measured, the preparation will be facilitated. The primary concern of protein chemists and enzymologists is that the material they ultimately isolate be in its native form—in other words, that it has not been denatured or degraded during any of the steps of the preparation.

In order to minimize the chances of denaturation, it is best to observe certain ground rules derived from experience with known proteins: (1) Temperatures should be kept as low as possible. This is particularly important when organic solvents such as ethanol and acetone are used. (2) Extremes of pH are to be avoided. (3) High concentrations of protein are preferable since most proteins are relatively more stable when concentrated. (4) Excessive agitation and foaming are to be avoided since proteins denature more rapidly at surfaces and interfaces.

In the first step of the preparation, mechanical disruption of the tissue or cell source is usually necessary for efficient extraction of the proteins. The tools used for this disruption can vary from a meat grinder, to a Waring blender, to an ultrasonic oscillator. Once the solution is made, any combination of the methods described below can be applied.

Salting out. High concentrations of neutral salt tend to precipitate proteins; the concentration necessary for such precipitation varies from protein to protein. The most commonly used salt for this purpose is ammonium sulfate, which has the

advantages of high solubility at low temperatures, and a low temperature coefficient of solubility. It is conventional to record the concentration of ammonium sulfate as the percentage of complete saturation at the given temperature rather than as the absolute molar concentration. By adding salt stepwise to a protein solution and centrifuging off the precipitate at each step, a series of arbitrary fractions is obtained in which the desired protein will generally be concentrated. For example, the addition of ammonium sulfate to serum to 34% saturation precipitates most of the γ-globulins and very little of the other protein components. This 34% "cut" can be centrifuged, redissolved, and subjected to further purification steps. At 50–60% saturation, the serum albumin that makes up 55% of the total serum proteins will precipitate. This fraction can be redissolved in distilled water and subsequently crystallized by the addition of ammonium sulfate to 55–65% saturation.

Salting out is a function not only of the molar concentration of salt but also of the charges on the ions. Thus, the effects of salts on protein solubility are better described in terms of ionic strength, defined by Eq. (1), where C_i denotes the molar

$$\mu = 1/2 \sum_i C_i Z_i^2 \qquad (1)$$

concentration of a given ionic species in the solution and Z_i denotes the charge on that species, and the sum is taken of all ionic species present. For example, the ionic strength of 1 M sodium chloride (NaCl) is 1; the ionic strength of 1 M ammonium sulfate $[(NH_4)_2SO_4]$ is 3. At a given pH, the change in solubility of a protein with change in salt concentration can be approximated by Eq. (2), where

$$\log S = \beta - K_s \mu \qquad (2)$$

μ is solubility in grams per liter; K_s is a salting-out constant, dependent on the nature of the protein and the salt used, but independent of pH and temperature; and β is the logarithm of the hypothetical solubility of zero ionic strength, a value strongly dependent on pH and temperature.

With sparingly soluble proteins such as myosin, purification is better achieved by first extracting the more readily soluble proteins, leaving the desired material in a partially purified form.

Isoelectric precipitation. At any given salt concentration, protein solubility varies with pH and is at a minimum at the isoelectric pH. By raising the salt concentration and adjusting the pH to the isoelectric point, it is often possible to obtain a precipitate considerably enriched in the desired material. In some cases, the desired component can be crystallized directly from a heterogeneous mixture of proteins by this simple procedure. Ovalbumin, for example, can be obtained in crystalline form from egg white in essentially two steps. First, the globulins are precipitated by adding ammonium sulfate to 40% saturation. The supernatant is then adjusted to pH 4.7, the isoelectric point of ovalbumin, and the ammonium sulfate concentration is gradually increased until a slight opalescence develops. Addition of seed crystals is frequently all that is necessary to initiate crystallization. Protein crystals obtained in this way are rarely completely free of contaminant proteins. Repeated recrystallization or application of other purification procedures is required to obtain a homogeneous protein.

Dialysis and dilution. Some proteins, the globulins, are relatively insoluble at very low ionic strengths and can be precipitated from a mixture simply by dialysis against water, thus progressively removing salt from the solution. Also, addition of large volumes of water will reduce the salt concentration (ionic strength) and effect precipitation.

Precipitation with organic solvents. Organic solvents, such as ethanol or acetone, reduce the solubility of most proteins. At room temperature, denaturation proceeds very rapidly in the presence of these reagents, but they can be and have been successfully employed by carrying out all operations at temperatures near or below 0°C. By appropriate selection of pH, ionic strength, temperature, and ethanol concentration, a series of precipitated fractions can be obtained which, although mixtures, represent a considerable degree of purification of each of the major groups of serum proteins. This separation can then be followed by subfractionation steps leading to progressively purer components.

Paper chromatography. This method is not widely used for purification of proteins, but it has been successful in a few instances, such as in the purification of insulin from pancreatic extracts on a small scale. It has been a key method, on the other hand, in the separation of peptides in connection with studies of protein structure.

Column chromatography. This procedure, using ion-exchange resins and chemically modified cellulose derivatives, is a powerful tool. Low-molecular-weight proteins, especially those with markedly acidic or basic isoelectric points, such as ribonuclease, histones, and lysozyme, can be separated from most other proteins in a mixture in a single experiment on an ion-exchange column. Powdered cellulose, chemically treated to introduce charged groups, is particularly suitable for protein fractionation, since the conditions of pH and ionic strength used are in a range in which most proteins are stable. By the use of eluants graded continuously in pH and ionic strength, remarkable resolution can be achieved, and the capacity of the columns permits the handling of gram quantities of protein.

Affinity chromatography. The resolving power of ion-exchange chromatography can, in some instances, be enhanced by the covalent attachment to the chromatographic matrix of a small molecule that has an affinity for the protein that is being purified. Where applicable, the technique has been successfully used in the purification of enzymes by attachment of the substrate for the enzyme to the solid phase. In a few cases total purification in one step has been achieved.

Countercurrent distribution. When two mutually immiscible solvent systems are available, countercurrent distribution is an effective system for purification, but the range of application has been narrow. The power of the method was shown by the successful separation by L. Craig of insulin into two components differing by only a single amide group. This method, however, has been much more widely utilized in fractionation of polypeptides than in fractionation of proteins.

Preparative ultracentrifugation. Proteins of high molecular weight can be concentrated at the bottom of a centrifuge tube by applying a high gravitational field for a prolonged time. It is therefore possible to achieve significant purification

only for the heaviest or the lightest components in a mixture, and the degree of purification will depend on the range of sedimentation velocities represented. Proteins with densities less than that of the solvent float to the surface under the influence of a strong gravitational field.

The latter principle has been applied with success to the study of serum lipoproteins, which, by virtue of their lipid content, have densities less than those of other serum proteins. Sufficient salt is added to the serum to raise its density above that of any of the lipoproteins, yet not above that of the other serum proteins. Centrifugation to equilibrium (100,000 g for 20 hr) brings the lipoproteins to the surface, where they can be collected. This technique has been refined by the use of repeated centrifugation steps at progressively rising salt densities so that subfractions of the lipoproteins in different density classes can be obtained on a preparative scale.

Gel filtration. Another technique for the purification of proteins that separates mainly on the basis of molecular weight is gel filtration. Dextran beads, micrometers in diameter, are selected that exclude proteins of high molecular weight but permit smaller protein molecules to diffuse in and out. With a column of such beads there is a continual distribution and eventual separation as the protein mixture moves through the column. Beads of different porosities are available to separate proteins of different molecular weights. For example, with one type of beaded dextran, proteins of molecular weight of about 10,000 can be easily separated from all those proteins whose molecular weights are greater than 50,000.

Preparative electrophoresis. In the classical free electrophoresis system of A. Tiselius, the mixture of proteins to be analyzed occupies one segment of a U-shaped vessel. When current is applied, the fastest-migrating component lags behind the body of proteins in the mixture. Thus, the proteins of maximum and minimum mobility can be isolated in a relatively pure form, but those of intermediate mobility can be only partially purified by this procedure. Therefore, modified methods, more suitable for preparative purposes, have been introduced.

In zone electrophoresis, the protein mixture is applied as a very narrow band on filter paper, on a block of starch, or on some other supporting medium wetted with an appropriate buffer solution. When current is passed through the supporting medium, each protein moves out from the line of origin with a characteristic velocity. Within a given time with a given current flow, each protein migrates a characteristic distance from the line of origin. At the end of the run, the proteins of the mixture are separated from one another. The supporting medium can then be divided into a number of separate zones, and the proteins in each zone can be eluted from the paper or starch for analysis and further purification. Electrophoresis on paper, using currents of 5000–10,000 V, is a most powerful tool for the separation of peptides obtained from partial enzymatic or acid hydrolysates of proteins.

Isoelectric focusing. In this procedure, which is usually carried out either in a vertical column of a solution that contains a gradient in sucrose concentration or in a semisolid phase of dextran, synthetic polymers of amino acids of varying isoelectric points are added to the protein mixture. In an electric field, these synthetic polymers migrate, and a gradient of these polyamino acids is eventually set up according to the pH values at which they have zero net charge (pI). The added proteins will also be distributed according to the pI of each protein in the mixture. Efficient separations can sometimes be achieved, but the technique suffers from the disadvantage that some proteins tend to precipitate at their isoelectric point, and thus the gradient can be disrupted.

Analysis. Because of the relatively high molecular weight of proteins, the classical methods of organic chemistry are not sensitive enough to establish purity. A more meaningful empirical formula for a protein is given in terms of the numbers of its constituent amino acids. Thus, the pure protein can be hydrolyzed in 6 N HCl to liberate the amino acids, which can be quantitatively estimated by amino acid analysis. These data, together with an independent measurement of the molecular weight of the protein, will yield the amino acid composition of the protein. In those few cases in which a protein is known to lack a particular amino acid (for example, tryptophan is absent from ribonuclease, and isoleucine is absent from human adult hemoglobin), the amino acid composition can also be an indication of the state of purity of the particular sample. Analysis for only one end group at the NH_2 terminus of a protein is suggestive evidence of purity. However, for most proteins, other criteria must be used to establish homogeneity. In the case of certain conjugated proteins that contain a stoichiometric amount of a prosthetic group, analysis for purity is simplified. For example, in the cytochromes, which contain an atom of iron, the iron content, which can be accurately determined, is an extremely sensitive index of purity. Crystallinity, once thought to be a rather good proof of purity, is now recognized to be inconclusive. Frequently a crystalline preparation, although very rich in the desired material, proves upon careful analysis by more sensitive methods to be a mixture of two or more proteins. Therefore, it has been necessary to develop special methods for protein characterization, and many of these methods are closely related to those used for isolation of pure proteins.

The most important generalization to be noted is that none of the methods commonly used will establish unequivocally the purity of a protein. A preparation that is pure by one criterion may prove to be inhomogeneous by another. The best that can be done is to accumulate negative evidence by applying a number of criteria. Electrophoresis and ultracentrifugation are the classical procedures for judging the purity of a protein. If the material migrates as a single component in an electric field and sediments as a single component in a centrifugal field, this is strong evidence of purity. Examination at different ionic strengths and pH values may reveal inhomogeneity in a protein that had been apparently pure under another set of conditions. What actually is demonstrated is that all of the proteins in the preparation have the same or very similar charge and molecular size and shape. Subtle differences in structure will not be detected. Insulin, for example, behaves as a homogeneous protein when examined by these methods, but

when the countercurrent distribution method is used, it is shown to be a mixture of two components which differ only by one amide group. *See* COLLOID.

The techniques of immunochemistry can be applied in several ways to the study of protein homogeneity. Antigen-antibody reactions, although highly specific, are not completely so. Consequently, the most sensitive methods utilize a combination of immunochemical properties and physical properties. For example, antibody prepared against a protein preparation can be incorporated into a gel, and the solution being tested for homogeneity can then be allowed to diffuse through the gel. If the preparation is pure, a single zone of precipitation will appear at the point in the advancing front at which the antibody-antigen ratio is optimal for the precipitin reaction. If more than one antigenic protein is present, more than one band will appear at points dependent on the diffusion constant of the proteins and on their immunochemical properties. Another highly sensitive method, immunoelectrophoresis, combines zone electrophoresis with immune precipitation.

Finally, during the determination of the sequence of a protein, significant amounts of impurities, if present, will become evident.

Structure. With the protein in a state of homogeneity, the problem of solving its structure could then be undertaken. This task required the development of many new techniques in protein chemistry. Pioneering contributions were made by F. Sanger, who determined the primary sequence of the protein insulin with its 51 amino acid residues, and by S. Moore and W. H. Stein, who determined the primary sequence of the enzyme ribonuclease with its 124 amino acid residues. The strategy in the sequencing of a protein has depended upon coupling of the free α-amino residue of the polypeptide with a chemical, particularly phenyl isothiocyanate, that will remove that residue under appropriate conditions and leave the remainder of the polypeptide chain intact.

At this point in the process it is possible to identify the cleaved derivative of the first amino acid residue or the remaining amino acids by a variety of techniques such as chromatography. The stepwise process, introduced by P. Edman, is then repeated in this manner as far as possible. The process has been automated, and the machinery is available commercially. Stepwise removal of amino acid residues from the carboxyl end of the molecule by enzymes called carboxypeptidases has also proved to be a useful technique. Usually it is necessary to partially degrade the protein, either with proteolytic enzymes that split at specific peptide bonds or by specific chemical cleavages within the polypeptide chain, for example, by splitting the protein at the methionine residues with cyanogen bromide to yield a mixture of smaller peptides. Each of these peptides can, in turn, be attacked by a combination of end-group methods, amino acid analysis, and some of the stepwise degradative procedures. By combining the results of a variety of such procedures, it is then possible to reconstruct the sequence within each peptide. Finally, by combining the results obtained by degrading the original protein with proteolytic enzymes of different bond specificity, the order of the peptide fragments in the protein and hence the total sequence can be deduced.

From the proteins that have been sequenced thus far, it is clear that proteins of similar function from different species and those with common genetic origins have similar sequences. When there are differences in the sequence, the changes are usually conservative, for example, the replacement of one aliphatic amino acid by a different aliphatic amino acid.

Proteins are not stretched polymers; rather, the polypeptide backbone of the molecule can fold in several ways by means of hydrogen bonds between the carbonyl oxygen and the amide nitrogen. As shown by C. B. Anfinsen, the folding of each protein is determined by its particular sequence of amino acids.

Largely as a result of x-ray diffraction studies, it is known that the long polypeptide chains of proteins, particularly those of the fibrous proteins, are in fact held together in a rather well-defined configuration. The backbone is coiled in a regular fashion, forming an extended helix. As a result of this coiling, peptide bonds separated from one another by several amino acid residues are brought into close spatial approximation. The stability of the helical configuration can be attributed to hydrogen bonds between these peptide bonds. The particular helical configuration which best fits the available x-ray data is that proposed by L. Pauling and R. B. Corey (see illustration). In this structure, each —NH group in peptide bond is

$$\overset{O}{\overset{\|}{-C-}}$$

hydrogen-bonded in the —C— group three residues removed from it.

The pitch of the helix is such that 3.7 amino acids are contained in one complete turn. There is no doubt of the importance of the helical configuration in fibrous proteins. There is also evidence for a similar orientation of the polypeptide chains in globular proteins. In addition to hydrogen bonds, there are electrostatic interactions, such as those between —COO⁻ and —NH₃⁺ groups of the side chains, and Van der Waals forces, that is, hydrophobic interactions, which help to determine the configuration of the polypeptide chain. The term secondary structure is used to refer to all those structural features of the polypeptide chain determined by noncovalent bonding of the types just discussed.

In addition to the α-helical sections of proteins, there are also segments that contain β-structures in which there are hydrogen bonds between two polypeptide chains that run in parallel or antiparallel fashion.

The third level of folding in a protein (that is, tertiary structure) comes about through various interactions between different parts of the molecule. The disulfide bridge formed between two cysteine residues at different linear locations in the molecule can stabilize parts of a three-dimensional structure by introducing a primary valence bond as a cross-link. Hydrogen bonds between different segments of the protein, hydrophobic bonds between nonpolar side chains of amino acids such as phenylalanine and leucine, and salt bridges such as those between positively charged lysyl side chains and negatively charged aspartyl side chains

all contribute to the individual tertiary structure of a protein.

Finally, for those proteins that contain more than one polypeptide chain per molecule, there is usually a high degree of interaction between each subunit, for example, between the α- and β-polypeptide chains of hemoglobin. This feature of protein structure is termed its quarternary structure.

Properties. The properties of proteins are determined in part by their amino acid composition. For example, the net charge on the macromolecule at any given hydrogen-ion concentration is largely a function of the relative number of basic (lysine, histidine, and arginine) and dicarboxylic amino acids (aspartic and glutamic acids). This net charge strongly influences the solubility of the protein at different pH values since the solubility depends in part on the proportion of polar groupings on the macromolecule. When the hydrogen-ion concentration is high (low pH), the net charge is positive; when the hydrogen-ion concentration is low (high pH), the net charge is negative. The pH at which the net charge of the protein is zero is defined as the isoelectric point (pI).

As macromolecules that contain many side chains that can be protonated and unprotonated depending upon the pH of the medium, proteins are excellent buffers. The fact that the pH of blood varies only very slightly in spite of the numerous metabolic processes in which it participates is due to the very large buffering capacity of the blood proteins.

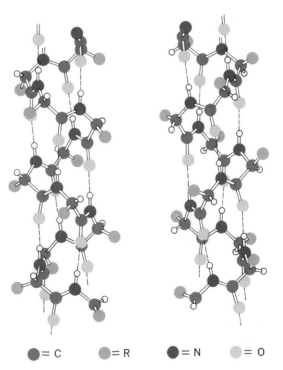

● = C   ● = R   ● = N   ● = O

The α-helix proposed by L. Pauling and R. B. Corey. The repeating —N—C—C— units form the backbone which spirals up in a left-handed or a right-handed fashion. Hydrogen bonds are indicated by the broken lines. Note that the side chains (R) are all directed out from the helix. The pitch of the helix is about 5.4 A (0.54 nm), and there are 3.7 residues contained in one complete turn. (From J. T. Edsall and J. Wyman, Biophysical Chemistry, vol. 1, Academic Press, 1958)

As mentioned above, it is the interaction of the side chains of amino acids that provides some proteins (enzymes) with their ability to catalyze essential reactions in body metabolism. Likewise, the specific binding of small ions to the side chains of proteins permits the transport of essential metal ions into and out of cells, as in the action of the sodium pump in the membrane of some cells.

Biosynthesis. Although a few proteins such as collagen are stable indefinitely in adulthood, most body proteins are in a continual process of degradation and synthesis (turnover). Thus, the half-life of serum proteins in humans is about 10 days. The processes by which proteins are synthesized biologically have been one of the central themes of molecular biology during the past 2 decades. The sequence of amino acid residues in a protein is controlled by the sequence of the DNA as expressed in a molecule called messenger RNA.

Each ingredient amino acid is first activated by adenosinetriphosphate in the presence of a specific enzyme. This activated amino acid is then transferred to a molecule of transfer RNA that possesses a triplet of nucleotides in its sequence (anticodon) that is unique for the amino acid it carries. The amino acid–transfer RNA complex then links up specifically to a segment of the messenger RNA on the ribosome through bonding between the anticodon on the transfer RNA and a complementary codon of three nucleotides on the messenger RNA. Two activated amino acid–transfer RNA complexes that are adjacent on the ribosome can then form a peptide bond and leave the ribosome. The process continues until the synthesis of the entire protein is complete. Although the general picture for the biological synthesis of proteins is now clear, the control mechanisms for the switching on and off of protein synthesis, as in cell differentiation, is an area of science that should generate enormous interest and excitement during the next few decades.

[GERTRUDE E. PERLMANN; JAMES M. MANNING]

Bibliography: M. L. Anson et al. (eds.), *Advances in Protein Chemistry*, 1944–1975; R. E. Dickerson and I. Geis, *The Structure and Action of Proteins*, 1969; C. H. W. Hirs and S. Timasheff, *Methods in Enzymology*, vol. 11, 1967, vol. 25, 1972; D. E. Koshland, Jr., *Sci. Amer.*, 229, 4:52–64, 1973; H. Neurath, *The Proteins*, vols. 1–4, 1963–1966, vol. 5, 1970.

Protein metabolism

The transformation and fate of food proteins from their ingestion to the elimination of their excretion products. Proteins are of exceptional importance to organisms because they are the chief constituents, aside from water, of all the soft tissue of the body. Special proteins have unique roles as structural and functional elements of cells and tissues. Examples are keratin of skin, collagen of tendons, actin and myosin of muscle, the blood proteins, enzymes in all tissues, and protein hormones of the hypophysis.

PROTEINS IN HEALTH AND DISEASE

Isotopic labeling experiments have established that body proteins are in a dynamic state, constantly being broken down and replaced. This is a rapid process in organs active in metabolism, such as liver, kidney, intestinal mucosa, and pancreas,

much slower in skeletal muscle, and extremely slow in connective tissue elements and skin.

Protein is digested to amino acids in the gastrointestinal tract. These are absorbed and distributed among the different tissues, where they form a series of amino acid pools that are kept equilibrated with each other through the medium of the circulating blood. The needs for protein synthesis of the different organs are supplied from these pools. Excess amino acids in the tissue pools lose their nitrogen by a combination of transamination and deamination. The nitrogen is largely converted to urea and excreted in the urine. The residual carbon products are then further metabolized by pathways common to the other major foodstuffs—carbohydrates and fats. *See* CARBOHYDRATE; LIPID.

The recommended daily protein intake is 1 g/kg body weight for adults, for example, 70 g for a 165-lb man. This is increased to 3.5 g/kg for infants up to 1 year, and from 1.5 to 2 g/kg for growing children and for women during the latter half of pregnancy and during nursing.

Role in diet. Ingestion of protein is needed primarily to supply amino acids for the formation of new and depleted body protein and as a source of various other body constituents derived from the amino acids. The amino acids of proteins fall into two nutritional categories: essential or indispensable, and nonessential or dispensable. For a number of amino acids, the category to which they belong changes between the periods of body growth and adulthood and changes also in different animal species.

The nutritional classification of the amino acids for the growth of the rat is shown in Table 1. It has been found to hold generally for a number of carnivores and omnivores. Such measurements have not been made on growing children. Ruminants synthesize practically all the amino acids through the action of the bacteria of the rumen.

The essential amino acids for maintenance of nitrogen equilibrium in healthy young men and the daily requirement are given in Table 2. This list comprises only eight amino acids. The remaining amino acids can be formed in the body from other materials. Only in this sense can the dietary dispensable amino acids be considered nonessential. All of the constituent amino acids are essential for protein formation, and certain of them are the precursors of such important body substances as creatine, thyroxin, adrenalin, histamine, and the purines and porphyrins. *See* AMINO ACIDS.

Table 1. Classification of amino acids with respect to growth effect in white rat*

Essential or indispensable		Nonessential or dispensable	
Lysine	Isoleucine	Glycine‡	Hydroxy-
Tryptophan	Methionine	Alanine	proline
Histidine	Valine	Serine	Citrulline
Phenyl-	Threonine	Aspartic acid	Cystine§
alanine	Arginine†	Glutamic acid	Tyrosine§
Leucine		Proline	

*After W. C. Rose, *Phys. Rev.*, 18:109, 1938.

†Arginine can be synthesized by the rat, but not at a sufficiently rapid rate to meet the demands of normal growth.

‡Glycine is essential for the growing chick.

§When adequate amounts of these amino acids are available in the diet, the requirement for methionine and phenylalanine, respectively, is diminished.

It might be expected that in conditions of augmented protein need, such as pregnancy and lactation and after trauma, or in specific pathological conditions, certain of the dispensable amino acids would become indispensable, due to overtaxing of the synthetic capacity. There is almost no information on this point. In the disease phenylketonuria, it has been indicated that tyrosine becomes indispensable because there is a block in the conversion of phenylalanine to tyrosine. *See* PHENYLPYRUVIC OLIGOPHRENIA.

Nutritive value of proteins. All proteins are not equally nutritious. Animal proteins are generally superior to vegetable proteins. Rarely, this may result from resistance to digestion, which usually is counteracted by cooking or heating. A well-known example is soybean meal. The nutritive value of its protein is improved by heating because this destroys a substance in the meal which inhibits digestion by trypsin. Overheating lowers the nutritional value of proteins by making lysine unavailable. This is a problem of some concern in connection with the manufacture of prepared breakfast cereals. The major cause of poor nutritional value, however, is a low content or unavailability of one or more of the indispensable amino acids. Vegetable proteins tend to be lacking in lysine and tryptophan. *See* FOOD ENGINEERING.

DIGESTION OF PROTEIN

This occurs to a limited extent in the stomach and is completed in the duodenum of the small intestine. The main proteolytic enzyme of the stomach is pepsin, which is secreted by the chief cells in an inactive form, pepsinogen. Its transformation to the active pepsin is initiated by the acidity of the gastric juice and accelerated and completed by pepsin. The activation process involves liberation of a portion of the pepsinogen molecule as a peptide. Pepsin preferentially hydrolyzes peptide bonds containing an aromatic amino acid, and it requires an acid medium to function. *See* DIGESTIVE SYSTEM.

A second proteinase in the stomach, rennin, present only in infancy, is particularly adapted to the digestion of milk protein. Digestion is initiated by the well-known milk-clotting reaction used in cheese manufacture. Rennin requires less acid than pepsin to be active. In infancy, hydrochloric acid secretion by the stomach is not fully developed. *See* CHEESE.

Digestion in intestine. The acid chyme is discharged from the stomach, containing partially degraded proteins, into a slightly alkaline fluid in the small intestine. This fluid is composed of pancreatic juice and succus entericus, the intestinal secretion. The pancreas secretes three known proteinases, trypsin, chymotrypsin, and carboxypeptidase. All three are secreted as inactive zymogens. Activation starts through the action of a substance present in the intestinal secretion, itself a specific enzyme — enterokinase. This transforms the inactive trypsinogen into the active trypsin. This conversion also is hastened by the autocatalytic activity of trypsin. Trypsin, in turn, activates chymotrypsin and carboxypeptidase. In all of these activation processes, certain peptide bonds are broken to yield the active enzymes. The mucosa of the small intestine contains various peptidases which are not liberated into the intestinal fluid, but apparently act by contact at the cell surface, or by absorption of the split products produced during intestinal digestion.

Trypsin and chymotrypsin are endopeptidases; that is, they cleave internal peptide bonds. The so-called peptidases are exopeptidases. They cleave terminal peptide bonds. Trypsin has a predilection for those containing the basic amino acid residues of lysine and arginine. These two proteinases perform the major share in hydrolyzing proteins to small peptides. Digestion to amino acids is completed by the exopeptidases. Carboxypeptidase acts on peptides from the free carboxyl end; aminopeptidases from the free amino end. Other peptidases act on di- or tripeptides, or peptides containing such special amino acids as proline.

The absorbed amino acids are carried by the portal blood system to the liver. From there, they are distributed to the rest of the body.

The amino acid digestion products of the proteins are absorbed as rapidly as they are liberated. The absorption is confined chiefly to the small intestine and is a process that involves the metabolic participation of the cells of the intestinal mucosa. Small amounts of the peptides formed during digestion escape further hydrolysis and may also enter the circulation from the intestine. This is shown by a rise in the peptide nitrogen in the blood.

The permeability of the intestinal mucosa for undigested protein appears greater in infancy. This, in combination with the low concentration of digestive enzymes, appears responsible for the immunological sensitization often observed in infants, particularly for milk and egg proteins. Thus, the digestion of protein is necessary not only to yield small, diffusible compounds that are readily absorbed from the intestine, but also to eliminate the antigenic properties of proteins, which could produce harmful allergic reactions.

To serve the needs for protein synthesis, all the constituent amino acids must be introduced into the body simultaneously. Withholding of an indispensable amino acid, even for a few hours, produces growth retardation or a negative nitrogen balance.

Protein in feces formation. The unabsorbed food residue in the small intestine is passed into the cecum, then the colon, and finally is eliminated as feces. Water is absorbed from the liquid mass, leading to a more solid consistency in the cecum and ascending colon. The fecal material is composed of undigested food residues, bile pigments,

Table 2. Essential amino acids for normal man when the diet furnishes sufficient nitrogen for the synthesis of the nonessentials*

Amino acid	Minimum requirement, g/day	Recommended intake,† g/day	Number of subjects tested
L-Tryptophan	0.25	0.5	37
L-Phenylalanine	1.10	2.2	28
L-Lysine	0.80	1.6	33
L-Threonine	0.50	1.0	24
L-Valine	0.80	1.6	29
L-Methionine	1.10	2.2	19
L-Leucine	1.10	2.2	14
L-Isoleucine	0.70	1.4	14

*After W. C. Rose, *Chem. Eng. News*, 30:2385, 1952.
†These figures represent in each case a safe intake and are not to be regarded as optimum.

leukocytes, bacteria, and the products of secretion of the intestine and pancreas—enzymes, mucus, and desquamated epithelial cells. The protein present in the feces comes from the above sources; as much as one-fourth of the dried feces may consist of bacteria. These bacteria also act on the amino acids liberated during digestion and produce degradation products useless for the metabolic needs of the body. The most conspicuous of these are indole and skatole, formed from tryptophan, which are chiefly responsible for the odor of feces. Roughly 1 g of nitrogen per day is carried by the feces, largely present in the bacteria.

UTILIZATION OF ABSORBED AMINO ACIDS

The absorbed amino acids that escape decomposition become part of the amino acid pools of the body. From these amino acids, new tissue proteins are synthesized to meet body needs.

Tissue protein synthesis. The need for new tissue protein is greatest in childhood during growth and in adults after protein depletion following fasting or convalescence from a wasting or debilitating disease. This is associated with a positive nitrogen balance, leading to an increase in body nitrogen.

In addition, turnover of tissue proteins occurs in the adult animal in nitrogen balance, with no net gain of body nitrogen. This is demonstrated by isotopic tracer experiments, and has led to the hypothesis that the body proteins are continually undergoing synthesis and degradation, but remain relatively constant in quantity. The rate of replacement varies greatly for different tissues. In man, it has been estimated that the average half-life of the total body protein is 80 days; that of lung, brain, bone, skin, and most muscle combined is 158 days; while that of liver and serum proteins combined is only 10 days. The difference in lability of tissue protein is supported by observations on the difference in protein loss by the tissues of the body in a 7-day fast by the rat. The liver lost 40% of its protein; the alimentary tract, pancreas, and spleen 29%; the heart 18%; muscle, skin, and skeleton together 8%; and the brain 5%.

Plasma protein synthesis. The plasma proteins offer the most readily available test material in determining the protein nutritional status of the individual. A blood sample is easily drawn, and estimation of the different plasma proteins is now becoming standard procedure. The plasma proteins are quite labile and show marked fluctuations in conditions associated with a disturbance of protein metabolism.

The major organ of plasma protein synthesis is the liver. It forms all of the plasma albumin and fibrinogen and a considerable proportion of the globulins. Advanced liver disease results in hypoalbuminemia and a lowered fibrinogen content. Prolonged protein deprivation both diminishes the albumin content and causes damage to the hepatic cells.

A portion of the total plasma globulin is synthesized in other tissues containing reticuloendothelial cells. The hormones and enzymes present in blood plasma are derived in the main from nonhepatic sources.

The plasma proteins have numerous important physiological functions. The albumin is the major factor in the regulation of the blood volume through its osmotic action, which counteracts the fluid expulsion effect of the hydrostatic pressure resulting from the contractions of the heart. Fibrinogen is only one component of a sequential process essential for coagulation of the blood. Other plasma components include the blood platelets and prothrombin. The globulins include fractions that are carriers of phospholipids and sterols and certain essential metal ions, iron, and copper. Other fractions, chiefly γ-globulin, contain the antibodies that are the defenses against numerous diseases.

Synthesis and utilization of the plasma proteins is a rapid process. Much of the knowledge of this has been learned from studies on the rate of renewal of the plasma proteins, and the albumin in particular, in health and in disease by isotopic labeling methods. These studies have shown that there is a complete turnover of the major plasma proteins in a period of a few days. The difference from normal in the turnover times in a variety of diseases provides an insight into the nature of the disease processes.

[DAVID M. GREENBERG]

Bibliography: B. T. Burton, *Heinz Handbook of Nutrition*, 2d ed., 1965; G. H. Beaton and E. W. McHenry, *Nutrition: A Comprehensive Treatise*, vols. 1–3, 1964–1966; A. White et al., *Principles of Biochemistry*, 5th ed., 1973.

Pumpkin

The term commonly applied to the larger, orange-colored fruit of the *Cucurbita* species, used when ripe as a table vegetable, in pies, or for autumn decoration. The flesh is somewhat coarse and strongly flavored, hence generally not served as a baked vegetable. Although some taxonomists would restrict the term pumpkin to the species *Cucurbita pepper* and *C. moschata*, it is also used in referring to *C. mixta*. Popular varieties (cultivars) are Connecticut Field and Small Sugar. Canned pumpkin is usually made from a blend of pumpkins and winter squashes. Cultural practices are similar to those used for squash. Harvesting generally begins when the fruits are mature, usually 4 months after planting. New Jersey, Illinois, and California are important producing states. *See* SQUASH; VEGETABLE GROWING.

[H. JOHN CAREW]

Quince

The tree *Cydonia oblonga*, originally from Asia, grown for its edible fruit. The deciduous, crooked-branched tree attains a height of about 20 ft. It is cultivated in either bush or tree form. The undersides of the leaves are densely tomentose (hairy); the solitary flowers (illustration *a*), up to 2 in. across, are snowy white or pale pink; the fruit is a pear-shaped or apple-shaped pome (illustration *b*), characteristically tomentose, up to 3 in. in diameter, aromatic, sour, astringent, and green, turning clear yellow at maturity. Used mostly for jam and jelly or as a stewed fruit, the fruit of the quince develops a pink color in cooking.

The quince is propagated on hardwood cuttings or by budding on quince seedlings. It may be used as stock for dwarfing the pear. The tree is only slightly hardier than the peach, the wood being severely injured at −15 to −20°F, and is subject to

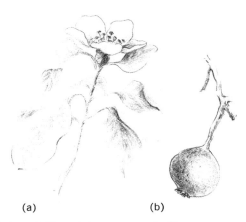

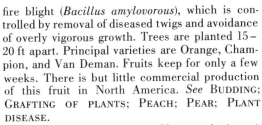

(a)   (b)

Quince. (*a*) Flower is borne on wood of the same season. (*b*) Short shoots start from the winter buds; flowers and fruits are produced on the ends of these shoots.

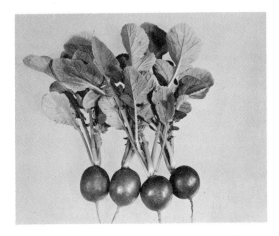

Radish (*Raphanus sativus*), cultivar Red Boy. (*Joseph Harris Co., Rochester, N. Y.*)

fire blight (*Bacillus amylovorous*), which is controlled by removal of diseased twigs and avoidance of overly vigorous growth. Trees are planted 15–20 ft apart. Principal varieties are Orange, Champion, and Van Deman. Fruits keep for only a few weeks. There is but little commercial production of this fruit in North America. *See* BUDDING; GRAFTING OF PLANTS; PEACH; PEAR; PLANT DISEASE.

The dwarf Japanese quince (*Chaenomeles japonica*), with orange-scarlet flowers, is grown as an ornamental shrub. *See* FRUIT, TREE; FRUIT (TREE) DISEASES; PLANT DISEASE CONTROL.

[HAROLD B. TUKEY]

Quinoa

An annual herb, *Chenopodium quinoa* (family Chenopodiaceae), 4–6 ft tall, a native of Peru, and the staple food of many people in South America. These plants, grown at high altitudes, produce large quantities of highly nutritious seeds used whole in soups or ground into flour, which is made into bread or cakes. The seeds are also used as poultry feed, in medicine, and in making beer. The ash is mixed with coca leaves to flavor them as a masticatory. In the United States the leaves are sometimes used as a substitute for spinach. *See* SPICE AND FLAVORING.

[PERRY D. STRAUSBAUGH/EARL L. CORE]

Radish

A cool-season annual or biennial crucifer, *Raphanus sativus*, of Chinese origin belonging to the plant order Capparales. The radish is grown for its thickened hypocotyl, which is eaten uncooked as a salad vegetable (see illustration). Propagation is by seed. Varieties (cultivars) are classified according to root shape and season or time of maturity. Colors include red, yellow, white, black, pink, and red-white combinations. Popular varieties are short-season (21–25 days), Early Scarlet Globe and Comet; medium-season (30–50 days), Crimson Giant; and long-season or winter varieties (50–70 days), Black Spanish. Commercial production, largely of the round red short-season varieties, is primarily in the field, but radishes are also produced commercially in greenhouses. Harvesting by hand or machine begins when the roots are ap-

proximately 1/2 to 1 in. in diameter, often only 21–23 days after planting. *See* VEGETABLE GROWING.

[H. JOHN CAREW]

Rape

Rape (*Brassica napus*) and turnip rape (*B. campestris*) plants are members of the Cruciferae family. The name is derived from the Latin *rapum*, meaning "turnip," to which these plants are closely related. The aerial portions of rape plants have been bred to produce oilseeds, fodder, and vegetable crops. Rape seed is small (2 to 5 g/1000 seeds), round, and usually black, although varieties with yellow seed coats are also grown. The plant germinates rapidly and forms a rosette of bluish-green leaves from which bolts an indeterminate race-

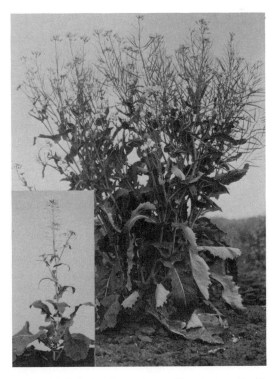

Well-podded plants of annual rape (*Brassica napus*) with insert detailing the characteristic inflorescence and basal leaves.

mose inflorescence (see illustration). Both annual and biennial forms of the crop are grown; the biennial form will not flower without extended exposure to freezing temperatures.

The seeds, borne in long slender pods or siliques, contain over 40% oil. Rapeseed contributes approximately 10–12% of the world's total edible vegetable oil supply and is one of the few edible oilseed crops that can be produced in northern Canada, Europe, and Asia, or, as a cool season crop, in subtropical areas. The oil is used as a salad and cooking oil and in the manufacture of margarines and shortenings. It also has industrial applications in lubricants and in the manufacture of a variety of products, including rubber, plastics, and nylon. Rapeseed meal, the by-product of oilseed extraction, is a high-quality protein feed supplement for livestock and poultry. In some Asian countries it is also used as a fertilizer and soil conditioner for specialty crops such as tobacco and citrus fruits.

Rape is widely used for forage. In some countries the whole plant is cut and fed to cattle, but more frequently biennial rape, such as the Dwarf Essex variety, is used as summer or late fall and winter pasture for sheep and swine. It is in the latter form that rape is most widely used throughout the United States and New Zealand. Some forms of turnip rape are used as leaf vegetables in Asia.
See TURNIP; VEGETABLE GROWING.

[R. K. DOWNEY]

Bibliography: E. A. Appelqvist and R. Ohlson (eds.), *Rapeseed: Cultivation, Composition, Processing and Utilization*, 1972; J. T. Harapiak (ed.), *Oilseed and Pulse Crops in Western Canada: A Symposium*, 1975.

Raspberry

The horticultural name for certain species of the genus *Rubus*, plant order Rosales. In these species the fruit, when ripe (unlike the blackberry), separates thimblelike from the receptacle. Raspberry plants are upright shrubs with perennial roots and prickly, biennial canes (stems). There are several species, both American and European, from which the cultivated raspberries have been developed. Varieties are grouped as to color of fruit—black, red, and purple, the last being hybrids between the red and black types. Red raspberries, with upright canes, are propagated by suckers or by root cuttings (Fig. 1); the black varieties, with long canes which arch over and touch the ground, are propagated by tip layers. The hybrid purple varieties are usually propagated by tip layers. Raspberry breeding has been carried on so extensively that all the important red and purple and most of the black varieties are the result of breeding experiments. Raspberries are grown extensively in home gardens over most of the United States. Leading states in commercial production are Michigan, Oregon, New York, Washington, Ohio, Pennsylvania, New Jersey, and Minnesota. Annual production usually grosses around $14,000,000 at the farm. The fruit is sold fresh for dessert purposes, is canned, and is made into jelly or jam, but quick freezing is the most important processing method.
See BREEDING (PLANT); FRUIT GROWING, SMALL.

[J. HAROLD CLARKE]

Raspberry and blackberry diseases. The diseases of raspberries and blackberries are similar, but there is a great difference between the two crops in the amount of damage sustained.

Anthracnose. This disease, caused by *Elsinoë veneta*, occurs on the canes (stems) of all berries, but is most destructive on black raspberries (Fig. 2). The disease appears on the lower parts of the stems as round or oval spots with raised, purple edges and sunken, grayish centers. Infected canes are brittle, are susceptible to winter injury, and may dry up and die. Anthracnose is controlled by removing the old canes, on which the fungus spends the winter, immediately after harvest, and by spraying with sulfur, copper, or dithiocarbamate fungicides. A somewhat similar disease, leaf and cane spot, caused by *Septoria rubi*, is common on raspberries in eastern North America and on blackberries in the western part. This disease is kept under control when the plants are sprayed for anthracnose.

Verticillium wilt. This disease, caused by *Verticillium albo-atrum*, which attacks all cane berries, is destructive on black raspberries but seldom causes serious damage to blackberries. It is most severe on plants grown in poorly drained soils. The disease causes a yellowing, wilting, and dropping of the leaves that progresses from the ground upward until the cane is defoliated. Frequently there is also a bluish discoloration of the canes, and eventually the plant dies. Only disease-free plants should be used, and they should be set out in a well-drained soil that has been free for at least 4 years from wilt-susceptible crops, such as potatoes, tomatoes, eggplants, peppers, and strawberries.

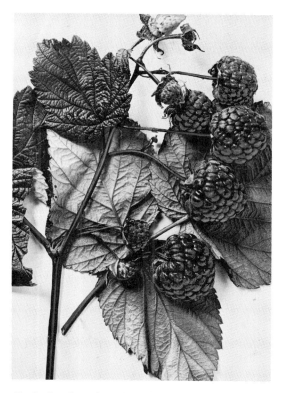

Fig. 1. A red raspberry branch, Loudon variety. (*USDA*)

Orange rust. This fungus disease, caused by *Gymnoconia interstitiales*, attacks blackberries and black raspberries, but not the red or purple raspberries. The disease first appears as tiny black dots on the upper surface of newly unfolded leaves. Later the under surface of infected leaves is covered with a conspicuous mass of orange-yellow waxy spores. The fungus invades all plant parts and diseased plants never recover. Infected plants should be destroyed promptly, and only disease-free nursery stock should be planted. Several other species of rust fungi are found on blackberries and raspberries.

Virus diseases. These diseases, including mosaics, ring spots, curls, and streaks, are the primary cause of loss of productivity, or running-out, of cane berries. Each of these diseases has distinctive symptoms, but all are systemic, and infected plants never recover. In addition to being spread by propagation from infected plants, the virus diseases usually are transmitted from diseased to healthy plants by insects or nematodes that feed on the plants. Viruses are not known to be spread by pruning or other cultural practices. Mosaics and leaf curls cause widespread damage in black and red raspberries, but seldom attack blackberries. The streaks affect black raspberries and blackberries. Measures used for control of all virus diseases of cane berries are use of disease-free planting stock; isolation, removal, and destruction of infected plants; spraying or dusting for control of insect vectors; and use of resistant or tolerant varieties. *See* PLANT VIRUS.

Other important diseases. Raspberries and blackberries are also susceptible to other important diseases, such as crown gall caused by *Agrobacterium tumefaciens*, spur blight caused by *Didymella applanata*, powdery mildew caused by *Sphaerotheca humuli*, cane blight caused by *Leptosphaeria coniothyrium*, and fruit rots caused by *Botrytis* sp. Development of new cultural techniques, particularly mechanical harvesting, is causing rapid changes in the relative importance of various diseases. *See* PLANT DISEASE; PLANT DISEASE CONTROL. [EDWARD K. VAUGHAN]

Redtop grass

One of the bent grasses, *Agrostis alba* and its relatives, which occur in cooler, more humid regions of the United States on a wide variety of soils. Redtop tolerates both wet and dry lands and acid and infertile soils, and it is used where other species of grasses do not thrive. Redtop is a perennial, spreads slowly by rootstocks, and makes a coarse, loose turf. Top growth is 2–3 ft tall, with moderately leafy, wiry stems. The inflorescence is a reddish open panicle. Redtop is used for pasture and hay and is fairly nutritious if harvested promptly when heading occurs. It is effective in preventing erosion by holding banks of drainage ditches, waterways, and terrace channels. *See* GRASS CROPS. [HOWARD B. SPRAGUE]

Reduced tillage agriculture

Recently developed herbicides which control weeds quite effectively are being substituted for tillage in the production of food, feed, and fiber crops. At the present time, terminology has not been standardized, and various reduced tillage systems are referred to as direct drilling, minimum tillage, no-tillage, sod planting, slot planting, eco-tillage, and mulch tillage, depending upon the operations used, the crops grown, and the locale. The ultimate in reduced tillage involves planting seeds of various crops into previously undisturbed soil and relying entirely upon herbicides for weed control.

Selective herbicides with adequate crop safety, effectiveness on a broad range of weedy plants, and season-long weed control have been available only since the early to mid 1960s. Before their introduction, moldboard plowing and other complete tillage operations were used to loosen the soil and destroy unwanted vegetation prior to planting crops. After emergence of row crops, such as corn, soybeans, or sugarbeets, the interrow spaces were cultivated one to several times to control weeds emerging after the primary tillage operations. Cultivation was not convenient for crops, such as wheat, barley, or oats, planted in rows as narrow as 15 to 20 cm apart. Earlier efforts to reduce tillage were not entirely successful. Modern herbicides paved the way for crop production without tillage.

Advantages. Reductions in the amount of tillage used to produce crops, if achieved without a sacrifice in crop productivity, have several advantages. Tillage operations demand relatively large amounts of time and power. Therefore, elimination of one or more operations results in fuel (energy) conservation and a potential for increased worker productivity.

But there is an even greater advantage to reduced tillage. Silt represents one of the most serious non-point-source pollutants in United States streams and waterways. Erosion of soil by wind and water is a serious and continuing problem in the agricultural sector, limiting land use and productivity on sloping sites because of measures required to minimize soil loss. Minimum tillage offers one solution to this problem. Some reduced tillage systems leave residue from the previous crop on the soil surface. Even under severe rainstorm conditions, erosion may be 50 to 100 times less from mulch-covered fields than from conventionally tilled fields. Mulch cover can practically eliminate wind erosion as well. Adoption of appropriate reduced tillage systems of crop production not only will decrease silt pollution in streams and waterways from agricultural sources, but will also increase the land base suitable for grain crop production to feed the expanding population by making possible more intensive crop production on rolling terrain.

Tillage and the crop environment. Weed control and crop establishment are important parts of any crop management system, and only recently have scientists been able to evaluate tillage systems with weed control removed as a reason for tillage. Differences in response of crops to tillage do exist on different soils, and tillage system selection should be tailored to specific soil characteristics. No-tillage is the most desirable system under some conditions, while moldboard plowing may be the most desirable system under others.

The residue from the previous crop is needed for moisture conservation and erosion control on cer-

RASPBERRY

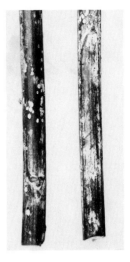

Fig. 2. Anthracnose disease on canes (stems) of black raspberry.

tain soils. If some soils are not covered with mulch, no-tillage crop yields may be depressed, and the best-choice tillage system will be one utilizing the moldboard plow. On these same soils, complete mulch cover may create conditions which result in a higher yield with no-tillage than with moldboard plowing. Mulch cover on poorly drained soils depresses soil temperatures and may cause slower crop growth early in the growing season in temperate areas. In more northern areas, this may reduce crop yields, making tillage systems that bury mulch more desirable. For temperate areas, tillage intensity may need to be increased for soils with poor drainage. Intermediate tillage systems that utilize disking or chisel plowing prior to planting may be more desirable on poorly drained soils than no-tillage.

Range of cultural practices. An entire spectrum of tillage practices, ranging from conventional tillage (plow, disk, cultivate) to no-tillage (spray, plant) is possible; these two systems, as well as a number of intermediate tillage systems, are currently being used. Typically, a no-tillage corn producer makes a broadcast application of herbicides and fertilizer on the surface of the field. The herbicides selected and rates used are tailored to the vegetation present on the site, and a mixture of as many as three different herbicides may be used. The herbicide may be mixed with liquid fertilizer, with both applied in a single operation. Crop seeds are planted with special machinery equipped to cut through mulch cover into the untilled soil, deposit the seeds at 3 to 4 cm depth, provide good seed-soil contact, and then cover the seed. Planting may be done either before or after herbicide application, and no more operations may be necessary until harvest time. While corn is the major crop produced with no-tillage, the techniques are applicable to other crops as well. Similar methods are used in planting wheat in Great Britain and in certain pasture renovation procedures employed in the United States, Australia, and New Zealand. In no-tillage pasture renovation, desirable forage species are introduced into the existing sward, and vegetation present is suppressed until seedlings of the forage species become established. This method is used to provide higher-quality forage for livestock.

In the Great Plains area of the United States, fallow periods may be necessary to conserve moisture for successive crops. Maintaining mulch cover on the soil surface minimizes wind erosion and helps conserve moisture. Combinations of tillage and herbicides are used to maintain fields weed-free during the fallow period and to produce successive crops.

Trends in tillage. At the present time, no-tillage methods are used on several million acres (2.47 acres = 1 ha) of cropland in the United States, less than 10% of the land area used for crop production. Reduced tillage systems using implements other than the moldboard plow occupy over 5×10^7 acres (2.024×10^7 ha). Together, reduced and no-tillage practices are used on about 30% of United States cropland. Rather than switching directly from moldboard plowing to no-tillage in one step, producers generally move gradually to systems that employ less tillage than their present system.

A U.S. Department of Agriculture technology assessment of tillage practices predicts that by the year 2000 most crops in the United States will be produced with reduced tillage methods of some type, and more than half of the acreage will be produced with no-tillage. Technology needed to make reduced tillage both practical and dependable in a wide range of crops and soil types is now being developed. See AGRICULTURE, SOIL AND CROP PRACTICES IN; HERBICIDE; MULTIPLE CROPPING. [GLOVER B. TRIPLETT, JR.]

Bibliography: Conservation Tillage, Proc. Nat. Symp. Soil Conserv. Soc. Amer., 1973; G. J. Musick (ed.), Crop production with reduced tillage, *Symp. Entomol. Soc. Amer. Bull.*, 22(2): 289–304, 1976; S. H. Phillips and H. M. Young, Jr., *No-tillage Farming*, 1973; G. B. Triplett, Jr., and D. M. Van Doren, Jr., *Sci. Amer.* 236(1): 28–33, 1977.

Rhizosphere

The soil region subject to the influence of plant roots. It is characterized by a zone of increased microbiological activity and is an example of the relationship of soil microbes to higher plants. Other examples are mycorhiza (a fungus-plant relationship) and bacterization (inoculation of soil or seed with microbes). A sharp boundary cannot be drawn between the rhizosphere and the soil unaffected by the plant (edaphosphere). At the root surface the rhizosphere effect is most intense, falling off sharply with increasing distance.

Growth of a plant markedly changes the microbial population of soil within its influence. In the rhizosphere there are more microorganisms than in soil distant from the plant (see illustration). This increase is most pronounced with bacteria but is evident with other groups, especially actinomycetes and fungi. Algae and protozoa increase less than other microorganisms. The effect may be revealed by plating methods and confirmed by examination of slides buried in contact with roots, which reveal accumulations of organisms near and at the root surface. The rhizosphere effect is seen in seedling plants; it increases with the age of the plant and usually reaches a maximum at the stage of greatest vegetative growth. Upon death of the plant the microbial population reverts to the level

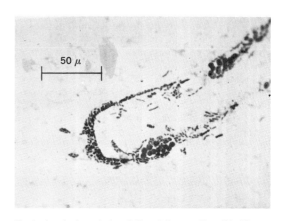

Bacteria clustered about tip of live rootlet. (*T. Gibson, World Crops, vol. 3, no. 4, 1951*)

of the surrounding soil. Within the range of soil moisture suited to plant growth, the number of rhizosphere organisms increases with decreasing moisture content. Leguminous plants support higher rhizosphere populations than nonlegumes. The stimulation of microorganism growth in the rhizosphere results chiefly from the liberation of readily available organic substances by the growing plant.

The plant exerts a characteristic effect by shifting the balance between groups of bacteria with respect to morphological and taxonomic type, physiology, and nutritional requirements. In the rhizosphere there is a preferential stimulation (increase in growth) of gram-negative rods and a relative suppression (decrease in growth) of gram-positive rods, coccoid rods, and aerobic sporeformers. Chief among those stimulated are species of *Pseudomonas*, *Agrobacterium*, and *Rhizobium*. *Rhizobium* is stimulated more particularly by legumes. *Arthrobacter*, *Azotobacter*, and nitrifying forms are less abundant in the rhizosphere than the aforementioned three species. Rhizosphere bacteria are physiologically more active than those in nonrhizosphere soil. Judged by oxygen consumption, isolates from the rhizosphere show a greater degree of metabolic activity than isolates from soil regions distant from the plant. In the rhizosphere, there are higher proportions of motile and chromogenic bacteria and of organisms able to decompose sugars, starches, and proteins. Cellulose-decomposing forms are stimulated by the presence of cellular debris sloughed off by the roots. Vitamin-synthesizing organisms are much more numerous in the rhizosphere.

From the standpoint of bacterial nutrition, the most characteristic rhizosphere effect is the preferential stimulation of organisms whose food needs are met by amino acids. This is mainly because amino acids are liberated from plant roots. Bacteria depending upon the more complex nutrients and growth factors provided by soil extract are less abundant in the rhizosphere.

The rhizosphere effect is related to certain aspects of plant disease. Varieties of flax, tobacco, and banana susceptible to certain pathogenic fungi exert a more pronounced rhizosphere effect than resistant varieties. Oat varieties susceptible to manganese deficiency disease show greater numbers of manganese-oxidizing organisms in the rhizosphere than resistant varieties. Some soil amendments (additives) are found to reduce the incidence of scab in potatoes by causing an increase in the rhizosphere of organisms antagonistic to the pathogen.

Mycorhiza. This is a special fungus-plant relationship in which fungi have a more intimate association with roots than that shown by the general rhizosphere population. Ectotrophic mycorhizal fungi do not penetrate root cells but form closely woven masses of hyphae about the rootlets and may enter root tissue between cells. This type of mycorhiza occurs commonly in forest trees. Endotrophic fungi penetrate more deeply into the tissues and invade the cells. This condition is more widespread and occurs in orchids, heather, fruit trees, and shrubs. The significance of the association is not well understood. The fungi obtain food partly from the plant. On the other hand, mycorhizas may function as an extension of the root system in extracting plant nutrients from soil. Thus mycorhizal fungi frequently stimulate plant growth.

Bacterization. The inoculation of soil or seed with microorganisms to stimulate plant growth or to protect plants against soil-borne pathogenic organisms is called bacterization. The value of inoculating seed of leguminous plants with cultures of symbiotic nitrogen-fixing bacteria adapted to the crop is established. There is no conclusive evidence that inoculation is of value for nonlegumes, for which purpose cultures of the nonsymbiotic nitrogen-fixing organism *Azotobacter* have been extensively tried. Attempts to control plant pathogenic fungi or bacteria by heavy inoculation of soil with cultures of antagonistic (antibiotic-producing) organisms have not been successful under field conditions. In natural soils the antagonist is in competition with other soil microorganisms; its numbers decline as the equilibrium is reestablished. More success has been achieved by modifying the environment to encourage antagonists normally present in the soil. *See* NITROGEN FIXATION (BIOLOGY); SOIL MICROBIOLOGY.

[ALLAN GRANT LOCHHEAD]

Rhubarb

A herbaceous perennial, *Rheum rhaponticum*, of Mediterranean origin, belonging to the plant order Polygonales. Rhubarb is grown for its thick petioles which are used mainly as a cooked dessert; it is frequently called the pieplant. The leaves, which are high in oxalic acid content, are not commonly considered edible. Propagation is by division of root crowns. Victoria, Macdonald, and Valentine are popular varieties (cultivars). Commercial production is generally limited to areas where crowns may become dormant for 2–3 months each year. Outdoor rhubarb is a common garden vegetable in most areas of the United States except the South. Harvesting begins in the spring and continues for 6–10 weeks. Commercial plantings are renewed every 4–8 years. Michigan and Washington are important centers for forced or hothouse rhubarb. Two- or three-year-old field-grown crowns are moved into darkened forcing structures in late winter and forced at 55–60°F to obtain petioles of a bright-red color. *See* VEGETABLE GROWING. [H. JOHN CAREW]

Riboflavin

Also known as vitamin B_2, riboflavin is widely distributed in nature, and is found mostly in milk, egg white, liver, and leafy vegetables. It is a water-soluble yellow-orange fluorescent pigment with the structural formula shown below. It is stable to acid

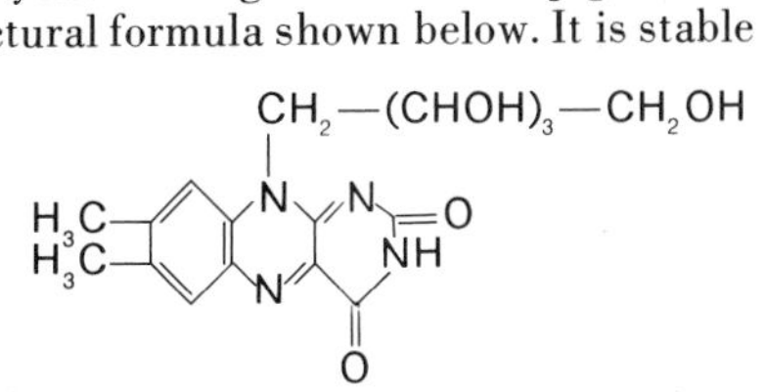

$$CH_2-(CHOH)_3-CH_2OH$$

and oxidation, but is rapidly destroyed by alkali at elevated temperatures and by light. Although little riboflavin is usually destroyed during cooking, half of the riboflavin in bottled milk exposed to the sun may be destroyed in 2 hr.

Riboflavin is determined by microbiological methods using the lactic acid-forming organism *Lactobacillus casei*, which requires it for growth. Riboflavin is also determined by chemical methods in which its fluorescent properties are used.

A dietary source of riboflavin is required by all nonruminant animal species studied. Riboflavin deficiency results in poor growth and other pathologic changes in the skin, eyes, liver, and nerves. Riboflavin deficiency in man is usually associated with a cracking at the corners of the mouth called cheilosis; inflammation of the tongue, which appears red and glistening (glossitis); corneal vascularization accompanied by itching; and a scaly, greasy dermatitis about the corners of the nose, eyes, and ears.

Riboflavin is found in all tissues with its concentration usually paralleling metabolic activity. The vitamin functions biochemically in two coenzymes, flavin mononucleotide (FMN) and flavin adenine dinucleotide (FAD). Enzymes containing these coenzymes are called flavoproteins. In general, these enzymes participate in oxidation-reduction reactions by accepting hydrogen ions (protons) and electrons from one substrate and transferring them to another. Over 14 riboflavin-containing enzymes have been studied.

Most of the energy-yielding oxidations of food to carbon dioxide and water occur through the cytochrome system, in which the flavoprotein cytochrome reductase is essential. L-Amino oxidase, another flavoprotein, is important in the interconversion of amino acids to nonnitrogenous metabolites of carbohydrate and fat metabolism.

Riboflavin requirements appear to be related to caloric requirements and muscular activity, and are affected by heredity, growth, environment, age, and health. Evidence in animals suggests a need for increased riboflavin in low-protein diets because of a decreased ability of the liver to retain the vitamin. There is also evidence that as a result of intestinal synthesis by bacteria, less riboflavin is required on diets high in carbohydrate than on those high in fat. Human requirements for riboflavin are based primarily on urinary excretion data and studies in which riboflavin deficiency has been experimentally produced. Riboflavin allowances of the National Research Council have been set at 0.07–0.1 mg/0.75 kg of body weight. Former allowances which employed a factor of 0.025 mg/g of protein allowance provided similar amounts of the vitamin.

[STANLEY N. GERSHOFF]

Industrial production. Riboflavin is produced commercially by either direct chemical synthesis or fermentation.

Chemical synthesis. Industrial syntheses of riboflavin generally proceed along the lines of the original Karrer method with modifications by individual producers. A typical manufacture starts with D-ribose, which is condensed with 1,3,4-xylidine and simultaneously hydrogenated to form *N*-D-ribitylxylidine. The ribitylxylidine is coupled with diazotized aniline to produce 1,2-dimethyl-4-D-ribitylamino-5-phenyl azo benzene. This azo compound is hydrogenated to 1,2-dimethyl-4-D-ribitylamino-5-aminobenzene, and then is con-

densed with a mixture of alloxan and alloxantin to riboflavin. By another method, the azo compound is condensed directly with barbituric acid.

[LEO A. FLEXSER]

Fermentation. Riboflavin produced commercially by fermentation utilizes the synthetic ability of bacteria, yeasts, or fungi. The outstanding organisms for production of riboflavin are the two closely related ascomycete fungi, *Eremothecium ashbyii* and *Ashbya gossypii*. The inoculum is started from slants or from spores dried on sand, and after one or two flask stages is carried through one or two tank inoculum stages.

The final fermentation is carried out in tanks with a capacity of 10,000–100,000 gal with a medium suitable for the organism being used. For *Eremothecium* usually stillage (still slops) from the ethyl alcohol fermentation with skim milk, soybean meal, or casein added is used as a proteinaceous source; a carbohydrate source, such as maltose, sucrose, or glucose, is added. For *Ashbya*, commercially used media may contain corn-steep liquor, and usually also some animal protein such as crude peptones, animal-stick liquor, or fish-stick liquor; the carbohydrate sources are similar to those used for *Eremothecium*. The medium is aerated and usually agitated during fermentation for 96–120 hr; optimum titers may be 3–6 g of riboflavin or more per liter. *See* CARBOHYDRATE; INDUSTRIAL MICROBIOLOGY; SOYBEAN.

Riboflavin may be recovered for animal feed supplements by evaporation of the whole broth in multiple-effect evaporators, followed by drum or spray drying. For drug and fine food uses, pure crystalline riboflavin is isolated by heating the fermentation broth, filtration, and precipitation of the riboflavin with dithionite (hydrosulfite) followed by several purification steps, including crystallization.

[RALPH E. BENNETT]

Bibliography: H. J. Peppler (ed.), *Microbial Technology*, 1967; L. A. Underkofler and R. J. Hickey (eds.), *Industrial Fermentations*, vol. 2, 1954.

Rice

The plant *Oryza sativa* is the major source of food for nearly one-half of the world's population. In China, Japan, Korea, the Philippines, India, and other countries of Asia, rice is far more important than wheat as a source of carbohydrates. In some countries of the Orient the consumption of rice per capita is estimated at 200–400 lb/year (90–180 kg). In contrast, the yearly per capita consumption of rice in the United States is only about 8 lb (3.6 kg). The most important rice-producing countries are mainland China, India, and Indonesia, but in many smaller countries rice is the leading food crop. Although the acreage planted in rice is only 60% of that planted in wheat, the total world production of rice is 85% of wheat because of higher average yields per acre. *See* CARBOHYDRATE; WHEAT.

Production and economic importance. In the United States rice is produced on approximately 2,000,000 acres (8092 km²), in contrast to more than 50,000,000 acres (202,300 km²) of wheat. Rice is largely concentrated in selected areas of Arkansas, California, Louisiana, and Texas. Although this represents less than 1% of the world rice acreage, the United States often is the world's largest exporter of rice, since most of the world rice crop is consumed in the countries where it is produced. Over half of the United States production is exported, largely to Asian countries.

Use. Over 95% of the world rice crop is used for human food. Although most rice is boiled, a considerable amount is consumed as breakfast cereals. Rice starch also has many uses. Broken rice is used as a livestock feed and for the production of alcoholic beverages. The bran from polished rice is used for livestock feed; the hulls are used for fuel and cellulose. The straw is used for thatching roofs in the Orient and for making paper, mats, hats, and baskets. Rice straw is also woven into rope and used as cordage for bags. This crop serves a multitude of purposes in countries where agriculture is dependent largely upon rice.

Origin and description. Rice apparently originated more than 6000 years ago in Southeast Asia, in the areas that are now eastern India, Indochina, and southern China. Rice was introduced to North America as early as 1609, and became established in South Carolina about 1690. Until about 1890 rice was grown mainly in the southeastern states. Louisiana became an important rice-producing state in the late 19th century. Early in the 20th century rice production spread to southeastern Texas, eastern Arkansas, and north-central California. Rice is a comparatively new crop in its present areas of greatest production in the United States.

Rice is unlike many other cereal grains in that all cultivated varieties belong to the same species and have 12 pairs of chromosomes, as do most wild types. The extent of variation in morphological and physiological characteristics within this single species is greater than for any other cereal crop. Although the chromosome number is the same, many of the ancient types have become so widely differentiated that hybrids between them are only partially fertile.

Rice is an annual grass plant varying in height from 2 to 6 ft (0.6 to 1.8 m). Plants tiller, that is, develop new shoots freely, the number depending upon spacing and soil fertility. Among the many types grown, some mature in 80 days; others require over 200 days. The inflorescence is an open panicle (Fig. 1). Flowers are perfect and normally self-pollinated, with natural crossing seldom exceeding 3–4%. A distinct characteristic of the flower is the six anthers rather than the customary three of other grasses. Spikelets have a single floret, lemma and palea completely enclosing the caryopsis or fruit, which may be yellow, red, brown, or black. Lemmas may be awnless, partly awned, or fully awned. Threshed rice, which retains its lemma and palea, is called rough rice or paddy. *See* GRASS CROPS.

Varieties. More than 30,000 varieties have been collected by the International Rice Research Institute in the Philippines. Relatively few of these varieties are widely grown. Thus in the United States only about 25 varieties are in commercial production. Cultivated rices are classified as upland and lowland. Upland types, which can be grown in high-rainfall areas without irrigation, produce relatively low yields. The lowland types,

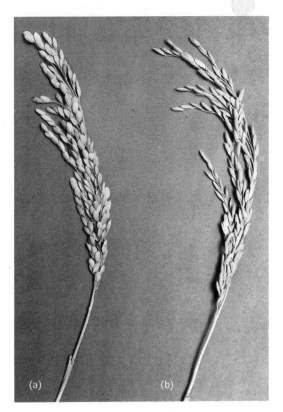

Fig. 1. Panicles of (a) short-grain and (b) long-grain rice. Each spikelet has a single caryopsis enclosed in the lemma and palea.

which are grown submerged in water for the greater part of the season, produce higher yields. In contrast to most plants, rice can thrive when submerged because oxygen is transported from the leaves to the roots. All rice in the United States is produced under lowland or flooded conditions. Rice varieties are also classified as long- or short-grain (Fig. 2). Most long-grain rices have high amylose content and are dry or fluffy when cooked, while most short-grain rices have lower amylose content and are sticky when cooked. In the United States a third grain length is recognized: medium-grain. The medium-grain rices have cooking qualities similar to short-grain varieties.

Plant breeders have been successful in developing high-yielding varieties that combine the vigor and disease resistance of typical tropical rices with the short stature of Taiwan varieties. The new "architecture" of these plants ensures their ability to stay erect until harvesting, thus preventing crop loss due to lodging (falling over) into the water.

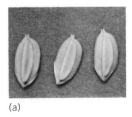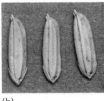

Fig. 2. Rice grains range from (a) short to (b) long.

Cultural practices. Because of the peculiar conditions of growing a crop submerged in water, rice land seldom becomes a part of a regular rotation system. Often two or more successive crops of rice are grown, and the land is then pastured or fallowed to control weeds. Rice is grown on heavy soils underlain by an impervious subsoil to prevent seepage of water. *See* SOIL.

In oriental countries and in many other countries, rice fields are established by transplanting seedlings from beds when the plants are 30–50 days old. Fields to be transplanted are flooded and worked into a soft mud. Clumps of three to four seedlings are pushed into the mud in rows to permit hand cultivation for control of weeds. This system of transplanting seedlings saves irrigation water and permits the field in which they are to be established to grow another crop while the smaller-sized seedling bed is being grown.

In the United States transplanting is impractical because of high labor costs. In California almost all rice seed is sown from airplanes directly into fields flooded with 4–6 in. (10–15 cm) of water. In the southern states rice is seeded either by airplane or by grain drill. In the latter case the rice is seeded into dry soil, which is gradually flooded to a depth of 4–6 in. as the rice emerges and grows. In all rice areas of the United States the water is kept at the 4–6 in. depth until the land is drained shortly before harvest.

The rice crop in oriental countries and some other countries is harvested by hand (Fig. 3). In the United States rice is harvested with large self-propelled combines similar to those used for wheat and other grain crops. The best stage for combine harvesting is at grain moisture content of 23–28%. Rice dried to a lower moisture content while standing in the field may break up in milling, resulting in lower grain quality. When harvested at this high moisture content, the grain is dried artificially to 14% moisture, care being taken to keep the drying temperature below 110°F (43°C) to avoid damage to the grain. *See* AGRICULTURAL SCIENCE (PLANT); AGRICULTURE, MACHINERY IN; GRAIN CROPS.

[J. N. RUTGER]

Diseases. Rice diseases are of great importance because large numbers of people in Asia depend mainly on this cereal for carbohydrate. Since population and rice production are in such close balance in countries like India, China, and Japan, relatively small losses can lead to conditions approaching famine. In 1934 famine in certain districts of Japan was caused by the rice blast disease. In 1943 the famine in Bengal, India, was attributed primarily to the loss in rice production caused by Helminthosporium leaf spot disease.

The major diseases of rice are the Helminthosporium leaf spot disease, blast or rotten neck caused by the fungus *Piricularia oryzae*, and the hoja blanca of Cuba and Venezuela. The hoja blanca is believed to be caused by a virus which is spread from diseased to healthy plants by an insect (Fig. 4). Losses is susceptible varieties caused by this disease have been reported to be as high as 60% of the crop. Control in these countries has not been satisfactorily obtained because the available resistant varieties do not yield well enough to be used.

Another disease of rice is the bakanae disease of Japan which is caused by *Gibberella fujikurae*. It is of particular interest, since this fungus is the producer of gibberellin, the plant growth stimulator, which has been recognized as a possible means of increasing plant growth and crop yields. *See* GIBBERELLIN; PLANT DISEASE.

[ST. JOHN P. CHILTON]

Processing. The four main parts of the rice kernel are the hull, bran, germ, and endosperm. The purpose of milling rice is to separate the outer portions from the inner endosperm with a minimum of breakage. The various steps followed in rice milling are illustrated in the flow diagram (Fig. 5).

Polished rice. Rough rice, or paddy rice, as it is known, is separated from foreign material by vibrating sieves and air currents. Various sizes of sieves separate seeds that are larger or smaller than rice, and air currents carry off chaff, dust, and other lightweight material. Rotating vertical cylinders containing indentations or perforations are also used to lift out and remove certain types of foreign seeds from rice.

The thoroughly cleaned rice is conveyed to shelling machines which loosen the hulls. The machines are similar to buhrstones used in wheat milling and consist of two steel plates usually 4 ft or more in diameter, mounted horizontally, with the inner surface of the plates lined with a mixture

RICE

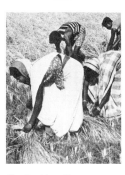

Fig. 3. Hand harvesting is common in many countries.

RICE

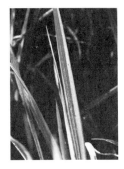

Fig. 4. Hoja blanca disease of rice. (*Inter-American Institute of Agricultural Sciences*)

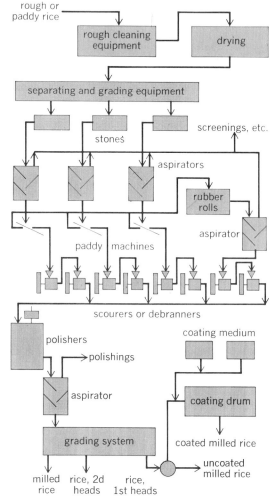

Fig. 5. Flow chart for the processing of rice.

of cement and coarse carborundum. One plate rotates, and the other, set at the proper distance to permit rice grains to assume vertical positions, remain stationary. As the plate revolves, the force on the ends of the kernels disengages the hulls. The great problem in rice milling is to remove the husk and bran without breaking the endosperm. After this first operation, approximately 20% of the rough rice remains unhulled and must be processed further.

The mixture of loose hull, bran, and germ, as well as the unhulled kernels, is conveyed to a stone reel. This consists of a large revolving octagonal framework covered with wire screens where fine material, known as stone-reel bran, is recovered. The large pieces of hull remaining are removed by suction in an aspirator, and the mixtures of hull and unhulled grains left are separated in a paddy machine, a large box shaker fitted with vertical plates to form zigzag divisions which separate the lighter unhulled paddy grains from the heavier hull grains. The plates and the shaking action cause the paddy grains to move gradually upward and over the machine into a trough, while the heavier, hulled grains are collected at the lower side. The unhulled grains are sent through auxiliary hulling stones, which are set to smaller clearances; from there, they reenter the main stream going to the stone reel.

Rice with hulls removed is called brown rice, because it retains a light-brown color from the bran coat. Removal of the bran layers is done in two sets of hullers generally referred to as first- or second-break operations. The term huller is a misnomer, since the function of this machine is to remove bran layers instead of hulls. The bran layers are removed by a scouring action between the inner walls of the huller and the rapidly revolving, grooved inner core. The mixture of scoured kernels and bran passes through the first-break bran reel where the bran is separated. Then the rice goes to the second-break hullers. Similar to the first, but adjusted for closer action, these remove the remaining part of the bran coat. After leaving the second set of hullers, the rice has lost much of its brown color. And it loses still more in the second bran reel.

Pearling cones are used in some mills as an adjunct to the hullers or in place of the last set of hullers. A pearling machine consists of a cone, coated with abrasive material, which revolves inside a heavy wire screen. The scouring action can be adjusted to suit requirements.

Rice passes from the second-break huller, or from the pearling cones, to a cooling bin and then to a brush machine. The brush machine consists of a vertical cylindrical frame covered with soft leather strips revolving at a high rate of speed within a cylinder of wire screening. The rice is rubbed smooth by friction during its travel through the machine. A considerable amount of heat is generated in a brush machine, and cooling is accomplished by a stream of air which travels countercurrent to the flow of the rice. From the brush machine, the rice passes through the brewers' reel, where the smallest fragments are removed. This reel usually is covered with a mesh screen of proper size to remove the rice fragments, known as brewers' rice because this material has a ready market in the manufacture of beer.

Often a coating of glucose or talc is applied in revolving tumblers. These are cylinders about 9 ft long and 4 ft in diameter, set on an incline of about 15° from the horizontal. Not all rice is coated with glucose or talc. In some markets an uncoated grade of rice is preferred, but the luster of the grains is greatly improved by coating.

Clean rice is graded by machines which consist of rows of vertical disks mounted on revolving shafts. The indented disks collect the smaller sizes, carry them over, and discharge them into a chute leading to cylinders where further separations take place. The kernel size can be changed by raising or lowering the edge of the apron on the stationary axis of the machine.

Many classes and grades of rice are marketed. The by-products of rice processing, such as hulls and bran, are generally sold for animal feed. Some rice hulls are used in the manufacture of purified alpha cellulose.

The common yields of the various products of rough rice are as follows: hulls, 20%; brown rice, 79%; whole grains, 58%; three-quarter to half-grains, 3%; and screenings, 6%. By-products are bran, 8%, and rice polishings, 2%.

Converted rice. In the course of manufacturing polished rice, much of the nutritive value, in both protein content and vitamins, is removed. Specifically, 76% of thiamine, 57% of riboflavin, and 63% of niacin are lost for human consumption. Because of this, efforts have been made to resupply the vitamins by a patented converted rice process, and by the Malek parboiling process. *See* NIACIN; RIBOFLAVIN; THIAMINE.

In the process of milling brown rice to white rice, there is a marked reduction in B vitamins and iron. Since customers prefer well-milled white rice to brown rice, there has been much interest in methods to retain more of the B vitamins in the milled rice. This problem has been approached in two ways: by removing less of the brown bran layers and germ in milling, and by processing the rice prior to milling in such a way as to transfer vitamins and other water-soluble nutrients from the outer portions of the grain into the endosperm.

The first method produces undermilled or unpolished rice. The outer bran is removed but the inner layers retained. Since the greatest decrease in B vitamins and minerals occurs in the first break, only limited improvement in nutritive value can be effected by decreasing the degree of refinement in subsequent stages of the milling process. Attention has therefore been focused on methods to increase the vitamin content of the milled rice by subjecting rough rice to a parboiling treatment prior to milling.

Converted rice is produced by the following process: Rough rice is cleaned and placed in steeping tanks which are sealed and evacuated to remove air from the tank and the interspaces of the rice kernels. Hot water is added and pressure is applied for a steeping treatment. This transfers the water-soluble vitamins from the bran and germ into the endosperm. Then the rice is subjected to live steam, dried under vacuum, and finally milled and polished. Converted rice is a highly milled, polished product of greatly improved nutritive value. Rice is among the cereals processed in the

form of flakes or puffed rice. *See* FOOD MANU-
FACTURING.

[JOHN A. SHELLENBERGER]

Bibliography: Agriculture Research Service,
USDA, *Rice in the United States: Varieties and
Production*, Agr. Handb. no. 289, 1973; J. R. Har-
lan, *Crops and Man*, American Society of Agron-
omy and the Crop Science Society of America,
1975; D. F. Houston (ed.), *Rice: Chemistry and
Technology*, American Association of Cereal
Chemists, Inc., 1972; International Rice Research
Institute, *Annual Report for 1973*, 1974; M. B.
Jacobs, *The Chemistry and Technology of Food
and Food Products*, 1951; M. A. Joslyn and J. L.
Heid, *Food Processing Operations*, vol. 3, 1964;
J. B. Reed, *The By-products of Rice Milling*, USDA
Bull. no. 570, 1917; United States Department of
Agriculture, *Agricultural Statistics*, 1975; J. C.
Walker, *Plant Pathology*, 3d ed., 1968; T. B.
Wayne, Modern rice milling, *Food Ind.*, 2:492–
495, 1930.

Rickets

A disorder of calcium and phosphorus metabolism,
primarily affecting bony structures, due to vitamin
D deficiency. Precursor substances from the diet
are normally converted to vitamin D by the action
of ultraviolet light (sunlight) on the skin. Therefore, infants are affected, especially in winter.
Dark-skinned peoples require additional vitamin D
as dietary supplement because their skin pigmen-
tations interfere with natural production. *See*
VITAMIN D.

In children, rickets consists of defective
calcification and excessive production of cartilage
at the ends of growing bones. Restlessness, constant movement often with hair loss from pillow
contact, and defects of the ribs and long bones are
typical symptoms. Bowlegs and pigeon breast may
result, in addition to craniotabes, or softening of
the flat skull bones, which later develop abnormally to form a square, boxlike skull. There is an increased susceptibility to fracture, delayed tooth
eruption and enamel defects, and other indications
of faulty mineral deposition.

In adults, vitamin D deficiency produces osteomalacia, or demineralization of bones. It is seen in
a softening of the spine, pelvis, and leg bones.
Fractures and deformities due to compression of
the defective bones are common. In addition, low
calcium levels in the blood may be present with
resulting irritability, spasms, and convulsions, particularly of the hands, face, and larynx.

Vitamin D regulates the absorption of calcium
and phosphorus from the gastrointestinal tract,
thereby maintaining blood levels.

[EDWARD G. STUART/N. KARLE MOTTET]

Root and tuber food crops

Crops cultivated for their edible roots and tubers.
In much of the humid tropics of America, Asia,
and Oceania, the carbohydrate basis of human
nutrition is provided not by grain crops, but by
vegetatively propagated root and tuber crops unfamiliar to the temperate world. Globally, the most
important is cassava, otherwise known as manioc,
mandioca, tapioca, or yuca *(Manihot esculenta;*
Euphorbiaceae; often incorrectly *M. utilissima)*. It
is grown almost throughout the tropics. In West

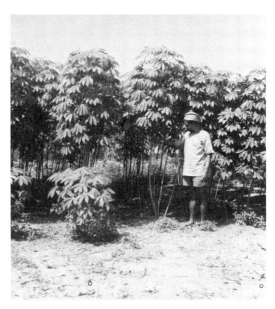

Fig. 1. Cassava plants in Sri Lanka.

Africa, the Pacific, and the Caribbean, the yams
(Dioscorea spp. Dioscoreaceae) are important food
crops. Throughout the Pacific, taro *(Colocasia esculenta;* Araceae) is a major staple crop; it is also
grown in Southeast Asia, under the name of coco-
yam in West Africa, and as dasheen or eddoe *(C.
esculenta* subsp. *antiquorum)* in the Caribbean.
The very similar tannia, ocumo, or yautia
(Xanthosoma sagittifolium; Araceae) is also now
grown throughout the tropics. Some other aroids
are of minor importance. The Irish potato
(Solanum tuberosum; Solanaceae) and the sweet
potato *(Ipomoea batatas;* Convolvulaceae) are also
grown in the tropics, but are primarily temperate
crops. Numerous other root and tuber crops grown
in various parts of the tropical world are of importance locally, but their production, viewed on the
global scale, is insignificant. These include arrowroot *(Maranta arundinacea;* Marantaceae), tacca
(Tacca leontopetaloides; Taccaceae), Hausa potato
(Solenostemon rotundifolius; Labiatae), oca
(Oxalis tuberosa; Oxalidaceae); ullucu *(Ullucus
tuberosus;* Basellaceae); and yacon *(Polymnia sonchifolia;* Compositae).

Production. The Food and Agriculture Organization (FAO) estimates indicated a total production of around $175{\times}10^6$ tonnes (T) in 1975, with
cassava accounting for almost two-thirds (see table). These crops thus provided the carbohydrate
basis for the diets of around 500,000,000 people.
This substantial contribution to the world's food is
largely derived from unimproved cultivars, grown
with minimal resource inputs by subsistence farmers cultivating small plots. These crops have been
neglected by agriculturalists until virtually the last
decade, and much greater potential should, therefore, exist for crop improvement than in other
crops already intensively studied. Yields under
present-day conditions are often low, only a few
tonnes per hectare, but recent experiments have
shown that with selected cultivars and an increase
in resource inputs yields of around 50 T/ha or
more can be obtained. Under humid tropical

Production of root crops in the developing world, in 10⁶ tonnes*

Region	Cassava	Potato	Yam	Sweet potato	Taro	Miscellaneous root crops	Total
Africa	42.844	2.039	19.279	5.539	3.569	1.446	74.716
Latin America	32.201	8.951	0.291	3.379	—	0.811	45.633
Near East	1.128	4.706	0.260	0.094	0.059	—	5.747
Far East	27.643	8.445	0.030	8.764	0.090	1.674	46.646
Other	0.221	0.006	0.700	0.560	0.262	0.390	1.639
Developing world total	104.037	23.647	20.060	18.336	3.980	4.321	174.381

*After FAO, 1975.

ecosystems even existing cultivars can often substantially outyield improved grain crop cultivars in terms of food calorie production.

Utilization. Root and tuber crops are used predominantly as food for the human populations in the areas of production. Recently, a substantial trade has developed in dried cassava products for use in animal feed formulation, mainly from Thailand and Indonesia to European Economic Community (EEC) countries; however, the proportion of total production so utilized is small. They primarily provide carbohydrate or energy food and are often criticized by nutritionists for having low-protein contents; this is true of cassava, but yams and aroids have protein contents at least comparable with grains on a dry-weight basis. Their nutritional value needs, in any case, to be reassessed in relation to the now widely accepted view that deficiency in food energy intake is the prime cause of malnutrition. Young leaves of cassava and the aroids are eaten and are a valuable source of protein.

Cassava. This has been a food crop for several thousand years among Amerindians in tropical South America. Its exact origins are obscure as it is unknown in the wild state, but Colombia or the borders of Brazil, Venezuela, and Guyana have been suggested as possible points of origin. Cassava appears to be a spontaneous hybrid, selected by early humans for its swollen roots. Before Columbus, it had reached its present limitations in cultivation, approximately 25°N and 25°S. It was carried to West Africa during the 16th century, and to East Africa, the Indian Ocean islands, India, and Sri Lanka shortly before 1800, but its rapid spread as a major food crop in Africa and Asia took place largely in the 20th century.

The cassava plant is a short-lived shrub, attaining up to 4 m in height, branching more or less according to cultivar, with palmate leaves (Fig. 1). The small, whitish flowers are borne in axilliary racemes, the female flowers followed by dehiscent three-seeded capsules. Although seed set and hybridization occur readily, propagation is normally by hardwood stem cuttings 200–400 mm long. A proportion of the roots develop by secondary thickening to cylindrical or tapering root tubers, arranged more or less radially around the base of the plant (Fig. 2). Size and form vary greatly with cultivar: 0.2 to 1.0 m long and up to 0.25 m diameter are common.

Cassava is a most adaptable crop; it cannot stand frost, but grows with as little as 500 mm or as much as 5000 mm rainfall, is resistant to drought, and is tolerant of poor or exhausted soils. Its recent rapid spread may be attributed to this adapta-

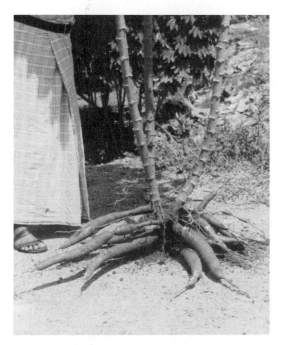

Fig. 2. Tubers of the cassava plant.

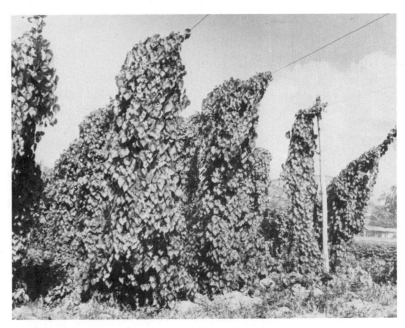

Fig. 3. Climbing vines of the yam *Dioscorea esculenta*, grown on a post and wire support in Trinidad. (*From D. G. Coursey and P. H. Haynes, World Crops, 22:261–265, 1970*)

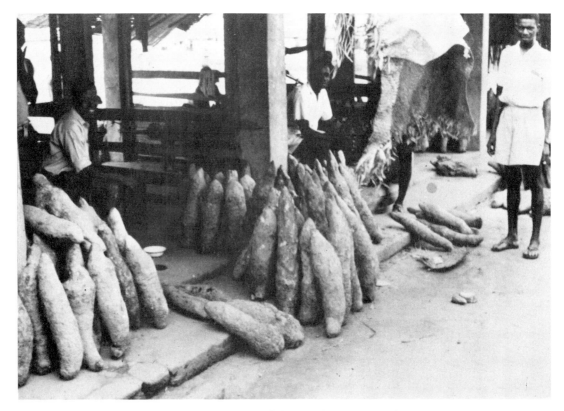

Fig. 4. Tubers of the yam *Dioscorea rotundata*. (*From D. G. Coursey, Yams, Longman Green, 1967*)

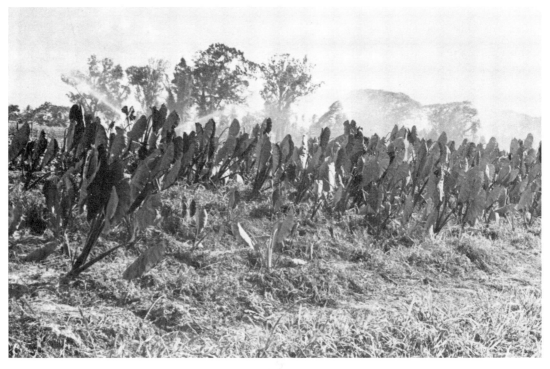

Fig. 5. Taro (*Colocasia*) crop in Trinidad. (*From D. G. Coursey and P. H. Haynes, World Crops, 22:261–265, 1970*)

bility, and to the fact that it yields more food per unit labor input than any other crop. Yield is seriously reduced by diseases, notably virus-induced cassava mosaic disease—almost universal in Africa but unknown in the Americas—and cassava bacterial blight (*Xanthomonas manihotis*)—of American origin but now pantropic; the latter is extremely destructive but can be controlled.

All cultivars contain the toxic hydrocyanic acid (HCN), as the glycoside linamarin, in all parts of the plant; the content ranges between 10 and about 500 parts per million (ppm). Both chronic or acute poisoning can occur, especially when the HCN concentration is above 150 ppm, and cassava-eating societies have traditional detoxication techniques, involving soaking, sun-drying, or fermentation. Sweet (low HCN) and bitter (high HCN) cultivars have been regarded, incorrectly, as separate species. Cassava roots have a very short storage life, and are usually left in the ground until required and processed immediately after harvest. *See* CASSAVA.

Yams. Only a few of the 600 *Dioscorea* spp. are major food crops. The primary area of cultivation is West Africa, where two closely related indigenous species, Yellow Yam *(D. cayenensis)* and White Guinea Yam *(D. rotundata)*, are grown. Yams are also grown in Southeast Asia and the Pacific, but here the White or Greater Yam *(D. alata)* and the Lesser Yam *(D. esculenta)* are the principal species. Asiatic Yams are grown to some extent in Africa, and both Asiatic and African species in the Caribbean, the tropical American *D. trifida* being much less cultivated. Several other species, including *D. bulbifera*, *D. dumetorum*, *D. hispida*, and *D. opposita*, are minor food crops. The term "yam" is often incorrectly applied in the United States to sweet potatoes.

The yams are climbing vines (Fig. 3), generally grown on stakes. The first three species form single, large tubers, weighing typically as much as 5 kg; the others form several smaller tubers (Fig. 4). Plants are normally dioecious, with the small flowers being born in racemes. Many cultivars are of limited seed fertility, and propagation is always by vegetative sets or tuber cuttings.

Most species grow best in temperatures above 25°C and cannot stand frost or temperatures below 10°C; rainfall of the order of 1500 mm is needed, with a marked dry season, when the plant tuberizes and becomes dormant. Yams need deep, fertile soil (they are often planted on mounds or ridges), and a high labor input. They respond well to fertilizer, especially nitrogen. Yam beetles (*Heteroligus* spp.) inflict much damage in Africa; scale insects and nematodes can be serious pests; and fungal diseases, *Colleototrichum* and *Cercospora*, are also locally serious, especially with *D. alata*. Yam tubers, being natural organs of dormancy, can be stored for several months, although decay and sprouting can cause loss. The main species are free from toxins, but some contain aklaloids or sapogenins.

Aroid root crops. Taro (*Colocasia*), one of the most ancient food crops, was domesticated in Southeast Asia and is still much grown in the Pacific (Fig. 5). The very similar tannia (*Xanthosoma*) is an Amerindian domesticate (Fig. 6); both are now pantropic in cultivation. They are herbaceous plants with cormous, more or less branching edible rootstocks, from which large peltate (taro) or sagittate (tannia) leaves rise up to 1 or 2 m. Inflorescences, of typically araceous form, consisting of spathe and many-flowered spadix, are rarely produced in most cultivars. There is much diversity in cultivated forms. Propagation is vegetative, by planting corm tops, or small cormels. Taro, especially, flourishes under moist conditions, or under irrigation, but some forms are adapted to upland rain-fed cultivation and need a growing season of eight months; they are not frost resistant. A virus disease of taro causes major destruction of

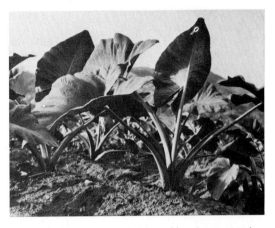

Fig. 6. Tannia (*Xanthosoma*), an aroid root crop, growing in Trinidad. (*From D. G. Coursey and P. H. Haynes, World Crops, 22:261–265, 1970*)

the crop in Melanesia; *Pythium* rots, leaf blight (*Phytophthora colocasia*), and attack by the beetle *Ligyrus ebenus* also cause problems.

Other aroids of local importance are the Giant Swamp Taros (*Cyrtosperma* spp.) in the coral atolls of Micronesia; the Elephant Yam (*Amorphophallus campanulatus*) in Southeast Asia and southern India; the Konjac (*A. rivieri*) in China and Japan; *Anchomanes dalzielli* in savannah Africa; and *Alocasia indica* and *A. macrorhiza*, which produce an edible stem used as a secondary or reserve crop in many tropical countries. *See* POTATO, IRISH; POTATO, SWEET.

[D. G. COURSEY]

Bibliography: D. G. Coursey and R. H. Booth, in C. L. A. Leakey and J. B. Wills (eds.), *Food Crops of the Lowland Tropics*, 1977; D. G. Coursey and P. H. Haynes, *World Crops*, 22:261–265, 1970; D. E. Kay, *TPI Crop and Product Digest No. 2, Root Crops*, 1973; J. W. Purseglove, *Tropical Crops: Dicotyledons*, 1968, and *Monocotyledons*, 1972.

Rutabaga

The plant *Brassica napobrassica*, a cool-season, hardy biennial crucifer of European origin, belonging to the order Capparales and probably resulting from the natural crossing of cabbage and turnip. Unlike turnip, it has smooth nonhairy leaves and 38 chromosomes. Propagation is by seed, commonly sown in early summer. The fleshy roots are cooked and usually eaten mashed as a vegetable. Rutabagas have been widely grown as a livestock feed in northern Europe and eastern Canada. Popular yellow-fleshed varieties (cultivars) are Laurentian and American Purple Top; a leading white variety is Macomber. Rutabagas have a high requirement for boron. High temperatures cause misshapen root growth. Commercial production is limited to Canada and the northern part of the United States. Harvesting generally begins after frost and when the roots are 4–6 in. in diameter, commonly 90–100 days after planting. The disease clubroot and the root maggot insect are the most common problems. For diseases of rutabaga *see* TURNIP. *See also* CABBAGE; PLANT GROWTH; VEGETABLE GROWING.

[H. JOHN CAREW]

Rye

A winter-hardy and drought-resistant cereal plant, *Secale cereale* L., in the grass family (Graminae). It resembles wheat, with which it intercrosses to a limited extent. Rye is propagated almost completely by cross-pollination; it is partly sterile if a plant is made to self-pollinate. The inflorescence is a spike or ear (Fig. 1a). Spikelets are arranged flatwise against a zigzag rachis (Fig. 2); they usually have two flowers, enclosed by a lemma and palea with two adjacent glumes. The young florets contain three stamens and a pistil. The fertilized pistil develops into a naked grain, or kernel (Fig. 1b and c), that is easily threshed. There are several recognized species of *Secale*, most of which have shattering spikes and small kernels. There are both perennial and winter-annual species of rye, with winter forms being favored over spring types for production. The only commercially cultivated species is the nonshattering *S. cereale*. Ergot sclerotia often are evident in the field and in threshed grain (Fig. 1d). See WHEAT.

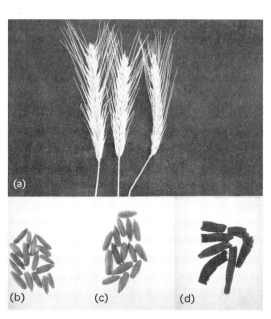

Fig. 1. Rye. (*a*) Spikes or ears. (*b*) Diploid kernels. (*c*) Tetraploid kernels. (*d*) Ergot.

Production. In 1974 world production was 32,690,000 metric tons (1,287,000,000 bu) or 9.7% as much as wheat. Rye production in 1974 was near its 10-year average, but wheat had increased rather steadily. Rye had lost nearly 40% of its area sown, while wheat gained. Barley increased in planted area and production, while oats remained nearly constant for 12 years.

Rye is more important in Europe and Asia than in the Western Hemisphere. The Soviet Union is the leading world producer, followed by Poland and West Germany. East Germany, Canada, and Argentina produce significant amounts, and Switzerland and northwest Europe have high yields.

Rye production in the United States fell after World War I and is still losing hectares (acres). In 1974, 498,000 metric tons (19,000,000 bu) were pro-

duced, mostly in South Dakota, North Dakota, Minnesota, and Georgia.

Uses. Rye grain is used for animal feed, human food, and production of spirits. Ground rye is mixed with other feeds for livestock. It is often fall-sown to provide soil cover and important pasturage for livestock. Egg yolks of chickens and butter from cows that are fed on rye have a rich yellow color. See DISTILLED SPIRITS.

Next to wheat, rye has the most desirable gluten for breadmaking. Rye bread is a staple food in certain sandy land areas of Europe and is favored by peoples of Slavic origin. In the United States, rye bread is made from blends of rye and wheat flour. Rye doughs lack gas retention, resulting in compact loaves or heavy bread. Rye flour contains several B vitamins and as many as 18 amino acids. Rye of different production conditions had 30% more lysine than spring wheats and durums, grown mostly in North Dakota, and somewhat more lysine than Triticales. Dark flours contain a higher content of amino acids than the lighter, refined flours.

Origin. N. I. Vavilov, a Russian plant scientist, believed that rye was introduced into cultivation simultaneously and independently at many localities in central Asia or Asia Minor. Great botanical diversity is found in Transcaucasia, Iran, Turkestan, and Asia Minor, where rye persists without being cultivated. Weedy rye types have closely investing lemmas with partially shattering spikes. Others resemble cultivated rye and are said to have high grain protein; their kernels are not well filled. Rye probably spread as mixtures of wheat.

Varieties. Compared to other small grains, rye has a fewer number of cultivars (agricultural varieties). Some common varieties grown in Europe and the Soviet Union are Belta, Danae, Dominant, Golden Dankow, Petkus, Petkus short straw, Sangaste, Toivo, Von Lochow, Vyatka, and Vyatka 2. Some common varieties in North America are Abruzzi, Adams, Cougar, Gator, Rymin, Von Lochow, and Weser. Short-strawed types are gaining favor. Plant and kernel characteristics of rye are variable, partly because of cross-pollination. Height may range from 4 to 6 ft (120 to 180 cm) under moderately fertile conditions. Kernel color may be amber, gray, green, blue, brown, or black.

Tetraploid forms, whose chromosome number has been doubled, are available. These kernels are large (Fig. 1c) and the straw is usually stiff, yet this type has not found much commercial use. Tetraploid wheat and rye have been hybridized and chromosomes doubled to form Triticales, which is increasing in usage. See BREEDING (PLANT).

Hybrid rye. Heterosis in rye, though not readily usable, has been recognized for several decades. Attempts to find cytoplasmic male sterility (cms) in cultivated types have been made since about 1960 in the Soviet Union and Europe. Progress has been reported, as well as finding fertility restorers. Hybridizing proper combinations of cms lines and restorers could enhance productivity and use of this crop.

Cultural practices. Culture of rye is similar to that of wheat. Seed-bed preparation is kept to a minimum, usually utilizing sandy soil. Plowing the land is preferable, but rye is sometimes drilled

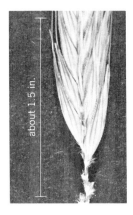

about 1.5 in.

Fig. 2. Florets and zigzag rachis of rye. (*Wisconsin Agricultural Experiment Station*)

directly into stubble. Seed can be sown by hand or with a regular drill at a rate of 56 to 85 lb/acre (25 to 83 kg/ha). Rye seed deteriorates during storage; therefore, it should be tested for germinability before sowing. Sowing in the Northern Hemisphere may be done from August to November, but before sustained freezing temperatures. Spring-sown rye is less important than winter rye. Rye may be plowed under for green manure, harvested for hay, or threshed for grain and straw. Grain should be 13.5% or lower in moisture and stored under dry conditions. *See* AGRICULTURE, SOIL AND CROP PRACTICES IN; GRAIN CROPS.

[H. L. SHANDS]

Processing. The selection of the proper type of grain is quite important in the manufacture of quality rye flour. Plumpness, soundness, and inside color are desirable characteristics. Sprout damage, ergot, and excessively thin rye should be avoided. In preparing rye for milling, separators, aspirators, disk machines, scourers, and brush machines are used to remove foreign material. It is desirable to remove as much of the outer covering of beeswing and germ as possible before milling. A short tempering before grinding is beneficial. Moisture of the rye at rolls should be about 14.5%.

The milling system for a rye mill is similar to that for a wheat mill, except that purifying and grading operations can be much simpler. Rye being tougher and more starchy than wheat, it requires more grinding and more bolting surface. Also, substantially more horsepower is required to reduce it to flour. Corrugated rolls are used throughout for all breaks and reductions. Smooth rolls have little value as they cause rye middlings to flatten and flake. Corrugations used are usually somewhat finer than for a wheat mill, with greater spiral and at least 2.5:1 differential on all grinding operations; that is, one of the rollers operates 2.5 times faster than the other.

Satisfactory white and dark rye flours can be made on a comparatively simple flow by proper selection and combining of basic mill-flour streams. White rye flours usually range from 0.58% to 0.64% ash, with dark rye running from 2.00 to 2.50% ash. Intermediate grades can be made by combinations of white and dark flours in the desired percentages. Rye-flour yields vary widely, according to the amount of dark flour made. A normal extraction ranges between 75 and 85% of the total grain ground.

Rye flours are usually blended with wheat flours to secure the desired results. The stronger types of wheat flour, such as clears, are usually used for this purpose. The offal of rye milling is called rye middlings, consisting of finely ground bran, germ, screenings, and a small amount of endosperm. *See* FOOD ENGINEERING. [JOHN A. SHELLENBERGER]

Bibliography: *FAO Production Yearbook*, vol. 26, 1972; *Foreign Agriculture Circular*, USDA FG5-75, March 1975; H. H. Geiger, and F. W. Schnell, Cytoplasmic male sterility in rye (*Secale cereale* L.), *Crop Sci.*, 10:590–593, 1970; V. D. Kobyljanskii, The production of sterile analogues of winter rye, sterility maintainers and fertility restorers, *Trud. po Pri. Bot. Gen. i Selek* (Russian), 44:76–84, 1971; W. H. Leonard and J. H. Martin, Rye, in *Cereal Crops*, 1963; H. L. Shands, Rye, in S. A. Matz (ed.), *Cereal Science*, 1969.

Saccharin

An organosulfur compound first prepared by Ira Remsen, and also called *o*-sulfobenzoic imide (I). The material used as a sweetening agent (about 500–700 times as sweet as cane sugar) is the sodium salt (II), which passes largely unchanged through the body and is excreted in the urine. The slightly bitter aftertaste of sodium saccharin is mainly that of impurities from the conventional synthesis and can be avoided by syntheses starting

$$\underset{\substack{o\text{-Toluene-}\\ \text{sulfonamide}}}{\overset{CH_3}{\underset{SO_2NH_2}{\bigcirc}}} \xrightarrow[\text{Heat}]{KMnO_4} \underset{(I)}{\overset{O}{\underset{S}{\overset{\parallel}{C}}}\!NH} \xrightarrow{NaOH}$$

$$\overset{O}{\underset{(II)}{\overset{\parallel}{C}}}N^-Na^+$$

from anthranilic acid or benzothiophene. Saccharin is used in food preparation for low-caloric diets and in diabetes therapy, where normal sugars cannot be tolerated.

[NORMAN KHARASCH]

Safflower

The plant *Carthamus tinctorius*, an annual thistle-like herb belonging to the family Compositae (see illustration). Probably originating as a cultivated plant in the Euphrates basin, safflower has become an oil crop in the western United States. Unique among the oil crops, safflower has been bred to have seeds (achenes) with an oil composition of more than three-fourths either oleic or linoleic fatty acid. This makes for versatile uses, either as an edible oil (cooking, salads, margarines, and so on) or an industrial oil (protective coatings, calks, putties, linoleums, and so on). In India, the leaves are sometimes used for salad. Prior to the advent of synthetic dyes, the red, yellow, or orange flowers were widely used to color cloth, cosmetics, and

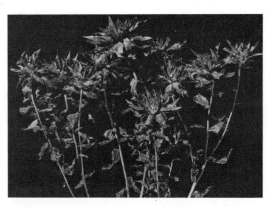

Safflower (*Carthamnus tinctorius*). (*USDA*)

food. *See* FAT AND OIL, EDIBLE.

[LEROY H. ZIMMERMAN]

Bibliography: E. A. Weiss, *Castor Sesame and Safflower*, 1971.

Saffron

SAFFRON

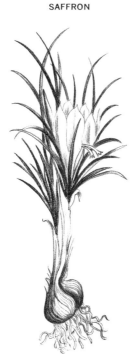

The plant *Crocus sativus*, a member of the iris family (Iridaceae). A native of Greece and Asia Minor, it is now cultivated in various parts of Europe, India, and China. This crocus (see illustration) is the source of a potent yellow dye used for coloring foods and medicine. The dye is extracted from the styles and stigmas of the flowers, which appear in autumn. It takes 4000 flowers to produce 1 oz of the dye.

[PERRY D. STRAUSBAUGH/EARL L. CORE]

Sage

The plant *Salvia officinalis*, a member of the mint family (Labiatae), the leaves of which yield a spice and an aromatic oil. It is a half-shrub (see illustra-

Saffron (*Crocus sativus*), of the family Iridaceae.

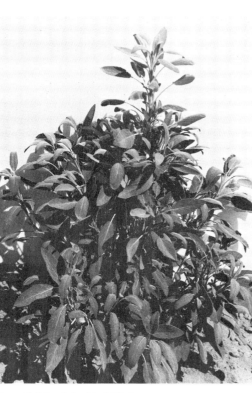

Sage (*Salvia officinalis*). (*USDA*)

tion) native to the Mediterranean region but is now widely cultivated. It is much used as a flavoring in stuffing for fowl and in meats, especially sausage. Oil of sage is used in making perfumes. *See* SPICE AND FLAVORING.

[PERRY D. STRAUSBAUGH/EARL L. CORE]

Salmonelloses

Diseases caused by *Salmonella*. These include enteritis (90–95% of all salmonelloses in the United States) and septicemia with or without enteritis (5–10%). *S. typhi*, *S. paratyphi A*, *B*, and *C*, and occasionally *S. cholerae suis*, cause particular types of septicemia called typhoid and paratyphoid fever, respectively; while all other types may cause enteritis or septicemia, or both together.

Typhoid fever. This type has an incubation period of 5–14 days. Typhoid fever is typified by a slow onset with initial bronchitis, diarrhea or constipation, a characteristic fever pattern (increase for 1 week, plateau for 2 weeks, and decrease for 2–3 weeks), a slow pulse rate, development of rose spots, swelling of the spleen, and often an altered consciousness; complications include perforation of the bowel and osteomyelitis. *S. typhi* can be isolated from the blood in the first 10 days and later from the feces and urine. The ileum shows characteristic ulcerations. Fecal excretion of *S. typhi* usually ends by the sixth week, but 2–5% of convalescents, mostly women, become chronic carriers. The organism may also persist in the gallbladder. The case fatality rate in the United States is now from 1 to 5%, with approximately 500 reported cases per year.

Typhoid fever leaves the individual with a high degree of immunity. Antibodies in the serum are detectable from the second week on: Anti-O antibodies signify a present infection, whereas anti-H antibodies, which appear later, are observed in convalescence, after vaccination, or after an earlier infection with an antigenically (H) related *Salmonella* species. Anti-Vi is often observed in carriers. Both anti-H and anti-Vi tend to persist.

Vaccine prepared from killed *S. typhi* gives an individual relative protection for about 3 years, which may be broken by large oral challenge doses.

The only effective antibiotic is chloramphenicol, although a few resistant strains have been reported in Mexico. Ampicillin may be helpful but is more useful in treating carriers. If gallbladder disease is present, cholecystectomy should be considered in carriers.

Preventive measures must concentrate on sanitation, since this exclusively human salmonella is transmitted most often by fecal contamination of water or foodstuffs.

Paratyphoid fever has a shorter course and is generally less severe than typhoid fever. Vaccination is an ineffective protective measure.

Enteric fevers. Enteric fevers, that is, septicemias due to types of *Salmonella* other than those previously mentioned, are more frequent in the United States than typhoid and paratyphoid fever but much less frequent than *Salmonella* enteritis. In children and in previously healthy adults, enteric fevers are most often combined with enteritis and have a favorable outlook. In certain predisposed individuals (for example, those under adrenocortical steroid treatment or those suffering from sickle cell anemia, malaria, or leukemia), septicemia with or without enteritis may occur; the prognosis then depends on the underlying illness. The organisms involved are the same as those causing *Salmonella* enteritis. Chloramphenicol or ampicillin are used in treatment. However, strains resistant to both drugs have been observed.

Enteritis. Inflammation of the small bowel due to *Salmonella* is one of the most important bacterial zoonoses. Approximately 22,000 cases are reported yearly in the United States, but the actual number, including mild, unreported cases may approach 2,000,000. The most frequent agents are *S. typhimurium*, *S. enteritidis*, *S. newport*, *S. heidelberg*, *S. infantis*, and *S. derby*. The incubation period varies from 6 hr to several days. Diarrhea and fever are the main symptoms; the intestinal epithelium is invaded, and early bacteremia is probable. Predisposed are persons with certain preexisting diseases (the same as for enteric fevers), very old and very young individuals, and postoperative patients. Chronic carriers exist but are rare in comparison with posttyphoid carriers. The main reservoir is animals, with transmission occurring chiefly through foodstuffs.

As would be expected, enteritides occur more frequently during the summer months. There is no immunity to this salmonellosis. Antibody determinations in the patient's serum may or may not yield positive results. In spite of laboratory effectiveness of many antibiotics, antimicrobial treatment serves only to prolong the carrier state and has no effect on the disease; neither has vaccination. Prevention must concentrate on improving sanitation in commercial food production (for example, improvements in slaughtering methods, slaughterhouse conditions, and transport facilities; and such measures as exclusion of carriers and decontamination of offal and powdered bulk food such as egg powder).

[ALEXANDER VON GRAEVENITZ]

Bibliography: E. J. Bowmer, The challenge of salmonellosis, *Amer. J. Med. Sci.*, 247:467, 1964; E. van Oye (ed.), *The World Problem of Salmonellosis*, 1964; F. H. Top and P. F. Wehrle (eds.), *Communicable and Infectious Diseases*, 7th ed., 1972.

Salt (food)

The chemical compound sodium chloride. It is used extensively in the food industry as a preservative and flavoring, as well as in the chemical industry to make chlorine and sodium. Historically, salt is one of the oldest materials used in man's food.

Manufacture. Salt was originally made by evaporating sea water (solar salt). This method is still in common usage; however, impurities in solar salt make it unsatisfactory for most commercial uses, and these impurities also lead to clumping. Salt, freshly produced from sea-water evaporation ponds, may contain large numbers of halophilic (salt-loving) microorganisms. These occasionally cause spoilage of meat, fish, vegetables, and hides when salt has been used in preservation.

In the United States refined salt is obtained from underground mines located in Michigan and Louisiana. Salt is usually handled during the refining processes as brine. These processes are discussed below.

Grainer salt. This type of salt is made by evaporation of brine in long shallow pans, as large as 18 ft wide, 1.5 ft deep, and 150 ft long. The daily capacity of such a grainer may be 80 tons. A scraping conveyor continually removes the crystallizing salt from the bottom of the grainer. The salt is then filtered, dewatered, dried, cooled, and rolled to break clumps. Grainer salt is usually the coarsest in grain and highest in impurities.

Vacuum pan salt. Salt brine is boiled at reduced pressure. A triple-effect evaporator is used; the first stage uses relatively light vacuum, but this is increased until in the third it is quite high and the salt solution boils at about 110°F. Production is continuous and the production cycle takes 48 hr. A 20% salt slurry is brought out from the bottom of the third evaporator at the same time fresh brine is admitted; thus impurities are washed from the surface of the outgoing crystals. The salt slurry is filtered, dewatered, and high-temperature-dried at 350°F before screening and packing.

Alberger process. Salt brine is heated to high pressures in heaters and then is passed to a graveller. A graveller is a large cylindrical vessel filled with stones which serves as a deposition site for calcium sulfate. The brine proceeds to flashers, where the pressure is gradually reduced to that of the atmosphere, and salt begins to crystallize. The brine and salt mixture is discharged to a large open pan; the crystallized salt is pumped to a centrifuge for dewatering, then dried in a rotary dryer.

Use. Large users of salt in the food industry are pickle makers and meat packers. In the pickle industry salt is used as brine to which fresh cucumbers are added. A selective fermentation then proceeds which is governed by salt concentration. Cost and time are dictating a movement toward "fresh-pack" pickles, in which salt and spices are added with the fresh cucumber, the jar is sealed, and the whole package is heated for pasteurization preservation. In the meat packing industry salt is added to fresh meat as a preservative, as in salt pork, or in combination with nitrates or nitrites as the first step in the production of cured meats, such as hams or bacon. *See* FOOD ENGINEERING; FOOD PRESERVATION.

Additives. Salt is liable to clumping during periods of high humidity, so preventives are added. Materials used include magnesium carbonate and certain silicates. Iodides are added in those areas where iodine deficiencies exist.

[ROY E. MORSE]

Bibliography: F. L. Hart and H. J. Fisher, *Modern Food Analysis*, 1970; S. C. Prescott and B. E. Proctor, *Food Technology*, 1937.

Sarsaparilla

A flavoring material obtained from the roots of at least four species of the genus *Smilax* (Liliaceae). These are *S. medica* of Mexico, *S. officinalis* of Honduras, *S. papyracea* of Brazil, and *S. ornata* of Jamaica, all tropical American vines found in the dense, moist jungles (see illustration). The flavoring is used mostly in combination with other aromatics such as wintergreen. *See* SPICE AND FLAVORING.

[PERRY D. STRAUSBAUGH/EARL L. CORE]

Scrapie

A transmissible, usually fatal disease of adult sheep characterized by degeneration of the central nervous system. The disease is known in Great Britain, France, Belgium, Iceland, the United States, Canada, and northern India. Scrapie has certain similarities with kuru, a human disease in New Guinea, and mink encephalopathy.

Clinical symptoms. Scrapie affects both sexes and is insidious in its onset, starting with hyperexcitability and progressive itch. Later, loss of wool occurs when the animal rubs against fixed objects or bites and nibbles its skin. Some animals do not rub but are either nervous and tremble when approached or appear sleepy. Incoordination of gait is constant and usually more evident in the hindquarters. In the final stages the sheep, being unable to stand, lie down, become emaciated, and die. In rare cases animals become fat before death. Most cases occur in sheep about 3–4 years old,

SARSAPARILLA

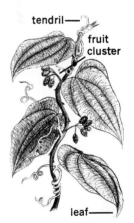

tendril—

fruit cluster

leaf—

Smilax aristolochiaefolia, which yields Mexican sarsaparilla.

although older animals may also be affected. It is extremely rare in sheep under 2 years of age.

Epidemiology. Scrapie spreads from ewes to offspring or by contact with unrelated sheep or goats. It is thought that animals become infected at birth or soon afterward and that the minimum incubation period under field conditions is about 2 years.

Pathology. On postmortem, constant and diagnostic changes are found only in the central nervous system, mainly in the brain. Apart from an increase in the amount of cerebrospinal fluid, all brain lesions are microscopic and are confined to subcortical centers, while the brain hemispheres remain unaffected. Lesions are most commonly found in the medulla or pons, but other parts such as midbrain, thalamus, hypothalamus, corpus striatum, cerebellum, and spinal cord may show pathological changes.

The lesions in scrapie are as a rule degenerative in character, symmetrically bilateral, diffuse or focal, and confined mainly to the gray matter. All forms of neuron degeneration may be found in the brain, ranging from chromatolysis to necrosis. However, of special interest are neuronal vacuoles because they form the basis for the diagnosis of the disease (Fig. 1). The vacuoles are very numerous, especially in the medulla, and consist of single or multiple cavities within the cytoplasm of the neurons. In addition to neuronal damage, areas of gray matter may show spongy degeneration in the form of empty spaces between the cellular elements and astrocytic gliosis. Astrocytes increase both in number and size and appear to fill the spaces occupied by degenerated neurons (Fig. 2).

Diagnosis and prognosis. Diagnosis is based on both the clinical symptoms and the characteristic pathological changes in the brain. Prognosis is unfavorable.

Etiology. Scrapie is caused by a transmissible self-replicating agent, which can be found in cell-free filtrates of the brain and other organs from scrapie-affected sheep. When inoculated into healthy sheep, the filtrate produces clinical scrapie in about 35% of animals after an incubation period of 4–12 months. The same filtrates given intracerebrally to goats, mice, hamsters, and rats gives rise to scrapie in all inoculated animals.

Two clinical syndromes, drowsiness and scratching, have been described in experimentally induced scrapie in goats. Subinoculations of brain filtrates from one syndrome produce the same syndrome in inoculated goats, but the brain lesions in the two forms are rather similar and resemble those in the brain of sheep affected with scrapie.

The transmission of scrapie from goats and sheep to mice gave rise to intensified research into the etiology of the disease. It was found that mice infected with goat or sheep material developed scrapie after 7–18 months, but when mice were inoculated with infected mouse brain or spleen the incubation period was reduced to 4–5 months. Mice appear to be very susceptible to scrapie and can develop the disease spontaneously after prolonged contact with affected mice. Clinically, mice might be either hyperexcitable or lethargic, and although the majority are very emaciated before death, a small proportion become very fat. Brain lesions in mice infected with sheep material resemble those seen in sheep brain, but in mice inoculated with filtrates of infected mouse brain or in mice that developed scrapie by contact, lesions can be found throughout the whole brain, including the hemispheres, where spongy degeneration and astrocytosis predominate. Similarly, when mouse brain material is inoculated into sheep or goats, although clinically the disease that ensues resembles scrapie of sheep or goats, the brain lesions resemble those of scrapie-infected mouse brain. The disease has been further transmitted to Chinese hamsters, mink, voles, and gerbils, and subsequently also to cynomolgus and squirrel monkeys. The transmission of scrapie to subhuman primates narrowed the gap between scrapie in animals and the spongiform encephalopathies of humans such as Kuru and Creutzfeldt-Jakob diseases.

Scrapie is classed as a slow virus disease, and the nature of its causative agent is still somewhat obscure. It can withstand physical and chemical treatment that would destroy all known viruses. Brain filtrates retain infectivity after boiling for more than 1 hr or after autoclaving for 30 min. Scrapie is not destroyed in brain tissue fixed in 4% formol for over 9 months, and substrates containing the agent remain infectious after exposure to ultraviolet irradiation or sterilizing doses of γ-radiation. Thus far, there has not been a consensus as to the identification of the scrapie agent in electron-microscopic preparations. While some authorities do not describe viral bodies in scrapie-affected tissues, others give illustrated accounts of tubular structures and sausage- and cucumber-shaped particles in the brain of scrapie sheep and rats. The particles described were 15–26 nm in diameter and 75 nm long.

The scrapie agent does not appear to stimulate an immune reaction in affected animals. None of the conventional serological and immunological tests, including fluorescent microscopy, are of any value in identifying scrapie. However, two tests were described alleging successful identification of the scrapie agent. The first is the polymorphonuclear (PMN) leukocyte depression test, based on the observation that brain and spleen homogenates from scrapie-affected animals when inoculated into normal mice reduced the percentage of circulating polymorphs. This claim has been strongly contested by some workers who could not obtain similar results, either with material from scrapie animals or with material from human spongiform encephalopathies. The second immunological reaction is the macrophage electrophoretic mobility (MEM) test, devised as a rapid method for diagnosing scrapie in sheep or goats. In this test the reactivity of the blood lymphocytes of the test animals to brain or spleen tissue from a mouse affected with scrapie is compared with that of lymphocytes of normal sheep.

[I. ZLOTNIK]

Bibliography: T. Alper et al., *Nature*, 214:764–766, 1967; J. G. Brotherston et al., *J. Comp. Pathol.*, 78:9–17, 1968; P. Brown and D. C. Gajdusek, *Nature*, 247:217–218, 1974; R. I. Carp et al., *J. Infect. Dis.*, 128:256–258, 1973; R. L. Chandler, *Res. Vet. Sci.*, 15:322–328, 1973, M. C. Clarke and D. A. Haig, *Res. Vet. Sci.*, 11:500–501, 1970; E. J. Field and B. K. Shenton, *Amer. J. Vet. Res.*, 35:

SCRAPIE

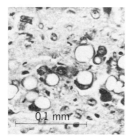

Fig. 1. Vacuoles in neurons of medulla of scrapie-infected animal.

SCRAPIE

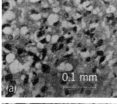
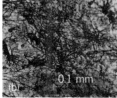
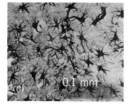

Fig. 2. Photomicrographs of the brain from scrapie affected animals. (a) Spongy degeneration. Astrocytic hypertrophy in (b) sheep and (c) mice.

393–395, 1974; C. J. Gibbs, Jr., and D. C. Gajdusek, in F. O. Schmitt and F. G. Worden (eds.), *Neurosciences*, 3d Study Program, pp. 1025–1041, 1974; H. K. Narang, *Acta Neuropath.*, 28:317–329, 1974; I. Zlotnik, *J. Comp. Pathol.*, 78:19–22, 1968; I. Zlotnik and J. C. Rennie, *Br. J. Exp. Pathol.*, 48:171–179, 1967.

Scurvy

An acute or chronic disease due to vitamin-C (ascorbic acid) deficiency. Vitamin C is a water-soluble vitamin, essential for the formation of collagen, ground substance, osteoid, dentine, and intercellular cement substance (connective tissues). Any tissues composed of these substances may be altered if a deficiency state occurs. *See* ASCORBIC ACID.

Infantile scurvy usually occurs between the sixth and twelfth months of life and is due to a lack of dietary vitamin, especially in artificially fed infants. The characteristic symptoms include irritability, failing appetite, and failure to gain weight. The child cries when moved or handled and may not move a limb. Bony malformations of the ribs and legs follow severe deficiency, often accompanied by a bleeding tendency. Hemorrhage, anemia, and infection are serious complications.

In adults scurvy is rarely due to dietary deficiency in normally fed populations, since 3–12 months of severe deficiency are required to produce symptoms. These include weakness, weight loss, irritability, and vague pains. Clinical signs include such things as delayed wound healing, tooth changes, gingivitis, petechial hemorrhages, and nosebleeds. Stress, infection, and hemorrhage may aggravate the situation. The disease is often related to chronic or severe gastrointestinal disease or to food idiosyncrasies. Any type of healing requires increased vitamin C supply, and infection similarly increases body demand.

Response to treatment is dramatic and effective if permanent bone and tissue damage has not prevailed. *See* VITAMIN.

[N. KARLE MOTTET]

Seed (botany)

A fertilized ovule containing an embryo which forms a new plant upon germination. Seed-bearing characterizes the higher plants—the gymnosperms (conifers and allies) and the angiosperms (flowering plants). Gymnosperm (naked) seeds arise on the surface of a structure, as on a seed scale of a pine cone. Angiosperm (covered) seeds develop within a fruit, as the peas in a pod.

Seed structure. One or two tissue envelopes, or integuments, form the seed coat which encloses the seed except for a tiny pore, the micropyle (Fig. 1). The micropyle is near the funiculus (seed stalk) in angiosperm seeds. The hilum is the scar left when the seed is detached from the funiculus. Some seeds have a raphe, a ridge near the hilum opposite the micropyle, and a bulbous strophiole. Others such as nutmeg possess arils, outgrowths of the funiculus, or a fleshy caruncle developed from the seed coat near the hilum, as in the castor bean. The fleshy, edible aril of the Philippine kamanchile completely encloses the seed to form a fruitlike structure. The embryo consists of an axis and attached cotyledons (seed leaves). The part of the axis above the cotyledons is the epicotyl (plumule); that below, the hypocotyl, the lower end of which bears a more or less developed primordium of the root (radicle). The epicotyl, essentially a terminal bud, possesses an apical meristem (growing point) and, sometimes, leaf primordia. The seedling stem develops from the epicotyl. An apical meristem of the radicle produces the primary root of the seedling, and transition between root and stem occurs in the hypocotyl.

Two to many cotyledons occur in different gymnosperms. The angiosperms are divided into two major groups according to number of cotyledons: the monocotyledons including orchids, lilies, grasses, and sedges; and the dicotyledons such as beans, roses, and sunflowers. Mature gymnosperm seeds contain an endosperm (albumen or nutritive tissue) which surrounds the embryo. In some mature dicotyledon seeds the endosperm persists, the cotyledons are flat and leaflike, and the epicotyl is simply an apical meristem (Fig. 2). In other seeds, such as the bean, the growing embryo absorbs the endosperm, and food reserve for germination is stored in fleshy cotyledons. The endosperm persists in common monocotyledons, for example, corn and wheat, and the cotyledon, known as the scutellum, functions as an absorbing organ during germination (Fig. 3). Grain embryos also possess a coleoptile and a coleorhiza sheathing the epicotyl and the radicle, respectively. The apical meristems of lateral seed roots also may be differentiated in the embryonic axis near the scutellum of some grains.

Monocotyledon and dicotyledon seeds also differ in seed coat structure. In grains, or caryopsis fruits, the mature fruit wall and seed coat may be fused and the outermost endosperm cells form an aleurone layer, rich in proteins. Flour brans consist of fragments of aleurone and fruit-seed coats. Most of the thiamine and riboflavin of grains occur

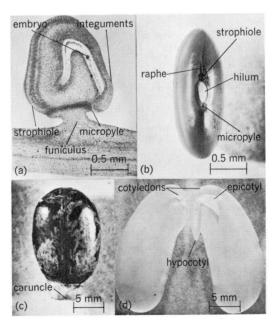

Fig. 1. Seed structures. (*a*) Median longitudinal section of pea ovule shortly after fertilization, showing attachment to pod tissues. (*b*) Mature kidney bean. (*c*) Mature castor bean. (*d*) Opened embryo of mature kidney bean.

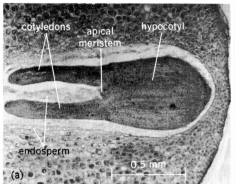
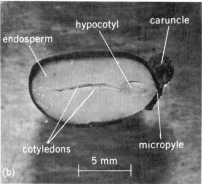
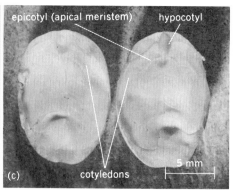

Fig. 2. Dicotyledon seeds. (a) Median longitudinal section of embryo of silk tassel bush (*Garrya elliptica*) embedded in endosperm which has been removed from mature seed. (b) Castor bean cut longitudinally. (c) Castor bean removed from seed coat and split longitudinally between cotyledons.

in these tissues and near the scutellum.

Cellular structure of the seed coat varies in the dicotyledons. An outer, water-impervious layer of wax or cuticle is usually present. The outermost cells in bean and pea seed coats, known as macrosclereids (Malpighian cells), have fluted, cellulosic wall thickenings; underlying them is a layer of osteosclereids, short bone-shaped cells. Two layers of macrosclereids occur at the hilum in peas and beans. Underlying them is a group of tracheary cells with reticulate (netted) wall thickenings, and a surrounding spongy tissue of branched cells and large air spaces. This structure appears to be well suited for water absorption during germination.

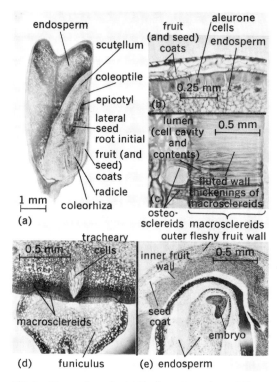

Fig. 3. Monocot seeds. (a) Section of corn kernel (*from M. J. Wolf et al., Cereal Chem., 29:321–382, 1952*). (b) Section of outer cell layers of wheat grain. (c) Section of outer cells of mature pea seed coat. (d) Section of hilum area of nearly mature pea. (e) Section through portion of young raspberry drupelet (segment of berry).

Many so-called seeds consist of hardened parts of the fruit enclosing the true seed which has a thin, papery seed coat. Among these are the achenes, as in the sunflower, dandelion, and strawberry, and the pits of stone fruits such as the cherry, peach, and raspberry. Many common nuts also have this structure.

Seed dispersal. Mechanisms for seed dispersal include parts of both fruit and seed. Some dry fruits have membranous air sacs which aid in seed dispersal by water. In cockleburrs and beggarticks the seeds are enclosed in spiny, barbed fruits which are readily carried in the fur of animals. Seed dispersal by wind is aided by hair tufts of dandelion achenes, wings of elm and maple fruits and of conifer seeds, and by seed-coat hairs of willow, cottonwood, and milkweed seeds. Cotton fibers consist of greatly elongated epidermal hairs of the seed coat as do also the kapok fibers of the silk-cotton tree (*Ceiba pentandra*).

Economic importance. Propagation of plants by seed and technological use of seed and seed products are among man's most important activities. Specializations of seed structure and composition provide rich sources for industrial exploitation apart from direct use as food. Common products include starches and glutens from grains, hemicelluloses from guar and locust beans, and proteins and oils from soybeans and cotton seed. Drugs, enzymes, vitamins, spices, and condiments are obtained from embryos, endosperms, and entire seeds, often including the fruit coat. Most of the oils of palm, olive, and pine seeds are in the endosperm. Safflower seed oil is obtained mainly from the embryo, whereas both the seed coat and embryo of cotton seed are rich in oils. *See* AGRICULTURE; FOOD ENGINEERING.

[ROGER M. REEVE]

Seed germination

The resumption of growth by the plant embryo when the proper conditions are provided. During the maturation of the seed on the parent plant, an embryo, or young plant, develops within the seed coats. Following maturation, there is a dormant phase during which the young embryo is usually quiescent. Technically, the germination process has begun when the seeds start to take up moisture. This imbibition period is a short one and is followed by biochemical or morphological changes or both. These changes, not apparent from the outside of the seed, permit cell multiplication and further growth and result in the penetration of the seed coats by the young radicle or root.

Two leading requirements for germination are suitable moisture supply and proper temperature. In addition, oxygen is usually essential, though there are seeds adversely affected by large amounts of it.

Testing and analysis of seeds. The quality of agricultural, vegetable, and tree seeds is of the utmost importance in planting programs that aim to provide the world's needs for food and other plant products. Because of this importance, official laboratories have been established throughout the world to conduct analysis of seed samples as to purity of the seeds (whether contaminated by weed seeds or those of other crops) and germinative capacity. Furthermore, certain rules have been agreed upon to ensure national and international uniformity in the testing and the reporting and evaluation of results. It has taken a great deal of research, much of which has been published in the Proceedings of the International Seed Testing Association, to arrive at these standard procedures.

Impermeable seed coats. Many seeds, especially those of the family Leguminosae, have coats which are impermeable to water. Most of these seeds germinate readily after the coats are treated to permit water absorption. Among such treatments are mechanical scarification or shaking and soaking in hot water, alcohol, or concentrated sulfuric acid.

Temperature and nondormant seeds. Some seeds, notably those of certain flowers, require special temperatures for germination. For example, wild columbine (*Aquilegia canadensis* L.), honeysuckle (*Lonicera tartarica* L.), and *Catalpa* sp. offer no special difficulties at temperatures of 15–25°C, but higher temperatures reduce or prevent germination.

The difficulties encountered by many rock garden enthusiasts in the germination of seeds may be attributed to any one of several factors. Seeds of *Primula obconica* Hance and *Ramonda pyrenaica* Rich. require light for germination. Although light is not essential for the germination of *Draba aizoides* L., *Gentiana lagodechiana* Kusn., *Mimulus langsdorfii* Donn, and *Primula denticulata* Sm., exposure of all of these seeds to light during the germination process permits seedling production at temperatures that would be inhibitive in darkness. Other rock garden seeds, such as *Calochortus macrocarpus* Dougl., *Camassia leichtlinii* Wats., and *Lewisia rediviva* Pursh, germinate only at temperatures of approximately 5°C. This is in contrast to *Draba alpina* L., *Meconopsis cambrica* Vig., and *Gentiana crinita* Froel., seeds of which possess dormant embryos and must be pretreated at low temperature, after which germination proceeds at ordinary greenhouse temperature.

Temperature and dormant embryos. There is a type of dormancy of low intensity that is exhibited by many seeds at maturity but that disappears after a period of dry storage. It is characteristic of many grain and flower seeds and of some vegetable seeds, notably lettuce. Such dormancy may be overlooked if no germination test is made until several months after harvest.

Many plants, especially those of the temperate zone, have seeds with dormant embryos. The method commonly used to break this dormancy is pretreatment in a moist medium at low temperatures. This process has long been used by nurserymen under the term "stratification," so called because of the practice of alternating layers of sand with layers of seeds for winter treatment. Stratification has come to mean any moist low-temperature pretreatment, whether the actual layering process is used or not. Mixing the seeds with some moist medium like granulated peat moss or vermiculite or just planting the seeds in soil in a regular manner are methods often used for the afterripening of embryos at low temperature.

The effective temperatures for bringing about the changes necessary for germination are usually between 1 and 10°C, with 5°C commonly effective. Many types of seeds respond to this treatment, from the delicate fringed gentian through aquatic plants to shrubs and large trees. Tables have been published listing some 100 species with the temperature and time requirements for satisfactory afterripening.

Unfavorable germination conditions often induce a secondary dormancy which also requires special treatment before germination can proceed.

Impermeable coats and dormant embryos. Some seeds with dormant embryos do not afterripen in a moist medium at low temperatures because their coats are impermeable to water. In these cases it is essential to make the coat permeable by mechanical or chemical treatment or a period in moist soil at about 25°C, after which a period in a moist medium at low temperature will break dormancy. This type of dormancy has been demonstrated for a number of forms, namely, *Aralia racemosa* L., *Arctostaphylos uva-ursi* (L.) Spreng., *Cornus canadensis* L., *Cotoneaster divaricata* Rehd. and Wils., *Cotoneaster horizontalis* Decne., several species of *Crataegus*, *Halesia carolina* L., *Rhodotypos kerrioides* Sieb. and Zucc., *Symphoricarpos racemosus* Michx., *Taxus cuspidata* Sieb. and Zucc., and *Tilia americana* L.

Epicotyl dormancy. All of the seeds described above as responding favorably to low-temperature pretreatment afterripen while still enclosed in seed coats, and once the embryo resumes growth, the green plant appears above ground in a short time. Another type of dormancy has been found in which the seed germinates to form a root without any pretreatment, but once the root is formed, low temperature is essential to break the dormancy of the shoot or the bud that forms it. This has been designated epicotyl dormancy. The so-called 2-year lilies, the tree peony (*Paeonia suffruticosa* Andr.), and several species of *Viburnum* belong to this category.

Dwarfs from nonafterripened embryos. When all of the coats surrounding seeds of *Rhodotypos kerrioides* Sieb. and Zucc., *Prunus persica* (L.) Stokes, *Pyrus malus* L., and some *Crataegus* sp. are removed, a certain percentage of the embryos that require cold stratification for normal development will grow at greenhouse temperatures to form dwarf plants. In such physiological dwarfs normal growth is initiated after some months of stunting or after exposure of the seedling to a cold period. This dwarf character is doubtless another expression of the phenomenon known as epicotyl dormancy.

Double dormancy. From the previous discussions it might be expected that there would be seeds that require pretreatment at low temperature to break the dormancy of the root, a period at high temperature to permit the root to grow, another period at low temperature to break epicotyl dormancy, and finally a second period at high temperature to permit the growth of the afterripened epicotyl. Such seeds do exist, for example, in *Caulophyllum thalictroides* (L.) Michx., *Convallaria majalis* L., *Smilacina racemosa* (L.) Desf., and *Trillium* sp.

Light. The influence of light on seed germination has been known for many years and has been reviewed by Michael Evenari, William Crocker, and E. H. Toole and coworkers. This influence takes the form of either inhibition or stimulation of germination, depending upon the wavelength of the light and the kind of seed. The specific action spectra responsible have been known since 1940, and the photoreaction controlling the germination of *Lactuca sativa* L. seeds was shown to be repeatedly photoreversible on the same seed in 1952. According to Toole and coworkers, this photoreversibility may be expressed by the formula below.

$$\text{Pigment} + \text{Reactant} \underset{\substack{7350\,A \\ \text{or} \\ \text{darkness}}}{\overset{6550\,A}{\rightleftharpoons}}$$
(Red-
absorbing)

Pigment + Changed
(Far-red-   reactant
absorbing)

The red portion of the spectrum stimulates and the far-red portion of the spectrum inhibits the germination of *Lactuca sativa* L. seeds. *See* PHOTOPERIODISM IN PLANTS.

It has been found further that the germination of seeds of many plants is controlled by a brief irradiation of low energy, whereas many other seeds, such as those of *Paulownia tomentosa* (Thunb.) Steud. and *Pinus taeda* L., need much longer exposures.

Still other kinds of seeds, whose germination response was not previously understood, really have high-energy light requirement. Inhibition of their germination is controlled by a combination of a reversible change of the pigment forms and their continued excitation. Examples of plants whose seeds require high-energy light are *Lactuca sativa* L., *Lamium amplexicaule* L., and *Nemophila insignis* Dougl.

Other factors. In certain cereals, including dormant wild oats, and in *Xanthium*, it has been shown that seed or fruit structures enclosing the embryos exclude oxygen and thus prevent germination. However, gaseous exchange is rarely a factor in germination.

The maturity of the seeds when they are shed or removed from the parent plants, the seed size, atmospheric pressure, electrical treatment, radioactivity, symbiotic relationship with other plants or plant parts, and even the Moon have been reported to affect seed germination. Chemicals of various kinds, applied externally or metabolized within the seeds, are also responsible for germination failure or stimulation.

Much work is being done in different laboratories on biochemical changes taking place in seeds during germination. Results of these investigations will contribute greatly to the elucidation of the germination process. *See* PLANT GROWTH; SEED (BOTANY).

[LELA V. BARTON/A. A. APP]

Bibliography: L. V. Barton, *Seed Preservation and Longevity*, in *Plant Science Monographs*, 1961; W. Crocker, *Growth of Plants*, 1948; W. Crocker and L. V. Barton, *Physiology of Seeds*, 1953; M. Evenari, Germination inhibitors, *Botan. Rev.*, 15(3):153–194, 1949; O. L. Justice (ed.), *Manual for Testing Agricultural and Vegetable Seeds*, USDA Handb.no. 30, 1952; A. M. Mayer and A. Poljakoff-Mayber, *The Germination of Seeds*, 1963; *Woody-Plant Seed Manual*, USDA Misc. Publ. no. 654, 1948.

Serine

An amino acid. The amino acids are characterized physically by the following: (1) the pK_1, or the dissociation constant of the various titratable groups; (2) the isoelectric point, or pH at which a dipolar ion does not migrate in an electric field; (3) the op-

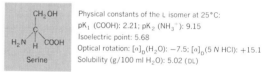

Physical constants of the L isomer at 25°C:
pK_1 (COOH): 2.21; pK_2 (NH_3^+): 9.15
Isoelectric point: 5.68
Optical rotation: $[\alpha]_D(H_2O)$: −7.5; $[\alpha]_D$(5 N HCl): +15.1
Solubility (g/100 ml H_2O): 5.02 (DL)

tical rotation, or the rotation imparted to a beam of plane-polarized light (frequently the D line of the sodium spectrum) passing through 1 dm of a solution of 100 g in 100 ml; and (4) solubility.

Serine reacts with periodate to yield glyoxylate, ammonia, and formaldehyde. Serine is a biosynthetic precursor of several important metabolites: glycine, cysteine, choline (and hence betaine), and the side chain of tryptophan. D-Serine is a constituent of the antibiotic polymyxin. Serine originates, biosynthetically, from 3-phosphoglyceric acid. Since glycine and serine are interconverted rapidly, the pathway glyoxylate → glycine → serine can furnish some serine also. *See* AMINO ACIDS; CYSTEINE; GLYCINE; TRYPTOPHAN.

During metabolic degradation serine deaminase (dehydrase) nonoxidatively attacks serine to yield pyruvate and ammonia. Another major pathway starts with transfer of the hydroxymethyl group to tetrahydrofolic acid, yielding glycine. Finally, a transaminase for serine exists, forming β-hydroxypyruvate. This compound may be convertible to glyceric acid, or the actual pathway may be the reversal of the biosynthetic one, involving phosphorylated intermediates.

[EDWARD A. ADELBERG]

Sheep

Sheep are members of the family Bovidae in the order Artiodactyla, the even-toed, hoofed mammals. Sheep were possibly the first animals to be domesticated about 11,000 years ago in southwestern Asia, a time when sheep were closely associated with the religious, civic, and domestic life of the people. They are referred to more often in the Bible than any other animal.

Wild sheep range over the mountainous areas of the Northern Hemisphere. They have long, curved, massive horns and mixed coats with a hairy outercoat and a woolly undercoat. Although wild sheep vary in size, they are usually larger than domestic sheep and have shorter tails.

Distribution. Over 1,000,000,000 domestic sheep extend over most of the land areas of the world. They are most heavily concentrated in the warmer parts of the temperate zones and are found in greatest numbers in the Southern Hemisphere in Australia, New Zealand, South Africa, and South America. Other countries with high sheep numbers include the Soviet Union, China, India, Iran, Turkey, and the United Kingdom. More common in drier regions and at high elevations, sheep are rarely found in the wet tropics and other humid areas.

Domestic sheep were first brought to the Americas by Spanish explorers. Sheep were introduced into the English colonies almost as soon as they were settled. By 1840, New England was the center for sheep production in the United States; the center moved westward to Ohio by 1850. This westward movement of sheep continued, encouraged by the availability of year-round grazing, and by 1860 there were many sheep in California and Texas. The sheep population reached a peak in 1884 with over 50,000,000 head. Since then numbers have declined to about 13,000,000 in the 1970s. Sheep are common in the north-central states and from Missouri to Virginia, but the bulk are found in the western states and Texas.

Terminology. Sheep are called lambs until about 12 months of age, from which time to 24 months they are referred to as yearlings, and thereafter as two-year-olds, and so on. The female sheep is called a ewe and the male, a ram or buck; the castrated male is called a wether. Sheep meat is called lamb or mutton depending on the age at slaughter. Young carcasses, where the forefeet are removed at the break joint or temporary cartilage just above the ankle, are sold as lamb; mutton carcasses are those of older animals where it is necessary to take the feet off at the ankle. Mutton is less desired and brings a lower price than lamb.

General description. A precise definition is difficult since sheep are so variable. Horns, if present, tend to curl in a spiral. If horns occur in both sexes, they are usually larger for the ram. In some breeds only the rams have horns but many breeds are hornless. The hairy outercoat common to wild sheep was eliminated by breeding in most domestic sheep. Wool may cover the entire sheep, or the face, head, legs, and part of the underside may be bare; or wool may be absent as in some breeds (bred for meat) with a short hairy coat or a coat which constantly sheds. Although domestic sheep are mostly white, shades of brown, gray, and black occur, sometimes with spotting or patterns of color. The faces and legs are white in some white breeds while black or mottled in others. The shape of the face and head varies from a small, dished face to one with a large, prominent nose. The ears may be small and pointed; somewhat straight and moderate-sized or long and pendulous; and erect or drooping. Body form varies from

the angular, uneven shape of wool-type breeds to the smooth, rounded, blocky appearance of meat-type breeds. The tail tends to be long in most domestic breeds but is often removed or docked soon after birth. It may be short in some breeds, but may be bare or completely covered with wool in others. Some desert breeds have large fat deposits on the rump or the tail.

The shape of the body of a sheep is determined by the bony skeleton and the amount and distribution of muscle and fat. The thoracic and lumbar vertebrae have both lateral and vertical extensions which contribute to the shape of the back. The front legs have no direct connections to the body skeleton, but the shoulder blades are attached by muscles. Body weights for mature animals may vary from well under 100 to 400 lb (45 to 181 kg) or more. Body measurements vary widely with breed, sex, age, and degree of fatness.

As in other ruminants the stomach of the sheep has four compartments and is adapted to regurgitation and cud chewing. Prior to regurgitation and further chewing, food is stored in the rumen, the largest compartment where roughages are broken down by microorganisms. When food is swallowed a second time, it passes into the third stomach or omasum, which is made up of lengthwise leaves and is connected to the abomasum or true stomach. *See* DIGESTIVE SYSTEM.

The sheep has 20 lamb or temporary teeth, and 32 permanent teeth of which 8 are incisors; a cartilaginous pad is found instead of incisors in the upper jaw. The sheep bites by clamping herbage between the incisor teeth and the dental pad and then jerking or twisting the head.

Although sheep mature in 1–2 years, they may not reach maximum weights and production until 3–5 years of age. The average life-span is about 6–7 years with the productive life sometimes being shorter; survival beyond 10–11 years is rare. Replacement of the lamb incisors with a pair of larger permanent incisors is generally used to estimate age of sheep, although this practice is quite inexact. The first central pair of permanent incisors appears around 1 year of age, and an additional pair is added approximately yearly until a full mouth of four pairs is obtained. After 4 years, age may be estimated from the spread, wear, or loss of the teeth. However, the only sure way to determine age is through individual or group identification from birth throughout life.

Wool and skin. Wool fiber is made up largely of insoluble, sulfur-containing proteins or keratins. The crimps or waves of the wool fiber vary from only 1–2 up to 25 or more per inch (1 up to 10 or more per centimeter), but the waves of adjacent fibers are generally parallel so that blocks of fibers in locks of wool or even over the entire fleece tend to be uniformly crimped. Fiber diameter varies from 10 to 70 micrometers (μm). The number of crimps per inch is greater in fine wool which has fibers of smaller diameters. Fiber length is generally recognized as length of staple, that is, length of wool as it grows on the sheep, and this may vary from about 1 up to 6 in. (2.5 up to 15 cm) or more for 1 year of growth. Length and diameter are associated to some extent and tend to vary with breed, and nutrition and possibly other environmental factors. Wool grows continually at a somewhat regular rate over the lifetime of the sheep even if it is not removed.

The skin of a sheep is about 1/12 in. thick, may be pigmented to various degrees, and contains sweat and sebaceous glands which, together with the hair and wool follicles, are generally arranged in a typical pattern. Those follicles which develop prenatally are called primary follicles, and each is associated with a sweat gland, oil gland, and a smooth muscle. Secondary follicles develop later and have only an oil gland. Primary follicles usually occur in groups of three with a variable number of secondary fibers. There are great variations within breeds and on individual animals regarding the total number of fibers per square inch; totals range from less than 5000 to more than 60,000 per square inch (775 to more than 9300 per square centimeter).

Reproduction. Sheep may reach puberty as early as 100–150 days although 5–10 months is more common. The first estrus in ewe lambs may occur somewhat later than the first sperm production in ram lambs. Sexual maturity may be more closely related to weight than to age and usually occurs when body weights reach 40–60% of mature weight; it may be delayed even beyond 1 year of age if nutrition is poor. Sexual maturity varies with breed, being earlier for fast-growing breeds such as the Suffolk than for slow-growing breeds such as the Merino, and is generally earlier for crossbred lambs than for purebreds. Ram lambs can be used successfully in breeding, but males are more commonly mated first at 18–20 months of age. Although ewes are often bred first to lamb at 2 years of age, it is not uncommon to breed ewe lambs. Ewes bred first as lambs generally will have greater lifetime lamb production than ewes bred first as yearlings. Conception rates for ewe lambs may vary 10–60% or more.

The breeding season is related to day length and generally commences as days become shorter; most domestic breeds of sheep have a breeding season restricted to the fall and winter months. There is considerable variation in estrous periods among breeds and among individuals, varying from a few periods to almost year-round breeding. The presence of rams near the beginning of the breeding season may stimulate the onset of the first estrus. Rams do not show a restricted breeding season, but semen production and quality are generally higher in the fall and may decline in the spring and summer; summer sterility may occur under continuous high temperatures.

Estrus. In the ewe estrus can only be recognized by willingness to stand and to allow the ram to mount. Sometimes the vulva is enlarged and there is usually a liquefaction and flow of mucus from the cervix. Cornified epithelial cells may be observed in the vaginal smear following estrus. Estrus may vary in duration from a few hours to 3 days or more with an average of 1–2 days; it may be shorter when rams are with ewes continuously. Ovulation normally occurs near the end of estrus.

The normal estrus cycle in the ewe varies from 14 to 19 days with an average of 17 days. Ovulation without estrus generally occurs one cycle before the first estrus. A postpartum estrus may occur within the first day or two after parturition but is not accompanied by ovulation. Ovulation and estrus may occur during lactation but both are more likely to occur after the first 4–10 weeks. Giving progesterone for 12–14 days during the breeding season may synchronize estrus, with estrus and ovulation usually occurring 1–5 days after the treatment is stopped. There may be some reduction in fertility if ewes are bred at the first synchronized estrus.

Ovulation. The number of eggs shed per heat period (ovulation rate) limits the number of lambs produced and therefore is an important aspect of productivity. It varies with year, season, age, breed, and nutrition. The most common ovulation rate as judged from the number of lambs born is one, although two occur often, three occasionally, and four sometimes, and five or six rarely; up to nine have been reported. Ovulation rate increases with age reaching a maximum at 3–6 years of age. It tends to be high in the early part to the middle of the breeding season but decreases toward the end.

Pregnancy. A number of reliable pregnancy tests may be used with sheep. Methods which are both rapid and accurate include palpation by laparotomy, observation with peritoneoscope, and ultrasonic detection of pregnancy either by echo or by the Doppler technique. This last method is highly accurate at about 60 days following conception or even earlier. Diagnosis with x-rays and with fetal electrocardiography is possible but of limited usefulness. Hormonal methods are coming into practical use with accurate diagnosis as early as 18 days after conception.

The average duration of pregnancy varies among breeds from 144 to 155 days; normal pregnancies may range from 138 to 159 days in individuals. Early-maturing breeds such as the Southdown and Shropshire have short gestation periods of about 145 days as do high-fertility breeds such as Finnsheep or Romanov with periods of 142–146 days, while late-maturing breeds such as the Merino or Rambouillet may have average periods as long as 151 days. Crossbred types such as the Columbia or Targhee tend to be intermediate. Pregnancy is shorter for twin lambs than for singles; it may be longer in older ewes.

The sex ratio is generally 49–50% males. Identical twins are rare. A few cases of freemartin lambs have been reported.

Parturition. The termination of pregnancy is determined in part by hormonal changes in which fetal adrenal activity initiates a series of hormonal trends culminating in parturition. The pelvic ligaments, vagina, and cervix tend to relax near the end of pregnancy. Parturition may be more common in the forenoon and late afternoon. The first signs of parturition are uneasiness, pawing and frequent turning, or lying down and standing up. The forefeet of the lamb generally appear first in front of the head; one or both front legs turned back are regarded as malpresentations. The lamb is licked dry by the mother following birth and sucks milk within an hour or two. The afterbirth is generally expelled 2–4 hr after parturition. The uterus normally returns to nonpregnant size in 2 weeks and is completely involuted by 4 weeks. Synchronization of parturition is feasible with hormonal treatments.

Male physiology. The spermatogenetic cycle in

the ram is about 49 days. The average sperm production has been measured at 5,500,000,000 per day. High-quality ram semen is characterized by having at least 2,000,000,000 sperm per cubic centimeter, a rapid swirling movement, a pH about 7.0 or with greater acidity, and with less than 25% abnormal sperm or less than 5% abnormal heads. Rams show wide variation in frequency of copulation from once in about 10 hr to over once an hour. The number of copulations increases in direct proportion to the number of available ewes in heat.

Altering reproductive cycles. Artificial insemination techniques have been developed for sheep, but fresh semen gives higher fertility than frozen semen. Practical use of artificial insemination generally requires synchronization of estrus, involvement of genetic improvement, and repeated reproductive cycles to reduce the length of dry periods.

Attempts to increase the reproductive rate of sheep have included selection for breeding at any time of the year and more often than once per year; use of the high-fertility Finnsheep in crossing; and improvement of the twinning rate through breeding, nutrition, and management. Complete control of reproduction in sheep is now feasible through synchronization of estrus, artificial insemination, early pregnancy diagnosis, and synchronization of parturition, but is not in practical use. *See* BREEDING (ANIMAL).

Adaptation. Although sheep are well adapted to cold climates, they have excellent tolerance to heat because of the excellent temperature regulation effected by their wool. Shearing may increase heat tolerance in summer and decrease it in cooler periods. Body temperature maintained at about 102°F may vary from about 98 to 106°F. The most important source of heat loss is evaporation from the respiratory tract; however, sheep do sweat to a limited extent.

Sheep are probably most productive in temperate climates. Hot climates are unfavorable for lamb meat production because of reduced fertility and reduced feed intake. Wool may usually be produced efficiently in hot, dry climates. Internal parasites become abundant and cause serious losses in warm, humid climates. Both lamb and wool are produced well in cold climates, but environmental protection may be necessary at lambing, after shearing, and under wet or stormy conditions.

Breeds. Hundreds of breeds of sheep of all types, sizes, and colors are found over the world; some of the more prominent breeds are shown in the illustration. Wool-type breeds, mostly of Merino origin, are important in the Southern Hemisphere, but both fine- and long-wool types are distributed all over the world. Sheep with fat tails or fat rumps are common in the desert areas of Africa and Asia. These usually produce carpet wool. Milk breeds are found mostly in central and southern Europe. Meat breeds from the British Isles are common over the world.

A total of 21 breeds of sheep, about half of which were imported from the British Isles, are represented with breed associations in the United States, although a few are inactive. The Suffolk and Hampshire breeds represent over half of the purebred registered sheep of the country and are used as sires of slaughter lambs. Other British breeds used for this purpose include Southdown, Shropshire, Dorset, Oxford, and Cheviot. The Dorset is favored for its ability to breed in the spring and fall. About 90% of registered Dorsets are polled.

In the United States fine wool breeds of the Merino from Spain and the Rambouillet from France and Germany have formed the basis for much of the western range sheep which are often crossed with meat-type rams to produce slaughter lambs. These two European breeds and the Debouillet resulting from their cross are used in the Southwest where wool production is important.

Breeds from long-wool—fine-wool breed crosses have spread over the entire United States and are truly dual-purpose in type, although they are often crossed with meat-type rams for commercial lamb production. The Corriedale, imported from New Zealand, was first used in the West but is now most common in the Midwest. The Columbia and Targhee breeds, developed by the Department of Agriculture, are large, rapidly growing, white-faced, polled sheep. The Columbia, which resulted from crossing Lincoln rams on Rambouillet ewes, produces heavy fleeces of 50–58s in spinning count while the Targhee, a three-quarter Rambouillet and one-quarter long-wool, produces fleeces of 60–62s in spinning count. Another crossbred type is the Montadale, from Columbia—Cheviot.

The Romney is the most numerous of the long-wool breeds although some Lincolns are maintained primarily for crossing with fine-wool sheep. The Cotswold and Leicester breeds have largely disappeared from the United States. The Tunis and Karakul breeds are quite minor in importance.

Breed improvement. Performance and progeny testing of rams both in central stations and on farms has been carried on in many states. The proportion of purebred sheep selected on production records is small but increasing. The Rambouillet and Hampshire breeds have led in development of plans for certifying rams on the performance of their offspring.

The average flock size for purebred flocks tends to be as small as 25–30 head with only one or two rams used per season. This small flock size limits selection so that breed improvement results from decisions made in only a very few flocks. Wool-type breeds tend to be kept in larger flocks than the meat-type breeds.

Crossbreeding for slaughter lambs has been used extensively for a number of years. Crosses of meat-type rams on wool-type or dual-purpose ewes not only produce desirable slaughter lambs but also result in hybrid vigor, which, from two-, three-, and four-breed crosses, has produced important increases in number and pounds of lambs weaned per ewe bred over comparable averages of the purebred parents.

Some exotic breeds might be used to advantage in the United States if disease restrictions on importation could be overcome. Finnsheep have shown their ability to increase lambing rates. Other desirable traits for improvement include adaptability to particular environments, less restricted breeding seasons, ability to produce more than one lamb crop per year, greater efficiency of feed use, and more desirable carcass traits.

Examples of prominent breeds of sheep. (a) Rambouillet ram (*Sheep and Goat Raiser*). (b) Dorset ram (*Continental Dorset Club*). (c) Hampshire ram. (d) Southdown ram (*Southdown Association*). (e) Suffolk ewe and ram (*photograph by A. L. Henley*). (f) Columbia ram (*photograph by A. Sponagel*). (g) Targhee ram (*Cook and Gormley*). (h) Finnsheep ewe and lamb (*Southwestern Range and Sheep Breeding Laboratory, Fort Wingate, N. Mex.*).

Nutrition and feeding. Forages make up about 95% of sheep diets and supply most of the energy needs. Diets should contain 10–15% protein, generally from leguminous plants. Sheep prefer fine forages but they eat a large variety of grasses, legumes, weeds, herbs, and shrubs. Legume hays are preferable, but corn or sorghum fodder, cereal or grass hays, and straws are often fed. Silages from corn, sorghum, cereal, and other plants may be used to replace part of the hay ration. Nonleguminous roughages may need protein and mineral supplements, but lack of energy may be the most common nutritional deficiency of sheep. Concentrates, including the common farm grains of oats, barley, corn, wheat, and sorghum are fed sparingly, usually in winter, also prior to and following lambing, and to growing and fattening lambs. Common protein supplements include cake or oil meal from soybeans, flaxseed, or cottonseed. Feeding of by-products, crop residues, and wastes such as poultry or other manures is increasing. *See* ANIMAL-FEED COMPOSITION.

Minerals such as calcium, phosphorus, iodine, copper, and cobalt may need to be supplied. Sheep may do without salt, but if supplied they will normally consume about 1 lb per month. Vitamins A, D, and E are required and may have to supplement certain rations. Vitamins C and the B complex are synthesized by sheep.

Feed required for maintenance and growth or production varies with age, weight, phase of reproduction, and climatic conditions. Nonlactating ewes and those in early gestation require 1.6–2.2% of body weight of air-dry feed. Requirements of mature ewes increase in late pregnancy and are greatest in early lactation with a range of 3.2–4.8% of body weight. Lambs and yearlings require 2.2–4.5% of their body weight with greater requirements per unit of body weight at lighter weights.

Pelleting of feeds reduces handling, storage space, and waste. Pelleting of high-roughage diets generally results in increased feed consumption and eliminates selection of the more palatable portions of the roughage. With pellets there is greater feed intake resulting from a more rapid passage of the finely ground material through the digestive tract.

Antibiotics may improve performance of growing and fattening lambs, particularly under conditions of stress. Supplemental or creep feeding of lambs from 2 to 6 weeks of age up to the time of weaning is often advantageous, particularly on ordinary pastures.

Production systems. Sheep under farm conditions are generally kept in fenced pasture from the spring to fall months. Housing, or some shelter, and harvested feed are usually provided in winter, especially in the colder and more humid climates. Flock size is typically small, ranging from 25 head or less, but may range up to 150 and sometimes up to several hundred.

Range sheep of the western states are often herded in bands of 700–1000 head of ewes with lambs and up to 2000 head or more of dry ewes. Some rangeland is fenced, and range sheep are sometimes herded only part of the year or not at all. Flock size is generally large with individual holdings often of several thousand up to 15,000 or 20,000. Lambing is often done in sheds although lambing on the range is not uncommon.

Intensive production involving large numbers of sheep in concentrated areas, generally with confinement for part or all of the year, may be practical. This system often involves lambing in the fall and winter months and may include lambing more often than once per year.

Management. Management practices are similar for different production systems although wide variations do exist. Breeding normally occurs in the fall for a period of 45–90 days. In purebred matings individual rams are mated to groups of ewes, while in commercial flocks rams are generally group mated, with from 2 or 3 rams per 100 ewes.

Extra care is usually provided at spring lambing time to increase the survival rate of the lambs. Ewes are commonly shorn or crutched just prior to lambing. The newborn lamb may be assisted in suckling and is often given extra protection from cold or wet weather. Docking and castrating may be done with rubber bands at birth or soon after, or by cutting within 6–10 days or up to 1 month after birth. The umbilical cord of the newborn lamb is dipped in iodine at birth to prevent infection. Vaccination for tetanus, overeating disease, and sore mouth may be done on the young lamb or sometimes later. Purebred lambs may be individually identified with ear tags at birth. Lambs are often identified with their mothers with paint brands.

Shearing to remove the annual growth of wool is usually done in the spring but may range from January to June. Fleeces are individually tied with paper string and are packed in bags holding about 20 to 40 fleeces. Average fleece weight is about 8.5 lb (3.8 kg).

Lambs may be weaned as early as three weeks but weaning under weights of 30–45 lb (13.6 to 20.4 kg) is not recommended. While weaning age may be extend up to 5 months, most ewes decline in milk production as lactation progresses. Lambs are often practically weaned by their mothers by 4 months more or less. The artificial rearing of lambs on cold milk from birth appears to be successful and reduces lamb mortality.

Culling is usually done in the fall. Ewes which are unsound, have bad udders, have poor or missing teeth, or are losing weight with age are eliminated. Ewes in their sixth year or older which fail to wean lambs should generally be culled. Ewes with low lamb production may be culled at any age. Ewes with light fleeces should generally be culled when young.

Diseases and parasites. Losses from diseases are moderate to low although sheep suffer from many diseases. Common diseases include abortion, pneumonia, and overeating disease. Foot rot can be eliminated or controlled by tedious trimming and treating of feet and isolation of infected animals. Vaccination is effective for some diseases, particularly blue tongue and sore mouth. Epididymitis may interfere with ram fertility.

External parasites such as lice or keds are troublesome and may be controlled by dipping, spraying, or dusting. Sheep scabies has been almost eradicated.

Internal parasites cause tremendous losses, particularly in warm humid areas. The stomach worm is probably the most common parasite. Weaning the lambs onto clean pasture from dry lot is generally effective in preventing or delaying the increase of parasites on summer pastures.

Products. Wool is an important source of income from sheep but it is less important than lamb meat. Wool is valued or graded chiefly on fineness or fiber diameter, staple length, clean yield, and freedom from contamination with foreign material. Color, strength handle, and crimp also are often considered. Wool is a superior fiber, even though synthetic fibers are often cheaper, and it is especially useful for warmth, moisture absorbability, and resistance to fire. It is unique in extensibility, resilience or wrinkle resistance, felting ability, and durability. Fine and medium wools are generally used for apparels and coarse wools are used for rugs and carpets.

Lamb meat is the most important product of sheep in the United States. High-quality carcasses are thick and blocky with a high proportion of lean, large loin-eye muscle, and with a thin covering of fat. The fat has a high melting point and the meat has a characteristic flavor. The loin chops, rib chops, and legs are the favored cuts. Consumption of lamb is about 2 lb (0.9 kg) per person per year. Lamb is not well distributed in the United States and therefore not available to many who would like to eat it.

Sheep are used for milk production as well as for meat and wool in many countries, particularly in southern Europe. Ewe milk averages about 6% fat. Sheep may yield up to 130 gal (492 liters) of milk annually. Sheep manure is valued in some areas. Skins are used for a variety of lightweight leathers. Pelts may be tanned with the wool on for items such as coats, rugs, and slippers. Fur pelts are produced from young Karakul lambs. Sheep have been used rarely for work and sport. *See* AGRICULTURAL SCIENCE (ANIMAL).

[CLAIR E. TERRILL]

Bibliography: H. H. Cole and M. Ronning, *Animal Agriculture*, 1974; M. E. Ensminger, *Sheep and Wool Science*, 1970; E. S. E. Hafez, *Reproduction in Farm Animals*, 1974; R. Jensen, *Diseases of Sheep*, 1974.

Soil

Freely divided rock-derived material containing an admixture of organic matter and capable of supporting vegetation. Soils are independent natural bodies, each with a unique morphology resulting from a particular combination of climate, living plants and animals, parent rock materials, relief, the groundwaters, and age. Soils support plants, occupy large portions of the Earth's surface, and have shape, area, breadth, width, and depth. Soil, as used here, differs in meaning from the term as used by engineers, where the meaning is unconsolidated rock material. *See* SOIL CHEMISTRY.

This article is divided into four parts: origin and classification of soils, physical properties of soil, soil management, and soil erosion.

ORIGIN AND CLASSIFICATION OF SOILS

Soil covers most of the land surface as a continuum. Each soil grades into the rock material below and into other soils at its margins, where changes occur in relief, groundwater, vegetation, kinds of rock, or other factors which influence the development of soils. Soils have horizons, or layers, more or less parallel to the surface and differing from those above and below in one or more properties, such as color, texture, structure, consistency, porosity, and reaction (Fig. 1). The horizons may be thick or thin. They may be prominent, or so weak that they can be detected only in the laboratory. The succession of horizons is called the soil profile. In general, the boundary of soils with the underlying rock or rock material occurs at depths ranging from 1 to 6 ft, though the extremes lie outside of this range.

Origin of soils. Soil formation proceeds in stages, but these stages may grade indistinctly from one into another. The first stage is the accumulation of unconsolidated rock fragments, the parent material. Parent material may be accumulated by deposition of rock fragments moved by glaciers, wind, gravity, or water, or it may accumulate more or less in place from physical and chemical weathering of hard rocks.

The second stage is the formation of horizons. This stage may follow or go on simultaneously with the accumulation of parent material. Soil horizons are a result of dominance of one or more processes over others, producing a layer which differs from the layers above and below.

Major processes. The major processes in soils which promote horizon differentiation are gains, losses, transfers, and transformations of organic matter, soluble salts, carbonates, silicate clay minerals, sesquioxides, and silica. Gains consist normally of additions of organic matter, and of oxygen and water through oxidation and hydration, but in some sites slow continuous additions of new mineral materials take place at the surface or soluble materials are deposited from groundwater. Losses are chiefly of materials dissolved or suspended in water percolating through the profile or running off the surface. Transfers of both mineral and organic materials are common in soils. Water moving through the soil picks up materials in solution or suspension. These materials may be deposited in another horizon if the water is withdrawn by plant roots or evaporation, or if the materials are precipitated as a result of differences in pH (degree of acidity), salt concentration, or other conditions in deeper horizons.

Other processes tend to offset those that promote horizon differentiation. Mixing of the soil occurs as the result of burrowing by rodents and earthworms, overturning of trees, churning of the soil by frost, or shrinking and swelling. On steep slopes the soil may creep or slide downhill with attendant mixing. Plants may withdraw calcium or other ions from deep horizons and return them to the surface in the leaf litter.

Saturation of a horizon with water for long periods makes the iron oxides soluble by reduction from ferric to ferrous forms. The soluble iron can move by diffusion to form hard concretions or splotches of red or brown in a gray matrix. Or if the iron remains, the soil will have shades of blue or green. This process is called gleying, and can be superimposed on any of the others.

The kinds of horizons present and the degree of their differentiation, both in composition and structure, depend on the relative strengths of the processes. In turn, these relative strengths are determined by the way man uses the soil as well as by the natural factors of climate, plants and animals, relief and groundwater, and the period of time during which the processes have been operating.

Composition. In the drier climates where precipitation is appreciably less than the potential for evaporation and transpiration, horizons of soluble salts, including calcium carbonate and gypsum, are normally found at the average depth of water penetration.

In humid climates some materials normally considered insoluble may be gradually removed from the soil or at least from the surface horizons. A part of the removal may be in suspension. The movement of silicate clay minerals would be an example. The movement of iron oxides is accelerated by the formation of chelates with the soil organic matter. Silica is removed in appreciable amounts in solution or suspension, though quartz sand is relatively unaffected. In warm humid climates free iron and aluminum oxides and silicate clays accumulate in soils, apparently because of low solubility relative to other minerals.

In cool humid climates solution losses are evident in such minerals as feldspars. Free sesquioxides tend to be removed from the surface horizons and to accumulate in a lower horizon, but mixing by animals and falling trees may counterbalance the downward movement.

Structure. Concurrently with the other processes, distinctive structures are formed in the different horizons. In the surface horizons, where there is a maximum of biotic activity, small animals, roots, and frost action keep mixing the soil material. Aggregates of varying sizes are formed and bound by organic matter, microorganisms, and colloidal material. The aggregates in the immediate surface tend to be loosely packed with many large biotic pores among them. Below this horizon of high biotic activity, the structure is formed chiefly by volume changes due to wetting, drying, freezing, thawing, or shaking of the soil by roots of trees swaying with the wind. Consequently, the sides of any one aggregate, or ped, conform in shape to the sides of adjacent peds.

Water moving through the soil usually follows root channels, wormholes, and ped surfaces. Accordingly, materials that are deposited in a horizon commonly coat the peds. In the horizons that have received clay from an overlying horizon, the peds usually have a coating or varnish of clay making the exterior unlike the interior in appearance. Peds formed by moisture or temperature changes normally have the shapes of plates, prisms, or blocks.

Horizons. Pedologists have developed sets of symbols to identify the various kinds of horizons commonly found in soils. The nomenclature originated in Russia, where the letters A, B, and C were applied to the main horizons of the black soils of the steppes. A designated the dark surface horizon of maximum organic matter accumulation, C the unaltered parent material, and B the intermediate horizon. The usage of the letters A, B, and C spread to western Europe, where the intermediate or B horizon was a horizon of accumulation of free sesquioxides or silicate clays or both. Thus the

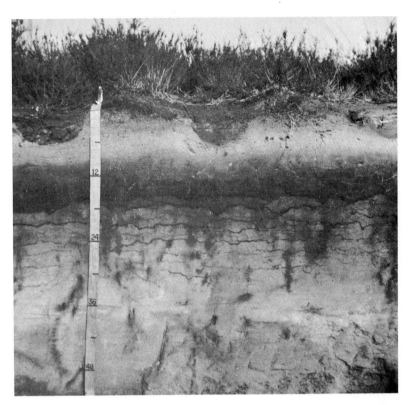

Fig. 1. Photograph of a soil profile showing horizons. The dark crescent-shaped spots at the soil surface are the result of plowing. The dark horizon lying 9–18 in. below the surface is the principal horizon of accumulation of organic matter that has been washed down from the surface. The thin wavy lines were formed in the same manner.

idea developed that a B horizon is a horizon of accumulation. Some, however, define a B horizon by position between A and C. Subdivisions of the major horizons have been shown by either numbers or letters, for example, Bt or B2. No internationally accepted set of horizon symbols has been developed. In the United States the designations shown in Fig. 2 have been widely used since about 1935, with minor modifications made in 1962. Lower-case letters were added to numbers in B horizons to indicate the· nature of the material that had accumulated. Generally, "h" is used to indicate translocated humus, "t" for translocated clay, and "ir" for translocated iron oxides. Thus, B2t indicates the main horizon of clay accumulation.

Classification. Systems of soil classification are influenced by concepts prevalent at the time a system is developed. Since ancient times, soil has been considered as the natural medium for plant growth. Under this concept, the earliest classifications were based on relative suitability for different crops, such as rice soils, wheat soils, and vineyard soils.

Early American agriculturists thought of soil chiefly as disintegrated rock, and the first comprehensive American classification was based primarily on the nature of the underlying rock.

In the latter part of the 19th century, some Russian students noted relations between the steppe and black soils and the forest and gray soils. They developed the concept of soils as independent natural bodies formed by the influence of environmental factors operating on parent materials over time. The early Russian classifications grouped soils at

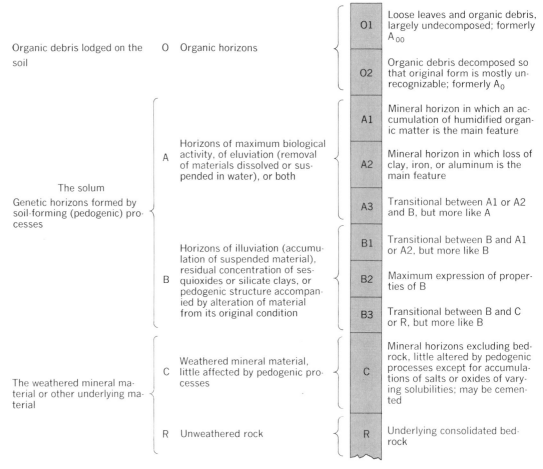

Organic debris lodged on the soil — O Organic horizons
- O1 Loose leaves and organic debris, largely undecomposed; formerly A_{00}
- O2 Organic debris decomposed so that original form is mostly unrecognizable; formerly A_0

The solum
Genetic horizons formed by soil-forming (pedogenic) processes

A Horizons of maximum biological activity, of eluviation (removal of materials dissolved or suspended in water), or both
- A1 Mineral horizon in which an accumulation of humidified organic matter is the main feature
- A2 Mineral horizon in which loss of clay, iron, or aluminum is the main feature
- A3 Transitional between A1 or A2 and B, but more like A

B Horizons of illuviation (accumulation of suspended material), residual concentration of sesquioxides or silicate clays, or pedogenic structure accompanied by alteration of material from its original condition
- B1 Transitional between B and A1 or A2, but more like B
- B2 Maximum expression of properties of B
- B3 Transitional between B and C or R, but more like B

The weathered mineral material or other underlying material

C Weathered mineral material, little affected by pedogenic processes
- C Mineral horizons excluding bedrock, little altered by pedogenic processes except for accumulations of salts or oxides of varying solubilities; may be cemented

R Unweathered rock
- R Underlying consolidated bedrock

Fig. 2. A hypothetical soil profile having all principal horizons. Other symbols are used to indicate features subordinate to those indicated by capital letters and numbers. The more important of these are as follows: ca, as in Cca, accumulations of carbonates; cs, accumulations of calcium sulfate; cn, concretions; g, strong gleying (reduction of iron in presence of groundwater); h, illuvial humus; ir, illuvial iron; m, strong cementation; p, plowing; sa, accumulations of very soluble salts; si, cementation by silica; t, illuvial clay; x, fragipan (a compact zone which is impenetrable by roots).

the highest level, according to the degree to which they reflected the climate and vegetation. They had classes of Normal, Abnormal, and Transitional soils, which later became known as Zonal, Intrazonal, and Azonal. Within the Normal or Zonal soils, the Russians distinguished climatic and vegetative zones in which the soils had distinctive colors and other properties in common. These formed classes that were called soil types. Because some soils with similar colors had very different properties that were associated with differences in the vegetation, the nature of the vegetation was sometimes considered in addition to the color to form the soil type name, for example, Gray Forest soil and Gray Desert soil. The Russian concepts of soil types were accepted in other countries as quickly as they became known. In the United States, however, the name soil type had been used for some decades to indicate differences in soil texture, chiefly texture of the surface horizons; so the Russian soil type was called a Great Soil Group. *See* SOIL, SUBORDERS OF; SOIL, ZONALITY OF.

Many systems of classification have been attempted but none has been found markedly superior; most systems have been modifications of those used in Russia. Two bases for classification have been tried. One basis has been the presumed genesis of the soil; climate and native vegetation were given major emphasis. The other basis has been the observable or measurable properties of the soil. To a considerable extent, of course, these are used in the genetic system to define the great soil groups. The morphologic systems, however, have not used soil genesis as such, but have attempted to use properties that are acquired through soil development.

The principal problem in the morphologic systems has been the selection of the properties to be used. Grouping by color, tried in the earliest systems, produces soil groups of unlike genesis.

The Soil Survey staff of the U.S. Department of Agriculture and the land-grant colleges adopted a new classification scheme in 1965. Although the new system has been widely tested, only time can tell how much more useful it will be than earlier systems. As knowledge of soil genesis increases, modifications of classification systems will continue to be necessary.

The system differs from earlier systems in that it may be applied to either cultivated or virgin soils. Previous systems have been based on virgin profiles, and cultivated soils were classified on the presumed characteristics or genesis of the virgin soils. The new system has six categories, based on both physical and chemical properties. These categories are the order, suborder, great group, subgroup, family, and series, in decreasing rank.

The nomenclature. The names of the taxa or classes in each category are derived from the classic languages in such a manner that the name itself indicates the place of the taxa in the system and usually indicates something of the differentiating properties. The names of the highest category, the order, end in the suffix "sol," preceded by formative elements that suggest the nature of the order. Thus, Aridisol is the name of an order of soils that is characterized by being dry (Latin *aridus*, dry, plus *sol*, soil). A formative element is taken from each order name as the final syllable in the names of all taxa of suborders, great groups, and subgroups in the order. This is the syllable beginning with the vowel that precedes the connecting vowel with "sol." Thus, for Aridisols, the names of the taxa of lower classes end with the syllable "id," as in Argid and Orthid.

Suborder names have two syllables, the first suggesting something of the nature of the suborder and the last identifying the order. The formative element "arg" in Argid (Latin argillus, clay) suggests the horizon of accumulation of clay that defines the suborder.

Great group names have one or more syllables to suggest the nature of the horizons and have the suborder name as an ending. Thus great group names have three or more syllables but can be distinguished from order names because they do not end in "sol." Among the Argids, great groups are Natrargids (Latin *natrium*, sodium) for soils that have high contents of sodium, and Durargids (Latin *durus*, hard) for Argids with a hardpan cemented by silica and called a duripan.

Subgroup names are binomial. The great group name is preceded by an adjective such as "typic," which suggests the type or central concept of the great group, or the name of another great group, suborder, or order converted to an adjective to suggest that the soils are transitional between the two taxa.

Family names consist of several adjectives that describe the texture (sandy, silty, clayey, and so on), the mineralogy (siliceous, carbonatic, and so on), the temperature regime of the soil (thermic, mesic, frigid, and so on), and occasional other properties that are relevant to the use of the soil.

Series names are abstract names, taken from towns or places near where the soil was first identified. Cecil, Tama, and Walla Walla are names of soil series.

Order. In the highest category 10 orders are recognized. These are distinguished chiefly by differences in kinds and amounts of organic matter in the surface horizons, kinds of B horizons resulting from the dominance of various specific processes, evidences of churning through shrinking and swelling, base saturation, and lengths of periods during which the soil is without available moisture. The properties selected to distinguish the orders are reflections of the degree of horizon development and the kinds of horizons present.

The orders, the formative elements in the names, and the general nature of the included soils

Table 1. Soil orders

Order	Formative element in name	General nature
Alfisols	alf	Soils with gray to brown surface horizons, medium to high base supply, with horizons of clay accumulation; usually moist, but may be dry during summer
Aridisols	id	Soils with pedogenic horizons, low in organic matter, and usually dry
Entisols	ent	Soils without pedogenic horizons
Histosols	ist	Organic soils (peats and mucks)
Inceptisols	ept	Soils that are usually moist, with pedogenic horizons of alteration of parent materials but not of illuviation
Mollisols	oll	Soils with nearly black, organic-rich surface horizons and high base supply
Oxisols	ox	Soils with residual accumulations of inactive clays, free oxides, kaolin, and quartz; mostly tropical
Spodosols	od	Soils with accumulations of amorphous materials in subsurface horizons
Ultisols	ult	Soils that are usually moist, with horizons of clay accumulation and a low supply of bases
Vertisols	ert	Soils with high content of swelling clays and wide deep cracks during some season

are given in Table 1.

Suborder. This category narrows the ranges in soil moisture and temperature regimes, kinds of horizons, and composition, according to which of these is most important. Moisture or temperature or soil properties associated with them are used to define suborders of Alfisols, Mollisols, Oxisols, Ultisols, and Vertisols. Kinds of horizons are used for Aridisols, compositions for Histosols and Spodosols, and combinations for Entisols and Inceptisols. *See* SOIL, SUBORDERS OF.

Great group. The taxa (classes) in this category group soils that have the same kinds of horizons in the same sequence and have similar moisture and temperature regimes. Exceptions to horizon sequences are made for horizons so near the surface that they are apt to be mixed by plowing or lost rapidly by erosion if plowed.

Subgroup. The great groups are subdivided into subgroups that show the central properties of the great group, intergrade subgroups that show properties of more than one great group, and other subgroups for soils with atypical properties that are not characteristic of any great group.

Family. The families are defined largely on the basis of physical and mineralogic properties of importance to plant growth.

Series. The soil series is a group of soils having horizons similar in differentiating characteristics and arrangement in the soil profile, except for texture of the surface portion, and developed in a particular type of parent material.

Type. This category of earlier systems of classification has been dropped but is mentioned here because it was used for almost 70 years and many references to it are found in the literature about soils. The soil types within a series differed primarily in the texture of the plow layer or equivalent horizons in unplowed soils. Cecil clay and Cecil fine sandy loam were types within the Cecil series. The texture of the plow layer is still indicated in published soil surveys if it is relevant to the use of the soil, but it is now considered as one kind of soil phase. Soil surveys are discussed in the next section of this article.

Classifications of soils have been developed in several countries based on other differentia. The principal classifications have been those of the Soviet Union, Germany, France, Canada, Australia, and New Zealand, and the United States. Other countries have modified one or the other of these to fit their own conditions. Soil classifications have usually been developed to fit the needs of a government that is concerned with the use of its soils. In this respect soil classification has differed from classifications of other natural objects, such as plants and animals, and there is no international agreement on the subject.

Many practical classifications have been developed on the basis of interpretations of the usefulness of soils for specific purposes. An example is the capability classification, which groups soils according to the number of safe alternative uses, risks of damage, and kinds of problems that are encountered under use.

Surveys. Soil surveys include those researches necessary (1) to determine the important characteristics of soils, (2) to classify them into defined series and other units, (3) to establish and map the boundaries between kinds of soil, and (4) to correlate and predict adaptability of soils to various crops, grasses, and trees; behavior and productivity of soils under different management systems; and yields of adapted crops on soils under defined sets of management practices. Although the primary purpose of soil surveys has been to aid in agricultural interpretations, many other purposes have become important, ranging from suburban planning, rural zoning, and highway location, to tax assessment and location of pipelines and radio transmitters. This has happened because the soil properties important to the growth of plants are also important to its engineering uses.

Soil surveys were first used in the United States in 1898. Over the years the scale of soil maps has been increased from 1/2 or 1 in. to the mile, to 3 or 4 in. to the mile for mapping humid farming regions, and up to 8 in. to the mile for maps in irrigated areas. After the advent of aerial photography, planimetric maps were largely discontinued in favor of aerial photographic mosaics. The United States system has been used, with modifications, in many other countries.

Two kinds of soil maps are made. The common map is a detailed soil map, on which soil boundaries are plotted from direct observations throughout the surveyed area. Reconnaissance soil maps are made by plotting soil boundaries from observations made at intervals. The maps show soil and other differences that are of significance for present or foreseeable uses.

The units shown on soil maps usually are phases of soil series. The phase is not a category of the classification system. It may be a subdivision of any class of the system according to some feature that is of significance for use and management of the soil, but not in relation to the natural landscape. The presence of loose boulders on the surface of the soil makes little difference in the growth of a forest, but is highly significant if the soil is to be plowed. Phases are most commonly based on slope, erosion, presence of stone or rock, or differences in the rock material below the soil itself. If a legend identifies a phase of a soil series, the soils so designated on a soil map are presumed to lie within the defined range of that phase in the major part of the area involved. Thus, the inclusion of lesser areas of soils having other characteristics is tolerated in the mapping if their presence does not appreciably affect the use of the soil. If there are other soils that do affect the use, inclusions up to 15% of the area are tolerated without being indicated in the name of the soil.

If the pattern of occurrence of two or more series is so intricate that it is impossible to show them separately, a soil complex is mapped, and the legend includes the word "complex," or the names of the series are connected by a hyphen and followed by a textural class name. Thus the phrase Fayette-Dubuque silt loam indicates that the two series occur in one area and that each represents more than 15% of the total area.

In places the significance of the difference between series is so slight that the expense of separating them is unwarranted. In such a case the names of the series are connected by a conjunction, for example, Fayette and Downs silt loam. In this kind of mapping unit, the soils may or may not be associated geographically.

It is possible to make accurate soil maps only because the nature of the soil changes with alterations in climatic and biotic factors, in relief, and in groundwaters, all acting on parent materials over long periods of time. Boundaries between kinds of soil are made where such changes become apparent. On a given farm the kinds of soil usually form a repeating pattern related to the relief (Fig. 3).

Because concepts of soil have changed over the years, maps made 30–50 years ago may use the same soil type names as maps made in recent years, but with different meanings. The older maps must therefore be interpreted with caution.

[GUY D. SMITH]

Nutrient element losses. Losses of most elements are normal to soil formation. Losses for a pair of soil orders are described below and the magnitudes indicated for others.

Ultisols are formed in strongly weathered regoliths from a variety of rocks, chiefly in warm, humid regions. The soils occupy old land surfaces. Major areas are in southeastern Asia and the United States.

Chemical and mineralogical composition of specimen Ultisols and their source rocks suggests that as much as 90% of the calcium, magnesium, and potassium disappears at the weathering front, where the rock decomposes. Losses continue as

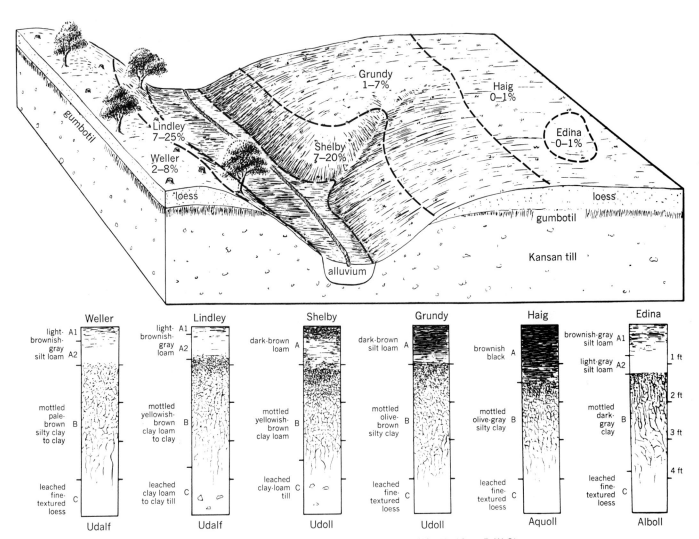

Fig. 3. Sketch showing the relation of the soil pattern to relief, parent material, and native vegetation on a farm in south-central Iowa. The soil slope gradient is expressed as a percentage. (*Modified from R. W. Simonson, F. F. Riecken, and G. D. Smith, Understanding Iowa Soils, Brown, 1952*)

the soils form. Quantities are eventually reduced to very low levels. Because of the low levels, people have thought that Ultisols were worn out by long cropping, whereas they were really "worn out" while being formed.

The approximate amounts of four nutrient elements carried by a pair of streams draining Ultisols in North Carolina are given in Table 2. Amounts of Ca and Mg are very low, whereas those of K, Na, and N are moderate to low.

Mollisols are formed in slightly weathered regoliths, chiefly in cool-temperate grasslands. The soils occupy young land surfaces. Major areas are in the north-central United States and adjacent Canada, the Ukraine and adjacent parts of the Soviet Union, and the pampas of Argentina.

Roughly a third of the Ca and K, a larger share of the Mg, and a very small part of the P in the source rocks disappear during formation of Mollisols. Hence, the soils have relatively high levels of these elements. Moreover, they have high levels of exchangeable Ca, Mg, and K, which are readily available to plants. Expressed as milliequivalents per 100 g of soil, average figures are 15 of Ca, 6 of Mg, and 0.8 of K. Amounts of phosphorus are also

high, with much in plant-available form.

High levels of nutrient elements in Mollisols are reflected in data for a pair of rivers in Iowa, given in Table 2. Quantities of Ca and Mg are about three times as large as in the streams in North Carolina. Quantities of K and Na are slightly lower, whereas that of N is about the same. A share of the amounts in the streams comes from the underlying rock, especially for Ultisols.

Ultisols and Mollisols are opposite extremes in losses of nutrient elements during soil formation. If the average chemical composition of the soils to

Table 2. Amounts of four nutrient elements carried by four rivers in one year*

River (state)	Ca	Mg	K	K + Na	N
Neuse (NC)	20	7	—	32	1.0
Hiwassee (NC)	33	11	9	—	—
Cedar (IA)	86	32	—	22	1.4
Iowa (IA)	78	29	—	22	1.0

*Expressed as pounds per acre of watershed.

a depth of 5 ft is compared, the ratios between Mollisols and Ultisols are 10:1 for Ca and Mg, 3:1 for K, 2:1 for P, and 5:1 for N. The ratios for elements in exchangeable form are even larger. As the ratios suggest, Mollisols are much more naturally fertile than Ultisols. Mollisols are at the top of the list, Ultisols near the bottom.

Losses of nutrient elements during formation of soils is well bracketed by the Mollisols and Ultisols. Similar to Mollisols in losses during their formation are Aridisols, Inceptisols of cold or dry regions, and Vertisols. If anything, losses are smaller for these soils than for Mollisols. Collectively, these groups of soils occupy about 40% of the Earth's land surface. Also similar to Ultisols in losses are the Oxisols and Inceptisols of the tropics and subtropics. Collectively, these soils plus Ultisols occupy about 25% of the land surface.

The remaining groups of soils, that is, Alfisols, Entisols, Spodosols, and some Inceptisols, fall between the two extremes. Mountain regions with their great variety of soils belong to this middle class. These soils are all intermediate in losses and also in present fertility levels. Collectively, these soils occupy about 35% of the land surface.

Losses of nutrient elements generally occur during formation of soils. The losses are small enough to be negligible for a few kinds of soils, very large for others, and intermediate for still others. The magnitude of past losses is reflected in the present fertility levels of all soils. The magnitude also directly affects soil usefulness for food and fiber production as well as the contributions of dissolved substances to lakes and streams.

[ROY W. SIMONSON]

PHYSICAL PROPERTIES OF SOIL

The physical properties of soil are important in agriculture because of their influence on plant growth and on the management requirements of the land. They influence plant growth from seeding to maturity by regulating the supply of air, water, and heat. The absorption of essential nutrients by plant roots is dependent upon an available supply of oxygen, water, and heat. Thus, physical properties indirectly regulate the nutrition of plants and their response to liming and fertilization. The more favorable the supply of air, water, and heat in each soil layer or horizon, along with the absence of mechanical impedance to root growth, the greater is the potential rooting system zone for plants.

Physical properties of the soil also determine the kind, amount, and ease of tillage, the runoff and erosion potential, and the type of plants which can or should be grown on a given soil.

Many people use the word tilth in referring to the physical condition of the soil. Tilth has been defined as the physical condition of the soil in its relation to plant growth. The physical condition of the soil is controlled by, or is the result of, whatever set of physical properties the soil has at any given time.

Soil physics is that branch of soil science which is concerned with the study of the physical properties of the soil. These physical properties include texture, particle density, structure, bulk density, porosity, water, air, temperature, consistency, compactibility, and color. Just as important as the amount of water, air, and heat in the soil at any one time is the soil's conductivity for these constituents. All of these properties are interrelated.

The four major components of the soil are inorganic particles, organic matter, water, and air. The proportions of these components vary greatly from place to place in a field, from one layer or horizon to another, and in different parts of the world. The amount of air, water, and heat in the soil changes from day to day and from season to season.

Soil texture. About one-half of the total volume of mineral soils consists of solid matter, of which 80–99% is inorganic and 1–20% is organic material. The inorganic fraction consists of rock and mineral particles of many sizes and shapes. They are classified into five major size groups called separates. The two largest separates are stone and gravel. Stone particles are greater than 76 mm (3 in.) and gravel particles are 2–76 mm along their greatest diameter. Sand particles are 0.05–2.00 mm in diameter. Sand particles may be graded by size as very fine, fine, medium, coarse, and very coarse. Silt has particles 0.002–0.005 mm in diameter. Clay, the smallest of the soil particles, has a diameter of less than 0.002 mm.

After separating the coarser separates by sieving, the amount of silt and clay is determined by methods that depend upon the rate of settling or sedimentation (based on Stoke's law) of these two separates from a water suspension in which they have been well dispersed with the aid of a dispersing agent. The stone, gravel, and sand separates of a soil can be seen with the naked eye. Clay can be examined only with an electron microscope.

Determination of the particle-size distribution in a soil is called a particle-size or mechanical analysis. The texture of a soil is determined by its content of sand, silt, and clay. The percentages of sand, silt, and clay in the 12 textural classes are shown in Fig. 4. With this texture triangle one can determine the textural class of a soil from its percentages of sand, silt, and clay. The textural class is combined with the series name of a soil to give

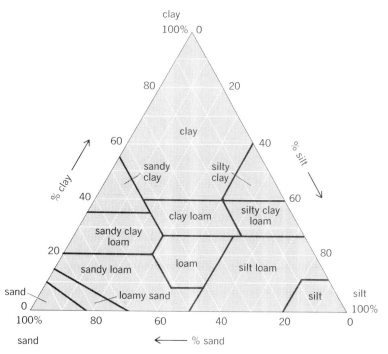

Fig. 4. Triangle showing percentage of sand, silt, and clay in each textural class.

the soil type, such as Sassafras sandy loam, Miami silt loam, or Houston clay loam.

The stone, gravel, and larger sand particles usually act as separate particles. They may be rounded, angular, or platelike in shape. They are composed of rock fragments and of primary minerals such as quartz. Soils with large amounts of stone, gravel, and coarse sand have low plant-nutrient and water-holding capacities, and permit rapid air, water, and heat movement through them. A high content of fine sand may increase water-holding capacity, but it also often increases a soil's susceptibility to wind and water erosion. Sand imparts a grittiness to the feel of a soil.

The clay fraction controls most of the important properties of a soil. In soils of the cold and temperate regions, clay is composed chiefly of secondary crystalline alumina silicates. These consist of the kaolinite, illite, and montmorillonite groups of clay minerals. Hydrated oxides of iron and aluminum are the main components of the clay in the more highly weathered soils typical of many parts of the tropics.

Because of their extremely small size, clay particles have a very large specific surface which is responsible for the great adsorptive capacity of clay soils for water, gases, ions, and organic molecules. Clays are well known for their plasticity and stickiness when wet. They also expand or swell with wetting and contract or shrink upon drying. Movement of air and water through clay soils is often very slow because of the small size of the pores between the clay particles. Clay particles are platelike in shape.

Silt particles exhibit some of the properties of sand and clay. They are usually angular in shape with quartz being the dominant mineral. The available water-holding capacity of soils often is proportional to their silt content. Many silt particles have a coating of clay particles. Without this clay coating silt has a floury or a talcum-powder feel when dry and loose. Soils with large amounts of silt and clay have very poor air and moisture relations and are very difficult to manage. They are often very erodible. The loam soils generally have the most desirable texture for crop growth and ease of management.

It is seldom feasible to try to change the texture of a soil in the field. However, sand often is mixed with clay soils to change their texture to a sandy loam for special uses, as in greenhouses. The texture of surface soils may change as a result of removal of the smaller particles by wind and water erosion or by eluviation (movement within the soil).

Organic matter. The organic matter in the soil is made up of the partially decomposed remains of plant and animal tissues as well as the bodies of living soil microorganisms and plant roots. Humus is the more or less stable fraction of the organic matter or its decomposition products remaining in the soil. Many good and some bad effects accompany the decomposition of organic matter. During decomposition of organic matter by the soil microorganisms, gluelike soil-aggregate bonding substances are produced. With knowledge of the great importance of these natural soil-conditioning materials, the chemical industry has produced a number of synthetic soil conditioners.

Much of the soil organic matter has colloidal properties. It has two to three times the absorptive capacity for water, gases, ions, and other colloids as the same amount of clay. Its superior water- and nutrient-holding capacity makes it an ideal substitute for clay in improving droughty, infertile sandy soils, and its good tilth-promoting qualities make it the universally recognized ameliorator of tight, sticky, or hard and lumpy clay soils.

Density of particles. The inorganic soil particles may consist of many kinds of minerals with a wide range in particle density. The average particle density for most mineral soils varies between 2.60 and 2.75 g/cm³. The average density of humus particles ranges between 1.2 and 1.4 g/cm³. For general calculations the average particle density of soil is taken to be 2.65 g/cm³. The pycnometer is used to determine soil particle density. The plowed layer weighs about 2,000,000 lb/acre.

Soil structure. Soil structure refers to the arrangement of soil particles into aggregates or peds of different sizes and shapes. Pure sands have single grain structure. Because of the adhesive and cohesive properties of clay and organic matter, the inorganic and organic particles have been combined to form the following types of structure as found in the A and B horizons of most soils: platy, prismatic, columnar, blocky, subangular blocky, granular, and crumb (Fig. 5).

These types of structure have been developed from the bonding together of the individual particles (accretion) or the breakdown of large massive

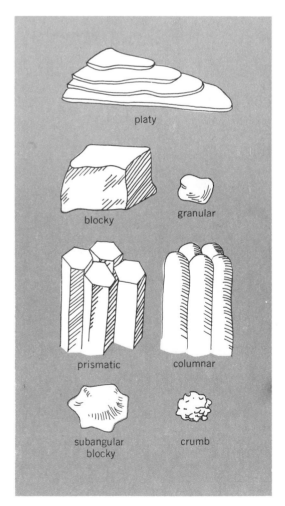

Fig. 5. Types of soil structure.

mixtures of gravel, sand, silt, clay, and organic matter (disintegration). The formation or genesis of a given type of structure and the stability of the aggregate produced seem to be associated with (1) the contraction and expansion resulting from hydration and desiccation of the clay-organic matter upon wetting and drying, as well as freezing and thawing; (2) the physical activity of roots and soil animals; (3) the influence of humus and decomposing organic matter and of the slimes and mycelia of the microorganisms that provide bonding substances with which aggregates are held together; and (4) the effect of absorbed cations which bring about flocculation or dispersion of the colloidal matter.

The prism, columnar, block, and sometimes the platelike types of structure are found mostly in subsoils. Granules and crumbs are found in largest numbers in surface soils (Fig. 6). Compacted layers in the soil often have a platy structure.

The size, shape, arrangement, and particularly the amount of overlap of soil aggregates and individual sand, gravel, and stone particles are extremely important because they largely determine the size, shape, arrangement, and continuity of pores in the soil.

There are a number of ways of attempting to characterize the structure of a soil. The first and most direct is by visual examination of an undisturbed section of soil. Much can be learned about the size, shape, and arrangement of the soil particles, and the pore space, by close inspection of each horizon with the naked eye or with a magnifying glass. Micromorphology is the microscopic observation and photography of soil structure.

A second method is to measure how much of the soil has been aggregated into granules or crumbs with diameters above a given dimension, 0.25 mm being the most common. In well-granulated soils 70–80% of the total mass may be aggregated into granules or crumbs greater than 0.25 mm, as determined by wet-sieving a sample of soil through a 60-mesh screen. Aggregation values of 40–50% are more commonly found in soils under ordinary management. Sandy soils or clay soils having poor structure may have only 10–20% aggregation. Except in very sandy soils, such a low amount of aggregation usually forecasts a physical condition very unsatisfactory for plant growth.

Measurement of the permeability of the soil to water and air provides another means of evaluating its structure.

Bulk density. Bulk density is the mass (weight) of a unit volume of dry soil usually expressed in grams per cubic centimeter. It is determined by the density of the particles and by their arrangement.

The soil structure is the major factor in accounting for changes in the bulk density of a soil from time to time or from layer to layer in the profile. Soils with many particles closely packed together have high bulk densities and correspondingly low total pore space. Bulk density is a measure of the amount of compaction in soils. Traffic by farm machinery in intensively cultivated soils, trampling of cattle in heavily grazed pastures, and foot traffic on lawns and recreational areas result in severe compaction as reflected in bulk densities of 1.7–2.0 g/cm³. Bulk densities of uncompacted, porous soils are about 1.2–1.3 g/cm³. In undisturbed forest or grassland soils densities may be 0.9–1.0 g/cm³. High amounts of organic matter will lower the bulk density.

Pore space. The voids or openings between the particles of the soil are spoken of collectively as the pore space. It makes up roughly one-half the volume of the soil. In very loose, fluffy soils with low bulk density it may occupy 60–65% of the total volume. In very compact soil layers it may be reduced to 35–40%. Pore space is calculated by Eq. (1).

$$\frac{\% \text{ total}}{\text{pore space}} = 100 - \left(\frac{\text{bulk density}}{\text{particle density}} \times 100 \right) \quad (1)$$

Pore space in a soil is occupied by air and water in reciprocally varying amounts. Very dry soils have most of their pore spaces filled with air. The opposite is true for very wet soils.

There is considerable variation in the size, shape, and arrangement of pores in the soil. The effective size of a pore can be estimated by the amount of force required to withdraw water from the pore. These suction values, expressed in centimeters of water, can be translated into equivalent pore diameters using the capillary rise equation, Eq. (2), where $r=$ radius of pore in centimeters,

$$r = \frac{2T}{hdg} \quad (2)$$

$T=$ surface tension of water, $d=$ density of water,

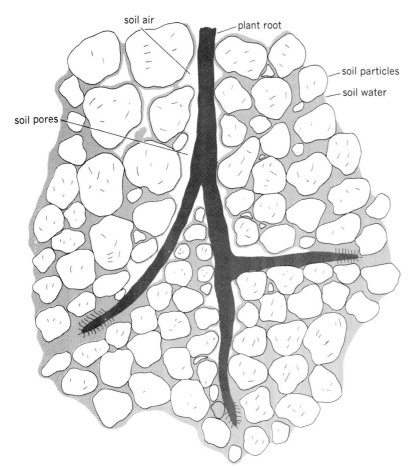

soil air

plant root

soil particles

soil water

soil pores

Fig. 6. Portion of surface soil with granular structure.

g = acceleration of gravity, and h = suction force in centimeters of water.

The ideal soil should have the proper assortment of large, medium, and small pores. A sufficient number of large or macro pores (with diameters greater than 0.06 mm), connected with each other, are needed for the rapid intake and distribution of water in the soil and for the disposal of excess water by drainage into the substratum or into artificial drains. When without water they serve as air ducts. Cracks, old root channels, and animal burrows may serve as large pores. Soils with insufficient functional macro porosity lose a great deal of rainfall and irrigation water as runoff. They drain slowly and often remain poorly aerated after wetting. One of the first effects of compaction is the reduction of the size and number of the larger pore spaces in the soil.

The primary purpose of the small pores (less than 0.01 mm in diameter) is to hold water. It is through medium-sized pores (0.06–0.01 mm in diameter) that much of the capillary movement of water takes place. Loose, droughty, coarse, sandy soils have too few small pores. Many tight clay soils could well afford to have a greater number of larger pores.

Soil water. The movement and retention of water in the soil is related to the size, shape, continuity, and arrangement of the pores, their moisture content, and the amount of surface area of the soil particles. Movement and retention of water may be characterized by the energy relationships or forces which control these two phenomena.

Water retention. Some water is held in the soil pores by the force of adhesion (the attraction of solid surfaces for water molecules) and by the force of cohesion (the attraction of water molecules for each other). Water held by these two forces keeps the smaller pores full of water and also maintains relatively thick films on the walls of many larger pores. Not until the pores in one layer of soil are filled with all the water they can hold does water move into the layer below.

Water is found in the soil in both the liquid and vapor state. The soil air in all the pores, except those in the surface inch or so of very hot, dry soils is saturated with water vapor.

The liquid water may be characterized by the suction force or tension with which it is held in the soil by adhesion or cohesion. These suction or tension values may be expressed as (1) height in centimeters of a unit water column whose weight just equals the force under consideration; (2) pF, the logarithm of the centimeter height of this column; (3) atmospheres or bars; or (4) pounds per square inch (psi). For example, 1000 cm water tension = pF_3 = 1 atm = 14.7 psi. The moisture content of the soil is determined by drying the soil at 105°C until it reaches constant weight and then dividing the weight of water lost by the weight of oven-dry soil. This value times 100 equals the percentage of water in the soil on a dry-weight basis. The percentage of moisture on the volume basis for a given depth of soil is calculated by Eq. (3). Tensiometers,

% soil moisture (dry weight basis) ÷ 100
　　　× bulk density × depth soil (in.)
　　　　　= in. of water per in. soil depth　　(3)

electrical resistance blocks, and neutron gages are

used to measure the moisture content of the soil in place. Thus changes in moisture content in the soil can be followed within the effective range of each instrument.

There are several soil-moisture "equilibrium" points. Water remaining at oven dryness is held at tensions above 10,000 atm. The hygroscopic coefficient is a rough measurement of the water held by air-dry soil at a tension of about 31 atm. The wilting point, or wilting percentage, represents that moisture content or moisture tension (15 atm) at which plant roots cannot absorb water rapidly enough to offset losses by transpiration, causing the plant to wilt, first temporarily and then permanently. Certain plants of desert and dry farming regions are able to stay alive and even grow on water held at tensions up to 25–30 atm by the soil. The field capacity represents the water remaining in a soil layer 2 or 3 days after having been saturated by rain or irrigation when the rate of downward movement of water held at low suction forces (0–1 atm) has decreased to a progressively slower rate of water removal. A definite tension value cannot be assigned to this equilibrium point, although the water held at a tension of 0.33 atm often is used to estimate the upper limit of a soil's available water-holding capacity. The maximum retentive capacity is the moisture content of a soil when all of its pores are filled or saturated with water, and under zero tension.

The moisture in a soil which is available for plant use is usually assumed to be that held between field capacity and the permanent wilting percentage. This is called the available soil moisture. Sandy loams hold 1–1½, loams 1½–2, and clay loams 1¾–2½ in. of available water per foot of soil. The retentivity of soils of different textures for moisture at different tensions is shown in Fig. 7. These are called soil moisture tension curves. Much of the water in sandy soils is held at low tensions. The opposite is true for water in clay soils.

Water held at tensions less than 1–2 atm is the most easily available for root absorption and plant growth. An adequate supply of this water should be maintained in the root zone by rainfall or irriga-

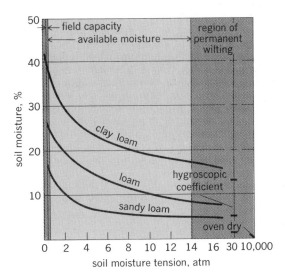

Fig. 7.　Soil moisture tension curves.

tion, especially during periods of critical water need by plants.

Water movement. Water moves in the soil as a gas and as a liquid. Vapor transfer takes place by diffusion in response to a vapor pressure gradient. Vapor movement is through air-filled pores from a moist to a dry layer and from a warm to a cool layer. Drying of a wet soil surface on a hot, dry, windy day and the condensation of water droplets on the undersurface of a plastic mulch on a cool, summer morning are the result of vapor transfer.

Liquid movement may be expressed by the equation $V = Ki$. V is the volume of water crossing the unit area perpendicular to the flow in the unit time. The proportionality factor K is the hydraulic conductivity or the permeability of the soil to water. It is controlled by the size, shape, arrangement, and moisture content of the soil pores. The value i is the water-moving force. It has two force components, the force of gravity and a suction or tension gradient force. The force or pull of gravity is of constant magnitude and always acts in a downward direction. The drainage or removal of most of the water from large pores is by this force, and the drainage is sometimes referred to as gravitational water. The suction or tension gradient force may vary both in magnitude and direction. The flow or capillary conduction of water in unsaturated soil is due to the gradient or difference in suction between two points in the soil. The flow is in the direction of the increase in suction. This accounts for the movement of water toward roots which have depleted the supply of water held at low tension in the soil at the soil-root interface, for the upward capillary conduction of water from an underlying saturated layer (water table), and for the slow downward movement of water after a rain or irrigation. Rate and amount of water movement by capillary conduction to the root system is not usually sufficient to meet the demands of the plant for water, except when a sufficient amount of water held at suctions less than 1 atm is present around the root. Since capillary conductivity decreases rapidly as the soil becomes drier, the water needs of plants are satisfied also by an extension of their root systems into fresh supplies of water held at low tension in hitherto untapped or recently refilled soil pores. It is very important, therefore, that soil structure be such as to permit the rapid extension of the root system through the whole soil mass.

Soil air and aeration. Soil air differs from the atmosphere above the soil in that it usually contains 5–100 times as much carbon dioxide (0.15–0.65%) and slightly less oxygen, and is saturated with water vapor. In deep, poorly drained soil layers or in heavily manured soils the CO_2 content may reach 10% and the O_2 content decrease to 1%. In water-logged soils, anaerobic conditions may result in methane and hydrogen sulfide production.

Aeration refers to the movement of gases in and out of each soil layer or horizon. The movement of gas within the soil as well as to and from the atmosphere is by diffusion in a direction determined by its own partial pressure. The rate of diffusion of each gas in and out of the soil depends on differences in concentration of each gas in the soil and in the atmosphere, and on the ability of the soil to transmit the gases. Diffusion or aeration is proportional to the volume of air-filled pores in any soil layer.

Temperature. The temperature of field soils shows rather definite changes at different depths, at different times during the day and night, and at different seasons of the year. These changes are determined by the amount of radiant energy that reaches the soil surface and by the thermal properties of the soil. Only that part of the heat energy which is absorbed causes changes in soil temperature. Heat produced by intense microbial decomposition of fresh organic matter mixed with the soil will also increase soil temperature. Dark-colored soils capture a much higher proportion of the radiant energy than do light-colored soils. The insulating effects of vegetative cover and surface mulches keeps the soil cooler than bare, fallow soil. Wet soils warm more slowly than dry soils because the heat capacity of water is five times that of the mineral soil particles. The energy absorbed by the soil surface is disposed of in one or more of the following ways: radiation to the atmosphere, heating of the air above the soil by convection, increasing the temperature of the surface soil, or conduction to the deeper soil layers.

Consistency and compactibility. As the moisture content of a soil changes from air dryness to saturation, its consistency varies from a state of hardness or brittleness, to loose, soft, or friable, to tough or plastic, to sticky or viscous. The reaction of the soil to physical manipulation, as in tillage, is primarily an expression of the properties of cohesion, adhesion, and plasticity. These properties are largely determined by the structure, organic matter content, kind and amount of clay, nature of adsorbed bases, and moisture content, which regulates the thickness of the water films around the soil particles. Tillage should be done only after the soil attains a soft, friable condition—when it breaks apart or can be worked into granules 1–5 mm in diameter. This is a very desirable range of particle size for good seed and root bed conditions.

Each soil has a critical moisture range, often near field capacity, at which pressure by foot or machinery traffic results in maximum compaction. Bulk density, permeability, porosity, and penetrometer measurements are used to indicate the degree of compaction as found in traffic pans in the surface soil, the plow sole, or natural hardpans. Soil compaction is a very serious problem because it reduces the permeability of the soil to air and water, and increases the resistance of the soil to root penetration. Hard, dry surface crusts may also prevent seedling emergence.

Color. Soil color may be influenced by, and indicates the kind of, parent material, chemical composition, organic matter content, drainage, aeration, or oxidation. A blotched or mottled yellow, gray, and blue subsoil indicates poor drainage, aeration, or oxidation. A clear red, yellow, or brown color indicates good drainage. The color of some soils is inherited from the parent material. Organic matter gives a brown to black color to that horizon where it is concentrated. Color of soils is determined by comparison with standard colors of known hue, value, and chroma in the Munsell soil color charts.

[RUSSELL B. ALDERFER]

SOIL MANAGEMENT

Soil management may be defined as the preparation, manipulation, and treatment of soils for the production of crops, grasses, and trees. Good soil management involves practices which will maintain a high level of production on a sustained basis. Ideally, these practices should provide the crop with an adequate supply of air, water, and nutrients; maintain or improve the fertility of the soil for subsequent crops; and prevent the development of conditions which might be injurious to plants.

Several systems of land-use classification have been developed which help a farmer to know the kinds of soils he has on his farm and their suitability for various types of farming. One of these systems, developed by the U.S. Soil Conservation Service, involves land-use capability ratings.

Land capability survey maps. Land capability survey maps are worked out in conjunction with the soil survey and serve as a guide to the suitability of land for cultivation, grazing, forestry, wildlife, watersheds, or recreation, with primary consideration given to erosion control. There are eight capability classes which describe the characteristics of the land and the difficulty or risk involved in using it for one kind of crop production or another. These eight classes are sometimes distinguished on land capability survey maps by roman numerals as well as by standard colors. Four of the eight classes include land that is suited for regular cultivation with varying degrees of erosion control measures and management practices required; three classes of land are not suited for cultivation but require permanent vegetation and impose severe limitations on land use; and one class includes lands suited only for wildlife, recreation, or watershed purposes. For a description of the land capability classes and the management practices recommended for each class see SOIL CONSERVATION.

Cropping system. A cropping system refers to the kind and sequence of crops grown on a given area of soil over a period of time. It may be a regular rotation of different crops, in which the sequence of crops follows a definite order, or it may consist of a single crop grown year after year in the same location. Other cropping systems include different crops but have no definite or planned sequence.

Cropping systems that involve the systematic rotation of different crops generally include hay and pasture crops, small grains, and cultivated row crops. Legumes, such as alfalfa, clover, and vetch, are usually grown alone or mixed with grasses in the hay and pasture sequence in the rotation because they supply nitrogen and contribute to good soil tilth. The beneficial effect of legumes and grasses on tilth may be attributed to the fact that (1) the soil is not tilled while these crops are being grown, and (2) the organic matter returned to the soil by the extensive root systems and in the plowed-under top growth is particularly suited to the development of a stable, porous soil structure.

Small grains function somewhat like legumes and grasses in giving protection against soil erosion, but they add no nitrogen and remove moderate quantities of plant food from the soil. Since small grains do not provide maximum economic return from the high nitrogen residues left in the soil by legumes, and are likely to lodge owing to the stimulation of growth from these residues, they are not planted in the rotation following legumes. Small grains are generally planted either at the end of a rotation following row crops or as a companion crop for legumes.

Row crops, such as corn, potatoes, cotton, and sugarbeets, are an excellent choice to follow legumes because they utilize the nitrogen supplied by the legumes and bring good cash returns. Since row crops in early stages of growth provide little protection against erosion and require considerable cultivation which breaks down soil structure, it is not considered desirable to plant them continuously.

A cropping system that involves growing the same crop year after year generally depletes the soil and results in lower crop yields. This is particularly true if the crop is cultivated frequently and returns little crop residue to the soil. Weeds, diseases, and insects also become more of a management problem when the cropping system does not involve rotation. Thus the farmer who intends to grow one crop year after year becomes completely dependent on disease-resistant varieties of plants, chemical insecticides and fungicides, soil fumigation, and other methods of controlling diseases, insects, and pests. Through the appropriate use of improved varieties, pesticides, and adequate amounts of fertilizers, farmers have succeeded in maintaining a high level of production on land repeatedly planted with the same crop. While such results are causing farmers to take another look at cropping systems that do not involve rotation, they are well aware that more intensive practices and costly supplements are required to maintain production.

Organic matter and tilth. The value of adding organic matter to the soil in the form of animal manures, green manures, and crop residues for producing favorable soil tilth has been known since ancient times. Research has provided information that helps to explain the mechanisms for this effect.

Experiments reveal that during the decomposition of organic matter in the soil, microorganisms synthesize a variety of gumlike substances, at least partly polysaccharide in nature which, when dried with the soil, bind the soil particles together into a porous, water-stable structure. While these binding substances are produced in relatively large quantities during stages of rapid organic-matter decomposition, they may in turn be decomposed by other organisms. Thus, to maintain a continuous supply of binding substances, organic matter must be added to the soil frequently.

In addition to the beneficial action of microbially synthesized binding substances, roots and fungal mycelia also contribute to the development of favorable soil tilth by molding the smaller gum-cemented granules into still larger aggregates. The aggregates adhering together form large pores that permit the rapid movement of air and water and form small pores that store water. Both conditions are essential features of good tilth.

Unfortunately not all the effects of organic matter on tilth are desirable. The growth of organisms in a fine-textured soil may interfere with the downward movement of water whenever the soil pores become clogged with microbial bodies. This condition is of particular significance where water is ponded to recharge underground water supplies or to leach excessive amounts of soluble salts from the soil.

Even the characteristic property of organic matter of promoting aggregate formation is not always desirable. Some surface mulches during decomposition induce the formation of a layer of small surface aggregates which are more susceptible to wind erosion than the fine soil particles initially present. In such cases, aggregation intensifies the hazard of severe wind erosion.

In spite of these negative effects of organic matter on the physical properties of soil, the incorporation of organic matter with soil is the most suitable and practical way of developing and maintaining good tilth.

Conditioners and stabilizers. Soil conditioners and stabilizers include a wide variety of natural and synthetic compounds that, upon incorporation with the soil, improve its physical properties. The term soil amendment also is applied to these compounds but is a more general term since it includes any material, exclusive of fertilizers, that is worked into the soil to make it more productive, regardless of whether it benefits the physical, chemical, or microbiological properties of the soil.

Soluble salts of calcium, such as calcium chloride and gypsum, or acid and acid formers, including sulfur, sulfuric acid, iron sulfate, and aluminum sulfate, have been used as conditioners to improve the physical properties of soils that were made unfavorable by excessive quantities of sodium ions adsorbed on the soil colloids.

The tilth of dense clay soils, which are slow to take water and have a marked tendency to become cloddy, may be improved by the addition of gypsum and by-product lime from sugarbeet processing factories. Limestone has improved the physical condition of acid soils, apparently by stimulating the activity of microorganisms to synthesize substances that bind soil particles into aggregates.

The discovery that soil microorganisms synthesize substances that improve soil structure stimulated the search for synthetic compounds that would be more effective than the natural products. While a wide variety of compounds have improved soil structure temporarily, three water-soluble, polymeric electrolytes of high molecular weight which are very resistant to microbial decomposition have been developed commercially for use in ameliorating poor soil structure. These are modified hydrolyzed polyacrilonitrile (HPAN), modified vinyl acetate maleic acid (VAMA), and a copolymer of isobutylene and maleic acid (IBMA). High cost relative to yield increase has limited these materials to experimental use.

Mixed with the soil in amounts ranging from 0.02 to 0.2% of soil by weight, these compounds are readily adsorbed by moist soils and tend to stabilize or fix the existing structure. They are therefore synthetic binding agents and should be added only to soils that have previously been worked into a desirable physical condition. These materials are not equally effective on all soils, and if improperly used can stabilize a poor physical condition.

Fertility. Soil fertility may be defined as that quality of a soil which enables it to provide nutrient elements and compounds in adequate amounts and in proper balance for the growth of specified plants, when other growth factors such as light, moisture, temperature, and the physical condition of the soil are favorable.

Testing. Even though relatively fertile and of good physical condition, a soil may be lacking in one or more of 16 elements presently known to be essential to plant growth, or it may be strongly acidic, alkaline, or salty, and thus unsuitable for plant growth. Fortunately, soil tests are available that indicate the existence of possible deficiencies or excesses in the soil. In most instances, these tests involve the use of various reagents for extracting from the soil the total or proportionate amount of the nutrient or compound in question. The amount of material extracted is then compared with values that have been correlated previously with crop response on the same or similar soil. No single test is reliable for all crops on all soils. *See* PLANT, MINERALS ESSENTIAL TO.

Control of pH. The availability of soil nutrients for plants is influenced greatly by the reaction of the soil. Soils may be classified as acid, neutral, or alkaline in reaction. The method commonly used in measuring and expressing degrees of acidity or alkalinity is in terms of pH. The pH value of soil may range from less than 4 to more than 8; the lower the value, the more acid the soil. Under most conditions lime is applied to acid soils to maintain their pH between 6.5 and 7.0. Under special conditions it may be desirable to maintain pH values either higher or lower than these. In any case the desirability of applying lime should be determined by the pH of the soil and the requirements of the plants to be grown.

It is occasionally necessary to make soils more acid. Materials commonly used to decrease pH are sulfur, sulfuric acid, iron sulfate, and aluminum sulfate.

Control of salinity. Restricted drainage caused by either slow permeability or a high water table is the principal factor in the formation of saline soils. Such soils may be improved by establishing artificial drainage, if a high water table exists, and by subsequent leaching with irrigation water to remove excess soluble salts.

Soils can be leached by applying water to the surface and allowing it to pass downward through the root zone. Leaching is most efficient when it is possible to pond water over the entire surface.

The amount of water required to leach saline soils depends on the initial salinity level of the soil and the final salinity level desired. When water is ponded over the soil about 50% of the salt in the root zone can be removed by leaching with 6 in. of water for each foot of root zone; about 80% can be removed with 1 ft of water per foot of soil to be leached; and 90% can be removed with 2 ft of water per foot of soil to be leached.

Because all irrigation waters contain dissolved salts, nonsaline soils may become saline unless water is applied in addition to that required to replenish losses by plant transpiration and evaporation, to leach out the salt that has accumulated during previous irrigations and through the addition of fertilizer.

Regulating nutrient supplies. The nutrients supplied to crops can be regulated by modifying the availability of nutrients already present in the soil. This can be accomplished by changing soil reaction, turning under green manure crops, including legumes which add nitrogen, and adding fertilizers. *See* FERTILIZER.

By changing soil reaction through the addition of lime, acidulating agents such as sulfur, or residually acid fertilizers such as ammonium sulfate, solubility and availability of compounds of phosphorus, iron, manganese, copper, zinc, boron, and molybdenum can be increased or decreased. Phosphorus compounds are generally more available in the slightly acid to neutral pH range, whereas compounds of iron, manganese, zinc, and copper become more available as the acidity of the soil increases. The activity of microorganisms responsible for the transformation of nitrogen, sulfur, and phosphorus compounds into forms available for plants also is influenced by soil reaction. A reaction which is too acid or too alkaline retards the activities of these organisms.

The decay of turned-under green manures and plant residues produces carbon dioxide, rendering soluble the nutrients from soil particles, and the nutrients which were absorbed from the soil during the growth of these crops are also made available. Although the turning under of a green manure affects the availability of nutrients, it does not add to the total nutrient supply unless the green manure is a legume which fixes atmospheric nitrogen.

The system of farming determines to a considerable extent the manner in which fertilizers are used to regulate nutrient supplies. Each system of farming depends upon the crop, soil, climate, kinds and rates of fertilizers applied, and available equipment; and for each system of farming there are many ways of applying fertilizers.

Common methods of applying fertilizers include broadcasting, banding, deep placement, and foliar applications. Broadcasting fertilizer on the soil is usually less desirable than localized placement of the fertilizer in relation to the seed or plant. Banding fertilizers to the side of the rows in furrow bottoms or beds and drilling fertilizer with the seed give the best response from limited quantities of fertilizer. Deep placement of fertilizers is effective in arid regions where soils dry out to a considerable depth or where deep-rooted crops are grown. Foliar applications of fertilizers, particularly those containing micronutrients, circumvent soil interactions. Such interactions within the soil may render the applied fertilizer unavailable to the crop. Foliar applications also make it possible for the farmer to supply his crops directly with a number of essential plant nutrients at critical stages of growth. *See* PLANT, MINERAL NUTRITION OF; PLANT, WATER RELATIONS OF.   [DANIEL G. ALDRICH, JR.]

Soils of the tropics. The tropics may be defined as that part of the Earth's surface between the Tropic of Cancer and the Tropic of Capricorn, about 23-1/2° north and south of the Equator. In this region three broad ecological zones may be recognized: evergreen and deciduous forests which cover about one-fourth of the land area; savanna and grasslands, about one-half; and semidesert and desert areas, about one-fourth. Because of the wide range of climate, vegetation, parent materials, and other factors affecting soil formation, there are as many if not more different kinds of soils in the tropics as in temperate regions. They range from fertile soils of alluvial valleys, through deep, highly weathered infertile acid soils of uplands through shallow stony soils of steep mountain slopes, to high lime soils of deserts. Though many soils of the tropics have formed from recently deposited alluvium and volcanic ash, most have developed from older weathered parent materials, and consequently are generally much less fertile than soils in temperate regions which are mostly formed from relatively recent glacial and loessial deposits.

Resources. Of the 12×10^9 acres (5×10^9 hectares) of land area in the tropics, about 2×10^9 acres are estimated to be potentially arable but as yet uncultivated. This is more than is now cultivated and represents about half of the world's uncultivated land which is potentially arable. Most of the potential for bringing new land under cultivation is in Africa and South America, where only about 22 and 11%, respectively, of the potentially arable soils are cultivated. Probably most potentially arable soils in the tropics not under cultivation are relatively infertile and require addition of nutrients and good management for economic crop production. The UN Food and Agriculture Organization and UNESCO have published soil maps of South America and Africa at a scale of 1:5,000,000 with accompanying texts. These are two volumes in a ten-volume series, *Soil Map of the World.* More detailed soil resource appraisals and expanded research efforts are required to provide necessary information for development of new lands and for improvement of soil management practices for intensification of production on presently cultivated soils. Substantial progress has been made in many tropical countries in making inventories of their soil resources.

Misconceptions. There are many misconceptions about soils of the tropics. One relates to the localized occurrence of laterite (irreversibly hardened ironstone) associated with the extensive red soils common in the tropics. These red soils have been called lateritic soils, and the mistaken notion arose that these soils when cleared of vegetation and cultivated would turn to hardened laterite and become worthless in a short time. Actually, extensive areas of red (so-called lateritic) soils in the tropics have been farmed for centuries without laterite forming. Probably only about 5% of soils in the tropics have laterite, and most are relics of previous geologic eras and not related to present use. Laterite forms under a particular set of conditions in localized areas and is of minor importance in the tropics.

A second prevalent misconception is that soils of the tropics have much less organic matter than those of temperate regions. This mistaken idea arose because of (1) warmer temperature in most of the tropics which accelerates organic matter decomposition and (2) widespread occurrence of reddish-colored soils in contrast to the generally dark-colored soils of the temperate regions. Analyses of soils from many different areas in the tropics have shown that, generally, the organic matter content is as high if not higher than that of soils in temperate regions. The long dry season in much of the tropics inhibits biological activity, just as winter temperatures do in temperate climates. In tropical areas with abundant rainfall there is much greater vegetative growth, which balances the increased biological activity in organic matter decomposition because of the warmer temperatures. Hence the soil organic matter content is maintained.

A third common misconception is that luxuriant forest growth in the low humid tropics is an indicator of fertile soils. More often than not, soils in tropical forests are relatively infertile. The nutrients are contained mostly in the vegetation and recycled as the decomposing organic matter releases them. The extensive roots of the forest vegetation prevent leaching of nutrients, and with abundant rainfall throughout the year luxuriant vegetation can be maintained on relatively infertile soils.

Agricultural systems. Though large areas of soils in the tropics are intensively cultivated for commercial export crops, most of the food for much of the population is produced under traditional, largely subsistence, shifting cultivation (slash-and-burn) systems. These are extensive systems supporting low-density populations, as the soil is usually cultivated with mixed crops for only a year or two followed by natural fallow for 5 to 15 years or more. With increased population pressure in many areas, the introduction of modern technology for more intensive use of the soils becomes necessary. Though substantial progress in this direction has been made, the intensification of traditional agriculture in the tropics within the limited resources of the farmers poses a major challenge to agricultural scientists.

[MATTHEW DROSDOFF]

Determining irrigation needs. Ideally, farmers should irrigate periodically before drought cuts crop growth and yield and then apply only the water required to refill the soil occupied by roots to its capacity to retain water against drainage. When necessary, more water (about 10%) is applied to leach excess salts to maintain low salinity in the root zone.

Three general approaches have been followed to assist farmers in the irrigation decision-making process: (1) measure soil water content or suction, (2) use plants as indicators, and (3) maintain a soil water budget.

Soil water content or suction. Various methods have been described for measuring soil water content or suction: the tensiometer and sorption block, the electrical resistance unit, the electrothermal unit, and the neutron moderation technique. The neutron meter measures soil water on a volume basis (cm^3/cm^3), which means that readings can be expressed in surface centimeters or inches of water per acre, a distinct advantage when considering water budgets for scheduling irrigations. However, the meter embodies a radiation hazard from fast neutrons and requires a competent technician to use it effectively.

Tensiometers equipped with vacuum gages measure soil water suction up to 0.8 bar (where 1 bar is equivalent to 10^{-5} Pa) and can be read quickly. Irrigation water is applied when the vacuum gage registers a prescribed limit of soil water suc-

tion at a specified depth for a given crop. For example, tensiometers used to irrigate avocados are placed in the active root zone and near the bottom of the root zone. Irrigation applied when the soil water suction at the 30-cm depth approaches 50 centibars does not penetrate to the 60-cm depth until the application time is nearly doubled (July 5, August 26, and September 16). Between irrigations, soil water suction at the lower depth gradually increases, indicating that loss of water below root zone is being controlled.

Plants as indicators. Farmers are using change of leaf color (from light to bluish green) as a practical guide for scheduling irrigations on field beans, cotton, and peanuts.

Measurement of the internal plant water condition by sophisticated techniques as a criterion for scheduling irrigation is impractical for two reasons: plant water status is difficult to measure, and variation in plant water stress with time of day is difficult to interpret.

Soil water budget. Use of the soil water budget approach to determine need for irrigation requires a knowledge of: (1) short-term evapotranspiration (ET) rates at various stages of plant development, (2) soil water retention characteristics, (3) permissible soil water deficits in relation to evaporative demand, and (4) the effective rooting depth of the crop grown.

Evaporation pans are being used to develop soil water budget schemes for scheduling irrigations for sugarcane in Hawaii and for cotton and orchard and vegetable crops in Israel. Evaporation from pans to schedule irrigations must be calibrated for a specific crop and geographic area.

Another advance in techniques to schedule irrigations has been made by using the modified Penman equation to estimate potential ET. Four basic meteorological parameters are required: solar radiation, mean temperature, wind speed, and vapor pressure (dew point). Crop characteristic curves are required.

Sophisticated solid-set and traveling-type sprinkler systems, dead-level automated surface irrigation systems, and graded furrow systems with tail-water reuse facilities provide a high degree of water control and are readily adapted to the irrigation-scheduling techniques described. Farmer acceptance of the computerized meteorological approach to irrigation scheduling has been far greater than any of the other methods discussed. Professional scheduling services were provided for a fee on about 250,000 acres of irrigated lands in Arizona, California, Idaho, Nevada, Washington, Nebraska, Kansas, and Colorado in 1974.

[HOWARD R. HAISE]

Soil conservation. Numerous studies continue to indicate that most herbicides and insecticides, when applied to soils at recommended dosage rates, exert little effect on most soil microorganisms or on soil properties. However, certain fumigants and fungicides may temporarily kill or reduce the numbers of nonparasitic soil organisms and may temporarily influence soil chemical properties. Generally the side effects of most pesticides are not detrimental or they may actually be beneficial, but occasionally they may retard or inhibit plant growth for a few weeks or a few months. The magnitude of these effects depends on dosage, soil type, temperature, moisture, and other factors.

Influence on soil organisms. When applied to soils or crops at normal field application rates, most herbicides or insecticides have little effect on the soil microbes, or they may slightly stimulate growth of some species. However, herbicides may kill soil algae, and insecticides may kill nonparasitic soil insects. Volatile soil fumigants, such as D-D (a mixture of dichloropropane and dichloropropene) and methyl bromide and many soil fungicides, on the other hand, kill numerous nonparasitic soil organisms, including bacteria, fungi, actinomycetes, yeasts, algae, protozoa, earthworms, and insects. After the initial kill, numbers of soil bacteria soon reach much higher numbers than were present in the original soil. In acid soil, fungi may quickly return in greater numbers than were originally present, whereas in alkaline soils they may return quickly or their numbers may be reduced for a year or longer. Although the total number of species may be greatly reduced, with time additional species recolonize the soil and total numbers slowly decline to normal. Fumigants and insecticides exert a similar effect on soil insects.

Factors responsible for the increased numbers of certain microbes following a soil treatment which initially kills large numbers of soil organisms are: (1) The pesticide chemical may be utilized as a food source by one or more organisms; (2) The bodies of the organisms killed by the treatment are utilized as a food source by surviving forms or by species that first recolonize the soil. (3) The organisms which survive or first become reestablished can reach very high numbers because the environment is less competitive.

Influence on soil chemistry. Pesticides which reach the soil or which are applied directly to the soil may influence soil chemical properties in the following ways: (1) The pesticide chemical or partial decomposition products represent a change in the chemical composition of the soil. (2) Upon decomposition of the pesticide chemical, the constituent elements are released as simple inorganic compounds such as ammonia, phosphate, hydrogen sulfide, sulfate, chloride, and bromide. Carbon is released as carbon dioxide. Some of the elements, especially carbon and nitrogen, are utilized for synthesis of cells and organic products of the soil population. Eventually about 10–20% or more of the added carbon is incorporated into the relatively resistant soil humus. The new humus, however, decomposes faster than older, stabilized humus. (3) Pesticidal chemicals which kill an appreciable percentage of the soil organisms often increase the water-soluble salt content of soils. Soluble calcium is especially increased; usually more soluble magnesium, potassium, and phosphorus are noted. (4) Fumigants and fungicides may increase soluble or extractable micronutrient elements, including manganese, copper, and zinc. (5) Most fumigants and fungicides and certain other pesticides kill or reduce numbers of the relatively sensitive nitrifying bacteria in the soil. These organisms oxidize ammonia to nitrites and nitrates. Until these bacteria become reestablished, relatively more of the available soil nitrogen will be in the form of ammonia. Reestablishment of nitrifying bacteria occurs generally within a few weeks to a few months. (6) Pesticides containing the benzene ring may be detoxified and altered with respect to side chains or groups, and may then undergo polymerization reactions with plant and microbial phenolic substances. In this way, parts of pesticide molecules may serve as constituent units in the formation of the beneficial soil humus. *See* SOIL CHEMISTRY.

Increased growth response. The microbiological and chemical effects (side effects) of pesticides in soils generally exert little influence on plant growth. Sometimes, however, growth may be temporarily enhanced or retarded. Increased growth may be related to fertilizer value of nitrogen or phosphorus released during decomposition of specific pesticides and cells of organisms killed by the pesticide treatments; increased availability of soil manganese, phosphorus, and other plant nutrient elements; a plant auxin-type action of some pesticide chemicals or of their partial decomposition products; and recolonization of the soil by microbial species that exert a strong antagonism against plant root parasites.

Reduced plant growth. Occasionally something seems to go wrong following application of a pesticide to soils, and plants may be injured or growth may be retarded for short periods of time. These unexpected results may be caused by various factors:

1. Many pesticide chemicals are toxic to some plant species, and a few, such as the fumigants, are toxic to most plants. If time is not allowed for these chemicals to decompose in the soil or volatilize from the soil, the residual chemical may injure or even kill crop plants. Continuous or frequent use of pesticides which decompose very slowly in the soil may increase soil levels of the pesticide to a point that growth of sensitive crops will be retarded.

2. Simple inorganic substances released during decomposition of certain pesticides may injure sensitive plants. Avocado plants, for example, are highly sensitive to soil chloride. Treatment of the soil with D-D, chloropicrin, or other chloride-containing chemicals may cause or increase chloride injury to this plant. Similarly, several plant species, including onions, carnations, and citrus, are sensitive to bromide. Bromide residues from certain pesticides may temporarily retard growth of these species. Other possibly toxic inorganic decomposition residues of pesticides include arsenic, iodine, copper, and mercury.

3. In greenhouse or ornamental operations, in which fertilization rates are high, the killing of bacteria which oxidize ammonia to nitrites and nitrates may result in the accumulation of toxic concentrations of ammonia from decomposing organic nitrogenous fertilizers.

4. In soils high in manganese, fumigation may increase the soluble manganese to toxic levels for a short period of time. Although extractable soil manganese is generally increased, soil fumigation may sometimes cause manganese deficiencies of cauliflower, brussel sprouts, and broccoli which may be related to increases in available potassium or other elements which reduce manganese uptake.

5. Sometimes treatment of the soil with any pesticide which kills large numbers of microbes will cause a temporary plant growth inhibition mani-

fested by reduced absorption of phosphorus, zinc, and sometimes copper. The growth inhibition is quite spotty, and healthy plants may grow next to severely injured ones. Young citrus, peach, and certain other tree seedlings are especially sensitive to this phenomenon.

Studies have shown that a primary factor in this type of plant growth inhibition is the killing of endotrophic mycorrhizal fungi which aid the plant roots in absorbing certain plant nutrient elements, especially phosphorus. The condition can be corrected, or partially corrected, by proper fertilization with phosphorus, zinc, and sometimes copper, by inoculation of seed or seedlings with an effective mycorrhiza strain, or by delaying the planting of a sensitive crop until the mycorrhizal fungi have become reestablished in the soil.

[JAMES P. MARTIN]

Fertilizer in semiarid grasslands. In the semiarid grasslands of temperate regions, lack of available nitrogen often limits production as much as does lack of available water. Consequently, use of nitrogen fertilizer is increasing on millions of acres of grasslands, particularly in the northern Great Plains of the United States and Canada. This practice immediately raises concern about the ecological impact of extensive nitrogen fertilization on pollution of surface and ground waters with nitrate. Results of recent research on the fate of fertilizer nitrogen applied to semiarid grasslands have greatly reduced the uncertainty that has surrounded this subject.

In addition to the nitrogen absorbed and translocated into plant tops, a semiarid grassland ecosystem can immobilize a fairly definite quantity of fertilizer nitrogen in the roots, mulch, residues, and soil organic matter. The quantity of nitrogen immobilized in these pools varies with soil type and texture, water availability, and possibly temperature, but is not influenced greatly by either grass species or most management schemes. Fertilizer nitrogen immobilized in these organic forms may later be mineralized by soil microorganisms and recirculated through the ecosystem. A relatively small quantity (10 to 40 lb per acre; 1 lb per acre equals 1.12 kg per hectare) of fertilizer nitrogen seems to be absorbed directly into the cells of the soil microbes and in a few weeks or months is mineralized and recirculated as successive generations of microbes are produced and die. Much more fertilizer nitrogen (up to about 200 pounds per acre) is immobilized in grass roots and mulches and seems to be recycled in 3 to 5 years. Typically, up to 350 pounds of fertilizer nitrogen per acre can be immobilized in various organic pools in the soil-plant system.

Nitrogen cycle. The nitrogen cycle in semiarid grassland ecosystems is essentially a closed system; that is, losses of nitrogen from the soil-plant system are relatively low. Ordinarily, no fertilizer nitrogen is leached below the root zone in semiarid grasslands, so leaching losses are generally inconsequential. Losses of fertilizer nitrogen in gaseous form (by ammonia volatilization or denitrification) also seem usually to be relatively small, except perhaps where urea-containing fertilizers are applied to semiarid grasslands at rates exceeding 80 to 100 pounds of nitrogen per acre. In such instances, available data suggest that volatilization losses may be relatively high. *See* NITROGEN CYCLE.

Typical data on the fate of fertilizer nitrogen applied to semiarid grasslands emerged in an experiment in which 80 pounds of nitrogen per acre (as ammonium nitrate) was applied annually for 11 years to mixed prairie (primarily *Agropyron smithii*, *Stipa viridula*, and *Bouteloua gracilis*) grazed by yearling steers. After 11 years, approximately 35% of the fertilizer nitrogen applied was found in the roots (19%) and vegetative mulch (16%) on the soil surface. A slightly larger quantity remained in the soil as inorganic (ammonium 2%, nitrate 39%) nitrogen, indicating that the fertilizer applied exceeded the nitrogen required by the ecosystem. Less than 3% of the fertilizer nitrogen was physically removed from the pasture in the form of beef. In total, about 82% (including standing tops 2%, crown 1%) of the fertilizer nitrogen applied was accounted for. The 18% not accounted for was immobilized in soil organic matter or lost to the atmosphere as gaseous nitrogen. Other research suggests that the gaseous loss was about 5% of that applied. Therefore, losses from the nitrogen cycle are relatively low, and a major part of the nitrogen applied to grasslands remains in forms that can be recycled and used for plant growth in later years. All of the nitrogen in the inorganic pool plus a major part of that in roots, residues, and mulches, and some in the soil organic nitrogen pool (included in the unaccounted-for fraction), may be recycled.

Plant debris. Research using the ^{15}N isotope shows that within hours after application, the isotope is found primarily in the senescent or dead plant material—mulches and decaying root materials. This suggests that fertilizer nitrogen is absorbed into the cells of the microorganisms as they rapidly multiply after addition of nitrogen fertilizer. The increased microbial population then decomposes the senescent and dead plant materials, mobilizing the nitrogen they contain. Thus, nitrogen immobilized in plant material is recirculated through the nitrogen cycle, illustrating the importance of plant debris both above and below the soil surface as a pool of potential plant-available nitrogen in semiarid grasslands.

[J. F. POWER]

SOIL EROSION

Soil erosion is that physical process by which soil material is weathered away and carried downgrade by water or moved about by wind. Two categories of erosion are recognized. The first, called geologic erosion, is a natural process that takes place independent of man's activities. This kind of erosion is always active, wearing away the surface features of the Earth. The second kind, referred to as accelerated erosion, occurs when man disturbs the surface of the Earth or quickens the pace of erosion in any way. It produces conditions that are abnormal and poses a problem for the future food supply of the world. To combat erosion successfully, it is important that man recognize the erosion processes and have a knowledge of the factors which affect erosion.

Types. Erosion by running water is usually recognized in one of three forms: sheet erosion, rill erosion, and gully erosion.

Sheet erosion. The removal of a thin layer of soil,

more or less uniformly, from the entire surface of an area is known as sheet erosion. It usually occurs on plowed fields that have been recently prepared for seeding, but may also take place after the crop is seeded. Generally only the finer soil particles are removed. Although the depth of soil lost is not great, the loss of relatively rich topsoil from an entire field may be serious (Fig. 8). If continued for a period of years, the entire surface layer of soil may be removed. In many parts of the world only the surface layer is suited for cultivation.

Rill erosion. During heavy rains runoff water is concentrated in small streamlets or rivulets. As the volume or velocity of the water increases, it cuts narrow trenches called rills. Erosion of this type can remove large quantities of soil and reduce the soil fertility rapidly (Fig. 9). This type of erosion is particularly detrimental because all traces of the rills are removed after the land is tilled. The losses which occurred are often forgotten and adequate conservation measures are not taken to prevent further loss of soil.

Gully erosion. This type of erosion occurs where the concentrated runoff is sufficiently large to cut deep trenches, or where continued cutting in the same groove deepens the incision. Gullying often develops where there is a water overfall. The stream bed is cut back at the overfall and the gully lengthens headward or upslope. Once started, gullying may proceed rapidly, particularly in soils that do not possess much binding material. Gully erosion requires intensive control measures (Fig. 10), such as terracing or the use of diversion ditches, check dams, sod-strip checks, and shrub checks.

Affective factors. The rate and extent of soil erosion depend upon such interrelated factors as type of soil, steepness of slope, climatic characteristics, and land use.

Type of soil. Soil types vary greatly in physical and chemical composition. The amounts of sand, silt, and clay constituents, colloidal material, and organic matter all have a bearing upon the ease with which particles or aggregates can be detached from the body of the soil. Such detachment is caused chiefly by the beating action of raindrops. The particles are then transported downgrade by moving water. Sandy or gravelly soils often have little colloidal material to bind particles together, and hence these materials are easily detached. However, because of their size, sand particles are more difficult to move than fine particles. For this reason sand particles are moved chiefly by rapidly flowing water on steep slopes or by streams at flood stage. Finer particles, such as silt, clay, and organic matter, can be carried by water moving at a slower rate. On gently sloping fields there is a tendency for more of the fine particles to be carried away, leaving the heavier sand particles behind. However, if rainfall is intense and the volume of runoff great, sand may be moved even on gentle slopes.

Slope. The relation of slope to the amount of erosion on different classes of soil is illustrated in Fig. 11. The amount of total runoff from rainfall increases only slightly with increase in the slope of the land above 1–2%, but the speed of the flowing water, or rate of runoff, may increase greatly.

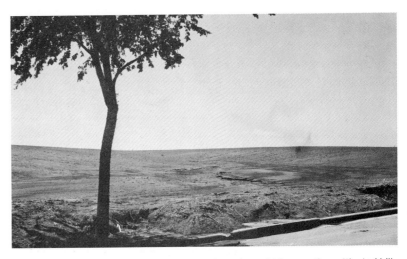
Fig. 8. Sheet erosion showing how soil has been brought from entire cultivated hillside. A large soil deposit has collected on flat area at bottom of slope. (*USDA*)

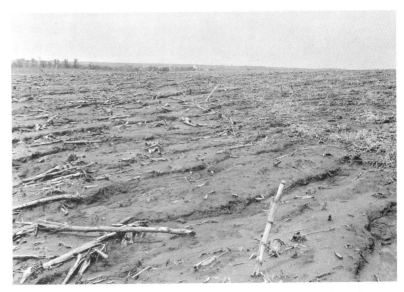
Fig. 9. Rill erosion showing how water has followed the old corn rows. (*USDA*)

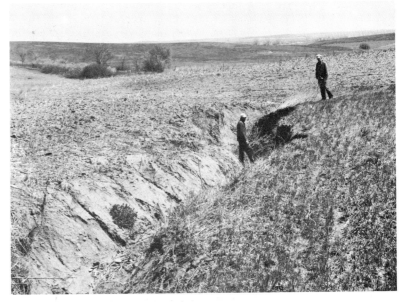
Fig. 10. Large gully could be repaired by plowing in and seeding to grass. (*USDA*)

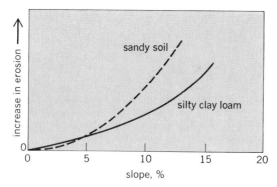

Fig. 11. Generalized diagram illustrating greater loss of fine-grained soil (silty clay loam) on gentle slopes (0–5%) and greater loss of sandy soil on steeper slopes.

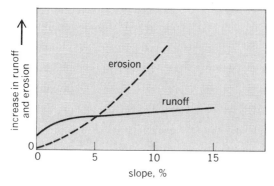

Fig. 12. Effect of slope on total amount of runoff and on rate of runoff and soil erosion.

Since the capacity of moving water to transport soil particles increases in geometric ratio to the rate of flow, the amount of erosion increases greatly with increase in the slope of the land (Fig. 12).

Climate. In cold climates the frozen soil is not subject to erosion for several months of the year. However, if such areas receive heavy snow, serious erosion may take place when the snow melts. This is particularly true if the snow melts as the ground gradually thaws. As the water moves over the thin unfrozen layer of soil, it transports much of this soil material downgrade.

In warm climates soils are susceptible to erosion any time there are heavy rains. Such soils are particularly vulnerable to erosion if rains fall in winter and there is little vegetative cover.

The amount of rainfall is an important factor in determining the erosion that occurs in a given region. However, the character of the rainfall is usually a much more important factor than the total amount in determining the seriousness of erosion. A rain falling at the rate of 2 in./hr may cause three to five times as much erosion as a rainfall of 1 in./hr. Regions where most of the precipitation comes in the form of mist or gentle rain may undergo little erosion, even though the total rainfall may be high and other conditions conducive to erosion.

In some areas of dry climates strong winds cause soil movement and serious loss of soil. Wind erosion is more common on sandy soils, but it is by no means confined to them. Heavier soils, which have a fluffy physical condition produced by freezing and thawing or drying, may be moved in great quantities by the wind.

Land use. The type of crops and the system of management influence the amount and type of erosion. Bare soils, clean uncultivated soils, or land in intertilled row crops permit the greatest amount of erosion. Crops that give complete ground cover throughout the year, such as grass or forests, are most effective in controlling erosion. Small-grain crops, or those that provide a fairly dense cover for only part of the year, are intermediate in their effect on erosion. Table 3 gives results of some of the earliest experiments in the United States on differences in land use and the effect on runoff and erosion. These results show that cultivated land, especially without a crop or protective cover of vegetation, is particularly vulnerable to erosion. In addition, excessive erosion usually occurs where cultivated crops like corn, cotton, and tobacco are grown on hilly or sloping land that is subjected to increased rates of runoff. In some areas where row crops have been grown continually the soil has been removed to the depth of the plow layer within a lifetime.

Pastures in humid areas usually have a tough continuous sod that prevents or greatly reduces sheet or surface erosion. Natural range cover, if in good condition, is usually effective in controlling erosion, but in areas of limited rainfall, where bunch grasses form most of the cover on range land, occasional heavy rain may cause severe erosion of the bare soil exposed between the bunches of grass. Forest lands, with their overhead canopies of trees and surface layers of decaying organic matter, have much greater water intake and much less surface runoff and erosion.

Wind erosion. In the western half of the United States and in many other parts of the world, great quantities of soil are moved by the wind. This is particularly so in arid and semiarid areas. Sandy soils are more subject to wind erosion than silt loam or clay loam soils. The latter, however, are easily eroded when climatic conditions cause the soil to break into small aggregates, ranging from 0.4 to 0.8 mm in diameter. The coarse particles usually are moved relatively short distances, but the fine dust particles may be carried by strong winds for hundreds or even thousands of miles.

In some areas the coarse, or sand, particles are moved by the wind and deposited over extensive areas as dunes. The dunes move forward in the same direction as the prevailing winds, the particles being moved from the windward side of the dune to the lee side. If dunes become covered with

Table 3. Relative runoff and erosion from soil under different land uses, with mean rainfall of 35.87 in.*

Land use and treatment	Runoff, %	Tons soil per acre eroded annually	Years required to lose surface 7 in. of soil
Plowed 8 in. deep, no crop; fallowed to keep weeds down	28.4	35.7	28
Plowed 8 in., corn annually	27.4	17.8	56
Plowed 8 in., wheat annually	25.2	6.7	150
Rotation: corn, wheat, red clover	14.1	2.3	437
Bluegrass sod	11.6	0.3	3547

*Missouri Res. Bull. no. 63, 1923.

grass or other vegetation, they cease to move. The sandhill region of Nebraska is a good example of such an area.

Control. The following are a few fundamental principles which will help control erosion and greatly reduce the damage done by soil erosion.

1. Keep land covered with a growing crop or grass as much time as possible. Cover increases intake of water and reduces runoff. The extent of erosion control will be roughly in proportion to the effective cover.

2. When there is no growing crop, retain a cover of stubble or crop residue on the land between crops and until the next crop is well started. This can be done by using a system known as stubble-mulch farming. It ultilizes the idea of preparing a seedbed for a new crop without burying the residue from the previous crop. Tillage tools that work beneath the surface and pulverize the soil without necessarily inverting it or burying the residue are used instead of moldboard plows. This system is best adapted to regions of low rainfall or warm climates.

3. Avoid letting water concentrate and run directly downhill. By doing this the soil is protected against water at its maximum cutting power. Construct terraces with gentle grades to carry the runoff water around the hill at slow speeds. These diversions should empty onto grassed waterways or on meadowland to prevent creation of gullies. See TERRACING (AGRICULTURE).

4. Plant crops and till the soil along the contours.

5. Control wind erosion by keeping land covered with sod or planted crops as much of the time as possible. Maintain crop residue on the land between crops and while the next crop is getting started.

6. If wind erosion begins on a bare field or where a crop is just getting started, the soil drifting may be stopped temporarily by cultivation. An implement with shovels that will throw up clods or chunks of soil to give a rough surface is usually effective. Often, only strips through the field need be so treated to stop erosion on the whole area.

7. Moving dunes may require artificial cover or mechanical obstructions on the windward side, followed by vegetative plantings, depending on climatic conditions. Along shorelines, beach grasses followed by woody plants and forests may be required.

For a discussion of the physical, economic, and social effects of soil erosion see SOIL CONSERVATION.

[FRANK L. DULEY]

Bibliography: L. D. Baver and W. H. Gardner, *Soil Physics*, 4th ed., 1972; P. W. Birkeland, *Pedology, Weathering, and Geomorphological Research*, 1974; C. E. Black (ed.), *Methods of Soil Analysis*, Amer. Soc. Agron. Monogr. no. 9, 1964; F. E. Broadbent and D. S. Mikkelsen, *Agron. J.*, 60: 674–677, 1968; E. T. Cleaves, A. E. Godfrey, and J. K. Coulter, Soil management systems, in *Soils of the Humid Tropics*, 1972; Food and Agriculture Organization–UNESCO, *Soil Map of the World*, 1971–1976; H. D. Foth and L. M. Turk, *Fundamentals of Soil Science*, 5th ed., 1972; R. M. Hagan, H. R. Haise, and T. W. Edminster (eds.), *Irrigation of Agricultural Lands*, 1967; H. R. Haise and

R. M. Hagan, in R. M. Hagan, H. R. Haise, and T. W. Edminster (eds.), *Irrigation of Agricultural Lands*, 1967; *International Rice Research Institute Annual Report*, 1970; D. D. Kaufman, in W. D. Guenzi (ed.), *Pesticides in Soil and Water*, pp. 135–202, 1974; C. E. Kellogg and A. C. Orvedal, Potentially arable soils of the world and critical measures for their use, *Advan. Agron.*, 21:109–170, 1969; G. D. Kleinschmidt and J. W. Gerdeman, *Phytopathology*, 62:1447–1453, 1972; H. Kohnke, *Soil Physics*, 1968; J. P. Martin, in C. A. I. Goring (ed.), *Organic Chemicals in the Soil Environment*, vol. 2, pp. 733–792, 1972; National Academy of Sciences, *Soils of the Humid Tropics*, 1972; C. H. Pair, in C. H. Pair et al. (eds.), *Sprinkler Irrigation*, 4th ed., 1975; J. F. Parr, in W. D. Guenzi (ed.), *Pesticides in Soil and Water*, pp. 315–340, 1974; W. H. Patrick and D. S. Mikkelsen, in *Fertilizer Technology and Use*, 1971; F. N. Ponnamperuma, in *Advances in Agronomy*, 1972; President's Science Advisory Committee, *The World Food Problem*, vol. 2, 1967; R. W. Simonson, Loss of nutrient elements in soil formation, in O. P. Englestad (ed.), *Nutrient Mobility in Soils: Accumulation and Losses*, Soil Sci. Soc. Amer. Spec. Publ. no. 4, 1970; Soil Survey Staff, *Soil Taxonomy: A Basic System of Soil Classification for Making and Interpreting Soil Surveys*, USDA Handb. 436, 1975; A. R. Thompson and C. A. Edwards, in W. D. Guenzi (ed.), *Pesticides in Soil and Water*, pp. 341–386, 1974; L. M. Thompson and F. R. Troeh, *Soils and Soil Fertility*, 3d ed., 1973; U. S. Department of Agriculture, *Soil: The Yearbook of Agriculture*, 1957.

Soil, suborders of

Broad classes at one level in the soil classification system adopted in the United States in 1965 are called suborders. A total of 47 suborders form the full set of classes in the second highest category (each category is a set of classes of parallel rank) in the system.

The number of local kinds of soils in a large country is also large. For example, 11,000 soil series have been recognized in soil surveys made in the United States through 1974. On the average, a series consists of six phases, which are the local kinds of soils. This means that approximately 66,000 local kinds have been defined up to the present time in a single large country, though all parts of that country have not been studied.

Despite the myriads of local kinds over the land surface of the Earth, all soils share some characteristics. They can all be related to one another in some way. The relationships are close for some pairs of local kinds and distant for others. The similarities and differences among the thousands of local kinds permit their grouping into sets of progressively broader classes in order to show degrees of kinship.

Though it is impossible for a single mind to retain concepts of 11,000 series or 66,000 phases, one can remember the salient features of a few dozen broad classes. Consequently, the nature of the 47 suborders is described in this article. The purpose is to provide a general picture of the kinds of soils in the United States and the world. A list of the 47 suborders grouped into the 10 orders is given in Table 1. For an explanation of the nomenclature

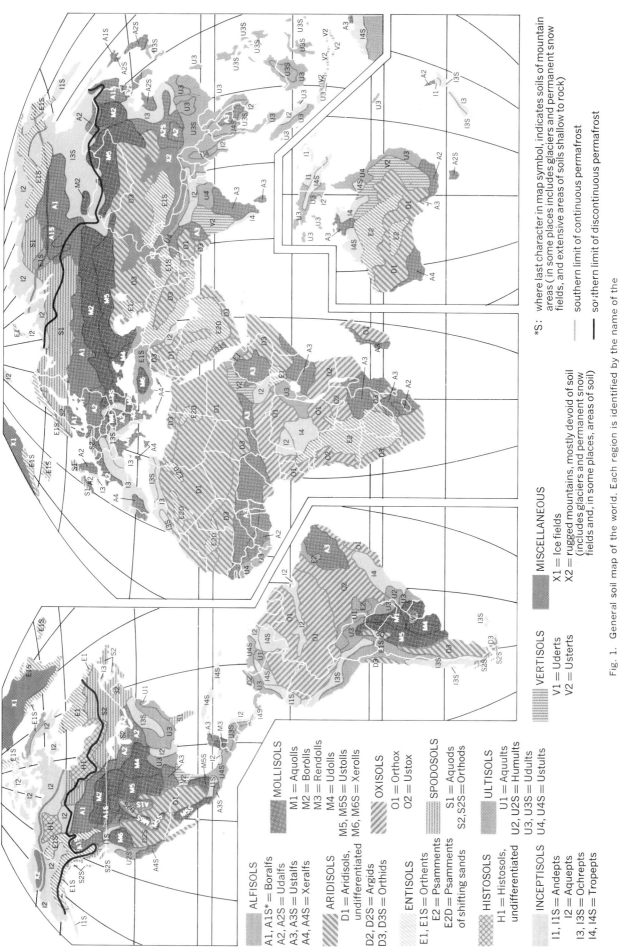

ALFISOLS
A1, A1S* = Boralfs
A2, A2S = Udalfs
A3, A3S = Ustalfs
A4, A4S = Xeralfs

ARIDISOLS
D1 = Aridisols,
undifferentiated
D2, D2S = Argids
D3, D3S = Orthids

ENTISOLS
E1, E1S = Orthents
E2 = Psamments
E2D = Psamments
of shifting sands

HISTOSOLS
H1 = Histosols,
undifferentiated

INCEPTISOLS
I1, I1S = Andepts
I2 = Aquepts
I3, I3S = Ochrepts
I4, I4S = Tropepts

MOLLISOLS
M1 = Aquolls
M2 = Borolls
M3 = Rendolls
M4 = Udolls
M5, M5S = Ustolls
M6, M6S = Xerolls

OXISOLS
O1 = Orthox
O2 = Ustox

SPODOSOLS
S1 = Aquods
S2, S2S = Orthods

ULTISOLS
U1 = Aquults
U2, U2S = Humults
U3, U3S = Udults
U4, U4S = Ustults

VERTISOLS
V1 = Uderts
V2 = Usterts

MISCELLANEOUS
X1 = Ice fields
X2 = rugged mountains, mostly devoid of soil
(includes glaciers and permanent snow
fields and, in some places, areas of soil)

*S: where last character in map symbol, indicates soils of mountain
       areas (in some places includes glaciers and permanent snow
       fields, and extensive areas of soils shallow to rock)
——————   southern limit of continuous permafrost
━━━━━━   southern limit of discontinuous permafrost

Fig. 1.   General soil map of the world. Each region is identified by the name of the
most extensive suborder. Other suborders are present in every region and are important in most of them. (*Soil Conservation Service, USDA*)

Table 1. Orders and suborders of United States soil classification system (adopted 1965)

Orders	Suborders	Orders	Suborders
Alfisols	Aqualfs	Mollisols	Albolls
	Boralfs		Aquolls
	Udalfs		Borolls
	Ustalfs		Rendolls
	Xeralfs		Udolls
Aridisols	Argids		Ustolls
	Orthids		Xerolls
Entisols	Aquents	Oxisols	Aquox
	Arents		Humox
	Fluvents		Orthox
	Orthents		Torrox
	Psamments		Ustox
Histosols	Fibrists	Spodosols	Aquods
	Folists		Ferrods
	Hemists		Humods
	Saprists		Orthods
Inceptisols	Andepts	Ultisols	Aquults
	Aquepts		Humults
	Ochrepts		Udults
	Plaggepts		Ustults
	Tropepts		Xerults
	Umbrepts	Vertisols	Torrerts
			Uderts
			Usterts
			Xererts

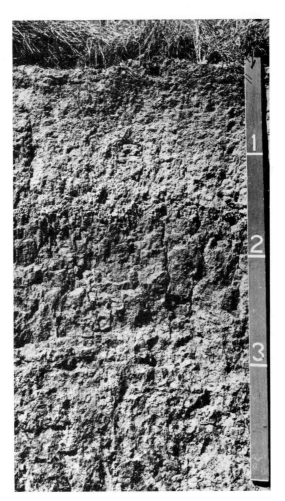

Fig. 2. Profile of an Aqualf with pale A horizon about 18 in. thick resting on B horizon high in clay which grades into C horizon at a depth of about 4 ft; numbers on scale indicate feet. (*Photograph by R. W. Simonson*)

for orders and suborders *see* SOIL.

The brief individual descriptions of the suborders are arranged in the same sequence as the list in Table 1. For a few suborders, no descriptions have been included because of the limited extent and importance or limited information on the soils.

The broad regional distribution of soils is shown for the world in Fig. 1. Each region outlined on the map is identified by the name of the most extensive suborder among the component soils. In every region, suborders other than the most extensive one are important. *See* SOIL, ZONALITY OF.

Alfisols. These soils have A horizons that are mostly pale in color and that have lost silicate clay, sesquioxides, and bases such as calcium and magnesium. For a detailed explanation of horizons *see* SOIL.

The soils have B horizons with accumulations of silicate clay and with moderate to high levels of exchangeable calcium and magnesium. The C horizons are usually lighter in color and lower in clay than the B horizons.

Alfisols are most extensive in humid, temperate regions but range from the edges of the tundra and the desert into the tropics. Mostly, the soils were under forest or savanna vegetation, though some were under prairie. All have been formed on land surfaces that are not old nor yet among the youngest in the world.

Occurring as they do in many parts of the world, these soils are used for a wide variety of crops. Some remain in forest, and those under drier climates are used chiefly for grazing.

Aqualfs. These are the seasonally wet Alfisols. They generally occur in depressions or on rather wide flats in local landscapes. In addition to the general morphology and composition shared with other soils of the order, Aqualfs are marked by gray or mottled colors reflecting their wetness (Fig. 2).

Boralfs. These are the well-drained Alfisols of cool or cold regions, such as west-central Canada

and the Soviet Union. The soils occur chiefly at high latitudes or high altitudes and barely extend into frigid zones.

In their morphology and composition, the soils are much like the Udalfs, though colors are more dull on the whole and the supply of calcium and magnesium a little higher.

Udalfs. These are the well-drained Alfisols of humid, temperate climates. The soils are important in the north-central part of the United States, in western Europe, and in eastern Asia. Udalfs differ from Aqualfs in that B horizons are characteristically brown or yellowish brown and lack marks of wetness. These have higher mean annual temperatures than do the Boralfs and are moist for higher proportions of the year than the Ustalfs and Xeralfs (Fig. 3).

Ustalfs. These are well-drained Alfisols occurring in somewhat drier and mostly warmer regions than Udalfs. On the whole, the soils have more reddish B horizons and are a little higher in calcium and magnesium than Udalfs. These soils are intermittently dry during the growing season.

Xeralfs. These are well-drained Alfisols found in regions with rainy winters and dry summers, in what are called mediterranean climates. Like the Ustalfs in nature of the B horizon, the soils have A horizons that tend to become massive and hard

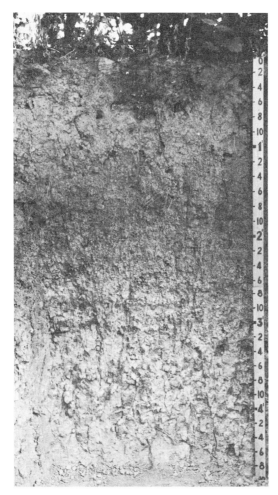

Fig. 3. Profile of a Udalf with A horizon 12 in. thick over darker B horizon with blocky structure grading into C horizon at a depth of about 4 ft; larger numbers on scale indicate feet. (*Photograph by R. W. Simonson*)

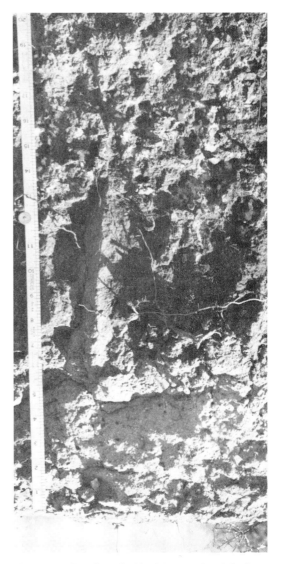

Fig. 4. Profile of an Argid with pale silty A horizon, darker B horizon higher in clay, and calcareous C horizon; profile shown is 20 in. deep; numbers on scale indicate inches. (*Photograph by R. W. Simonson*)

during the dry season. Some of the soils have duripans (cemented layers at depth of 2 or 3 ft) that interfere with root growth.

Aridisols. These are major soils of the world's deserts, which form about one-fourth of the land surface. Soils of other orders, especially the Entisols, are also present but less extensive in the deserts.

Formed under low rainfall, Aridisols have been leached little and are therefore high in calcium, magnesium, and other more soluble elements. The low rainfall has also limited growth of plants, mostly shrubs and similar species, so that the soils are low in organic matter and nitrogen. The combined A and B horizons are no more and frequently less than 1 ft thick. The A horizons are light-colored, as a rule, whereas B horizons are similar or slightly darker in color. The C horizons are light-colored and usually calcareous. All horizons are neutral or mildly alkaline in reaction.

Most Aridisols in use provide some grazing for nomadic herds. On the other hand, if water and other resources, including adequate skills, are available and climate is favorable, some Aridisols will support a large variety and produce high yields of crops.

Argids. These well-drained Aridisols have B horizons of silicate clay accumulation. The B horizons are characteristically brown or reddish in color and grade into lighter colored C horizons marked by carbonate accumulation. On the whole, these soils occupy the older land surfaces in desert regions (Fig. 4).

Orthids. These Aridisols lack B horizons of clay accumulation. Many are free of carbonates in the A and part of the B horizon; most are well drained. Common colors are gray or brownish gray with little change from top to bottom of the profile. A few Orthids are fairly high in soluble salts such as sodium sulphate and sodium chloride, whereas others are high in calcium carbonate throughout. More extensive than the Argids, generally, Orthids occupy younger but not the youngest land surfaces in deserts.

Entisols. These soils have few and faint horizons, with reasons for the limited horizonation differing among suborders. Reasons for the practical absence of horizons are indicated for individual suborders.

Entisols occur in all parts of the world and may be found under a wide variety of vegetation. Most,

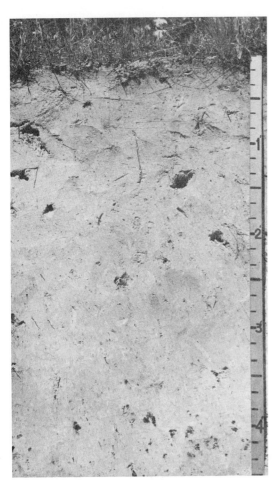

Fig. 5 Profile of a Psamment lacking evident horizons and consisting of sand throughout; numbers on scale indicate feet. (*Photograph by R. W. Simonson*)

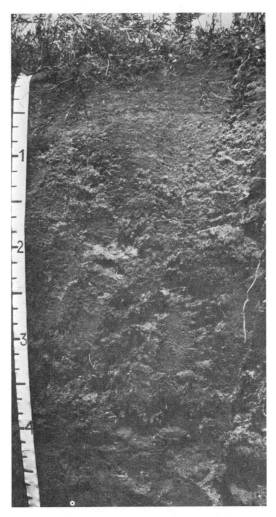

Fig. 6. Profile of a Fibrist with little or no change from the surface to a depth of 5 ft; soil consists of partly decayed plant residues; numbers on scale indicate feet. (*Photograph by R. W. Simonson*)

though not all, are on young land surfaces, distributed from the tundra to the tropics and from the deserts to the rainiest climates. Entisols have a wide range in usefulness. Some are highly productive and others are not.

Aquents. These Entisols have been under water at the margins of oceans, lakes, or seas until very recent time. The wetness is reflected in the bluish-gray or greenish-gray colors. Examples are the soils in recently reclaimed polders of the Netherlands. The total extent of Aquents in the world is very small.

Arents. These are Entisols because of severe disturbance of soils formerly classifiable in other orders. The sequence of horizons has been disrupted completely, and remnants of those horizons can be found randomly distributed in the profiles of Arents.

Fluvents. These well-drained Entisols are in recently deposited alluvium. The soils occur along streams or in fans where the rate of sediment deposition is high. The marks of sedimentation are still evident, and identifiable horizons are lacking, except for a slightly darkened surface layer or A1 horizon. Small bodies of these soils are scattered over all parts of the world.

Orthents. These well-drained Entisols are of medium or fine texture, mostly on strong slopes. For an explanation of texture *see* SOIL.

The soils may have A1 horizons or slightly darkened surface layers an inch or so thick but otherwise lack evidence of horizonation. Many of the soils are shallow to bedrock.

Psamments. These Entisols are of sandy texture. Like the Orthents, these may have thin A1 horizons, which grade into thick C horizons. The sandiness is the distinctive character of the suborder (Fig. 5).

Histosols. These are wet soils consisting mostly of organic matter, popularly called peats and mucks. Most have restricted drainage and are saturated with water much of the time. A few are wet but not saturated. Widely distributed over the world, these soils may occur in small or large bodies, with the latter occurring chiefly at high latitudes. A large proportion of the total area is idle. Where the climate is favorable, some of the soils have been drained and are producing vegetables and other crops.

Fibrists. These Histosols consist mainly of recognizable plant residues or sphagnum moss. They are saturated with water most of the year unless drained (Fig. 6).

Folists. These Histosols consist of forest litter resting on rock or rubble. Drainage is not restricted, but a combination of rainfall, fog, and low

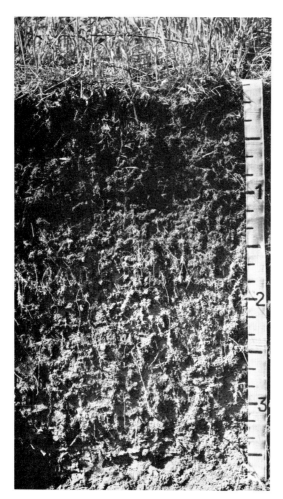

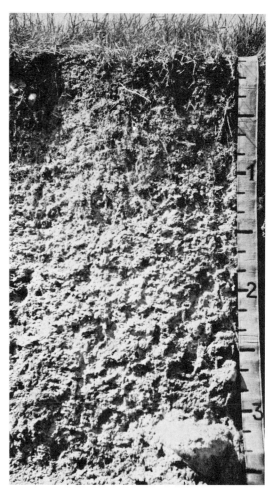

Fig. 7. Profile of an Andept with thick, dark A horizon, faint B horizon, and lighter C horizon; fine plant roots are numerous; numbers on scale indicate feet. (*Photograph by R. W. Simonson*)

Fig. 8. Profile of an Aquept with thin, dark A horizons, fairly thick, light-gray B horizon, and stone in C horizon beside tape; numbers on scale indicate feet. (*Photograph by R. W. Simonson*)

temperatures keeps the litter wet.

Hemists. These Histosols consist of partially decayed plant residues. Plant structures have largely been destroyed but an appreciable share of the mass remains as fibers when rubbed vigorously. The soils are saturated with water much of the time unless drained.

Saprists. These Histosols consist of residues in which plant structures have been largely obliterated by decay. A very small part of the mass remains as fibers after vigorous rubbing. The soils are saturated with water much of the time unless drained. Most Saprists in the United States are known as muck.

Inceptisols. These soils have faint to moderate horizonation but lack horizons of accumulation of translocated substances other than carbonates and silica. Two of the suborders have distinct dark A horizons, and most of them have B horizons formed by losses and transformations without corresponding gains in substances. Thus, the Inceptisols are in some ways intermediate in horizonation between the Entisols and Vertisols on the one hand, and the Alfisols, Mollisols, Spodosols, Ultisols, and Oxisols on the other.

Inceptisols are widely distributed, ranging from the arctic region to the tropics and from the margins of the desert into regions of heavy rainfall.

They may consequently be found under a wide variety of vegetation. Usefulness of the soils has as wide a range as does their distribution. Some are highly productive and others are of little or no value.

Andepts. These Inceptisols are formed chiefly in volcanic ash or in regoliths with a high component of ash. Mostly, the soils are light and tend to be fluffy. They have thick dark A horizons, rather high levels of acidity, and poorly crystalline clay minerals. The soils are widely distributed but seem to be restricted to regions of fairly recent volcanic activity (Fig. 7).

Aquepts. These Inceptisols are wet or have been drained. Like the Aqualfs, the soils have gray or mottled B and C horizons, but they lack silicate clay accumulation in their profiles. The A horizon may be dark and fairly thick or it may be thin, as it is in many of the soils (Fig. 8).

Ochrepts. These Inceptisols have pale A horizons, darker B horizons, and lighter colored C horizons. The B horizons lack accumulations of translocated clay, sesquioxides, or humus. The soils are widely distributed, occurring from the margins of the tundra region through the temperate zone but not in the tropics. Ochrepts also occur in the fairly dry regions though not in deserts (Fig. 9).

Plaggepts. These Inceptisols have very thick

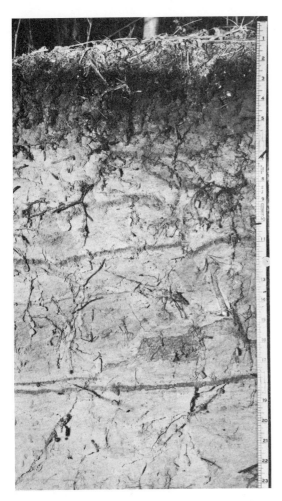

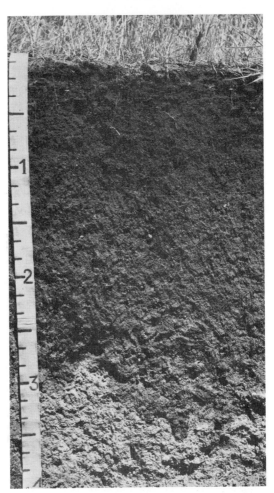

Fig. 9. Profile of an Ochrept with litter on the surface, dark A horizon 4 in. thick, thin B horizon, and pale C horizon; deeper profile is marked by plant roots and traces of former roots; numbers on scale indicate inches. (*Photograph by R. W. Simonson*)

Fig. 10. Profile of an Aquoll with very thick, dark A horizon, signs of mixing and burrowing by animals at depths between 3 and 3½ ft, and lighter C horizon at the bottom; the numbers on the scale to the left indicate feet. (*Photograph by R. W. Simonson*)

surface horizons of mixed mineral and organic materials added as manure or as human wastes over long periods of time. For the world as a whole, such soils are of negligible extent, but they are conspicuous where found.

Tropepts. These Inceptisols have moderately dark A horizons with modest additions of organic matter, B horizons with brown or reddish colors, and slightly paler C horizons. The soils are less strongly weathered than the geographically associated Ultisols and Oxisols. In general appearance, the profiles are much like that of the Orthox shown in Fig. 12. Tropepts are restricted to tropical regions, largely to those of moderate and high rainfall.

Umbrepts. These Inceptisols have dark A horizons more than 10 in. thick, brown B horizons, and slightly paler C horizons. The soils are strongly acid and the silicate clay minerals are crystalline rather than amorphous as in the Andepts. The Umbrepts occur under cool or temperate climates, are widely distributed, and are of moderate extent.

Mollisols. These soils have dark or very dark, friable, thick A horizons high in humus and bases such as calcium and magnesium. Most have lighter colored or browner B horizons that are less friable and about as thick as the A horizons. All but a

few have paler C horizons, many of which are calcareous.

Major areas of Mollisols occur in subhumid or semiarid cool and temperate regions. They meet the desert along their drier margins and meet soils such as the Alfisols at their more humid margins. Mollisols were formed under vegetation consisting chiefly of grasses and are thus the major ones of former prairies and steppes. The soils occupy rather young land surfaces.

Though they produce a variety of crops, Mollisols are largely used for cereals. These soils now produce a major share of the world's output of corn and wheat. Topography is generally favorable for the operation of large machinery, and many Mollisols are therefore in large farms. Yields have a wide range, depending on climatic conditions. Wide fluctuations in yield with wet and dry years are normal for the Mollisols marginal to arid regions. On the other hand, yields are consistently high for those under more humid climates.

Albolls. These are Mollisols with dark A1 horizons, bleached A2 horizons, distinct B horizons marked by clay accumulation, and paler C horizons. The soils are wet, especially in the upper part, for some part of the year. Mostly, the soils occur on upland flats and in shallow depressions.

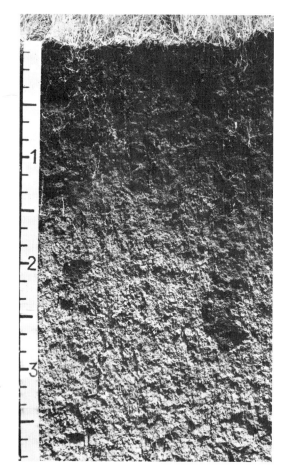

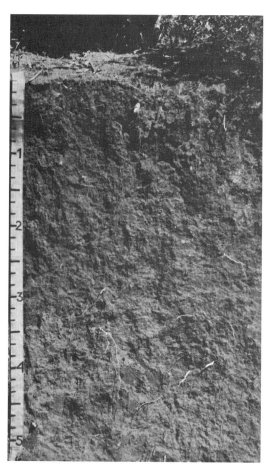

Fig. 11.   Profile of a Udoll with thick, dark A horizon, B horizon gradational in color, and rather pale C horizon; filled former animal burrows in B horizon; numbers on scale indicate feet. (*Photograph by R. W. Simonson*)

Fig. 12.   Profile of an Orthox with slightly darkened A horizon about 1 ft thick, little further change to depth of profile, and deep penetration by fine plant roots; scale in feet. (*Photograph by R. W. Simonson*)

Aquolls. These are wet Mollisols unless they have been drained. Because they were formed under wet conditions, the soils have thick or very thick, nearly black A horizons over gray or mottled B and C horizons. If they have not been drained, the soils may be under water for part of the year, but they are seasonally rather than continually wet (Fig. 10).

Borolls. These are the Mollisols of cool and cold regions. Most areas are in moderately high latitudes or at high altitudes. The soils have fairly thick, nearly black A horizons, dark grayish-brown B horizons, and paler C horizons that are commonly calcareous. The B horizons of some soils have accumulations of clay. These soils are extensive in Canada and the Soviet Union.

Rendolls. These are the Mollisols formed in highly calcareous parent materials, regoliths with more than 40% calcium carbonate. The soils may be calcareous to the surface and must have high levels of carbonates within a depth of 20 in. Rendolls do not have horizons of carbonate accumulation. The profiles consist of dark or very dark A horizons grading into pale C horizons. For the most part, Rendolls are restricted to humid, temperate regions.

Udolls. These are Mollisols of humid, temperate and warm regions where maximum rainfall comes during the growing season. The soils have thick,

very dark A horizons, brown B horizons, and paler C horizons. Throughout the profile these soils are browner than the Borolls and are not as cold. Udolls lack horizons of accumulation of powdery carbonates. Some of the soils have B horizons of clay accumulation and others do not. These soils are major ones of the Corn Belt of the United States (Fig. 11).

Ustolls. These are the Mollisols of temperate and warm climates with lower rainfall than the Udolls. The soils are therefore dry for an appreciable part of each year, usually more than 90 cumulative days. Horizons and their sequence are much the same as for Udolls except that most Ustolls have accumulations of powdery carbonates at depths of 40 in. or less.

Xerolls. These are Mollisols of regions with rainy winters and dry summers. The nature and sequence of horizons are much like those of the Ustolls. The soils are completely dry for a long period each year.

Oxisols. These soils have faint horizonation, though formed in strongly weathered regoliths. The surface layer or A horizon is usually darkened and moderately thick, but there is little evidence of change in the remainder of the profile. Because of the intense or long weathering, the soils consist of resistant minerals such as kaolinite, forms of sesquioxides, and quartz. Weatherable minerals such as feldspars have largely disappeared. Moreover, the clay fraction has limited capacity to retain bases such as calcium and magnesium.

The soils are porous and readily penetrated by water and plant roots. A distinctive feature of Oxisols is the common occurrence of tubular pores about the diameter of ordinary pins extending to depths of 6 ft or more.

Oxisols are largely restricted to tropical and subtropical regions, low to moderate altitudes, and old land surfaces. Those occurring elsewhere in the world seem to be relicts from earlier geologic ages. The soils are formed mostly under humid climates, grading toward semiarid ones in places. Most of the soils were under forest vegetation with some under savanna cover.

The amount of study of soils of tropical regions thus far has been small as compared to the great extent of those regions. Far fewer man-years per 1000 mi² have been given to soil studies in the tropics than in Europe, the United States, or the Soviet Union. As a result, the soils of the tropics are not well known, and this is reflected in the tentative nature of proposed suborders of Oxisols.

Five suborders have been proposed, namely, Aquox, Humox, Orthox, Torrox, and Ustox. These five differ from one another mainly in moisture regimes. The Aquox are wet and the others are not. Humox and Orthox are both moist, but the former is relatively cool with high accumulations of humus. Torrox and Ustox are dry for some part of the year with the former dry for much longer periods (Fig. 12).

Most Oxisols are in forest or savanna and produce little. Many areas are sparsely inhabited, with people largely dependent on shifting cultivation for their food. Some Oxisols are cultivated by operators with access to complex technology and are productive. Even so, methods of management to ensure sustained high yields are still to be developed for the more strongly weathered Oxisols.

Spodosols. These soils have B horizons with accumulations of one or both of organic matter and compounds of aluminum and iron. The accumulated substances are amorphous in nature. They impart red, brown, or black colors to the B horizons, which may have irregular lower boundaries with tongues extending downward a foot or more. If the soil has not been disturbed, the surface layer consists of both fresh and partly decayed litter. This rests on a very pale, leached A2 horizon overlying a highly contrasting B horizon. The Spodosols formed from sands under boreal coniferous forests have some of the most striking profiles in the world. Mostly, the soils are strongly acid because of the small supplies of bases.

Spodosols are most extensive in humid, cool climates, but some occur at low elevations under tropical and subtropical climates. The soils were largely under forest. The bulk of the Spodosols have been formed in sandy regoliths with others in loamy regoliths. Land surfaces are fairly young.

Most Spodosols remain in forest, but some are cultivated in both cool and tropical regions. The variety of crops produced is large because of the wide climatic range under which the soils occur. The range in yields is also wide, being dependent on the combination of climatic conditions and prevailing level of technology. Production is modest

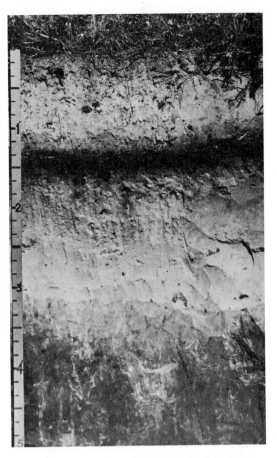

Fig. 13. Profile of an Aquod with distinct A2 horizon, dark B horizon at depth of 18 in., pale C horizon below, and part of a buried profile below 4 ft; soil consists of sand; numbers on scale indicate feet. (*Photograph by R. W. Simonson*)

for most Spodosols under cool climates and simple management. Production is high from some soils cultivated with complex management in tropical climates.

Aquods. These are seasonally wet Spodosols unless drained. The soils may be wet most of each year but not all of the time. The B horizons are black or dark brown in color and some are cemented. Aquods occupy depressional areas or wide flats from which water finds it hard to escape (Fig. 13).

Ferrods. These are well-drained Spodosols having B horizons of iron accumulation with little organic matter. Appearance of the profile is much like that of Orthods.

Humods. These are well-drained Spodosols, having B horizons of humus accumulation, usually black or dark brown in color. Aluminum usually accumulates with the humus but iron is lacking, especially from the upper part of the B horizon. Where formed in white or nearly white sands, the soils have striking profiles, as in parts of western Europe.

Orthods. These are well-drained Spodosols having B horizons of humus, aluminum, and iron accumulation. The B horizons are mostly red or reddish in color and are friable. They grade downward into lighter-colored C horizons which are commonly less friable and may be very firm. Orthods form

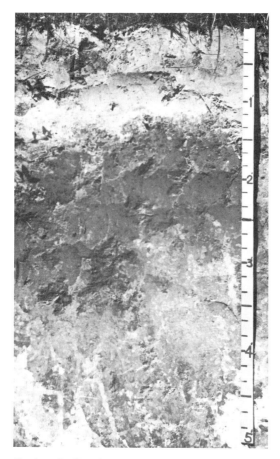

Fig. 14. Profile of a Udult with pale A horizon 16 in. thick, darker B horizon higher in clay and iron oxides, and C horizon near bottom; numbers on scale indicate feet. (*Photograph by R. W. Simonson*)

Fig. 15. Profile of a Ustert with thick, dark A horizon, which is due in part to mixing and churning of soil mass and which grades into the lighter-colored C horizon; scale in feet. (*Photograph by E. H. Templin*)

the most extensive suborder among the Spodosols, being extensive in Canada and the Soviet Union.

Ultisols. Like Alfisols, these soils have A horizons that have lost silicate clays, sesquioxides, and bases. Most A horizons are pale, though not all are. The B horizons have accumulations of silicate clays and low levels of exchangeable calcium and magnesium. The C horizons are usually lighter in color and lower in clay than the B horizons. Combined thickness of the A and B horizons is greater, on the average, for Ultisols than for Alfisols. Ultisols are strongly acid throughout their profiles, reflecting the low levels of exchangeable bases.

Ultisols are most extensive under humid, warm-temperate climates but extend through the tropics. They are not found in cold regions. The largest bodies of the soils are in southeastern Asia, nearby islands, and the southeastern United States. The soils were usually· under forest but some were covered by savanna vegetation. All were formed in strongly weathered regoliths on old land surfaces.

Many Ultisols remain in forest. Among those producing crops, a majority are used under some method of shifting cultivation. Production is limited in such circumstances. On the other hand, the variety of crops and yields obtained can be large if cultivators are in position to apply complex technology to Ultisols.

Aquults. These are seasonally wet Ultisols, saturated with water an important part of the year un-

less drained. Usually the soils have thin, dark A horizons, but they may be as thick as 20 in. Deeper profiles are gray, with or without red mottles. Aquults occur in depressions or on wide upland flats from which water moves very slowly.

Humults. These are well-drained Ultisols formed under rather high rainfall distributed evenly over the year. The soils are high in humus throughout their profiles, and most have darkened A horizons of moderate thickness. Deeper profiles tend to be brown, reddish-brown, or yellowish-brown in color. Humults are common in southeastern Brazil.

Udults. These are well-drained Ultisols of humid, warm-temperate and tropical regions. The soils are low or relatively low in humus and typically have thin, darkened A horizons. The B horizons are yellowish-red, red, brown, or yellowish-brown in color and are fairly thick. Rainfall is high enough and distributed evenly enough over the year so that the soils are dry for only short periods. Udults are major soils in the southeastern parts of the United States and Asia (Fig. 14), and their total extent is large.

Ustults. These are well-drained Ultisols of warm-temperate and tropical climates with moderate or low rainfall. The soils are like the Udults in general appearance but are dry for appreciable periods each year. Examples of Ustults may be found in northeastern Australia. Total extent of the suborder is appreciably less than that of Udults.

The Xerults are similar to Ustults in general appearance and composition but occur in regions with rainy winters and dry summers. The soils become dry every summer for a long period.

Vertisols. These soils have faint horizonation for two main reasons. In the first place, Vertisols are formed in regoliths that are high in clay and therefore resistant to change.

In the second place, the clay fraction in the soils has high levels of activity. The soils are therefore subject to marked swelling and shrinking as they wet and dry. Cracks extending to the surface are formed as the soil becomes dry. When rains come again, soil materials from the surface are washed into such cracks. As the mass rewets and swells, it cannot reoccupy the space of the partially filled cracks. Part of the mass must therefore move upward. As such movement continues over long periods, overturning and mixing of the soil tends to offset horizon differentiation. Vertisols have therefore been called "self-swallowing," and it has also been said that the soils "plow themselves."

Vertisols exhibit little change from top to bottom of the profile. Most have darkened surface layers that are thick, and many are calcareous at some depth. All are low in organic matter and high in bases. Most of the Vertisols are neutral or mildly alkaline in reaction because of the high supplies of bases.

Vertisols occur in warm-temperate and tropical climates with one or more dry seasons. The soils were under savanna vegetation for the most part with a few in forest. Land surfaces are old or fairly old. Large bodies of Vertisols are found on the Deccan Plateau of India and in the Gezira Plain of the Sudan.

Because they are high in active clays, Vertisols are hard to cultivate. The soils therefore remain in savanna in many places, and the savannas are used for grazing or left alone. Large areas of the soils are cultivated, some with simple, bullock-drawn implements and others with large machinery. A wide variety of crops is produced, but yields are generally modest, especially for cultivators dependent on simple technology. The soils will, however, produce crops indefinitely under simple management.

The Vertisols are subdivided into four suborders, namely, Torrerts, Uderts, Usterts, and Xererts. These are set apart by differences in moisture regimes. Torrerts are restricted to arid regions and are dry most of the time, becoming wet occasionally. Uderts are formed under humid climates but are dry for short periods of time. Usterts are dry for an appreciable period or for more than one period each year, though not as long as Torrerts. Xererts are restricted to regions with rainy winters and dry summers. They become wet each winter and dry again each summer. Soils of the several suborders are alike in the general appearance of their profiles and also similar in many ways in their composition (Fig. 15).

Great soil groups. The great soil groups were a widely used set of broad classes in the classification system followed in the United States from 1938 to 1965. The principal great soil groups were described briefly in the first edition (1960) of this encyclopedia. For the benefit of those familiar with the great soil groups of the earlier system, the proximate distribution among present suborders and orders of the great soil groups is given in Table 2. Major soils of each great soil group were considered in preparing the table.   [ROY W. SIMONSON]

Soil, zonality of

Many soils that are geographically associated on plains have common properties that are the result of formation in similar climates with similar vegetation. Because climate determines the natural vegetation to a large extent and because climate changes gradually with distance on plains, there are vast zones of uplands on which most soils have many common properties. This was first observed in Russia toward the end of the 19th century by V. V. Dokuchaev, the father of modern soil science. He also observed that on floodplains and steep slopes and in wet places the soils commonly lacked some or most of the properties of the upland soils. In mountainous areas, climate and vegetation tend to vary with altitude, and here the Russian students observed that many soils at the same altitude had many common properties. This they called vertical zonality in contrast with the lateral zonality of the soils of plains.

Zonal classification of soils. These observations led N. M. Sivirtsev to propose about 1900 that major kinds of soil could be classified as Zonal if their properties reflected the influence of climate and vegetation, as Azonal if they lacked well-defined horizons, and as Intrazonal if their properties resulted from some local factor such as a shallow groundwater or unusual parent material.

This concept was not accepted for long in Russia. It was adopted in the United States in 1938 as a basis for classifying soil but was dropped in 1965. This was because the Zonal soils as a class could not be defined in terms of their properties and because they had no common properties that were not shared by some Intrazonal and Azonal soils. It

Table 2. Proximate distribution of soils of former great soil groups among suborders and orders

Great soil group	Principal suborders or orders
Alluvial soils	Fluvents, Orthents, Aquepts, Aquolls, Borolls, Udolls, Ustolls
Alpine Meadow soils	Umbrepts, Aquolls, Borolls
Ando soils	Andepts
Bog soils	Histosols
Brown soils	Ustolls, Borolls, Argids, Orthids, Ochrepts
Brown Forest soils	Ochrepts, Rendolls, Udolls
Brown Podzolic soils	Orthods, Ochrepts
Brunizems	Udolls, Xerolls
Calcisols	Orthids, Ochrepts, Aquolls, Borolls
Chernozems	Borolls, Ustolls, Udolls, Xerolls
Chestnut soils	Ustolls, Borolls, Xerolls
Desert soils	Argids, Orthids
Gray-Brown Podzolic soils	Udalfs, Udults
Gray Wooded soils	Boralfs
Groundwater Podzols	Aquods
Groundwater Laterite soils	Oxisols, Ultisols
Grumusols	Vertisols
Humic-Gley soils	Aquolls, Aquepts, Aquults
Latosols	Inceptisols, Oxisols, Ultisols
Lithosols	Entisols, Inceptisols, Mollisols
Low Humic-Gley soils	Aquepts, Aquults, Aqualfs, Aquox
Noncalcic Brown soils	Xeralfs
Planosols	Aqualfs, Albolls
Podzols	Spodosols
Reddish-Brown soils	Argids, Orthids, Ochrepts
Reddish-Brown Lateritic soils	Humults, Udults
Red-Yellow Podzolic soils	Udults
Reddish Chestnut soils	Ustalfs, Ustolls, Xeralfs, Ochrepts
Red Desert soils	Argids, Orthids
Reddish Prairie soils	Udolls, Ustolls
Regosols	Entisols, Inceptisols, Mollisols
Rendzinas	Rendolls
Sierozems	Orthids, Argids
Solonchak soils	Orthids, Orthents
Solonetz soils	Aridisols, Alfisols, Mollisols
Soloth soils	Mollisols
Sols Bruns Acides	Ochrepts, Orthents
Subarctic Brown Forest soils	Ochrepts
Tundra soils	Inceptisols, Spodosols
Yellowish-Brown Lateritic soils	Humults, Udults

was also learned that many of the properties that had been thought to reflect climate were actually the result of differences in age of the soils and of past climates that differed greatly from those of the present.

Zonality of soil distribution is important to students of geography in understanding differences in farming, grazing, and forestry practices in different parts of the world. To a very large extent, zonality is reflected but is not used directly in the soil classification currently being used in the United States. The Entisols include most soils formerly called Azonal. Most of the soils formerly called Intrazonal are included in the orders of Vertisols, Inceptisols, and Histosols and in the aquic suborders such as Aquolls and Aqualfs. Zonal soils are mainly included in the other suborders in this classification. For a discussion of this classification *see* SOIL.

The soil orders and suborders have been defined largely in terms of the common properties that result from soil formation in similar climates with similar vegetation. Because these properties are important to the native vegetation, they have continuing importance to farming, ranching, and forestry. Also, because the properties are common to most of the soils of a given area, it is possible to make small-scale maps that show the distribution of soil orders and suborders with high accuracy. For an example of such a map *see* SOIL, SUBORDERS OF.

Zonal properties of soils. A few examples of zonal properties of soils and their relation to soil use follow. The Mollisols, formerly called Chernozemic soils, are rich in plant nutrients. Their natural ability to supply plant nutrients is the highest of any group of soils, but lack of moisture often limits plant growth. Among the Mollisols, the Udolls are associated with a humid climate and are used largely for corn (maize) and soybean production. Borolls have a cool climate and are used for spring wheat, flax, and other early maturing crops. Ustolls have a dry, warm climate and are used largely for winter wheat and sorghum without irrigation. Yields are erratic on these soils. They are moderately high in moist years, but crop failures are common in dry years. The drier Ustolls are used largely for grazing. Xerolls have a rainless summer, and crops must mature on moisture stored in the cool seasons. Xerolls are used largely for wheat and produce consistent yields.

The Alfisols, formerly a part of the Podzolic soil group, are lower in plant nutrients than Mollisols, particularly nitrogen and calcium, but supported a permanent agriculture before the development of fertilizers. With the use of modern fertilizers, yields of crops are comparable to those obtained on Mollisols. The Udalfs are largely in intensive cultivation and produce high yields of a wide variety of crops. Boralfs, like Borolls, have short growing seasons but have humid climates. They are used largely for small grains or forestry. Ustalfs are warm and dry for long periods. In the United States they are used for grazing, small grains, and irrigated crops. On other continents they are mostly intensively cultivated during the rainy season. Population density on Ustalfs in Africa is very high except in the areas of the tsetse fly. Xeralfs are used largely for wheat production or grazing because of their dry summers.

Ultisols, formerly called Latosolic soils, are warm, intensely leached, and very low in supplies of plant nutrients. Before the use of fertilizers, Ultisols could be farmed for only a few years after clearing and then had to revert to forest for a much longer period to permit the trees to concentrate plant nutrients at the surface in the leaf litter. With the use of fertilizers, Udults produce high yields of cotton, tobacco, maize, and forage. Ustults are dry for long periods but have good moisture supplies during a rainy season, typically during monsoon rains. Forests are deciduous, and cultivation is mostly shifting unless fertilizers are available.

Aridisols, formerly called Desertic soils, are high in some plant nutrients, particularly calcium and potassium, but are too dry to cultivate without irrigation. They are used for grazing to some extent, but large areas are idle. Under irrigation some Aridisols are highly productive, but large areas are unsuited to irrigation or lack sources of water.   [GUY D. SMITH]

Bibliography: M. Baldwin, C. E. Kellogg, and J. Thorp, Soil classification, in USDA, *Soils and Men: The Yearbook of Agriculture*, 1938; B. T. Bunting, *The Geography of Soil*, 1965; H. C. Byers et al., Formation of soil, in USDA, *Soils and Men: The Yearbook of Agriculture*, 1938; C. E. Kellogg, Soil and society, in USDA, *Soils and Men: The Yearbook of Agriculture*, 1938.

Soil balance, microbial

The equilibrium between the diverse types of microorganisms in soil. Although the qualitative and quantitative composition of the soil microflora and microfauna fluctuates with temperature, moisture, and treatment (such as fertilization, cultivation, and cropping) of the soil, a balance exists which is characteristic of a given soil. The balance is determined chiefly by the available supply of nutrients required by groups of microorganisms of different nutritional needs. The numbers and types of the microorganisms also depend on the available nutrient supply. Associative and antagonistic effects exerted by certain organisms on others are factors in establishing the balance. The equilibrium is not easily upset. Natural soil resists balance change when organisms are introduced.

Associative action. The process whereby one type of microorganism produces a substance required by another is widespread in soil. This action may be extended through successive groups to give a chain effect. Thus ammonia formed through decomposition of proteins by proteolytic microorganisms is used by nitrite-forming bacteria. Nitrite is required by nitrate-forming bacteria. Many cellulose-decomposing organisms utilize nitrate in hydrolyzing cellulose, and form glucose and organic acids which may be used by still other forms. Many soil bacteria synthesize vitamins needed by other organisms. Syntrophism is a form of associative action in which two organisms are mutually dependent, each producing a factor needed by the other.

Antagonisms between soil microbes. These are a factor in maintaining the equilibrium and are manifested in different ways. Many protozoa depend upon bacteria for food and ingest certain species in preference to others. Antagonism may rest on a competition for nutrients. It may also depend upon the production of substances inhibitory to other organisms, particularly antibiotics. Though synthesized only in small amounts, the antibiotics exert their effects in the microenvironments in which soil microbes are active. The advantage possessed by such microorganisms does not lead to their predominance, since capacity for antibiotic production is but one factor in the competition with other microbes. *See* RHIZOSPHERE; SOIL MICROBIOLOGY.   [ALLAN G. LOCHHEAD]

Soil chemistry

The study of the composition and chemical properties of soil. Soil chemistry involves the detailed investigation of the nature of the solid matter from which soil is constituted and of the chemical processes that occur as a result of the action of hydrological, geological, and biological agents on the solid matter. Because of the broad diversity among soil components and the complexity of soil chemical processes, the application of a wide variety of concepts and methods employed in the chemistry of aqueous solutions, of amorphous and crystalline solids, and of solid surfaces is required. For a general discussion of the origin and classification of soils *see* SOIL; SOIL, SUBORDERS OF.

Elemental composition. The elemental composition of soil varies over a wide range, permitting only a few general statements to be made. Those soils that contain less than 12–20% organic carbon are termed mineral. (The exact percentage to consider in a specific case depends on drainage characteristics and clay content of the soil.) All other soils are termed organic. Carbon, oxygen, hydrogen, nitrogen, phosphorus, and sulfur are the most important constituents of organic soils and of soil organic matter in general. Carbon, oxygen, and hydrogen are most abundant; the content of nitrogen is often about one-tenth that of carbon, while the content of phosphorus or sulfur is usually less than one-fifth that of nitrogen (Table 1). The number of organic compounds into which these elements are incorporated in soil is very large, and the elucidation of the chemistry of soil organic matter remains a challenging problem.

Besides oxygen, the most abundant elements found in mineral soils are silicon, aluminum, and iron (Table 2). The distribution of chemical elements will vary considerably from soil to soil and, in general, will be different in a specific soil from the distribution of elements in the crustal rocks of the Earth. Often this difference may be understood in terms of pedogenic weathering processes and the chemical reactions that accompany them. Some examples are the illuvial accumulation of aluminum and iron oxides in the B horizon of a Spodosol and of $CaCO_3$ in the calcic horizon of a Mollisol. The most important micro or trace elements in soil are boron, copper, manganese, molybdenum, and zinc, since these elements are essential in the nutrition of green plants. Also important are cobalt, which is essential in animal nutrition, and selenium, cadmium, and nickel, which may accumulate to toxic levels in soil. The average distribution of trace elements in soil is not greatly different from that in crustal rocks (Table 3). This indicates that the total content of a trace element in soil usually reflects the content of that element in the soil parent material and, generally, that the trace element content of soil often is not affected substantially by pedochemical processes.

The elemental composition of soil varies with depth below the surface because of pedochemical weathering. The principal processes of this type that result in the removal of chemical elements from a given soil horizon are: (1) soluviation (ordinary dissolution in water), (2) cheluviation (complexation by organic or inorganic ligands), (3) reduction, and (4) suspension. Soluviation, cheluviation, and reduction include leaching by water into lower horizons; suspension involves removal by erosion or by translocation downward along soil pores. The principal effect of these four processes is the appearance of illuvial horizons in which compounds such as aluminum and iron oxides, aluminosilicates, or calcium carbonate have been precipitated from solution or deposited from suspension.

Minerals. The minerals in soils are the products of physical, geochemical, and pedochemical weathering. Soil minerals may be either amorphous or crystalline. They may be classified further, approximately, as primary or secondary minerals, depending on whether they are inherited from parent rock or are produced by chemical

Table 1. Average percentages of total carbon, total nitrogen, and organic phosphorus in selected soils

Soil	% C	% N	% P
Sand	2.5	.23	.04
Fine sandy loam	3.3	.23	.06
Medium loam	2.3	.22	.05
Clay loam, well drained	4.6	.36	.10
Clay loam, poorly drained	8.0	.43	.05
Peat	46.1	1.32	.03

Table 2. Average percentages of the major and some micro elements in subsurface soil clays and crustal rocks

Soil order:	Alfisol	Inceptisol	Mollisol	Oxisol	Spodosol	Ultisol	Crustal rocks
Si	19.20	24.69	23.01	12.43	5.79	16.02	27.72
Al	12.38	19.61	10.29	19.33	15.86	17.49	8.13
Fe	8.04	3.81	6.83	10.83	3.29	11.96	5.00
Ca	.69	.00	3.59	.10	.29	.15	3.63
Mg	1.26	.40	1.62	.46	.15	.08	2.09
Na	.18	2.52	.04	.00	.27	.06	2.83
K	3.63	n.d.	1.20	.07	.40	.22	2.59
Ti	.40	.28	.44	1.32	.16	.50	.44
Mn	.06	n.d.	.06	.08	.06	.05	.10
P	.14	n.d.	.14	.27	.17	.12	.11

Table 3. Average amounts of trace elements commonly found in soils and crustal rocks

Trace element	Soil, ppm*	Crustal rocks, ppm
As	6	1.8
B	10	10
Cd	.06	.2
Co	8	25
Cr	100	100
Cu	20	55
Mo	2	1.5
Ni	40	75
Pb	10	13
Se	.2	.05
V	100	135
Zn	50	70

*ppm = parts per million.

weathering, respectively.

Primary minerals in soil. The bulk of the primary minerals that occur in soil are found in the silicate minerals, such as the olivines, garnets, pyroxenes, amphiboles, micas, feldspars, and quartz. The feldspars, micas, amphiboles, and pyroxenes commonly are hosts for trace elements that may be released slowly into the soil solution as weathering of these minerals continues. Chemical weathering of the silicate minerals is responsible for producing the most important secondary minerals in soil. The general scheme of the weathering sequence is shown in Fig. 1.

Secondary minerals in soil. The important sec-

ondary minerals that occur in soil are found in the clay fraction. These include aluminum and iron hydrous oxides (usually in the form of coatings on other minerals), carbonates, and aluminosilicates. The term "allophane" is applied to the x-ray amorphous, hydrous aluminosilicates that are characterized by variable composition, the presence of Si-O-Al bonds, and a differential thermal analysis curve displaying only a low-temperature endotherm and a high-temperature exotherm. The significant crystalline aluminosilicates possess a layer structure; they are chlorite, halloysite, kaolinite, montmorillonite (smectite), and vermiculite. These clay minerals are identified in soil by means of the characteristic x-ray diffraction patterns they produce after certain pretreatments, although their positive identification may be difficult if two or more of the minerals are present at once.

The distribution of secondary minerals varies among different soils and changes with depth below the surface of a given soil. However, under a leaching, well-oxidized environment, soil minerals do possess a differential susceptibility to decomposition, transformation, and disappearance from a soil profile. This has made possible the arrangement of the clay-sized soil minerals in the order of increasing resistance to chemical weathering. Those minerals ranked near the top of the following list are present, therefore, in the clay fractions of slightly-weathered soils; those minerals near the bottom of the list occur in extensively weathered soils.

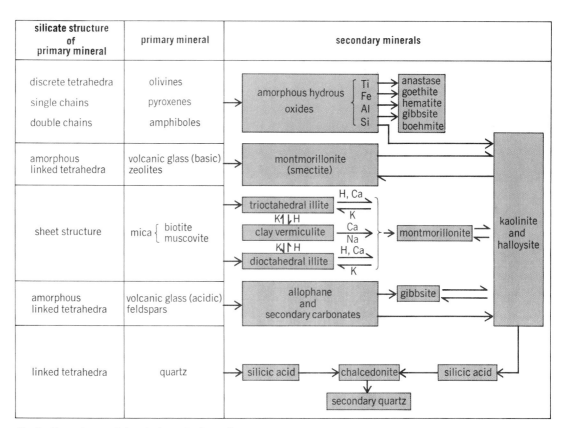

Fig. 1. The scheme of chemical weathering to form secondary minerals from primary silicate minerals. (*Modified from M. Fieldes and L. D. Swindale, Chemical weathering of silicates in soil formation, J. Sci. Tech. New Zealand,* 56:140–154, 1954)

Weathering index	Clay-sized minerals
1	Gypsum, halite
2	Calcite, apatite
3	Olivine, pyroxene
4	Biotite, mafic chlorite
5	Albite, microcline
6	Quartz
7	Muscovite, illite, sericite
8	Vermiculite
9	Montmorillonite, Al-chlorite
10	Kaolinite, allophane
11	Gibbsite, boehmite
12	Hematite, goethite
13	Anatase, rutile, zircon

Table 4. CEC values in meq/100 g for some soil textural classes and clay mineral compounds

Soil texture	CEC	Soil mineral	CEC
Sand	1–5	Allophane	25–70
Fine sandy loam	5–10	Chlorite	10–40
Loam or silt loam	5–25	Halloysite	5–50
Clay loam	15–30+	Illite	10–40
Clay (mineral soil)	≥25	Kaolinite	3–15
Clay (14% organic)	23	Smectite	80–150
Clay (39% organic)	76	Vermiculite	100–150+
Clay (100% organic)	150–600	Al, Fe hydrous oxides	≃4

In zonal soils of humid-cool to subhumid-temperate regions, illite is the predominant clay mineral. Mixtures of kaolinite, vermiculite, and interstratified clay minerals are found in humid-temperate regions. In humid-warm regions, kaolinite, halloysite, allophane, gibbsite, and amorphous analogs of goethite are found. The mineralogical composition of the highly weathered and leached soils of the humid tropics is a subject of active investigation, in part because these soils (the Oxisols and Ultisols) constitute approximately one-third of the world's potentially arable land. The soil minerals are dominated by iron and aluminum hydrous oxides, kaolinite, halloysite, and quartz. Amorphous weathering residues of kaolinite and halloysite also are found in thin coatings on clay particle surfaces, and Al-chlorite (montmorillonite with interlayer Al-hydroxy polymers) is frequently encountered.

The chemical conditions favoring the genesis of kaolinite are the removal of Na^+, K^+, Ca^{2+}, Mg^{2+}, and Fe^{2+} by leaching, the addition of H^+ in fresh water, and a high Al-Si molar ratio. Smectite (montmorillonite) is favored by the retention of the basic cations (arid conditions or poor drainage) and of silica.

Cation exchange. A portion of the chemical elements in soil is in the form of cations that are not components of inorganic salts but that can be replaced reversibly by the cations of leaching salt solutions or acids. These cations are said to be exchangeable, and their total quantity, usually expressed in units of milliequivalents (meq) per 100 g of dry soil, is termed the cation exchange capacity (CEC) of the soil. The CEC ordinarily is measured by leaching a known amount of soil with a salt solution, such as 1 N ammonium acetate at pH 7.0, followed by an additional leaching with isopropyl alcohol to remove the residual salt, then determining the quantity of replacing cation (such as NH_4^+) in the soil. However, this is an arbitrary procedure, since the quantity of cation remaining after such treatment does not have a unique value characteristic of the soil alone, but depends as well on the concentration, the ionic composition, and the pH of the leaching solution. The CEC of a soil generally will vary directly with the amounts of clay and organic matter present and with the distribution of clay minerals (Table 4).

Soils which are less weathered because of recent origin, low precipitation, or temperate to cold climate have as exchangeable cations largely calcium and magnesium. Some soils of dry areas contain significant amounts of exchangeable sodium. Extensively weathered soils, unless formed from basic parent material, have 20–95% of their exchangeable cations as aluminum. Prolonged leaching with fresh water supplies H^+ ions that eventually penetrate and disrupt the structures of soil aluminosilicates, thereby releasing aluminum cations, some of which remain in exchangeable form. The distributions of exchangeable cations for representative soils are shown in Fig. 2.

The chemical equilibrium between exchangeable cations and cations in a leaching solution may be expressed by Eq. (1), where ν is a stoichiometric

$$\nu_A A(ex) + \nu_B B \rightleftharpoons \nu'_A A + \nu'_B B(ex) \qquad (1)$$

coefficient, and A or B refers to a cation species, such as Na^+ or Ca^{2+}. Generally speaking, the equilibrium will shift to the right if cation B has a greater charge or a smaller hydrated radius than cation A. The relative affinity of a soil for cation species B may be described formally by the law of mass action as applied to exchange equilibrium equation (2), where K is an equilibrium constant and a is a

$$K = \frac{a_{B(ex)}^{\nu'_B} a_A^{\nu'_A}}{a_{A(ex)}^{\nu_A} a_B^{\nu_B}} \qquad (2)$$

thermodynamic activity. The applicability of this equation to soils depends on whether it is possible (1) to divide the soil-solution system into "solution" and "exchanger" phases and (2) to define unambiguously the meaning of the activity ratio $a_{B(ex)}^{\nu'_B}/a_{A(ex)}^{\nu'_A}$. Different forms of the expression for

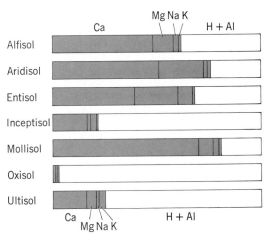

Fig. 2. The typical distributions of exchangeable cations in some soil orders. The shaded regions refer to exchangeable bases.

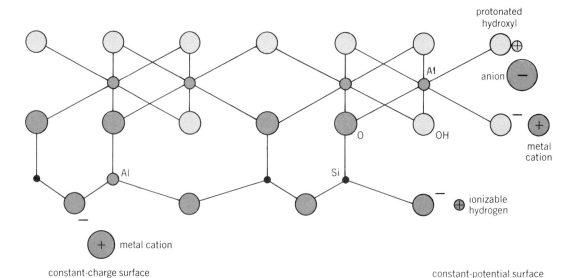

Fig. 3. An idealized diagram of the kaolinite structure showing exchange sites at constant-charge absorbing surfaces (isomorphous-substitution) and constant-potential absorbing surfaces (pH-dependent).

K have been developed on the basis of different interpretations of requirements 1 and 2. For example, if the activities of the exchangeable cations are set equal to mole fractions and the activity ratio $a_A^{\nu'A}/a_B^{\nu'B}$ is set equal to its value in the leaching solution, the expression for K is known as Vanselow's equation. The parameter K then is termed a selectivity coefficient and, in principle, may vary with the solution activity ratio. If the exchangeable cation activities are replaced by equivalents per unit mass of dry soil and the activities in solution are replaced by molar concentrations, the expression for K (again a selectivity coefficient) becomes Gapon's equation. Published data on these kinds of special cases demonstrate that the selectivity coefficients take on constant values only over a limited range of solution concentrations. The development of practicable cation exchange equations with broad applicability remains a challenging problem in soil chemistry.

Isomorphic substitution in clay minerals. One of the most important sources of cation exchange capacity in soils is the negative charge that occurs on clay mineral surfaces because of isomorphic substitution (see Fig. 3). The replacement of Si^{4+} in the tetrahedral sheet by Al^{3+} or of Al^{3+} in the octahedral sheet by Mg^{2+} and Fe^{2+} results in a permanent, negative surface charge on the clay mineral structure. This charge can be balanced by the creation of structural OH groups out of O ions or by the filling of more than two-thirds of the cation positions in the octahedral sheet; however, more commonly charge neutrality is achieved by the adsorption of cations between structural layers on the mineral cleavage surfaces. In kaolinite and illite, isomorphous substitution occurs primarily in the tetrahedral sheet. Because the extent of this substitution is very small in kaolinite and because, in general, cations bonded through a charge deficit in the tetrahedral sheet are held very strongly, the CEC of kaolinite and illite is not large. On the other hand, the CEC of the smectites and vermiculite is relatively large. Extensive isomorphous substitution occurs in the octahedral sheets of these

clay minerals, and the resultant electrostatic force bonding the cations adsorbed on the cleavage surface is weak, since it must act through a relatively greater distance than in the case of substitution in a tetrahedral sheet. Interlayer potassium ions in soil micas, illite, and vermiculite, however, usually are not readily exchangeable, both because of the source of the negative charge binding them and because K^+ does not hydrate easily and fits almost perfectly into the hexagonal cavities in the cleavage surfaces of these minerals.

Ionizable hydroxyl groups in clay minerals. At the edges of the structural layers in the crystalline clay minerals and on the surfaces of the amorphous clay minerals, OH groups may be found bonded to exposed Si^{4+} or Al^{3+} cations (Fig. 3). These hydroxyl groups can act as weak Brönsted acids, ionizing in aqueous solution when the pH is sufficiently high. Thus a pH-dependent, negative surface charge can develop that will contribute to the CEC. The mineral surfaces for which this pH-dependence occurs are termed constant-potential adsorbing surfaces, as opposed to the constant-charge adsorbing surfaces generated by isomorphous substitution. The pH value at which the surface charge on a constant-potential adsorbent vanishes is called the zero point of charge (ZPC). ZPC for any soil mineral depends on its composition and defect structure, as well as on the nature of the surrounding electrolyte solution; a value of ZPC between 4 and 6 is common. The maximum negative charge generally is observed at about pH 10. The magnitude of the negative charge developed at a given pH value depends on the extent to which the clay mineral particles possess surfaces bearing ionizable OH groups. For montmorillonite the pH-dependent CEC may be 20% of the total CEC; for illite it may be 50%, while for kaolinite and allophane it may be essentially 100%.

Ionizable functional groups in organic matter. The organic matter in soil contains two types of functional groups that contribute importantly to the CEC: aromatic and aliphatic carboxyls and phenolic hydroxyls. When the pH is greater than 6, these acidic groups ionize in aqueous solution and provide a source of negative charge for metal cation adsorption. The cations of metals in groups IA and IIA (for example, Na^+ and Ca^{2+}) of the periodic table are readily exchangeable after adsorption by soil organic matter, whereas those of the transition metals and of the metals in groups IB and IIB (for example, Fe^{3+} and Cu^{2+}) often are not. The contribution to the CEC from organic functional groups can be as large as 600 meq per 100 g organic matter at high pH values.

Anion exchange. The stoichiometric exchange of the anions in soil for those in a leaching salt solution is a phenomenon of relatively small importance in the general scheme of anion reactions with soils. Under acid conditions (pH < 5) the exposed hydroxyl groups at the edges of the structural sheets or on the surfaces of clay-sized particles become protonated and thereby acquire a positive charge. The degree of protonation is a sensitive function of pH, the ionic strength of the leaching solution, and the nature of the clay-sized particle. The magnitude of the anion exchange capacity (AEC) usually varies from near 0 at pH 7 for any soil colloid to as much as 50 meq per 100 g of allophanic clay at about pH 4. Smectite and other clay minerals with high, pH-invariant CEC values do not adsorb exchangeable anions to any degree unless the ionic strength of the leaching solution is very large. The AEC may be measured conveniently by shaking a 5 gm sample of soil for 1 hr in 20 ml 0.17 N $AlCl_3$, filtering, and determining the amount of Cl in the filtrate. AEC is then the difference, per 100 g of soil, between the initial amount of Cl and that in the filtrate.

Negative anion adsorption. Soils whose CEC is approximately independent of pH often display a significant negative adsorption of anions: The concentration of anions in a solution separated from a soil suspension by a membrane permeable to electrolyte is larger than that of the anions in the liquid phase of the suspension. This phenomenon may be understood simply on the basis of the presence of a permanent negative charge on the surface of the solid-phase particles in the suspension. This surface charge attracts cations and repels anions. The principal effects of this repulsion are to reduce the AEC and to increase the ease with which anions may be leached from a soil. If the solution concentration of anions becomes very high, the ionic strength will be high and the concentrations of anion in solution and in the suspension will tend to become equal, if the activity of the anion in solution decreases more than that of the anion in the suspension.

Specific anion adsorption and reprecipitation. Anion exchange in the classic sense applies primarily to halide and nitrate ions. For other ions, in particular, borate, molybdate, sulfate, and orthophosphate, the reaction with the solid matter in soil involves an irreversible specific adsorption or decomposition-reprecipitation. The *o*-phosphate ion, for example, can react with the accessible aluminum hydroxy ions of clay minerals and with hydrous aluminum and iron oxides in soil to form x-ray amorphous analogs of the known crystalline aluminum and iron phosphate minerals. The nature and extent of this reaction are strongly dependent on pH, the metal cations in solution, the acidi-

ty of the added phosphate compound, and the structure of the solid phase with which the phosphate ion reacts. Under conditions of a relatively high pH, low acidity of the added phosphate, or high degree of crystallinity of the solid phase reactant, PO_4^{3-} will tend to be "specifically adsorbed" by Al or Fe ions at the surface of the solid. If these conditions are reversed, the combination of PO_4^{3-} with the solid phase may result in a nearly complete destruction of the reactant solid and the formation of an amorphous Al- or Fe-phosphate. In this case, the reaction is more properly termed a "reprecipitation" of the Al or Fe. With either case, the fundamental chemical process is the same. This is an area of active research in soil chemistry.

Soil solution. The solution in the pore space of soil acquires its chemical properties through time-varying inputs and outputs of matter and energy that are mediated by the several parts of the hydrologic cycle and by processes originating in the biosphere (Fig. 4). The soil solution thus is a dynamic and open natural water system whose composition reflects the many reactions that can occur simultaneously between an aqueous solution and an assembly of mineral and organic solid phases that varies with both time and space. This type of complexity is not matched normally in any chemical laboratory experiment, but nonetheless must be amenable to analysis in terms of chemical principles. An understanding of the soil solution in terms of chemical properties has proven to be essential to progress in the maintenance of soil fertility and the quality of runoff and drainage waters.

Chemical speciation of macrosolutes. The macrosolute composition of a soil solution will vary depending on pH, pε (negative common logarithm of the electron activity), organic matter content, input of chemical elements from the biosphere (including humans), and effectiveness of leaching. Under conditions of near-neutral pH, high pε, low organic matter content, no solute input from agriculture, and good but not excessive drainage, the expected macrosolutes are Ca, K, Mg, Na, Cl, HCO_3, $Si(OH)_4$, and SO_4. If the pH is low, H and Al should be added to this list; if it is high, CO_3 should be added. If the soil has been fertilized, NO_3 and H_2PO_4 become important. If the drainage is excessive, Al may be abundant and one or more of the solutes in the original list may be insignificant. If the drainage is poor and, therefore, the pε is low, SO_4 will be replaced by S and CO_3 should be added. If the organic matter content is high,

Table 5. Chemical speciation in percent of the macrosolutes in the soil solution of a well-drained, sandy soil as computed from data on total concentrations and pH using complex stability constants

Metal	Free	Complexed with		
		Cl	HCO_3	SO_4
Ca	68.9	0	1.0	30.1
K	94.1	0	0	5.9
Mg	73.5	0	1.0	25.5
Na	96.8	0	0.2	3.1

*Input data: $pCa_T = 1.47$, $pK_T = 4.10$, $pMg_T = 1.74$; $pNa_T = 1.94$, pH = 6.8, $pCl_T = 1.92$; $pCO_{3T} = 2.51$, $pSO_{4T} = 1.35$.

Table 6. Trace element concentration ranges and median values in the saturation extracts of 30 California soil series

Element	Range, ppm*	Median value, ppm
B	<.1 – 26.0	<.1
Co	<.01 – .14	<.01
Cr	<.01 – .017	<.01
Cu	<.01 – .2	.03
Fe	<.01 – .8	.03
Hg	.0002 – .011	.001
Mn	<.01 – .95	<.01
Mo	<.01 – 22.0	<.01
Ni	<.01 – .09	<.01
Pb	<.01 – .30	<.01
Ti	<.1	<.1
Zn	.01 – .40	.04

*ppm = parts per million.

organic solutes become important. Combinations of these different environmental conditions will change the original list of solutes in still other ways (for example low pϵ and nitrogen fertilizer addition would add NH_4 to the list).

The chemical speciation of the macrosolutes (that is, their distribution among the free-ionic, complexed, precipitated, and adsorbed forms) depends on the nature of the solid matter in the soil, the composition of metals and ligands in solution and their concentration, and the pϵ value. Clearly the macrosolutes themselves are interdependent in determining their speciation, and even

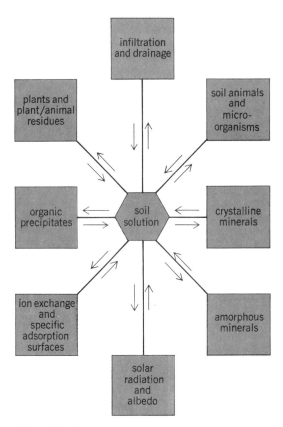

Fig. 4. The factors influencing the chemistry of the soil solution. (*Modified from J. F. Hodgson, Chemistry of the micronutrients in soils, Adv. Agron., 15:141, 1963*)

the three factors just mentioned cannot be considered in complete isolation from one another. Nevertheless, it is possible to make some very broad statements about the macrochemical species to be expected by employing the principle of hard and soft acids and bases (HSAB).

The macrosolute metal cations are hard acids. This means that they generally tend to form chemical bonds of a simple electrostatic type and, therefore, that their reactivities with any ligand (including a mineral surface) should be predictable on the basis of ionic charge and radius along with their common property of low polarizability. In a soil solution, the macrosolute metal cations will tend to: (1) form complexes and sparingly soluble precipitates primarily with oxygen-containing ligands (hard bases), such as H_2O, OH^-, HCO_3^{2-}, CO_3^{2-}, $H_2PO_4^-$, PO_4^{3-}, SO_4^{2-}, and constant-charge, nonhydroxylated mineral surfaces, the stabilities of these complexes will tend to increase with the ratio of ionic charge to ionic radius (or hydration radius) of the metal; usually no reaction will occur with soft or nearly soft bases such as S^{2-} and Cl^-; (2) form complexes with carboxyl groups, but not with organic ligands containing only nitrogen and sulfur electron donors.

These generalizations make it possible to enumerate the probable complexes and precipitates of the macrosolute metals in a soil solution of known composition (including adsorbing surfaces). The exact speciation of the metals then can be calculated if stability constants are available for the expected chemical reactions. A simple example of this type of calculation is shown in Table 5. Usually a large set of nonlinear equations must be solved on a digital computer and ionic strength corrections must be performed.

Chemical speciation of microsolutes. The important microsolutes in the soil include the trace metals, such as Fe, Cu, and Zn, and the trace element oxyanions, such as those formed by As, B, Mo, and Se. The common ranges and median values of trace element concentrations in soil solutions are listed in Table 6. The tableau of microsolutes in a given soil solution is more dependent on inputs from the lithosphere and the biosphere (particularly humans) and less on proton or electron activity and hydrologic factors than is the composition of macrosolutes. The trace metals present, for example, usually are derived from the chemical weathering of specific parent rocks, from the application of fertilizers, pesticides, and urban wastes, and from air pollution.

The most general features of the chemical speciation of the microsolutes also may be predicted on the basis of the HSAB principle. The trace metal cations are soft or nearly soft acids, and the trace element anions are hard or nearly hard bases. The exception to this statement is Fe^{3+}, which is a hard acid. This means that the trace metal cations, except for Fe^{3+}, will tend to form chemical bonds of a covalent type whose strength will depend much more on detailed electronic structural considerations than on cationic size or charge. For the anions, the implication is that they will combine strongly with hard-acid metal cations, just as do other oxygen-containing ligands. The trace metal speciation thus presents a more complicated problem than does that of the macrosolute metals.

Generally, the trace metal cations in a soil solution will: (1) form complexes and insoluble precipitates more readily with the inorganic ligands Cl^- and S^{2-} and with sites on mineral surfaces that can bind covalently, than with oxyanions; stronger complexes also will form more readily with organic functional groups containing S, P, and N donors than with carboxyl groups; (2) tend to follow the Irving-Williams order in regard to the stabilities of strong complexes: $Mn^{2+} < Fe^{2+} < Co^{2+} < Ni^{2+} < Cu^{2+} > Zn^{2+} > Cd^{2+}$.

These broad predictions imply that the trace metal speciation in soil solutions will depend sensitively on the content and type of organic matter, the percentage of kaolinitic and amorphous hydrous oxide minerals, the pH, the pϵ, and the ionic strength. For example, a low solubility of the micronutrients Cu and Zn should occur for soils high in immobile organic matter (but not too low in pH) or for soil solutions with low pϵ values. Moreover, the solubilities of the trace metals should increase significantly with an increase in chloride concentration or in organic solutes. Since the complexes formed in these cases would reduce the ionic charge on the soluble trace metal species, a decrease in the affinity of a constant-charge adsorbing surface (for example, that of montmorillonite) should also occur (Fig. 5). It is evident that the detailed speciation of the trace metals presents a formidable problem. Much information still is needed on the important reactions and corresponding stability constants before definitive predictions can be made.

Clay-organic complexes. The clay minerals in soils often are observed to be intimately associated with carbonaceous materials. These materials may be residues from plant or animal decomposition, herbicides or other pesticides, organic polymers and polyelectrolytes, surfactant compounds, or microbial metabolites. The complexes which they form with clay minerals bear importantly on soil fertility, soil structure, soil moisture and aeration characteristics, the biological activity of organic compounds applied or disposed on soil, and the degradation of solid and liquid organic wastes in the soil environment. Generally, the organic component of a naturally occurring clay-organic complex will be of a very complicated nature that defies a conclusive structural determination. Therefore, in order to obtain fundamental information about the mechanisms of bonding between clay minerals and organic matter in soil, a major line of research has involved the study of the reactions of known organic compounds with single types of clay mineral. On the basis of these studies, some important bonding mechanisms have been identified. They are expected to apply to the associations between clay minerals and organic matter in nature whenever the appropriate mineral species and organic functional groups are present.

Bonding mechanisms. The principal mechanisms through which organic compounds may bind to clay minerals have been elucidated largely by spectroscopic and x-ray diffraction studies. They may be classified as follows:

1. Organic cation adsorption can occur, through protonated amine or carbonyl groups, onto any constant-charge clay mineral surface. The protonation of the functional groups may be either a

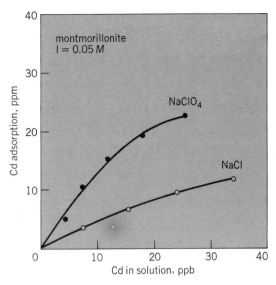

Fig. 5. The adsorption of Cd by montmorillonite at fixed pH and ionic strength as influenced by chloride complexing. In the NaCl system, the amount of adsorption is reduced because of the formation of $CdCl^+$, $CdCl_2^0$, and $CdCl_3^-$, which have smaller positive charges than Cd^{2+}, the only Cd species present in the $NaClO_4$ system.

pH effect or an acceptance of a proton that was formerly occupying an exchange site, was associated with a water molecule hydrating a metal cation, or was bound on another adsorbed organic cation. The affinity of an organic cation for a constant-charge surface depends on the molecular weight, the nature of the functional groups present, and the molecular configuration. Steric effects can be particularly significant because of the localized character of exchange sites and the quasi-rigid hydration envelope built up on a clay mineral surface. The stability of the water structure on a smectite (montmorillonite) surface is, in fact, great enough to require interstratified layers of either adsorbed metal cations or adsorbed organic cations when the clay mineral surfaces are only partially saturated with the organic compound. A mixture of the two types of cation in a single interlayer region disrupts the water structure too much to be stable.

2. Polar organic functional groups can bind to adsorbed cations through simple ion-dipole forces or complex formation involving covalent bonds. The ion-dipole mechanism is to be expected, of course, for hard-acid metal cations, such as Ca^{2+} and Al^{3+}, while the formation of covalent bonds is to be expected for soft-acid metal cations, such as Cu^{2+}. As the organic functional groups often would have soft-base character, the strength of binding by this mechanism should be greatest for exchangeable transition metal cations. A sharp exception to this rule could occur with "complexable" Al^{3+} (or Fe^{3+}) in amorphous aluminosilicates that bind organic matter containing large numbers of carboxyl groups.

3. Large organic molecules can bind effectively to a clay mineral surface through hydrogen bonding. This bonding can involve a water bridge from a hydrated exchangeable cation to an oxygen-containing functional group, a hydrogen bond from a more acidic functional group adsorbed directly on

the clay mineral surface to a less acidic free one containing oxygen, or a direct hydrogen bond to a surface oxygen or hydroxyl plane in the clay mineral. If the exchangeable metal cation is a hard acid, the first type of hydrogen bond will by far dominate the third type in importance. Direct hydrogen bonds to a plane of surface atoms would be accompanied by weaker dipole-dipole (that is, van der Waals) interactions, in general. This type of binding should be most important when very large organic molecules associate with a clay mineral surface containing relatively few exchange sites.

Catalysis reactions. Constant-charge surfaces of clay minerals have been shown often to catalyze reactions involving organic compounds. This catalytic function appears to be connected intimately with the presence of exchangeable metal cations and may be separated into two distinct types. The first type relates to the fact that the water molecules hydrating the exchangeable cations tend to dissociate very readily and, therefore, to endow the clay mineral surface with a pronounced acidity that increases markedly with desiccation. The enhanced proton-donating capability of the clay mineral, which will be greater the harder an acid the exchangeable cation is, serves a catalytic function in, for example, the formation of unsaturated and saturated hydrocarbons during transalkylation of alkylammonium cations and the surface protonation of amines and amino acids.

A second type of catalytic function derives from the formation of organic complexes with the exchangeable cations. This mechanism, which should be more significant the softer an acid the adsorbed metal cation is (again excepting Al^{3+} and Fe^{3+}), appears to play a basic role in, for example, the decarboxylation reaction of fatty acids, carboxyl activation prior to the polymerization of amino acids, and the stabilization of humic compounds against degradation. These and other reactions

catalyzed by clay minerals may prove to be very important in understanding how soil organic matter forms and how molecules of biological significance can be synthesized abiotically.

[GARRISON SPOSITO]

Nutrients. Plants tolerate larger amounts of molybdenum than do animals and, except for legumes, do not need cobalt for growth. Ruminant animals require a minimum of about 0.07 ppm (parts per million) of cobalt in feed and, under grazing conditions, cannot tolerate much more molybdenum than 10–20 ppm. Areas where common forage plants have too little cobalt for grazing animals occur principally in the eastern United States, and areas of plants with too much molybdenum are in the West (Fig. 6). Soil and geologic materials determine the distribution of cobalt deficiency and molybdenum toxicity in grazing animals.

Molybdenum. Molybdenum toxicity is a problem among ruminant animals principally in parts of California, Nevada, Oregon, and Montana. The problem areas are largely wet, narrow floodplains and alluvial fans of small streams. The extent of the problem areas tends to be exaggerated because the problem areas are interspersed locally with broad areas of productive soils.

Size of streams and the rock areas they drain determine how much molybdenum is present in alluvium. Most areas of molybdenum toxicity in the western United States are on granitic alluvium that is not mixed with materials from other streams. Small areas also occur on alluvium derived from some shales in northwestern Oregon. Because all alluvium from granite and shales does not give rise to molybdenum-toxic areas, there must be a source of the molybdenum in the higher-lying areas that the streams drain. Broad floodplains of large rivers have materials from many streams, and the large amounts of molybdenum that any stream may contribute are diluted. Thus, molybdenum toxicity is not a problem on broad floodplains.

The molybdenum in alluvium is readily released to plants if soils are wet. If soils are well drained, the release of molybdenum to plants is slow; and plants do not accumulate large amounts of molybdenum, even though the soil may contain large amounts. Molybdenum is also more available to plants in alkaline than in acid soils. Thus, the incidence of molybdenum toxicity is greatest in wet, neutral-to-alkaline soil areas; but molybdenum toxicity can also occur in wet, acid soil areas if the soils have enough molybdenum. The release of molybdenum from these acid soils may not be as rapid as from alkaline soils, but plants may have from 10 to 20 ppm or more of molybdenum.

Cobalt. Cobalt deficiency occurs in the eastern United States. Unlike molybdenum-toxic areas, cobalt-deficient areas cover broad glacial-drift plains in New England and the lower coastal plain from North Carolina to Florida.

Geology also plays an important role in the distribution of areas where deficiencies of cobalt occur. In New England the glacier that overrode the White Mountains left drift deposits on broad plains to the southeast that contribute very little cobalt to soils. The small amounts of cobalt contributed by granites of the White Mountains are today trace-

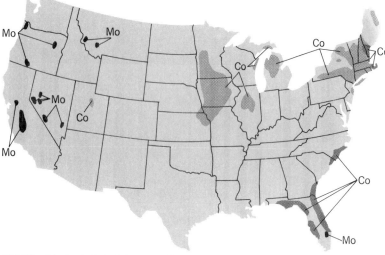

critical cobalt deficiency (neither legumes nor grasses meet minimum requirements for cobalt)

sporadic cobalt deficiency (legumes but not grasses meet minimum requirements for cobalt)

molybdenum toxicity (legumes have 10 ppm or more of molybdenum)

Fig. 6.   Areas of cobalt deficiency and molybdenum toxicity.

able through the low cobalt content in soils on floodplains of the Saco and Merrimac rivers, both of which originate in the White Mountains. Cobalt deficiency in this part of New England was a problem for the earliest settlers who tried to raise cattle.

Only very small amounts of cobalt were contributed by the sandy coastal-plain deposits of the southeastern United States. Here the cobalt deficiency probably resulted from weathering and loss of cobalt as the sandy materials which were weathered in the Piedmont and mountains were carried to the sea to form coastal-plain deposits.

The development of spodosols (podzols) in granitic deposits of New England and humaquods (humus groundwater podzols) in sandy coastal-plain deposits has caused further loss of whatever cobalt these sandy materials had. Cobalt is leached from these soils much as are iron and organic matter. The humaquods especially have very small amounts of reactive forms of cobalt left because of intense leaching. The cobalt leached from humaquods contrasts strikingly with an apparent biopedogenic recycling of soil cobalt from the subsoil to the ground surface in ultisols (red-yellow podzolic soils) of the southeastern United States. Cobalt deficiency is not a problem in ruminant animals on farms with ultisols, because plants have adequate amounts of cobalt to meet their nutritional requirements.

[JOE KUBOTA]

Bibliography: F. E. Bear (ed.), *Chemistry of the Soil*, 2d ed., 1964; J. J. Fripiat and M. I. Cruz-Cumplido, Clays as catalysts for natural processes, *Annu. Rev. Earth Planet. Sci.*, 2:239–256, 1974; J. E. Gieseking (ed.), *Soil Components*, vol. 1: *Organic Components*, vol. 2: *Inorganic Components*, 1975; M. M. Mortland, Clay-organic complexes and interactions, *Adv. Agron.*, 22:75–117, 1970; J. J. Mortvedt, P. M. Giordano, and W. L. Lindsay (eds.), *Micronutrients in Agriculture*, 1972; M. Schnitzer and S. U. Khan, *Humic Substances in the Environment*, 1972; W. Stumm and J. J. Morgan, *Aquatic Chemistry*, 1970; K. Wada and M. E. Harward, Amorphous clay constituents of soils, *Adv. Agron.*, 26:211–260, 1974.

Soil conservation

The practice of arresting and minimizing artificially accelerated soil deterioration. Its importance has grown because cultivation of soils for agricultural production, deforestation and forest cutting, grazing of natural range, and other disturbances of the natural cover and position of the soil have increased greatly in the last 100 years in response to the growth in world population and man's technical capacity. Accelerated soil deterioration has been the consequence.

Erosion extent and intensity. Accelerated erosion has been known throughout history wherever men have tilled or grazed slopes or semiarid soils. There are many evidences of the physical effects of accelerated erosion in the eastern and central parts of the Mediterranean basin, in Mesopotamia, in China, and elsewhere. Wherever the balance of nature is a delicate one, as on steep slopes in regions of intense rainstorms, or in semiarid regions of high rainfall variability, grazing and cultivation eventually have had to contend with serious or disabling erosion. Irrigation works of the Tigris and Euphrates valleys are thought to have suffered from the sedimentation caused by quickened erosion on the rangelands of upstream areas in ancient times. The hill sections of Palestine, Syria, southern Italy, and Greece experienced serious soil losses from grazing and other land use mismanagement many centuries ago. Accelerated water erosion on the hills of southern China and wind erosion in northwestern China also date far back into history. Exactly what effects these soil movements may have had on history has been a debated question, but their impact may have been serious on some cultures, such as those of the Syrian and Palestinian areas, and debilitating on others, as in the case of classical Rome and the China of several centuries ago.

The exact extent of accelerated soil erosion in the world today is not known, particularly as far as the rate of soil movement is concerned. However, it may be safely said that nearly every semiarid area with cultivation or long-continued grazing, every hill land with moderate to dense settlement in humid temperate and subtropical climates, and all cultivated or grazed hill lands in the Mediterranean climate areas suffer to some degree from such erosion. Thus recognized problems of erosion are found in such culturally diverse areas as southern China, the Indian plateau, south Australia, the South African native reserves, the Soviet Union, Spain, the southeastern and midwestern United States, and Central America.

Within the United States the most critical areas have been the hill lands of the Piedmont and the interior Southeast, the Great Plains, the Palouse area hills of the Pacific Northwest, southern California hills, and slope lands of the Midwest. The high-intensity rainstorms of the Southeast, and the cyclical droughts of the Plains have predisposed the two larger areas to erosion. The light-textured A horizon formed under the Plains grass cover was particularly susceptible to wind removal, while the high clay content of many southeastern soils predisposed them to water movement. These natural susceptibilities were repeatedly brought into play by agricultural systems which stressed corn and cotton in the Southeast, corn in the Midwest, and intensive grazing and small grains on the Plains, Palouse, and California. The open soil surface left in the traditional cotton, corn, and tobacco cultivation of the Southeast furnished almost ideal conditions for water erosion, and at the same time caused heavy nutrient depletion of soils thus cropped. The open fields of seasons between crops have also been susceptible to soil depletion. Open fields have been especially disastrous to maintenance of soil cover during the droughts of the Plains. Soil mismanagement thus has been a common practice in parts of the United States where the stability of soil cover hangs in delicate balance.

Types of soil deterioration. Soil may deteriorate either by physical movement of soil particles from a given site or by depletion of the water-soluble elements in the soil which contribute to the nourishment of crop plants, grasses, trees, and other economically usable vegetation. The physical movement generally is referred to as erosion. Wind, water, glacial ice, animals, and man's

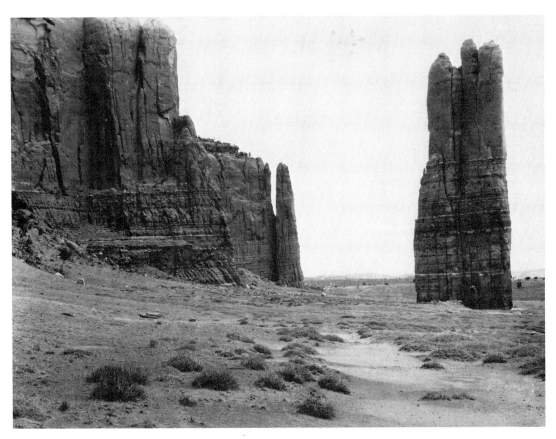

Fig. 1. Erosion of sandstone caused by strong wind and occasional hard rain in an arid region. (*USDA*)

tools in use may be agents of erosion. For purposes of soil conservation, the two most important agents of erosion are wind and water, especially as their effects are intensified by the disturbance of natural cover or soil position. Water erosion always implies the movement of soil downgrade from its original site. Eroded sediments may be deposited relatively close to their original location, or they may

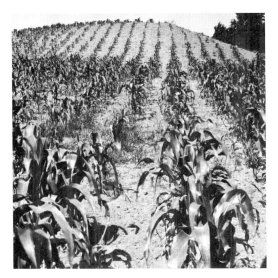

Fig. 2. Improper land use. Corn rows planted up and down the slope rather than on the contour. Note better growth of plants in bottom (deeper) soil in foreground as compared to stunted growth of plants on slope. (*USDA*)

be moved all the way to a final resting place on the ocean floor. Wind erosion, on the other hand, may move sediments in any direction, depositing them quite without regard to surface configuration. Both processes, along with erosion by glacial ice, are part of the normal physiographic (or geologic) processes which are continuously acting upon the surface of the Earth. The action of both wind and water is vividly illustrated in the scenery of arid regions (Fig. 1). Soil conservation is not so much concerned with these normal processes as with the new force given to them by man's land use practices.

Depletion of soil nutrients obviously is a part of soil erosion. However, such depletion may take place in the absence of any noticeable amount of erosion. The disappearance of naturally stored nitrogen, potash, phosphate, and some trace elements from the soil also affects the usability of the soil for man's purposes. The natural fertility of virgin soils always is depleted over time as cultivation continues, but the rate of depletion is highly dependent on management practices. *See* PLANT, MINERAL NUTRITION OF; SOIL.

Accelerated erosion may be induced by any land use practice which denudes the soil surfaces of vegetative cover (Fig. 2). If the soil is to be moved by water, it must be on a slope. The cultivation of a corn or a cotton field is a clear example of such a practice. Corn and cotton are row crops; cultivation of any row crop on a slope without soil-conserving practices is an invitation to accelerated erosion. Cultivation of other crops, like the small grains, also may induce accelerated erosion, espe-

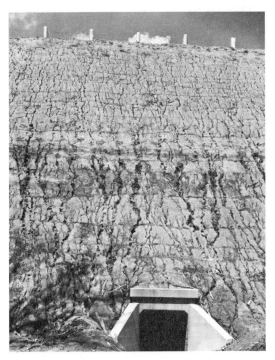

Fig. 3. Rill erosion on highway fill. The slopes have been seeded (horizontal lines) with annual lespedeza to bind and stabilize soil. (*USDA*)

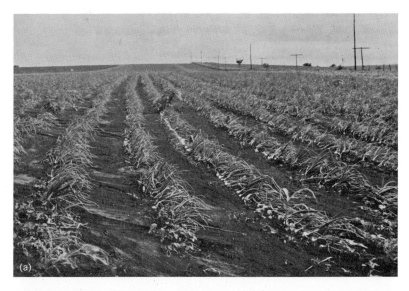

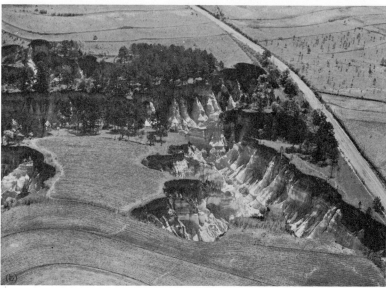

Fig. 4. Two most serious types of erosion. (*a*) Sheet erosion as a result of downhill straight-row cultivation. Note onions washed completely out of ground. (*b*) Gully erosion destroying rich farmland and threatening highway. (*USDA*)

cially where fields are kept bare between crops to store moisture. Forest cutting, overgrazing, grading for highway use, urban land use, or preparation for other large-scale engineering works also may speed the natural erosion of soil (Fig. 3).

Where and when the soil surface is denuded, the movement of soil particles may proceed through splash erosion, sheet erosion, rill erosion, gullying, and wind movement (Fig. 4). Splash erosion is the minute displacement of surface particles caused by the impact of falling rain. Sheet erosion is the gradual downslope migration of surface particles, partly with the aid of splash, but not in any defined rill or channel. Rills are tiny channels formed where small amounts of water concentrate in flow. Gullies are V- or U-shaped channels of varying depths and sizes. A gully is formed where water concentrates in a rivulet or larger stream during periods of storm. It may be linear or dendritic (branched) in pattern, and with the right slope and soil conditions may reach depths of 50 ft or more. Gullying is the most serious form of water erosion because of the sharp physical change it causes in the contour of the land, and because of its nearly complete removal of the soil cover in all horizons. On the edges of the more permanent stream channels, bank erosion is another form of soil movement.

Causes of soil mismanagement. One of the chief causes of erosion-inducing agricultural practices in the United States has been ignorance of their consequences. The cultivation methods of the settlers of western European stock who set the pattern of land use in this country came from a physical environment which was far less susceptible to erosion than North America, because of the mild nature of rainstorms and the prevailing soil textures in Europe. Corn, cotton, and tobacco,

moreover, were crops unfamiliar to European agriculture. In eastern North America the combination of European cultivation methods and American intertilled crops resulted in generations of soil mismanagement. In later years the plains environment, with its alternation of drought and plentiful moisture, was also an unfamiliar one to settlers from western Europe.

Conservational methods of land use were slow to develop, and mismanagement was tolerated because of the abundance of land in the 18th and 19th centuries. One of the cheapest methods of obtaining soil nutrients for crops was to move on to another farm or to another region. Until the 20th century, land in the United States was cheap, and for a period it could be obtained by merely giving assurance of settlement and cultivation. With low capital investments, many farmers had little stimulus to look upon their land as a vehicle for permanent production. Following the Civil War, tenant cultivators and sharecroppers presented another

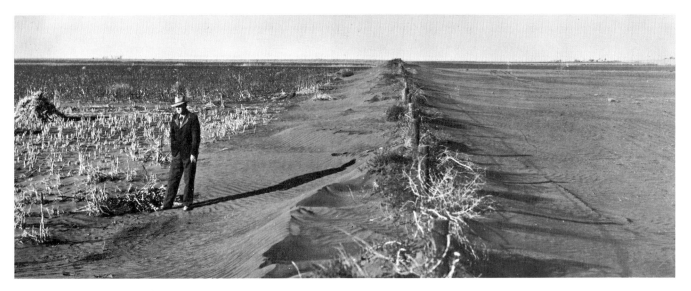

Fig. 5.   Wind erosion. Accumulation of topsoil blown from bare field on right. (*USDA*)

type of situation in the Southeast where stimulus toward conservational soil management was lacking. Management of millions of acres of Southeastern farmland was left in the hands of men who had no security in their occupancy, who often were illiterate, and whose terms of tenancy and meager training forced them to concentrate on corn, cotton, and tobacco as crops.

On the Plains and in other susceptible western areas, small grain monoculture, particularly of wheat, encouraged the exposure of the uncovered soil surface so much of the time that water and wind inevitably took their toll (Fig. 5). On rangelands, the high percentage of public range (for whose management little individual responsibility could be felt), lack of knowledge as to the precipitation cycle and range capacity, and the urge to maximize profits every year contributed to a slower, but equally sure denudation of cover.

Finally, the United States has experienced extensive erosion in mountain areas because of forest mismanagement. Clearcutting of steep slopes, forest burning for grazing purposes, inadequate fire protection, and shifting cultivation of forest lands have allowed vast quantities of soil to wash out of the slope sites where they could have produced timber and other forest values indefinitely. In the United States the central and southern Appalachian area and the southern part of California have suffered severely in this respect, but all hill or mountain forest areas, except the Pacific Northwest, have had such losses.

Economic and social consequences. Where the geographical incidence of soil erosion has been extensive, the damages have been of the deepest social consequence. Advanced stages of erosion may remove all soil and therefore all capacity for production. More frequently it removes the most productive layers of the soil—those having the highest capacity for retention of moisture, the highest soil nutrient content, and the most ready response to artificial fertilization. Where gullying or dune formation takes place, erosion may make cultivation physically difficult or impossible. Thus, depending on extent, accelerated erosion may

affect productivity over a wide area. At its worst, it may cause the total disappearance of productivity, as on the now bare limestone slopes of many Mediterranean mountains. At the other extreme may be the slight depression of crop yields which may follow the progress of sheet erosion over short periods. In the case of forest soil losses, except where the entire soil cover disappears, the effects may not be felt for decades, corresponding to the growth cycle of given tree species. Agriculturally, however, losses are apt to be felt within a matter of a few years.

Moderate to slight erosion cannot be regarded as having serious social consequences, except over many decades. As an income drepressant, however, it does prevent a community from reaching full productive potentiality. More severe erosion has led to very damaging social dislocation. For those who choose to remain in an eroding area or who do not have the capacity to move, or for whom migration may be politically impossible, the course of events is fateful. Declining income leads to less means to cope with farming problems, to poor nutrition and poor health, and finally to family existence at the subsistence level. Communities made up of a high proportion of such families do not have the capacity to support public services, even elementary education. Unless the cycle is broken by outside financial and technical assistance or by the discovery of other resources, the end is a subsistence community whose numbers decline as the capacity of the land is further reduced under the impact of subsistence cultivation. This has been illustrated in the hill and mountain lands of southeastern United States, in Italy, Greece, Palestine, China, and elsewhere for many millions of peasant people. Illiteracy, short life-spans, nutritional and other disease prevalence, poor communications, and isolation from the rest of the world have been the marks of such communities. Where they are politically related to weak national governments, idefinite stagnation and decline may be forecast. Where they are part of a vigorous political system, their rehabilitation can be accomplished only through extensive investment contributed by the nation at large. In the absence of rehabilitation, these communities may constitute a continued financial drain on the nation for social services such as education, public health, roads, and other public needs.

Effects on other resources. Accelerated erosion may have consequences which reach far beyond the lands on which the erosion takes place and the community associated with them. During periods of heavy wind erosion, for example, the dust fall may be of economic importance over a wide area beyond that from which the soil cover has been removed. The most pervasive and widespread effects, however, are those associated with water erosion. Removal of upstream cover changes the regimen of streams below the eroding area. Low flows are likely to be lower and their period longer where upper watersheds are denuded than where normal vegetative cover exists. Whereas flood crests are not necessarily higher in eroding areas, damages may be heightened in the valleys below eroding watersheds because of the increased deposition of sediment of different sizes, the rapid lifting of channels above floodplains, and the choking of irrigation canals.

A long chain of other effects also ensues. Because of the extremes of low water in denuded areas during dry seasons, water transportation is made difficult or impossible without regulation, fish and wildlife support is endangered or disappears, the capacity of streams to carry sewage and other wastes safely may be seriously reduced, recreational values are destroyed, and run-of-the-river hydroelectric generation reaches a very low level. Artificial storage becomes necessary to derive the services from water which are economically possible and needed. But even the possibilities of storage eventually may disappear when erosion of upper watersheds continues. Reservoirs may be filled with the moving sediment and lose their capacity to reduce flood crests, store flood waters, and augment low flows. For this reason plans for permanent water regulation in a given river basin must always include watershed treatment where eroding lands are in evidence.

Conservation measures and technology. Measures of soil management designed to reduce the effects of accelerated erosion have been known in both the Western world and in the Far East since long before the time of Christ. The value of forests for watershed protection was known in China at least 10 centuries ago. The most important of the ancient measures on agricultural lands was terrace construction, although actual physical restoration of soil to original sites also has been practiced. Terrace construction in the Mediterranean countries, in China, Japan, and the Philippines represents the most impressive remaking of the face of the Earth before the days of modern earth-moving equipment (Fig. 6). Certain land management practices which were soil conserving have been a part of western European agriculture for centuries, principally those centering on livestock husbandry and crop rotation. Conservational management of the soil was known in colonial Virginia and by Thomas Jefferson and others during the early years of the United States. However, it is principally since 1920 that the technique of soil conservation has been developed for many types of environ-

ment in terms of an integrated approach. The measures include farm, range, and forest management practices, and the building of engineered structures on land and in stream channels.

Farm, range, and forest. A first and most important step in conservational management is the determination of land capability—the type of land use and economic production to which a plot is suited by slope, soil type, drainage, precipitation, wind exposure, and other natural attributes. The objective of such determination is to achieve permanent productive use as nearly as possible. The United States Soil Conservation Service has developed one of the more easily understood and widely employed classifications for such determination (Fig. 7). In it eight classes of land are recognized within United States territory. Four classes represent land suited to cultivation, from the class 1 flat or nearly flat land suited to unrestricted cultivation, to the steeper or eroded class 4 lands which can be cultivated only infrequently. Three additional classes are grazing or forestry land, with varying degrees of restriction on use. The eighth class is suited only to watershed, recreation, or wildlife support. The aim in the United States has been to map all lands from field study of their capabilities, and to adjust land use to the indicated capability as it becomes economically possible for the farm, range, or forest operator to put conservational use into force.

Once the capability of land has been determined, specific measures of management come into play. For class 1 land few special practices are necessary. After the natural soil nutrient minerals begin to decline under cultivation, the addition of organic or inorganic fertilizers becomes necessary. The return of organic wastes, such as manure, to the soil is also required to maintain favorable texture and optimum moisture-holding capacity. Beyond these measures little need be added to the normal operation of cultivation.

On class 2, 3, and 4 lands, artificial fertilization will be required, but special measures of conserva-

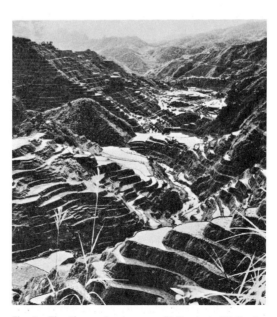

Fig. 6.   The Ifugao rice terraces, Philippines. (*Philippine Embassy, Washington, D.C.*)

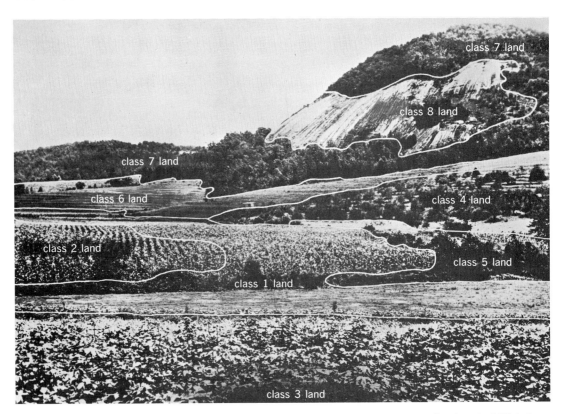

Fig. 7. Land capability classes. Suitable for cultivation: 1, requires good soil management practices only; 2, moderate conservation practices necessary; 3, intensive conservation practices necessary; 4, perennial vegetation—infrequent cultivation. Unsuitable for cultivation (pasture, hay, woodland, and wildlife): 5, no restrictions in use; 6, moderate restrictions in use; 7, severe restrictions in use; 8, best suited for wildlife and recreation. (*USDA*)

tional management must be added. The physical conservation ideal is the maintenance of such land under cover for as much of the time as possible. This can be done where pasture and forage crops are suited to the farm economy. However, continuous cover often is neither economically desirable nor possible. Consequently, a variety of devices has been invented to minimize the erosional results from tillage and small grain or row crop growth. Tillage itself has become an increasingly important conservational measure since it can affect the relative degree of moisture infiltration and soil grain aggregation, and therefore erosion. Where wind erosion is the danger, straw mulches or row or basin listing may be employed and alternating strips of grass and open-field crops planted. Fields in danger of water erosion are plowed on the contour (not up- and downslope), and if lister cultivation is also employed, water-storage capacity of the furrows will be increased. Strip-cropping, in which alternate strips of different crops are planted on the contour, may also be employed. Crop rotations that provide for strips of closely planted legumes and perennial grasses alternating with grains such as wheat and barley and with intertilled strips are particularly effective in reducing soil erosion. Fields may also be terraced, and the terraces strip-cropped. The bench terrace, which interrupts the slope of the land by a series of essentially horizontal slices cut into the slope, is now comparatively little used in the United States in contrast to the broad-base terrace, which imposes comparatively little impediment to cultivation. A broad-base terrace consists of a broad, shallow surface channel, flanked on the downward slope by a low, sloping embankment. If the terrace is constructed with a slight gradient (channel-type or graded terrace), it serves to reduce erosion by conducting excess water off the slope in a controlled manner. If it is constructed on the contour (level or ridge-type terrace), its primary purpose is to conserve moisture. The embankment on the downslope side of a broad-base terrace may be constructed from soil taken from the upper side only (sometimes referred to as a Nichols terrace) or from both sides (Mangum terrace).

Design of conservational cultivation also includes provision for grass-covered waterways to collect drainage from terraces and carry it into stream courses without erosion. Where suitable conditions of slope and soil permeability are found, shallow retention structures may also be constructed to promote water infiltration. These are of special value where insufficient soil moisture is a problem at times. Additional moisture always encourages more vigorous cover growth.

The measures just described may be considered preventive. There are also measures of rehabilitation where fields already have suffered from erosion and offer possibilities of restoration. Grading with mechanical equipment and the construction of small check dams across former gullies are examples.

For the remaining four classes of land, whose principal uses depend on the continuous maintenance of cover, management is more important than physical conditioning. In some cases, however, water retention structures, check dams, and other physical devices for retarding erosion may be applied on forest lands and rangelands. In the United States such structures are not often found in forest lands, although they have been commonly employed in Japanese forests. In forestry the conservational management objective is one of maximum production of wood and other services while maintaining continuous soil cover. The same is true for grass and other forage plants on managed grazing lands. For rangelands, adjustment of use is particularly difficult because grazing must be tolerated only to the extent that the range plants still retain sufficient vitality to withstand a period of drought which may arrive at any time.

A last set of erosion-control measures is directed toward minimizing stream bank erosion which may be large over the length of a long stream. This may be done through revetments, retaining walls, and jetties, which slow down current undercutting banks and hold sand and silt in which soil-binding willows, kudzu, and other vegetation may become established. Sediment detention reservoirs also reduce the erosive power of the current, and catchment basins or flood-control storage helps reduce high flows (Fig. 8).

Conservation agencies and programs. Whereas excellent soil-conserving soil management was maintained for generations by some farmers and farm groups, as in Lancaster County, Pa., a major amount of the soil-conservation activities in the United States is derived from Federal government assistance. The Soil Conservation Service of the USDA has been a focal agency in spreading knowledge of soil conservation in farmland and rangeland management and aiding in its application. In practice, the local administration of a soil-conserving program is within a Soil Conservation District, which usually is coincident with a county, and is organized under state law. The district is the liaison unit between the farmer and public assistance agencies at the state and Federal levels. It is managed by a board or committee, generally composed of five members, and usually elected by farmers within the district. Other local public bodies which may have soil-conservation objectives include conservancy districts, wind-erosion districts, drainage or irrigation districts,

Agricultural Stabilization and Conservation Service County Committees, and Farmers' Home Administration County Committees. In addition there are private groups with conservational interests, such as the farmers' cooperatives and national farm organizations like the Farm Bureau Federation.

The local districts may be aided technically and financially in their program. Much of the financial aid stems from Federal sources, and theoretically it is on a matching fund basis. In actual practice, however, a major part of the expenditures for special soil-conserving programs is from Federal funds. Technical aid is provided throughout the nation by the Soil Conservation Service, and also by the U.S. Forest Service for its special fields of forestry and grazing-land management. Technical aid also has been provided by the Agricultural Extension Services and the Land Grant Colleges of the several states. The Tennessee Valley Authority has maintained a program of its own design, with the cooperation of the colleges and the Extension Services. The Soil and Moisture Conservation Operations Office of the Indian Service, U.S. Department of the Interior, likewise has conducted a program limited to specific Indian lands.

Financial assistance for soil-conservation measures has been provided by the Federal government through the Soil Conservation Service, the Agricultural Stabilization and Conservation Service, the TVA, and the Farmers' Home Administration. Assistance has been particularly in the form of loans from the FHA, in low-cost fertilizer from the TVA, and as direct cash outlay from other agencies. Over the years, the program of the Agricultural Stabilization and Conservation Service has been the largest single source of financial aid for these purposes.

In addition to technical and financial aid, the farmers or other land operators of the United States are given valuable indirect assistance through the many research programs, basic and applied, which treat the fields related to soil conservation. The work of the Agricultural Research Service, of the Soil Conservation Service, of the Tennessee Valley Authority, and of the Land Grant Colleges has been especially helpful. Through these works new soil-conserving plants, new fertilizers, improved means of physical control, and new methods of management have been developed. Through them soil conservation has not only become important but also an increasingly efficient public activity in the United States. *See* AGRICULTURE.

[EDWARD A. ACKERMAN; DONALD J. PATTON]

Bibliography: I. Burton and R. W. Kates, *Readings in Resource Management and Conservation*, 1965; R. B. Held, *Soil Conservation in Perspective*, 1965; R. M. Highsmith, J. G. Jensen, and R. D. Rudd, *Conservation in the United States*, 1962; G. O. Schaub et al., *Soil and Water Conservation Engineering*, 2d ed., 1966.

Soil microbiology

A study of the microorganisms in soil, their functions, and the effect of their activities on the character of soil and the growth and health of plant life, particularly cultivated crops. It embraces the biology of microorganisms—their morphology, physiology, and taxonomy—as well as their biochemis-

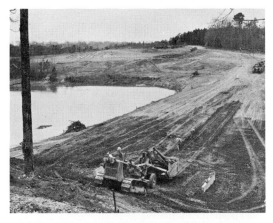

Fig. 8. Stream bank erosion control. Construction of a new conservation pool which will help reduce flooding, retard downstream erosion, and store water. (*USDA*)

try. It is related to soil chemistry and physics and, in its application, to agronomy, plant physiology, and plant pathology.

Microorganism characteristics. The soil microorganisms are viruses, Myxomycetes (slime fungi), protozoa, algae, yeasts, fungi, actinomycetes, and bacteria (see illustration). Soil is distinguished from subsoil chiefly by the presence of organic matter in the soil. The organic matter is composed of dead plant and animal tissues and the products of their decomposition by microorganisms. The microorganisms derive their energy by oxidizing plant and animal residues. Plants depend upon nutrients made available by microorganisms which form an essential link in the cycle of food in nature.

The soil is the greatest natural reservoir of microorganisms. These take part in many reactions in the soil. Some microorganisms are specific, taking part only in certain reactions (*Nitrosomonas*, which oxidize ammonia to nitrite). Some are more general in their metabolism (heterotrophic types, which depend on organic material for energy source) and take part in many reactions. One group of organisms may use the products of another, for example, during the course of decomposition of complex nitrogenous material to nitrate. In addition to forming simpler degradation products, microorganisms synthesize many complex substances. These are bound up in microbial protoplasm, while excess amounts may be liberated to provide essential substances for other groups of microorganisms. In contrast to this associative action are antagonisms caused by competition for the same food or by the ability of many organisms to produce antibiotics.

The net result of such associations and antagonisms is the establishment of a microbial equilibrium, which varies with the geological origin and evolutionary history of the soil. Although the equilibrium is ever shifting under the influences of season, temperature, moisture, and state of cultivation, the micropopulation of a soil of definite type has a characteristic composition, consisting of organisms that have become adapted to the particular environment.

Microorganisms are not uniformly distributed throughout the soil, because soil is not homogeneous but comprises a variety of microenvironments. The organisms congregate in colloidal films about the surface of soil particles and are particularly abundant around fragments of decaying plant and animal debris.

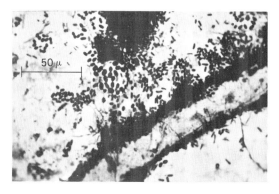

Bacteria attacking fragments of dead plant material in soil. (*T. Gibson, World Crops, vol. 3, no. 4, 1951*)

The majority of soil microorganisms are most active at pH 6.0–6.8. Some sulfur-oxidizing bacteria tolerate a pH as low as 2.0 and other organisms a pH as high as 10. A supply of free oxygen is important to most organisms. Almost all fungi, actinomycetes and protozoa as well as most bacteria, are aerobic. With abundant oxygen, decomposition proceeds rapidly to completion. However, in close-textured and wet soils where anaerobic conditions (molecular oxygen not available) prevail, organic matter is decomposed slowly and incompletely. The number of microorganisms is highest in spring and fall. Proximity to growing plants markedly increases the number of soil organisms.

The soil micropopulation may be divided into two groups, autochthonous and zymogenous microorganisms. The autochthonous organisms, making up the great majority, are the indigenous forms responsible for the processes occurring under normal conditions. Their character is relatively uniform in soil of definite type, and they are little affected by amendments (changes in soil organic matter). In contrast, the zymogenic microorganisms, much less numerous and normally quiescent, increase temporarily to participate in primary decomposition processes upon addition of readily decomposable organic material.

Microbiological soil analysis. The enumeration of soil microorganisms is carried out by culture and microscopic methods. Culture methods depend upon the growth of organisms and permit their isolation for detailed study. In microscopic methods counts are made from stained films, but since the organisms are killed no cultures can be made.

Culture methods. These include plate and elective culture procedures. Plate cultures are used for counts of bacteria, actinomycetes, and fungi, and are prepared by suspending a definite weight of soil in sterile water. Dilutions are made of the soil suspension with sterile water. Aliquots (representative portions) of these dilutions are placed in petri plates with an agar medium which will support the growth of the microorganisms in the soil sample. For counts of protozoa the soil aliquots are placed on the surface of agar plates, and after incubation wet mounts are examined microscopically. In order to group soil bacteria on the basis of taxonomy, nutritional requirements, and ability to synthesize substances such as vitamins or antibiotics, isolates (individual bacterial colonies) are taken nonselectively from plate cultures. The relative incidence in soil of a given category of bacteria can be estimated from a study of the individual isolates.

Elective culture methods are used to count microorganisms of special physiological groups, such as algae and the nitrifying, denitrifying, sulfur-oxidizing, and cellulose- or protein-decomposing bacteria. Portions of successive soil dilutions are added to liquid media selected to promote growth of the group in question. The presence of organisms is determined by visual or microscopic observation or by chemical tests for by-products. The use of replicates (that is, more than one sample of the particular soil) permits the calculation of the most probable numbers.

Microscopic methods. Such methods are based on the examination of a definite amount of soil spread over a definite area of a slide and stained.

From the known area of the microscope field numbers of organisms may be estimated. As this procedure involves mixing the soil, the "contact-slide" method is used to observe the localized distribution of the organisms. A glass slide is inserted in the soil and later removed, stained, and examined for organisms adhering to the surface.

Plating methods, which are more commonly used for counting soil microorganisms, give too low values because there is no medium on which all will grow. Microscopic methods give far higher numbers than plate counts but suffer from the disadvantage that they do not distinguish readily between living and dead cells. The two methods are complementary. *See* HUMUS; MANURE; NITROGEN CYCLE; RHIZOSPHERE; SOIL BALANCE, MICROBIAL; SOIL MICROORGANISMS; SOIL MINERALS, MICROBIAL UTILIZATION OF; SOIL PHOSPHORUS, MICROBIAL CYCLE OF; SOIL SULFUR, MICROBIAL CYCLE OF; YEAST.

[ALLAN G. LOCHHEAD]

Bibliography: M. Alexander, *Introduction to Soil Microbiology*, 1961; A. Burges and F. Raw (eds.), *Soil Biology*, 1967; S. D. Garrett, *Soil Fungi and Soil Fertility*, 1963; N. A. Krasilnikov, *Soil Microorganisms and Higher Plants*, transl. by Y. Halperin, 1958.

Soil microorganisms

Microorganisms in the soil include protozoa, fungi, slime molds, green algae, diatoms, blue-green algae, and bacteria. The bacteria are a heterogeneous group and include the procaryotic mycelial forms called actinomycetes as well as the simple unicellular forms called eubacteria.

Bacteria, actinomycetes, and fungi are the groups most active in decomposing organic residues and in rendering inorganic nutrients soluble. The final result of this activity is the liberation of such elements as carbon, nitrogen, phosphorus, potassium, and sulfur in forms available to plants.

Eubacteria. The eubacteria exceed all other soil microorganisms in numbers and in the variety of their activities. Numbers may surpass 100,000,000/g of soil by plate count or 1,000,000,000/g by microscopic count. The bacteria vary in size, shape, growth requirements, energy utilization, and function. Morphologically they are divided into straight or irregular rods, of both spore-forming and non-spore-forming types, thin flexible rods, cocci, vibrios, and spirilla. Short rods and cocci are most frequent, but many of the cocci are the coccoid stage of pleomorphic (varying in shape and size) rods or spores of actinomycetes.

Members of most taxonomic groups, with the exception of certain animal and human parasites, occur in soil. Some taxonomic groups are characteristic of soil alone. Although the identity of many bacteria engaged in specific processes, such as nitrification and nitrogen fixation, is known, a large proportion of the indigenous (autochthonous) organisms have not been classified. Of these, many have not been grown in any culture medium, a requisite for systematic study. Thus, taxonomic knowledge of these microflora is imperfect.

On the basis of their nutrition, soil bacteria are divided into autotrophs and heterotrophs. Autotrophs are able to use carbon dioxide as the sole source of carbon for their body tissues; heterotrophs must obtain carbon from organic foods.

Autotrophic bacteria. These comprise two groups (photosynthetic and chemosynthetic) according to their source of energy. Purple and green sulfur bacteria are photosynthetic because of their bacteriochlorophyll or chlorobium chlorophyll pigments. Like chlorophyll-containing algae and higher plants, they obtain energy from sunlight.

Other autotrophs are chemosynthetic, deriving energy from various oxidation reactions. Their requirements for food and energy are met by inorganic sources. These autotrophs carry out the process of nitrification, in which two stages are distinguished, the oxidation of ammonia to nitrite and that of nitrite to nitrate. Autotrophic sulfur bacteria derive energy from the oxidation of elemental sulfur, sulfides, sulfites, thiosulfates, and thiocyanates to sulfuric acid, which reacts with soil bases to form sulfates.

Heterotrophic bacteria. Heterotrophic bacteria, which constitute the great majority of soil bacteria, derive both food and energy from the decomposition of organic substances. They embrace a wide variety of morphological and taxonomic types including spore-formers or zymogenous forms, which are bacteria that develop in soil in response to the addition of certain substances like organic matter, or certain processes like aeration. Also included are the far more numerous non-spore-formers which make up the great majority of the autochthonous microflora. The most abundant forms are short rods and pleomorphic rods.

The majority of the heterotrophs require combined nitrogen to build cell substance. The nitrogen-fixing bacteria utilize elemental nitrogen of the air. These bacteria include symbiotic organisms, such as species of the genus *Rhizobium* that live in symbiosis with leguminous plants, and nonsymbiotic organisms, such as species of the aerobic genera *Azotobacter, Beijerinckia,* and *Azotomonas,* and the anaerobic genus *Clostridium.* The indigenous heterotrophic bacteria may be classified according to their nutritional requirements. Though all require a source of energy, such as a simple sugar, the additional needs of some are satisfied by inorganic salts. Other soil bacteria require amino acids or more complex food sources, and some more exacting bacteria require factors present in soil extract. The proportion of each of the nutritional groups is fairly constant in soil of definite type. However, increased fertility, such as that resulting from fertilizer treatment, is reflected in an increase in the proportion of bacteria with complex requirements at the expense of those with simple nutritional needs. Although there is no precise correlation between nutritional requirements and morphological type or taxonomic grouping, *Pseudomonas* species are more abundant among the nutritional group with simpler needs; the pleomorphic types, particularly *Arthrobacter* species, are relatively more numerous in the group with the most complex requirements.

As much as 25% of the indigenous soil bacteria capable of being isolated may require one or more vitamins for growth. The vitamins most essential are, in order of frequency, thiamine, biotin, and vitamin B_{12}. A smaller percentage require other B vitamins as well as the terregens factor, a substance found only in soil that promotes bacterial growth. *See* NITROGEN CYCLE; SOIL SULFUR, MICROBIAL CYCLE OF.

Actinomycetes. Next to the bacteria in numbers, the actinomycetes range from hundreds of thousands to several millions per gram of soil. They are more abundant in dry and warm soils than in wet and cold soils. With increasing depth of soil, their numbers are reduced proportionately less than those of bacteria. Actinomycetes are particularly abundant in grassland soil. The three genera of Actinomycetales occurring most commonly in soil are *Nocardia*, *Streptomyces*, and *Micromonospora*. Thermophilic forms, represented by the genus *Thermoactinomyces*, are active in rotting manure and also may be present, though inactive, in normal soil. *Streptomyces* species are the dominant types. Although they are largely saprophytes, a few species, such as those associated with potato scab, are parasitic.

Less is known of the function of the actinomycetes in soil than of the bacteria. They are heterotrophic and are nutritionally an adaptable group, less demanding in growth requirements than many bacteria. They take part in the decomposition of a wide range of carbon and nitrogen compounds, including the more resistant celluloses and lignins, and are important in humus formation. Actinomycetes are responsible for the earthy or musty odor characteristic of soil rich in humus. *See* HUMUS.

As much as 60% of the actinomycetes isolated from soil by plating methods may show antagonism toward bacteria or fungi in artificial culture. The importance of this antibiotic-producing capacity under normal soil conditions is not known. However, although antibiotics can rarely be detected in soil and then only under abnormal conditions, they may be important in microenvironments where intense microbial activity takes place.

Fungi. Fungi are present in numbers ranging from several thousand to several hundred thousand per gram of soil. They occur extensively in the mycelial state, as well as in the form of spores. Since plate colonies may develop from fragments of mycelium or from spores, plate counts give only an approximation of the abundance of fungi in soil. As with bacteria, some fungi do not grow on plates; consequently plating methods give minimum counts. Most fungi require humid, aerobic conditions for growth and spore formation. They are most common near the surface of soil and are more abundant in lighter, well-aerated soils than in heavier soils. Because the optimum pH range for fungi is 4.5–5.5, they are more prevalent in acid soils which are less favorable to bacteria and actinomycetes.

Ecologically, two broad groups of soil fungi may be recognized, the soil-inhabiting and the root-inhabiting types. The soil-inhabiting fungi are able to survive indefinitely as saprophytes and have a general distribution in soil. They include not only obligate saprophytes but also some unspecialized parasites which are able to infect plant roots, but whose parasitism is only incidental to their saprophytic existence. Root-inhabiting fungi are specialized parasites that invade living root tissues. Their distribution in soil is localized and depends upon the presence of the host plant. Their activity diminishes following death of the plant and they persist in soil only as resting spores or sclerotia. Mycorrhizal fungi are included among the root-inhabiting fungi.

Soil fungi are heterotrophic and have a wide variety of food requirements. All obtain their carbon entirely from simple carbohydrates, alcohols, or organic acids. But although some fungi can utilize inorganic nitrogen, others require more complex forms or vitamins, chiefly thiamine and biotin.

Soil fungi do not comprise as many physiological groups as do the bacteria, but as a group they are more versatile in their ability to decompose a great variety of organic compounds. The saprophytes, the true soil inhabitants, may be divided into groups depending upon the nature of the substrate favoring their development. Two such groups are the sugar fungi and the cellulose-decomposing fungi. Other groups attack some of the most resistant substances, such as lignins, vegetable gums, and waxes. When plants die, or when fresh plant material is added to soil, the growth of fungi is greatly stimulated. Those able to attack the more soluble constituents, such as sugars and other simpler carbon compounds, develop rapidly. Chief among such forms are the Phycomycetes. As the special substrate is exhausted, other types flare up and attack progressively more resistant components of organic residues. Cellulose and hemicelluloses are decomposed by a variety of fungi including species of *Penicillium*, *Aspergillus*, *Sporotrichum*, and *Fusarium*. Fungi are the predominant lignin-decomposing organisms. Various simple fungi can attack the lignin of straw and leafy plant material, although the higher Basidiomycetes are most active in decomposing lignin-rich residues.

Although polysaccharide-forming bacteria play a part, fungi are chiefly responsible for improving the physical structure of soil by exerting a binding effect on loose particles, thus forming water-stable aggregates. This binding effect is caused by the growth of mycelia which form fine networks that entangle the smaller particles. The soil-binding effect is favored by addition of fresh organic material whose decomposition products provide cementing substances. *See* RHIZOSPHERE.

Yeasts. A group of simple fungi, yeasts occur in soil only to a limited extent in the surface layers. In field soils their numbers are small, some samples being devoid of yeasts. They are found most frequently in the soils of orchards, vineyards, and apiaries where special conditions, particularly the presence of sugars, favor growth of yeasts which invade the soil. Soil is not a favorable medium for the growth of yeasts, and they do not play a significant part in soil processes.

Algae. These are widely distributed in soils, developing most abundantly in moist, fertile soils well supplied with nitrates and available phosphates. They contain chlorophyll and in the soil surface layers, where they are chiefly confined, function as green plants converting carbon dioxide and inorganic nitrogen into cell substance by means of energy derived from sunlight. Smaller numbers occur at lower depths where, in the absence of sunlight, they exist heterotrophically. The soil algae comprise the green algae (Chlorophyceae), the blue-green algae (Myxophyceae), and the diatoms (Bacillariaceae). In acid soils green algae predominate, whereas in neutral or alkaline soils the other groups are more prominent. Numbers of algae in soil vary widely, ranging from a few hundred to several hundred thousand per gram of soil.

As autotrophs, algae are of importance in adding to the organic matter of soils. They play a fundamental ecological role on barren and eroded lands by colonizing such areas and synthesizing protoplasm from inorganic substances. Several blue-green algae are able to fix atmospheric nitrogen and are of agricultural significance, particularly in rice culture. Under the water-logged conditions needed for this crop, blue-green algae develop abundantly and may increase the nitrogen supply by as much as 20 lb/acre.

Protozoa. Occurring in all arable soils, protozoa are largely confined to the surface layers although in drier, sandy soils they may penetrate more deeply. Numbers usually range from a few hundred in dry soil to several hundred thousand per gram in moist soils rich in organic matter. Most soil protozoa are flagellates and amebas; ciliates are less frequent although they are often found in wet soils and swamps. Protozoa are active in soil only when living in a water film. The majority are able to form cysts, and in this inactive state they can withstand desiccation.

Although a few flagellates, such as *Euglena*, have chlorophyll and are autotrophic and others can live saprophytically by absorbing nutrients from solution, the majority of soil protozoa feed by ingesting solid particles, mainly bacteria. Not all bacteria are suitable as food. Amebas have decided preferences for certain bacterial species and will not ingest others, particularly pigmented bacteria. The formation of cysts by protozoa is favored by some bacterial types, not by others. Excystment of some amebas requires the presence of bacteria; others are independent of bacteria. Though protozoa are a factor in maintaining the microbial equilibrium in soil through their selective action on bacteria, their effect is limited and is not considered detrimental to the activities of the micropopulation as a whole. *See* PROTOZOA.

Myxomycetes. Myxomycetes, or slime fungi, form a minor group of soil microorganisms intermediate in character between the flagellated protozoa and the fungi. They possess a motile, flagellated stage in their life cycle, and later form large aggregates of cells or coalesce into jellylike masses of naked protoplasm. These eventually form spores which give rise to flagellated forms. Like the protozoa, myxomycetes feed on various species of bacteria.

Viruses and phages. Although these ultramicroscopic organisms exist in soil, little is known of the part they play in soil processes. Viruses that attack plants and animals can in some cases be transmitted from the soil. Phages, which are active against bacteria and actinomycetes, limit susceptible microorganisms and thus affect the microbial balance. Those that attack the various species of symbiotic nitrogen-fixing bacteria may prevent effective inoculation of legumes, particularly in soils in which the same crop has been repeatedly grown. The deleterious effect of phage on the nitrogen-fixing bacteria was formerly ascribed to direct lytic action (dissolution of the bacterial cell). However, this is now considered to result from the development of phage-resistant mutants which are less effective in fixing nitrogen than are the parent strains. *See* SOIL MICROBIOLOGY.

[ALLAN G. LOCHHEAD]

Soil minerals, microbial utilization of

Microorganisms utilize soil minerals for their own growth, and also help make the essential nutrients available to higher plants. A soil is fertile mainly because it can supply growing plants with nutrients (calcium, magnesium, potassium, and phosphate) in forms which can be readily taken up by plants. The conversion of the nutrients in soil minerals into forms available to plants is of course partly carried out by the plant roots themselves, but experiments have begun to show that microorganisms play a part in this conversion.

Soil formation. New soil is perpetually being formed all over the world by the breaking up of rocks into fine particles and the dissolving out of minerals from them. This process, the so-called weathering of rocks, was at one time supposed to be caused entirely by physical and chemical agents—heat, frost, water, and the oxygen of the air. It is now known that exposed rocks are subject also to microbial attack. When the island of Krakatau was visited 3 years after the great volcanic explosion which blew off its top, microscopic blue-green algae were found growing on the bare rocks, the first living things to appear there. These blue-green algae are the most self-supporting of all forms of life; they are photosynthetic, obtaining carbon from the carbon dioxide in the air, and also nitrogen-fixing, obtaining nitrogen from the atmosphere. In 1946, Soviet microbiologists found that the blue-green algae on freshly exposed rocks are soon accompanied by bacteria, among which nitrogen fixers and autotrophic nitrifiers are prominent. The nitrogen fixers add to the nitrogen supply, and the nitrifiers, because they fix carbon dioxide, add to the carbon supply in the film of growth on the rock. The two groups pave the way for other bacteria and fungi. The film of organic growth, which is continually dissolving mineral nutrients from the rock below it, increases until it can support the growth first of lichens, then of mosses, and finally of higher plants.

Buried rocks are also broken down to form new soil; if they are not buried too deeply, there is probably a succession of microbial growth on them. This has not been proved, because plant roots, at depths which they can reach, also break up rocks. Rock minerals are dissolved by carbon dioxide and by organic acids; both of these are given off by plants and by microorganisms. Since it is impossible to distinguish between them, in most cases it must be assumed that both plant roots and microorganisms are taking part in soil formation.

Utilization of minerals in formed soils. In soil which is already formed, microorganisms may release nutrients from the soil minerals and make them available to plants. In soil where a particular nutrient is scarce, they may render it unavailable by assimilating the nutrient as fast as they release it from the minerals; in this case they may be said to be competing successfully with the growing plants.

The mechanism of release of nutrients consists in dissolving out the nutrient from the soil mineral and converting it into a soluble salt or (in the case of heavy metals) into a complex with a chelating compound. Carbon dioxide is probably the most abundant dissolving agent, as all microorganisms and plant roots produce it in respiration. Organic acids such as lactic acid are also important dissolving agents which are secreted into the soil by plant roots and microorganisms, particularly fungi. Some fungi and bacteria from podzols (relatively infertile soils) are evidently adapted to dissolve minerals in a poor soil because in cultures of them more acid is formed in poor than in rich nutrient media. The gum, or slime, produced by some bacteria can take up phosphate, sulfate, and possibly potassium from culture media; if the same mechanism operates in soil, it should supply the bacteria with more of these nutrients.

Inorganic acids are produced by some autotrophic soil bacteria. For example, the nitrifiers *Nitrosomonas* and *Nitrobacter* produce nitric acid as the end result of their combined activity, and the sulfur-oxidizing *Thiobacillus* species produce sulfuric acid. These acids quickly combine with metals in the soil minerals to form nitrates and sulfates. The autotrophic bacteria are useful to plants not only because they supply nitrogen or sulfur in an assimilable form but also because they make soluble salts of most of the metals essential for plant growth, such as potassium and magnesium. Hydrogen sulfide, produced during the bacterial decomposition of proteins, may render tertiary phosphates soluble. Even if it causes the precipitation of iron and other metals, the sulfides are subject to bacterial oxidation, with the formation of soluble sulfates.

Some of the bacteria that reduce ferric hydroxide convert the iron into a chelated form held in an organic complex, but the nature of these organic complex-forming substances is quite unknown.

Phosphates. The most definite evidence for the beneficial effect of soil microorganisms on plant growth has been obtained in work with phosphates in the Netherlands, the Soviet Union, and Australia since 1950. Most of the phosphate in soil is combined with calcium or iron in insoluble compounds; many soil bacteria and fungi, when they are first isolated from soil, can dissolve these insoluble phosphates, though they lose this ability when kept in artificial culture. These phosphate dissolvers are commoner in the rhizosphere (the zone immediately surrounding plant roots) than elsewhere, and it has been found that plants grow better and take up more phosphate from insoluble calcium phosphate in soil with rhizosphere organisms present than in sterile soil. Cultures of phosphate-dissolving microorganisms are added to compost heaps in the Soviet Union and are said to improve the quality of the compost.

The mycorhiza fungi on the roots of pine trees are supposed to supply the trees with phosphate, but this is unlikely since trees without mycorhiza, such as oaks, also increase soluble phosphate in the soil around their roots. It is more probable that phosphate is brought up from the subsoil by the tree roots themselves.

Microorganisms may deprive plants of phosphate under certain conditions. All microorganisms need phosphate, and some soil species, the nitrogen-fixing *Azotobacter* sp. for instance, need quite large amounts. Fungi have a particularly high phosphate requirement; if much organic matter with a low phosphate content is added to soil, the fungi that develop on it may fix so much phosphate in organic compounds that a temporary phosphate starvation is induced in plants which are growing in the area.

Potassium, calcium, and magnesium. Very little is definitely known about the effect of microorganisms on the supply of these three elements to plants. It may reasonably be assumed that all three are turned into soluble salts through the action of the sulfur oxidizers and the nitrifying bacteria. Potassium is liberated in the breakdown of complex silicates by the so-called silicate-decomposing bacteria. It is quite probable that the breakdown of silicates is not a specific enzymatic process carried out by a special group of bacteria, but is caused rather by acids produced by many different soil bacteria and fungi.

Iron and manganese. Bacteria which reduce oxides of iron and manganese to soluble ferrous and manganous salts are very common in soil. The most efficient of them appear to be so because they make either organic acids or chelating substances. It is probable, but by no means proved, that these bacteria improve the supply of iron and manganese to plants. They also induce movement of both metals in the soil profile.

Microbial oxidation of iron and manganese compounds to insoluble oxides and hydroxides also takes place in soil. It has been claimed that the autotrophic iron bacteria, which are common in water and in bogs, also occur in drier soils. They may make the iron concretions and hardpans in tropical lateritic soils, but there is no experimental evidence for this claim.

It is therefore probable, though not yet proved, that soil microorganisms can increase the supply of essential nutrients to plants. A great deal more experimental work will be necessary to decide how much microbes contribute to plant nutrition by modifying soil minerals. *See* NITROGEN CYCLE; RHIZOSPHERE; SOIL MICROBIOLOGY; SOIL MICROORGANISMS.

[JANE MEIKLEJOHN]

Soil phosphorus, microbial cycle of

This microbial cycle is essentially a phosphate cycle. Plants assimilate phosphorus as phosphate, the $H_2PO_4^-$ ion, and build it into organic compounds such as phytin, nucleic acids, and phospholipids. The microbial breakdown of dead plant tissues liberates the phosphate again, so that there is an alternation in the soil between organic and inorganic phosphate. Microorganisms themselves assimilate phosphate, and consequently much of the organic phosphate in soil is contained in microbial cells. Plants may be deprived of phosphate by the addition of phosphate-deficient organic wastes to soil because the fungi which develop on the waste assimilate all the available phosphate.

There is also an alternation in soil between soluble and insoluble inorganic phosphates. Microorganisms can increase the phosphate supply to plants by dissolution of insoluble, tertiary phosphates through acid production; such microbes are particularly active in the rhizosphere. Others may precipitate soluble primary or secondary phosphates as tertiary salts as a result of the production of alkali. *See* SOIL MICROBIOLOGY; SOIL MINERALS, MICROBIAL UTILIZATION OF.

[JANE MEIKLEJOHN]

Soil sulfur, microbial cycle of

Plants and microorganisms assimilate sulfur from soil sulfates and convert it into organic sulfur compounds. Sulfates are formed in soil by oxidation of sulfides (see illustration), which are derived from

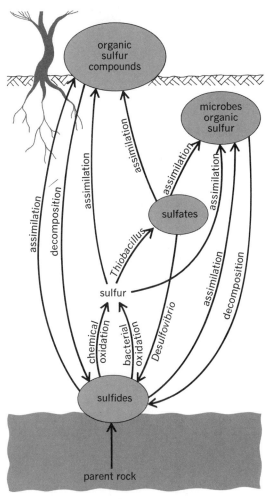

The microbial cycle of soil sulfur.

(1) the parent rock from which the soil is formed, (2) the breakdown of organic sulfur compounds, and (3) the reduction of sulfates by anaerobic bacteria of the genus *Desulfovibrio*. Corrosion of water pipes and other buried iron structures is caused by species of *Desulfovibrio*. The oxidation of sulfides to sulfur in soil is probably not a microbial process but a purely chemical one. The sulfur is oxidized microbially to sulfates by the autotrophic *Thiobacilli*. See SOIL MINERALS, MICROBIAL UTILIZATION OF.

[JANE MEIKLEJOHN]

Sorghum

Sorghum includes many widely cultivated grasses having a variety of names. Sorghum is known as guinea corn in West Africa, Kafir corn in South Africa, mtama in East Africa, and durra in the Sudan. In India sorghums are called juar, jowar, or cholam; in China, kaoliang; and in America, milo. Cultivated sorghums in the United States are classified as a single species, *Sorghum bicolor*, al-

though there are many varieties and hybrids. The two major types of sorghum are the grain, or non-saccharine, type, cultivated primarily for grain production and to a lesser extent for forage, and the sweet, or saccharine, type, used for forage production and for making syrup and sugar.

GRAIN SORGHUM

Grain sorghum is grown in the United States chiefly in the Southwest and the Great Plains. It is a warm-season crop which withstands heat and moisture stress better than most other crops, but extremely high temperatures and extended drought may reduce yields. Sorghum responds well to optimum growing conditions, fertility, and management to produce large grain yields. It is most extensively grown in Texas, Kansas, Nebraska, Oklahoma, Missouri, Colorado, and South Dakota. The average acreage planted to grain sorghum during the period 1970–1974 was 18,471,000 (1 acre = 4046 m²), with an average yield of 3016 lb/acre (1 lb = 0.45 kg). This grain production is fed to cattle, poultry, swine, and sheep primarily, with less than 2% going into nonagricultural markets such as starch, dextrins, flour, and industrial preparations. Sorghum is considered nearly equal to corn in feed value.

Origins and description. Sorghums originated in the northeastern quadrant of Africa. They have been grown in Africa and Asia for more than 2000 years. Introduction of a sorghum called chicken corn was made on the southern Atlantic coast in Colonial American times, but it was not successfully cultivated. The variety escaped and became a weed. Practically all grain sorghums of importance until recent years introduced to the United States were tall, late maturing, and generally unadapted. Since its introduction into the United States, the crop has been altered in many ways, these changes coming as a result of naturally occurring genetic mutations combined with hybridization and selection work of plant breeders. The rapid expansion in acreage came with the development of widely adapted varieties and later higher-yielding hybrids. The fact that hybrid grain sorghums with high yield potential could be produced with stems short enough for harvesting mechanically (Fig. 1) made the crop appealing to many farmers.

Grain sorghum is difficult to distinguish from corn in its early growth stages, but at later stages it becomes strikingly different. Sorghum plants may tiller (put out new shoots), producing several head-bearing culms from the basal nodes. Secondary culms may also develop from nodal buds along the main stem. The inflorescence (head) varies from a dense to a lax panicle, and the spikelets produce perfect flowers that are subject to both self- and cross-fertilization. The amount of natural cross-pollination ranges from 25 to 0% but averages about 5%. Mature grain in different varieties varies in size and color from white to cream, red, and brown. Color pigments are located in the pericarp (outer covering) of the grain or in a layer of cells beneath the pericarp called the testa. In some varieties the testa is absent; when the testa is present, however, the seed color is brown or some variation of brown. The endosperm (starch portion of the seed) is either white or yellow. There are endosperm modifications which cause the starch to be sugary or waxy, or to process a higher lysine con-

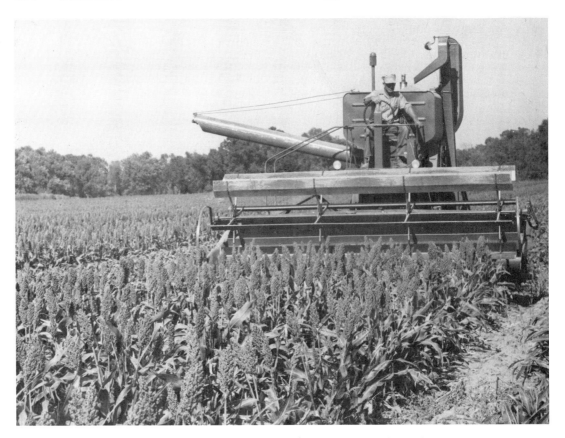

Fig. 1. Dwarf grain sorghum hybrids are grown throughout the sorghum belt of the United States because their
short stems make them adaptable to mechanical harvesting.

tent. The texture of the endosperm may vary from
completely corneous to full floury. Most sorghums
are intermediate in endosperm texture.

Grain sorghums are classified into types designated as milo, kafir, feterita, hegari, durra, shallu,
kaoliang, and zerazera. This classification is based
on morphological rather than cytological differences, since all types (including forage sorghums,
broomcorn, and Sudangrass) have 10 pairs of chromosomes and freely cross.

Varieties and hybrids. A combine-height grain
sorghum was developed before World War I but
was not accepted by farmers or agriculturalists.
Acceptance of combine grain sorghums was stimulated by the drought of the 1930s and by a farm
manpower shortage during World War II. A number of widely adapted productive varieties were
developed during this period. Nonetheless, varieties disappeared rapidly when hybrids were introduced in the mid-1950s (Fig. 2).

The commercial production of seed of sorghum
hybrids was made possible by the discovery of cytoplasmic male sterility in the early 1950s. This
type of sterility, as used in corn and a few other
crops, prevents the development of normal pollen
grains and makes possible the formation of hybrid
seed by cross-pollination. Because the flowers of
sorghum are perfect, containing both staminate
(male) and pistillate (female) parts, the production
of commercial quantities of hybrid seed was not
possible without a workable male-sterility mechanism. The first hybrid seed in quantity was sold to
farmers in 1957, and within a period of less than 5
years hybrids had replaced most of the varieties

previously grown. Hybrids yield at least 20% more
than varieties, and concurrent improvements in
cultural practices have combined to boost per-acre
yield over 50% since their development. Increased
emphasis on research in fertilization, irrigation,
insect and disease control, and other areas has
provided information to help account for the remarkable yield and production increases over the
years.

Through a process of conversion many of the
best varieties from around the world are being
changed from tall, late, unadapted types to short,
early, very useful cultivars. From this program
plant breeders are expanding germ-plasm utilization and are developing parents of hybrids for the
entire sorghum-producing world. *See* BREEDING,
PLANT.

Planting. Grain sorghum seeds are small and
should not be planted too deep since sorghum
lacks the soil-penetrating ability of corn. A seeding
depth of 1 in. (2.5 cm) is acceptable in moist and
friable soil, but 2 in. (5 cm) may be necessary under dry soil conditions. The seeds are planted either in rows wide enough for tractor cultivation or
in narrower rows if cultivation is not intended.
Row planters for corn, cotton, field beans, and
sugarbeets may be used when equipped with the
proper seed plates. When wheat farming is practiced, much grain sorghum is planted with a grain
drill with alternate or various feeder holes plugged
to provide the desired row spacing. Soil temperature largely determines when the seed should be
planted, assuming soil moisture conditions are
adequate. Being tropical in origin, sorghum should

not be planted in the spring until soil temperature is 65–70°F (18–22°C) at the planting depth and until there is little chance of subsequent lower temperatures. Dry-land grain sorghum is planted at a rate of 3–5 lb/acre, and the rate is increased up to 10 lb/acre when planted under more favorable moisture conditions and irrigation.

Cultivation. Good seedbed preparation is essential for full stands and for weed control. Tilling fields improves soil structure in most cases and often aids in warming the soil. A rotary hoe is effective in controlling weeds when the plants are small. Subsequent cultivations are made as needed with the same equipment used for cultivating corn. Minimum tillage is practiced in many areas where control of weeds with chemicals is a part of the technology of sorghum production. When used correctly, heribicides are a boon to sorghum culture, but when used carelessly, disappointment may result. There are several chemical herbicides registered and approved for weed control in sorghum.

Harvesting. Nearly all grain sorghum is harvested standing in the field with a combine (Fig. 1). Harvest begins in southern Texas in early June and slowly proceeds northward. In the central and northern Great Plains, the crop is usually harvested after frost. The grain threshes freely from the head when the seed moisture content is 20–25% or lower. The grain should not contain more than 12% moisture to ensure safe storage after harvest. Grain dryers are often used when the grain at harvest is not dry enough for optimum storage. Proper storage must be maintained until the grain can be marketed. The industry's economic health lies in the ability to provide grain of the right quality in the right quantity at the proper time and place.   [FREDERICK R. MILLER]

SWEET SORGHUM

Commonly known as sorgo, sweet sorghum was introduced into North America from China in 1850, although its ancestry traces back to Egypt. It is an annual, rather drought-resistant crop. The culms are from 2 to 15 ft tall, and the hard cortical layer, or shell, encloses a sweet, juicy pith that is interspersed with vascular bundles. At each node both a leaf and a lateral bud alternate on opposite sides; the internodes are alternately grooved on one side. Leaves are smooth with glossy or waxy surfaces and have margins with small, sharp, curved teeth. The leaves fold and roll up during drought. The inflorescence is a panicle of varying size having many primary branches with paired ellipsoidal spikelets containing two florets in each fertile sessile spikelet. The plant is self-pollinated.

Seed is planted in cultivated rows and fertilized similarly to corn. Maturity varies between 90 and 125 days. The juice contains about 12% sugar. The main sorghum-syrup-producing area is in the south-central and southeastern United States (Fig. 3).   [LEONARD D. BAVER]

DISEASES

Diseases frequently are limiting factors in production and may be classified in four general categories: (1) those that rot the seed and kill seedlings; (2) those that attack the leaves, making the plants less valuable for forage; (3) those that attack

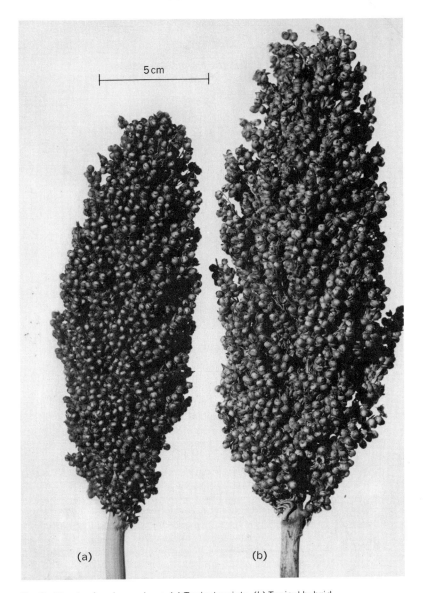

Fig. 2. Heads of grain sorghum. (a) Typical variety. (b) Typical hybrid.

and destroy the grain in the heads; and (4) those that attack the roots and stalks.

Fungi causing seed rotting and seedling diseases may be seed-borne or soil-inhabiting and are most destructive when the soil is cold and wet after planting. Species of *Fusarium*, *Pythium*, *Helminthosporium*, and one of *Penicillium* are the most important fungi involved. Damage may be considerably reduced by planting sound seed of recommended varieties treated with a good disinfectant in soil warm enough to ensure prompt germination.

Leaf and sheath diseases caused by at least three species of bacteria and eight fungus species are generally favored by high temperature and humid conditions. Disease lesions occurring as discolored spots or streaks may coalesce to involve the entire leaf. Sanitation, seed treatment, and the use of resistant varieties are recommended control measures.

Three smuts—covered kernel, loose kernel, and head smut—are the principal diseases attacking the grain (Fig. 4). Kernel smuts are distinguished by the replacement of the grain with a dark, sooty

SORGHUM

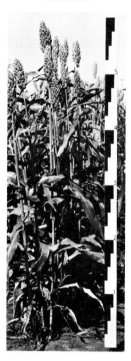

Fig. 3. Sweet sorghum in Oklahoma. (*USDA*)

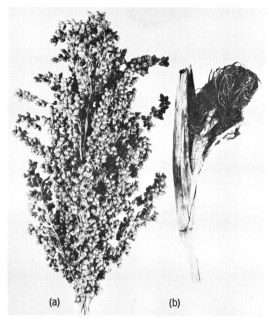

Fig. 4. Head smut on *Leoti sorgo.* (*a*) Healthy head. (*b*) Smutted head.

mass of spores, the covered type contained in a semipermanent membrane in contrast to the easily ruptured gall of the loose smut. Head smut destroys the entire head. Resistant varieties control kernel and head smuts to some extent, and seed treatment controls the kernel smuts.

Three diseases of the roots and stalks are of primary importance. Periconia root rot infecting the roots and crown caused extensive damage to milo and darso sorghums until it was controlled by resistant varieties. Charcoal rot, most evident as the plant approaches maturity under extreme conditions of heat or drought, causes shredding of the stalks and extensive lodging. Development of resistant varieties appears to be the only effective method of control. *See* BREEDING (PLANT); PLANT DISEASE CONTROL.   [HERMAN A. RODENHISER]

Bibliography: H. Doggett, *Sorghum,* 1970; J. R. Quinby, *Sorghum Improvement and the Genetics of Growth,* 1974; J. S. Wall and W. M. Ross, *Sorghum Production and Utilization,* 1970.

Soybean

Glycine max, a legume native to China that has become a major source of vegetable protein and oil for human and animal consumption and for industrial usage. Introduced into the United States in the late 1700s, soybeans were first grown as a curiosity and then as a forage and soil-building crop. The valued portion of the plant is the seed, which contains about 40% protein and 21% oil. There were 4.94×10^7 acres (2×10^7 ha) of soybeans harvested in the United States during 1976 with the greatest acreage in Illinois, followed by Iowa, Arkansas, Missouri, Indiana, Mississippi, Minnesota, Ohio, Louisiana, and Tennessee. The soybean production area of the United States is similar to that of corn and cotton because it can be grown interchangeably with either crop.

Economic importance. In 1975–1976 the United States was the world's largest producer of soybeans, followed by Brazil, the People's Republic of China, Mexico, Indonesia, and Argentina. About 59% of the soybeans produced in the United States were crushed or processed domestically, 35% were exported as whole beans, 5% were used for seed, and 1% had miscellaneous uses. Soybeans shipped from the United States in 1975–1976 as unprocessed whole beans, soybean meal, and oil accounted for 50% of total United States production and ranked with corn as the two agricultural commodities of highest monetary value for export. Countries that import large quantities of whole beans for processing include Japan, the Netherlands, West Germany, Spain, Italy, and Canada. West Germany, France, the Netherlands, and Italy import large quantities of soybean meal, and Pakistan, Bangladesh, Canada, and Iran are major importers of soybean oil.

Livestock consume about 98% of the soybean protein utilized in the United States. There is a limited use of the protein for human consumption as soy flours, grits, and texturized proteins in combination with other foods. Soybean oil is widely used throughout the world for human consumption as margarine, salad and cooking oils, and shortening.

In the People's Republic of China, Taiwan, Japan, Korea, and Indonesia, soybeans are a regular part of the human diet as a source of protein and oil. Soybean milk, made by soaking beans in water, grinding the soaked beans, and filtering the insoluble pieces out, is directly consumed primarily by the Chinese, but is the starting material for preparation of a soybean curd, probably the most important and popular soybean food in the Orient. The soft cheeselike curd, known as "tou fu," "tofu," "tubu," and other local names, has a bland taste and can be flavored with seasonings or blended with other foods. It contains about 53% protein, 26% fat, 17% carbohydrate, and 4% minerals, vitamins, and fiber. Soybean curd is made into a variety of products by frying, dehydration, and freezing, and is consumed daily in the same manner as high-protein foods in Western cultures. Soybeans also are prepared by fermentation with microorganisms to form highly flavored foods and seasonings such as soy sauce and fermented soybean paste. Soybean sprouts, immature green seed, and deep-fried mature seed provide additional sources of food for human consumption.

Plant characteristics. The soybean is an annual plant that reaches a mature height of 25 to 50 in. (64 to 127 cm). The cotyledons are the part of the seed that emerge from the soil as the seedling develops. Two unifoliolate leaves (single leaflet) develop opposite each other above the cotyledonary nodes. Other leaves produced on the plant generally are trifoliolate (three leaflets). Branches develop from the main stem in response to the amount of space between adjacent plants. A plant may produce few branches and only a few seeds in close spacings or many branches and over a thousand seeds in wide spacings.

Flowers of soybeans are self-fertilized and white or varying shades of purple. Pubescence (hair) on the stems, leaves, and pods is brown or gray. Pod color of commercial varieties in the United States is brown or tan, although genetic types are available with black pods. The pods generally contain one to four seeds ranging in size from about 800 to 10,000 seeds per pound (1800 to 22,000 seeds per kilogram); however, most commercial varieties have two or three seeds per pod with a size of 1600 to 3600 seeds per pound (3600 to 8000 seeds per kilogram). The seedcoat of commercial varieties is yellow, and the common colors of the hilum (seed scar showing point of attachment to pod) are yellow, gray, buff, brown, imperfect black, or black. Varieties of soybean native to Asia have yellow, green, black, brown, and varicolored seedcoats.

As a legume, soybeans can obtain nitrogen needed for growth from nitrogen-fixing bacteria that live in their roots. The bacteria can be applied at the time of planting by mixing them with the seed or by direct application to the soil. They can survive in most soils for several years and do not have to be reapplied when soybeans are grown in a field every 2 or 3 years. *See* LEGUME; NITROGEN FIXATION (BIOLOGY).

The growing season for soybean varieties is controlled by their response to photoperiod and temperature; consequently, the most productive varieties for the northern United States are different from those grown in the South. The number of days from planting to maturity can range from about 90 to 180 days, depending on the variety and environmental conditions.

Several thousand varieties and selections of soybeans have been introduced into the United States from other areas of the world, and in the past some of them were grown commercially. Current production, however, is entirely devoted to varieties produced by the breeding programs conducted by the U.S. Department of Agriculture, state agriculture experiment stations, and private companies.

Most soybeans in the United States are planted in a well-prepared seedbed, although in some locations they are planted in unplowed fields to reduce soil erosion. In areas where the growing season is long enough, soybeans are planted as a second crop immediately after wheat or similar crops are harvested. Planting is done in rows ranging in width from 7 to 40 in. (18 to 102 cm) with equipment also used to plant corn, cotton, wheat, and similar crops. Weed control includes the use of chemical herbicides, mechanical cultivation, and hand labor. Harvest of soybeans with combines begins when the leaves have dropped and moisture in the seed is at or below the 13% level required for safe storage.   [WALTER R. FEHR]

DISEASES

Most diseases of soybean that occur throughout the world can be found in the United States. Diseases tend to be chronic in nature, occurring with some regularity from year to year and taking a small (and often unnoticed) toll. Annual losses from all diseases have been estimated at 12%, and this figure can fluctuate considerably, depending upon environmental conditions in any one particular season. Many diseases are usually found in any one field, and a disease-free field is rare indeed.

Although the term disease is often difficult to define, it is usually considered that soybean diseases can be caused by both living and nonliving entities. In the first category are the parasitic diseases caused by fungi, nematodes, bacteria, and

viruses. The nonliving causes of disease include conditions of weather and soil and the deficiency or excess of various minerals. Iron, potassium, and manganese deficiencies are common, and varying degrees of chlorosis accompany such deficits. Herbicide and lightning damage are also often reported by growers.

Fungus diseases. Fungi cause more diseases than other parasitic organisms. Leaves can be attacked by *Peronospora manshurica* and become severely spotted with yellowish-green areas on upper leaf surfaces. If the case is severe enough, the leaves can fall prematurely; the leaves more often remain intact, and the spots take on a dark-brown appearance with fungus growth apparent on the lower side of leaves. This symptom gives rise to the common term mildew. The fungus spreads rapidly from plant to plant and may overwinter in fallen leaves or invade pods and survive on seeds as a white crust. Many pathogenic variants of this fungus are found, and resistant varieties of soybean are being developed. Up to 8% reduction in yield has been reported from this disease alone in Iowa.

In the Midwest, brown spot, caused by *Septoria glycines*, is another disease of importance on leaves. It appears early in the season as angular lesions on primary leaves and may continue to move up the plant and cause defoliation, attack pods, and ultimately invade seed. Target spot, a disease caused by *Corynespora cassiicola*, is found further south in the soybean-growing region and has caused losses in the range of 18–32% in Mississippi. Its name is derived from concentric dark rings formed as large brown and often irregular spots develop on leaves. Fungus leaf spots of minor importance include those caused by *Cerco-*

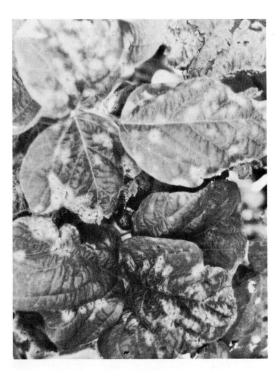

Fig. 1. Bacterial blight symptoms on soybean leaves under field conditions. The condition results principally in chlorate spots and malformations.

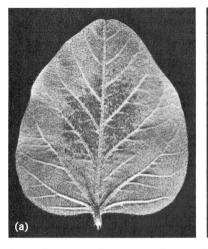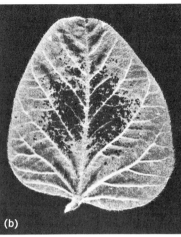

Fig. 2. Response of soybean varieties to bacterial blight. (a) Complete resistance. (b) Complete susceptibility.

spora sojina, Phyllosticta sojicola, and *Alternaria atrans.*

A series of fungus root and stem rots may plague soybeans. Root rot, caused by *Phytophthora megasperma,* is probably the most spectacular and serious disease in areas where it occurs. Plants die in all stages of growth, usually in low places in fields and along end turn rows. Several states and Canada have reported damage from this disease, and control is now effected by the use of resistant varieties. Inheritance of resistance is controlled by a single factor, thus making it relatively simple to incorporate this resistance into promising (or preexisting) varieties of soybeans. The pathogen is not seed-borne.

Brown stem rot, caused by *Cephalosporium gregatum,* is a disease of major concern in the Midwest. No resistance is known, and the fungus is widespread in Minnesota, Illinois, Iowa, and Indiana. Crop rotation (on a 3–4-year basis) is the only known control. Seed rot and root rot by *Pythium* and *Rhizoctonia* are common and chronic on seedlings over vast areas of the soybean region. Plants able to emerge usually outgrow this problem; however, stand reduction may be severe enough to warrant replanting. Stem canker and pod and stem blight are two stages of an important disease caused by *Diaporthe phaseolorum* which are favored by high humidity and can be controlled to some extent by chemical seed treatment.

Soybean rust, a fungus-induced disease, is assuming more importance as acreages expand in traditional soybean growing areas and as production moves into new areas. The disease is serious in the Orient, especially in tropical and subtropical areas. In Taiwan, Thailand, the Philippines, and Java it is the most damaging fungal disease affecting soybean crops. The pathogen, *Phakopsora pachyrhizi* Sydow, can infect and sporulate on species in 17 known legume genera but is economically important only on soybean. The pathogen has been reported in Africa on cowpea but not on soybean. In 1976 soybean rust was found on soybean cultivars Biloxi, Hardee, Santa Rosa, and Williams in an experimental planting in the highlands of western Puerto Rico. This was the first record of rust on soybean in the Western Hemis-

phere, and is cause for concern in the Americas. It is likely that the pathogen will be found on soybean plantings elsewhere in the Caribbean area.

Bacterial diseases. Bacterial diseases usually are not epidemic, being more of a chronic problem of this crop. They are exceedingly widespread, bacterial blight (Fig. 1) caused by *Pseudomonas glycinea* being found primarily in the upper Midwest and bacterial pustule caused by *Xanthomonas phaseoli* predominating in the southern United States. These pathogens enter plants through pores or injuries in leaves and are spread rapidly by windblown rain. Seed-borne infection is common and constitutes the major means of overwintering. Infected seedlings can thus emerge, and the disease cycle begins again. Antibiotic sprays are impractical, and resistant strains of the blight pathogen develop rapidly during their use. Some varieties of soybean are more resistant to blight than others (Fig. 2), and inheritance of resistance in the soybean host depends upon the particular strain of the pathogen being tested.

A chlorisis (yellowing of leaves) may develop from strains of *Rhizobia,* which are abnormal in that they cannot fix nitrogen but are aggressive in entering soybean roots. These bacteria thus occupy space that efficient nitrogen fixers would otherwise occupy. A bacterial wilt caused by *Corynebacterium flaccumfaciens* has been reported in certain areas of the Midwest but is not of great economic importance.

Virus diseases. The viruses may enter soybean plants by any of several methods, although each virus usually is very specific in its mode of entrance. They may be injected into the plant by insects or nematodes or through wounds or may go from one generation to the next via the seed. Only a few of the viruses of this crop have been studied extensively.

Soybean mosaic is common and is easily transmitted mechanically or by insects or seeds. It usually appears on leaves as crinkling and distortion of young tissues, and damage is similar to that produced by sprays used in weed control. It affects the seed by producing a "mottled" appearance; the seed becomes discolored when pigments from the seed scar appear to streak across seed coat surfaces during their development. Control is difficult, but yield losses have not been excessive.

Bud blight, on the other hand, is a very destructive virus disease, and no resistance is known. It, too, is seed-borne; it is apparently transmitted by insects, but this vector has not been discovered. Usually, isolated plants in a field are found scattered at random (originating from infected seed), or plants along the edge of fields bordering alfalfa or fence rows may be heavily infected. This phase is thought to be due to an insect vector moving the virus from other plants to soybeans. Loss in yield can be 100% of the crop. This virus causes the plant to produce a rank green stem which stays green after frost, and seed pods are either absent or small; if infected while young, the growing point of plants die and curve downward, giving rise to the common name bud blight. The same virus causes ring spot in tobacco. *See* PLANT VIRUS.

Nematodes. These pathogens are microscopic, eellike worms in the soil. Members of the genus *Meloidogyne* cause root knots or galls which form as large swellings and cause severe yellowing and stunting of aboveground portions of the plant. Crop rotation and the use of resistant varieties constitute the usual control methods. The soybean cyst nematode *Heterodera glycines* represents a real threat to soybean production and is under strict quarantine. It was first found in 1952 in North Carolina and since then has been found in isolated places in Virginia, Mississippi, Arkansas, Illinois, Kentucky, Missouri, and Tennessee. Symptoms vary but are not very dissimilar to root knot symptoms on aboveground parts of the plants. Below ground, small white cysts are noted and few or no nodules are associated with nitrogen fixation. Yield loss may be severe. *See* PLANT DISEASE; PLANT DISEASE CONTROL.

[BILL W. KENNEDY]

PROCESSING

Processing of soybeans into oil and defatted cake or meal began in the Orient. The oil was used primarily in foods, whereas the meal was used as a fertilizer and in animal feed. Today, the soybean processing industry converts the oil and meal from the soybean seed into numerous food and indus-

trial products. The products can be generally classified into three categories: soybean oil, soybean meal, and soybean protein products.

In the United States, soybeans have been processed primarily to obtain oil. The oil was processed for use in shortenings, margarines, and salad dressings. The defatted cake or soybean meal, once a by-product of soybean processing, is now the principal product from soybeans because of its protein value for livestock feeding. Soybean protein products are prepared primarily for direct human consumption. Direct food usage has been limited, but is expected to increase dramatically due to population pressure on the food supply and limited land and energy resources available for expansion of the livestock industry.

Statistics. The United States production of soybeans in 1975 was 1.546×10^9 bu ($5.45\ 10^7$ m^3). Approximately 8.65×10^8 bu (3.05×10^7 m^3) were processed, 5.4×10^8 bu (1.9×10^7 m^3) were exported, and 8.5×10^7 bu (3×10^6 m^3) were used for feed and seed. The remainder (about 5.6×10^7 bu or 1.97×10^6 m^3) was carried into the 1976 crop year.

Approximately 9.6×10^9 lb (4.36×10^9 kg) of soybean oil and 2.07×10^{10} lb (9.4×10^9 kg) of soy-

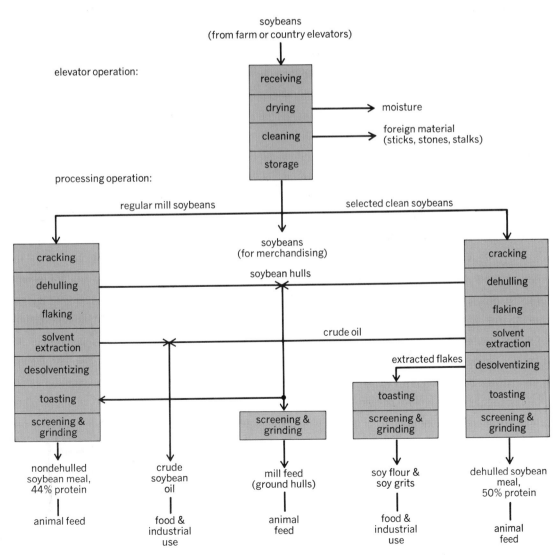

Fig. 3. Solvent extraction method.

bean meal were produced in 1975. Most of the meal (2.04×10^{10} lb or 9.3×10^9 kg) was used for animal feeds. The average price of crude soybean oil during 1975 was 18.3¢ lb (40.3¢/kg), and meal (44% protein) was $147.75/ton ($162.90/metric ton).

The combined processing or crushing capacity of all soybean mills in the United States is estimated at 1.2×10^9 bu (4.23×10^7 m³). Since there is more processing capacity than soybeans milled, plant utilization is estimated at 66%.

Oil extraction. The basic processing of soybeans consists of separation of the oil and meal. The equipment used varies considerably from plant to plant although the general process, solvent extraction of the oil, remains the same. Older, obsolete methods used either continuous screw presses or hydraulic presses to squeeze out the oil. Solvent extraction has almost universally been adopted because of its efficiency and low operating cost.

The steps involved in the solvent extraction of soybeans are outlined in Fig. 3. Storage of soybeans in elevators or silos is included as part of the processing since it ensures a continuous, year-round supply of beans for processing without the day-to-day price fluctuations of the commodity market. The soybeans, prior to storage, are cleaned and dried to 12–14% moisture for improved stability until processed.

Preparation. The processing operation consists of preparation, extraction, and meal-finishing phases. Preparation for extraction consists of steam-conditioning the beans, cracking, dehulling, and flaking. Cracking the beans into small particles, usually six to eight pieces, loosens the hulls from the soybean meats and assists in the flaking operation. Corrugated rollers are used for the cracking operation. Dehulling or separation of the hull material from the cracked meats is necessary to increase extraction efficiencies. Dehulling is performed by a combination of air aspiration, screening, centrifugal separation, and density separation methods. Flaking the cracked, dehulled soybean meats facilitates the extraction process by disruption of the internal cellular structure of the bean and by allowing better contact of the extracting solvent with the internal parts of the seed. Flaking is done by heating and steaming the cracked meats and passing them through differential roller mills. The resulting flakes are paper-thin (0.25–0.40 mm).

Extraction. This operation consists of washing the flakes with a petroleum solvent, usually hexane. The solvent is kept near 50°C during extraction to speed the solubilization of oil from the flakes into the solvent. The oil-laden solvent, called micella, is then separated from the flakes and distilled for recovery of the solvent for further use. The crude soybean oil is then pumped to storage tanks for further processing or to be sold as crude soybean oil.

Finishing. The solvent-wet, defatted flakes are desolventized by steam and heat. The severity of the desolventizing depends upon subsequent uses for the meal. If the extracted flakes are to be utilized in animal feeds, moisture is adjusted and the flakes are heat treated (toasted) to increase their feeding value. Flakes to be used for edible soy flour or protein products are subjected to less severe heating to prevent heat damage to the pro-

teins present. After desolventizing, the flakes are screened and ground to the desired particle size. The protein content may also be adjusted. Anti-caking agents are sometimes added to ensure ease in handling.

Yields. The processing yields based on a 60-lb (27.2 kg) bushel are 10.2–11.6 lb (4.6–5.3 kg) of crude oil and 48.4–49.8 lb (22–22.6 kg) of meal and feed products. The maximum yield of crude oil is always attempted. The meal from the extraction contains 49–50% protein. The hulls, accounting for about 5% of the beans, are ground and may be added back to the extracted meal for production of a 44% protein meal. The quantities of each meal prepared depend upon the market value at the time of production. The ground hulls may be stored for later use, sold as mill feed to be used as a source of fiber in mixed livestock feed products, or used in a patented process as a carrier for molasses in feed concentrates.

Soybean oil processing. Soybean oil is used in salad dressings, shortenings, and margarines and in various nonfood applications such as paints and varnishes. Most (93%) is used in foods. To be suitable for edible products, crude oil from the extraction requires further processing.

The processing of soybean oil, generally referred to as refining, is outlined in Fig. 4. Individual processes are degumming, alkali refining, bleaching (decolorizing), hydrogenation, deodorization, and winterization. Semirefined oils are also marketed, depending upon the customer's demands. Hydrogenation is varied, depending upon the final use of the oil. All edible oils are deodorized.

Degumming. During degumming, the soybean phospholipids are removed from the crude oil. Degumming itself refers to the gummy consistency of the wet phospholipids. The process involves the addition of a small amount of water or steam to the crude oil, resulting in the hydration of the phospholipids and their subsequent precipitation. Acidic catalysts are sometimes added with the water to improve the hydration. The precipitated phospholipids are then separated by centrifugation and are vacuum-dried. The dried phospholipids are sold as soybean lecithin.

Lecithin. Commercial soybean lecithin is widely used in foods, particularly chocolate, margarine, shortening, and greaseless frying compounds. Soybean lecithin from the degumming step contains 60–65% phospholipids and 30–35% entrained soybean oil. The principal phospholipids present are phosphatidylcholine, phosphatidylethanolamine, and phosphatidylinositol. The crude lecithin is dark-colored and may be bleached with hydrogen peroxide to produce a light, straw-colored product. Fatty acids may be added to make a fluid product, or the lecithin may be treated with ammonia to form a firm, plastic consistency. More refined grades (pharmaceutical lecithin) are produced by acetone extraction of the entrained soybean oil. The phospholipids are insoluble and precipitate. Further processing consists of desolventizing and granulating.

Alkali refining. The degummed soybean oil is next alkali-refined to remove the residual phospholipids, free fatty acids, and color from the oil. Alkali refining consists of addition of caustic soda, soda

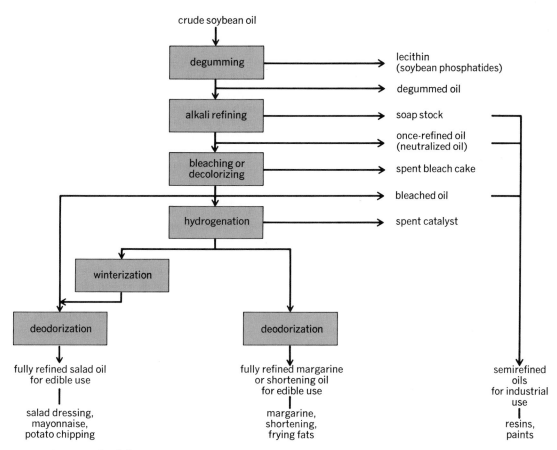

crude soybean oil

degumming → lecithin
(soybean phosphatides)

→ degummed oil

alkali refining → soap stock

→ once-refined oil
(neutralized oil)

bleaching or
decolorizing → spent bleach cake

→ bleached oil

hydrogenation → spent catalyst

winterization

deodorization

deodorization

fully refined salad oil
for edible use

fully refined margarine
or shortening oil
for edible use

semirefined
oils
for industrial
use

salad dressing,
mayonnaise,
potato chipping

margarine,
shortening,
frying fats

resins,
paints

Fig. 4. Soybean oil refining process.

ash, or a combination of the two to neutralize the free fatty acids present. Careful addition of the alkali is required to prevent further degradation of the oil. The neutralized free fatty acids or soaps are removed from the oil by centrifugation or settling. The soaps, referred to as soapstock, are sold to soap manufacturers, fatty acid industries, or livestock feed formulators in the alkaline form, or in an acidulated form after treatment with sulfuric acid. The alkali refined oil is further washed with water to remove all traces of alkali and soaps present and then dried. The neutralized oil is often sold to industrial users for nonfood applications.

Bleaching. Bleaching (decolorizing) removes the pigments present in the oil by adsorption on activated earth or carbon. The bleaching agent is simply dispersed in the oil and removed by filtration. The bleached oil is sent to the hydrogenation unit or to the deodorizers, depending upon the final use. Foods requiring plastic fats such as margarines or bakery shortenings require hydrogenation.

Hydrogenation. Development of the hydrogenation process for vegetable oils has permitted the substitution of vegetable oils for animal-derived fats and the substitution of the various types of vegetable oils with soybean oil. Variations in the hydrogenation conditions can be used to produce high-stability soybean oil, hardened soybean oils that melt rapidly at body temperature, and shorteninglike fats.

Hydrogenation is performed by purging the oil with hydrogen gas at an elevated temperature and pressure in the presence of a catalyst. Nickel catalysts are generally used. The addition of hydrogen

to the fat saturates the molecular structure. The degree of saturation depends upon the time, temperature, and pressure of hydrogenation.

Deodorizing. Deodorization of the oil removes the undesirable flavor and odor constituents. Oils must be odorless and bland in flavor to be suitable for food use. Deodorization is carried out under high temperature and vacuum with steam injected to assist volatilization of the undesirable components.

Winterization. Winterization is performed on lightly hydrogenated soybean oil that is to be used as a salad oil. The oil, in addition to conforming to oxidative stability requirements, must remain clear at refrigerator temperatures. Winterization consists of cooling of the oil and filtering off the cloudy haze that forms.

Reversion. Refined soybean oil is a highly unsaturated oil and will develop, after storage, characteristic flavors and odors described as "painty" or "fishy." The development of these flavors is called reversion, and is possibly a result of the oxidation of the linolenic acid component of the oil. Care in the exposure of the oil to air during processing and controlled hydrogenation to partially saturate the linolenic acid minimizes the tendency of soybean oil to reversion. Metal sequestrants, such as citric acid, are sometimes added during deodorization to inactivate the prooxidant metals such as iron and copper. Antioxidants may also be added. *See* FAT AND OIL, EDIBLE; LINOLENIC ACID.

Soybean protein products. The soybean protein products are prepared from the extracted meal. Three distinct product types are prepared: soy

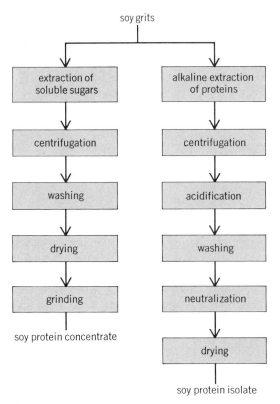

Fig. 5. Production of soy protein concentrates and isolates.

flour and grits, soy protein concentrates, and soy protein isolates. These are used both in foods and in nonfood applications.

Flour and grits. Soy flour and grits production in the United States has risen to 9×10^8 lb (4.1×10^8 kg). Numerous products are prepared, each containing approximately 50% protein based on the nonlipid fraction. Flours and grits are used in processed meats, bakery mixes, cereals, breads, and baby foods. A large amount has been utilized in nutrients for export to undeveloped, underfed countries.

The term "soy flour" refers to an extremely fine powdered product, whereas "grits" refer to a granular product. Various products are prepared varying in oil content, oil type, particle size, and water solubility of the protein. In general, the oil content varies from less than 1% (defatted) to 18–20% (full fat); the oil source is soybean oil or lecithin. Particle size varies from powders that pass a 200-mesh screen (flour) to those that pass a 14-mesh (grits). Water solubility of the protein ranges from 10% (toasted) to 80% (untoasted).

Soy flour or grits is produced similarly to soybean meal, except with thorough removal of the hulls before extraction. Desolventizing and toasting are varied to alter the water solubility of the protein, with minimum heating being required for high protein solubility. The defatted, desolventized flakes are ground and screened to the desired particle size.

The oil-containing products are generally prepared by blending soybean oil or lecithin back to the extracted meals. Full-fat soy flour may also be prepared by steaming the unextracted, dehulled

flakes to remove the bitter flavors, and then drying, grinding, and screening them to the desired particle size.

Concentrates. Soybean protein concentrates and soybean protein isolates are generally prepared from soy flour or grits. The processing methods vary considerably between processors. A generalized process is shown in Fig. 5.

Soybean protein concentrates contain 70% protein. Concentrates are prepared by washing the water-soluble carbohydrates from the meal under conditions designed to ensure minimum protein solubility. Dilute acids or aqueous alcohol solutions have been used. The washing is performed in agitated tanks. The remaining insoluble proteins and carbohydrates are removed from the extraction by centrifugation or filtration, washed, dried, and ground. Products are marketed with ranges of particle sizes and protein solubilities similar to soy flour and grits. Soy protein concentrates are usually bland in flavor, possess a lighter color, and are more functional than soy flour (having emulsification, water-binding, gelling, and other properties).

Isolates. Soy protein isolates are the purest form of soy proteins marketed (90% protein minimum). The isolates are prepared by solubilizing the protein present in the grits by using mildly alkaline solutions, separating the protein solution from the firbrous residue by centrifugation or filtration, and acidifying the protein solution to precipitate the protein as a curd. The curd is recovered, washed, and resolubilized, and the spray is dried into a fine, flourlike powder.

Soy protein isolates are manufactured to possess specific functional properties such as gelling, whipping, foaming, emulsifying, thickening, and binding. Isolates are used in meats, simulated dairy products, and bakery products.

Textured proteins. Each of the soybean protein products can be used to form textured soy proteins. Textured soy proteins have a meatlike texture and appearance when hydrated and can be used for extension of ground and comminuted meats (such as ground meat and bologna) and for the preparation of simulated meats. When used as extenders, the textured proteins increase cook yield, aid in binding of meat constituents, and improve emulsion stability.

Two general processes (with variations) are used for texturizing soy proteins: extrusion cooking and spinning. Extrusion cooking consists of moistening the protein, working the doughlike mass under high temperature and pressure, and forcing the cooked mass through an orifice, which permits the heated compressed mass to expand. The product is then dried and sized. Colored and flavored extruded soy protein products are prepared by addition of these additives either before or after extrusion. Imitation bacon bits based on extruded soy flour are widely marketed.

Soy protein isolates are required for spinning. Spun proteins are somewhat more adaptable to simulated meat production than extruded proteins. Spun proteins are produced by solubilizing the isolates in an alkaline solution and forcing this solution through a multiholed die immersed in an acid bath. The solubilized protein immediately coagulates in the acid bath, forming a continuous filament. The filaments are stretched to orient the protein molecules within the filament. Toughness of the filaments is dependent upon the degree of protein orientation. Filament diameters are approximately 0.003 in. (0.076 mm). Groups of filaments when combined with egg white, flavors, and colors, followed by compression and heat setting, form imitation meats such as ham, chicken, or beef. *See* FOOD ENGINEERING; FOOD MANUFACTURING.

[F. T. ORTHOEFER]

Bibliography: L. P. Hanson, *Vegetable Protein Processing*, 1974; A. K. Smith and S. J. Circle, *Soybeans Chemistry and Technology*, vol. 1, 1972; D. Swern (ed.), *Bailey's Industrial Oil and Fat Products*, 1964; W. J. Wolf and J. C. Cowan, *Soybeans as a Food Source*, 1971.

Spice and flavoring

Substances added to food to enhance savoriness. Spices are aromatic vegetable materials used for food seasoning. Flavorings are compounded blends of materials used to produce particular flavors or simulate other known flavors.

A spice may be derived from any part of the plant: leaf (bay), flower bud (cloves), fruit (pimento), bark (cassia), rhizome (turmeric), root (horseradish), or seed (anise). Spices may be used whole as are caraway and poppy seed or ground as is cinnamon bark. With the exception of red peppers and a few others, spices used in the United States are imported, since most grow in tropical or subtropical climates. In the food industry spices are used in many physical states. Besides in the whole and ground conditions, spices are procured as mixed materials ready for use. There has been a growing use of spice extracts, or oleoresins, either as such, or spread on the surface of sugar, salt, or dextrose to make so-called "soluble spices." These have the advantage of showing no specking in light-colored foods. Premixed oleoresins are available for use in such products as canned foods and pickles.

The oleoresins are prepared by solvent extraction of the spice and may be separated into two fractions by steam distillation. The volatile fraction which comes over in steam distillation is called the essential oil; the oleoresin portion remaining behind is called the fixed oil. Spices vary markedly in their proportion of volatile to fixed oils as well as in their total oleoresin content.

In the preparation of oleoresins and essential oils it is usual commercial practice in the United States to remove the active flavoring constituents by solvent percolation. The essential oil is then

Economically important spices

Spice	Plant and source	Plant part used	Principal use
Allspice* (*Pimenta*)	Evergreen of myrtle family from Jamaica and Guatemala	Dried fruit	Pickles, roast meat, ketchup
Anise*	Parsley family from Mediterranean	Seed	Baked goods, anisette (a liqueur)
Basil	Mint family grown in U.S. and other parts of world	Leaves and tender stems	Sauces and soups, especially tomato-based
Bay	Evergreen of laurel family from Mediterranean, Turkey, Greece, and Portugal	Leaf	Pickles, stews, soups, sauces
Caraway*	Biennial of parsley family from north-central Europe and southern England	Seed	Bread and baked goods, cheese, sauces, kummel (a liqueur)
Cardamon*	Ginger family from Guatemala and India	Seed	Baked goods, coffee blends, curry powders
Cayenne	Capsicum family grown over most of the world (name used for those high in pungency)	Pod or fruit	Many foods, pickles, sauces, meats, curry powder
Celery*	Parsley family principally from France and India	Seed	Sauces, salads, pickles, soups
Cinnamon*	Evergreen member of laurel family from Ceylon	Bark	Baked goods, pickles, candy
Clove*	Evergreen tree of the myrtle family from Madagascar and Zanzibar	Unopened bud flower	Pork products, pickles, stews, meats, and gravies
Coriander*	Plant of parsley family from Yugoslavia and Morocco	Dried fruit	Frankfurters, bologna, baked goods
Cumin*	Annual plant of parsley family from Iran and Morocco	Dried fruit	Chili powder
Dill*	Member of parsley family from India and domestic sources	Seed and leaves	Pickles, soups, sauces
Fennel*	Perennial of parsley family from India and Rumania	Seed	Baked goods, salad dressings, meat products
Garlic*	Member of lily family from U.S. and Mediterranean	Bulb	Baked meats, sauces, dressings, soups
Ginger*	Tuberous perennial from Jamaica, India, and Africa	Rhizome	Soft drinks, baked goods, pickles, puddings

*See individual articles for further information.

Economically important spices (cont.)

Spice	Plant and source	Plant part used	Principal use
Mace	Tropical tree similar to rhododendron from Indonesia and West Indies	Aril covering nutmeg	Baked goods, processed meats
Marjoram	Perennial of mint family from France, Peru, and Chile	Leaves	Soups, stews, sauces
Mint	Perennial herb of many varieties grown in U.S.	Leaves	Confections, sauces, jellies, gums
Mustard*	Annual of mustard family from U.S. in Montana and California	Seeds	Sauces, baked meats, processed meats and gravies
Nutmeg*	Tropical tree similar to rhododendron from Indonesia or West Indies	Seed	Baked goods, processed meats, meat, fruit sauces
Oregano	Perennial of mint family from U.S., Mexico, Italy, and France	Leaves	Sauces and stews, especially tomato-based
Paprika*	Member of capsicum family from Spain, U.S., and Hungary	Pod or fruit	Red-colored dressings, sauces, meats, condiments as ketchup
Pepper* black white	Perennial climbing vine from India, Borneo, Malaya, and Indonesia	Berry (black): berry with cortex removed (white)	Virtually all food products, table use
Poppy seed	Annual of poppy family from Poland, Argentina, Iran, and Turkey	Seed	Toppings for baked goods and confections
Rosemary	Evergreen of mint family from France, Spain, and Portugal	Leaf	Meats, sauces, gravies
Saffron*	Plant of crocus family from Spain	Stigma of flower	Coloring rice and other specialties
Sage*	Member of mint family from Dalmatia, Greece, and Yugoslavia	Leaf	Sausage, poultry, poultry stuffing
Savory	Member of mint family from France and Spain	Leaf	Meats, stuffings, salads, sauces
Sesame	From sesame plant in U.S., Nicaragua, Salvador, Egypt, Brazil	Seed	Baked goods and confections
Thyme	Perennial of mint family from France and U.S.	Leaf	Sauces for shellfish and with fresh tomato
Tumeric*	Member of ginger family from India, Haiti, Jamaica, and Peru	Rhizome	Yellow color in pickles, sauces, and fish

*See individual articles for further information.

removed from the oleoresin by steam distillation. It is not uncommon, however, to remove the oil from the flavor-bearing substance by direct steam distillation. In solvent extraction for oleoresin the spice material is usually ground to increase extraction efficiency. Particle size is extremely important as in all solvent extraction procedures. The time of extraction and solvent used are determined by the material being extracted. Hexane, perchlorethylene, trichlorethylene, acetone, and ethyl and propyl alcohols are used as solvents. Each spice presents a peculiar problem; for example, cassia extract polymerizes readily and if not treated promptly will "set up" in the receiver so that it is virtually impossible to remove.

Spices. The economically important spices are shown in the table.

Flavoring. A great deal has been written on the use of various flavoring materials, but much of the field remains in the art state and reliance is placed on experienced personnel with knowledge of the materials available and of the nature of the finished products desired.

Flavor ester mixtures are flavoring materials which closely resemble the flavor and odor of natural herbs, nuts, fruits, and seeds. A solution of flavor ester mixtures in alcohol is known as a flavor extract; a flavor ester mixture in a solvent other than alcohol is termed a flavor.

Blended flavorings are mixtures of natural and synthetic compounds. These may be naturally occurring substances, such as lemon oil; substances like eugenol, isolated from naturally occurring flavoring materials; substances like vanillin, prepared synthetically but also occurring in natural material; or synthetic substances, such as methyl anthranilite used in grape essence. Methyl anthranilite is also used in banana, currant, and melon flavors. Compounding these materials calls for careful balancing of the ingredients. *See* CITRUS FLAVORING; FOOD ENGINEERING; FOOD MANUFACTURING; SALT (FOOD); VANILLA EXTRACT.

[ROY E. MORSE]

Bibliography: E. Guenther, *The Essential Oils*, vols. 1–6, 1948–1952; F. L. Hart and H. J. Fisher, *Modern Food Analysis*, 1970; R. Hemphill, *Fra-*

grance and Flavor, 1960; M. B. Jacobs, *Synthetic Food Adjuncts,* 1947; L. W. Jones (ed.), *A Treasury of Spices,* 1956; J. W. Parry, *Spices,* 1969.

Spinach

A cool-season annual of Asiatic origin, *Spinacia oleracea,* belonging to the plant order Caryophyllales. It is grown for its foliage (see illustration) and served as a cooked vegetable or as a salad. New Zealand spinach (*Tetrogonia expansa*) and Mountain spinach (*Atriplex hortense*) are also called spinach but are less commonly grown. Spinach plants are usually dioecious.

Propagation is by seed, commonly planted in rows 10–20 in. apart. Cool weather favors maximum production. High temperatures and long daylight periods encourage seedstalk formation and reduce vegetative growth. Fall-seeded spinach is overwintered and harvested in the spring in areas where the weather is mild or the crop is protected by snow cover. *See* PHOTOPERIODISM IN PLANTS; SEED (BOTANY); VEGETABLE GROWING.

Varieties (cultivars) are classified according to seed (smooth or prickly), leaves (smooth or savoyed), and seeding tendencies (early or late, or long standing). Popular varieties are Long Standing Bloomsdale, Eary Hybrid 7, Hybrid 424, Savoy Hybrid 621, and Viroflay.

Harvesting by hand or machine begins when the plants have reached full size and before seedstalks form, usually 40–50 days after planting.

In the United States the average annual value of spinach for the fresh market from about 10,000 acres is approximately $9,000,000. Texas and California are the important producing states. The nation's average annual farm value of spinach for processing from approximately 27,000 acres is about $9,000,000, with California and Oklahoma being the principal producing states.

[H. JOHN CAREW]

Squash

The common name for edible fruits of several species of the genus *Cucurbita: C. pepo, C. moschata, C. maxima,* and *C. mixta.* Those species originated in the Americas but are now grown in most countries around the world. Within squash there is tremendous variation is size, shape, color, and usage (see Fig. 1).

Summer squash. The most clearly defined group is summer squash, fruit of any species of *Cucurbita* eaten as a vegetable when immature. It is most commonly *C. pepo,* and its plants are usually bushy rather than having long runners. In some countries fruits may be picked as early as the day the flowers open, but they are eaten at all stages up to the time when the rind starts to harden. Fruit color may be white, yellow, or light or dark green, and the green may be solid or striped. Shapes may be flattened disks as in Pattypan, cylindrical as in Zucchini and Cocozelle, or with necks as in the straightneck and crookneck types. Summer squash has mild flavor, high water content (about 95%), and relatively low nutritional value. It is not especially high in any one nutrient but contributes modest amounts of several vitamins and minerals.

Winter squash. Winter squash is fruit of *Cucurbita* eaten when mature and derives its name from

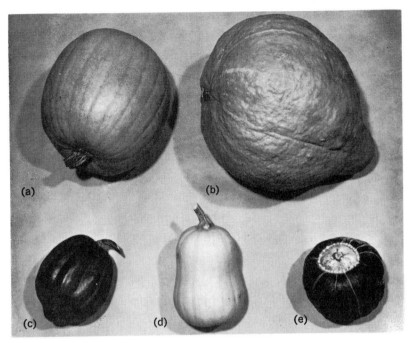

Fig. 1. Five varieties of squash (*a*) Young's Beauty pumpkin; (*b*) Boston Marrow squash; (*c*) Table Queen squash; (*d*) Butternut squash; (*e*) Buttercup squash.

its ability to be stored for several weeks or months before consumption. Varieties of winter squash are found in all four species. The Table Queen group, synonymous with Acorn, is *C. pepo,* Butternut belongs to *C. moschata,* Green-striped Cushaw is *C. mixta,* while *C. maxima* has the widest range of types, including Buttercup, Hubbards, and Delicious of various colors, Banana, and Boston Marrow. Flesh color varies from light yellow to dark orange, and the edible portion ranges from thin to very thick, depending on variety.

Characteristics. The percentage of soluble solids, which are mostly sugars, in cooked winter squash is commonly 8–10% and may be as high as 16%, putting squash in the same range as good melons. Squash is a good source of calories and of vitamin A, particularly those with dark orange flesh, which are high in carotene. Varieties tend to have their own characteristic flavors: the greatest difference is between the Table Queen group and the other winter squashes. Plants of winter squash are characteristically viny in habit with runner lengths of 12 to 20 ft (3.6 to 6 m) under good growing conditions, but bush or semiviny forms have been developed in some of the types. The bush forms of winter squash tend to be lower in solids and in quality, especially if they set a heavy load of fruit.

There is some confusion in terminology between winter squash and pumpkin, and the use of these names differs from place to place. Both names refer to mature fruits, and varieties called squash and others called pumpkins may be found in all four *Cucurbita* species. In the United States, varieties eaten as a vegetable are generally called squash, while those used for pies, stock feed, or autumn decorations are usually called pumpkins. Pumpkins tend to be round with orange exterior color and flesh that is paler, more fibrous, and less sweet than squash. *See* PUMPKIN.

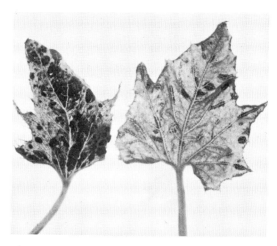

Fig. 2. Squash leaves, mottled by mosaic virus.

Propagation. Squash is propagated by seed and its flowering habit is monoecious, that is, with separate male and female flowers on the same plant. Male flowers usually appear several days before the first female. Pollination is done naturally by insects, and within a species types which look very different cross readily with each other. However, the fruit is not affected in the year crossing occurs. Natural crossing occurs only rarely between the different species. Separation of the sexes makes controlled crossing relatively easy, and first-generation hybrids are increasingly being used as varieties, especially in summer squash where hybrid vigor is manifested in earlier flowering. One result of hybridization is that Butternut, Table Queen, Zucchini, and others which were originally single varieties have become groups of varieties with similar fruit shape but differing fruit sizes, colors, times of maturity, and plant sizes. *See* BREEDING (PLANT).

Squash seed is usually planted directly in the field after the soil is warm, in rows 4–6 ft (1.2–1.8 m) apart for bush types and 6–9 ft (1.8–2.7 m) apart for vining types. Plants may be spaced from 2–3 ft (0.6–0.9 m) apart in both cases. In cool re-

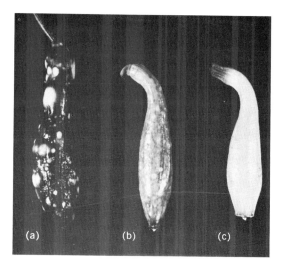

Fig. 3. Crookneck squash. (*a, b*) Fruit mottled by mosaic virus. (*c*) Healthy fruit.

gions, plants may be started in a greenhouse, provided they are grown in containers which permit transplanting without much disturbance of roots and before they become too large. The best size for transplanting may be reached in 10–14 days under good growing conditions.

Harvesting and storage. Summer squash begins to bear in 50–60 days from planting. The fruit grows very rapidly and must be harvested at frequent intervals (3–4 times per week) if one wishes the plants to continue bearing for an extended period.

Winter squash should be harvested when fully mature for best quality. Unless planted very early, it is often left in the field until the first light frost occurs, then harvested before the exposed fruit can be damaged by subsequent frost. Storage temperatures of 50–60°F (10–16°C) are best because chilling injury occurs at lower temperatures and shortens storage life. For all varieties except Table Queen, a curing period of 1–2 weeks at 70–80°F (21–27°C) may improve quality by hastening conversion of starch to sugar. *See* VEGETABLE GROWING.   [H. M. MUNGER]

Diseases. Diseases cause about a $250,000 loss in the 50,000 acres of squash annually grown in California, Texas, Florida, the Midwest, and the mid-Atlantic states. The value of the squash crop in these areas exceeds $4,000,000. Seed decay occurs when soils are wet and below 75°F. Seedling growth is good when seeds are shallow-sown with adequate soil moisture and are protected with either 6 oz of chloranil or 4 oz of thiram per 100 lb of seed. Plants infected with the fungus *Fusarium solani* are stunted, yellowed, and wilted and produce few fruits. The tops sometimes break off because the fungus weakens and girdles the crowns. Infected squash seed should be soaked for 5 min in 1:1000 mercuric chloride and rinsed well before planting. Seed should not be sown in infested soil, as the fungus lives in the soil for years and attacks both squash and melons. Mosaic viruses, which are both seed-borne and insect-transmitted, mottle the leaves (Fig. 2) and distort the fruits (Fig. 3). Virus-free seed, clean weed-free culture, and insect control assure satisfactory yields. *See* FUNGISTAT AND FUNGICIDE; INSECTICIDE; PLANT VIRUS.
                                  [JOHN T. MIDDLETON]

Bibliography: See AGRICULTURAL SCIENCE (PLANT); PLANT DISEASE.

Starch

The reserve carbohydrate stored usually in the seeds, roots, or stems of plants. It is second in abundance only to cellulose as a source of carbohydrates. For many centuries, corn, wheat, potato, and rice have supplied the basic carbohydrate needs of mankind. *See* CARBOHYDRATE.

Although starch is widespread in plants, only a few sources are sufficiently abundant to make the extraction of the starch commercially feasible. These sources are corn, tapioca, potato, sago, waxy maize, wheat, sorghum, rice, and arrowroot. The naturally occurring starch is separated from the seed, as in corn, wheat, waxy maize, sorghum, and rice; from the root, as in tapioca, potato, and arrowroot; or from the stem, as in sago, by a variety of methods. The usual procedure consists in cleaning the plant material, which is then ground,

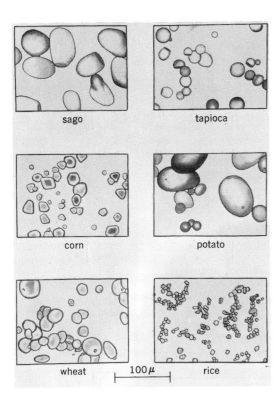

Fig. 1. Microscopic views of starch granules. (*National Starch Products, Inc.*)

sago

tapioca

corn

potato

wheat   100μ   rice

soaked, washed, sieved, and filtered. The washed starch is recovered as a filter cake before it is dried and ground.

Starch in this form is a white powder, and the unaided eye can detect little difference between the various starches extracted from different plants. All the starches are insoluble in alcohol, most solvents, and cold water. A dilute solution of iodine stains starch a blue to bluish-red.

Under the microscope, the starches appear as cellular or granular material with shapes varying with the botanical origin (Fig. 1).

Molecular structure. Granular differences are related to the basic differences in molecular structures which the various plants build for their individual needs. Starch and cellulose, the two principal carbohydrates of plant origin, are very similar in molecular structure. Both are natural polymers of glucose. The glucose units are joined by β-1,4-glucoside linkages to form cellulose straight-chained molecules; α-1,4-glucoside linkages bond the straight-chained starch polymers together. In addition to straight-chained starch molecules, known as amylose, there are branched starch molecules, known as amylopectin. The branches are formed occasionally in treelike fashion from the 1,6-glucoside linkage in a normal 1,4-glucoside straight-chained polymer. *See* GLUCOSE.

Thus, there are two basic types of starch molecules: the linear starch polymer and the branched starch polymer. Amylose molecules vary in size from about 100 to over 1000 glucose units (Fig. 2). Amylopectin molecules are three or more times larger (Fig. 3). The sizes of the molecules and the amounts of each type present in the starch granule determine the specific properties of the individual starch. Both types are normally synthesized by,

and are present in, plants. Most starch granules, as produced by nature, contain approximately 20–30% of the amylose-type molecule, and the balance of the amylopectin type. Starches from the so-called waxy grains contain only amylopectin molecules. Some special hybrids produce granules high in amylose content.

Forms of processed starch. The starch granules are formed by attractive forces between these large carbohydrate molecules. The linear portions of the molecules tend to associate together into micelles which bind the various molecules together into a crystallinelike structure. Such a structure is fairly rigid and insoluble in cold water. However, when the temperature of a suspension of starch in water is increased to a critical point, called the gelatinization temperature, water penetrates the granules to hydrate and swell them to produce a viscous mass. Gelatinization temperatures vary (60–75°C) from starch to starch. Further swelling, with more thickening, occurs as the temperature is increased, and the starch is cooked. Starches lose their unique microscopic appearance or shape as gelatinization proceeds and they become fully cooked. The characteristics of the viscous solutions vary from starch to starch. The root-type starch solutions, after cooling to room temperature, are clearer, more fluid, and cohesive in texture, while the cereal-type starches produce cloudy, less fluid starch pastes that tend to be jellylike in texture.

The natural starches find a variety of uses as thickeners in foods and industrial processes. Many times, however, these starches are processed further to obtain viscosity or texture differences of even greater use. For example, starch may be converted with enzymes (amylases) to produce lower-viscosity types for sizing purposes. In the presence of acid, and at temperatures below the gelatinization point, starch may be converted in water suspension by breaking some of the molecules to obtain starches which give less viscous solutions. These thin boiling-type starches find many uses where increased concentration is desirable without more viscosity. These cooked starch pastes usually set on cooling with increased jellylike textures. The molecular size of starch may also be

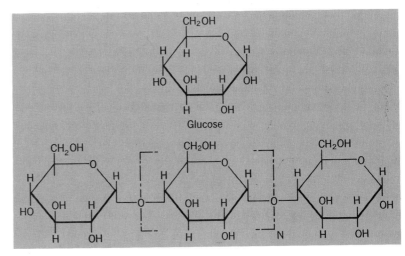

Fig. 2. Linear amylose starch molecule.

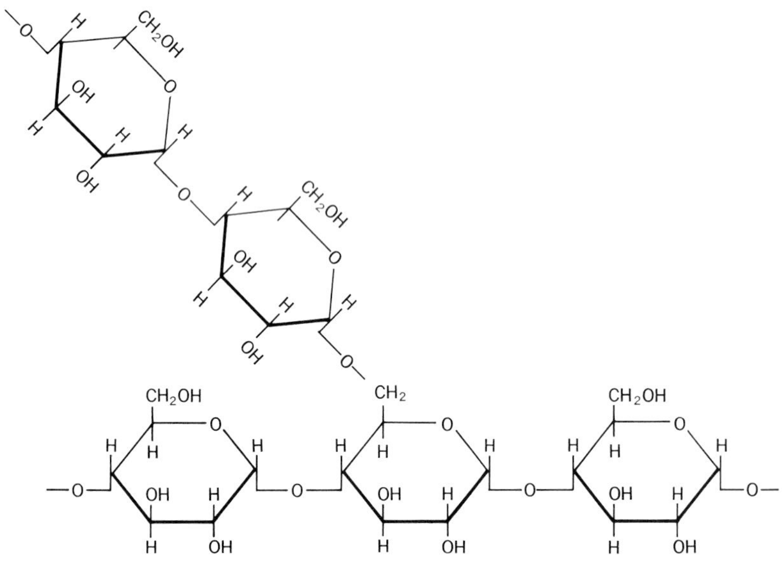

Fig. 3. Branched amylopectin starch molecule.

reduced with oxidizing agents. Carboxyl groups are introduced into the molecules in this way, and cooked starch pastes of these types are less jelly-like in texture.

When starch is roasted in dry form, usually in the presence of a small amount of acid, a wide variety of starch products is obtained. The color usually darkens to shades of tan to brown, and the viscosity is reduced with increased roasting. This dextrinization process is a complex chemical reaction, and consists of a combination of hydrolysis, oxidation, and transglucosidation of the starch molecule, as well as repolymerization of some of the reaction products. The normally insoluble (in cold water) starch granule is converted with increasing dextrinization into smaller molecules which are soluble in cold water. Some common names for dextrins are British gums, white dextrins, and canary or yellow dextrins. These products find many industrial uses. Concentrated solutions of dextrins are sticky and have wide adhesive applications.

If the starch molecule is depolymerized further, usually by acid hydrolysis, a variety of sugars and dextrose or glucose is obtained. These in syrup or dry form find wide application in food products as sweeteners. *See* CORN.

Carboxyl (COOH) groups are introduced into the starch molecule on oxidation. Other groupings or radicals, such as ethers or esters, can be introduced to produce different properties in the individual starch. Starch molecules also may be joined to form larger molecules. Thus, a wide variety of starch properties may be obtained to suit the needs of industry.

Use of modified starches in foods or food containers is regulated in the United States by Food Additives Regulation 121.1031 for Food Starch—Modified and 121.2506 for Industrial Starch—Modified, respectively, under the Federal Food, Drug, and Cosmetic Act. *See* FOOD; FOOD ENGINEERING; FOOD MANUFACTURING.   [T. A. WHITE]

Bibliography: Corn Industries Research Foundation, *Corn Starch*, 1964; F. H. Frost et al., *Starch and Starch Products in Paper Coating*, Tech. Ass. Pulp Pap. Ind. Monogr. Ser. no. 17, 1957; R. D. Guthrie and J. Honeyman, *An Introduction to the Chemistry of Carbohydrates*, 1964; F. L. Hart and H. J. Fisher, *Modern Food Analysis*, 1970; R. W. Kerr, *Chemistry and Industry*, 2d ed., 1950; National Starch Products, Inc., *The Story of Starches*, 1953; J. A. Radley, *Starch and its Derivatives*, 4th ed., 1968; R. L. Whistler, *Methods in Carbohydrate Chemistry*, vol. 4: *Starch*, 1965; R. L. Whistler and E. F. Parchall, *Starch: Chemistry and Technology*, vol. 1, 1965, and vol. 2, 1967.

Starvation

A physiological condition associated with a prolonged unavailability of food or inadequate amounts of food. It involves generalized wasting of body tissues with progressive development of biochemical abnormalities and changes in the function of vital organs until ultimately death occurs. The onset of death is usually associated with a severe infectious process of rapid deterioration of a significant organ system, such as the central nervous, cardiovascular, gastrointestinal, or pulmonary system. As in most nutritionally related problems, starvation has its greatest impact on the physiologically sensitive groups, particularly infants and young children, the rapidly growing adolescent, the pregnant and lactating female, and the elderly.

People in developing countries with very limited incomes and a hand-to-mouth existence are far more prone to suffer from the vagaries of food supplies brought on by drought, floods, or other climatic calamities. Millions of people are in a very precarious position with regard to the adequacy of their food supply, and their risk of starvation is more immediate when any adverse event limits food. Moreover, in inadequately fed populations the nutritional quality of the food supply is usually restricted, with emphasis on carbohydrate and reduced availability of quality protein, which is essential for balanced nutrition and good health. *See the feature article* FEEDING THE WORLD; *see also* AGRICULTURAL GEOGRAPHY; NUTRITION.

Biochemical adaptation. The human body can accommodate itself to food deprivation for remarkably prolonged periods of time. The body is helped in adapting by its metabolic regulatory system, which seeks to maintain a constant lean body mass, that is, to preserve the protein tissues. One of the first adaptations during starvation or prolonged fasting is the reduction in basal metabolic rate. Examples on a huge scale were documented in the study of World War II prisoners whose diets provided only 400–600 kilocalories (1700–2500 megajoules) per day. Their basal metabolic rate dropped dramatically as a physiological adaptation to the imparied availability of food calories. Along with this was observed lethargy, fatigability, irritability, and chilliness, which are commonly seen in the hypothyroid individual.

Feedback loops. Other metabolic regulation characteristics have been recognized in the fasting or starving individual. There are evidently three feedback loops integrated through the function of insulin. First, insulin lowers blood glucose levels by facilitating glucose uptake by muscle as glycogen and by adipose tissue as fat. Conversely, increased glucose concentrations stimulate insulin release. The primary set point of this negative feedback loop seems to be a fasting blood glucose level near the physiological norm. *See* INSULIN.

The second feedback loop involves insulin–fatty acid–glucose. Insulin decreases the release of free fatty acid from adipose tissue by reducing cyclic AMP–mediated activation of a hormone-sensitive lipolytic enzyme and increasing glycerol phosphate availability for free fatty acid reesterification. Insulin also exerts an antiketogenic action on the liver. Because free fatty acids and ketone bodies can be used as substrates for energy production by most tissues, their elevation will spare glucose from consumption, elevate glucose plasma levels, and thus indirectly promote insulin secretion. However, this feedback can function only to the extent of reducing blood glucose to normal levels.

Third, in the insulin–amino acid–glucose loop, insulin enhances the uptake of amino acids by peripheral tissues as protein. It also reduces protein catabolism. At the same time, glucogenic amino acids increase glucose formation, elevate blood glucose levels, and thus stimulate insulin release. In addition, certain amino acids directly stimulate the release of insulin. *See* CARBOHYDRATE METABOLISM; PROTEIN METABOLISM.

Fat reserves. In order to keep the lean body mass constant, excesses in caloric balance are translated into changes in the amounts of fat stored in adipose tissue, causing obesity. The nitrogen balance remains close to zero and amino acid oxidation is rapid, in spite of the anabolic high insulin levels. However, during periods of severe caloric deprivation or starvation and low insulin levels, metabolic fuel consumption shifts to minimize amino acid breakdown and to preserve body protein mass. It can be concluded that all aspects of energy metabolism are significantly a function of insulin level, which is in turn influenced by glucose. Maintenance of normal fasting blood glucose level appears to provide the fundamental set point in the overall metabolic regulatory system. During starvation or fasting there is a progressive decrease in nitrogen lost in the urine, again suggesting an increased conservation of lean body protein mass and an increasing reliance on fat as fuel. The capability of utilizing these mechanisms for conserving the lean body mass or the vital protein stores depends to a great extent on the initial level of fat reserves in the body. In poverty-stricken nations, where the food supply is generally marginal, there is very little obesity and few individuals have significant levels of fat reserves to fall back on to conserve body protein. Consequently, a vanishing food supply takes its toll more rapidly with the fatal results coming sooner.

Glucose metabolism. As in normal circumstances, insulin is the dominant hormone in controlling fuel mobilization and biochemical homeostasis during starvation. During fasting or starvation, glucose and insulin levels tend to decrease, while free fatty acid and ketone body levels increase. This resultant state of ketosis is considered responsible for the diminished hunger sensations that are reported in prolonged fasts and severe starvation. During the first day with no or very little food, basal glucose demands are primarily satisfied by the combustion of glucose derived from amino acids. With more prolonged fasting, glucose metabolism begins to be excluded from the majority of tissues, particularly from muscle tissue. This spares the need for glucose synthesis. An adaptive mechanism then takes place in which energy derived from the oxidation of fatty acid in the liver is used to shuttle glucose to peripheral glycolytic tissues, where it is metabolized to lactate and then cycled back to the liver and resynthesized into glucose. This process has an important sparing effect on the breakdown of protein to form glucose, by limiting complete oxidation of glucose to carbon dioxide.

The most important adaptation, however, is the brain's ability to utilize ketone bodies that are able to cross the blood-brain barrier and require no insulin for entrance into the cell. This has a sparing action on glucose, and thus ultimately spares body protein from breakdown into glucose.

Therefore, with prolonged fasting, there is a progressive shift to preferential and almost exclusive utilization of fat and fat-derived fuels. However, before this shift can be completed and particularly when there is little fat reserve, substantial losses occur in protein, derived from muscle tissues predominantly.

Problems with starvation. In addition to robbing the body of proteins in increased protein catabolism, other hazards relating to vital organs occur. A major impact of starvation is on the cardiovascular system, particularly the heart. Significant breakdown and fragmentation of the contractile muscle fibers of the heart are commonly associated with starvation. Other physiological problems during starvation include severe hypotension, especially in the erect position, severe thermocytic-thermochromic anemia (iron deficiency anemia), and gouty arthritis.

The starving individual suffers a reduction of plasma blood volume, which in turn produces a functional impairment of renal activity of glomerular filtration and hepatic perfusion. Transient rises in serum creatinine and alterations in liver function occur, as manifested by serious elevations in liver enzymes in the blood and biopsy evidence of fatty infiltration of the liver with subsequent cirrhotic and fibrotic degeneration.

The depletion of body proteins results in hair loss and dry, scaly skin. Some have attributed the hair loss to associated reduction in intake of certain essential fatty acids, such as linoleic acid, and also the possible adverse effects of progressive zinc deficiency. Certainly, mineral losses always take place during starvation, which can lead to marked sodium depletion and potassium loss. The latter is relatively slow, and usually seen after 2 weeks. The acceleration of potassium loss is noted particularly with increased protein breakdown, and occurs more rapidly when fat stores are minimal.

Other side effects associated with starvation include headaches, nervousness and tension, increasing sensitivity to cold (probably related to hypometabolism), dizziness, fatigue, apathy, and indifference. The starving person is almost totally unable to work, thus further limiting the individual's ability to gain food.

The problems of starvation are obviously the concern of all nations of the world, as well as of the World Health Organization and the Food and Agricultural organizations. A world food bank is essential to make food available to deprived nations during times of deprivation. Another consideration is the disaster that would be produced should adverse climatic circumstances occur simultaneously in the three great food-producing areas of the world: the north-central portion of North America, the Eurasian Belt across Europe and southern Russia, and southeastern Asia.

[W. A. KREHL]

Sterilization

An act of destroying all forms of life on and in an object. A substance is sterile, from a microbiological point of view, when it is free of all living microorganisms. Sterilization is used principally to prevent spoilage of food and other substances and to prevent the transmission of diseases by destroying microbes that may cause them in man and animals.

Microorganisms can be killed either by physical agents, such as heat and irradiation, or by chemical substances. Regardless of the manner in which they are killed, they generally die at a constant rate under specified environmental conditions. If the logarithm of the number of survivors is plotted against time, the resulting curve is a straight line.

When testing a substance for sterility, care must be taken to employ appropriate techniques. A bacterial cell is considered to be killed when it is no longer capable of reproducing itself under suitable environmental conditions. If an inadequate medium is employed to subculture the treated bacteria, the substance being tested may be wrongly considered to be sterile.

By far the most resistant of all forms of life, to both physical and chemical killing agents, are some of the bacterial endospores. If they did not exist, sterilization of such materials as bacteriological media and equipment, hospital supplies, and canned foods would be much simpler.

Heat sterilization. This is the most common method of sterilizing bacteriological media, foods, hospital supplies, and many other substances. Either moist heat (hot water or steam) or dry heat can be employed, depending upon the nature of the substance to be sterilized. Moist heat is also used in pasteurization, which is not considered a true sterilization technique because all microorganisms are not killed; only certain pathogenic organisms and other undesirable bacteria are destroyed. See PASTEURIZATION.

Moist-heat sterilization. Some bacterial endospores are capable of surviving several hours at 100°C. Therefore, for moist-heat sterilization, an autoclave, pressure cooker, or retort, with steam under pressure, is required to achieve higher temperatures (Fig. 1).

Most bacteriological media are sterilized by autoclaving with steam at 121°C, with 15 lb pressure, for 20 min or more, depending upon the volume of material being heated. Some spores are capable of

surviving moist-heat sterilization equivalent to at least 7 min at 121°C.

Steam under atmospheric pressure in an Arnold sterilizer is sometimes employed for specialized bacteriological media that are easily heat damaged. Because many bacterial spores survive this treatment, it is obviously inadequate to ensure sterility.

Tyndallization. The food or medium is steamed for a few minutes at atmospheric pressure on three or four successive occasions, separated by 12- to 18-hr intervals of incubation at a favorable growing temperature. In theory the intervals of incubation allow any surviving bacterial spores to germinate into more heat-sensitive, vegetative cells, which then would be killed during the next heat treatment. However, spores like vegetative cells may require special conditions such as an appropriate medium, proper oxygen tension, or proper temperature to germinate and reproduce. These conditions may not be realized during the intervals between heat treatment and no matter how often the steaming is repeated ungerminated spores may survive and eventually germinate when conditions have been changed. The survival of ungerminated spores reduces the effectiveness of this method and it has been supplanted by other methods.

Hot-air sterilization. Glassware and other heat-resistant materials which need to be dry after treatment are usually sterilized in a hot-air sterilizer. Dry sterilization requires heating at higher temperatures and for longer periods of time than does sterilization by steam under pressure. Temperatures of 160–165°C for at least 2 hr is generally employed in hot-air sterilization. Dry heat kills the germs through denaturation of protein which may involve oxidative processes.

Radiation sterilization. Many kinds of radiations are lethal, not only to microorganisms but to other forms of life. These radiations include both high-energy particles as well as portions of the electromagnetic spectrum. The mechanism of the lethal action of these radiations is not entirely clear. It may involve a direct energy absorption at some vital part of the cell (direct target theory), or the production of highly reactive, ionized, free radicals near some vital part of the cell (indirect effect). Bacterial endospores are relatively resistant to all types of radiation.

Ultraviolet radiation. Radiant energy in the ultraviolet region of the spectrum is highly bactericidal, especially at wavelengths of approximately 2650 A. Lamps which generate ultraviolet radiation in this region are useful for the sterilization of air and smooth surfaces. Ultraviolet rays have very low penetrative capacity, since even a thin layer of glass absorbs a high percentage of the rays. Some irradiated cells that are presumably dead may be photoreactivated with visible light.

Gamma rays. These are high-energy, electromagnetic radiations similar to x-rays. They have great penetrative capacity, and their energy is dissipated in the production of ionized particles from the material being irradiated. Radioactive isotopes, such as cobalt-60, are a common source of gamma rays (Fig. 2). Gamma irradiation of foods has received much attention as a means of sterilizing foods without cooking them. Sterilization requires a radiation dose of approximately 5,000,000 rads (5×10^8 ergs of energy absorbed per gram).

Cathode rays. These high-speed electrons (beta rays) may be generated with various types of electron accelerators. This type of radiation has relatively low penetrative capacity, depending upon the energy level of the emitted electron beam. Cathode rays sterilize in a manner identical to gamma rays and without significantly raising the temperature of the material being irradiated. They have received some application in the sterilization of surgical supplies and drugs and in the experimental sterilization of foods (Fig. 3).

Filtration sterilization. This is the physical removal of microorganisms from liquids by filtering through materials having relatively small pores. Sterilization by filtration is employed with liquid that may be destroyed by heat, such as blood serum, enzyme solutions, antibiotics, and some bacteriological media and medium constituents. Examples of such filters are the Berkefeld filter (diatomaceous earth), Pasteur-Chamberland filter (porcelain), Seitz filter (asbestos pad), and the sintered glass filter. Most of these filters are available in different pore sizes.

The mean pore size of bacteriological filters is not the only determinant in their effectiveness. The electric charge of the pore surfaces tends to adsorb the bacteria and thus prevent their passage. Most bacteria have a net negative electrical charge on their surfaces. Usually, bacteriological filters will permit the passage of viruses, which are then called filterable.

A Millipore filter is a specially prepared membrane molecular filter designed to remove bacteria from water, air, and other materials, for the purpose of estimating quantitatively the bacterial population. A sterile filter disk is assembled in a filtration unit, and a specified volume of water or solution is drawn through the disk which then retains the bacteria. The filter disk is removed and placed in a sterile petri dish containing an absorbent pad, previously saturated with an appropriate bacteriological medium. Upon incubation, colonies will develop on the filter disk wherever bacteria were entrapped at the time of filtering. Special differential, or selective, media can be employed for the purpose of detecting quantitatively specific types of bacteria from the original material.

Chemical sterilization. Chemicals are used to sterilize solutions, air, or the surfaces of solids. Such chemicals are called bactericidal substances. In lower concentrations they become bacteriostatic rather than bactericidal; that is, they prevent the growth of bacteria but may not kill them. Other terms having similar meanings are employed. A disinfectant is a chemical that kills the vegetative cells of pathogenic microorganisms but not necessarily the endospores of spore-forming pathogens. An antiseptic is a chemical applied to living tissue that prevents or retards the growth of microorganisms, especially pathogenic bacteria, but which does not necessarily kill them.

The death of microorganisms subjected to bactericidal substances can be expressed exponentially, in that a straight-line graph is produced when the logarithm of survivors is plotted against time.

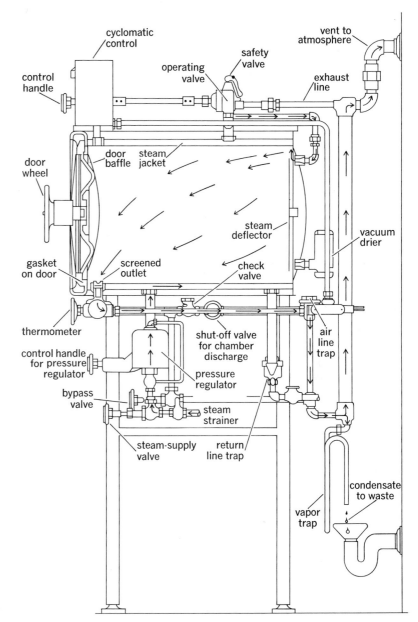

Fig. 1. Diagrammatic sketch of an autoclave. (*American Sterilizer Co.*)

The more concentrated the chemical employed, the greater is the rate of death.

There are hundreds of chemicals that may be considered to have sterilizing or bactericidal properties, depending upon the particular use for which they are intended. A chemical may be particularly useful for one purpose but not for another. Many are widely used for sterilization or disinfection of air, water, tabletops, surgical instruments, and so on.

The desirable features sought in a chemical sterilizer are toxicity to microorganisms but nontoxicity to man and animals, stability, solubility, inability to react with extraneous organic materials, penetrative capacity, detergent capacity, noncorrosiveness, and minimal undesirable staining effects. Rarely does one chemical combine all these desirable features.

Among chemicals that have been found useful

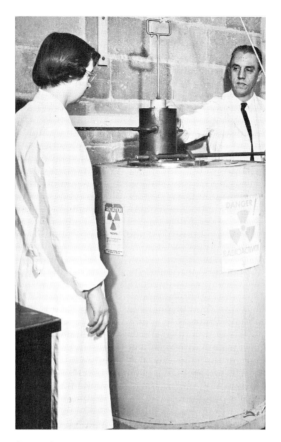

Fig. 2. Cobalt-60 furnace which is designed for experimental food sterilization.

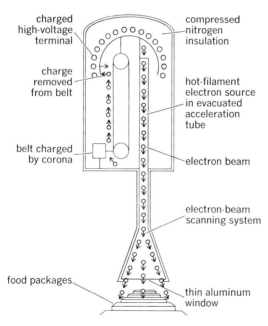

Fig. 3. Van de Graaff generator principle; packaged products sterilized by means of high-intensity electron beam which penetrates packages. (*From W. M. Urbain, Food Eng., vol. 25, February, 1953*)

Chlorine. Chlorine and chlorine-containing compounds represent the most widely used group of disinfectants. Chlorine gas is often used to purify municipal water supplies.

Various compounds of chlorine, such as the hypochlorites and chloramine, have many industrial and domestic uses as disinfectants or antiseptics.

Ozone. This is a highly oxidizing gas (O_3) used as a deodorizer, and also for disinfection of air and water. It has found some use in the food fields, but effective bactericidal concentrations may be irritating and toxic to humans.

Hydrogen peroxide. This chemical (H_2O_2) has high oxidizing and bleaching qualities and is usually employed in a 3% solution for topical application and disinfection of cuts, scratches, and minor wounds. It decomposes into water and oxygen and therefore is used where no taste, odor, or toxic residues are permitted.

Volatile organic compounds. Such compounds as formaldehyde and ethylene oxide have been used for the disinfection of sickrooms occupied by patients suffering from contagious disease (terminal disinfection), and of solids that do not permit heat treatment. These volatile substances have the advantages of effective penetrative capacity and ease of removal after treatment.

Volatile organic substances are sometimes employed as bacteriostatic agents to preserve bacteriological medium constituents until they are heat-sterilized. An example is a mixture of chlorobenzene, dichloroethane, and *n*-butyl chloride, as employed by S. H. Hutner.

[CHARLES F. NIVEN, JR.]

Bibliography: M. J. Pelczar and R. D. Reid, *Microbiology*, 3d ed., 1972: G. F. Reddish (ed.), *Antiseptics, Disinfectants, Fungicides, and Chemical and Physical Sterilization*, 2d ed., 1957.

Strawberry

Low-growing perennials, spreading by stolons, with fruit consisting of a fleshy receptacle, and "seeds" in pits or nearly superficial on the receptacle.

The strawberry in the United States is derived from two species: *Fragaria chiloensis*, which grows along the Pacific Coast of North and South America, and *F. virginiana*, the eastern meadow strawberry, both members of the order Rosales. These species were apparently crossed in Europe in the early 18th century, and some of the hybrid offspring were brought back to North America, where they have been crossed and recrossed until the characteristics of the original parental types are hard to see. The European strawberry is a smaller-fruited type, usually grown from seed. *See* SEED (BOTANY).

Distribution and importance. The strawberry (see illustration) is the most universally grown of the small fruits, both in the home garden and in commercial plantings. Home garden production is possible in nearly all of the states, provided water can be supplied where rainfall is insufficient. Commercial production is important in probably three-fourths of the states. Although the acreage may vary greatly from year to year, the following states are large producers: Oregon, California, Tennessee, Michigan, Louisiana, Washington, Arkansas,

as sterilizing agents are the phenols, alcohols, chlorine compounds, iodine, heavy metals and metal complexes, dyes, and synthetic detergents, including the quaternary ammonium compounds.

Kentucky, and New York. *See* FRUIT GROWING, SMALL.

Propagation and harvesting. Strawberries are propagated by transplanting plants which were produced vegetatively as runners in the previous growing season. In many cases a new planting is made each year, produces fruit the following year, and is then plowed under. However, two annual crops may be produced from one planting, and sometimes as many as three or four. Harvesting is mostly done by hand, although mechanical harvesting is being researched intensively. A large part of the crop is sold fresh, a small amount is made into preserves, and a large quantity is frozen. *See* FOOD ENGINEERING.

Most varieties produce a crop in early summer, the picking season lasting about 2 weeks in the North, but much longer in the South. In Florida, and to some extent in the other Gulf states, plants may be set in the fall and produce fruit throughout the winter. In California the picking season extends over several weeks. Other varieties, usually limited to home garden production, produce flowers more or less continuously in the North, hence the term "ever-bearing" strawberry.

Strawberry breeders have been active since the earliest introduction of the present cultivated fruit, all of the important varieties now being the result of controlled crosses. Strawberry varieties are usually adapted to rather limited areas so that different varieties are grown in each producing section, although a few seem adapted to more than one area. Varieties commonly grown in the South will produce during the short days of winter, whereas northern varieties will not fruit normally during short days. *See* BREEDING (PLANT); PHOTOPERIODISM IN PLANTS.   [J. HAROLD CLARKE]

Diseases. Strawberries are afflicted with root rots, leaf spots, and fruit rots, which vary in geographic distribution, destructiveness, and economic importance.

Root diseases. Black root, most common of the fungus root rots, may be caused by species of *Fusarium*, *Rhizoctonia*, and *Verticillium* or by *Coniothyrium fuckellii* and *Hainisia lythri*. No single organism is implicated as the primary pathogen, but *Rhizoctonia* and *Fusarium* are the most frequent. *Verticillium* also causes a wilt of strawberry in England and in California.

The most dangerous root disease, red stele, is caused by *Phytophthora fragariae*. Diseased plants have "rattail" root systems with few rootlets. Root tips die and turn brown, while the central cylinder, or stele, of the root is red. A field once infested with the fungus is useless for strawberry production for many years. Resistant varieties are available. *See* PLANT DISEASE CONTROL.

Nematodes cause root lesions and root knot and such diseases as spring and summer dwarf. Their importance. in commercial production is not known.

Foliage diseases. Prevalent fungus diseases of strawberry are common leaf spot caused by *Mycosphaerella fragariae*, leaf scorch caused by *Diplocarpon earliana*, and leaf blight caused by *Dendrophoma obscurans*. Leaves, leaf and fruit stalks, stolons, calyxes, and fruit caps are attacked. Leaf blight occasionally causes fruit deterioration. Powdery mildew caused by *Sphaerotheca macu-*

laris is of minor importance in the United States. Leaf-spot diseases reduce yield and grade of marketable berries and weaken the runner plants.

Viruses occur in all commercial strawberry varieties and in wild species of *Fragaria*. Certain virus strains and combinations of strains deform foliage and reduce plant vigor, stolon formation, and yield. Virus-free varieties can be grown. *See* PLANT VIRUS.

Fruit diseases. Greater losses result from fruit rots than from all other diseases combined. Gray mold caused by *Botrytis cinerea*, tan rot caused by *Pezizella lythri*, leathery rot caused by *Phytophthora cactorum*, and brown rot caused by *Rhizoctonia* sp. may be common and severe in the field. Leak, caused by *Rhizopus nigricans*, probably is the most important market disease. *See* AGRICULTURAL SCIENCE (PLANT); PLANT DISEASE.   [THOMAS H. KING]

Sucrose

An oligosaccharide, α-D-glucopyranosyl-β-D-fructofuranoside, also known as saccharose, cane sugar, or beet sugar. The structure is shown in the illustration. The sugar occurs universally through-

Structural formula for sucrose.

out the plant kingdom in fruits, seeds, flowers, and roots of plants. Honey consists principally of sucrose and its hydrolysis products. Sugarcane and sugarbeets are the chief sources for the preparation of sucrose on a large scale. Another source of commercial interest is the sap of maple trees. The consumption of sucrose in the United States is more than 100 lb per capita per year. *See* OLIGOSACCHARIDE; SUGARBEET; SUGARCANE.

The specific rotation of sucrose $[\alpha]_{D}^{20}$ is $+66.5°$ and melting point (mp) 186°C. It is nonreducing and is not fermentable by yeast. Sucrose is very soluble in water and crystallizes from that medium in the anhydrous form.

The bacterium *Pseudomonas saccharophila* contains an enzyme, sucrose phosphorylase, which catalyzes the synthesis of sucrose from α-D-glucose-1-phosphate and D-fructose. In plants, sucrose is synthesized from uridine diphosphate D-glucose and D-fructose or D-fructose-6-phosphate. In the latter case the resulting sucrose phosphate is hydrolyzed by an enzyme, phosphatase, to yield free sucrose.

The specific rotation of sucrose is $+66.5°$ in water; it is readily hydrolyzed by acids and by the specific enzyme sucrase (invertase) to yield equal amounts of D-glucose and D-fructose, as in the equation below. As the levorotation due to D-fructose exceeds the dextrorotation due to D-glucose, the hydrolysis results in a change in sign. The process is therefore called inversion, and the

The strawberry (*a*) flower and (*b*) fruit.

$$\text{Sucrose} + \text{water} \rightarrow \text{D-glucose} + \text{D-fructose}$$
$$[\alpha]_D^{20} + 66.5° \qquad [\alpha]_D^{20} + 52.2° \quad [\alpha]_D^{20} - 93°$$

Invert sugar
$$[\alpha]_D^{20} - 20.4°$$

equimolar mixture of the two sugars is known as invert sugar.   [WILLIAM Z. HASSID]

Bibliography: L. Machlis, *Annual Review of Plant Physiology*, vol. 18, 1967; E. G. V. Percival, *Structural Carbohydrate Chemistry*, rev. by E. Percival, 1962.

Sugar

Most usually, sucrose, the common sugar of commerce. This sugar is a disaccharide, $C_{12}H_{22}O_{11}$, which is split, as shown by Eq. (1), by hydrolysis

$$C_{12}H_{22}O_{11} + H_2O \rightarrow C_6H_{12}O_6 + C_6H_{12}O_6 \qquad (1)$$
$$\text{Sucrose} \quad \text{Water} \quad \text{Glucose} \quad \text{Fructose}$$

into two monosaccharides, or simple sugars: glucose (dextrose) and fructose (levulose). Sucrose rotates the plane of polarized light to the right, as does glucose, but fructose is so strongly levorotatory that it overcomes the effect of glucose. Thus mixtures of equal amounts of glucose and fructose are levorotatory. The hydrolytic reaction is called inversion of sugar, and the product is invert sugar or, simply, invert. *See* CARBOYHDRATE.

Sucrose is widely distributed in nature, having been found in all green plants that have been carefully examined for its presence. The total quantity of all sugars formed each year has been estimated at a colossal 400,000,000,000 tons. Commercial sugar of fairly high purity, which has been centrifuged to separate molasses, totals about 72,000,000 tons a year, and the amount is rapidly increasing.

In spite of its availability in all green plants, sucrose is obtained commercially in substantial amounts from only two plants: sugarcane, which supplies about 56% of the world total, and the sugarbeet, which provides 44%.

Cane sugar manufacture. The manufacture of cane sugar is usually done in two series of operations. First, raw sugar of about 98% purity is produced at a location adjacent to the cane fields. The raw sugar is then shipped to refineries, where a purity that is close to 100% is achieved.

Raw cane sugar. The production of raw cane sugar begins with growing the cane in tropical or subtropical areas. The cane is harvested after a season varying from 7 months in subtropical areas to 12–22 months in the tropics. The cane stalks are harvested either mechanically or by heavy hand-knives. The trend is toward mechanization. The stalks are transported to a mill by oxcart, rail, or truck. *See* SUGARCANE.

At the mill the stalks are crushed and macerated between heavy grooved iron rollers while being sprayed countercurrently with water to dilute the residual juice. The expressed juice contains 95% or more of the sucrose present. The fibrous residue, or bagasse, is usually burned under the boilers, although increasing amounts are being made into paper, insulating board, and hardboard as well as furfural, which is a chemical intermediate for the synthesis of furan and tetrahydrofuran.

Cane juice. The cane juice is treated with lime to bring its pH to about 8.2. This pH prevents the inversion reaction, which is favored by heat and acid and would lower the yield of crystallizable sugar. The juice is then heated to facilitate the precipitation of impurities, which are removed by continuous filtration.

The purified juice is concentrated by multiple-stage vacuum evaporation (usually four or five stages) and, when sufficiently concentrated, is boiled to grain or seeded with sucrose crystals in a single-stage vacuum pan. Usually three successive crops of crystals are grown, cooled, and centrifuged. The final mother liquor, which is resistant to further crystallization, is called blackstrap molasses. It is used principally as a feed for cattle. Relatively small amounts are still fermented to produce industrial alcohol and rum.

Raw cane sugar refining. The refining of raw sugar begins with dissolution of the molasses which remains in a thin film on the crystals in spite of the centrifugation. This step, called affination, brings the purity from about 98 to about 99%. The crystals are dissolved in hot water and percolated through bone char columns to remove color by adsorption. The sucrose is finally concentrated by vacuum evaporation, crystallized by seeding, centrifuged, and dried.

A major step forward has been the use of bone char in a continuous countercurrent manner (Grosvenor patent). The bone char is washed, dried, and burned to remove impurities; it is reused until it wears out mechanically and is discarded as fines. Even the fines have value as fertilizer because of their high calcium phosphate content.

In some plants, in place of bone char, activated vegetable charcoal is used. The fragility of this material requires the employment of filter presses rather than char columns. An activated char made from coal that is sufficiently strong to be used in columns has become available. Ion-exchange resins reduce the ash content of sugar solutions and thus increase sucrose recovery with a lowering of molasses production. They are employed to a limited but increasing extent.

Beet sugar. In the United States, sugarbeets are grown under contract by farmers from seed supplied by a beet sugar company. Because sugarbeets, like other temperate-zone crops, thrive best under crop rotation, they are not well adapted to one-crop agriculture. *See* SUGARBEET.

Beet processing. When beets are delivered to a factory, they are washed and sliced, and the slices are extracted countercurrently with hot water to remove the sucrose. The resulting solution is purified by repeatedly precipitating calcium carbonate, calcium sulfite, or both, in it. Colloidal impurities are entangled in the growing crystals of precipitate and removed by continuous filtration. The resulting solution is nearly colorless, and the sucrose is concentrated by multiple-effect vacuum evaporation. The syrup is seeded, cooled, and centrifuged, and the beet crystals are washed with water and dried.

Beet molasses differs from cane molasses in having a much lower content of invert sugar. It is, therefore, relatively stable to the action of alkali and, in the United States, is usually treated with calcium oxide to yield a precipitate of calcium sucrate. This is a mixture of loose chemical aggregates of sucrose and calcium oxide which are relatively insoluble in water. The precipitate is filtered, washed, and added to the incoming crude sugar syrup, where it furnishes calcium for the precipitations of calcium carbonate and sulfite referred to above, which remove impurities. Carbon dioxide in the form of flue gas is the other reagent, and sulfur dioxide from burning sulfur is used to produce sulfite.

Beet residue use. The beet tops and extracted slices, as well as the molasses, are valuable as feeds. More feed for cattle and other ruminants can be produced per acre-year from beets than from any other crop widely grown in the United States. This is independent of the food energy in the crystallized sucrose, which exceeds that available from any other temperate-zone plant. It is for these reasons that the densely populated countries of Europe have expanded their beet sugar production, in spite of the ready availability of cane sugar from the tropics.

The increased use of nitrogenous fertilizer has resulted in augmenting the protein content of the molasses and other beet by-products.

Nutritional value of sugar. Sucrose has, in the past, been attacked by some nutritionists on the ground that it provides only "empty calories," without protein, minerals, or vitamins. This argument lost much of its force when it was shown that all the vitamins and minerals recommended by the National Research Council can be obtained by consuming any of a great variety of foods in amounts that yield a total of only one-half of the caloric requirements of an average person. The wide use by the public of vitamin supplements has caused some nutritionists to express an opposite worry over excessive vitamin consumption.

The problem of sugars and tooth decay is not so easily disposed of, however, and continues to be the subject of active research. It is currently believed that dental plaque is a dextran, formed from sucrose and important to the etiology of caries. If this theory is confirmed, the systematic application of dextranases should be effective in preventing tooth decay in humans as it has been in animals.

The discovery that sugars have an effect in diminishing appetite has led to their inclusion in reducing diets.

A charge leveled against sugar is that it may be involved in the etiology of atherosclerosis. Certainly there is a strong correlation between sugar consumption in a population and the prevalence of atherosclerosis. This fact alone, however, is far from establishing a cause-and-effect relationship (telephones also correlate well with atherosclerosis). Research is actively under way on the relation of diet to atherosclerosis with the prospect of definitive results in the near future.

Use in organic synthesis. Since 1952 active research has been under way on the use of sucrose as an inexpensive, pure, and readily available starting material for organic synthesis. This research has led to the commercial production of sucrose-based detergents, emulsifiers, and plasticizers.

Other sources of sugar. In Hawaii, the pineapple industry recovers both sucrose and citric acid from the rinds. The residue is fed to cattle. The total quantity of sucrose obtained from waste fruits is statistically negligible. On the other hand, a substantial fraction of the total sucrose consumed is that naturally present in a large number of fruits, vegetables, and nuts. *See* SUCROSE; SUGAR CROPS.

Lactose. Cow's milk, on a dry basis, is about 38% lactose or milk sugar. In the United States about 13 lb of lactose per year for each person is consumed in milk products. This compares to 97 lb for sucrose. When milk is converted into cheese, the lactose remains in the whey, from which it may easily be isolated and purified. Lactose is a disaccharide which is split by hydrolysis into glucose and galactose. It is about one-tenth as soluble in water as sucrose and one-sixth to one-half as sweet, depending on concentration. Uses are actively being sought. *See* CHEESE; LACTOSE.

Starch. Starches can be hydrolyzed either by dilute acid or by enzymes. The product of acid hydrolysis varies with time and conditions but contains glucose, maltose, maltotriose, maltotetrose, and other sugars up to the dextrins. Only glucose, a monosaccharide, is readily isolated. Crystallized as the monohydrate and used in foods, it has captured about 4% of the sweetener market. *See* CORN; GLUCOSE.

Syrups high in maltose, a disaccharide, can be obtained by the action of amylases on starch. This hydrolysis has been of great importance for thousands of years in splitting starches for alcoholic fermentation. As yet, there is no large-scale production of pure maltose. *See* MALTOSE; STARCH.

Maple sugar. When America was discovered by the white man, the Indians were collecting and concentrating the juice of the hard maple (*Acer saccharum*), thus making maple syrup. The practice was quickly accepted by the new settlers, and the production of maple syrup has been an industry ever since in the regions where hard maples are common, principally the northeastern United States.

Research has disclosed the curious fact that the maple flavor does not exist in the sap but is developed by heating it. By additional heating at about 120°C, a flavor four or five times more intense can be developed. Maple syrup so produced is of special value for adding flavor to the less expensive products of the sucrose industry. Maple sugar is sucrose of about 95–98% purity; the delicious flavor, delight of gourmets, makes up only a small percent. Fairly satisfactory imitation maple flavors are available.

Honey. Honey is a form of relatively pure invert sugar dissolved in water to form a concentrated solution. However, honey also contains precious flavors derived from the nectar of the flowers from which it was obtained by the bee. Nutritionally, it is nearly equivalent in invert sugar but contains an excess of fructose over glucose. The sucrose found in the flowers is inverted by the enzyme honey invertase. Tupelo honey is remarkable in containing about twice as much fructose as glucose, and hence has little tendency to deposit glucose crystals.

The ready availability of the food energy in honey was known to athletes in ancient Greece. Only in recent times has it been discovered that, paradoxically, the energy of sucrose is still more quickly available. The flavors of various honeys run a wide gamut. That from the Mount Hymettus region, which is flavored by wild thyme, has been known and treasured since the poems of Homer.

Molasses. Virtually all molasses is distributed in the form of concentrated viscous solution, but it can be reduced to a powder by means of spray-drying. It can then be handled without an investment by the consumer in tanks, pipes, and pumps. Unfortunately, later contact with moisture converts the dried molasses to a gummy mass. The availability of vaporproof bags (for example, those lined with polyethylene) has provided one solution to this problem. There are also various additives which, when mixed with molasses, reduce its tendency to pick up moisture. So far (1970) dried molasses has made little headway against the practice of handling concentrated solutions.

Comparison with synthetic sweeteners. In recent years sugars, particularly sucrose, have had to face competition with synthetic sweeteners. The first of these was saccharin, which is about 300 times as sweet as sucrose. After dulcin and certain other sweeteners had failed to win approval by the U.S. Food and Drug Administration, the salts of cyclohexylsulfamic acid (cyclamates) were permitted under various trade names. In 1969, however, very high doses of the cyclamates were shown to cause bladder tumors in laboratory animals. Because of these experiments the use of cyclamates in soft drinks and a number of drugs was banned in the United States.

Cyclamates are only about 30 times as sweet as sucrose, but lack the bitterness that many people notice in saccharin. Cyclamates are also more resistant than saccharin to the action of hot water; therefore they can be used to prepare canned fruit with lower caloric content than that sweetened with sucrose. Tests have shown that such fruit is much preferred to that canned in plain water but not equal in flavor to a sucrose pack.

Despite the increased use of artificial sweeteners, the per capita consumption of sugar in the United States has held remarkably steady over the decade ending in 1967. It averaged 96.1 lb/year in 1957–1959 and was 96.9 in 1967.

Syrups. Syrups are relatively concentrated, somewhat viscous, solutions of various sugars, frequently in admixture to hinder crystallization. The Dutch word for syrup is *stroop*, which, in altered form, has entered the language in the term blackstrap molasses.

Approximately a quarter of the sucrose sold in the United States is in the form of syrups of high purity. These so-called liquid sugars have the double advantage of economy of handling (being moved with pumps, pipes, tank trucks, and tank cars) and of a high degree of sanitation because closed containers are used. It is necessary, however, to pay freight on the water content, which limits the distance between a refinery and a liquid sugar user. This problem has been met in two ways. First, some sugar manufacturers have established centers for the distribution of liquid sugars at places remote from the refinery. Granulated sugar is transported to the distribution center in a densely populated area and there dissolved in water and delivered to customers. Second, granulated sugar may be distributed to a customer in tank cars and dissolved in water after delivery. A minimum water content, compatible with not too great

a tendency to deposit crystals, can be maintained when the sucrose is about one-half inverted. Where inverted sugar is acceptable, as in the manufacture of bread, this product makes for economy; a water content of only 22% in the syrup is standard.

It is the aim of the sugar refiner and the beet processor to eliminate color and all flavors other than sweetness. The manufacture of table syrups, which are widely used on waffles and pancakes, aims at a broader spectrum of flavor. Corn syrup, which is somewhat lacking in sweetness, ordinarily has about 15% sucrose added. The high viscosity of the corn syrup, resulting from the content of dextrins, tends to hinder crystallization and is an advantage in the manufacture of certain candies.

Some sugar refiners reduce the color of their molasses and remove much of the characteristic strong flavor, thus producing an acceptable table syrup. Another source of table syrup is the juice of sorghum, which is expressed and concentrated by evaporation in open pans at atmospheric pressure. The dark, strongly flavored product seems to be declining in production. *See* FOOD ENGINEERING; FOOD MANUFACTURING.

[H. B. HASS]

Bibliography: W. M. Grosvenor, Purification of Sugar Solutions, U.S. Patent 2,954,305, *Chem. Abstr.*, 55:4020c, 10:932g; O. Lyle, *Technology for Sugar Refinery Workers*, 3d ed., 1957; G. Meade, *Cane Sugar Handbook*, 1963; Research Corp., *Sugar Esters*, 1968; Saccharin and cyclamates safety: FDA would like another look, *Oil Paint Drug Rep.*, 193(13):4–34, 1968; J. Yudkin, Why blame sugar?, *Chem. Ind.*, pp. 1464–1466, Sept. 2, 1967.

Sugar crops

Crops produced as major sources of sugar, syrup, and other sugar substances.

Sugarbeet and sugarcane. These are crops which serve as a source of sucrose, the sugar of commerce. Sugar is a broad term applied to a large number of carbohydrates that have a more or less sweet taste. The primary sugar, glucose, is a product of photosynthesis and occurs in all green plants. Through chemical union, diverse sugars and starches are elaborated and become the major reserve food in storage organs, fruits, and sap of plants. In most plants the sugars occur as a mixture that cannot be readily separated into the components. In the sap of some plants the sugar mixtures are condensed into syrup. The juices of sugarcane and sugarbeet are unusually rich in pure sucrose. These two sugar crops serve as the sources of commercial sucrose. Sugar production from sugarbeet is about 3,700,000 tons and from sugarcane, about 2,600,000 tons. The remainder of United States total consumption of about 11,000,000 tons is imported. *See* CARBOHYDRATE; PHOTOSYNTHESIS; SUCROSE; SUGARBEET; SUGARCANE.

Other sugar crops are sweet sorghum, sugar maple, sugar palm, honey, and corn sugar. These are discussed briefly below.

Sweet sorghum. *Sorghum bicolor*, introduced into the United States during the mid-19th century as a potential sugar crop, has been grown primarily for syrup production (approximately 2,500,000 gal annually) and for forage. Although most of the sugar is sucrose, initial attempts to use sweet sorghum as a source of sugar were hindered by low yield varieties, in comparison to sugarcane, and by problems in processing the sugar. Modern varieties which are disease-resistant and high in quality and yield, as well as new processing techniques, have increased the potential of sweet sorghum for sugar production, especially as a supplementary sugar crop in sugarcane- and sugarbeet-producing areas. *See* SORGHUM.

Sugar maple. Colonists learned from the American Indian the art of making sugar and syrup from the sap of certain maple trees of the Great Lakes and St. Lawrence River regions. The techniques, once used only for maple sugaring at home, have been for many years the basis for commercial production of sugar and syrup.

There are about 12 species of maple (*Acer*) in North America, but *A. saccharum* is the major source of sugar. The farm woodlot of maple trees is known as a sugar bush. The trees are tapped for sap in early spring before the buds open. A large tree may be tapped each spring for many years. Trees vary greatly in yield of sap and sugar, with an average yield per tree of 2 lb of sugar, which is equivalent to 1 qt of syrup. The annual production in the United States is about 1,000,000 gal of syrup which, in terms of sugar, amounts to 8,000,000 lb. The sugar in maple sap is almost 100% sucrose.

Sugar palm. Palm sugar is obtained from the sap of several species of palm in tropical regions of the world. In eastern Asia and Malaysia, where the production of palm sugar is an important village industry, the sugar palm is the major source of sap. The sap is collected from the stalk of the male flower rather than by tapping the bole or trunk of the palm, as practiced with the maple tree. The sap contains 10–16% sucrose. In processing, the sap is condensed by heating until it becomes a thick syrup in which the sucrose crystallizes. The viscous mass is poured into molds to form small cakes of sweet substance. In some regions this product is known as jaggery.

Honey. Honey is a sugar substance collected and condensed by bees from the nectaries of flowering plants. The sugar of nectar consists of sucrose, glucose, and fructose, the last being reducing sugars that result from the inversion of sucrose, a chemical reaction induced by the bees. The percentage of these sugars in the nectar varies widely among plants, but the sugar in clover nectar, a favorite source of honey, consists roughly of 60% sucrose, 20% glucose, and 20% fructose. In contrast, in clover honey the glucose and fructose amount to about 75% and the sucrose is reduced to 1 or 2%. Beekeepers of the United States harvest a honey crop of more than 200,000,000 lb annually. Approximately 75% of this crop is a mixture of sugars gathered as nectar from many flowering plants by innumerable bees. *See* BEEKEEPING.

Corn sugar and syrup. These are produced by the inversion of starch to its component sugar. Corn sugar, known as dextrose in its granular form, amounts to about 500,000 tons annually in the United States. These sweeteners have wide use in bakery, confectionery, and beverage industries.

Some varieties of corn have a sweet juice in the stalks. Cornstalk juice is reported to have been a source of a sweet substance used by Indians of Central America. Occasionally, the possibility of obtaining a liquid sweetener from cornstalk juice is reexamined in the United States.

[DEWEY STEWART]

Bibliography: K. C. Freeman, D. M. Broadhead, and N. Zummo, *Culture of Sweet Sorghum for Sirup Production*, USDA Agr. Handb. no. 441, 1973; W. G. Hammond, *Sugar From Farm to Market*, 1967; R. H. Miller, The versatile sugar palm, *Principles*, *J. Palm Soc.*, 8(4):115–147, 1964; F. E. Winch and R. R. Morrow, *Production of Maple Sirup and Other Maple Products*, Cornell Ext. Bull. no. 974, 1967.

Sugarbeet

The plant *Beta vulgaris*, developed in modern times to fill the need for a sugar crop that could be grown in temperate climates (Fig. 1). During Napoleon's struggle to control Europe, ports were closed to English ships and to colonial trade that had been the source of cane sugar from tropical regions. The desire for sugar and the urge to be self-sufficient in the production of this food motivated the development of the sugarbeet and the establishment of a beet sugar industry in central Europe.

Production. The sugarbeet was the source of only 5% of the world's commercial sugar in 1840, but by 1890 it supplied almost 50%. Since about 1920 the ratio of commercial sugar from sugarcane and sugarbeet plants has fluctuated, but the production has been generally about 40% from the sugarbeet and 60% from sugarcane. *See* SUGARCANE.

European countries produce most of their sugar from sugarbeet, with some countries having surplus sugar for export. The Soviet Union is the world's largest sugar-producing country, and all its

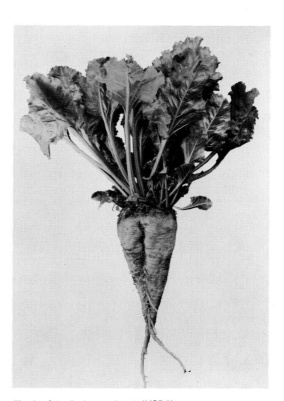

Fig. 1. A typical sugarbeet. (*USDA*)

sugar is produced from the sugarbeet. Beet sugar is produced in Morocco, Algeria, Syria, Israel, Turkey, Iran, Pakistan, Chile, Uruguay, China, Japan, Canada, and the United States.

The desire for home-grown sugar led to the production of sugarbeet in the pioneer West of the United States, where land for crops was plentiful but where sugar was scarce and expensive. Due to lack of processing know-how, several early attempts at beet sugar production failed in the midwestern United States. The first successful production of beet sugar in the United States began in 1870 at Alvarado in the San Francisco Bay area of California. A big expansion in sugarbeet production occurred about 1890 with the development of new, irrigated districts. By 1920 sugarbeets supplied almost 25% of the needs for sugar in the United States.

In the United States, sugar importation and sugar production from sugarbeet and sugarcane have been regulated since the 1930s by acts of Congress. The grower receives benefit payments for compliance with minimum labor rates and restricted acreage. The Sugar Act of 1948 was amended in 1965; it expired in 1974. In 1968 the sugarbeet quota amounted to 3,300,000 tons of sugar, or 30% of the national need of 11,000,000 tons. Domestic sugarcane, plus that grown in Puerto Rico, has about the same basic quota of production. The remainder of the United States sugar requirement (40%) is imported from the tropics.

The sugarbeet production in the United States varies from 23,000,000 to 28,000,000 tons produced on 1,000,000 to 1,400,000 acres that are grown in 17 states where soil and climate are favorable for the crop. The per acre yield of beets is approximately 18–20 tons, or roughly 5000 lb of sugar.

Processing. Recovery of crystalline sugar from the sugarbeet is not a simple procedure. In its life processes, the sugarbeet forms many organic substances other than sucrose and takes up inorganic nutrient elements from the soil. In the process of diffusing sucrose from the beet tissue, these non-sucrose substances are also brought into solution and enter the processing stream. Some are re-moved by liming and filtering, but those that remain inhibit the crystallization of sucrose and promote the formation of molasses, a by-product of low value. Since payment to the grower is based directly or indirectly on the crystalline sugar recovered from the beets, production of a crop of excellent quality and technological value is advantageous.

Field practices. The maximum sugar yield is generally obtained from approximately 25,000 plants per acre. In the humid region, where the sugarbeet is grown under rainfall, the rows are usually 24 or 28 in. apart. In California and other irrigated regions, beds are formed on which two rows of sugarbeet seed are planted. The furrow between the beds, or between the rows if planted on a level seedbed, is used for the flow of irrigation water. The seeds are planted 1 in. deep and 2–6 in. apart along the row. The seedlings are thinned to leave plants 10–12 in. apart. By midseason the plants have a large foliage and the field is covered with a mass of green leaves. See AGRICULTURE, SOIL AND CROP PRACTICES IN; IRRIGATION OF CROPS.

Since 1955 the entire acreage of sugarbeet in the United States has been harvested by machine. The spring season operations of sugarbeet production were more difficult to mechanize before because of the nature of the "seed" or "seedball," which is a round, multiple fruit containing one to seven seeds. Clumps of seedlings emerge from these seedballs, which require thinning and singling by hand. The advantages of single-seeded fruits were recognized many years ago, and attempts were made to develop monogerm sugarbeet seed as early as 1903. In 1948 a sugarbeet with heritable single-seeded fruits was discovered; and by 1957 a small experimental acreage was planted with a monogerm variety. Since 1966, essentially all American sugarbeet acreage has been planted with seed of adapted monogerm hybrids. Field practices of planting monogerm seed 5–6 in. apart along the row eliminate singling and thinning. Cultivation and selective herbicides provide weed control (Fig. 2).

Monogerm hybrids have reduced, by fully 50%, hand labor requirements for sugarbeet production in the United States. In 1967 and 1968 thousands of acres of sugarbeet were produced without hand labor. Complete mechanization of production is on the increase. The development of adapted monogerm varieties has been the outstanding accomplishment in sugarbeet production during the past century.

Botany. The sugarbeet is a biennial plant. Under natural conditions it completes a generation in 2 years. Flowering and seed formation may be induced by exposure to low temperatures (45–60°F) for about 90 days. Long days also promote flowering. If light and temperature treatments are properly applied, the biennial tendency of the sugarbeet can be overcome. In the United States, seed is produced from autumn plantings that overwinter in the field. The plants flower the following spring, and seed is harvested in June and July. Rigid control of environment enables the sugarbeet breeder to obtain a full generation each year and, with special treatments, even two generations are possible. See PHOTOPERIODISM IN PLANTS.

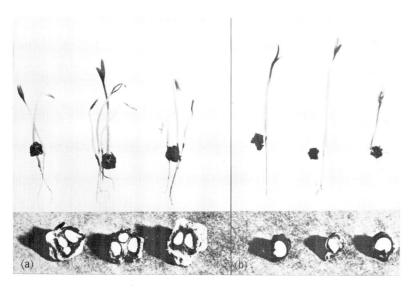

Fig. 2.   Sugarbeet germination. (a) Clumps of sugarbeet seedlings emerging from multigerm seed. (b) Single seedling from monogerm seed.

The sugarbeet, fodder beet, garden beet, and leaf beet (Swiss chard) are cultivars of *B. vulgaris* and are genetically related. The basic number of chromosomes of the sugarbeet and related cultivars is 9. Diploid plants ($2n = 18$) have been converted to tetraploid lines with 36 chromosomes. These two ploidy types have been crossed to produce triploid or polyploid varieties. *See* BEET.

In addition to *B. vulgaris*, which includes all cultivated forms of beet, there are 12 species of wild beet in the Mediterranean and Middle Eastern regions. These wild beets are of interest in sugarbeet improvement as sources of disease resistance. *See* PLANT DISEASE CONTROL.

Most varieties of sugarbeet in the United States are hybrid. Three-way hybrids, which involve three parental lines, are the most productive. Hybridization of parental lines is controlled by male sterility in the seed-bearing plant. *See* BREEDING (PLANT); SUGAR.

[DEWEY STEWART]

Diseases. Major diseases affecting the sugarbeet in the United States are curly top, *Cercospora* leaf spot, and black root. Epidemics of these may occur over wide areas when climatic conditions favor their development and spread. Other diseases, such as rusts, mildews, root rots, and bacterial and virus infections, although serious, are more localized.

Curly top. This virus disease occurs chiefly in sugarbeet-growing districts west of the Rocky Mountains. Affected plants are dwarfed and have curled, upturned leaves. Susceptible varieties may fail almost completely. The virus is transmitted by the beet leafhopper (*Circulifer tenellus*). This insect overwinters on weeds such as Russian thistle, various mustards, alfilaria, and halogeton that have invaded western rangelands. Many of these weeds harbor the curly top virus. When range plants dry in the spring, virus-carrying insects move to irrigated fields, thereby starting the cycle of curly top in sugarbeets. This disease, once a threat to the western beet sugar industry, has been controlled by the introduction of curly top–resistant varieties bred by the U.S. Department of Agriculture (Fig. 3).

Leaf spot. This disease, caused by the fungus *Cercospora beticola*, may be serious in Colorado and Nebraska and in eastern United States if rainfall throughout the growing season is above normal. The pathogen is seed-borne; early spring infections develop on emerging seedlings. If rainy periods are frequent, spores of the fungus spread from these primary foci, bringing about new infections which, in turn, produce new crops of spores. Thus a leaf spot epidemic may develop by mid-July from repeated sporulations and infections. Blighted foliage of the sugarbeet is replaced by the new leaves produced at the expense of root growth. Hence sugar storage in the roots is reduced. Susceptible varieties produce low yields of low-quality roots that are unprofitable for both the farmer and the factory. Leaf spot–resistant varieties bred by the Department of Agriculture control this disease.

Black root. This is a general name given to the seedling diseases that bring about decimation of stands of sugarbeets in humid areas. Several soil-inhabiting fungi are responsible. One group known as the cause of damping-off (stem rot near soil sur-

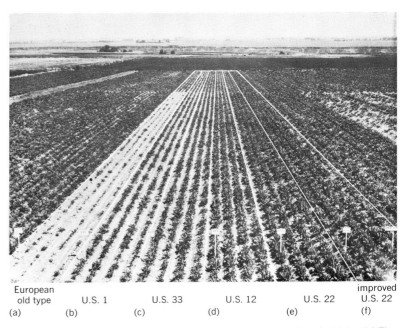

European old type (a); U.S. 1 (b); U.S. 33 (c); U.S. 12 (d); U.S. 22 (e); improved U.S. 22 (f)

Fig. 3. Demonstration of curly top–resistant varieties of sugarbeet in Idaho. (a) The susceptible European variety, Old Type. (b) The first curly top–resistant variety, U.S. 1. (c–f) Various improvements up to the second release of U.S. 22. (*From A. G. Norman, ed., Advances in Agronomy, vol. 7, Academic Press, 1955*)

face) of vegetable crops brings about, on poorly drained fields, an acute disease of sugarbeet seedlings whenever the spring season is wet. Treatment of seed with a fungicide and improvement of soil conditions usually control damping-off. The control of the chronic black root caused by water mold (*Aphanomyces cochlioides*) is much more difficult. This fungus not only causes damping-off, which may reduce the stand, but also attacks the feeding roots of the sugarbeet throughout the season, dwarfing affected plants. Seasonal conditions and degree of soil infestation determine extent of loss from *Aphanomyces*. Crops such as legumes, grown directly before the sugarbeet crop, increase the fungus infestation, whereas corn preceding sugarbeets exerts a sanitative effect. Proper crop sequences, good fertilizer practice, and use of black root–resistant varieties bred by the Department of Agriculture have given good control.

Virus yellows. This disease is extremely important in Europe, and it threatens to be equally serious in California and in the other sugarbeet-producing districts of the United States. Various aphids, especially the green peach aphid, are vectors of the virus. Research to develop adequate control measures is under way. *See* PLANT DISEASE; PLANT VIRUS.   [GEORGE H. COONS]

Bibliography: C. A. Browne and F. W. Zerban, *Physical and Chemical Methods of Sugar Analysis*, 1941; G. H. Coons, F. V. Owen, and D. Stewart, Improvement of the sugarbeet in the United States, in A. G. Norman (ed.), *Advances in Agronomy*, vol. 7, 1955; N. Deerr, *The History of Sugar*, 2 vols., 1950; U.S. Beet Sugar Association, *The Beet Sugar Story*, 1959.

Sugarcane

Saccharum officinarum L., a member of the grass family. This crop originated in New Guinea about 8000–15,000 B.C., and was later moved by primi-

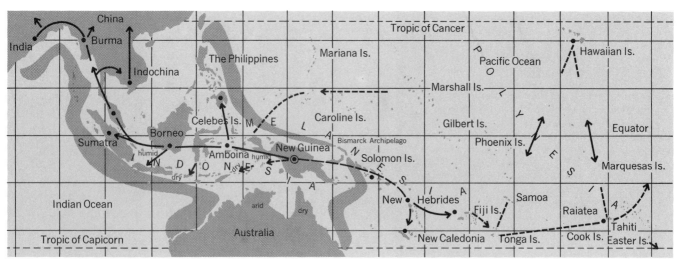

location of the *Saccharum officinarum,* derived from
S. robustum, which occurred 8000-15,000 B.C.

- - - first track of migration of *S. officinarum,* beginning about 8000 B.C.

second tracks of migration, beginning about 6000 B.C.

- - - - third tracks of migration, about A.D. 500–1100

• satellite centers of diversity along tracks of migration

Fig. 1. Origin, migration, and diversification centers of noble sugarcanes. (*USDA*)

tive man westward into Southeast Asia and India and eastward into Polynesia (Fig. 1). The original sugarcane, so-called noble canes, have $2n = 80$ chromosomes, although there are some exceptions. The noble canes probably evolved from a wild ancestor, *Saccharum robustum* Brandes and Jesweit ex Grassl, with $2n = 60 - 194$ chromosomes (Fig. 2). *S. officinarum* hybridized with wild species, especially *S. spontaneum* L., in Asia, giving rise to new types that were variable in morphology and ecological tolerance and that extended the distribution of sugarcane into the subtropics. Two additional species, *S. sinense* and *S. barberi,* are recognized in botanical literature.

Most current commercial varieties are interspecific hybrids involving primarily two or more of the following species: *S. officinarum, S. robustum,* and *S. spontaneum.* Extensive breeding programs, in the tropics where sugarcane flowers under natural conditions and in the subtropics in climate-controlled structures (Fig. 3), sponsored by public and private research agencies provide a continuous supply of new varieties adapted to major sugarcane-producing areas of the world. *See* BREEDING (PLANT).

Structure. Every new variety of sugarcane begins as a single shoot (stalk) that develops from a seed. The cylindrical stalk is divided into nodes and internodes (Fig. 4) with a lateral bud at each node. The lateral buds occur alternately on opposite sides of the stalk, and there is an apical bud. A root band at each node includes several rows of root primordia. The internodes are covered with wax and are filled with parenchyma or storage cells (pith) and the vascular bundles. The leaf consists of a sheath (Fig. 5) attached to the stalk at the node, an auricle, a ligule, a dewlap, and a blade which tapers gradually from the base to the tip and is supported by a midrib extending almost its entire length. Edges of leaves of most varieties are serrate. The inflorescence is a silky panicle at the

apex of the stem (Fig. 6) bearing many small spikelets which are arranged in pairs on the branches. Each spikelet contains a bisexual flower with three anthers and a single ovary surmounted by two plumelike stigmas (Fig. 7). The flower primordium is differentiated under the influence of short days or long nights. *See* PHOTOPERIODISM IN PLANTS; SEED (BOTANY).

Reproduction and cultivation. Sugarcane is propagated asexually with cuttings having one to several lateral buds that give rise to shoots that develop into a stool of cane (Fig. 8) consisting of roots and both primary and secondary stalks (Fig. 9). In most countries the crop is started during the fall, winter, or spring and harvested by cutting the stalks at the surface of the ground and at the topmost mature internodes, at 11–16 months of age in the tropics and at 8–12 months in the subtropics (Fig. 10). In Hawaii the crop periods range from about 24 months at lower elevation to 30 months or more above 2000 ft. The stalks are harvested by hand cutting or machine cutting and piling into windrows. From the windrow the cane is mechanically loaded into either field wagons or larger conveyors for direct transport to the factory. In some areas combine-type harvesters directly cut and load the stalks for transport. After harvest, lateral buds on the stubbles (Fig. 9) develop new shoots and shoot roots that produce a ratoon (stubble) crop. A crop cycle usually includes one crop from planted cane followed by one to three from ratoons. The crop requires 60 in. or more annual rainfall or irrigation. Irrigation is accomplished by applying water in furrows or by overhead sprinklers. Sugarcane requires large quantities of nitrogen, phosphorus, and potassium. *See* IRRIGATION OF CROPS.

Processing. Sugar is generally removed from sugarcane in large factories by either the milling or the diffusion process. Milling crushes the stalks as they pass between a series of large metal rollers

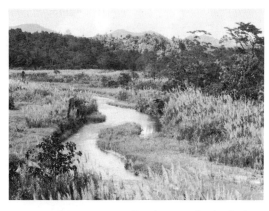

Fig. 2. Wild sugarcane (*Saccharum robustum*) along Screw River near Maprik, New Guinea. (*USDA*)

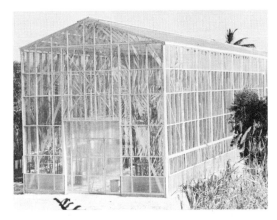

Fig. 3. Plastic-covered crossing house at the U.S. Sugarcane Field Station, Canal Point, Fla. (*USDA*)

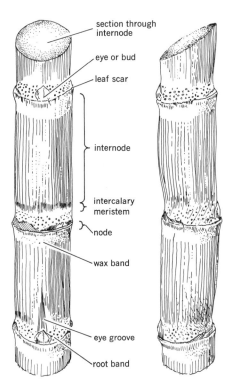

Fig. 4. Cuttings of sugarcane stalks showing nodes, internodes, and lateral buds. (*From J. P. Martin et al., eds., Sugar Cane Diseases of the World, Elsevier, 1961*)

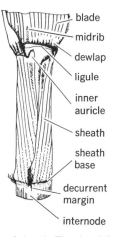

Fig. 5. Structure of sheath. The sheath is drawn without part of the stem that it normally encloses. (*USDA*)

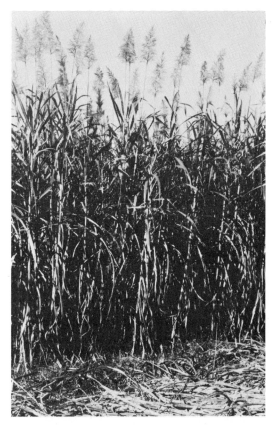

Fig. 6. Flowering sugarcane in Florida. (*USDA*)

separating the fiber (bagasse) from the juice laden with sugar. The diffusion process separates sugar from finely cut stalks by dissolving it in hot water or hot juice. Processing of the juice is completed by clarification to remove nonsugar components, by evaporation to remove water, and by removal of molasses in high-speed centrifuges to produce centrifugal sugar.

In some countries sugarcane is processed in small factories without use of centrifuges, and a dark-brown product, noncentrifugal sugar, is produced.

In 1974 sugarcane accounted for almost 63% of

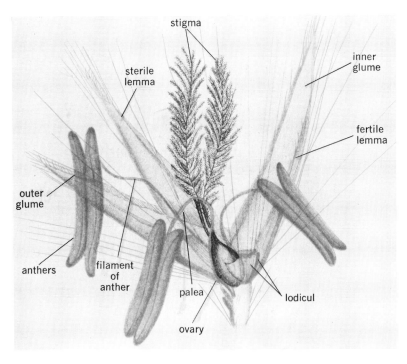

Fig. 7. Sugarcane flower. (*USDA*)

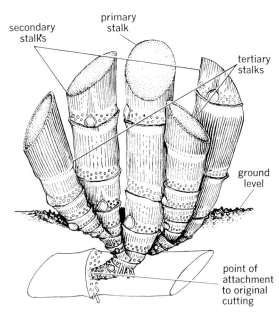

Fig. 9. Underground portion of sugarcane stubble (ratoon) showing primary, secondary, and tertiary stalks. (*From J. P. Martin et al., eds., Sugar Cane Diseases of the World, Elsevier, 1961*)

the world's sugar (see table). Centrifugal sugar was produced in more than 60 countries, noncentrifugal sugar in about 20 countries.

By-products. Bagasse and molasses are the principal by-products from processing sugarcane. Bagasse is used primarily as fuel for factories and for the manufacture of building boards and paper products. Molasses is used primarily as feed for

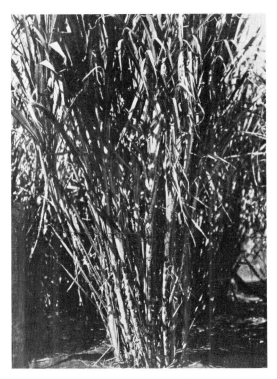

Fig. 8. Stool of sugarcane, variety H. 109, in Hawaii; age 14 months. (*From J. P. Martin et al., eds., Sugar Cane Diseases of the World, Elsevier, 1961*)

livestock and for the production of alcohol and for high-protein yeast products that are useful as livestock feed and for human consumption. Other by-products produced in some areas include ammoniated bagasse pith used for cattle feed as well as such products as crude wax and aconitic acid recovered during the processing of sugar. *See* SUGAR: SUGARBEET.

Diseases. Sugarcane is subject to over 60 diseases, of which 9 have caused, or are causing, serious losses in susceptible varieties. Diseases become of particular importance in sugarcane because of (1) the use of the stalk (vegetative part) for commercial plantings, a practice that spreads disease into new plantings if the propagative stalks are diseased; (2) the relatively small number of varieties grown in a country, which exposes large areas to a disease if the dominant variety is susceptible; and (3) the production of several crops from one original planting, which may result in the accumulation of disease in a field. Fortunately, the distribution of each of the major diseases is not worldwide, and control of all the diseases in any one country is not necessary. If not brought under control, a major disease can cause losses as high as 50%.

The important diseases of sugarcane are caused by viruses, bacteria, and fungi. Viruses cause mosaic and Fiji disease. Ratoon stunting disease (Fig. 11), gummosis, and leaf scald are caused by bacteria. Red rot, smut, downy mildew, and root rot are caused by fungi. Except for root rot, all diseases are carried in the seed piece (stem node) and are spread in the field by insect vectors, mechanical means such as harvesting, or rain. *See* BACTERIA; FUNGI; PLANT VIRUS.

Resistant or tolerant varieties provide the most satisfactory means for controlling disease. Such varieties are available for all important diseases. At present ratoon stunting disease is controlled by

World cane sugar production in 1974, in short tons (and metric tons)

Region	Type of sugar			
	Centrifugal		Noncentrifugal	
North America, including Central America and the Caribbean area; Hawaii	15,853,000	(14,382,000)	263,000	(239,000)
South America	13,573,000	(12,313,000)	1,150,000	(1,043,000)
Europe (Spain and Madeira)	44,000	(40,000)		
Africa	5,753,000	(5,219,000)		
Asia, including Philippines	16,705,000	(15,155,000)	10,006,000	(9,077,000)
Oceania (Australia and Fiji)	3,617,000	(3,281,000)		
World total	55,545,000	(50,390,000)	11,419,000	(10,359,000)

Fig. 10. Field of sugarcane in Louisiana at harvest; age approximately 9 months. (*USDA*)

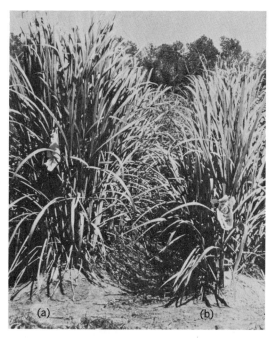

Fig. 11. Effect of ratoon stunting disease on sugarcane. (*a*) Healthy plants. (*b*) Diseased plants.

immersing cane in hot water at 50°C for 2 hr before planting, or by hot-air treatment at 58–59°C for 8 hr.

[ROBERT E. COLEMAN]

Bibliography: E. Artschwager and E. W. Brandes, *Sugarcane (Saccharum officinarum L.): Origin, Characteristics, and Descriptions of Representative Clones*, USDA Handb. no. 122, 1958; R. P. Humbert, *The Growing of Sugarcane*, 1963; S. Price, *Cytology of Saccharum robustum and Related Sympatric Species and Natural Hybrids*, USDA Tech. Bull. no. 1337, 1965; G. L. Spencer and G. P. Meade, *Cane Sugar Handbook*, 9th ed., 1963; U.S. Department of Agriculture, *Sugar*, F.A.S. Circ. FS 2-75, July 1975.

Sunflower

This plant, *Helianthus annuus*, is one of the very few annual cultivated species which evolved and was domesticated within the continental limits of the United States. Its culture was at an advanced state by American Indians when they were first contacted by Europeans. The most common wild weed sunflower of North America belongs to the same species. There are many varieties of cultivated sunflower. Most of these have broad, ovate leaves growing from a single stem which varies from 3 to 20 ft in height. Large, composite flowers have yellow petals and produce flat, round seed heads (the capitulum) 6–15 in. in diameter (see illustration). Sunflower seed (actually a fruit called an achene) vary greatly in size and are usually black or gray with white or dark gray stripes. Ornamental sunflowers are usually much branched, with each branch terminating in a flower which may have all shades of yellow, orange, or red petals; some of the most attractive have double (chrysanthemum-type) flower heads. *See* SEED (BOTANY).

Distribution. Sunflowers have become distributed to all parts of the world. Traditionally, North Dakota, Minnesota, and California have produced the bulk of the domestic commercial crop. Until 1967, large-seeded, low-oil-content varieties were grown for the confectionery (35%) and wild bird food (65%) trades.

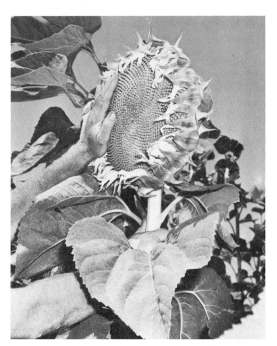

Maturing sunflowers on a farm in California. (*U.S. Department of Agriculture*)

Economic importance. Sunflowers are an important oilseed in world trade (being grown on about 20,000,000 acres), usually ranking third in importance and being lower in tonnage than soybeans and similar to peanuts. Sunflower seed production exceeded that of peanuts in 1967. The Soviet Union ranks first in world sunflower seed production, with more than 9,000,000 tons produced on 11,800,000 acres in 1967. Argentina is usually the second largest producer, but sunflowers are also grown in many eastern European countries and in Asia, South Africa, and Canada. The oil is a high-quality edible oil, being high in the polyunsaturated fatty acid linoleic acid; it is used in cooking, salad dressing, margarine, and soap and as a drying oil in paint. The high-protein meal remaining after extraction of the oil from the seed is a high-quality supplement in animal nutrition and has promise in human nutrition. In the Soviet Union threshed sunflower heads are used as cattle feed and as a source of pectin; alcohol and furfural are manufactured from the seed hulls. Sunflower plants were formerly used for livestock feed in the form of silage in the northern United States and Canada, but this practice has practically disappeared.   [MURRAY L. KINMAN]

Diseases. Sunflowers are subject to destructive disease throughout the world.

Causal organisms. Rust, caused by an airborne fungus (*Puccinia helianthi*), reduces seed yields and may kill the plants. Root rot and wilt, caused by a soilborne fungus (*Sclerotinia sclerotiorum*), affects sunflowers and also many other broadleaved plant species. Other sunflower diseases caused by soilborne fungi include downy mildew, caused by *Plasmopara halstedii*, leaf mottle, caused by *Verticillium dahliae*, both of which are worldwide in distribution, and black root rot, caused by *Sclerotium bataticola*, which is most common in tropical and subtropical regions.

The virus diseases of sunflowers include mosaics and aster yellows. They are still somewhat restricted in geographical distribution. *See* PLANT VIRUS.

Control measures. Chemical control of both rust and leaf mottle is possible, but it is not economically feasible. Cultural measures, such as weed removal and rotation with other crops which are disease resistant, help reduce losses from most of the sunflower diseases, and these measures are the only controls available against some of them. Sunflowers resistant to rust have been produced in Manitoba, Canada, and varieties resistant to downy mildew, leaf mottle, and aster yellows are being developed there. *See* AGRICULTURAL SCIENCE (PLANT); PLANT DISEASE; PLANT DISEASE CONTROL.

[WALDEMAR E. SACKSTON]

Swine production

An agricultural business which is usually located in proximity to sources of high-energy feedstuffs; in the United States particularly, the geographical distribution of swine production is closely related to corn and milo production. Swine, as nonruminants, utilize large quantities of concentrate feeds; for instance, it is estimated that 30% of the corn grain produced is fed to swine. Swine can utilize only limited quantities of roughage in the diet.

The United States has about one-fourth of the world hog population. The leading states expressed as number of hogs per state and number per square mile on Jan. 1, 1974, are indicated in Table 1. These inventory values reflect a total United States yearly production of about 90,000,000 hogs.

Swine production industry is evolving from the status of a supplement to farm income to that of intensified units in which swine production is a major enterprise. The total number of swine producers is decreasing at the rate of 5% per year, but the volume per unit is increasing sufficiently to maintain the total volume of production. Ninety-eight percent of all hogs are produced by independent producers. The other 2% are produced by totally integrated enterprises. This trend is expected to continue. Intensified swine production in modern confinement facilities requires highly trained biological managers capable of applying the principles of breeding, nutrition, physiology, environmental control, and economics.

Swine products. The primary products of swine are pork, lard, hides, and innumerable by-products of a pharmaceutical nature. Pork and lard supply approximately 15% of the total calories consumed as food in the United States. Pork is more successfully cured and stored than many other meats, and it is estimated that about 60% of the swine carcass is cured by various methods.

Swine breeding. Market hogs are produced with emphasis on red meat production while minimizing fat or lard production. Breeders of purebred, hybrid, and crossbred swine provide the seed stock for commercial hog production and are entrusted with the responsibility of changing the carcass to better meet the demands of the consumer. The purebred breeds of major significance include the following: Berkshire, Chester White, Duroc, Hampshire, Landrace, Poland China, Spotted Poland China, and Yorkshire. A typical example of a modern meat-type hog is illustrated in Fig. 1.

Most commercial producers of swine practice a system of crossbreeding, mating individuals from two, three, or four different breeds. Research has shown that crossbreeding increases the vigor and feeding qualities of the offspring. This effect is called heterosis or hybrid vigor. Crossbred dams mated to a boar of a third breed farrow and wean larger and heavier litters than purebred dams. In practical swine operations a system of rotation

Table 1. Hog inventory, January 1974

State	Pigs raised per square mile	Total pigs
Iowa	261	14,700,000
Illinois	134	7,350,000
Indiana	134	4,875,000
Missouri	62	4,325,000
Minnesota	47	3,978,000
Nebraska	45	3,445,000
Ohio	55	2,274,000
South Dakota	28	2,175,000
Kansas	21	2,000,000
North Carolina	35	1,950,000
United States total	33	61,022,000

breeding is recommended to realize the advantages of crossbreeding. Rotation breeding is accomplished by using male "seed" stock from three or four breeds in rotation and retaining female stock sired by the boar. *See* BREEDING (ANIMAL).

Swine normally reach puberty between the ages of 5 and 7 months. Females exhibit sexual maturity at a slightly earlier age but are not usually bred until they are 8 months old and weigh at least 100 kg. Boars are not used for breeding until they are at least 8 months of age.

Estrus, or the time of sexual excitement in the sow, lasts 48–72 hr and occurs approximately every 21 days. Ovulation normally occurs during the latter part of the estrous period. Female swine shed an average from 15 to 18 ova at each estrous period although only 60–70% survive the gestation period of 114 days. The heavy mortality has not been explained. With first litter gilts the number of ova ovulated may be increased by feeding a high-energy ration for 2–3 weeks before breeding. Once a gilt is bred embryonic mortality is reduced by limiting energy intake during gestation. Maternal weight gain of 32 kg for gilts and 18 kg for sows during gestation is sufficient to produce a healthy littler of pigs and form a nutrient reserve for lactation.

Litter size, which averages 9.8 pigs, is influenced by a number of factors. The age of the female at mating is the most important factor; the number of pigs per litter increases up to the fifth litter or the time the sow is about 3 years of age. Breeds differ, and within breeds the short, compact sows usually have smaller litters than the larger individuals.

The majority of sows in the United States is bred by natural service, though the use of artificial insemination is rapidly increasing.

Swine nutrition. Feed costs comprise about 65–75% of the total cost of production. Feeding programs of today are scientifically formulated to obtain optimum rate and maximum efficiency of weight gain. The performance of pigs fed rations which were characteristic of designated times in the history of the swine industry is illustrated in Fig. 2. These littermates were housed and managed similarly, only the diets (1908 versus 1958 formulations) differed. Since 1958, further refinement of diet formulation has improved efficiency of converting feed into pork.

Nutritionally the period during the growth of the baby pig is considered critical. The nutritional needs of the other periods of the life cycle—gestation, lactation, growing, and finishing—are easily met by fortifying natural feedstuffs. Requirements of swine may be classified as water, energy (carbohydrate, fat, and protein), amino acids (protein), minerals, and vitamins. It is essential that these nutrients be in proper balance and that the minimum requirement be met to promote optimum performance.

Water serves as a medium for digestion absorption, transportation, and excretion of other nutrients. The water requirements of swine decrease from about 12% of the liveweight for young swine to 5% for mature swine or about 2 lb of water per pound of feed consumed.

Most of the energy need of the pig is supplied by dietary carbohydrate. Fat usually plays a minor

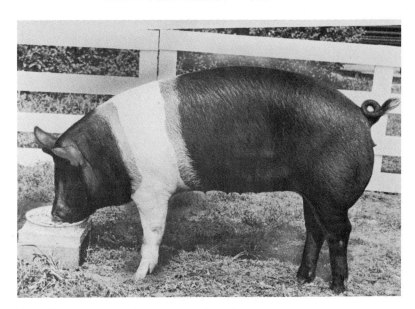

Fig. 1. Typical example of a modern meat-type hog.

role. In general, carbohydrates such as starch, dextrins, disaccharides (except lactose), and monosaccharides are equally metabolizable by the weanling pig. Lactose is an excellent energy source for the baby pig but may cause diarrhea in older pigs. This results from a developmental shift with increasing age in intestinal enzyme activities. Energy requirements of swine are usually expressed as a daily need for total feed or digestible nutrients. Feed intake increases as nutrient requirements for maintenance and weight gain increase. The increase in energy requirement with increasing size is shown in Table 2. *See* CARBOHYDRATE; FAT AND OIL, EDIBLE.

Amino acids, required for maintenance, growth,

Table 2. Energy needs of swine

Body weight, kg	Daily gain, kg	Daily feed, kg	Net energy per day, cal
5	0.23	0.34	1,141
14	0.45	0.86	2,774
18	0.55	1.20	3,854
36	0.75	2.10	6,745
45	0.82	2.54	8,119
54	0.86	2.85	9,123
72	0.91	3.18	10,185
90	0.95	3.91	12,528
100	0.98	4.30	13,764

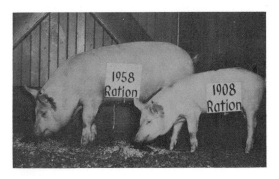

Fig. 2. Performance of 1908 and 1958 swine.

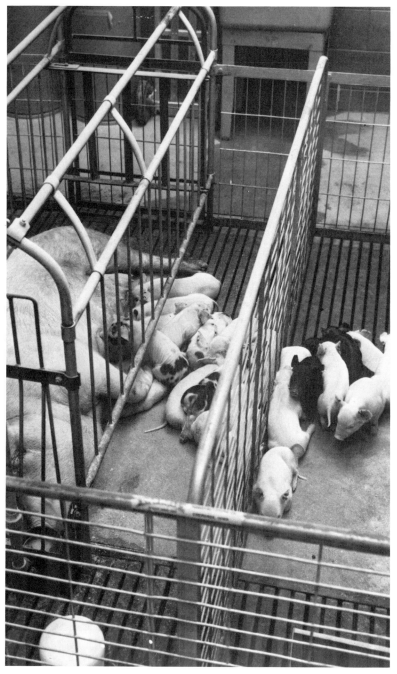

Fig. 3. Farrowing stall with sow and litter.

gestation, and lactation, are chemically linked as proteins in feedstuffs. An essential amino acid is one that swine cannot synthesize at a sufficiently rapid rate to permit normal performance. Ten of the amino acids found in feedstuffs are considered essential for growing swine.

The essential amino acids for growing swine are arginine, histidine, isoleucine, leucine, lysine, methionine, phenylalanine, threonine, tryptophan, and valine. Cystine can supply up to 56% of the need for methionine. Tyrosine can satisfy 30% of the need for phenylalanine. Additional dietary nitrogen is needed by the body to form the remaining amino acids found in the body. The amino acids of most practical importance are lysine and tryptophan, which are most severely deficient in cereal grains (corn, milo, and wheat). Although there is increasing emphasis on the amino acid needs of swine, it is still customary to formulate rations by providing ample quantities of protein. Soybean oil meal is the most common dietary supplement used for the correction of the amino acid deficiences in cereal grains. See AMINO ACIDS.

The mineral and vitamin requirements of weanling pigs are described in Table 3. Cereal grains and soybean oil meal lack vitamins and minerals; hence, practical diets normally require supplementation. See VITAMIN.

Calcium, phosphorus, sodium, and chloride are normally added as ground limestone, dicalcium phosphate or defluorinated rock phosphate, and trace mineralized salt. The salt serves as a carrier for trace minerals including iron, copper, manganese, selenium, iodine, and zinc. The trace minerals may not always be dietary essentials since they may be obtained from extra dietary sources. Supplemental vitamins are most economically provided as synthetically produced vitamin supplements. A typical ration for growing swine is shown in Table 4.

Feed additives, such as antibiotic supplements, are ingredients of swine rations for swine up to 35 kg in weight and during late gestation and throughout lactation. Antibiotic supplements containing sources such as chlortetracycline, oxytetracycline, tylosin, or penicillin are added to rations to provide 10–20 ppm in the ration. Copper sulfate and arsenicals are also included in rations as antibacterial compounds. These products stimulate the rate of gain apparently by improving the health of the pigs. See ANIMAL-FEED COMPOSITION.

Table 3. Nutrient needs of weanling pigs (15–35 kg)

Mineral	Amount	Vitamin	Amount
Calcium, %	0.6	Vitamin A, IU/kg	3300
Phosphorus, %	0.5	Vitamin D, IU/kg	330
Sodium chloride, %	0.5	Vitamin E, IU/kg	11
Copper, ppm*	6.0	Vitamin K, ppm	2.2
Iron, ppm	70	Thiamin, ppm	1.1
Iodine, ppm	0.22	Riboflavin, ppm	2.2
Manganese, ppm	20	Niacin, ppm	17.8
Zinc, ppm	50	Pantothenic acid, ppm	11
Selenium, ppm	0.10	Pyridoxine, ppm	1.1
		Choline, ppm	890
		Vitamin B_{12}, ppb†	15

*ppm = parts per million.   †ppb = parts per billion.

Table 4. Typical ration for growing swine

Ingredient	Amount, %
Yellow corn	79.3
Soybean oil meal	18.0
Dicalcium phosphate	1.0
Ground limestone	1.0
Trace mineralized salt	0.5
Vitamin supplement*	0.1
Antibiotic supplement	0.1

*Supplies per kilogram of ration: 3333 IU vitamin A; 333 IU vitamin D; 22 IU vitamin E; 1.1 mg riboflavin; 5.5 mg pantothenic acid; 16.5 mg niacin; 110 mg choline; 17.8 μg vitamin B$_{12}$.

Most swine rations are completely mixed and self-fed to growing-finishing swine to conserve labor and maximize feed intake. The breeding herd is limit-fed either by hand or mechanically in order to reduce feed cost and keep herds in excellent physical condition for optimum reproductive performance.

Swine management. Items included as management are primarily directed at minimizing adverse environmental factors of swine and providing maximum opportunity for survival and growth. About 25% of the pigs farrowed fail to survive to 6 weeks of age. The mortality is caused primarily by crushing by the sow, enteric infections, and starvation. Modern climatically controlled farrowing quarters (Fig. 3) with farrowing crates are being used to minimize losses. The newborn pig is incapable of maintaining body temperature and is dependent on supplemental heat from the environment. Other biological management practices for the newborn pig include clipping needle teeth, applying antiseptic to the navel, and providing iron to compensate for its severe deficiency in milk.

Since the pig has very limited ability to dissipate body heat by sweating, finishing pigs or breeding stock must be protected during periods of high temperature. Shades and water mists have been used in the past, but today many confinement buildings are being constructed for finishing hogs and breeding stock in which the environmental extremes are minimized. The reduction of temperature extremes encourages more rapid and more efficient gains, particularly in finishing swine. These buildings include slotted floors to reduce or practically eliminate floor cleaning.

Swine are particularly susceptible to diseases and parasites. Due to a well-planned and executed course of action, hog cholera has essentially been eliminated from the United States. This required close teamwork of the national, state, and local governments with swine organizations and individual producers. This will save millions of dollars previously spent on vaccines and eliminate extensive death losses due to cholera. Erysipelas, dysentery, leptospirosis, atrophic rhinitis, and transmissible gastroenteritis are some of the other important diseases. Several diseases can be prevented by use of appropriate vaccines or other medication. However, for many diseases specific control has not been realized. Thus, preventative and control measures of proven value are recommended.

Swine are especially subject to infestations with ascarids, which are parasites primarily of the intestinal tract that impair metabolism and growth. Following ingestion of the embryonated ascarid eggs by the pig, the larvae burrow through the intestinal wall and migrate through the body causing considerable damage to the liver and lungs. Passing from the lungs to the mouth the larvae are ingested and develop into mature ascarids in the intestine.

The use of confinement facilities, particularly those with slotted floors, reduces the spread of disease and parasites and allows rapid removal of excreta from the pens, thereby reducing opportunities for contact with the many vectors of the diseases. Excellent sanitation is part of any sound biological management system.

Swine marketing. Swine normally attain a market weight of 90–100 kg at approximately 6 months of age. Of the swine slaughtered under Federal inspection, 87% consists of barrows and gilts and the remainder is sows, boars, and stags. The market hogs move from farm to the slaughter plants through terminal public markets, country buying stations, and auction markets or by direct sale to the packer. The type of marketing varies considerably in different areas, although terminal public markets and country buying stations' are the most popular channels.

Market grades of slaughter barrows and gilts have been developed according to a scheme which places a premium on the four major lean cuts— ham, loin, and picnic and Boston butt. In addition, market grades penalize excess finish and lard. Barrow and gilt carcasses are graded as U.S. No. 1, U.S. No. 2, U.S. No. 3, U.S. No. 4, and utility. Utility grade is characterized by a low degree of finish.

Market price of hogs is largely determined by the prevailing commodity price level and by supply and demand. Keen competition from other meats is particularly important to the marketing of pork. *See* AGRICULTURAL SCIENCE (ANIMAL).

[ALDON H. JENSEN; DONALD E. BECKER]

Tea

A small tree (in cultivation, constant pruning makes it a shrub 3–4 ft, or 0.9–1.2 m, tall); a preparation of its leaves dried and cured by various processes; and a beverage made from these leaves. The plant, *Camellia sinensis* (or *Thea sinensis*), is an evergreen tree of the Theaceae family, native to southeastern Asia, and does best in a warm climate where the rainfall averages 90–200 in. (2200–5000 mm). The slower growth at higher altitudes improves the flavor. China, Japan, Taiwan, India, Sri Lanka, and Indonesia are among the leading tea-producing countries, with China contributing about one-half of the world's supply. According to Chinese folklore, the Chinese emperor Shen-mung discovered the use of tea about 2500 B.C.

Tea leaves contain caffeine, various tannins, aromatic substances attributed to an essential oil, and other materials of a minor nature, including proteins, gums, and sugars. The tannins provide the astringency, the caffeine the stimulating properties.

The tea plant normally produces a full crop of leaves (flush) about every 40 days. In China and Japan the leaves are plucked when the flush has

TEA

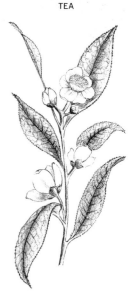

Flowering branch of tea plant (*Thea sinensis*).

mostly completed its growth, but in India and Indonesia the leaves are picked every week or two, resulting in most of the leaves being gathered at the best time. The leaves are named, beginning with the topmost, as pekoe tip, orange pekoe, pekoe, first souchong, second souchong, first congou, and second congou.

In its natural state the tea plant grows to a height of 15–30 ft (4.5–9 m). The leaves vary from 1½ to 10 in. (4–25 cm) long and are thick, smooth, and leathery. The white, fragrant flowers are produced in the axils of the leaves (see illustration). The fruits are dark brown capsules.
[EARL L. CORE]

Tea production technology depends on whether black, green, or semifermented tea is to be manufactured. The characteristic appearance and flavor of each arise more from different processing and manufacturing methods than from type of leaf.

Black tea. This tea requires quick transportation of the green leaf from garden to factory, where it is carefully spread on withering tats. The leaf loses moisture and becomes flaccid within 24 hr. Circulation of conditioned air during withering shortens the time substantially. The next process, called rolling, ruptures the leaf cells and releases their juices. This is accomplished in a brass roller box, equipped with an adjustable pressure cap and an open base. The box is filled with withered leaf and rotated eccentrically over a brass table fitted with curved battens. During a 30-min period the leaf cells rupture under the pressure and the rubbing action. In a second rolling period the leaf is twisted and coated with juices, leading to balling. The leaf changes to a bright copper color, and a characteristic tea aroma develops. A roll breaker is subsequently employed to disintegrate the balls for fermentation.

In fermentation, enzyme action and oxidation occur. The rolled leaf is spread to a 2- or 3-in. depth on fermenting beds and held under high humidity at 75–80°F. Since the body, or strength, of the tea depends on this fermentation, careful attention to its progress is required. Approximately 3½ hr are needed for the rolling and fermentation operations.

Firing or drying of fermented tea leaf conventionally is carried out by passing it through heated ovenlike chambers. Temperatures of 170–180°F arrest fermentation and develop the familiar blackish color. Drying is practically completed in one pass, but further heat is applied to produce the "case hardening" that protects quality. The leaf is sieved, graded, and packed into chests lined with aluminum foil. Each chest contains about 100 lb of finished tea.

Green tea. Green tea manufacture requires that the plucked leaves be steamed as quickly as possible. Such processing at 160°F makes them soft and pliable and, by inactivating the natural enzymes, prevents fermentation. After steaming, the leaf is alternately rolled and dried until it becomes too stiff for further manipulation. For export, green tea is refired in pans with mechanical stirring to produce a luster.

Oolong teas. Oolong teas are midway between black and green teas in that they are semifermented. After a short sun-withering in the garden, the leaf is gently rolled in the plucker's hands, whereupon a slight fermentation is initiated. After a short period this leaf is sent to the factory to be fired and packed for shipment.

Instant tea. This type of tea is obtained by spray-drying of a black tea extract, with or without the admixture of maltodextrins. The technology is patterned closely after that followed in manufacturing of instant coffee. Concentrated tea extract also may be combined with a heavy sugar syrup and marketed as a liquid. Solubility of instant tea powder can be varied by manipulations in processing. See FOOD ENGINEERING. [JOHN H. NAIR]

Terracing (agriculture)

A method of shaping land to control erosion on slopes of rolling land used for cropping and other purposes. In early practice the land was shaped into a series of nearly level benches or steplike formations. Modern practice in terracing, however, consists of the construction of low-graded channels or levees to carry the excess rainfall from the land at nonerosive velocities. The physical principle involved is that, when water is spread in a shallow stream, its flow is retarded by the roughness of the bottom of the channel and its carrying, or erosive, power is reduced. Since direct impact of rainfall on bare land churns up the soil and the stirring effect keeps it in suspension in overland flow and rills, terracing does not prevent sheet erosion. It serves only to prevent destruction of agricultural land by gullying and must be supplemented by other erosion-control practices, such as grass rotation, cover crops, mulching, contour farming, strip cropping, and increased organic matter content.

In areas of low rainfall and absorbent soils, nearly level terraces are used to retain the runoff and conserve soil moisture, thus preventing wind erosion of the soil. See EROSION; SOIL CONSERVATION.

Types of terraces. The two major types of terraces are the bench and the broadbase (see illustration).

Bench. This is essentially a steep-land terrace and consists of an almost vertical retaining wall,

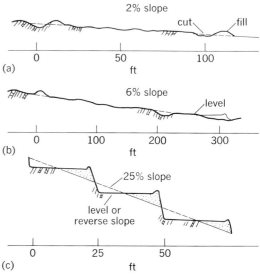

Types of terraces. (a) Broadbase. (b) Conservation bench. (c) Bench. (*From Soil and Water Conservation Engineering, 2d ed., The Ferguson Foundation Agricultural Engineering Series, Wiley, 1966*)

called a riser, or a steep vegetative slope to hold the nearly level surface of the soil for cultivation, orchards, vineyards, or landscaping. The bench terrace has been in use all over the world for the past several thousand years, particularly in Europe, Australia, and Asia. Bench terraces are adaptable to slopes of 25–30% and are costly to construct. For the most part, bench terraces have been abandoned for general farming because they are not adaptable to the efficient use of modern-day farm equipment.

Modern mechanized farming greatly increased the need for erosion control; at the same time, however, modern machinery furnished the power for increased terracing. The early United States practice of constructing hillside ditches across the slopes of fields to prevent up- and downhill gullying was followed by the development of the more easily controlled levee or ridge. This was called a narrow-base ridge terrace and was, in some cases, vegetated and developed into a bench terrace. By plowing to this narrow levee and maintaining the drainage channel, its base was widened until it became known as a broadbase terrace.

Broadbase. This terrace has the distinguishing characteristic of farmability; that is, crops can be grown on this terrace and worked with modern-day machinery. These terraces are constructed either to remove or retain water and, based on their primary function, are classified either as graded or level.

A graded broadbase terrace is constructed from the upper side only with a variable or uniform grade in the channel to remove water at an acceptable rate. This is sometimes called the Nichols or channel terrace.

A level broadbase terrace is constructed on the contour and from both sides. It is recommended in areas where the soil is permeable to prevent overtopping. This terrace is sometimes called the Mangum or ridge terrace.

Another terrace in use today in semiarid regions where maximum moisture conservation is needed is the Zingg conservation bench terrace. It consists of an earthen embankment and a very broad, flat channel resembling a level bench. The runoff store in the channel comes from the sloping area above the bench which extends upslope to the next terrace.

The design of any type terrace must take into consideration factors such as soil characteristics, the cropping system to be used, soil management practices, climatic conditions, and others. All influence the effectiveness of the terrace system.

Terrace outlets. Since terrace channels concentrate rainfall on hillsides, outlets are a major feature of any successful terrace system. There are many different schemes for outlet construction. Masonry structures, such as storm sewers, concrete flumes, or drop inlets, may be used on steep land. Vegetation, such as grass or other thick-growing crops, may be used on gentle slopes. Modern practice in outlet construction calls for the use of natural channels with careful shaping and vegetating before large concentrations of water are turned into them.

Parallel terraces. Parallel terraces have been a major change in the layout of the terracing system. The object of parallel terracing is to facilitate the use of modern farm machinery by the elimination of point rows. Point rows in a field cause an excessive loss of productive time because of the turning of equipment. They also cause the destruction of crops and terraces by making it necessary for machinery to pass over them in their course of turning. Parallel terraces are made possible by a relatively small amount of land forming, such as moving land from high to low spots in the field and smoothing. This allows the efficient use of 4-, 6-, and 8-row cultivating equipment.

Construction equipment. Terracing equipment may be classified according to the method by which it moves the soil: lift and roll, throw, scrape and push, and carry.

The ideal terracing machine will meet certain requirements, such as (1) displacement of soil laterally to the desired position in the ridge; (2) placing the topsoil on or near the top of the ridge; (3) high work speed; (4) operation on slopes up to 15–20%; and (5) low initial and operating cost. *See* AGRICULTURE, SOIL AND CROP PRACTICES IN; LAND DRAINAGE (AGRICULTURE).

[CHARLES B. OGBURN]

Thiamine

A water-soluble vitamin found in many foods; pork, liver, and whole grains are particularly rich sources. It is also known as vitamin B_1 or aneurin. The structural formula of thiamine is shown in the illustration.

Chemistry. The vitamin is heat-labile, and considerable amounts are destroyed during cooking. Thiamine is unstable in alkaline solutions but stable in acid solutions. It acts like a weak base and can be absorbed on basic ion-exchange materials such as decalso and fuller's earth, a property used in its chemical determination. Biological and microbiological methods for its estimation are available but are seldom used, and a chemical assay based on the production of thiochrome, a fluorescent reaction product of thiamine, is the chosen method.

Biochemistry. Thiamine functions in enzyme systems as thiamine pyrophosphate, a coenzyme known as cocarboxylase. Thiamine-containing enzymes decarboxylate α-keto acids such as pyruvic acid and α-ketoglutaric acid. Thiamine pyrophosphate is also involved in the transketolation of pentose to heptulose in the hexose monophosphate shunt system which is an alternative to the conventional glycolytic pathway of anaerobic glucose metabolism. *See* CARBOHYDRATE METABOLISM.

Deficiency. Thiamine deficiency is known as beriberi in humans and polyneuritis in birds. Muscle and nerve tissues are affected by the deficiency, and poor growth is observed. People with beriberi are irritable, depressed, and weak. They often die of cardiac failure. Wernicke's disease observed in alcoholics is associated with a thiamine deficiency. This disease is characterized by brain lesions, liver disease, and partial paraly-

Structural formula for thiamine.

sis, particularly of the motor nerves of the eye. As is the case in all B vitamin diseases, thiamine deficiency is usually accompanied by deficiencies of other vitamins.

Dietary requirements. A dietary source of thiamine is required by all nonruminant animals that have been studied. Thiamine is the most poorly stored of the B vitamins. Individuals eating vitamin-deficient diets are likely to develop beriberi symptoms first. Approximately 5 mg of thiamine can be absorbed per day by normal adults. Excess thiamine given by mouth or parenterally is usually lost through excretion in the urine and feces. Thiamine requirements are related to caloric intake. More thiamine is required in high-carbohydrate diets than in high-fat diets, but the reason for this is still not clear. Some foods, particularly raw fish, contain enzymes which destroy thiamine. More thiamine is needed in altered physical states, such as hyperthyroidism, pregnancy, and lactation. Thiamine requirements of humans are primarily estimated by means of urinary excretion data. The recommended dietary allowances of the National Research Council provide 0.5 mg of thiamine for each 1000 cal for adults.

[STANLEY N. GERSHOFF]

Manufacture. Industrial synthesis of this vitamin is accomplished by linking chloromethylpyrimidine with 4-methyl-5-(β-hydroxyethyl)-thiazole to give aneurin. Another way to build up the thiamine molecule on a commercial scale is to convert 4-amino-5-cyanopyrimidine into the thioformyl-aminomethyl derivative via catalytic hydrogenation and reaction with sodium dithioformate. This compound is then treated with 1-acetoxy-3-chloro-4-pentanone to form the thiazole ring in situ connected to the pyrimidine ring via a methylene bridge. (U.S. Patents 2,193,858 and 2,218,350.) See VITAMIN.

[FERNAND DE MONTMOLLIN]

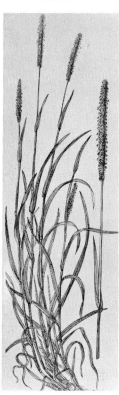

TIMOTHY

Timothy (*Phleum pratense*).

Threonine

An amino acid which is considered essential for normal growth of animals. The amino acids are characterized physically by the following: (1) the pK_1, or the dissociation constant of the various titratable groups; (2) the isoelectric point, or pH at which a dipolar ion does not migrate in an electric field; (3) the optical rotation, or the rotation imparted to a beam of plane-polarized light (frequently the D line of the sodium spectrum) passing through 1 dm of a solution of 100 g in 100 ml; and (4) solubility.

Physical constants of the L isomer at 25°C:
pK_1 (COOH): 2.71; pK_2 (NH_3^+): 9.62
Isoelectric point: 6.16
Optical rotation: $[\alpha]_D (H_2O)$: −28.5; $[\alpha]_D$ (5 N HCl): −15.0
Solubility (g/100 ml H_2O): 20.5 (DL)

Threonine reacts with periodate to form glyoxylate, ammonia, and acetaldehyde, and is a biosynthetic precursor of isoleucine in microorganisms. Threonine is biosynthesized from aspartic acid. See AMINO ACIDS.

The major pathway in metabolic degradation starts with the nonoxidative deamination to α-ke-

tobutyric acid. This keto acid may be oxidatively decarboxylated to propionyl-CoA, or transaminated to form α-aminobutyric acid. Another pathway of threonine degradation involves an initial cleavage to glycine and acetaldehyde.

[EDWARD A. ADELBERG]

Timothy

A plant, *Phleum pratense*, of the order Cyperales, long the most important hay grass for the cooler temperate humid regions. It is easily established and managed, produces seed abundantly, and grows well in mixtures with alfalfa and clover. It is a short-lived perennial, makes a loose sod, and has moderately leafy stems 2–4 ft tall and a dense cylindrical inflorescence (see illustration). Timothy responds to fertile soils with high yield and nutritive content. Cutting promptly after heading improves the feed quality. Timothy-legume mixtures still predominate in hay and pasture seedings for crop rotations in the northern half of the United States, but orchard grass and bromegrass have increasingly replaced timothy in such mixtures in many areas since about 1950. See ALFALFA; CLOVER; GRASS CROPS.

[HOWARD B. SPRAGUE]

Tomato

An important vegetable grown for its edible fruit belonging to the genus *Lycopersicon*, especially *L. esculentum*. *Lycopersicon* species are native to South America, especially Peru, and the Galapagos Islands. The tomato was first domesticated in Mexico, where it received its name from the Aztec word *xitomate*.

It was introduced to Europe in the mid-16th century, and was prominently featured in the early herbals. Known as the "love apple" and "poma d'ora," it was grown for the beauty of its fruit but was not often eaten, except in Italy and Spain, because many considered it to be poisonous like its distant relative the deadly nightshade. But today the tomato is one of the most popular vegetables in the world.

Although native to the New World, the tomato was introduced to America from Europe. It has been grown in the United States since colonial days, but it has become an important vegetable there only in the past century.

Classification and structure. The genus *Lycopersican* (Greek, "wolf peach") is a member of the Solanaceae, the nightshade family. *L. esculentum*, the familiar tomato, can be hybridized with each of the eight other species of *Lycopersicon*. It can be easily crossed with *L. pimpinellifolium*, the red currant tomato. Crosses with the more distantly related, green-fruited *Lycopersicon* species are more difficult; usually the tomato must be the maternal parent, embryo culture is sometimes required, and the hybrids have varying degrees of fertility. Despite these obstacles, tomato breeders have transferred many genes, particularly for disease resistance, from wild *Lycopersicon* species to the tomato. See BREEDING (PLANT).

Lycopersicon is allied to *Solanum*, a diverse genus that includes potato, eggplant, and over 2000 other species. Two *Solanum* species, *S. pennellii* and *S. lycopersicoides*, have been crossed with the tomato.

The tomato, and all other species it can be crossed with, has 12 pairs of chromosomes. There is good homology between chromosomes of each species. Tomato chromosomes differ in length, centromere position, and heterochromatin distribution, and each of the chromosomes of the tomato can be distinguished cytologically.

The tomato is a herbaceous perennial, but is usually grown as an annual in temperate regions since it is killed by frost. Originally it had an indeterminate plant habit, continuously producing three nodes between each inflorescence. Many modern varieties, however, are determinate; they have the self-pruning (sp) gene, and therefore have fewer than three nodes between inflorescences with the stem terminating in an inflorescence.

The compound leaves are usually alternate and odd-pinnate. The branches are procumbent or partly erect, and the weak stem is sometimes supported by a stake in cultivation.

The inflorescence is a monochasial cyme of 4 to 12 perfect and hypogynous flowers (Fig. 1). Primitive tomatoes have the solanaceous trait of five flower parts, but modern tomato varieties often have more than five yellow petals and green sepals. The five anthers are joined around the pistil in *Lycopersicon*, one of the key distinctions from the closely related *Solanum* genus. Wild *Lycopersicon* species which are self-incompatible, and therefore are obligate cross pollinators, have their style exserted beyond the anther cone. Cultivated tomatoes are self-fertile, and their style length is more similar to the anther length, a characteristic that favors self-pollination.

The fruit is a berry with 2 to 12 locules containing many seeds. Most tomato varieties have red fruit, due to the red carotenoid lycopene. Different single genes are known to produce various shades of yellow, orange, or green fruit. There is no basis for the common belief that yellow-fruited tomatoes are low in acidity. Many greenhouse varieties have pink fruit, due to a single gene (y) that prevents formation of the yellow pigment in the epidermis of the fruit.

Distribution and economic importance. The tomato is the most important processed vegetable, constituting over 23 lb (10.4 kg) of the 54 lb (24.3 kg) of processed vegetables the average American consumes each year. Commercial tomato growers in the United States received more than $800,000,000 for their crop in 1976, a value greater than that for any other vegetable except potatoes.

Over three-quarters of the 375,407 acres (152,000 ha) of processing tomatoes grown in the United States in 1976 were in California. Other leading states, in order of acreage of processing tomatoes, were Ohio, Indiana, and New Jersey. Florida was the leading state for fresh market tomatoes, with 28,300 acres (11,460 ha) in 1976, followed by California, South Carolina, Alabama, and Texas. Sizable amounts of fresh market tomatoes are imported to the United States from Mexico in winter months. Tomatoes are grown in every state, including Alaska. Although most tomato varieties prefer a long, warm season, very early varieties have been bred for northern areas.

Much of the world's production of tomatoes is in the United States. The Soviet Union has the largest acreage of tomatoes, but its production is second to the United States. Other leading countries, in order of acreage, are Italy, Egypt, Mexico, Turkey, and Spain. Tomatoes are often grown in greenhouses in northern Europe, especially in the Netherlands and England. The greenhouse tomato production in the United States is centered in Cleveland, Ohio.

Cultural practices. Tomatoes prefer warm weather. Cool temperature, 10°C (50°F) and below, delays seed germination, inhibits vegetative development, reduces fruit set, and impairs fruit ripening. High temperature, above 35°C (95°F), reduces fruit set and inhibits development of normal fruit color. Tomato plants cannot tolerate frost, and home gardeners often cover plants to protect them when frost threatens.

The tomato plant is day-neutral, flowering when grown with either short or long days. This makes it possible to grow tomatoes outdoors during the short days of winter in frost-free areas, such as southern Florida and the Imperial Valley of California, as well as in more northern areas during the long days of summer.

In California, seeds for most commercial tomatoes are planted directly in the field. Transplants are used in shorter-season areas, with plants grown for about 6 weeks in a local greenhouse or shipped from a southern state where they are grown in the field. Home gardeners often grow their own transplants in a warm, sunny location, then harden them in a cold frame before transplanting.

A "starter solution," soluble fertilizer applied when transplanting, is often beneficial. Tomatoes prefer fertile soil, but can be grown on a variety of soils with proper fertilization. Heavy nitrogen fertilization does not make plants vegetative, as is often believed, but rather delays maturity and promotes rank vine growth. Nitrogen fertilizer and irrigation are often withheld late in the season when tomatoes are to be mechanically harvested,

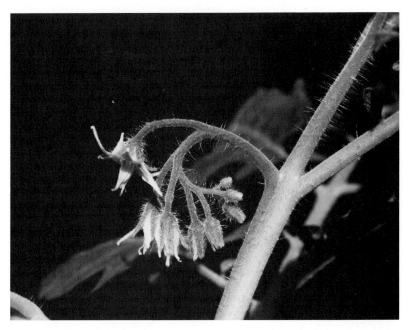

Fig. 1. Inflorescence of tomato (*Lycopersicon esculentum*) with open flowers and flower buds in different stages of development.

since this increases the proportion of ripe fruit in a single harvest. Phosphorus is often applied in a band near the seed when direct-seeding.

Level, uniform fields with few stones are best for mechanical harvesting. Heavy soils should be avoided when direct-seeding because of the danger of the soil crusting before the seedlings emerge. Soil pH of 6.0 to 6.5 is recommended.

Tomatoes respond to irrigation in many areas. A uniform supply of soil moisture is needed to prevent excessive losses from cracking and blossom-end rot. Good drainage is essential for high yields.

Better fruit set is often obtained with greenhouse tomatoes if the flowers are vibrated to ensure pollination. This is usually not necessary in the field, since the wind suffices.

Disease. Some diseases can be controlled by the use of resistant varieties. The letters V, F, and N in the name of a variety or its catalog description indicate that it is resistant to verticillium wilt (V), fusarium wilt (F), or root knot nematodes (N). Genetic resistance has also been achieved for other diseases, including tobacco mosaic virus, early blight, late blight, anthracnose, gray leaf spot, black spot, septoria blight, nailhead spot, bacterial wilt, tobacco etch, spotted wilt, curly top, and leaf mold, as well as to aphids, red spider mites, flea beetles, and white flies. No one variety is resistant to all diseases afflicting tomatoes, and most commercial growers apply a fungicide. *See* PLANT DISEASE CONTROL.

Harvesting. Tomatoes for processing are harvested when red ripe and are soon sent to a nearby cannery. Tomatoes for fresh market, however, are often harvested at an earlier stage of maturity when they are still firm and better able to tolerate shipment to distant markets. Mature green fruits will ripen normally, but more immature fruits should not be harvested since their quality will be inferior.

Ethylene, a gas that is the natural ripening hormone in tomatoes and other fruit, is sometimes applied to stimulate green fruit to ripen after harvest. Recently, ethephon (2-chloroethylphosphonic acid), a growth regulator that liberates ethylene, has been extensively used commercially to promote ripening of tomatoes.

Most tomatoes for fresh market are harvested by hand, but almost all of the processing tomatoes in California are harvested mechanically. Mechanical harvesting is less common in other areas, but is increasing. The harvester cuts the vine off at ground level, elevates it on an inclined chain, then shakes the fruit off and discards the vine (Fig. 2). Workers on the machine remove most of the immature and defective fruit, and the rest are conveyed to a bulk container. Since only a single harvest is possible with mechanical harvesting and bruising is possible, varieties and cultural practices are used that favor (1) a maximum proportion of simultaneously ripe fruits, (2) the ability of fruits to remain in sound condition for a prolonged period after ripening, (3) tight attachment of fruits to prevent them from falling off when the plant is lifted by the machine, and (4) resilient fruits that are not easily bruised. *See* AGRICULTURE, MACHINERY IN.

Culinary and biological uses. The tomato is highly esteemed as a source of vitamin C. Tomato varieties differ in ascorbic acid content, and many tomato breeders are striving to increase the content of vitamin C. Most tomato varieties have about 20–25 mg ascorbic acid per 100 g, and one medium-sized tomato provides about half of the required daily allowance of vitamin C for adults. *See* ASCORBIC ACID.

Tomatoes are also a significant source of vitamin A. Red tomatoes have about 1000 international units (IU) of vitamin A per 100 g. Some orange-fruited varieties which have the *B* gene, such as

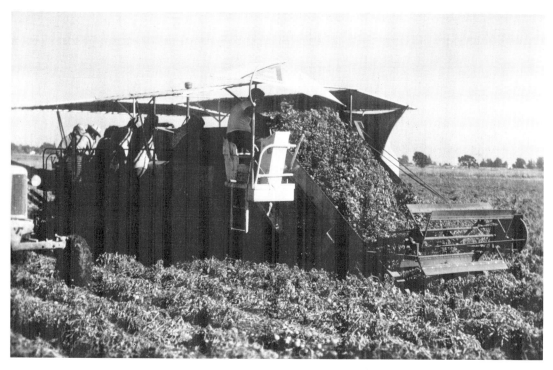

Fig. 2. Mechanical harvesting of tomatoes.

Caro Red and Caro Rich, have 10 times as much β-carotene (pro vitamin A) as red tomatoes, and a single fruit will provide more than the required daily allowance of vitamin A. See VITAMIN A.

Tomatoes are a good source of protein, but most of it is in the seeds. Tomato juice contains 19 amino acids, principally glutamic acid.

Most tomato varieties have 4.5 to 7.0% soluble solids, much of it as fructose or glucose. Citric acid is the predominant acid in tomato juice. The pH of tomatoes for processing should be below 4.5 to prevent spoilage, but the belief that modern hybrid varieties are lower in acidity than older varieties and more susceptible to botulism is unfounded. The ratio of sugar to acid is important for tomato flavor. The biochemistry and genetics of several of the aromatic organic compounds that contribute to tomato flavor have been determined.

The tomato has been a favored organism for genetic studies. Over a thousand genes are known for the tomato, and several hundred of these have been located on their respective chromosomes. Features of the tomato plant that make it very desirable for genetic and physiological studies include its high rate of natural self-pollination, the ease of controlled cross pollination, the large number of seeds per fruit and per plant, its ease of propagation by seed and cuttings and of culture in the field and the greenhouse, the relatively short time for each generation to reach maturity, the economic importance of the crop, and the wide assortment of available mutants, some of them with known effects on vitamin formation, carotenoid biosynthesis, hormones, mineral nutrition, water relations, and other physiological processes. See AGRICULTURAL SCIENCE (PLANT); FOOD MANUFACTURING; PLANT PHYSIOLOGY.

[R. W. ROBINSON]

Tryptophan

An amino acid considered essential for normal growth of animals. The amino acids are characterized physically by the following: (1) the pK_1, or the dissociation constant of the various titratable groups; (2) the isoelectric point, or pH at which a

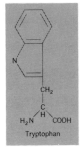

Physical constants of the L isomer at 25°C:
pK_1 (COOH): 2.38; pK_2 (NH_3^+): 9.39
Isoelectric point: 5.89
Optical rotation: $[\alpha]_D(H_2O)$: −33.7; $[\alpha]_D(1\ N\ HCl)$: +2.8
Solubility (g/100 ml H_2O): 1.14
Absorption spectrum: peak at 280 mμ (ultraviolet)

dipolar ion does not migrate in an electric field; (3) the optical rotation or the rotation imparted to a beam of plane-polarized light (frequently the D line of the sodium spectrum) passing through 1 dm of a solution of 100 g in 100 ml; (4) solubility; (5) absorption spectrum, or the wavelength at which maximum absorption occurs.

Tryptophan forms a blue-violet color when treated with glyoxylic acid in the presence of concentrated sulfuric acid (Hopkins-Cole test). Tryptophan is the precursor of the several important substances, including the plant growth hormone, indoleacetic acid; the animal hormone, serotonin (5-hydroxytryptamine); the vitamin, nicotinic acid; and certain eye pigments of insects.

The biosynthesis of tryptophan begins with phosphoenolpyruvic acid and D-erythrose-4-phosphate, and proceeds by way of shikimic acid, anthranilic acid, and indoleglycerol phosphate. See AMINO ACIDS.

During metabolic degradation, several pathways exist, including the following:

1. Peroxidation of the heterocyclic ring to formylkynurenine, which is deformylated to kynurenine. Kynurenine then is metabolized further by any of three alternative routes: (a) deamination to the α-keto acid, which spontaneously cyclizes to kynurenic acid; (b) cleavage to alanine and anthranilic acid; anthranilic acid is oxidized, in certain bacteria, to succinate and acetyl coenzyme A; (c) oxidation to 3-hydroxykynurenine, which is converted to nicotinic acid via 3-hydroxyanthranilic acid (see illustration).

A major pathway for the metabolic degradation of the amino acid tryptophan.

2. Cleavage of the side chain by the enzyme tryptophanase, forming indole, pyruvic acid, and ammonia.

3. Decarboxylation to tryptamine, and oxidation of the latter to indoleacetic acid.

4. Oxidation to 5-hydroxytryptophan, followed by formation of 5-hydroxytryptamine and 5-hydroxyindoleacetic acid.   [EDWARD A. ADELBERG]

Turmeric

A dye or a spice obtained from the plant *Curcuma longa*, which belongs to the ginger family (Zingiberaceae). It is a stout perennial with short stem, tufted leaves, and short, thick rhizomes which contain the colorful condiment (see illustration). As a natural dye, turmeric is orange-red or

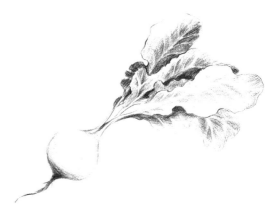

A turnip, member of the Brassicaceae family.

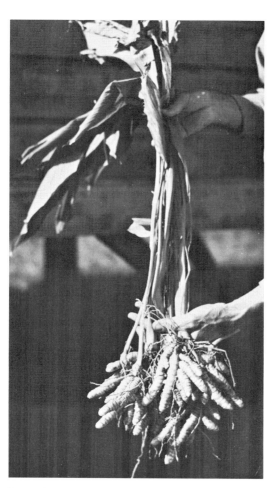

Turmeric plants (*Curcuma longa*) cultivated in Tela, Honduras. (*Photograph by W. H. Hodge, USDA*)

reddish brown, but it changes color in the presence of acids or bases. As a spice, turmeric has a decidedly musky odor and a pungent, bitter taste. It is an important item in curry and is used to flavor and color butter, cheese, pickles, and other food. *See* SPICE AND FLAVORING.

[PERRY D. STRAUSBAUGH/EARL L. CORE]

Turnip

The plant *Brassica rapa*, or *B. campestris* var. *rapa*, a cool-season, hardy crucifer of Asiatic origin belonging to the order Capparales which is grown for its enlarged root and its foliage, which are eaten cooked as a vegetable (see illustration). The plant is an annual when planted early, a biennial if seeded late in the summer. Propagation is by seed. Popular white-fleshed varieties (cultivars) grown for their roots are Purple Top Globe and White Milan; Yellow Globe and Golden Ball are common yellow-fleshed varieties. Shogoin is a popular variety grown principally in the southern United States for turnip greens. Turnip harvesting begins when the roots are 2–3 in. in diameter, usually 40–70 days after planting. Principal areas of production in the United States are in the South. *See* RUTABAGA; SEED (BOTANY); VEGETABLE GROWING.   [H. JOHN CAREW]

Disease of turnip and rutabaga. Turnip and rutabaga (a hybrid form probably derived from crossing turnip with cabbage) are affected by many of the same diseases that attack cauliflower and cabbage. Blackleg and black rot are two of the most important. The former infects the roots but causes little damage until the roots are harvested and stored; then a destructive dry rot ensues. Similarly, black rot invades the xylem vessels in the roots and is followed by bacterial soft rot in storage. Rotation, clean seed, and hot-water seed treatment will control these diseases.

Even light infections of clubroot, another disease, are objectionable in turnip and rutabaga because the roots are the parts used for food. After much work, resistant varieties of these crops have been produced in Denmark, Sweden, and Great Britain. Boron deficiency is frequently important in turnip and rutabaga, causing internal breakdown of the root tissues. *See* AGRICULTURAL SCIENCE (PLANT); CABBAGE; CAULIFLOWER; PLANT DISEASE.   [CARL J. EIDE]

Tyrosine

An amino acid. The amino acids are characterized physically by the following: (1) the pK_1, or the dissociation constant of the various titratable groups; (2) the isoelectric point, or pH at which a dipolar ion does not migrate in an electric field; (3) the optical rotation, or the rotation imparted to a beam of plane-polarized light (frequently the D line of the sodium spectrum) passing through 1 dm of a solution of 100 g in 100 ml; and (4) solubility; (5) absorption spectrum, or the wavelength at which maximum absorption occurs.

Tyrosine is a precursor of the hormones epinephrine (adrenalin), norepinephrine (noradrenalin), thyroxin, and triiodothyronine, and of the

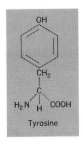

Physical constants of the L isomer at 25°C:
pK$_1$ (COOH): 2.20; pK$_2$ (NH$_3^+$): 9.11
Isoelectric point: 5.66
Optical rotation: [α]$_D$(5 N HCl): −10.0
Solubility (g/100 ml H$_2$O): 0.05
Absorption spectrum: peak at 275 mμ (ultraviolet)

Tyrosine

black pigment melanin. The amino acid is formed from phosphoenolpyruvic acid and D-erythrose-4-phosphate, by way of shikimic acid and prephenic acid. In animals, tyrosine is formed by the oxidation of dietary phenylalanine. The major pathway for metabolic degradation leads to fumaric and acetoacetic acids, as shown below.

Tyrosine → p-Hydroxyphenyl pyruvic acid → Homogentisic acid →

Maleylacetoacetic acid

Fumarylacetoacetic acid

Fumaric acid   Acetoacetic acid

See AMINO ACIDS; PHENYLALANINE.

[EDWARD A. ADELBERG]

Valine

An amino acid considered essential for normal growth of animals. The amino acids are characterized physically by the following: (1) the pK$_1$, or the dissociation constant of the various titratable groups; (2) the isoelectric point, or pH at which

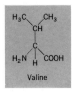

Physical constants of the L isomer at 25°C:
pK$_1$ (COOH): 2.32; pK$_2$ (NH$_3^+$): 9.62
Isoelectric point: 5.96
Optical rotation: [α]$_D$(H$_2$O): +5.6; [α]$_D$(5 N HCl): +28.3
Solubility (g/100 ml H$_2$O): 8.85

Valine

a dipolar ion does not migrate in an electric field; (3) the optical rotation, or the rotation imparted to a beam of plane-polarized light (frequently the D line of the sodium spectrum) passing through 1 dm of a solution of 100 g in 100 ml; and (4) solubility.

The biosynthetic precursor, as well as the deamination product of valine, is α-ketoisovaleric acid. It is also a precursor of leucine and of the pantoic acid moiety of pantothenic acid.

Valine is biosynthesized from pyruvic acid. Most or all of the enzymes concerned also catalyze the analogous reactions in isoleucine biosynthesis. *See* AMINO ACIDS; ISOLEUCINE.

During metabolic degradation the first steps are the deamination and oxidative decarboxylation to form isobutyrylcoenzyme A (isobutyryl-CoA). The final steps in metabolic degradation are the conversion of isobutyryl-CoA to CO$_2$ and propionyl-CoA by the formation of the following compounds: methacrylyl-CoA, β-hydroxyisobutyryl-CoA, and methylmalonic acid semialdehyde.

[EDWARD A. ADELBERG]

Vanilla

A choice flavoring obtained from a climbing orchid, *Vanilla fragrans*, a native of tropical American forests. Its fruits are pods called vanilla beans (see illustration). These are picked at the proper

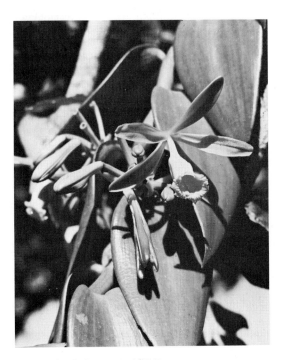

Vanilla (*Vanilla fragrans*). (USDA)

time before they have fully matured and then subjected to a prolonged and critical curing process. During the curing, enzymatic action converts a glucoside into vanillin which has the characteristic odor and flavor. Vanilla is used in cookery, confectionery, and beverages. Vanilla extract, most used, is prepared by extracting the crushed beans with alcohol. A synthetic vanillin is made from eugenol occurring in clove oil, but the natural product is preferred. Several plants have been used as substitutes for true vanilla but these are of little value. *See* SPICE AND FLAVORING.

[PERRY D. STRAUSBAUGH/EARL L. CORE]

Vanilla extract

Flavoring prepared from vanilla beans with or without one or more of the following added: sugar, dextrose, glycerol. Vanilla extract contains the soluble matters from not less than 10 g of vanilla beans in 100 ml. To be legally called vanilla extract, 1 U.S. gal of vanilla extract must contain the soluble matter from not less than 13.35 oz of vanilla beans. The finished flavoring should contain at least 35% alcohol by volume to keep the solubles in solution. *See* VANILLA.

The vanilla plant belongs to the orchid family and is indigenous to southeastern Mexico, where it was used by the Aztecs to flavor their cocoa. In 1510 *vagnuila* first appeared in Spain. The principal types of commercially used vanilla beans are the Mexican, Bourbon (Bourbon comes mainly from Madagascar, but was named after the Island of Reunion in the Indian Ocean, formerly known as the island of Bourbon, where the French started the cultivation of vanilla), South American, Javan, and Tahitian.

Vanillin (4-hydroxy-3-methoxybenzaldehyde) is the principal component of vanilla, although other components contribute to the distinctive flavor of the extract compared to synthetic vanilla. When they are harvested, the beans contain no free vanillin; it develops during the curing period from glucosides that break down during the fermentation and sweating of the beans. The sweating process consists of alternately drying the beans in sunlight and bunching them so that they heat and ferment. Sweating boxes are used in Mexico, whereas the shorter Madagascar method starts out by wilting green pods in hot water and uses blankets on which the beans can first be spread out and later rolled up for the enzymatic reactions and fermentation to take place. Further curing and dehydration occur in a warehouse. Periods of 4 weeks to 4 months may be required to develop the proper flavor and reduce the moisture content of the beans sufficiently to prevent molding. Beans can be artificially dried in ovens, but frequently an inferior-quality product results. *See* FERMENTATION; FOOD ENGINEERING.

After curing, the pods are sorted into grades based on quality. The best cured beans are 8–10 in. long, with drawn-out ends and curved bases. They are soapy or waxy to the touch, dark brown, and coated with fine crystals of vanillin, termed frost. Vanillin constitutes 1.2–3.5% of the bean, but other compounds contribute also to the aroma. In addition to the flavoring materials, vanilla beans contain fat, wax, sugar, gum, resin, and tannin.

In the alcoholic extraction of the vanilla flavor, the color of the extract is influenced by the quality of the beans, the strength of the alcoholic menstruum, the duration of the extraction, and the presence of glycerin, which is added to retard evaporation and to retain the flavor in the extract. Best results are obtained with three consecutive extractions at room temperature, each requiring a minimum of 5 days. The first should have a maximum alcohol content of 65%; the second, 35%; the third, 15%. To improve aroma, extracts are aged, using stainless steel or glass containers.

A standard vanilla extract is equivalent in flavoring strength, though not in quality, to a 0.7%

vanillin solution; thus 1 lb of vanilla beans has a flavoring strength equivalent to about 1.12 oz of vanillin. The vanillin content of pure extracts range from 0.11 to 0.35 g/100 ml, with the average at about 0.19 g/100 ml. Ash content, soluble ash, lead number, alkalinity of total ash, alkalinity of soluble ash, total acidity, and acidity other than vanillin are among the conventional indices used to detect adulteration.

The approximate average maximum levels of usage (in ppm) for vanilla extract in foods are:

Beverages	200	Baked goods	1900
Ice cream, ices	3000	Syrups	54
Candies	4000	Icings	4800
Toppings	2700		

[GIDEON E. LIVINGSTON; MYRON SOLBERG]
Bibliography: L. W. Jones (ed.), *A Treasury of Spices*, 1956; J. Merory, *Food Flavorings*, 2d ed., 1968.

Vegetable growing

A branch of horticulture relating to the production of a number of herbaceous plants or plant parts, commonly referred to as vegetables. No concise definition of the term is possible; for example, such so-called vegetables as tomatoes, corn, and beans are technically fruits. The term olericulture, referring to vegetable production, is used occasionally. *See* FRUIT (BOTANY).

Vegetables are excellent sources of minerals and vitamins. Wider recognition of this fact has resulted in greater per capita consumption of carrots, lettuce, sweet corn, and many other highly palatable crops. More than 40 vegetables are grown by commercial farmers and home gardeners for fresh consumption and for processing. *See* FOOD ENGINEERING; VITAMIN.

Home gardening. A large assortment of vegetables can be raised in all parts of the United States if adapted varieties (cultivars) are selected and plantings are made to coincide with favorable climatic periods. A home garden can reduce family food costs, provide vegetables of higher quality than those available in many stores, and serve as recreation.

Commercial practices. The vegetable industry has undergone dynamic changes since World War II. As a result of vastly improved production, handling, and transportation techniques, a wide variety of fresh and processed vegetables from distant areas is available in all parts of the United States throughout the year.

In the past, the term market gardening referred to the production of vegetables for local markets; truck farming described the production of crops in large volume for shipment to distant markets. Small acreages, low transportation costs, and a diversity of crops characterized the market garden operation, whereas low labor and land costs were typical of the distant shipping regions. These distinctions are no longer valid.

Rapid growth of chain stores and food-processing companies and changes in consumer buying habits have resulted in a concentration of purchasing power in the hands of comparatively few produce buyers. Emphasis on a steady supply and large volume of uniform-quality vegetables has favored the long-season areas having favorable climate and large acreages that usually are great distances from the centers of dense population. Individual vegetable farms are generally large and heavily mechanized.

The availability of selective chemical weed killers and the development of vastly improved equipment for planting, spraying, mechanical harvesting, and grading have made possible the farming of large acreages in areas where a supply of labor had been limited. California, Florida, Texas, and Arizona account for 60% of the total fresh vegetable production in the United States despite the higher transportation costs involved. Smaller vegetable farms near cities are declining in importance but still compete by selling at roadside stands, on farmers' markets, or through group-marketing organizations. *See* AGRICULTURE, MACHINERY IN.

Consumption of canned and frozen vegetables is increasing. The West Coast, Wisconsin, and Minnesota lead in production. In many areas crops for processing are grown by farmers who produce for the fresh market also; in other areas, processing vegetables are raised by grain or livestock farmers in addition to their other products. Dehydrated onions and potatoes are becoming more popular, although dehydration is currently not an important means of preserving vegetables.

Smaller acreages of a few crops are "forced" in special structures at times other than their normal season of growth; for example, tomatoes and cucumbers are produced in greenhouses during the winter in Ohio, Michigan, and other northern states.

Additional commercial vegetable-growing activities include production of vegetable seeds and of young tomato, cabbage, and similar plants for sale to other growers. The plant-growing industry is well developed in Georgia and Texas, while seed production is confined mainly to Idaho, Washington, Oregon, and California.

See separate articles on vegetables listed under their common names.

[H. JOHN CAREW]

Bibliography: *See* AGRICULTURAL SCIENCE (PLANT).

Vetch

Any of a group of plants which are mostly annual legumes with weak viny stems terminating in tendrils. The leaves are compound with many leaflets. Vetches are used mainly for green manure, cover crops, hay, and pasture. Cool temperatures promote best development. Seed is sown in the fall in the South and in early spring in the Northern states. Inoculation of seed with nodule-forming bacteria for symbiotic nitrogen fixation is necessary unless vetch previously has been grown in the field. *See* LEAF (BOTANY); SOIL MICROBIOLOGY.

Hairy vetch (*Vicia villosa*) is winter hardy and is most widely grown. Smooth vetch (*V. villosa* var. *glabrescens*) and woollypod vetch (*V. dasycarpa*) are similar to hairy vetch; seeds of the three may be found in mixtures. Bird vetch (*V. cracca*) is a winter-hardy perennial. Identification of vetches is difficult until pods and seeds develop. Common vetch (*V. sativa*) and purple vetch (*V. bengalensis*) are less winter-hardy than hairy vetch.

Hungarian vetch (*V. pannonica*) is confined to the Pacific Northwest. Monantha vetch (*V. articulata*) has fine leaves and stems but, lacking winter hardiness, is confined to warm regions. Bitter vetch (*V. ervilla*) is not grown commercially. Narrow-leaf vetch (*V. angustifolia*) occurs mostly as a weed in waste places in the United States. It spreads by volunteering and makes excellent pastures. Bard vetch (*V. monantha*) is of minor importance and is grown only in irrigated valleys of the southwestern United States. Horsebeans (*V. faba*), which produce coarse, upright plants with large leaves and pods, are only one of several of the vetches that are important sources of food for human beings. Some varieties are grown as vegetables. *See* VEGETABLE GROWING.

Vetch seed is produced commercially along the Pacific Coast and in the southern Great Plains. Much hairy vetch seed is imported from Europe. Vetch is grown alone and with small grains which give mechanical support to the weak stems of the vetch. Seed retains vitality for 5 years or longer. *See* SEED (BOTANY).

Diseases and insect pests. Diseases of vetch include anthracnose, gray mold, downy mildew, black stem, stem rot, root rot, rust, ovularia leaf and stem spot, and septoria scald. Root-knot nematodes attack all varieties. Control is aided by using uninfected seed of resistant varieties on clean land. *See* PLANT DISEASE.

Insect pests include aphids, corn earworm, grasshoppers, cutworms, fall armyworm, weevils, and leafhoppers. Aphids are the most troublesome and destructive.

Crown vetch. This plant, *Coronilla varia*, is a long-lived, winter-hardy perennial legume, but it is not a true vetch. It spreads by seeds and rhizomes to form a dense, weed-free, erosion-resisting ground cover. Its greatest use is for erosion and weed control on unmowed slopes of highways, industrial developments, and military installations. Its forage value is being studied. Crownvetch has wide adaptation to variations in climate and soils. It is highly regarded for its resistance to fire. Rose, pink, and white blossoms enhance its attractive-

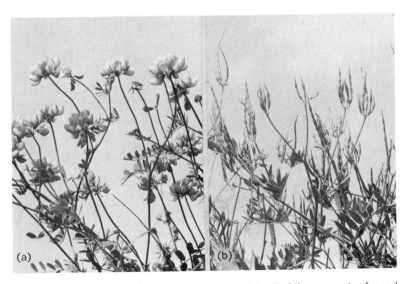

Crown vetch. (*a*) The plant in flower and (*b*) in seed. Each of the segments of a pod contains a seed.

ness throughout most of the growing season (see illustration). It thrives best on well-limed and well-drained soils, requires no mowing, and rarely needs fertilization. Plantings are made with crowns (roots) or with seed that require special bacterial inoculation.

Crown vetch is slow to germinate and become established. Diseases and insects are of minor importance. Neither spittlebug nor weevil attacks crownvetch. Grazing animals do not bloat on it. Seed originally was produced only in Pennsylvania, starting in 1946; now it is grown in several states, including Ohio, New York, Nebraska, Iowa, and West Virginia. The first variety named and released was Penngift; later the Emerald (Iowa) and the Chemung (New York) varieties were named and released. *See* COVER CROPS; SOIL CONSERVATION.

[FRED V. GRAU]

Bibliography: See AGRICULTURAL SCIENCE (PLANT); PLANT DISEASE.

Vinegar

The product of the incomplete oxidation to acetic acid of ethyl alcohol produced by a primary fermentation of vegetable materials. The oxidation, often called secondary fermentation, proceeds under the influence of various kinds of so-called vinegar bacteria, species of the genera *Acetobacter* and *Acetomonas*.

The overall chemical equations for the production of vinegar are given below:

$$Sugar \xrightarrow{Yeast} 2CH_3CH_2OH + 2CO_2$$

$$2CH_3CH_2OH + 2O_2 \xrightarrow[\text{Bacteria}]{\text{Vinegar}} 2CH_3COOH + 2H_2O$$

Vinegar contains not less than 4 g of acetic acid (CH_3COOH) per 100 ml. The production of vinegar in the United States exceeds 100,000,000 gal annu-

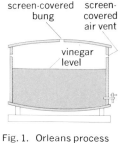

Fig. 1. Orleans process barrel for making the wine vinegar. (*From L. A. Underkofler and R. J. Hickey, eds., Industrial Fermentations, 2 vols., Chemical Publishing, 1954*)

ally. It is used in the preparation of pickled fruits and vegetables or other large-scale food manufacture such as salad dressings, and as a seasoning agent for table use.

Types. Vinegars are classified as to raw materials used in their manufacture: there are products designated as wine, cider, malt, and sugar vinegar. Wine vinegar is the product obtained from the acetous souring of grape wine. Cider vinegar is derived from the alcoholic fermentation of other fruit juices, usually apple juice, followed by acetous fermentation. Malt vinegar is obtained by the alcoholic fermentation of starchy materials, such as cereal grains or potatoes saccharified, or converted to sugar, by the enzymes of malt, followed by acetous fermentation. Distilled vinegars usually belong to the malt vinegar class. Sugar vinegar is obtained by the alcoholic fermentation of sugars such as syrups of glucose, blackstrap molasses, or refiners' molasses. In the preparation of distilled vinegar, the alcohol is distilled off the fermented vegetable mashes before it is fermented by the vinegar bacteria. Nondistilled vinegars are characterized by distinctive flavors and odor. Seasoned vinegars are prepared by soaking vegetable seasoning agents, such as tarragon leaves, onions, garlic, peppers, or various spices, in vinegar.

Processes. Vinegar is made by the older French or Orleans process, the quick vinegar process, and the continuous process.

Orleans process. In the Orleans process, wine or hard cider is fermented in wooden barrels or small covered vats (Fig. 1). Air vents, with screens to exclude vinegar flies, are located in the top and upper walls of the vessel. A starter culture of about equal volumes of good, nonpasteurized vinegar and fresh wine is introduced into the barrel, and the fermentation is continued until acetification is complete. About three-fourths of the vinegar is then drawn off and replaced with fresh wine. The

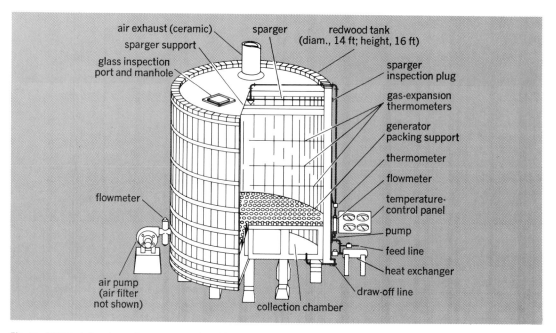

Fig. 2. Recirculating-type vinegar generator. Above the collection chamber is the large chamber for percolation.

(*From L. A. Underkofler and R. J. Hickey, eds., Industrial Fermentations, 2 vols., Chemical Publishing, 1954*)

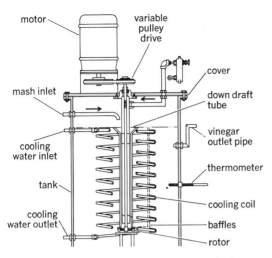

Fig. 3. Continuous process generator. *(From R. F. Cohee and G. Steffen, Food Eng., 31(3):58–59, 1959)*

process is repeated for as many times as a good quality vinegar can be withdrawn. Failure to produce a good vinegar is usually due to the gradual replacement of the desirable types of vinegar bacteria by other microorganisms, including some species of vinegar bacteria themselves, which oxidize acetic acid to carbon dioxide and water. The Orleans process is slow and can be operated only in small vessels. The vinegar so produced is of superior flavor and aroma, due to the fact that the conditions under which the conversion of alcohol to acetic acid proceeds permit the accumulation of larger quantities of products of side reactions leading to such materials as ethyl acetate and acetoin. Such vinegars are usually reserved for table use. The Orleans process may be applied on a household scale.

Quick vinegar process. Nearly all the vinegar of commerce is now made by the quick vinegar process. Here the fermentation is conducted in a recirculatory-type vinegar generator, a vessel composed of two chambers (Fig. 2). The larger upper chamber is packed to within about 8 in. of the top with solid materials having a very large surface area. Beechwood shavings are preferred for distilled vinegar production and corncobs or coke for the production of wine, cider, or sugar vinegar. The packed upper chamber is separated from the lower chamber by a screen. Air is blown upward through the screen and packing material, and escapes from the top of the generator. Fermenting liquids are distributed intermittently over the top of the packing, allowed to percolate through the mass, collected in the lower chamber, then pumped back to the top and recirculated until the alcohol content is reduced to 1/2%. The vinegar is drawn off, and fresh alcoholic solution is added. This process is repeated until bacterial slimes or contamination results in reduced yield of acetic acid or poor percolation. If cider, sugar, or wine vinegar is being made, a vinegar generator is cleaned and restarted twice a year, but a distilled vinegar generator may operate satisfactorily for several years without loss of efficiency.

On the completion of fermentation of a batch of vinegar for table use, it is aged in well-filled, air-tight wooden barrels or tanks for several weeks, then filtered, bottled, and pasteurized. Vinegars for pickling or other large-scale food manufacture may be filtered and pasteurized immediately after the fermentation is completed.

Continuous process. The use of an air-incorporation principle, known as a cavitator, in the generator has made possible continuous production of vinegar with 98% efficiency. The beechwood shavings are eliminated, and the mash is aerated by a rotor and by air which is drawn down through the hollow shaft when rotor speed exceeds a predetermined value (Fig. 3). The intimate air-mash mixture, produced by the rotor's nozzles, spreads out toward the tank's walls before rising. When it reaches the surface of the generator, the mash is recycled by going down through the draft tube to combine with air. Vinegar generation produces an increase in temperature which is controlled by cooling coils. When the rate of conversion of alcohol to acetic acid has been stabilized and the fermentation is nearly finished, additional dilute alcohol is pumped continuously into the fermentor at exactly the rate at which alcohol is oxidized to acetic acid, thus maintaining the alcohol supply. The liquid level is kept constant by withdrawal of vinegar from the fermentor. See INDUSTRIAL MICROBIOLOGY.

[LEWIS B. LOCKWOOD]

Bibliography: R. F. Cohee and G. Steffen, *Food Engineering,* 31(3):58–59, 1959; C. L. Duddington, *Microorganisms as Allies: The Industrial Use of Fungi and Bacteria,* 1961; H. J. Peppler, *Microbial Technology,* 1967; S. C. Prescott and C. G. Dunn, *Industrial Microbiology,* 3d ed., 1959; L. A. Underkofler and R. J. Hickey (eds.), *Industrial Fermentations,* vol. 1, 1954.

Vitamin

An organic compound essential for the normal functioning of the body, and usually obtained from foods. Vitamins are present in food in minute quantities compared to the other utilizable components of the diet—proteins, fats, carbohydrates, and minerals. The average adult eats about 600 g of food per day on a dry-weight basis, of which less than a gram are vitamins.

Almost all knowledge of the vitamins has been obtained during the 20th century. The discovery of the vitamins has primarily been the result of two lines of investigation: the study of nutritional disease in people and the feeding of purified diets of known composition to experimental animals. In this way vitamin deficiency diseases, known as avitaminoses, have been described. The production of specific avitaminoses has usually been followed by the chemical synthesis of the protective vitamin after its isolation and characterization from natural food materials.

Synthetic and natural vitamins usually have the same biological value. The use of vitamins has been subject to many false claims by quacks and food faddists. The vitamins are often not related chemically or functionally. They are conventionally divided into a fat-soluble group consisting of vitamins A, D, E, and K, and a water-soluble group

Vitamin sources and deficiencies

Vitamin*	Best sources	Deficiency	Areas primarily affected
Fat-soluble			
α-, β-carotene	Fish-liver oils, green plants, carrots	Xerophthalmia, nyctalopia	Eyes, skin, mouth, respiratory and urogenital tracts
D	Fish oils	Rickets, osteomalacia	Bones, teeth
E	Grains and vegetable oils		Reproductive tract, muscles, red blood cells, liver, brain
K	Green vegetables		Blood prothrombin
Water-soluble			
Thiamine	Pork, liver, whole grains	Beriberi	Brain, nerves, heart
Riboflavin	Milk, egg white, liver, leafy vegetables		Skin, mouth, eyes, liver, nerves
Niacin	Yeast, wheat germ, meats	Pellagra	Gastrointestinal tract, skin, brain
Pantothenic acid	Liver, kidneys, green vegetables, egg yolk		Adrenals, kidneys, skin, brain, spinal cord
B_6	Whole grains, yeast, egg yolk, liver		Skin, red blood cells, brain, kidneys, adrenals
Inositol	Whole grains, liver		
Biotin	Liver, kidney, yeast		Skin, muscles
Choline	Egg yolk, brain, grains		Liver, kidneys, pancreas
p-Aminobenzoic acid	Yeast		
Folic acid	Liver, deep green leafy vegetables	Various macrocytic anemias	Red blood cells
B_{12}	Liver, meats	Pernicious anemia	Red blood cells
Ascorbic acid	Citrus fruits, fresh vegetables, potatoes	Scurvy	Bones, joints, mouth, capillaries

*See individual articles on each vitamin, except α-,β-carotene. The lettered vitamins will be found as separate articles under Vitamin.

consisting of the various B vitamins, including thiamine, riboflavin, nicotinic acid, B_6, pantothenic acid, biotin, folic acid, B_{12}, *p*-aminobenzoic acid, inositol, and choline, as well as vitamin C, or ascorbic acid.

The vitamins, particularly the water-soluble ones, are found spread almost universally throughout the animal and plant kingdoms (see table), functioning in essentially the same type of biochemical systems in the lowest and highest forms of life. Variations in the dietary requirements of different animal species for vitamins are usually related to the varying abilities of the animal's tissues or gastrointestinal flora to synthesize them.

Vitamins exhibit varied site preferences for uptake in the small intestine; for example, ascorbic acid is absorbed in the duodenum and vitamin B_{12} in the ileum. It is therefore likely that there cannot be a common mechanism for the absorption of all vitamins. Vitamin absorption may be hampered by certain events within the intestinal tract. For example, uptake of the fat-soluble vitamins is generally impaired by disease of the biliary tract, due in part to the lack of adequate emulsification which results from lack of bile salts. Thiaminases in some foods may destroy thiamin within the intestinal lumen. Biotin may be rendered unabsorbable in the presence of avidin, a protein which binds biotin.

The gut is also a region of vitamin excretion, and this activity may increase following x-radiation of the intestine. Some of the vitamins are absorbed into the gut, pass to the liver, and pass out into the bile. This enterohepatic cycling can also be deranged in diseases of the gut or liver.

The vitamins function as coenzymes, active parts of enzyme systems, which catalyze many of the various anabolic and catabolic reactions of living organisms necessary for the production of energy, the synthesis of tissue components, hormones, and chemical regulators, and the detoxification and degradation of waste products and toxins. Because of their role in metabolism, the vitamins are generally concentrated in those animal and plant tissues which are most active metabolically. For this reason, liver or kidneys are a more potent source of vitamins than muscle or skin, and the germ of a seed contains more vitamins than its other components. *See* NUTRITION.

[STANLEY N. GERSHOFF]

Hypervitaminosis. The Food and Nutrition Board of the National Academy of Sciences publishes tables of recommended dietary allowances, that is, the levels of intake of essential nutrients considered in its judgment, on the basis of available scientific knowledge, to be adequate to meet the nutritional needs of practically all healthy persons. The recommended daily allowances (RDA) do not cover the therapeutic nutritional needs of individuals who may have illnesses such as infections, metabolic disorders, chronic diseases, or other abnormalities that may require special nutritional management, such as total parenteral nutrition. Special nutritional needs may also relate to certain genetic difficulties, such as vitamin B_6 and vitamin B_{12} enzyme problems, and to the use of certain drug preparations, such as oral contraceptives.

Some people choose to take large doses of vitamins—especially believers in the megavitamin concept—in the expectation that the excess will be beneficial to health. However, it must be cautioned that this practice is controversial, and can even have toxic effects. Fortunately, the excessive ingestion of the water-soluble vitamins, including the B complex vitamins and vitamin C, offers little proved hazard. These substances are rapidly excreted by the kidney when their renal threshold is exceeded in the blood. Also, there is little evidence that they are accumulated in any tissue or storage site and hence have little opportunity to exert a specific toxic effect at the tissue or cellular level. Whether or not the excessive use of the B complex vitamins exerts an adverse effect at the cellular or metabolic level has not yet been clearly demonstrated. However, the toxic potential of fat-soluble vitamins A and D are very significant and the hazard very real.

Vitamin A. The RDA for vitamin A for the adult male is 5000 international units (IU). This is about 25% higher than the recommended allowance level of other Western countries and of the Food and Agriculture Organization and World Health Organization. The RDA for the adult female is somewhat less, but during pregnancy is increased to 5000 units; and an even somewhat larger allowance is recommended during lactation to provide for the vitamin A secreted in milk.

The Food and Nutrition Board cautions that the regular ingestion of more than 6700 IU of preformed vitamin A above that already in the diet should be carefully monitored by a physician. Interestingly, the toxic manifestations of vitamin A are somewhat like those of deficiency. Loss of appetitie, lethargy, and apathy are common, and hair loss and bone fragility may be noted in severely toxic situations. The documentation of the exact level of vitamin A that does produce consistent toxic symptoms is vague. Vitamin A in doses of 50,000 IU per day may often be prescribed by dermatologists in the treatment of certain skin conditions, and apparently this does not produce significant toxicity, at least over reasonable periods of time. However, this is a highly individual matter and should be under the supervision of a physician. *See* VITAMIN A.

Vitamin D. The importance of vitamin D in human nutrition is based on its function as a regulator of the metabolism of calcium and phosphorus. It promotes the intestinal absorption of calcium and may directly influence bone mineralization. When it is inadequate or lacking, mineralization of bone matrix suffers and collagen synthesis is defective, resulting in rickets in children and osteomalacia in adults. *See* RICKETS.

Since vitamin D can readily be formed by the action of sunlight on the skin, the minimum requirement of vitamin D is difficult to establish and is dependent on a number of variables, including length and intensity of exposure to the sun and skin color. Heavily pigmented skin significantly reduces the penetration of ultraviolet radiation and minimizes the synthesis of vitamin D. Normally, the adult requirement of vitamin D is adequately met by exposure to sunlight. An intake of about 400 IU of vitamin D per day is recommended for pregnant and lactating women, infants, children, and adolescents. No specific dietary recommendation for vitamin D is given for the normal healthy adult.

The excessive ingestion of vitamin D is highly toxic, and the margin of toxicity seems to be relatively small. The initial signs and symptoms in young children and infants are poor appetite, lassitude, lethargy, and increased irritability. The prolonged use of vitamin D at levels of 2000 IU or more per day has produced hypercalcemia in infants and small children and calcification of the kidney in infants and adults. There is no evidence of distinct benefit from large doses of vitamin D.

Megavitamin concept. Stimulated by the reports of Linus Pauling that vitamin C in very large doses may exert a preventive effect against colds, many people have become very enthusiastic about ingesting large doses of vitamins. The megavitamin concept is based on the philosophy of orthomolecular medicine, proposed by Pauling, which suggests potential benefit by consuming a nutrient commonly present in the body at large levels so that there is a beneficial effect on enzymatic activity at the cellular level. The concept of utilizing huge doses of vitamin C is reminiscent of the earlier recommendations for the use of vitamin E to minimize atherosclerotic impact and risk of myocardial infarction.

It should be emphasized that there is no evidence in the scientific literature that one may achieve "supernutrition." Very large doses of any of the water-soluble vitamins have a finite upper limit that may be maintained in the blood, largely because the excess is excreted by the kidney. Proponents of the orthomolecular concept and megavitamin treatment of such diseases as cancer and schizophrenia have had enthusiastic support. However, it should be emphasized that any possible benefits derived from huge doses of vitamins do not appear to be related to the traditional nutritional effect, but appear to be of a pharmacological nature, the mechanism of which remains unclear.

With regard to the common cold, it would appear that there are doubts concerning the preventive effect of large doses of vitamin C, but seemingly vitamin C does reduce the seriousness of the symptomatology and permits individuals to return to their normal activities more quickly. Megavitamin doses of vitamin E have been demonstrated to produce benefits for individuals suffering from intermittent claudication (severe lower leg cramps). The beneficial claims for vitamin E in relation to angina and myocardial infarction remain controversial The beneficial effects of niacin (nicotinic acid), vitamin B_6, and other vitamins in the treatment of schizophrenia remain uncertain.

Apparently there is a place for megavitamin nutritional therapy, although it certainly must be developed under a much more controlled and carefully supervised program than currently exists.

Hypovitaminosis. Vitamin-deficiency disease underlines the importance of nutritional factors in human well-being. Clinical manifestations of diseases such as scurvy, rickets, beriberi, and pellagra are based on fundamental abnormalities at the cellular level, involving specific enzymes and coenzymes through which the vitamins function. Modern developments in biochemistry point to the important role of many of the B complex vitamins, particularly in metabolic reactions at the cellular level. The results of nutritional surveys in many sectors of the United States reveal significant shortcomings in the nutritional status of the American people, suggesting that the availability of an adequate food supply containing the necessary vitamins does not, in fact, guarantee good nutritional status. There is also an increasing realization that a considerable variability exists among individuals regarding nutrient needs. Today, in modern society, the overt deficiency diseases are rarely seen, and great difficulty rests in identifying "latent nutritional deficiency."

Latent nutritional deficiency. Vitamin malnutrition cannot be separated from the overall problem of malnutrition. There can be a graded spectrum of nutritional deficit, which may be initiated by occasional aberrant nutritional patterns of food intake, for varying periods of time, with probably little evidence of biochemical alteration. The recent nutrition survey in the United States indicates an alarming prevalence of the characteristics associated with undernourished groups. There is substantial evidence of unacceptable levels of nutrients that have traditionally been associated with latent nutritional deficiencies. These deficiencies are most commonly noted in the highly physiologically sensitive groups, such as young children, rapidly growing adolescents, females during pregnancy and lactation, and older individuals. The nutrients of greatest concern with respect to finding unacceptable levels are iron, vitamin A, folic acid, and vitamin C.

Relation to other factors. Primary nutritional deficiency disease due solely to inadequate intake is rare, but it does occur if faulty dietary habits persist over a long period of time. Marginal nutritional deficits are usually not evident at the clinical level, but may occur in relation to such factors as inadequate nutrient intake, poor absorption, decreased utilization, increased excretion, increased destruction, and increased nutritional requirements based on individual variability.

Biochemical changes. Metabolic limitations and the rapid excretion of vitamins, particularly the B complex, make nutritional replenishment of the tissues a daily task. No cell in the body is immune to inanition or improper vitamin supply, and none can long survive the rigors of nutritional deprivation without losing some viability.

Unfortunately, as the tissue depletion of vitamins proceeds, biochemical lesions may be increasingly manifested by a reduction in enzyme activity at the cellular level and altered metabolite levels. These biochemical changes in blood do not develop in clear-cut stages, but by gradations, in which the time factor is most important. Nutritional deficiency seldom is an easily discernible problem until, after a long enough period of time, the classical anatomical lesions of scurvy, pellagra, beri-beri, rickets, and so on, become evident. At this stage of nutrient deficiency the complete responses to full vitamin therapy are often slow.

It is important, therefore, to diagnose problems of malnutrition before these overt diseases develop.

Difficulty in diagnosis. One reason that nutritional problems are so difficult to identify is the conglomerate of nonspecific complaints that coincide in time with the latent phase of nutritional deficiency. The most common complants associated with hypovitaminosis are anorexia, abdominal discomfort, anxiety, backache, confusion, decreased work output, depression, dyspepsia, fatigue, headache, insomnia, irritability, lassitude, muscle pain, muscle weakness, nervousness, palpitation, heightened nerve sensitivities, and poor concentration. The pattern of symptoms varies significantly among patients and in the same patient at different times. This makes the identification of specific nutrient deficiency very difficult.

Vitamin-deficiency diseases. An outstanding discovery in the 1970s was the observation that vitamin B is transformed into a hormone before it functions. Vitamin D is first converted to 25-hydroxy-vitamin D in the liver and subsequently to the hormone 1,25-hydroxy-vitamin D in the kidney. This hormonal form of vitamin D is very biologically active, and its discovery has provided important therapies in bone and calcium disorders and holds great promise in the treatment of other metabolic bone problems.

A variety of genetic diseases that appear to stem from the reduced affinity of essential vitamins for B vitamin–derived enzymes have been observed, but the frequency and medical significance of many such conditions are still not clear. Genetic diseases relating to increased needs for vitamin B_6 and vitamin B_{12} are being investigated.

In the United States, alcoholism is probably the most common disease that causes clinical deficiencies of thiamine, folic acid, vitamin B_6, and vitamin B_{12}.

Interrelationships of vitamin deficiency and drug action have also been discovered. Isoniazid, used extensively as an antituberculosis drug, is also known for its effects on mental outlook and is a vitamin B_6 antagonist in humans. Depression observed in women ingesting steroid contraceptives may be related to a changed metabolism and increased need for vitamin B_6.

Effect on central nervous system function. Biochemical disorders significantly affect function of the central nervous system. This observation dates back to the early 1930s, when it was noted that the dementia characteristic of advanced pellagra could be rapidly cured by the vitamin nicotinic acid (subsequently, the dementia was noted to be affected favorably by the amino acid tryptophane, which is convertible in the body to nicotinic acid). Other B complex vitamins are known to have great significance in nerve function. Vitamin B_6, for example, is involved in the metabolism of almost all of the amino acids and therefore in the synthesis of many of the neurohormones (such as dopamine and serotonin). Since all of these compounds are intimately involved in neurofunction, the rationale for a prominent role for vitamin B_6 in brain function is evident. Similar arguments can be made in connection with many other vitamins, all of which are intimately involved in metabolic changes in the brain. Thiamine triphosphate has been reported to serve as a neurotransmitter. Possibly, a breakthrough is coming in psychopharmacology relating to the central nervous system, insofar as it is involved in psychiatric disorders.

[W. A KREHL]

Vitamin A

A pale-yellow alcohol, soluble in fat but not in water. It is readily destroyed by oxidation, which causes significant losses during storage and cooking. The structural formula is shown in the illustration.

Structural formula for vitamin A (retinol).

Source. There are three sources of vitamin A activity. Vitamin A itself is found in all animal tissues. It is particularly concentrated in the liver and viscera, and the most important natural sources of the vitamin are the fish-liver oils. The livers of some fresh-water fish contain vitamin A_2, which differs slightly from vitamin A in structure. Plants contain a number of carotenoid pigments, which can be converted to vitamin A in the tissues of animals such as in the rat intestinal wall.

Bioassay. The vitamin A activity of these carotenoids varies with their chemical structure. β-Carotene has the most activity. One international unit (IU) of vitamin A has been set at 0.3 microgram (μg) of vitamin A or 0.6 μg of β-carotene. This is confusing since the efficiency of conversion of β-carotene to vitamin A becomes greater in a deficiency state. Although biological rat assays are used, vitamin A and carotene are usually determined chemically by spectrophotometric techniques.

Physiological activities. In vitamin A deficiency the epithelial tissues of many organs are affected. Growth failure occurs, particularly in the bones and teeth. In young animals this can result in neurological symptoms resulting from pressures on the central nervous system. Changes occur in the skin, mouth, respiratory tract, urogenital tract, and some glands. The changes in epithelial tissues increase the susceptibility of the deficient organism to infection. Vitamin A does not affect the bacteria. It protects the integrity of the mucous membrane. Besides severe inflammation of the eyes, or xerophthalmia, vitamin A–deficient animals suffer from night blindness, a condition known as nyctalopia. This condition is common in many parts of the world and can be diagnosed by means of a biophotometer, which measures ability to adapt to changes in light. The role of vitamin A in sight has been related to a retinal pigment called rhodopsin, which is composed of a protein, opsin, and vitamin A. Under the stimulus of light this pigment breaks down to opsin and vitamin A aldehyde, retinene. Resynthesis of rhodopsin, which is necessary for normal vision, is poor in vitamin A deficiency.

Except for its function in the retina, the metabolic role of vitamin A is obscure. If animals are fed vitamin A acid instead of vitamin A, they grow normally but become blind and sterile. It has been suggested that vitamin A acid is converted into other compounds which may be "active" forms of vitamin A.

Chemistry. Vitamin A appears to be necessary for normal mucoprotein synthesis. It has been reported that it is necessary for the incorporation of sulfate into mucopolysaccharide. It is thought that vitamin A deficiency labilizes biological membranes, particularly those of lysosomes, mitochondria, and erythrocytes.

Requirements. Studies of many mammalian species have related the vitamin A requirement to body size. Approximately 40 IU of β-carotene or 20 IU of vitamin A per kilogram of body weight will support growth and prevent symptoms of deficiency. In estimating human requirements, it has been assumed that two-thirds of the vitamin A consumed is in the form of carotenoid pigments. There is evidence that it is of value to ingest considerably more vitamin A than the amount necessary to prevent deficiency signs. The recommended dietary allowances of the National Research Council are approximately twice the minimal requirements. These daily allowances vary from 1500 IU for infants to 5000 IU for normal adults and 8000 IU for lactating women. Diseases which upset the normal digestion and absorption of the intestines and the presence of large amounts of mineral oil interfere with the absorption of the fat-soluble vitamins. *See* VITAMIN.

In many parts of the world there is widespread vitamin A deficiency, resulting in thousands of cases of blindness and untold human suffering. The cost of enough vitamin A to meet the requirements of a man for a year is a nickel.

The misuse of vitamins by laymen and physicians has resulted in cases of vitamin A toxicity in people receiving 25 to several hundred times their requirement over prolonged periods. Symptoms of excessive intake include anorexia, hyperirritability, skin lesions, bone decalcification, and increased intracranial pressure. Discontinuance of vitamin A supplementation in these individuals usually has been followed by a dramatic disappearance of symptoms in a few days.

[STANLEY N. GERSHOFF]

Industrial production. There are three approaches to the industrial preparation of vitamin A and its esters. In one method β-ionone is converted to the 14-carbon aldehyde (C_{14}-aldehyde), a key intermediate, by a glycidation reaction. This aldehyde is condensed by an acetylenic Grignard reaction with a 6-carbon fragment, obtained by the ethynylation of methylvinyl ketone and by the rearrangement of the resulting carbinol. The condensed product is preferentially reduced, acetylated, dehydrated, and rearranged to give esters of vitamin A.

The industrial synthesis of β-carotene is based on the work of H. H. Inhoffen and F. Bohlmann and of O. Isler and his coworkers. In this method, the C_{14}-aldehyde, an intermediate in the vitamin A synthesis, is acetalized, then condensed with ethylvinyl ether and hydrolyzed to C$_{16}$-aldehyde. This process is repeated using ethylpropenyl ether to give C$_{19}$-aldehyde. Two moles of C$_{19}$-aldehyde are condensed with acetylene-dimagnesium bromide to yield a C$_{40}$-acetylenic glycol. Dehydration, rearrangement, and preferential hydrogenation of this glycol yield β-carotene.

[ALFRED OFNER]

Vitamin B$_6$

A vitamin which exists as three chemically related and water-soluble forms found in food: pyridoxine, pyridoxal, and pyridoxamine. The structural formulas of these compounds are shown in the illustration. All three forms have equal activity for animals and yeast, but pyridoxal and pyridoxamine have several thousand times the activity of pyridoxine for some bacteria. Vitamin B$_6$ is stable in acid, but is rapidly destroyed by light in alkaline or neutral solutions.

Bioassay. Chemical assays for vitamin B$_6$ are laborious; microbiological assays are commonly used. They often give results which appear much too high when compared to animal-feeding tests. This is because vitamin B$_6$ is conjugated with other substances in foods, and the acid hydrolysis procedures used in preparing samples for microbiological assay release quantities of the vitamin not released by normal digestive processes.

Dietary requirements. Most studies of vitamin B$_6$ deficiency have been done on animals, since a deficiency of this vitamin in humans is very rare. Vitamin B$_6$ deficiency is accompanied by poor growth, dermatitis, microcytic anemia, epileptiform convulsions, and kidney and adrenal lesions. There is evidence that some women in the third trimester of pregnancy may have a special requirement for vitamin B$_6$ in that its administration often relieves the nausea of pregnancy. Some types of human dermatitis respond to local application of this vitamin. Experimental studies have suggested that vitamin B$_6$–deficient animals are deficient in available insulin and growth hormone. Marked abnormalities in lipid, carbohydrate, and protein metabolism are caused by this deficiency.

Vitamin B$_6$–deficient animals are oxaluric and may form kidney stones. Atherosclerosis and impaired antibody formation have been reported. Vitamin B$_6$–responsive anemias have been reported in man, and it has been suggested that supplemental vitamin B$_6$ may protect against dental caries, particularly during pregnancy.

It is difficult to set requirements for vitamin B$_6$, since no single set of assay conditions or criteria has received universal acceptance. Based on animal experiments, a number of dietary factors probably affect the vitamin B$_6$ requirement. High-protein diets increase the requirement. High-carbohydrate diets probably increase intestinal synthesis of vitamin B$_6$, while unsaturated fatty acids decrease the requirement. Adults probably require about 1.5–2 mg per day, and a dietary intake of 0.4 mg per day would probably be satisfactory for most infants.

Biochemistry. Vitamin B$_6$ functions as a coenzyme in the form of pyridoxal 5-phosphate. The value of pyridoxine and pyridoxamine lies in the ability of tissues to convert them into pyridoxal. Vitamin B$_6$–containing enzymes are included in aminotransferase reactions (transamination) which are important mechanisms for the synthesis of amino acids by the tissues from α-keto acids. An example would be:

Glutamic acid + pyruvic acid $\rightleftharpoons$
α-ketoglutaric acid + alanine

Vitamin B$_6$ is also involved in amino-acid decarboxylation reactions. The transformations of histidine to histamine and of aspartic acid to β-alanine are examples of these. This vitamin has a special function in the metabolism of tryptophan and is necessary for the conversion of tryptophan to niacin. In most vitamin B$_6$–deficient animals, xanthurenic acid, a metabolite of tryptophan, is excreted in abnormal quantities, and this has been used as the basis for tests of the adequacy of vitamin B$_6$ nutrition. This vitamin also has a special function in the metabolism of the sulfur-containing amino acids.

[STANLEY N. GERSHOFF]

Industrial production. Two prominent processes of the many industrial syntheses of vitamin B$_6$, called pyridoxine or adermin, are based on the publication of S. A. Harris and K. Folkers and the publications of other workers.

Both syntheses form pyridone rings by condensation of β-diketones with cyanoacetamide. With the first method, the ring is first nitrated in the 5 position, then the hydroxyl group is replaced in the 2 position by chlorine. In the second method, the ester in the 4 position is treated with ammonia to form the carbamide and dehydrated to the dinitrile, followed by nitration and chlorination. These compounds are then reduced to the corresponding di- or triamines which, upon diazotization, yield the vitamin.

[MARC COLE]

Structural formulas for the three naturally occurring forms of vitamin B$_6$. (a) Pyridoxine (pyridoxol). (b) Pyridoxal. (c) Pyridoxamine.

Bibliography: S. A. Harris and K. Folkers, Synthesis of vitamin B_6, *J. Amer. Chem. Soc.*, 6: 1245–1247, 1939; J. H. Mowat, F. J. Pilgrim. and G. H. Carlson, *J. Amer. Chem. Soc.*, 65:954–955, 1943; W. H. Sebrell (ed.), *Vitamins: Chemistry, Physiology, Methods*, 2d ed., 1967.

Vitamin B_{12}

A group of closely related polypyrrole compounds containing trivalent cobalt. It is often called cobalamin, and its structural formula is shown in the illustration. The vitamin is a dark-red crystalline compound; in aqueous solution and at room temperature it is most stable at pH 4–7.

Source and assay. In general, vitamin B_{12} is synthesized by microorganisms, not by plants, and is found in animal tissues as a result of intestinal synthesis or ingestion. It is now thought that the animal-protein factor, which was studied widely, is at least in part vitamin B_{12}. Vitamin B_{12} is usually determined microbiologically at the present time, although rat and chick growth assays are also available.

Physiology and requirements. Vitamin B_{12} deficiency in animals is characterized primarily by anemia and neuropathy. In man, this deficiency is called pernicious anemia. People suffering from this disease lack a factor secreted in normal gastric juice which, by affecting absorption directly and by protecting vitamin B_{12} from intestinal destruction, enables the vitamin to be absorbed. This factor, called intrinsic factor, appears to be one or more mucoproteins. Its action in facilitating the absorption of vitamin B_{12} is calcium-dependent. Vitamin B_{12} deficiency in man may be caused by a genetically controlled lack of intrinsic factor, gastrectomy, malabsorption disease, or vegetarianism. Body stores of the vitamin are such that it takes approximately 5 years for a deficiency state to appear clinically after a gastrectomy has been performed.

Structural formula for vitamin B_{12}.

Requirements for vitamin B_{12} are increased by reproduction or hyperthyroidism. Of the known vitamins, B_{12} is the most active biologically. A daily injection of 1 μg of vitamin B_{12} will prevent the recurrence of symptoms in people with pernicious anemia. For normal people a diet containing 3–5 μg per day (providing 1–1.5 μg absorbed) will satisfy vitamin B_{12} requirements. Some of the vitamin B_{12} requirement is probably met by intestinal synthesis.

Biochemistry. Several coenzymes of vitamin B_{12} exist. They are included in isomerization reactions (methylmalonyl–CoA mutase, glutamate mutase), conversion by dioldehydrases of 1, 2-diols to deoxaldehydes, methylation reactions (formation of methionine and thymidine 5′-phosphate), and conversion of ribose to deoxyribose.

[STANLEY N. GERSHOFF]

Commercial production. Processes for the commercial production of vitamin B_{12} utilize the synthetic ability of either bacteria or streptomycetes. Yeasts and higher fungi are, for the most part, nonsynthesizers, as are higher plants and animals.

Most commonly, *Propionibacterium freudenreicheii* or a similar organism is grown by the usual fermentation techniques, such as are employed to produce riboflavin, penicillin, or streptomycin. The organism is grown in 10,000- to 50,000-gal tanks in a medium of yeast extract, minerals, and sucrose or other carbohydrate for a period of 72–120 hr after inoculation. Optimum vitamin titers of 2–6 mg/liter are obtained under conditions of mild aeration, though the organism can grow anaerobically.

Since the vitamin is almost entirely contained in the cells, it can be recovered by centrifugation of the final broth. The cells can be dried, and used directly as a food or animal-feed supplement. The product is further purified for drug uses.

Vitamin B_{12} has sometimes been produced as a by-product during the production of streptomycin and certain other antibiotics. Relatively large quantities of the vitamin are produced by microorganisms which grow during the reduction of sewage by the activated sludge process, but it is not recovered for use. *See* INDUSTRIAL MICROBIOLOGY.

[RALPH E. BENNETT]

Bibliography: W. W. Umbriet (ed.), *Advances in Applied Microbiology*, vol. 1, 1959.

Vitamin D

The term vitamin D refers to two chemically similar fat-soluble, sterol-like compounds, calciferol, or vitamin D_2, and activated 7-dehydrocholesterol, or vitamin D_3 (see illustration). Vitamins D_2 and D_3 have about the same potency for most mammals including man, but vitamin D_3 is 30–100 times as effective as vitamin D_2 for birds and some monkeys.

Source. In animals 7-dehydrocholesterol is secreted at the surface of the skin, where it is activated by sunlight, and the vitamin D_3 formed is reabsorbed. Vitamin D_2 is prepared by the ultraviolet irradiation of ergosterol, a vitamin D precursor found in plants. Most naturally occurring foods have little vitamin D activity. Fish oils are an exception, being highly potent sources of the vitamin. It is common practice to give children vitamin D supplements, and much of the milk marketed in

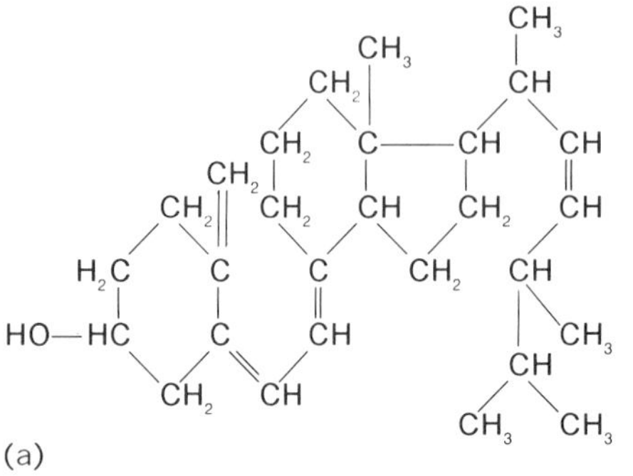

(a)

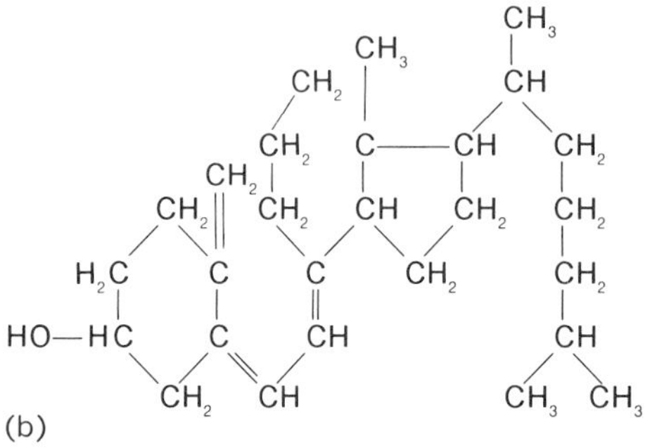

(b)

Structural formulas for the two vitamin D compounds. (a) Vitamin D$_2$ (calciferol). (b) Vitamin D$_3$ (activated 7-dehydrocholesterol).

the United States has been enriched with 400 IU per quart.

An international unit (IU) of vitamin D is equal to 0.025 microgram (μg) of vitamin D$_3$.

Assay. There are no satisfactory physical or chemical methods for the determination of vitamin D in food. Rats or chicks are used in biological assays. In these, measurements are made of the ash content of bones or beaks or the rate at which new bone is being formed.

Physiological activities. Vitamin D deficiency in growing animals is called rickets and has been produced in a large number of species. In adult animals the disease is called osteomalacia. Vitamin D deficiency is associated with skeletal pathology. Bones and teeth are soft and fracture easily. Poor growth accompanied by malformations of the bones, particularly the long bones and the ribs, occurs. The disease is seldom fatal, but predisposes to other diseases, particularly bronchopneumonia. *See* RICKETS.

Biochemistry. Little is known of the metabolic role of vitamin D. It increases the intestinal absorption of calcium, but the process is not clear. Studies suggest that vitamin D stimulates the production of a protein essential for the transport of calcium across the intestinal mucosa. There is evidence that vitamin D mobilizes bone mineral to help maintain serum levels of calcium and phosphate. Vitamin D also affects mitochondrial metabolism. In vitamin D deficiency there is a failure of deposition of Ca salts in the cartilaginous matrix of the bones. Two new compounds having vitamin D–like activity, 25-hydroxycholecalciferol and 25-hydroxyergocalciferol, have been reported to have greater antirachitic properties than vitamin D.

It has been suggested that in some small children hypersensitivity to vitamin D exists since intakes of as little as 1000 IU per day have led to hypercalcemia with attendant complications.

Dietary requirements. The recommended daily dietary allowance of the National Research Council for children and pregnant or lactating women is 400 IU. Normal adults can probably depend on sunshine and the small amount of the vitamin from their food to meet their needs. Because vitamin D is readily stored, single doses of 600,000 units two times a year, orally or intramuscularly, may be used if it is impractical to give children daily supplements or to enrich the milk. Massive doses of vitamin D have been used in the treatment of diseases having no relation to rickets, in some cases with favorable results. Doses of vitamin D 500–1000 times the recommended allowance, if continued over a long period of time, can result in extensive calcification of the kidneys, heart, arteries, stomach, and other soft tissues, accompanied by nausea, weakness, and even death. *See* VITAMIN.

[STANLEY N. GERSHOFF]

Commercial production. Commercial vitamin D is available in several forms. Irradiated yeast is a source of vitamin D$_2$ and is used in supplementing rations of livestock. Provitamin ergosterol is extracted from yeast and, when irradiated and purified, yields crystalline vitamin D$_2$. Vitamin D$_3$ is obtained from fish-liver oils, which are refined for use in foods, or it is produced from lanolin by extraction of the provitamin 7-dehydrocholesterol, which is irradiated and from which crystalline D$_3$ is derived.

Foods are generally fortified with vitamin D standardized concentrates of the vitamin in suitable carriers. One form consists of the vitamins taken up in milk carriers which are canned and sterilized and which are used primarily for milk products. Other carriers consist of propylene glycol, alcohol, or oils containing added emulsifying agents which are used for dairy products and other foods, and stabilized beadlets in which the vitamin D is encased in a gelatin matrix.

[KENNETH G. WECKEL]

Vitamin E

A group of compounds called tocopherols. There are eight of these, each differing slightly in its chemical configuration.

Chemistry. These structural differences have a decided effect on the biological activity of the compounds. When the rat is used as a test animal, and the activity of α-tocopherol (see illustration) is set at 100, the activities of the β-, γ-, and δ-tocopherols are 40, 8, and 1, respectively. In addition to the tocopherols, many synthetic compounds with similar structures and a number of antioxidants unrelated chemically to the tocopherols also have vitamin E activity.

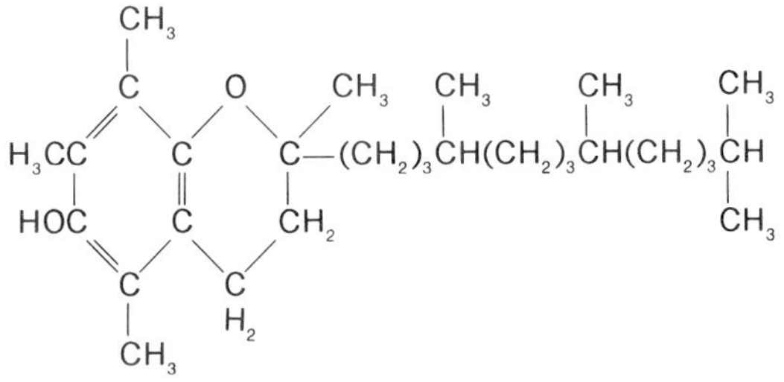

Structural formula for α-tocopherol.

The tocopherols are fat-soluble. They are widespread in nature and are particularly concentrated in vegetable oils. They are stable to heat, acids, and alkalies, but they are easily destroyed by ultraviolet light or oxidizing agents.

Assay. Chemical and physical analyses for tocopherols are difficult, often expensive, and may not differentiate between the different tocopherols. Vitamin E activity can be determined biologically, but these methods are also disappointing.

Physiological activities. Vitamin E deficiency in animals has often been associated with reproductive failure and irreversible testicular damage. This aspect of vitamin E deficiency has resulted in many unfounded claims as to the role of vitamin E in reproduction. There is no good evidence that vitamin E deficiency is associated with any human reproduction problems. In vitamin E deficiency, dystrophy of both striated and cardiac muscles occurs, and death often occurs as a result of cardiac failure. Vitamin E therapy has not been of value in treating muscular dystrophy in humans. Vitamin E–deficient rats develop liver necrosis, and chicks develop encephalomalacia and subcutaneous edema. The rat-liver necrosis and the edema of chicks can be cured by traces of selenium as well as vitamin E. The relation between vitamin E and selenium is not clear. The fat of some vitamin E–deficient animals becomes brown because of the deposition of ceroid pigments. The red blood cells of deficient animals are more subject to hemolysis, and this characteristic of vitamin E deficiency is used in biological assays for the vitamin. Anemia and other hematological problems have been reported in vitamin E–deficient monkeys. Poorly nourished Jordanian children with macrocytic anemia responded to vitamin E therapy when other forms of treatment failed. Sclerema neonatorum, a type of edema found in premature infants, can be cured by oral administration of α-tocopherol acetate.

Biochemistry. Practically nothing is known of how vitamin E functions in metabolism, although it seems reasonably certain that it functions as a biological antioxidant. In this capacity, it has been shown to have a sparing effect on the vitamin A content of tissues. It appears to have a function in maintaining the integrity of biological membranes. Vitamin E requirements increase with increased intakes of polyunsaturated fatty acids. Conditions interfering with fat absorption reduce the amount of vitamin E absorbed.

Dietary requirements. There are few good data concerning the vitamin E requirements of humans. Adult requirements may vary between 10 and 30 mg per day. The amount usually obtained from human milk, 0.5 mg α-tocopherol per kilogram, has been suggested as a minimum requirement for infants.

[STANLEY N. GERSHOFF]

α-**Tocopherol production.** Racemic dl-α-tocopherol is synthesized industrially by development of a basic procedure described by P. Karrer in 1938. By this method, trimethylhydroquinone is condensed with phytyl bromide in the presence of zinc chloride. The technical variations include the use of isophytol, phytol, and phytadiene with other catalysts.

The product is purified by a short-path, high-vacuum distillation. The synthetic tocopherol is used mostly as the acetate, which is as active as the free phenol, but has greater stability toward oxidation. Tocopherol acetate is manufactured by direct acetylation of free tocopherol with acetic anhydride, followed by a high-vacuum distillation.

[ALFRED OFNER]

Vitamin K

A naturally occurring vitamin consisting of two chemically similar yellowish oils known as K_1 and K_2, which are fat-soluble, nonsteroid, nonsaponifiable, and unstable to light. Many compounds with vitamin K activity have been synthesized. The most important of these is menadione or K_3. The structural formulas for vitamins K_1, K_2, and K_3 are shown in the illustration.

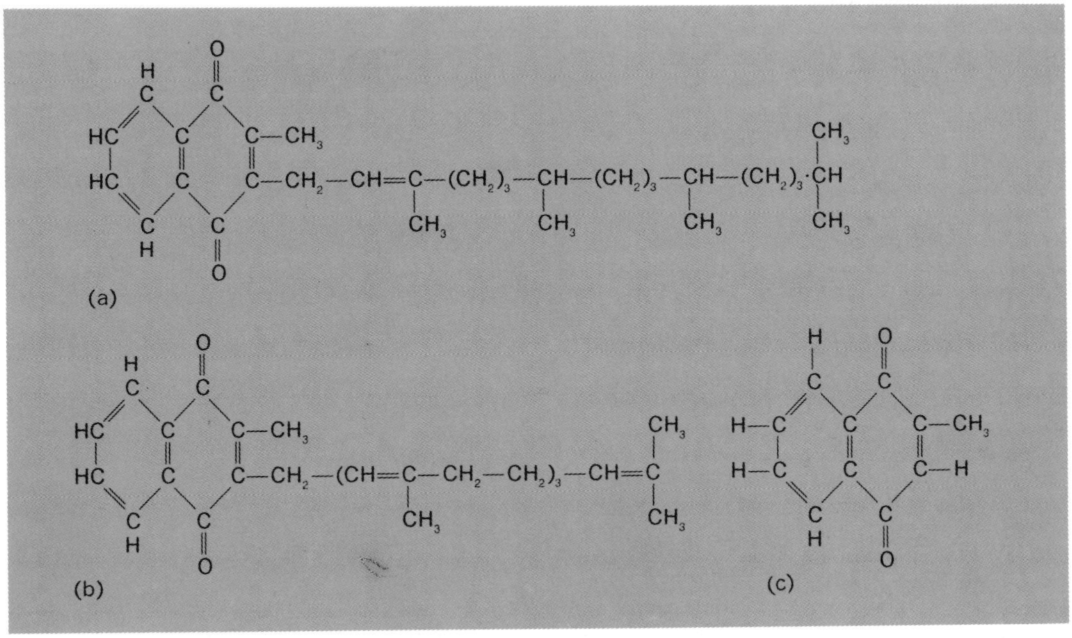

Structural formulas for (*a*) vitamin K_1, (*b*) vitamin K_2, and (*c*) vitamin K_3 (menadione).

Physiological activities. Vitamins K_1, K_2, and K_3 have equal activities for most species, except the dog, when fed on an equimolecular basis. The only major effect of a vitamin K deficiency in animals is a decrease in blood prothrombin, resulting in prolonged clotting time. Thus, vitamin K deficiency results in subcutaneous and intramuscular hemorrhages. The role of vitamin K in the production of prothrombin by the liver is not known. It may act as a prosthetic group or activator for some enzyme necessary for the production of the prothrombin, or it may even be incorporated to some extent in the prothrombin molecule.

Vitamin K is so widespread in nature in green leafy vegetables, and its synthesis by intestinal microorganisms is so great that vitamin K deficiency is rare. Liver disease, which may result in decreased prothrombin formation and bile secretion, can result in vitamin K deficiency, because bile secretion is necessary for its absorption. Intestinal disease or the ingestion of large amounts of mineral oil or antibiotics can also affect vitamin K economy. Relatively little is known about the biochemistry of vitamin K. It has been shown that vitamin K_1 is involved as a coenzyme in both electron transport and oxidative phosphorylation systems.

Assay. There are no good chemical or physical assays for vitamin K. The vitamin is usually determined by measuring its effect on the prothrombin or coagulation time of blood from depleted chicks.

In therapy. Two to three days prior to surgery, individuals with low prothrombin values are often given vitamin K therapy. The newborn infant has very low prothrombin values because of poor placental transfer, an undeveloped intestinal flora, and the low vitamin K content of milk. It is customary to give prospective mothers large doses of vitamin K a day or two before delivery and to give the newborn infant some also. A vitamin K antagonist, dicumarol, which lowers blood prothrombin levels, is used to reduce the possibility of thrombosis complications in some selected patients. *See* VITAMIN.   [STANLEY N. GERSHOFF]

Industrial production. The industrial synthesis of vitamin K_1 depends upon the condensation of phytyl moiety with 2-methyl-1,4-naphthoquinone. The phytyl moiety may be phytol or a phytyl halide.

In a typical synthesis, 2-methyl-1,4-naphthoquinone is converted to a stable derivative, such as 2-methyl-1,4-naphthalenediol-1-monoacetate or 1-monobenzoate by reductive esterification. The ester is condensed with the phytyl moiety in the presence of an acid catalyst, such as zinc chloride, oxalic acid, aluminum chloride, or boron trifluoride. The dihydro-vitamin K_1 ester thus produced is then saponified to dihydro-vitamin K_1, which is easily oxidized to vitamin K_1.

[ALFRED OFNER]

Walnut

This name is applied to about a dozen species of large deciduous trees widely distributed over temperate North and South America, southeastern Europe, and central and eastern Asia. The genus (*Juglans*) is characterized by pinnately compound aromatic leaves and chambered or laminate pith (Fig. 1). The staminate (male) flowers are borne

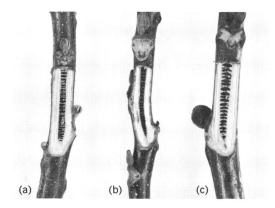

Fig. 1. Pith of (a) black walnut (*Juglans nigra*), (b) butternut (*J. cinera*), (c) English walnut (*J. regia*).

in unbranched catkins on the previous season's growth, and the pistillate (female) flowers are terminal on the current season's shoots. Pollination is by wind. The shells of the nuts of most species are deeply furrowed or sculptured.

The plants fall into two natural groups, one characterized by a prominent band of hairs on the upper edge of the leaf scar, pointed buds, and usually elongate nuts. The leaf scars of the other group lack the cushion of hairs, and the nuts are spherical or nearly so. Of the six North American species, five are in the latter group and one, the butternut or white walnut (*J. cinera*), in the former (Figs. 1 and 2).

Two species, the black walnut (*J. nigra*) and the Persian or English walnut (*J. regia*), are of primary importance for their timber and nuts. The butternut finds local use in the northeastern United States. The other species are sparingly used as shade trees, as grafting stocks, and as sources of nuts.

Black walnut. The black walnut is a large tree, sometimes reaching a height of over a hundred feet and 4–5-ft diameter. It is native to the hardwood forests of the Central Mississippi Valley and the Appalachian region of North America.

Walnuts thrive on rich, well-drained, alluvial soils well supplied with moisture and are most abundant in the river valleys and along streams. They have, however, been planted beyond their

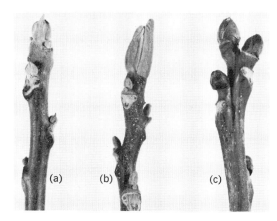

Fig. 2. (a) Black walnut (*Juglans nigra*). (b) Butternut (*J. cinera*). (c) English walnut (*J. regia*).

natural range and succeed on good agricultural soils over a wide area. The roots produce a toxic substance, juglone, which under some conditions is injurious to tomatoes, alfalfa, and some other crops.

The pinnately compound leaves have 15–20 leaflets, and the stamens and pistils are borne separately (monoecious) as in other members of the genus. The drupelike spherical fruit $1\frac{1}{2}$–$2\frac{1}{2}$ in. long is borne singly or in clusters of two or three. It consists of an outer indehiscent fleshy husk about $\frac{1}{2}$ in. thick enclosing the hard, rough-shelled nut $1\frac{1}{4}$–$1\frac{1}{2}$ in. in length. The kernels formed from the cotyledons are enclosed in membraneous seed coats which turn brown if nuts remain in husks (Fig. 3). The dark-brown, strong, durable wood is rated as North America's best for gunstocks, fine furniture, and veneer. Although the stand of black walnut is estimated at over 1,000,000,000 board feet, with an annual cut of around 50,000,000 board feet, the demand for high-quality logs exceeds the supply. This is in part due to the export of walnut logs, which in 1963 was 16,000,000 board feet. Unless conditions change, a greater shortage is anticipated, and planting walnut for lumber is being encouraged.

Nut production is mostly confined to the millions of trees in the forests and farmsteads. Formerly the nuts were gathered in large quantities, hulled, dried, and cracked for home use, or the operation was a cottage industry. With the advent of cracking machines about 1935, shelling and processing plants have developed in the Central Mississippi Valley. These handle about 50,000,000 lb of nuts in shell yearly, which yield about 6,000,000 lb of kernels. Also, there is the beginning of a black walnut orchard industry which aims at production of both timber and nuts. Under orchard conditions, the culture and harvesting of the crop will undoubtedly be mechanized as with the Persian or English walnut.

Black walnut kernels were an important source of food for the American Indians and the early settlers in the United States. Now they are extensively used in ice cream, candy, and baked goods. Kernels are graded at the processing plant according to size of the pieces. In the cracking process part of the kernels are recovered as whole quarters and, with the fragments larger than $\frac{1}{6}$ in., are sold in plastic bags, glass jars, or metal cans. The dense hard shells of the nuts are ground and used for drilling mud in oil fields and for abrasive in polishing metal castings.

English walnut. The most important of the nut-bearing trees belonging to the genus *Juglans* is the English walnut. Native to central Asia and Asia Minor, the tree was distributed widely in ancient times throughout the temperate and subtropical climatic zones of the Old World. It is also called Persian walnut, which is considered a more appropriate name. The large, round-headed, long-lived trees produce the circassian walnut lumber of commerce that is valued for gunstocks, furniture, veneer, and paneling. In France, the Balkans, and elsewhere the trees are raised for both nuts and lumber.

The leaves are pinnately compound with five to nine entire leaflets, variable in shape and size. The trees are monoecious, with the staminate flowers borne in catkins and the nutlets terminal on the current season's growth. Securing adequate pollination may be a problem because pollen shedding by the catkins may not overlap the receptive period of the pistils; hence several varieties should be planted together.

The wild-type nuts of central Asian origin are small and hard-shelled. Through centuries of selection, large thin-shelled types have been developed. The oval fruit, about 2 in. long in good varieties, consists of a fleshy outer hull about $\frac{1}{4}$ in. thick which at maturity splits irregularly, freeing the nut (Fig. 4).

Production in the world other than in the United States and western Europe is mostly from seedling trees which receive little care. In central and northern California and in Oregon, where more than 150,000 acres are grown, high-yielding grafted varieties are planted and given the best modern culture. Requirements are for a well-drained soil 8–10 ft deep, a climate cold enough in winter to break dormancy of the trees yet without winter temperatures below about 15°F, and freedom from late-spring frosts. Temperatures about 100°F may cause damage to the nuts from sunburn. Some varieties from the Carpathian Mountains of central Europe may withstand winter temperatures of −25°F, but these often suffer from late frosts, and consistent high yields have not been secured from the trees in the eastern United States where they are being tried.

Harvesting and processing in most of the producing countries is done with local hand labor. In California, however, operations are highly mechanized. Before harvest, the ground under the trees is cleaned and leveled. Machines shake the nuts from the trees and sweep them into windrows, from which they are picked up mechanically and taken in bulk to the processing plant, where they are hulled, washed, and dried. About 42% of the crop to be marketed in the shells is sized and bleached. The others are machine-shelled, and the kernels are graded for color by electronic machines, sized, and packaged for the retail trade. The Diamond Walnut Growers, Inc., handles over 80% of the crop and determines quality and grade. The Walnut Control Board decides the amounts available for export and the proportion to be shelled.

California and Oregon produce a 5-year average of 80,200 tons of walnuts in shells, with 96,000 tons reported in 1966 and 76,800 in 1967. Other

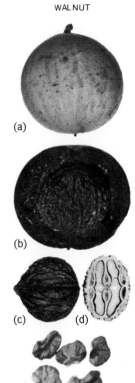

Fig. 3. Black walnut (*Juglans nigra*). (*a*) Mature fruit. (*b*) Nut with half of hull cut away. (*c*) Nut without husk. (*d*) Nut cut transversely to show shell structure. (*e*) Kernels in quarters.

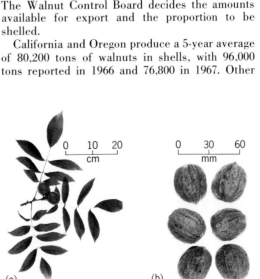

Fig. 4. English walnut (*Juglans regia*). (*a*) Twig with leaves and fruit. (*b*) Hulled nuts.

producing countries are France (28,600 tons in 1965), Italy (24,900), and Turkey (8400). The Soviet Union and China also produce commercial quantities of walnuts.

More than half of the English walnuts are shelled, and the kernels are used in a great variety of ways in baking and confectionery, and are also salted. The others are sold in shell to the consumer. In foreign countries many of the nuts are used locally as food.

Butternut. The butternut, or white walnut, is the hardiest of the American species of *Juglans*, its range extending from Maine and New Brunswick, westward to Ontario, south to Arkansas and the mountains of Georgia. The trees are adapted to upland soils and in the northeastern United States are one of the few nut-bearing species. Distinguishing characters are the pointed buds and the cushion of hairs above the leaf scar (Figs. 1 and 2). The nuts, which are borne in clusters of two or three, are ellipsoid and pointed and are enclosed in a tight indehiscent husk which is covered with sticky hairs. The shell is deeply sculptured with jagged ridges.

The butternut, as compared with the black walnut, has a shallow root system and a more spreading crown. Trees are often short-lived because of defoliation by fungus disease. The wood is lighter-colored and less dense than the black walnut, and is used for interior finish and furniture. The husks of the nuts were formerly used in dying cloth greenish yellow.

At the present time, butternuts are used locally for their highly flavored oily kernels. Nuts from most of the wild trees are difficult to crack. Some progress has been made in selecting clones with good cracking quality.

[LAURENCE H. MAC DANIELS]

Watermelon

The edible fruit of *Citrullus lanatus*, of the family Cucurbitaceae. The plant is an annual prostrate vine with multiple stems alternating from short nodes near the base of the main axis, reaching lengths of 10 to 15 ft (3 to 4.5 m). Short vine or "bush" type cultivars exist but are not commercially useful. In a typical monoecious plant, pistillate flowers occur at every seventh node, with staminate flowers at intervening nodes. Cultivated plants range from 250 to 1000 hills per acre (4047 m^2) according to variety and region. Commercially, an average yield of one mature melon per plant is acceptable.

Varieties and productions. The numerous open-pollinated cultivars of watermelon are highly diverse in fruit size (5–85 lb; 2.3–38.3 kg), shape (round, oval, oblong-cylindrical), rind color (very light to very dark green and often striped or mottled), flesh color (red, pink, orange, yellow, white), and seed size and color. The flesh contains 6–12% sugar, depending upon variety and condition of growth, with 8% sugar being acceptable on most markets, corresponding to juice refractometer readings of 9 or 10% total soluble solids. A few low-sugar cultivars called citrons are planted only for livestock. Such citron types grow wild in parts of Africa and are probably a significant factor in the survival of native animals in drought periods.

Seedless watermelons were introduced in 1948 in Japan. These are more difficult and costly to produce, yet they have become popular in some Oriental countries. Seedless triploid watermelons are notably superior in flesh quality. Equally superior flesh quality occurs in some tetraploid varieties originated in the United States which are semiseedless and have extra firm flesh and hard rinds. Due to the extra stable flesh quality, these crops may be left on the vine for a single harvest.

The watermelon species is native to Africa, where it still occurs in the wild state in semiarid areas and is also widely cultivated by native farmers, both for human consumption and for livestock. Watermelons are grown in most tropical and subtropical and many temperate climates. They are grown locally in most of the United States, but in large volumes for interstate shipment primarily in the southern states and in California, Indiana, and Texas. Areas harvested annually in the United States ranged from 241,000 to 268,000 acres (97,570 to 108,500 ha), from 1971 to 1973. Meaningful estimates of worldwide volume of watermelons are not available *See* MELON GROWING.

Food products. Watermelon juice of the sweet cultivars can be reduced to edible sugar and syrup. Watermelon rinds are either hard or soft, and this affects the handling performance of different cultivars. Varieties that best resist breakage in transit have firm interior flesh although the rind may be neither very thick nor very hard. Sweet pickles made from rinds have some commercial importance. Soft-rind varieties are best for that purpose.

Watermelon seeds are relished as food in some Near East countries and in China, and certain varieties are grown primarily for that purpose. There is a small industry in Iran where grilled (roasted) watermelon seeds are bagged and sold like popcorn. Salt-preserved watermelon seeds are often eaten in China.

Health value. Fresh watermelon flesh has a unique melting quality that has proved impossible to preserve in palatable form through any processing technique. The flesh consists of water (91%), fiber, and sugar, and little else of obvious nutritional value, but may have some as yet unproved health-promoting value. It is said to have diuretic properties, and both frozen concentrate and canned juice have been available for the treatment of nephritis. The seeds also are said to contain substances effective in the control of hypertension.

[C. F. ANDRUS]

Bibliography: C. F. Andrus, V. S. Seshadri, and P. C. Grimball, *Production of Seedless Watermelons*, U.S. Dept. Agr. Tech. Bull. no. 1425, 1971; I. S. Barksdale, Studies on the blood-pressure lowering principle in the seed of watermelon, *Amer. J. Med. Sci.*, 171(1):111–123, 1926; R. A. Bliss, R. W. Morrison, and E. O. Prather, An investigation of the diuretic properties of watermelon juice, *Amer. J. Pharm.*, 105:5358, 1933; W. E. DuPree, J. G. Woodroof, and S. Siewert, *Watermelon Rinds in Food Products*, Ga. Agr. Exp. Sta. Bull. no. 285, 1953; H. Kihara, Triploid watermelons, *Proc. Amer. Soc. Hort. Sci.*, 58:217–230, 1951; J. E. Webster and F. A. Romshe, Watermelon sirup: Its composition and the composition of juice from which it was made, *Proc. Amer. Soc. Hort. Sci.*, 57: 302–304, 1951.

Wheat

A food grain crop. Wheat is the most widely grown food crop in the world, and is increasing in production. It ranks first in world crop production and is the national food staple of 43 countries. At least one-third of the world's population depends on wheat as its main staple. The principal food use of wheat is as bread, either leavened or unleavened.

In 1967, world wheat production passed the 10^{10} bu (2.72×10^8 metric tons) mark, and recent annual wheat crops have exceeded 1.2×10^{10} bu (3.72×10^8), or about 3 bu (.082) for every person in the world. Recent crops in the United States have exceeded 2×10^9 bu (0.54×10^8). The United States is second to the Soviet Union in total production, but the average yield per acre in the United States is about twice that of the Soviet Union.

Other major wheat-producing countries in the world are Canada, China, India, France, Argentina, and Australia. Highest per acre yields (60 bu, or 1.63 metric tons, and above) are produced in Western Europe. The change to day-length-insensitive, short straw and stiff straw varieties which can be heavily fertilized and irrigated has resulted in yield increases, especially in food-deficit countries from about 35°N latitude to the Equator (Fig. 1). Wheat is an important commodity of international trade. Of the total wheat production, about one-fifth moves in world trade. The United States leads in exports. Other leading export countries include Canada, Australia, France, and Argentina.

Adaptation. Wheat is best adapted to a cool dry climate, but is grown in a wide range of soils and climates. Much of the world's wheat is seeded in the fall season and, after being dormant or growing very slowly during winter, it makes rapid growth in the spring and develops grain for harvest in early summer. In the United States, about 80% of the wheat is fall-seeded. Wheat competes with other crops where the fall-seeded type makes good use of limited rainfall and where the spring-seeded type makes good use of the short frost-free growing season. Medium-textured and well-drained soils are best for wheat since it cannot withstand long periods of wet ground.

General cultural practices. Clean, weed-free seed of an adapted variety treated to control seedborne diseases, along with good germination, increases the prospect of a satisfactory crop. Wheat is usually seeded at a depth of 1–2 in. (2.5–5 cm), or deeper when topsoil is dry. A firm seed bed, together with soil firmly packed over the seed, improves stands and reduces losses from winter kill and similar hazards. Wheat may be seeded as part of a rotation following corn, soybeans, or other small grain crops in humid regions; a year of fallow during which moisture is accumulated and weeds kept under control often precedes wheat in areas of low rainfall. Seeding time depends on soil moisture, soil temperature, presence of certain insects and disease organisms, and other factors. Seeding rate averages about 60 lb/acre (67 kg/ha) in the United States but may be as high as 120 lb/acre 134 kg/ha) in the eastern United States and as low as 30 lb/acre (33 kg/ha) in the arid West.

Most wheat is harvested directly from the field with a combined harvester-thresher, or it may be windrowed first and then combined when dry. Wheat grain should contain no more than 13% moisture for safe storage, should be cool, and free from insects. Forced-air dryers are used to reduce the moisture content of grain harvested at above 13%.

Market classes. Wheat for milling is classified according to hardness, color, and best use. In the United States, there are seven official market classes of which the following five are the most important: (1) hard red winter, for bread; (2) hard red spring, for bread and rolls; (3) soft red winter, for cake and pastries; (4) white, for bread, breakfast foods, and pastries; and (5) durum, for macaroni products.

Distribution of types and varieties. Variety adaptation, production practices, and crop hazards are widely different in the major areas of production in the United States. Therefore, the United States can be divided into six wheat-growing regions (Fig. 2), although the boundaries overlap. These are: region I, the Northeast and Ohio Valley; region II, the Southeast; region III, the Northern Plains; region IV, the Central Plains; region V, the Pacific Northwest; and region VI, California and Arizona.

Regions I and II have the highest rainfall of the six, and wheat of soft texture with low protein generally is grown. The crop is fall-seeded. General crop rotations are used in which corn and soybeans take prominent places. Yorkstar, Genesee, and Ionia, all white grains, are the leading varieties in region I. In region II, Arthur, a soft red winter type, is the leading variety in most of the states.

In region III, spring-sown wheat predominates. The leading varieties of durum wheat are Rolette and Leeds, while the leading hard red spring vari-

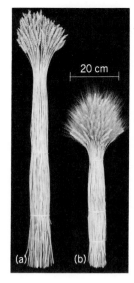

Fig. 1. Sheaves of wheat: (a) tall, awnless variety; (b) short, awned or bearded variety. Both tall and short types have awns.

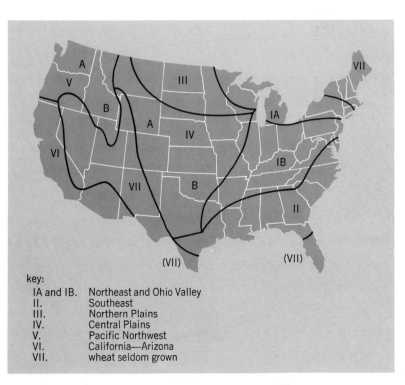

key:
IA and IB. Northeast and Ohio Valley
II. Southeast
III. Northern Plains
IV. Central Plains
V. Pacific Northwest
VI. California—Arizona
VII. wheat seldom grown

Fig. 2. Adaptation regions for wheat in the United States. (USDA)

eties are Era, Waldron, and Olaf. Some fall-sown wheat is grown in the western portion of this region, but the winters are severe and the crop often is lost. In general, the region has low rainfall, hence tillage and rotations are designed to conserve as much moisture as possible.

In region IV, little else but hard red winter wheat is grown. Subregion IVA requires a cold-hardy variety, and subregion IVB, with its hot summers, requires an early maturing variety for most dependability. In subregion IVA, leading varieties in recent years have been Winalta and Cheyenne; in subregion IVB, Scout, Centurk, Triumph, and Sturdy. This region has rather low rainfall, and tillage, including summer fallow, is especially timed to conserve moisture for the next crop.

In region V, wheat of several types is grown but soft white and hard red winter predominate. Much of region V uses summer fallow in the cropping sequence. A small acreage is irrigated. Nugaines and Hyslop have been the most important white wheat varieties in this region. Paha and Moro, club wheats with white grain, have been grown also. Wanser is the leading hard red winter variety, and Komar and Thatcher hard red spring wheats continue to be found on a small acreage.

Region VI grows day-length-insensitive common wheats with red or white grain, or amber durum. Irrigation is common for wheat in this region. The mild winters allow nonhardy varieties to be utilized from fall seeding. The leading varieties in recent years have been Anza and Inia 66.

In all of these regions, variety changes occur every year as improved forms are introduced; hence, the varieties named here represent types but may not continue to be the particular varieties actually produced in a given year. Some wheat is irrigated in regions IV, V, and VI, but the major acreage is rain-fed.

Northwestern Mexico grows varieties similar to those found adapted in region VI and utilizes similar production methods. In Canada the varieties used are similar to those used in region III. Production practices in Canada are also similar to those used in region III, with heavy emphasis on dry-land farming. The leading variety of hard red spring wheat in Canada is Neepawa.

Characteristics. The wheat inflorescence is a spike bearing sessile spikelets arranged alternately on a zigzag rachis. Two, three, or more florets may develop in each spikelet and bear grains. The florets are composed of three stamens and a single ovary with its style and stigma enclosed by a lemma and palea (Fig. 3). The lemma may be awned or awnless. The grain may be white, red (brown), or purple, and it may be hard or soft in texture. Size of the grain or caryopsis may be large, as in durum, or very small, as in shot wheat *(Triticum sphaerococcum)*. Wheats vary in plant height and in the ability to produce tillers. The stems are usually hollow.

Wheat is normally a self-pollinating plant, although out-crosses do occur. When a breeder deliberately makes crosses, the anthers must be removed before they shed pollen, and fresh pollen must be transferred from the second parent in the cross to the stigmas while they are receptive. Certain breeding stocks of wheat have been found that are male-sterile and shed no pollen. These have been used successfully to develop hybrid wheats without resorting to hand pollination procedures.

The wheat grain is composed of the endosperm and embryo enclosed by bran layers. The endosperm portion is principally starch and is therefore used as energy food. Wheat is also an important protein source, especially for those people who use wheat as their main staple. Since wheat protein is deficient in lysine and some of the other essential amino acids that are important in human nutrition, breeding for improved amino acid balance or nutritional value is a primary objective in many breeding projects. *See* SEED (BOTANY).

Origin and relationships. Wheat was gathered for food in prehistoric times and has been grown as a crop for perhaps 7000 years. The exact center of origin of cultivated wheat has not been established, but the most likely area is the foothills of southwestern Iran, southeastern Turkey, and adjacent parts of Iraq and Syria with an extension to Israel. Wild *Aegilops* and *Triticum* are still found in these regions.

Botanically, wheat is a member of the grass family to which rice, barley, corn, and several other cereal grain crops also belong. The *Triticum* genus includes a wide range of wheat forms (Fig. 4). They are often grouped by their polyploid chromosome number series of 7, 14, and 21 pairs. In Fig. 4, *a* and *b* have 7 pairs (diploid), *c* to *l* have 14 pairs (tetraploid), and *m* to *q* have 21 pairs (hexaploid) of chromosomes.

Recent taxonomic studies place the goat grasses *(Aegilops)* and wheat *(Triticum)* in one genus, *Triticum.* They intercross to some extent, and it is believed that *Aegilops* species have contributed one or more groups of chromosomes to the tetraploid and hexaploid species of *Triticum*. Breeders have transferred individual genetic characteristics from goat grasses to wheat. The forms illustrated in Fig. 4 have been intercrossed, and in this way resistance to wheat rusts has been transferred from durum and emmer to common wheat. Wheat has been crossed with rye *(Secale)* and with *Agropyron*

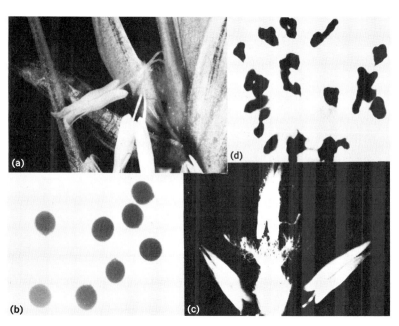

Fig. 3. Flower parts of a male fertile wheat plant: (*a*) three stamens; (*b*) pollen grains; (*c*) a single ovary with feathery stigma; and (*d*) normal chromosomes.

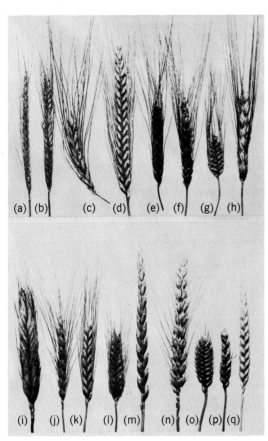

Fig. 4. Spikes of some representative varieties of wheat. (a) Wild and (b) cultivated forms of einkorn (*Triticum monococcum*); (c) wild emmer (*T. dicoccoides*); (d) emmer (*T. dicoccum*); (e) durum (*T. durum*); (f) poulard (*T. turgidum*); (g, h) durum (*T. durum*); (i) Polish (*T. polonicum*); (j) Persian (*T. carthlicum*); (k) emmer (*T. dicoccum*); (l) timopheevi (*T. timopheevi*); (m) spelt (*T. spelta*); (n) bread or common (*T. aestivum*); (o) club (*T. compactum*); (p) shot (*T. sphaerococcum*); and (q) spelt (*T. spelta*). (*Courtesy of H. Kihara*)

(a grass), and by the use of irradiation, segments of alien chromatin have been transferred to wheat, sometimes with beneficial results. New forms, called *Triticale*, have been derived from crossing rye and wheat followed by doubling the chromosomes in the hybrid. The most successful of these is based on a cross of rye and durum wheat in which there are 14 pairs of wheat and 7 pairs of rye chromosomes in the new species. Several variations occur.

Since there is much genetic similarity among the three genomes (sets of 7) of common wheat, the loss of a chromosome of one genome is partially compensated by similar chromosomes in the other genomes. This allows the development of 21 different genetic stocks, each deficient for one chromosome or one chromosome pair. The use of such stocks has greatly accelerated genetic studies and has made work more precise. An extension of this technique permits the substitution of a whole chromosome in one variety for the same chromosome in another variety. This has value in genetic studies and is also useful in variety improvement. *See* BREEDING (PLANT).

Variety development. Most countries in which wheat is grown have wheat breeding programs in which the objective is to develop more productive and more stable varieties (cultivars). Many methods are combined in these programs, but in nearly all of them specially selected parent types are crossbred followed by pure-line selection among the progeny to develop new combinations of merit. Varieties and genetic types from all over the world become candidate parents to provide the desired recombinations of good quality, winter and drought hardiness, straw strength, yield, and disease resistance. Wheats must be bred for specific milling processes and to provide quality end-use products. Many new varieties have complex pedigrees.

A number of worldwide collections of diverse wheats are available to breeders. The collection maintained by the U.S. Department of Agriculture contains about 35,000 items. Teams of breeders, geneticists, entomologists, plant pathologists, and cereal chemists are found at major breeding centers to give comprehensiveness to the breeding of the new varieties. *See* GRAIN CROPS.

[LOUIS P. REITZ]

DISEASES

It is estimated that in the United States more than 76,000,000 bu of wheat are destroyed annually by diseases. Some diseases, such as stem rust and scab, become epidemic only in certain years; others, such as root rots, are prevalent every year. When diseases like leaf and stem rusts, smuts, and scab become epidemic, they may destroy 25–50% of the potential crop, both locally and regionally.

Thus in the years 1935 and 1937 stem rust nearly ruined the wheat crop in the Upper Mississippi Valley and in the prairie provinces of Canada. In 1953 and 1954 durum wheats were almost annihilated by race 15B of wheat stem rust in Minnesota and the Dakotas.

Etiological agents. Diseases of wheat are caused chiefly by fungi, bacteria, nematodes, and viruses. The more important ones are stem rust, caused by *Puccinia graminis tritici*; leaf rust, caused by *P. recondita*; bunt, caused by *Tilletia* sp.; scab or fusarial head blight, caused by many species of *Fusarium*, particularly *F. roseum* (Fig. 5); and seedling blight and root rot, caused by many species of fungi, especially *Fusarium* sp., *Helminthosporium sativum*, *Ophiobolus graminis*, *Leptosphaeria herpotrichoides*, and *Pythium* sp. Most of these pathogens comprise many races that differ greatly in their parasitic capabilities on wheat. For example, stem rust of wheat consists of more than 300 distinct races. Throughout history, bunt has been a scourge to agriculture by decreasing yields, lowering seed quality, and interfering with threshing and processing operations. Bunt and smut spores coat surfaces of threshed grain, making necessary washing before milling; the cost of this extra operation is reflected in lower prices offered the farmer for smutted grain. Fusarial head blight is more prevalent in the Corn Belt, where the temperature and relative humidity are high during the blossoming period. Infected kernels contain substances toxic to man and certain animals. *See* PLANT VIRUS.

Root rots of wheat are ubiquitous diseases. They are debilitating and insidious, but usually inconspicuous. Most of the root-rotting pathogens live in

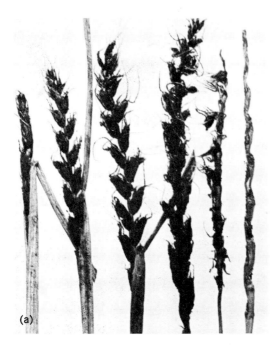

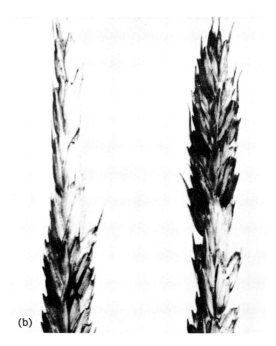

Fig. 5. Diseased spikes of cultivated wheat. (a) Loose smut, caused by *Ustilago nuda.* (b) Fusarial head blight, caused by *Fusarium* sp. (*Minnesota Agricultural Experiment Station*)

or on the seed, in soil, and on dead plants. They attack all underground parts of plants, blight the seedlings, rot the roots, and kill adult plants prematurely. *See* SOIL MICROBIOLOGY.

Wheat kernels are frequently discolored by fungi and bacteria, which often serve as the forerunners of infection for seedling blights and root rots, and which may also make dirty-looking flour or semolina (for macaroni). Moreover, storage molds, such as *Aspergillus.* and *Penicillium*, may invade wheat kernels after harvest and make the grains unsuitable for milling and baking.

Control measures. Although diseases of wheat cannot be prevented completely, they can be reduced substantially by good agricultural practices. The use of sound seed, treated with fungicides, eliminates the pathogens from the seed and protects them from soil-borne organisms. A good cropping sequence, coupled with the use of disease-resistant varieties, is highly recommended. Although most varieties may be only temporarily resistant, this greatly reduces the danger of destructive epidemics, particularly of stem rust and bunt. *See* FUNGISTAT AND FUNGICIDE; PLANT DISEASE.

[J. J. CHRISTENSEN/MILTON F. KERNKAMP]

PROCESSING

The milling process breaks open the wheat kernel and reduces the particles formed so as to separate the outer and inner portions of the kernel. Bran and germ are almost completely separated from the white interior portions of the kernel in the milling of refined flour. Milling of wheat was brought about through efforts to remove impurities and foreign material and after the discovery that the inside of the wheat kernel tastes better than the outside. Grinding wheat also aids mastication, and milling is necessary to produce flour for use in fabricated foods, such as bread.

Sifted meal keeps better than unsifted and pro-

duces a whiter product, which is usually preferred.

When the entire kernel is ground and no separations are made, the product is whole wheat flour.

Flour milling has become one of the principal industries in terms of value of product processed and of value added to the product during processing. Milling is a mechanical process; therefore, the number of persons employed per unit investment is less than for most industries.

The following steps are involved in milling wheat: wheat selection, blending, cleaning, conditioning or tempering, breaking, bolting, sieving, purifying, reducing, classifying, and some combination of maturing, bleaching, and diastatic or enriching treatment of the flour.

Cleaning is done with machines that use sieves and air currents to separate dirt, chaff, and foreign seeds from wheat. Other devices are available to remove metal or stone contamination and to wash wheat before it is milled. Water and often heat are added in the process called tempering or conditioning before the actual milling operation begins, to prevent the bran from fragmenting unduly during milling and to maintain proper milling conditions.

The initial step in actual milling, after the cleaning and tempering, is cracking wheat to small pieces between steel rolls that are corrugated with small grooves. This is called the breaking system. The pieces of broken kernel of various sizes and dimensions are separated by rotating sieves and by purifiers which combine sieves and air current to separate particles on the basis of size and density. The stocks thus produced are directed to either additional break rolls or smooth steel reduction rolls. The flow of material in a typical flour mill is as shown in Fig. 6.

Note that the flour produced comes from many different machines in the milling process. These flour streams can differ in quality. By combining

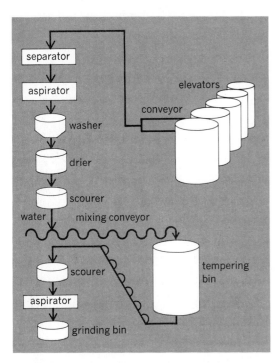

Fig. 6. Flow sheet of wheat cleaning. (*From M. E. Parker, E. H. Harvey, and E. S. Stateler, Elements of Food Engineering, vol. 1, Reinhold, 1952*)

starch granules have a particle size range from about 1 to 50 μ, while protein particles range from about 1 to 5 μ. Particles in these size ranges can be separated by air classification, whereby they are activated by a strong centrifugal force, produced by a rapidly rotating disk. As the particles are thrown toward the perimeter, they are met by strong air currents moving in the opposite direction. The airstream exerts a drag on the moving particles, first slowing the movement of the smaller, lighter material, eventually bringing them to a stop, and then reversing the direction of movement. Adjustment of either the rotating force or the velocity of the airstream makes possible a selection in the size of the particles separated.

Bulgur is a special processed-wheat product which is exported in large quantities. It is a partly debranned, parboiled wheat used either whole or cracked in many foods, such as soups, main dishes similar to rice, and desserts. Through sieving and fine grinding, the high-protein, nutritionally valuable portions of the wheat kernel are made available for food use, especially in developing countries. These take the form of meatlike foods, fermented products, and beverages for children.

[JOHN A. SHELLENBERGER]

Bibliography: I. Hlynka, *Wheat Chemistry and Technology*, 1964; G. E. Inglett, *Wheat: Production and Utilization*, 1974; M. A. Joslyn and J. A. Heid, *Food Processing Operations*, vol. 3, 1964; J. Lockwood, *Flour Milling*, 4th ed., 1960; W. Q. Loegering, J. W. Hendrix, and L. E. Browder, *The Rust Diseases of Wheat*, USDA Agr. Handb. no. 334, November 1967; E. S. Miller, *Studies in Practical Milling*, 1941; R. F. Peterson, *Wheat: Botany, Cultivation, and Utilization*, 1965; K. S. Quisenberry and L. P. Reitz (eds.), *Agronomy Monograph No. 13*, 1967; L. P. Reitz, *Wheat in the United States*, USDA Agr. Inform. Bull. no. 386, 1976; B. Sullivan, Wheat-based products for world use, *Cereal Sci. Today*, October 1967; Wheat Flour Institute, *From Wheat to Flour*, 1965.

Wine

Alcoholic beverages made by fermentation of the juice of fruits or berries. As defined by United States government agencies, wine is essentially the fermented alcoholic beverage made from grape juice. Wines from other materials are always required to show their source on the label, for example, apple wine, berry wine, and cherry wine. California produces over 80% of the grape wine made in the United States, and well over a hundred varieties of the cultivated grape (*Vitis vinifera*) are used.

Classification. This depends on the color, relative sweetness, alcoholic content, presence of carbon dioxide, the variety of grape, and the region where the grapes are grown. Wines may be red or white. In the production of red wines, the red anthocyanin pigments are extracted from the skins of blue grapes by allowing the fermentation to take place in contact with the skins. When white wines are made from dark grapes, the skins are separated before fermentation. The terms dry and sweet refer to the relative sugar content of a wine. Table wines contain less than 14% alcohol by volume, and dessert wines contain over 14%, usually 20%, alcohol. The higher alcohol content of dessert

flour streams, flour of different grades is produced. "Patent" grade is that flour portion freest from bran and germ contamination. The portions of the total flour not included in the patent grade are called "clears." A "straight" grade represents the total flour yield. The feed portion is about equally divided between bran and shorts.

Flours are milled for many purposes such as bread, pastries, cakes, cookies, or macaroni. This necessitates wheat selection and different processing to some extent, although the basic principles are not changed. Flours are manufactured from hard, soft, or durum wheat or combinations of these. The yield of 100 lb of wheat is usually 72 lb of flour and 28 lb of feed.

One of the newer developments in wheat processing is fine grinding and air classification of flour particles. Through this process, the flour produced by conventional milling systems can be more finely ground and fractionated into products having different compositions and properties. Grinding is accomplished in high-speed centrifugal machines, sometimes with centrifugal rotors having pins or blades rotating in opposite directions. The flour particles are projected at high velocities against hard blades or pins or the surface of the machine where the force of impact causes the particles to break into smaller pieces; correct use of airstreams can help increase particle impact force.

Wheat flour contains a low-protein, high-starch fraction and a high-protein, low-starch fraction; thus a protein shift can be accomplished by the separation of these two fractions. Particle size separations at cut points of 15–40 μ will separate fractions consisting principally of starch granules. Below 15 μ are principally broken starch granules and much of the protein matrix. Fine grinding makes the "shift" more complete because free

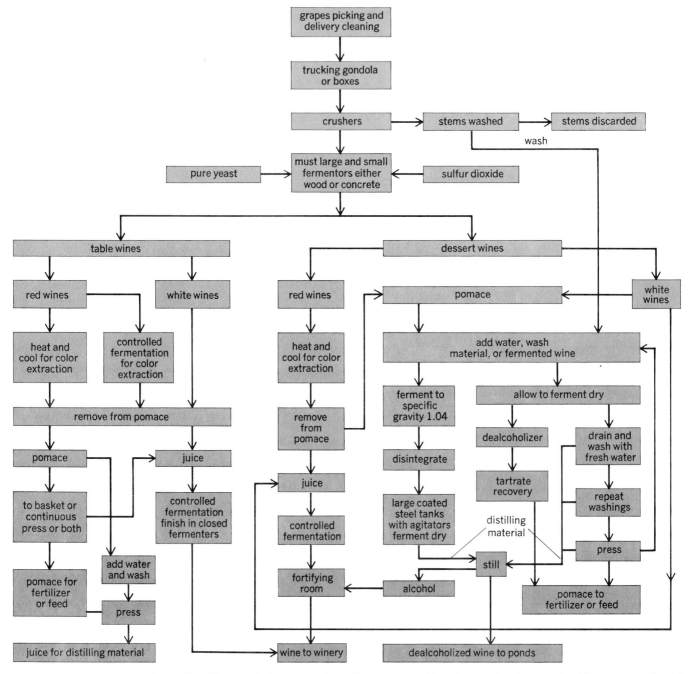

Fig. 1. Flow diagram of wine manufacture. The operations vary widely according to the type of wine produced.

(From L. A. Underkofler and R. J. Hickey, eds., Industrial Fermentations, vol. 1, Chemical Publishing, 1954)

wines is obtained by the addition of brandy, which is called fortification. Sparkling wines such as champagne and sparkling Burgundy contain carbon dioxide. Examples of red, dry, table wines are Burgundy, claret, Chianti, cabernet, barbera, and zinfandel. The first three wines are made from various grape varieties, and each has a characteristic color, body, and flavor. The last three are made of the corresponding grape varieties. Some important white table wines are Rhine wines (such as Moselle, Riesling, Traminer), Chablis, white Chianti, dry sauterne, and sweet sauterne.

Examples of dessert wines are angelica, an amber- or yellow-colored sweet wine without mus-

cat flavor, of California origin; muscatel, a sweet wine made in part from muscat grapes, with a pronounced muscat flavor; port, a deep-red color; tawny port, an amber-tinted sweet wine; white port, a light-colored sweet wine without muscat flavor; sherry, a wine with a characteristic flavor and aroma and varying sugar content, but less than 7%; and Tokay, a sweet wine with a pink tint.

Production. Grapes are harvested when they have reached the desired sugar and acid content; they are taken to the winery in boxes or in bulk. Several pickings are required to produce fine wines. The grapes go through a crusher-stemmer, which crushes the berries, but not the seeds, and

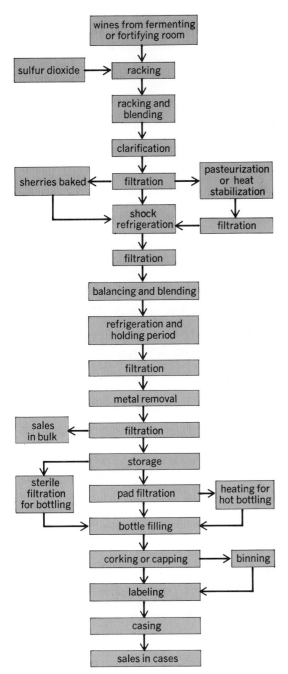

Fig. 2. Cellar operations in a winery. (*L. A. Underkofler and R. J. Hickey, eds., Industrial Fermentations, vol. 1, Chemical Publishing, 1954*)

removes the stems. The must, still containing seeds and skins, is pumped to fermentation tanks where it receives about 100–150 ppm of sulfur dioxide, SO_2, gas. This controls, to a large extent, the growth of bacteria and wild yeasts, whereas the various strains of wine yeast are adapted to this amount of SO_2. A pure yeast starter, consisting of various strains of *Saccharomyces cerevisiae*, is then added. In the production of white wines, the juice is separated from the skins and seeds at an early stage of the fermentation, often after 4–8 hr. The residue may be pressed and extracted for the manufacture of lower-quality wines, or it may be fermented to completion and used for distillation.

Many variations are in use in different wineries, depending on the type of wine to be made. The fermentation tanks, especially the large ones, are cooled in order to maintain the temperature of the wine at 23.9–29.4°C (Fig. 1). *See* FERMENTATION.

After the initial fermentation is over, the wine is transferred to the storage cellar for completion of fermentation, clarification, aging, stabilization, and bottling. These operations are called cellar practices (Fig. 2). The sediment of yeast and other insoluble matter is called lees. The new wine is drawn off, or racked, from the lees to avoid picking up undesirable flavors from the lees. Aging is then continued. Wines are often chilled to precipitate excess cream of tartar, the potassium acid tartrate from the grape, which otherwise might precipitate upon chilling of bottled wine. Champagne is made by allowing a secondary fermentation to occur with a special flocculating type of yeast, either in bottles, by the original French procedure, or in bulk, using pressure tanks followed by bottling. The carbon dioxide, CO_2, of sparkling wines is produced by yeast fermentation. Most sherry wines of California obtain their characteristic flavor and aroma by a heating process, called baking, over an extended period of time. Spanish sherries are made by the "flor" process, involving the participation of a film-forming yeast growing for many months at the surface of the wine in partially filled oak barrels. The yeast imparts the characteristic sherry flavor to the wine. No heating is used in this process.

Spoilage organisms. Wines, especially the sweet wines, are susceptible to spoilage by wild yeasts and bacteria. Growth of wild yeasts may occur in unpasteurized bottled wines, causing the wine to become turbid or form a sediment. In the absence of air, bacterial spoilage is caused principally by species of *Leuconostoc* and *Lactobacillus*. In the presence of air, species of *Acetobacter* may oxidize the alcohol of table wines to vinegar. Control measures are pasteurization of about 1 min at 62.8°C, use of SO_2, and sterilization by filtration through special filters. *See* FOOD SPOILAGE.

[EMIL M. MRAK; HERMAN J. PHAFF]

Bibliography: M. A. Amerine, H. W. Berg, and W. V. Cruess, *The Technology of Wine Making*, 3d ed., 1972; M. A. Amerine and V. L. Singleton, *Wine: An Introduction for Americans*, 1965; M. A. Joslyn and M. A. Amerine, *Dessert, Appetizer and Related Flavored Wines*, 1964; L. A. Underkofler and R. J. Hickey (eds.), *Industrial Fermentations*, vol. 1, 1954.

Xylitol

Xylitol is a natural sweetener found in many fruits and vegetables such as berries, yellow plums, and mushrooms. It is a white, odorless, crystalline powder with sweetness and caloric content equal to that of sucrose.

Metabolism. Xylitol is a normal intermediate in the metabolism of carbohydrates and is produced in humans at the rate of 5–15 g per day. It is metabolized in humans via the glucuronic acid–xylulose cycle, which requires very little insulin. Xylitol is absorbed slowly compared with glucose. As a result, peaks in blood glucose levels are avoided. Therefore, it is used as a sugar substitute for diabetics in a number of European countries. It is also used extensively in infusion solutions for parenteral nutrition in Japan and Germany. Animal tests have shown xylitol to exert inhibiting effects on fatty acid synthesis.

Xylitol is generally well tolerated when taken orally. Transient laxation has been observed at high doses; however, continued intake results in rapid adaptation.

Physical and chemical properties. The negative heat of solution of xylitol is 10 times higher than that of sucrose. As a result, xylitol provides a marked cooling effect when dissolved in the mouth. It also enhances mint-type flavors because of its sweet, cool taste.

Xylitol is stable to air and heat and is slightly hygroscopic, especially at relative humidities above 75%. At 76% relative humidity, xylitol has approximately the same hygroscopicity as sucrose, slightly less than mannitol, and much less than dextrose and sorbitol. It is very stable both in crystalline and aqueous solutions under the thermal processing conditions prevailing in the food industry. Generally, no fermentation caused by yeasts occurs in solutions containing xylitol. It is a poor substrate for most microorganisms.

Xylitol does not participate in the sometimes undesirable nonenzymatic browning (Maillard) reactions occurring when reducing sugars are heated in the presence of amino acids. If Maillard-type aromatics or flavoring agents are desirable, the reaction can be controlled by adding a small quantity of fructose.

Xylitol is easily soluble in water (approximately 160 g/100 ml) and sparingly soluble in 94% alcohol (approximately 1.7 g/100 ml). Its low melting point of about 94°C can be an advantage in confectionery production.

Production. Xylitol is commercially produced in Finland, with birch wood chips used as raw material. Xylans from wood chips are acid-hydrolyzed to xylose which is purified by using ion-exchange and chromatographic techniques and is subsequently hydrogenated to xylitol. This is purified and crystallized to produce pure food-grade xylitol. The production of xylitol is not, however, limited to birch wood as the raw material since a number of waste products such as oat hulls, corncobs, and bagasse can be used. The complex manufacturing process and the relatively low yields from bulky raw materials result in a high cost of production for xylitol.

Regulatory status. The use of xylitol in the United States is permitted by the Food and Drug Administration (FDA) under a regulation published in 1963 which states: "Xylitol may safely be used in foods for special dietary purposes, provided the amount used is not greater than that required to produce its intended effect."

Clinical research. A number of research scientists have reported in clinical experiments conducted in animals as well as humans that xylitol does not promote tooth decay since it cannot be utilized by oral microorganisms to produce acids which are primarily responsible for the formation of dental caries. Since sugar consumed between meals in the form of snacks or confectionery is believed to be highly cariogenic, the use of xylitol in such products could be beneficial.

Product development. The replacement of sucrose by xylitol in many foods may require certain minor process modifications because of minor differences in the properties of xylitol and sucrose. Xylitol does not exist in a glasslike state like sucrose, and its crystallization properties are somewhat different from sucrose. However, these differences in properties are not very significant, as a variety of baked goods, confectionery products, desserts, canned fruits and vegetables, jams and jellies, beverages, spices and relishes have been prepared with xylitol.

Confectionery. Extensive product development trials have been carried out at a number of food research laboratories in Europe to formulate confectionery products such as chewing gum, hard candy, caramels, toffee, and chocolate. In normal sucrose confectionery, corn syrups are added to control the crystallization characteristics of sucrose. Although corn syrups may serve a similar purpose in xylitol confectionery, they are not preferred because of their cariogenic nature. Research has been directed toward addition of other ingredients of lower cariogenicity to achieve desirable crystallization properties with xylitol.

The "sugarless" confectionery products on the market now contain sorbitol or mannitol, which are only about half as sweet as sucrose. It is, therefore, necessary to add artificial sweeteners such as saccharin to achieve the desired sweetness. Xylitol, being as sweet as sucrose, does not require the addition of artificial sweeteners, and sugarless confectioneries produced with xylitol have excellent taste and flavor properties.

A procedure for the manufacture of hard candies from xylitol has been developed by using the basic method of depositing liquid masses into molds. This is the preferred method since xylitol does not lend itself to being made into a plastic mass which can be pressed or cut into desired shapes. The candies formed are hard, glossy, and opaque with a pleasant sweet, cool taste.

Different varieties of sugarless chewing gum containing xylitol are now being produced commercially in many countries. Processing is slightly different from conventional methods. Depending on the gum base used, the kneading operation can be controlled with an aqueous xylitol solution or with glycerol. Xylitol should be used in a powder form with a median particle size corresponding to that for confectioners' sugar. It may be necessary to cool the grinder to avoid caking, which may result due to the low melting point of xylitol.

Xylitol-containing chocolates are presently being marketed in Scandinavia. Some changes have to be made in traditional production process to account for the lower viscosity of xylitol-containing products.

It is possible to produce xylitol-coated confectionery products such as chewing gum, chocolate, and tablets. The use of gelatin in warm coating with xylitol syrup appears to be indispensable to obtain a regular coating. The drying time for xylitol coating is longer than that for sucrose, which would require appropriate adjustments in the manufacturing process.   [AJIT K. KOTHARI]

Bibliography: M. Brin and O. N. Miller, The safety of xylitol, in H. L. Sipple and K. W. McNutt (eds.), *Sugars in Nutrition,* Nutrition Foundation,

Washington, 1974: U. Manz, E. Vanninen, and F. Voirol, Xylitol: Its properties and use as a sugar substitute in foods, *Food: R. A. Leatherhead Symposium on Sugar and Sugar Replacements*, London, Oct. 10, 1973: O. Touster, The metabolism of polyols, in H. L. Sipple and K. W. McNutt (eds.), *Sugars in Nutrition*, Nutrition Foundation, Washington, 1974.

Yeast

A collective name for those fungi which possess, under normal conditions of growth, a vegetative body (thallus) consisting, at least in part, of simple, individual, single cells. In addition, the cells making up the thallus may occur in pairs, in groups of three, or in straight or branched chains consisting of as many as 12 or more cells. Yeast plays a large part in industrial fermentation processes such as the production of ethanol, malt beverage, and wine and also in diseases of man, animals, and plants. *See* DISTILLED SPIRITS; WINE; YEAST, INDUSTRIAL.

Morphology. The shape and size of the individual cells of some species vary slightly, but in other species the cell morphology is extremely heterogeneous. The shape of yeast cells may be spherical, globose, ellipsoidal, elongate to cylindrical with rounded ends, more or less rectangular, pear-shaped, apiculate or lemon-shaped, ogival or pointed at one end, or tetrahedral (Fig. 1). The dimension of a spherical cell may vary from 2 to 10 microns (μ) in diameter. The length of cylindrical cells is often 20–30 μ and, in some cases, even greater.

The asexual multiplication of yeast cells occurs by a budding process, by the formation of cross walls or fission, and sometimes by a combination of these two processes. Yeast buds are sometimes called blastospores. When yeast reproduces by a fission mechanism, the resulting cells are termed arthrospores.

In some genera of yeast true septate mycelium is formed, for example, in some species of *Candida* and always in *Trichosporon*. In *Candida*, the mycelium, if present, remains intact; that is, it does not break up at the septa. In *Trichosporon*,

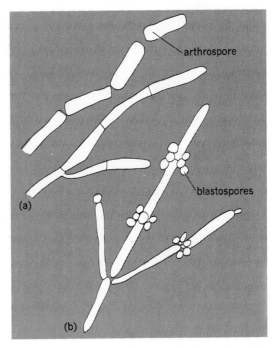

Fig. 2. Yeast mycelia. (*a*) True septate showing break to form arthrospore. (*b*) Pseudomycelium.

the mycelium breaks apart into arthrospores which at first are rectangular but often develop rounded ends when mature (Fig. 2a). Many yeasts produce a type of thallus which is termed a pseudomycelium. In a pseudomycelium the component cells are formed by elongation of buds and not by the formation of septa. Usually a group of characteristically arranged blastospores develops at the junctions of cells making up a pseudomycelium (Fig. 2b).

Yeasts are also characterized by certain macromorphological features. These are studied as slant cultures and as giant colonies. Slant cultures are made by inoculating the yeast as a thin line on the center of an agar slope in a medium which may be malt extract or synthetic. After several weeks of growth the culture may be described with respect to: color—for example, cream, pink, yellow, brown, black, white, and intermediate shades; surface—smooth, wrinkled, warty, glossy, dull; texture—pasty, shiny, tough; cross section—flat, raised, hemispherical, extent of spreading; and border—entire, hairy, irregular. Giant colonies are usually inoculated on malt gelatin, by a light, pinpoint inoculation. Macromorphological features usually develop more characteristically on gelatin than on agar media (Fig. 3). The description of the growth after about 3 weeks of growth is similar to that which is employed for the description of streak cultures.

Yeast cytology. Yeast cells are surrounded by a wall, which in the case of bakers' yeast and many other species consists of polysaccharides such as glucan and mannan, a small amount of chitin, protein, lipids, and minerals. The filamentous yeasts have a higher chitin content than the budding yeasts. Some species contain as yet unidentified components. With the electron microscope bud scars can be observed in the walls of yeast. Suc-

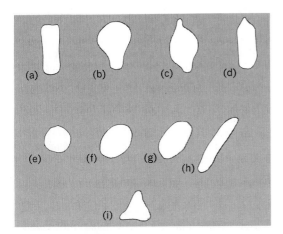

Fig. 1. The cell shapes of yeasts can be extremely varied. (*a*) Rectangular. (*b*) Pear-shaped. (*c*) Apiculate. (*d*) Ogival. (*e*) Spherical. (*f*) Globose. (*g*) Ellipsoidal (oval). (*h*) Elongate. (*i*) Tetrahedral.

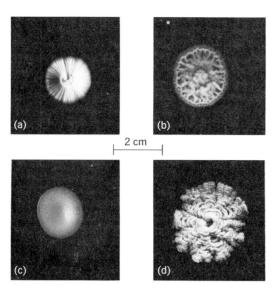

Fig. 3. Giant yeast colonies. (a) *Saccharomyces rouxii*, (b) *Sporobolomyces pararoseus*, (c) *Rhodotorula glutinis*, and (d) *Saccharomyces cerevisiae*, all after 6 weeks of growth on wort gelatin at 20°C.

cessive buds, 20–40 from one bakers' yeast cell, are always formed at different places on the cell surface. A cell also contains a birth scar, which differs in appearance from a bud scar. Yeast cells are generally uninucleate. The cytoplasm may contain one or more vacuoles. In addition the cytoplasm may contain lipid globules, volutin (polyphosphate) granules, mitochondria, and submicroscopic particles. When yeast cells are treated with iodine, they usually stain deep brown, because of their high glycogen content.

Sexual reproduction of yeasts. Yeasts are divided into sporogenous and asporogenous groups, or perfect and imperfect yeasts.

Ascospores. The sexual spores of yeasts are ascospores, which are formed in simple structures, often a vegetative cell. Such asci are called naked asci because of the absence of an ascocarp, which is a more complex fruiting body found in the higher Ascomycetes. If the vegetative cells are diploid, a cell may transform directly into an ascus after the

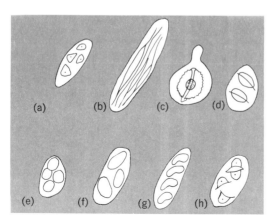

Fig. 4. Shapes of ascospores of various yeasts. (a) Helmet. (b) Needle. (c) Walnut. (d) Saturn. (e) Spherical. (f) Oval. (g) Kidney or crescent. (h) Hat.

$2n$ nucleus undergoes a reduction or meiotic division.

In the case of haploid yeasts, a conjugation or fusion between two cells normally occurs. The fusion of the cytoplasmic contents of the two cells is called plasmogamy. This is followed by fusion of the two haploid nuclei, or karyogamy. Meiosis then follows. Each of the haploid nuclei resulting from meiosis gathers cytoplasmic material around it and finally develops into a characteristically shaped ascospore. The spores in such a process are formed by "free cell formation," in contrast to spore delineation by cleavage of the cytoplasm. The shape of ascospores may be spherical, oval, kidney- or crescent-shaped, hat-shaped, helmet-shaped, hemispherical, needle-shaped, walnut-shaped, or saturn-shaped (Fig. 4).

The number of ascospores per ascus varies with the species. Some contain a single spore, others one or two, two to four, or four to eight. In rare cases, more than eight spores are formed. In some yeasts the asci rupture soon after maturation, and the spores are liberated into the medium. In others, the spores remain in the ascus until they germinate. The heat resistance of ascospores is only slightly greater than that of the vegetative cells. The number and shape of the ascospores are important characters in generic descriptions. The species of most genera have only one type of ascospore, but sometimes more than one shape is found among the species of a genus, for example, in *Endomycopsis* and *Hansenula*.

The ease with which yeasts form ascospores varies enormously with the species. In some, an abundance of ascospores is formed on nearly all media of growth. In others, special sporulation media must be used, and often the percentage of asci is small. Another complication is that certain yeasts lose the ability to sporulate upon prolonged cultivation in pure culture.

Imperfect and perfect yeasts. Certain haploid yeasts have been shown to be heterothallic; that is, sporulation can occur only if strains of opposite mating type (sometimes indicated by + and − strains) are mixed on sporulation media. If no mating type is known, a yeast is considered to be imperfect. The perfect yeasts are classified in the order Saccharomycetales (Endomycetales), and the imperfect yeasts belong in the class Fungi Imperfecti, order Cryptococcales (Torulopsidales). Besides these there are yeasts which produce spores on a short stalk, or sterigma. After maturation these so-called ballistospores are shot off by a drop-excretion mechanism. Vegetative reproduction occurs by budding, true mycelium, pseudomycelium, arthrospores, or by various combinations of these mechanisms. These yeasts are members of the order Sporobolomycetales. There is evidence that they belong to the class Basidiomycetes and that ballistospores are thus a type of basidiospore.

Physiological properties. Some yeasts have the ability to carry out an alcoholic fermentation. Other yeasts lack this property. In addition to the fermentative type of metabolism, fermentative yeasts as a rule also have a respiratory type of metabolism whereas nonfermentative yeasts have only a respiratory, or oxidative, metabolism. Fermentation may be represented by Eq. (1), respiration by Eq. (2). Both reactions produce energy,

$$C_6H_{12}O_6 \rightarrow 2C_2H_5OH + 2CO_2 \qquad (1)$$

$$C_6H_{12}O_6 + 6O_2 \rightarrow 6CO_2 + 6H_2O \qquad (2)$$

with respiration producing by far the most, which is used in part for synthetic reactions, such as assimilation and growth. Part is lost as heat. In addition, small or sometimes large amounts of by-products are formed, including organic acids, esters, aldehydes, glycerol, and higher alcohols. When a fermenting yeast culture is aerated, fermentation is suppressed and respiration increases. This phenomenon is called the reaction of Louis Pasteur.

Fermentation. Yeasts cannot ferment pentose, or five-carbon sugars. In the case of disaccharides, trisaccharides, and polysaccharides, hydrolysis by hydrolytic enzymes, or hydrolases, must precede fermentation. There is evidence that some hydrolytic enzymes are located in the peripheral layer of the cell. Such hydrolases may be secreted into the medium as extracellular enzymes. Species of yeasts are often differentiated on the basis of the various hydrolases which they possess. *See* CARBOHYDRATE.

Some simple rules of fermentation have been formulated. If a yeast cannot ferment glucose, it cannot ferment any other sugar. If a yeast can ferment glucose, it can also ferment fructose and mannose (although often at different rates), but not always galactose. If a yeast ferments maltose, it usually cannot ferment lactose and vice versa.

Respiration and assimilation. Yeasts differ greatly in their ability to respire and to assimilate organic substrates. Depending on the species, yeasts can utilize such compounds as pentoses (D-xylose, D-arabinose, L-arabinose, D-ribose), methyl-pentoses (L-rhamnose), sugar alcohols (mannitol, sorbitol, dulcitol, erythritol, adonitol), organic acids (lactic, acetic, succinic, citric, gluconic, 2-ketogluconic, 5-ketogluconic, and many other acids), polysaccharides (soluble starch, inulin), and even such compounds as i-inositol.

The source of nitrogen may be organic or inorganic. All yeasts, with rare exceptions, can use ammonium ion for the synthesis of proteins. Others can utilize nitrate, and still others can use nitrite but not nitrate. Yeasts also can absorb intact amino acids from the medium. There is considerable variation in the ability of yeasts to deaminate individual amino acids. Lysine, as a single nitrogen source, is used by few yeasts. Glutamic acid is utilized by nearly all yeasts. Sulfur is ordinarily supplied as sulfate, although some yeasts grow better when the sulfur is supplied as cysteine or methionine. The following mineral salts and concentrations are required by yeasts in a medium: monobasic potassium phosphate, KH_2PO_4, 0.1%; magnesium sulfate, $MgSO_4$, 0.05%; sodium chloride, NaCl, 0.01%; and calcium chloride, $CaCl_2$, 0.01%. In addition, the following trace elements should be added to a synthetic medium: boron, copper, zinc, iron, manganese, molybdenum, and iodine.

Special synthetic products are carotenoid pigments, produced by species of *Rhodotorula* and *Sporobolomyces* (β-carotene is responsible for a yellow color; torulin and torularhodin are responsible for pink colors). Some species of the genus *Cryptococcus* produce a starchlike polysaccharide in acidic media. In addition, species of *Cryptococcus*, *Rhodotorula*, and some other yeasts produce capsules, consisting of various polysaccharides.

Yeast ecology. Yeasts are not as ubiquitous in nature as are bacteria. Many species have highly specific habitats, whereas others are found on a greater variety of substrates in nature.

Soil. Soil may be considered as a reservoir of yeasts. Active growth in soil occurs only under favorable conditions, such as those found in fruit orchards and meadowlands. However, small numbers of a great variety of yeasts are found in many types of soil. Yeasts belonging to the genera *Lipomyces* and *Schwanniomyces* have been isolated only from soil.

Trees. Other yeasts have their natural habitat in the exudates or slime fluxes of trees. The yeasts found in exudates of coniferous trees generally differ from those in exudates of deciduous trees. Species of *Nadsonia* have been found only in tree exudates; certain species of *Hansenula*, *Saccharomycodes*, *Pichia*, *Saccharomyces*, and *Endomyces* are specifically associated with certain trees.

Insects. Since insects, such as *Drosophila*, frequently use sap exudates for breeding and sometimes for feeding purposes, yeasts can be found in appreciable numbers in the intestinal tract of such insects. Bark beetles, which live in the cambium layer of coniferous as well as deciduous trees, and the wood-boring ambrosia beetles also have been shown to have a specific yeast flora associated with them. Many species of yeast have been found in nature only in association with certain insects. Yeasts are rapidly digested by insects, and in this way they form an important part of their diet. The nectar of flowers is another habitat for yeasts. Those flowers which are much frequented by bees are especially likely to contain large numbers of yeast. The intestinal tract of warm-blooded animals is also a habitat for yeasts. In some cases the yeast is so dependent on its host that it has lost the ability to grow at room temperature and in the common media used for propagation of yeasts. An example is the monospecific genus *Saccharomycopsis*, which has been found only in the intestinal tract of rabbits. *S. guttulata* grows only at about 37°C and in very complex media. Interestingly, in the presence of about 15% free carbon dioxide its minimum temperature for growth is lowered to 30°C.

Pathogens. Whereas most yeasts associated with warm-blooded animals are nonpathogenic, a number of at least potentially pathogenic yeasts are known. With the expanding use of antibiotics, the natural balance of microbes in the gastrointestinal tract of mammals appears to have been disturbed, and yeast infections are on the increase. The most common locations of infections by yeasts are the skin, especially the mucosa, and the respiratory tract, but occasionally systemic infections occur.

Candida albicans is the most common cause of yeast infections in man. In medical literature, it is often referred to as *Monilia*. The basic cause of pathogenicity of *C. albicans* is not clear, since many normal individuals, while carriers of this yeast, experience little if any ill effects. Diseases caused by *C. albicans* include thrush in the oral cavity of infants, infections of the skin, nails, bronchi, lungs, vagina, and the intestinal tract. Other species of *Candida*, such as *C. tropicalis*, *C. parapsilosis*, and *C. guilliermondii*, are more rarely associated with yeast infections. In general, the diseases in which species of *Candida* are involved are called candidiasis or moniliasis.

Cryptococcus neoformans (*Torulopsis histolytica*, *Cryptococcus hominis*) causes a disease called cryptococcosis or torulosis. It is relatively rare, but often fatal. In man, the yeast develops in the central nervous system and induces a chronic and often fatal meningitis. Sporadic cases have been reported from all continents, but no epidemic has ever been reported, and thus the disease does not seem to be contagious. It is difficult to find *Cr. neoformans* in nature, but it has been found rather regularly in pigeon droppings and rarely in soil. Another yeast which may occasionally become pathogenic is *T. glabrata*. It has been found associated with diseases similar to those caused by *Candida albicans*, and occasionally it may cause a systemic infection. *Pityrosporum ovale* (bottle bacillus) can frequently be found on the skin, especially the scalp, of persons suffering from seborrheic dermatitis or pityriasis (dandruff). Although some believe that this yeast is responsible for these diseases, most of the evidence points to the fact that *P. ovale* is a harmless saprophyte of man and that it occurs on the scalp because of its requirement of oils or fats for growth.

Some mycotic infections by true fungi are characterized by yeastlike cells in the infected tissues (yeast phase), whereas in culture the causative organisms produce hyphae and look like molds (mycelial saprophytic phase). This is called the phenomenon of dimorphism. An example is *Blastomyces dermatitidis*, the causal agent of North American blastomycosis.

Plant pathogenic yeasts are limited to a few species. These are *Nematospora coryli*, a yeast with needle-shaped ascospores, and a yeastlike fungus, *Ashbya gossypii*, producing similar ascospores. The diseases which result from infection by *N. coryli* are yeast spot in lima beans and soybeans; stigmatomycosis of the fruits of tomatoes, citrus fruits, and others; and discoloration of cotton bolls. The last plant is also the principal host for *A. gossypii*. The yeast is transmitted by plant bugs and other biting insects. *See* PLANT DISEASE.

Yeasts in food spoilage. Yeasts are important as spoilage organisms of a great variety of foods. Specific types occur, depending primarily on the composition of the food. Sugar-tolerant, or osmophilic, yeasts occur on dried fruits, syrups, honey, and the like. Examples are *Saccharomyces rouxii*, *Schizosaccharomyces octosporus*, and the yeastlike fungus *Eremascus albus*. Species of *Debaryomyces* are usually highly salt-tolerant and occur in brines and on processed meats, such as bacon, hams, and sausage. Dairy products may be spoiled by lactose-fermenting yeasts. Some species of *Torulopsis* and of *Zygosaccharomyces* (haploid forms of *Saccharomyces*) may spoil salad dressing and similar products because of their great tolerance to vinegar. *Endomycopsis fibuliger* forms starch-splitting enzymes and can cause spoilage of cereal products and grains. *See* FOOD MICROBIOLOGY; FOOD SPOILAGE.

[EMIL M. MRAK; HERMAN J. PHAFF]

Bibliography: A. H. Cook (ed.), *The Chemistry and Biology of Yeasts*, 1958; J. Lodder and N. J. W. Kreger-Van Rij, *The Yeasts: A Taxonomic Study*, 1952; H. J. Phaff, M. W. Miller, and E. M. Mrak, *The Life of Yeasts*, 1966.

Yeast, industrial

Those yeast strains used for the commercial production of fermented beverages or other fermented foods, baking purposes, and the production of vitamins, enzymes, proteins (food and feed yeasts), alcohol, and glycerol. In most instances, definite species of yeast are employed for each of these processes. In many cases, induced mutant strains or genetic hybrids of yeast are selected for optimal results.

Fermented beverages. The processes involved in alcoholic fermentation will not be discussed in detail. These beverages are generally classified by the two broad classes of raw materials which serve as substrates for the yeast activity. The first of these is based on a substrate which contains a supply of directly fermentable sugars. These are principally fruits and berries for the production of wine. The second involves substrates which are a potential source of fermentable sugars, mainly in the form of starches which must be converted either by plant enzymes (amylases of germinated barley) or from fungi (such as *Aspergillus oryzae*). Conversion of starches to fermentable sugars is necessary because most industrial yeasts cannot ferment starch and other polysaccharides directly. Beer and sake are examples of alcoholic beverages produced from the second group of substrates. *See* DISTILLED SPIRITS; FERMENTATION; WINE.

Baker's yeast. This product, during the course of history, has undergone many changes.

Leaven. This, as used for the fermentation of dough in breadmaking, was mentioned in the Bible, and was probably a mixture of yeast and lactobacilli propagated in a dough medium. Leaven is still used in some remote areas, as well as being the basis of the French sour dough process, and relies upon the use of a starter or mother sponge, which consists primarily of a portion of the previously fermented batch of dough. In the sourdough process, this starter contains a mixture of a yeast (*Saccharomyces exiguus*) and a heterofermentative lactic acid bacterium (*Lactobacillus sanfrancisco*), which propagate side by side in the dough. This symbiotic growth depends upon the fact that the yeast involved utilizes only glucose but not maltose in the dough, whereas the bacterium does not use glucose but maltose, thus creating no competition for an energy source in the dough.

Barm. From the Middle Ages until the beginning of the 19th century, excess yeast from brewing and winemaking industries, called barm, was employed. Barm was relatively unsatisfactory because of its variable quality and unstable nature, although the source was quite dependable, since virtually every center of population had a brewery and, in season, winemaking operations.

Production. The specific production of yeast for breadmaking as a distinct manufacturing operation and with some degree of control depended upon several innovations. The first was the growth of baker's yeast on a grain mash, which was improved by the passage of a gentle stream of air.

From the researches of Louis Pasteur the need for intense aeration was recognized, resulting in further improvement in yeast yield accompanied by a reduction in the production of ethanol. During World War I a shortage of grain led to the introduction of molasses, a by-product of sugar production, as the fermentable substrate. This was supplemented by phosphate and ammonia to form the growth medium for the baker's yeast. The last improvement was to change the so-called batch process, in which all of the nutrients are supplied initially, to the use of incremental feeding schedules, where the rate of substrate addition is carefully matched to follow the growth curve of the yeast. In this process, a low sugar concentration is maintained so that the respiratory activity is maximized to greatly increase the yield of yeast and to suppress alcohol formation which, in the production of baker's yeast, is an undesirable by-product.

Yeast strain. Today, baker's yeast is composed almost exclusively of cells of one or more selected strains of *S. cerevisiae*. It is marketed in the form of cakes of compressed fresh yeast cells whose moisture content is about 70% or as granules of yeast masses which have been dehydrated to about 7.5% moisture content. Different strains are used for the two forms, and production schedules differ so that the stability and dough-raising properties of each form are maximized. Usage of the dried form has increased, although the moist compressed yeast is still commonly used in areas with temperate climates and relatively short distribution times.

Nutrient sources. Molasses has essentially replaced mashed grain and other substrates as a source of carbon, energy, and other essential nutrients. Depending upon cost, availability, and composition, beet molasses, refiner's cane molasses, and blackstrap cane molasses are used. Less frequently, high-test cane molasses, which is a concentrate of the original cane juice, may be used. The molasses is diluted, clarified, and decolorized before use. Blending of the various types is common, depending upon their composition. For example, in the case of beet molasses most of the assimilable sugar is sucrose, whereas in the various types of cane molasses appreciable portions of glucose and fructose are present. Sterilization of the molasses is necessary and is accomplished by heating to 100–110°F (38–43°C) for about 1 hr with the pH value between 6.0 and 8.0 to prevent carmelization of the sugars. Since beet molasses is deficient in biotin, a vitamin generally required for growth of *S. cerevisiae*, blackstrap molasses, which is rich in this growth substance, is generally added. It is usually advantageous to use as high a proportion of blackstrap molasses as possible, as it is usually richer in the various growth substances required. When blackstrap or other types of cane molasses are not available, other materials such as malt and grain extracts, corn-steep liquor, and yeast extract may be added to beet molasses to supply essential nutrients.

Nitrogen is supplied in the form of ammonium sulfate and ammonium hydroxide to maintain a pH of 3.8–4.5 since at higher pH values the danger of bacterial infection increases markedly. Potassium is usually present in sufficient amounts in molasses substrates, although phosphate is usually supplied as dibasic sodium phosphate and magnesium as magnesium sulfate.

Culture aeration. In the presence of sufficient oxygen, the yeast metabolism is chiefly oxidative, and the crop per unit amount of raw material used may be increased by a factor of 20; thus the fermentation tanks are vigorously aerated. Cooling is necessary since oxidative metabolism also creates much heat. The temperature is kept at 26–30°C, because higher temperatures influence the keeping and baking qualities of the yeast unfavorably. Foaming of the culture liquid during the period of aeration is controlled by the periodic addition of various antifoam compounds. After all of the nutrients have been added, permitting a sufficient degree of multiplication (usually three or four generations of the last stepwise inoculum), aeration is continued and carbohydrate is still added to ripen the yeast. During the ripening period, young buds mature and the yeast increases its content of reserve carbohydrates (glycogen and trehalose) and improves its storage stability.

Moist cake form. For the manufacture of compressed moist cake baker's yeast, after the completion of the growth and ripening phases, the wort is centrifuged and concentrated about tenfold. This resulting concentrate, containing about 4 lb of yeast per gallon (0.74 kg/liter), is washed, recentrifuged, and pressed in a filter press. The yeast scraped from the press is placed in a mixer with a small amount of vegetable oils, which are added to facilitate extrusion of the yeast into a bar and to improve appearance. Handling the yeast after growth at reduced temperatures improves the stability of the yeast cake and also aids in the reduction of contamination.

Active dry form. Active dry yeast manufacturing utilizes specially selected strains of *S. cerevisiae*, and the feeding schedule in the fermentor is such that the reserve carbohydrate becomes as high as possible. The compressed yeast from this operation is usually extruded from a machine into thin threads, which are dried on trays in an airflow of carefully controlled temperature and humidity to a final moisture content of approximately 7.5%. The yeast is then packed into moisture-proof containers, with oxygen excluded, and refrigerated. Dried yeast is stable for many months under refrigeration, especially when packaged under a nitrogen atmosphere. Dried yeast must be rehydrated in warm water (approximately 43°C), since lower temperatures cause an excessive leaking of cell contents and a definite loss in baking quality.

Baking tests. With both compressed cake baker's yeast and active dried baker's yeast, standardized baking tests are conducted to evaluate the quality of the product. While much lower in moisture content, dried baker's yeast must be used in amounts between 40 and 50% of the weight normally used for pressed yeast, which means that, on a dry weight basis, active dried yeast has approximately 65% of the activity of the compressed moist cake yeast. While possessing a much longer shelf life than the compressed yeast, the dried yeast's lower activity may be due to a number of causes. Among these are the different yeast strains employed, difference in the method of multiplication, loss of viability during drying and in reconstitution, and excretion of various enzymes and cofactors during reconstitution.

Food and feed yeasts. These yeasts are produced for human and animal consumption, and represent valuable dietary additions of proteins, vitamins of the B complex, and minerals. They are produced from a variety of raw materials and by widely different processes. Some, known as secondary yeasts, represent a by-product of the brewer and distillery industries; others, the primary yeasts, are grown specifically as food or feed sources from cane or beet molasses, hydrolyzed starch, cheese whey, spent sulfite waste liquor of the paper industry, acid-hydrolyzed wood, and various agricultural wastes. Food yeasts differ from feed (fodder) yeasts in quality characteristics. Generally, food yeasts exhibit lower bacterial and mold counts; higher levels of vitamins; higher protein content; a bland flavor; light color; and the absence of obnoxious microorganisms, added food ingredients, or fillers than do feed yeasts. Because food yeasts are intended for human consumption, rigid chemical and microbiological standards have been established by professional groups and government agencies and may be augmented by individual food processers and formulators to meet specific processing conditions and desired dietary standards.

Raw materials. The choice of raw materials for the manufacture of food or feed yeasts usually depends upon cost and availability. Excellent sources of carbohydrates are beet molasses, blackstrap molasses of the sugarcane industry, and hydrol, the residual syrup from the corn sugar industry. Another inexpensive substrate is spent sulfite liquor, the waste product of the sulfite pulping process of the paper industry. About 400 lb (180 kg) of carbon compounds which are utilizable by yeasts are contained in the waste liquor from each ton (0.9 metric ton) of paper pulp. These carbon compounds consist mainly of hexoses, pentoses, and acetic acid. The proportions vary greatly with the type of wood. Since sulfur dioxide is toxic to yeast, steam stripping or neutralization by lime is commonly employed to prevent inhibitory concentrations of sulfur dioxide in the raw material. Acid-hydrolyzed wood as a source of fermentable sugar is fairly costly, and thus the manufacture of food yeasts from this source is less economical than that from sulfite waste liquor or the other sources. The use of agricultural wastes, such as milk whey, fruit wastes, citrus peel hydrolyses, and cull potatoes, has the disadvantage of being seasonal in supply. Some wastes also are impractical because of the inability to collect sufficient quantities in a central location to provide a reliable supply year-round.

Yeast strain. The choice of yeast depends upon the substrate, availability, and growing conditions. Yeasts of the genus *Saccharomyces* are suitable only with those substrates with readily fermentable hexoses, such as molasses and corn syrup hydrol. The pentose sugars present in wood are not utilizable by *Saccharomyces* species; however, *Candida utilis* (*Torulopsis utilis*, Torula yeasts) can utilize a much greater array of compounds than *S. cerevisiae*, and have the ability to respire pentoses as well as hexoses. This ability to utilize pentoses makes it the yeast of choice to grow on substrates of wood hydrolysate and sulfite waste liquor from the paper industry. *Kluyveromyces fragilis* has the ability to utilize the disaccharide lactose present as the primary sugar in cheese whey.

Production process. Regardless of the substrate used and the yeast species or strain selected, growth is conducted in large fermentors under highly aerated conditions with carbohydrate sources, nitrogen, phosphate, and potassium supplements added at a rate which parallels the growth rate of the yeast. Some of these processes operate on a continuous basis, where the rate of substrate addition equals the rate of withdrawal of yeast-containing effluent. In others, the batch process is commonly used. At least six different commercial processes are presently in use. After growth, the yeast suspension is concentrated by centrifugation and is usually dried on drum driers. The inactivated yeast product is then used for supplementation of human diets or in animal feed mixtures. Although these yeasts contain all of the essential amino acids needed by higher animals and humans, the sulfur-containing amino acids L-cysteine and L-methionine, as well as tryptophan, occur in suboptimal concentrations. For this reason, microbial or single-cell proteins are most effective as supplements (up to 50%) in animal diets, rather than as a sole source of protein.

Vitamin production by yeasts. A number of yeasts (for example, *C. utilis* and *Hansenula anomala*) can synthesize all of the necessary vitamins required for growth from simple substrate precursors. However, many yeasts, among them most of the species of *Saccharomyces*, require one or more vitamins in the medium to supplement the nutrients which they can synthesize themselves. However, although requiring an exogenous source of several vitamins, *S. cerevisiae* is able to concentrate and absorb quite large quantities of the B vitamin complex from the medium during growth and thus form enriched products. Therefore, by supplementing the medium with crude sources of these particular vitamins (thiamin, nicotinic acid, and biotin) or sometimes even their precursors, yeasts of exceptionally high vitamin content can be made. Dried yeasts enriched in this manner are sold for therapeutic uses. Baker's and brewer's yeasts, as well as *C. utilis*, are good sources of thiamin, riboflavin, pyridoxin, and biotin; pantothenic, nicotinic, folic, and *para*-aminobenzoic acids; and choline and inositol.

Some yeasts produce exceptionally large amounts of a particular vitamin; for example, *Ermothecium ashbyi* and *Ashbya gossypii* can oversynthesize, and selected strains are known to produce 4.5–5 g of riboflavin per liter of growth medium. Strains for the production of riboflavin are genetically selected, grow optimally under aerobic conditions at 26–28°C, and utilize lipids (for example, corn oil or soybean oil) preferentially as a carbon source. Organic nitrogen and accessory factors supplied by the addition of corn-steep liquor, yeast extract, or distiller solubles are required. Most of the overproduction of riboflavin occurs after active growth ceases, and maximum yields have been reported in 6–7 days. High yields of this magnitude can compete very well with the synthetically produced vitamins.

Strains of *Saccharomyces* can produce as much as 7–10% of the dry weight as ergosterol. This sterol can be transformed by ultraviolet radiation into vitamin D_2 (calciferol), a valuable feed supplement for mammals.

Production of β-carotene is known for yeasts belonging to the genera *Cryptococcus* and *Rhodotorula*. The concentration, however, is too low to be economically important when compared with the production of this vitamin by other fungi (*Blakeslea trispora*).

Yeast sources of enzymes. Invertase, an enzyme which splits sucrose into a mixture of glucose and fructose (invert sugar), is produced in excess by baker's yeast, *S. cerevisiae*. When grown aerobically on a sucrose substrate, the enzyme is induced and the yeast may contain 50–100 times the concentration of invertase needed to maintain fermentation at its maximal rate. Invertase, a mannan-containing glycoprotein, is associated with the yeast cell walls and can be obtained in soluble form by treating the cells with either toluene or chloroform followed by cell autolysis. The purified enzyme is used in the production of artificial honey and invert sugar, and in the manufacture of cream-center chocolate confections.

Kluyveromyces fragilis, a lactose-fermenting yeast, is the primary supply of the enzyme lactase. This enzyme is also inducible. In ice cream, lactase prevents crystallization of lactose and, in other dairy products, reduces the content of this sugar. A very significant proportion of the world's population is lactose-sensitive, due to the absence of lactase in the intestinal tract. Such individuals experience gastrointestinal disturbances when lactose-containing dairy products are ingested. Some strains of *K. fragilis* produce an exocellular pectic enzyme, polygalacturonase, of high purity. Commercial application of this yeast-produced enzyme is, at the present, limited.

Lipid materials. Some species of yeasts produce remarkably high levels of lipid materials, but commercial production by yeasts has not been economical except during periods of war. A number of yeast species have been used experimentally or commercially for fat production, for example, *Trichosporon pullulans*, *Lipomyces* species, *Metschnikowia reukaufii*, *Oospora lactis* (*Geotrichum candidum*), and *Rhodotorula* species. They have primarily an oxidative metabolism and can convert carbohydrates to lipid materials. Production is maximum under conditions where protein synthesis is limited, usually when the nitrogen or phosphate content of the medium is low. Under such conditions, while the yield of cells is not maximized, the fat content may be up to 50–60% of the dry weight. The lipids produced include triglycerides, fatty acids, phospholipids, and sterols. The bulk of the fatty acids are unsaturated, and the main sterol is ergosterol. Up to 15–18 g of lipid material can be produced from 100 g of sugar substrate under suitable growth conditions.

Glycerol and other polyhydroxy alcohols. The formation of glycerol by wine yeasts and other species of *Saccharomyces* has been known for many years, where 2–3% of the weight of the sugar fermented consists of this trihydric alcohol. However, in nonaerated cultures supplied with calcium sulfite and a pH of 6.7–7.0, yeasts can produce glycerol up to 27% of the fermentable sugar weight. Increased yields of glycerol can also be obtained when fermentation is carried out in the presence of 30% sodium carbonate. High yields of glycerol are highly dependent upon the selection of suitable yeast strains. Recovery under conditions of sulfite addition or alkaline conditions is complicated by the presence of the large amounts of salt.

As production of glycerol by yeast was in great demand only during wartime, a more recent discovery has potential commercial application. Under highly aerobic conditions, many haploid, osmoduric species of *Saccharomyces*, *Pichia*, and related imperfect yeasts belonging to the genus *Torulopsis* produce, in the absense of steering agents such as sulfite or carbonate, various combinations of glycerol, erythritol, D-arabitol, and sometimes D-mannitol. Under optimum conditions, where a low phosphate level in the medium favors a synthesis of these compounds, as much as 40% of the glucose supplied can be converted to polyhydric alcohols.

Polysaccharides. In recent years, there has been a considerable interest developed in the use of microbial polysaccharides for various industrial purposes, including use in crude oil recovery and as modifiers of texture and consistency in food products. Phosphomannans, produced by certain species of *Hansenula*, *Pichia*, and *Pachysolen*, are among the most interesting and promising products. Selected strains of these yeasts have the remarkable ability to convert up to 50% of the glucose in the medium into extracellular, capsular polysaccharides, which are subsequently released into the culture medium. Virtually all these polymers contain only mannose in addition to phosphate. Isolated phosphomannans form highly viscous, clear solutions, which are quite resistant to bacterial attack. They have been used experimentally for controlling the consistency of various food products. See INDUSTRIAL MICROBIOLOGY.

[MARTIN W. MILLER]

Bibliography: H. J. Phaff, M. W. Miller, and E. M. Mrak, *The Life of Yeasts*, 2d ed., in press; G. Reed and H. J. Peppler, *Yeast Technology*, 1973; A. H. Rose and J. S. Harriston (eds.), *The Yeasts*, vol. 3: *Yeast Technology*, 1970.

CONTRIBUTORS

List of Contributors

A

Ackerman, Dr. Edward A. *Carnegie Institution of Washington.* SOIL CONSERVATION—coauthored.

Adams, Dr. Elijah. *Professor and Head, Department of Biological Chemistry, School of Medicine, University of Maryland.* HYDROXYPROLINE; PROLINE.

Adams, Prof. M. W. *Department of Crop and Soil Sciences, Michigan State University.* BEAN—in part.

Addicott, Prof. Fredrick T. *Department of Agronomy, University of California, Davis.* ABSCISIC ACID; ABSCISSION.

Adelberg, Dr. Edward A. *Department of Microbiology, Yale University.* AMINO ACIDS—in part, coauthored; ARGININE; CYSTEINE; SERINE; articles on other amino acids.

Albert, Dr. W. W. *Department of Animal Science, College of Agriculture, University of Illinois.* CATTLE PRODUCTION, BEEF.

Alderfer, Dr. Russell B. *Professor of Soils and Crops Department, College of Agriculture and Environmental Science, Rutgers University.* SOIL—in part.

Aldrich, Dr. Daniel G., Jr. *Chancellor, University of California, Irvine.* SOIL—in part.

Alikonis, Justin J. *Director of Research, Paul F. Beich Company, Bloomington, IL.* FOOD MANUFACTURING—in part.

Allen, Dr. L. H., Jr. *University of Florida.* MICROMETEOROLOGY, CROP.

Andrus, Dr. C. F. *Agricultural Consultant; formerly, U.S. Department of Agriculture, Charleston, SC.* WATERMELON.

App, Dr. A. A. *Boyce Thompson Institute for Plant Research, Inc., New York.* Validator of SEED GERMINATION.

Arbuckle, Prof. Wendell S. *Department of Dairy Science, University of Maryland.* ICE CREAM—in part.

B

Ball, Dr. C. Olin. *Food and Container Laboratory, New Brunswick, NJ.* FOOD ENGINEERING—in part, coauthored.

Barton, Dr. Lela V. *Deceased; formerly, Plant Physiologist, Boyce Thompson Institute for Plant Research, Inc., New York.* SEED GERMINATION.

Baver, Dr. Leonard D. *Agronomy Department, Ohio State University.* SORGHUM—in part.

Beachell, William A., Jr. *Consumer and Marketing Service, Portland.* PEA—in part.

Becker, Dr. Donald E. *Head, Department of Animal Science, University of Illinois.* SWINE PRODUCTION—coauthored.

Bennett, Dr. Ralph E. *Director, Science Information Department, Squibb Institute for Medical Research, New Brunswick, NJ.* RIBOFLAVIN; VITAMIN B_{12}—both in part.

Biggs, Dr. Robert H. *Professor (Biochemist), Department of Fruit Crops, University of Florida.* AUXIN; PLANT HORMONES.

Billings, Dr. William D. *Department of Botany, Duke University.* ECOLOGY, PHYSIOLOGICAL (PLANT).

Black, Dr. Clanton C. *Department of Biochemistry, University of Georgia.* PHOTORESPIRATION.

Black, Prof. Richard D. *Department of Agricultural Engineering, New York State College of Agriculture, Cornell University.* LAND DRAINAGE (AGRICULTURE).

Blanc, Milton L. *Research Climatologist, Office of Climatology, U.S. Weather Bureau, Tempe, AZ.* AGRICULTURAL METEOROLOGY—coauthored; GROWING SEASON.

Borgstrom, Dr. Georg. *Department of Food Science and Human Nutrition, Michigan State University.* AGRICULTURAL GEOGRAPHY.

Boswell, Dr. Victor R. *Retired; Plant Industry Station, Beltsville, MD.* HONEY DEW MELON; PERSIAN MELON.

Bradfield, Dr. Richard. *Emeritus Professor, Cornell University.* MULTIPLE CROPPING.

Bradley, Dr. Robert L., Jr. *Department of Food Science, College of Agricultural and Life Sciences, University of Wisconsin.* MILK.

Brantley, Dr. Blake B., Jr. *Department of Horticulture, University of Georgia College of Agriculture.* COWPEA—in part.

Bressler, Dr. Glenn O. *Department of Poultry Science, Pennsylvania State University.* POULTRY PRODUCTION.

Brody, Aaron L. *Mead Packaging, Atlanta.* FOOD ENGINEERING—in part.

Brooks, Dr. Stanley N. *Assistant Chief, Oilseed and Industrial Crops Research Branch, Agricultural Research Service, U.S. Department of Agriculture.* HOP.

Broyer, Prof. Theodore C. *Department of Soils and Plant Nutrition, University of California, Berkeley.* FERTILIZING—in part.

Bruhn, Dr. Hjalmar D. *Agricultural Engineering Department, University of Wisconsin.* AGRICULTURE, SOIL AND CROP PRACTICES IN—in part.

Buettner, Dr. Konrad J. K. *Deceased; formerly, Pierce Foundation, Yale University.* BIOCLIMATOLOGY.

C

Carew, Dr. H. John. *Professor of Horticulture, Michigan State University.* ASPARAGUS; BEET; CARROT; VEGETABLE GROWING; articles on various vegetables.

Chen, Dr. Wei-Jen. *Department of Pathology, University of Washington.* DIGESTIVE SYSTEM.

Chilton, Dr. St. John P. *Head, Department of Plant Pathology, Louisiana State University.* RICE—in part.

Christensen, Dr. Clyde M. *Professor of Plant Pathology, University of Minnesota.* PLANT DISEASE—in part.

Christensen, Dr. J. J. *Deceased; formerly, Professor of Plant Pathology, University of Minnesota.* WHEAT—in part.

Clarke, Dr. J. Harold. *Horticulturist, Clarke Nursery, Long Beach, WA.* BLACKBERRY; BLUEBERRY; CURRANT—in part; FRUIT GROWING, SMALL; articles on various fruits.

Cole, Marc. *Senior Chemist, Production and Development, Hoffmann-LaRoche, Inc., Nutley, NJ.* VITAMIN B_6—in part.

Coleman, Dr. Robert E. *Staff Scientist, Sugar Crops Production, National Program Staff, BARC-WEST, Beltsville, MD.* SUGARCANE.

Conner, Dr. Herbert W. *Deceased; formerly, William*

Wrigley Jr. Company, Chicago. FOOD MANUFACTUR-ING—in part.

Coons, Dr. George Herbert. *Collaborator, Tobacco and Sugar Crops Research Branch, Agricultural Research Service, U.S. Department of Agriculture, Beltsville, MD.* SUGARBEET—in part.

Core, Dr. Earl L. *Professor of Botany, Department of Biology, West Virginia University.* BREADFRUIT; TEA—in part. Validator of ALLSPICE; BAMBOO; COLCHICINE; GINGER; articles on various spice and medicinal plants.

Coursey, Dr. D. G. *Assistant Director, Plant Food Commodities Department, Tropical Products Institute, London.* ROOT AND TUBER FOOD CROPS.

Court, Dr. Arnold. *Professor of Climatology, Department of Geography, San Fernando Valley State College.* FROST.

Crafts, Dr. Alden S. *Department of Botany, University of California, Davis.* DEFOLIANT AND DESICCANT.

Cross, Dr. Chester E. *Agricultural Experiment Station, University of Massachusetts.* CRANBERRY.

Culbertson, Dr. Joseph O. *Assistant Chief (retired), Oilseed and Industrial Crops Research Branch, Crops Research Division, U.S. Department of Agriculture, Beltsville, MD.* FLAX—in part, coauthored.

D

Davis, Charles H. *Assistant Director of Chemical Development, Tennessee Valley Authority.* FERTILIZER.

DeBach, Dr. Paul. *Professor of Biological Control, University of California, Riverside.* INSECT CONTROL, BIOLOGICAL.

Desrosier, Dr. Norman W. *Research Center, National Biscuit Company, Fair Lawn, NJ.* FOOD MANUFACTUR-ING—in part.

Dollear, Frank G. *Head, Peanut Products Investigation, Southern Utilization Research and Development Division, U.S. Department of Agriculture, New Orleans.* BUTTER—in part; FAT AND OIL, EDIBLE.

Doudoroff, Dr. Michael. *Deceased; formerly, Department of Bacteriology, University of California, Berkeley.* CARBOHYDRATE METABOLISM.

Downey, Dr. R. K. *Agricultural Research Station, Saskatoon.* RAPE.

Doyle, Edwin S. *National Canners Association Research Laboratory, Berkeley.* FOOD ENGINEERING—in part.

Drosdoff, Dr. Matthew. *Professor of Soil Science, Department of Agronomy, Cornell University.* SOIL—in part.

Duley, Dr. Frank L. *Principal, Agricultural College, University of Peshawar.* SOIL—in part.

Dunegan, John Clymer. *Agricultural Consultant, Sarasota, FL.* APRICOT; CHERRY; PEACH; PLUM—all in part.

Dunn, Dr. J. Avery. *Formerly, Sales Manager, Atlantic Gelatin, General Foods Corporation.* GELATIN.

E

Eide, Dr. Carl J. *Department of Plant Pathology, Institute of Agriculture, University of Minnesota.* CABBAGE; PLANT DISEASE (coauthored); PLANT DISEASE CONTROL; POTATO, IRISH; TURNIP—all in part.

Einset, Dr. John. *Professor of Pomology, Cornell University.* GRAPE CULTURE—in part.

Erickson, Dr. David R. *Director of Research, Unitech Chemical Inc.* LINOLEIC ACID; LINOLENIC ACID.

F

Fehr, Prof. Walter R. *Department of Agronomy, Iowa State University.* SOYBEAN—in part.

Fellers, Dr. Carl R. *Formerly, Food Consultant.* FOOD ENGINEERING—in part.

Finberg, Alfred J. *Consultant in Food Technology, New York.* FOOD MANUFACTURING—in part.

Flexer, Dr. L. A. *Vice President of Chemical Production, Hoffmann-LaRoche, Inc., Nutley, NJ.* RIBOFLAVIN—in part.

Forsythe, Dr. Richard H. *Vice President, Research and Development Center, Henningsen Foods, Inc., Springfield, MO.* EGG PROCESSING.

Fratianne, Douglas G. *Department of Botany, Ohio State University.* PHOTOSYNTHESIS.

French, Dr. Orval C. *Department of Agricultural Engineering, Cornell University.* AGRICULTURAL ENGINEERING; AGRICULTURE, MACHINERY IN.

Frey, Dr. Kenneth. *Department of Agronomy, Iowa State University.* OATS—in part.

Futral, Prof. J. G. *Department of Agricultural Engineering, Georgia Agricultural Experiment Station.* FERTILIZING—in part.

G

Gardner, Dr. Frank E. *Horticulturist, Agricultural Research Service, U.S. Department of Agriculture, Orlando, FL.* KUMQUAT; MANDARIN.

Gauch, Dr. Huch G. *Department of Botany, College of Agriculture, University of Maryland.* PLANT, MINERAL NUTRITION OF; PLANT, MINERALS ESSENTIAL TO.

Geiger, Dr. Donald. *Department of Biology, University of Dayton.* PLANT TRANSLOCATION OF ORGANIC SOLUTES.

Gemmill, Arthur V. *Consultant, Food Engineering, Morristown, NJ.* FOOD ENGINEERING—in part.

Gershoff, Prof. Stanley N. *Department of Nutrition, Harvard School of Public Health, Boston.* ASCORBIC ACID; BIOTIN; VITAMIN A; articles on other vitamins—all in part.

Gigg, Dr. Roy H. *Chemistry Division, National Institute for Medical Research, London.* LIPID.

Goss, Dr. Harold. *Professor Emeritus of Animal Husbandry, University of California, Davis.* ANIMAL-FEED COMPOSITION.

Grau, Dr. Fred V. *Consulting Agronomist, College Park, MD.* VETCH.

Greenberg, Prof. David M. *Department of Biochemistry, School of Medicine, University of California, San Francisco.* PROTEIN METABOLISM.

Grierson, Dr. William. *Institute of Food and Agricultural Sciences, University of Florida.* CITRON.

Gunckel, Prof. James E. *Department of Botany, Rutgers College, Rutgers University.* BUDDING; GRAFTING OF PLANTS.

H

Hader, Rodney N. *Secretary, American Chemical Society, Washington, DC.* AGRICULTURAL CHEMISTRY.

Hagood, Mel A. *Irrigated Agriculture Research and Extension Center, Washington State University.* IRRIGATION OF CROPS.

Haise, Dr. Howard R. *Northern Plains Branch Headquarters, Soil and Water Conservation Research Division, Agricultural Research Service, U.S. Department of Agriculture, Fort Collins, CO.* SOIL—in part.

Haley, Dr. Leanor D. *Chief, Mycology Training Unit, Department of Health, Education and Welfare, National Communicable Disease Center, Atlanta.* FUNGISTAT AND FUNGICIDE—in part.

Hall, Dr. Carl W. *Dean, College of Engineering, Washington State University.* AGRICULTURE, SOIL AND CROP PRACTICES IN—in part; DAIRY MACHINERY.

Halvorson, Dr. H. Orin. *Retired; Department of Biochem-*

istry, University of Minnesota. FOOD MICROBIOLOGY—in part.

Hanson, Dr. Clarence H. *Agricultural Research Service, U.S. Department of Agriculture, Beltsville, MD.* ALFALFA.

Harrar, J. George. *Rockefeller Foundation, New York.* PLANT DISEASE CONTROL—in part.

Haskins, Dr. R. H. *Head, Physiology and Biochemistry of Fungi Section, National Research Council, Prairie Regional Laboratory, Saskatoon.* INDUSTRIAL MICROBIOLOGY.

Hass, Dr. H. B. *Director of Chemical Research, M. W. Kellogg Company, Piscataway, NJ.* SUGAR.

Hassid, Prof. William Z. *Deceased; formerly, Department of Biochemistry, University of California, Berkley.* CARBOHYDRATE; FRUCTOSE; GLUCOSE; MONOSACCHARIDE; articles on other carbohydrates and sugars.

Havighorst, Carl R. *Western Contributing Editor, "Food Engineering."* FOOD ENGINEERING—in part.

Hayakawa, Dr. Kan-ichi. *Department of Food Science, Rutgers University.* FOOD ENGINEERING—in part, coauthored.

Heyne, Prof. E. G. *Professor of Plant Breeding, Department of Agronomy, Kansas State University.* GRAIN CROPS.

Hirst, Dr. J. M. *Rothamsted Experimental Station, Harpenden, England.* PLANT DISEASE—in part.

Hollowell, Eugene A. *Consultant in Agronomy, Port Republic, MD.* CLOVER—in part.

Hooker, Dr. Arthur L. *Department of Plant Pathology, University of Illinois.* PLANT DISEASE CONTROL—in part.

Hooker, Prof. William J. *Department of Botany and Plant Pathology, Michigan State University.* ATMOSPHERIC POLLUTION.

Horsfall, Dr. James G. *Director, Connecticut Agricultural Experiment Station, New Haven.* FUNGISTAT AND FUNGICIDE (coauthored); PLANT DISEASE CONTROL—both in part.

Hubbell, Dr. David H. *Department of Soil Science, University of Florida.* NITROGEN FIXATION (BIOLOGY).

I

Ibrahim, Dr. Aly M. *Agricultural Research Service, Western Region, U.S. Department of Agriculture, Salinas, CA.* ARTICHOKE.

Israel, Dr. Yedy. *Department of Pharmacology, University of Toronto.* ALCOHOLISM.

J

Jacobs, Dr. Woodrow C. *Director, Environmental Data Service, Environmental Science Services Administration.* AGRICULTURAL METEOROLOGY—coauthored.

Jensen, Dr. Aldon H. *Department of Animal Science, University of Illinois.* SWINE PRODUCTION—coauthored.

Johnson, Howard W. *Plant Pathologist (retired), U.S. Department of Agriculture, Stoneville, MS.* COWPEA—in part.

Johnson, Prof. Ronald R. *Department of Animal Science, Institute of Agriculture, University of Tennessee.* AGRICULTURAL SCIENCE (ANIMAL).

Johnstone, Prof. Francis E., Jr. *Director, University of Georgia Botanical Garden.* PEACH—in part.

K

Kallio, Dr. R. E. *School of Life Sciences, University of Illinois.* Validator of NITROGEN CYCLE.

Katznelson, Dr. Harry. *Deceased; formerly, Director,*

Research Branch, Microbiology Research Institute, Canada. NITROGEN CYCLE.

Kayan, Prof. Carl F. *Professor of Mechanical Engineering, School of Engineering, Columbia University.* COLD STORAGE.

Keller, Prof. Walter D. *Department of Geology, University of South Florida, Tampa.* EROSION.

Kempf, Norman W. *Consultant, Harvard, MA.* COCOA POWDER AND CHOCOLATE.

Kennedy, Dr. Bill W. *Department of Plant Pathology, Institute of Agriculture, University of Minnesota.* SOYBEAN—in part.

Kernkamp, Dr. Milton F. *Head, Department of Plant Pathology, University of Minnesota.* BARLEY; FLAX; validator of WHEAT—all in part.

Kharasch, Prof. Norman. *Department of Biomedicinal Chemistry, University of Southern California, Los Angeles.* SACCHARIN.

King, Dr. Donald W. *School of Medicine, Yale University.* MALNUTRITION; METABOLIC DISORDERS.

King, Dr. Frederick J. *Gloucester Laboratory, U.S. Department of Commerce, Gloucester, MA.* FOOD FROM THE SEA—feature.

King, Dr. Thomas H. *Department of Plant Pathology and Physiology, University of Minnesota.* PEA; STRAWBERRY—both in part.

Kinman, Dr. Murray L. *Crops Research Division, U.S. Department of Agriculture; and Department of Soils and Crop Science, Texas A & M University.* SUNFLOWER—in part.

Kinne, Dr. Ivan L. *Manager, Development Programs Office, Battelle Memorial Institute, Columbus, OH.* ENERGY IN THE FOOD SYSTEM—coauthored feature.

Knightly, William H. *Specialty Chemical Division, Imperial Chemical Industries—United States, Wilmington.* FOOD MANUFACTURING—in part.

Korab, Harry E. *National Soft Drink Association, Washington, DC.* FOOD MANUFACTURING—in part.

Kothari, Dr. Ajit. *Product Planning Manager, Hoffmann-LaRoche, Inc., Nutley, NJ.* XYLITOL.

Kott, Dr. Maurice G. *Director, Division of Mental Retardation, Department of Institutions and Agencies of the State of New Jersey.* PHENYLPYRUVIC OLIGOPHRENIA.

Krehl, Dr. Willard A. *Chairman, Department of Community Health and Preventive Medicine, Jefferson Medical College, Thomas Jefferson University, Philadelphia.* CALORIE; OBESITY; STARVATION; VITAMIN—in part.

Kreitlow, Dr. Kermit W. *Assistant Chief, Forage and Range Research, Crops Research Division, Agricultural Research Service, U.S. Department of Agriculture, Beltsville, MD.* CLOVER; GRASS CROPS—both in part.

Kritchevsky, Dr. David. *Department of Biochemistry, Wistar Institute, University of Pennsylvania.* PLANT FIBER, DIETARY.

Kubota, Dr. Joe. *Research Soil Scientist, Soil Survey Investigations, Plant, Soil and Nutrition Laboratory, U.S. Department of Agriculture, Ithaca, NY.* SOIL CHEMISTRY—in part.

Kuc, Dr. Joseph. *Department of Biochemistry, Purdue University.* PLANT DISEASE CONTROL—in part.

Kupchan, Prof. S. Morris. *Department of Chemistry, University of Virginia.* CAFFEINE.

L

Lagler, Prof. Karl F. *School of Natural Resources, University of Michigan.* FISHERIES CONSERVATION.

Lamb, Dr. Robert C. *Department of Pomology and Viticulture, New York State Agricultural Experiment Station, Geneva.* APRICOT—in part.

Landsberg, Dr. H. E. *Professor and Director, Institute for Fluid Dynamics and Applied Mathematics, University of Maryland.* Validator of BIOCLIMATOLOGY.

Lapedes, Daniel N. *Editor in Chief, "McGraw-Hill Encyclopedia of Science and Technology," McGraw-Hill Book Company, New York.* AMYLASE.

Larsen, Dr. R. Paul. *Superintendent and Horticulturist, Tree Fruit Research Center, Washington State University.* APPLE; CHERRY—in part; FRUIT, TREE; PLUM—in part.

Lawler, Frank K. *Editor in Chief, "Food Engineering," Philadelphia.* FOOD ENGINEERING; FOOD MANUFACTURING—both in part; FOOD TECHNOLOGY.

Lindenmaier, Dr. Werner A. *Hoffmann-LaRoche, Inc. Nutley, NJ.* ASCORBIC ACID—in part.

Linsley, Prof. Ray K. *Professor of Civil Engineering, Stanford University.* EVAPOTRANSPIRATION.

Livingston, Dr. Gideon E. *Food Science Associates, Rye, NY.* FOOD SCIENCE; VANILLA EXTRACT—both coauthored.

Lochhead, Dr. Allan G. *Canada Department of Agriculture, Microbiology Research Institute, Ottawa.* MANURE; RHIZOSPHERE; SOIL BALANCE, MICROBIAL; SOIL MICROBIOLOGY; SOIL MICROORGANISMS.

Lockhart, Ernest E. *Coca-Cola Company, Atlanta.* COFFEE—in part.

Lockwood, Dr. Lewis B. *Assistant Director of Microbiological Research, Union Division, Miles Laboratories, Elkhart, IN.* VINEGAR.

Ludvik, Dr. George F. *Insecticide Application Research, Agricultural Research and Development Department, Monsanto Company, St. Louis.* MITICIDE; PESTICIDE.

Luttrell, Dr. E. S. *Georgia Experiment Station, Athens.* GRAPE CULTURE—in part.

M

McClung, Dr. Leland S. *Professor of Microbiology, Indiana University.* BLACKLEG; BOTULISM.

McClure, Dr. Thomas A. *Development Programs Office, Battelle Memorial Institute, Columbus, OH.* ENERGY IN THE FOOD SYSTEM—coauthored feature.

MacDaniels, Dr. Laurence H. *Professor Emeritus of Floriculture and Ornamental Horticulture, Ithaca, NY.* ALMOND; BRAZIL NUT; CASHEW; NUT CROP CULTURE; articles on other nuts.

McHugh, Dr. J. L. *Professor of Marine Resources, Marine Sciences Research Center, State University of New York, Stony Brook.* MARINE FISHERIES.

McQuigg, Dr. James D. *Certified Consulting Meteorologist, Columbia, MO.* CLIMATE AND CROPS—feature.

Magee, Paul T. *Assistant Professor, Department of Microbiology, School of Medicine, Yale University.* AMINO ACIDS—in part, coauthored.

Mahoney, Dr. Lee R. *Chemistry Department, Ford Motor Company, Dearborn, MI.* ANTIOXIDANT.

Mandava, Dr. N. *Plant Pathologist, Plant Hormone and Regulators Laboratory, Agricultural Research Service, U.S. Department of Agriculture, Beltsville, MD.* BRASSIN—coauthored.

Manning, Dr. James M. *Rockefeller University.* ALBUMIN; PEPTIDE; PROTEIN—coauthored.

Manning, Dr. Paul D. V. *Professor of Chemical Engineering (retired), California Institute of Technology.* MONOSODIUM GLUTAMATE.

Marshall, Dr. H. G. *Crops Research Division, Agricultural Research Service, Department of Agronomy, Pennsylvania State University.* BUCKWHEAT—in part.

Martin, Franklin W. *Mayaguez Institute of Tropical Agriculture, Mayaguez, PR.* CASSAVA; LEREN.

Martin, Prof. James P. *Professor of Soil Science, Department of Soils and Plant Nutrition, College of Biological and Agricultural Sciences, University of California, Riverside.* SOIL—in part.

Martin, R. G. *National Institutes of Health, Bethesda.* AMINO ACIDS—in part.

Martin, Dr. Weston J. *Professor of Plant Pathology, Louisiana State University.* POTATO, SWEET—in part.

Mayhall, Temple R. *Director of Education, American Institute of Baking, Chicago.* FOOD ENGINEERING; FOOD MANUFACTURING—both in part.

Meiklejohn, Dr. Jane. *Senior Research Fellow, University College, Salisbury, Rhodesia.* SOIL MINERALS, MICROBIAL UTILIZATION OF; SOIL PHOSPHORUS, MICROBIAL CYCLE OF; SOIL SULFUR, MICROBIAL CYCLE OF.

Melnick, Dr. Joseph L. *Department of Virology and Epidemiology, Baylor College of Medicine.* FOOT-AND-MOUTH DISEASE; LOUPING ILL.

Mercanton, Dr. Roger A. *Hoffmann-LaRoche, Inc., Nutley, NJ.* BIOTIN—in part.

Meyer, Dr. Bernard S. *Professor of Botany, Ohio State University.* PLANT, WATER RELATIONS OF; PLANT PHYSIOLOGY.

Middleton, Dr. John T. *Commissioner, National Air Pollution Control Administration.* CUCUMBER; SQUASH—both in part.

Miller, Dr. Carlos O. *Department of Botany, Indiana University.* CYTOKININS.

Miller, Dr. Frederick R. *Department of Soil and Crop Sciences, Texas A & M University.* SORGHUM—in part.

Miller, Dr. Julian C. *Department of Horticulture, Louisiana State University.* POTATO, SWEET—in part.

Miller, Dr. Lawrence. *Department of Plant Pathology, Virginia Polytechnic Institute.* PEANUT—in part.

Miller, Prof. Martin W. *Department of Food Science and Technology, College of Agricultural and Environmental Sciences, University of California, Davis.* YEAST, INDUSTRIAL.

Milner, Dr. Reid T. *Department Head, Food Science, University of Illinois.* FOOD ENGINEERING—in part.

Minges, Dr. Philip A. *Department of Vegetable Crops, Cornell University.* GARLIC.

Moore, Dr. M. B. *Department of Plant Pathology, Institute of Agriculture, University of Minnesota.* OATS—in part.

Morrison, Dr. Kenneth J. *Cooperative Extension Service, Washington State University.* LENTIL; PEA—in part.

Morse, Dr. Roger A. *Department of Entomology, Cornell University.* BEEKEEPING.

Morse, Dr. Roy Earl. *Director of Research, Pepsico, New York.* CITRUS FLAVORING; SALT (FOOD); SPICE AND FLAVORING.

Mottet, Dr. N. Karle. *Professor of Pathology and Director of Hospital Pathology, University Hospital, University of Washington.* BERIBERI; SCURVY. Validator of PELLAGRA; RICKETS.

Mrak, Dr. Emil. *Office of Chancellor Emeritus, University of California, Davis.* DISTILLED SPIRITS; WINE; YEAST—all coauthored.

Munger, Prof. H. M. *Department of Plant Breeding and Biometry, New York State College of Agriculture and Life Sciences, Cornell University.* SQUASH—in part.

Murray, Dr. Merritt J. *Formerly, A. M. Todd Company, Kalamazoo, MI.* PEPPERMINT.

Musgrave, Dr. R. B. *Department of Agronomy, Cornell University.* AGRICULTURE, SOIL AND CROP PRACTICES IN—in part, coauthored.

N

Nair, Dr. John H. *Consultant to Food Industry, Raleigh, NC.* FOOD; FOOD MANUFACTURING; TEA—all in part.

Namias, Jerome. *Chief, Extended Forecast Division, Weather Bureau, Environmental Science Services Administration, Washington, DC.* DROUGHT.

Nelson, Dr. Curtis J. *Department of Agronomy, University of Missouri.* AGRICULTURAL SCIENCE (PLANT).

Nelson, Elton G. *Collaborator (WOC), Crops Research Division, U.S. Department of Agriculture.* FIBER CROPS; FLAX—in part, coauthored.

Nichols, Dr. Mark L. *Deceased; formerly, U.S. Depart-

ment of Agriculture, Auburn, AL. AGRICULTURE, SOIL AND CROP PRACTICES IN—in part.

Niven, Dr. Charles F., Jr. *Director of Research, Del Monte Research Center, Walnut Creek, CA.* PASTEURIZATION; STERILIZATION.

O

Ofner, Dr. Alfred. *Director of Technical Development (retired), Hoffmann-LaRoche, Inc., Nutley, NJ.* VITAMIN A; VITAMIN E; VITAMIN K—all in part.

Ogburn, Charles B. *Cooperative Extension Service, Auburn University.* TERRACING (AGRICULTURE).

Olson, Dr. Norman F. *Department of Food Science, University of Wisconsin.* CHEESE—in part.

Ordal, Dr. Z. John. *Department of Food Science, University of Illinois.* FOOD PRESERVATION.

Orthoefer, Dr. F. T. *A. E. Staley Manufacturing Company, Decatur, IL.* SOYBEAN—in part.

Ourecky, Dr. Donald K. *Department of Pomology and Viticulture, New York State Agricultural Experiment Station, Cornell University.* GOOSEBERRY.

P

Paleg, Dr. L. G. *Department of Chemistry, University of California, Los Angeles.* GIBBERELLIN.

Patton, Dr. Donald J. *Carnegie Institution of Washington.* SOIL CONSERVATION—coauthored.

Perlmann, Dr. Gertrude E. *Deceased; formerly, Rockefeller University.* GLUTELIN; PROTEIN—coauthored.

Perry, Astor. *Extension Agronomy Specialist, North Carolina State University.* PEANUT—in part.

Phaff, Dr. Herman J. *College of Agriculture, University of California, Davis.* DISTILLED SPIRITS; WINE; YEAST—all coauthored. FOOD MICROBIOLOGY—in part.

Philip, Dr. Cornelius B. *Principal Entomologist, U.S. Public Health Service, Hamilton, MT.* HEARTWATER DISEASE.

Power, Dr. James F. *Northern Great Plains Research Center, Agricultural Research Service, U.S. Department of Agriculture, Mandan, ND.* SOIL—in part.

R

Radke, Dr. Rodney O. *Agricultural Product Research Laboratory, Monsanto Company.* HERBICIDE.

Ramsey, Dr. Glen Blaine. *Principal Pathologist, Agricultural Marketing Service, U.S. Department of Agriculture.* LETTUCE; ONION—both in part.

Reeve, Dr. Roger M. *Western Regional Research Laboratory, U.S. Department of Agriculture, Albany, CA.* SEED (BOTANY).

Reid, Dr. David A. *Agricultural Research Service, U.S. Department of Agriculture, Tucson.* BARLEY—in part.

Reitz, Dr. Louis P. *Retired; Crops Research Division, Agricultural Research Service, U.S. Department of Agriculture.* CEREAL; WHEAT—in part.

Rich, Dr. Saul. *Chief, Department of Plant Pathology and Botany, Connecticut Agricultural Experiment Station, New Haven.* FUNGISTAT AND FUNGICIDE—in part, coauthored.

Riley, Dr. Ralph. *Plant Breeding Institute, Cambridge, England.* BREEDING (PLANT).

Rizack, Dr. Martin A. *Rockefeller University.* LIPID METABOLISM.

Robinson, Prof. Richard W. *Department of Seed and Vegetable Sciences, New York State Agricultural Experiment Station, Cornell University.* TOMATO.

Rockett, Frank H. *Engineering Consultant, Charlottesville, VA.* BAKING POWDER; LINSEED OIL.

Rodenhiser, Dr. Herman A. *Deputy Administrator, Agri-*

cultural Research Service, U.S. Department of Agriculture. MILLET; SORGHUM—both in part.

Ross, Douglas N. *The Conference Board, Inc., New York.* FEEDING THE WORLD—feature.

Rowell, Dr. John B. *U.S. Department of Agriculture; and Department of Plant Pathology and Botany, University of Minnesota.* PLANT DISEASE—in part.

Rutger, Dr. J. Neil, *Department of Agronomy, University of California, Davis.* RICE—in part.

S

Sackston, Prof. Waldemar E. *Department of Plant Pathology, McGill University, Macdonald Campus.* SUNFLOWER—in part.

Salisbury, Dr. Frank B. *Chairman, Plant Science Department, Utah State University.* PHOTOPERIODISM IN PLANTS.

Schmidt, G. H. *Dairy Science Department, Ohio State University.* CATTLE PRODUCTION, DAIRY.

Schroeder, Dr. Charles A. *Department of Botanical Sciences, University of California, Los Angeles.* AVOCADO; BANANA—in part; DATE; FIG; OLIVE.

Seeley, Dr. John G. *Department of Floriculture and Ornamental Horticulture, Cornell University.* FLORICULTURE.

Sequeira, Prof. Luis. *Department of Plant Pathology, University of Wisconsin.* BANANA—in part.

Shands, Dr. H. L. *Department of Agronomy, University of Wisconsin.* RYE—in part.

Sharvelle, Eric G. *Department of Botany and Plant Pathology, Lilly Hall of Life Sciences, Purdue University.* FRUIT (TREE) DISEASES—in part.

Shellenberger, Dr. John A. *Department of Grain Science and Industry, Kansas State University.* BARLEY; CORN; FOOD MANUFACTURING; articles on other grains—all in part. CEREAL CHEMISTRY.

Sidransky, Dr. Herschel. *Department of Experimental Biology, Weizmann Institute.* KWASHIORKOR DISEASE.

Silliker, Dr. John H. *President, Silliker Laboratories, Chicago Heights, IL.* FOOD MICROBIOLOGY—in part; FOOD SPOILAGE.

Silver, Dr. Edward A. *Agricultural Engineer, Columbus, OH.* AGRICULTURE, SOIL AND CROP PRACTICES IN—in part, coauthored.

Simonson, Dr. Roy W. *Director (retired), Soil Classification and Correlation, U.S. Department of Agriculture, Hyattsville, MD.* SOIL—in part; SOIL, SUBORDERS OF.

Smith, Dr. David W. E. *Associate Professor of Microbiology and Pathology, Indiana University.* AMINO ACIDS—in part; HISTIDINE; LYSINE.

Smith, Dr. Guy D. *Soil Conservation Service, U.S. Department of Agriculture.* SOIL—in part; SOIL, ZONALITY OF.

Smith, Dr. Harry. *Department of Microbiology, University of Birmingham.* ANTHRAX.

Smith, Dr. Kenneth M. *Cell Research Institute, Department of Botany, University of Texas.* PLANT VIRUS.

Smith, Dr. Ora. *Department of Agricultural Sciences, Cornell University.* POTATO, IRISH—in part.

Smith, Prof. Paul G. *Department of Vegetable Crops, College of Agricultural and Environmental Sciences, University of California, Davis.* PEPPER.

Solberg, Dr. Myron. *Department of Food Science, Rutgers University.* FOOD SCIENCE; VANILLA EXTRACT—both coauthored.

Soost, Dr. Robert K. *Department of Plant Science, University of California, Riverside.* GRAPEFRUIT; LEMON; LIME; ORANGE.

Spink, Dr. Wesley W. *Regents' Professor of Medicine, School of Medicine, University of Minnesota.* BRUCELLOSIS.

Sposito, Dr. Garrison. *Department of Soil Science and Agricultural Engineering, University of California, Riverside.* SOIL CHEMISTRY—in part.

Sprague, G. F. *Department of Agronomy, University of Illinois.* CORN — in part.

Sprague, Dr. Howard B. *Agricultural Consultant, Washington, DC.* AGRICULTURE; FARM CROPS; GRASS CROPS — in part; articles on various grasses.

Stakman, Dr. E. C. *Professor Emeritus, Institute of Agriculture, University of Minnesota.* PLANT DISEASE (coauthored); PLANT DISEASE CONTROL — both in part.

Stern, Joseph A. *Bionetics Corporation, Hampton, VA.* FOOD MANUFACTURING — in part.

Stewart, Dewey. *Crops Research Division, Agricultural Research Service, U.S. Department of Agriculture, Beltsville, MD.* SUGAR CROPS — coauthored; SUGARBEET — in part.

Stokes, Dr. I. E. *Crops Research Division, Agricultural Research Service, U.S. Department of Agriculture, Beltsville, MD.* SUGAR CROPS — coauthored.

Strausbaugh, Dr. Perry D. *Deceased; formerly, Professor Emeritus of Botany, West Virginia University.* ALLSPICE; BAMBOO; COLCHICINE; GINGER; articles on various spice and medicinal plants.

Stuart, Dr. Edward G. *Deceased; formerly, West Virginia School of Medicine.* PELLAGRA; RICKETS.

T

Tabor, Paul. *Soil Conservation Service, Athens, GA.* KUDZU; LEGUME FORAGES; LESPEDEZA; LUPINE.

Terrill, Dr. Clair E. *Chief, Sheep and Fur Animal Research Branch, U.S. Department of Agriculture, Beltsville, MD.* SHEEP.

Thomas, Dr. Walter I. *Agricultural Experiment Station, Pennsylvania State University.* AGRONOMY.

Thomsen, L. C. *Professor Emeritus of Food Science, University of Wisconsin.* BUTTER — in part.

Tracy, Dr. Paul H. *Consultant to the Dairy Industry, DeLand, FL.* CASEIN; CHEESE.

Trauberman, Leonard. *Food Engineering Consultant.* FOOD ENGINEERING — in part.

Trearchis, George. *Manager, Food Industry Division, Foxboro Company, Foxboro, MA.* FOOD ENGINEERING — in part.

Triplett, Dr. Glover B., Jr. *Department of Agronomy, Agricultural Research and Development Center, Wooster, OH.* REDTOP GRASS — in part.

Tukey, Dr. Harold. *Deceased; formerly, Professor Emeritus, Department of Horticulture, Michigan State University.* QUINCE.

Turner, Dr. Richard J. *Technical Director, American Cyanamid Company, New York.* FOLIC ACID — in part.

V

Van Niel, Dr. C. B. *Hopkins Marine Station, Pacific Grove, CA.* FERMENTATION.

Van Vleck, Dr. L. D. *Department of Animal Science, New York State College of Agriculture & Life Science, Cornell University.* BREEDING (ANIMAL).

Vaughan, Dr. Edward K. *Agricultural Experimental Station, Oregon State University.* CURRANT; RASPBERRY — both in part.

Vierheller, Prof. Albert F. *Retired; College of Agriculture, University of Maryland.* HORTICULTURAL CROPS.

Von Graevenitz, Dr. Alexander W. C. *Director of Clinical Microbiology, Yale – New Haven Hospital.* SALMONELLOSES.

W

Wallace, James M. *Professor Emeritus, Citrus Research Center, University of California, Riverside.* FRUIT (TREE) DISEASES — in part.

Weckel, Dr. Kenneth G. *Department of Food Science, University of Wisconsin.* VITAMIN D — in part.

Weiss, Dr. Theodore J. *Technical Manager, Industrial Department, Hunt-Wesson Foods, Inc.* MARGARINE.

Wellman, Dr. Frederick L. *Visiting Professor of Tropical Plant Pathology, Department of Plant Pathology, North Carolina State University.* COCONUT — in part.

Went, Dr. Frits W. *Professor of Botany, Desert Research Institute, University of Nevada.* PLANT GROWTH.

Whistler, Prof. Roy L. *Department of Biochemistry, Purdue University.* GUM.

White, Dr. T. A. *Formerly, Technical Director for Foods, National Starch and Chemical Corporation, Plainfield, NJ.* STARCH.

Wiesman, Clarence K. *Director, Research and Development Division, John Sexton and Company, Chicago.* FOOD ENGINEERING; FOOD MANUFACTURING — in part.

Wilbur, Donald A., Sr. *Emeritus Professor of Entomology, Kansas State University.* FUMIGANT.

Wilkes, Dr. H. Garrison. *Department of Biology, University of Massachusetts, Harbor Campus, Boston.* THE GREEN REVOLUTION — feature.

Williams, Dr. Lansing E. *Ohio Agricultural Research and Development Center, Wooster.* CORN — in part.

Williams, Dr. Roger J. *Department of Chemistry, University of Texas.* NUTRITION.

Winder, Dr. William C. *Department of Food Science, University of Wisconsin.* ICE CREAM — in part.

Wodicka, Dr. Virgil O. *Consultant in Food Technology and Quality Assurance, Fullerton, CA.* FOOD; FOOD ENGINEERING — in part.

Woodroof, Dr. Jasper G. *Consultant, Food Science Division, Georgia Experiment Station.* PEANUT — in part; PECAN.

Wooley, Prof. John C. *Professor Emeritus in Agricultural Engineering, University of Missouri.* AGRICULTURE, STRUCTURES IN.

Worley, Dr. J. F. *Plant Pathologist, Plant Hormone and Regulators Laboratory, Agricultural Research Service, U.S. Department of Agriculture, Beltsville, MD.* BRASSIN — coauthored.

Y

Yermanos, Dr. D. M. *Department of Plant Sciences, University of California, Riverside.* JOJOBA.

Z

Zaumeyer, Dr. William J. *U.S. Department of Agriculture, Beltsville, MD.* BEAN — in part.

Zimmerman, Dr. Leroy H. *Agricultural Research Service, U.S. Department of Agriculture; and Department of Plant Sciences, University of Arizona.* SAFFLOWER.

Zink, Dr. Frank W. *Department of Vegetable Crops, University of California, Davis.* CANTALOUPE; MELON GROWING; MUSKMELON.

Zlotnik, Dr. I. *Microbiological Research Establishment, Wilts, England.* SCRAPIE.

Zwerman, Prof. Paul J. *Department of Agronomy, Cornell University.* COVER CROPS.

APPENDIX

Composition of foods, showing constituents of 100 g of edible portion[a]

Food	Calories[b]	Water, g	Protein, g	Fat, g	Ash, g	Total carbohydrates, g	Crude fiber, g	Ca, mg	P, mg	Fe, mg	Na, mg	K, mg	A, IU	B_1, mg	B_2, mg	Niacin, mg	C, mg	Total calories[b]	Measure[e]	Weight, g
Almonds (dry)	597	4.7	18.6	54.1	3	19.6	2.7	254	475	4.4	160[c]	710[c]	0	0.25	0.67	4.6	Tr.	850	1 cup	140
Angel food cake	270	31.6	8.4	0.3	1	58.7	0	6	24	0.3	0.2		0	0.01	0.14	0.2	0	110	2 in. sec. of 8 in. cake	41
Apple, raw	58	84.1	0.3	0.4	0.3	14.9	1	6	10	0.3		74	90	0.04	0.03	0.2	5	87	1 medium (2½ in. diam.)	150
Apple, dry	277	23	1.4	1	1.4	73.2	3.9	19	48	1.4			0	0.10	0.10	1	12	315	1 cup	114
Apple juice	50	85.9	0.1	0	0.3	13.8		6	10	0.5	4	100	40	0.02	0.03	Tr.	1	124	1 cup	249
Apple pie	246	47.8	2.1	9.5	1.1	39.5	0.7	7	24	0.4			160	0.03	0.02	0.2	1	330	4 in. sec. of 9 in. pie	220
Apple sauce	72	79.8	0.2	0.1	0.2	19.7	0.6	4	8	0.4	0.3	55	30	0.02	0.01	Tr.	1	185	1 cup	254
Apricot, raw	51	85.4	1	0.1	0.6	12.9	0.6	16	23	0.5	0.6	440	2,790	0.03	0.05	0.8	7	54	3	114
Apricot, canned	80	77.3	0.6	0.1	0.6	21.4	0.4	10	15	0.3	2	65	1,350	0.02	0.02	0.3	4	97	4 medium halves, 2 tbsp syrup	122
Apricot, dry	262	24	5.2	0.4	3.5	66.9	3.2	86	119	4.9	11	1,700	7,430	0.01	0.16	3.3	12	280	40 halves	150
Apricot nectar	52	86.1	0.3	0.1	0.5	12.4	0.2	9	13	0.3	2.9	98	1,090	Tr.	0.01	Tr.	1	170	1 cup	254
Artichoke	63	83.7	2.9	0.4	1.1	11.9	3.2	47	94	1.9	43	430	390	0.15	0.03		11	33	1, 3 in. diam.	50
Asparagus, raw	21	93	2.2	0.2	0.7	3.9	0.7	21	62	0.9	2	240	1,000	0.16	0.19	1.4	33	16	6, 6 in. stalks	75
Asparagus, cooked	20	92.5	2.4	0.2	1.3	3.6	0.8	19	53	1			1,040	0.13	0.17	1.2	23	36	1 cup cut spears	175
Asparagus, canned	18	93.6	1.9	0.3	1.3	2.9	0.5	18	43	1.7	410	130	600	0.07	0.10	0.9	15	22	6 medium spears	126
Avocado	245	65.4	1.7	26.4	1.4	5.1	1.8	10	38	0.6	3	340	290	0.06	0.13	1.1	16	280	½, 3½ × 3¼ in.	114
Bacon (fried)	607	13	25	55	6	1	0	25	255	3.3	2,400	390	0	0.48	0.31	4.8	0	97	2 slices	16
Banana	88	74.8	1.2	0.2	0.8	23	0.6	8	28	0.6	0.5	420	430	0.04	0.05	0.7	10	132	1 medium, 6 × 1½ in.	150
Barley, pearled	349	11.1	8.2	1	0.9	78.8	0.5	16	189	2	3	160	0	0.12	0.08	3.1	0	710	1 cup	204
Beef (cooked), chuck	309	51	26	22	0.7	0	0	11	117	3.1	51	360	0	0.05	0.20	4.1	0	265	3 oz	86
Beef, porterhouse	342	49	23	27	1.1	0	0	11	170	3	69	334	0	0.06	0.18	4.7	0	293	3 oz	86
Beef, rib roast	319	51	24	24	1.2	0	0	10	185	3	107	345	0	0.06	0.18	4.3	0	266	3 oz	86
Beef, round	233	59	27	13	1.3	0	0	11	224	3.4	68	400	0	0.08	0.22	5.5	0	197	3 oz	86
Beef, dried or chipped	203	47.7	34.3	6.3	11.6	0	0	20	404	5.1	4,300	200	0	0.07	0.32	3.8	0	115	2 oz	56
Beef, roast beef	224	60	25	13	2	0	0	16	116	2.4	8		0	0.02	0.23	4.2	0	189	3 oz	86
Beer (4% alcohol)	20–48	90.2	0.6	0	0.2	4.4		4	26	0		46	0	Tr.	0.03	0.2	0	72–173	12 oz	360
Beet, raw	42	87.6	1.6	0.1	1.1	9.6	0.9	27	43	1	54	350	20	0.02	0.05	0.4	10	56	1 cup diced	134
Beet, cooked	41	88.3	1	0.1	0.8	9.8	0.8	21	31	0.7			20	0.02	0.04	0.3	7	68	1 cup diced	165
Beet, canned	34	90.3	0.9	0.1	0.8	7.9	0.5	15	29	0.6	36	120	20	0.01	0.02	0.1	5	82	1 cup	246
Beet greens, raw	27	90.4	2	0.3	1.7	5.6	1.4	118	45	3.2	130	570	6,700	0.08	0.18	0.4	34	27	1 cup	100
Beet greens, cooked	27	90.4	2	0.3	1.7	5.6	1.4	118	45	3.2			7,440	0.05	0.16	0.4	15	39	1 cup	145
Blackberries	57	84.8	1.2	1	0.5	12.5	4.2	32	32	0.9		150	200	0.04	0.04	0.4	21	82	1 cup	144
Blue mold cheese	368	40	21.5	30.5	6	2	0	315	339	0.5			1,240	0.03	0.61	0.2	0	104	1 oz	28
Blueberries, raw	61	83.4	0.6	0.6	0.3	15.1	1.2	16	13	0.8	0.6	89	280	0.02	0.02	0.3	16	85	1 cup	140
Blueberries, canned	98	73	0.4	0.4	0.2	26	1	41	6	0.5			40	0.01	0.01	0.2	13	245	1 cup	249
Bluefish (baked)	155	69.2	27.4	4.2	1.9	0	0	23	293	0.7				0.12	0.11	2.2		178	4 oz	115

Composition of foods, showing constituents of 100 g of edible portion[a] (cont.)

	Proximate composition							Minerals					Vitamins[d]					Total calories[b]	Average portion	
	Calories[b]	Water, g	Protein, g	Fat, g	Ash, g	Total carbohydrates, g	Crude fiber, g	Ca, mg	P, mg	Fe, mg	Na, mg	K, mg	A, IU	B₁, mg	B₂, mg	Niacin, mg	C, mg		Measure[c]	Weight, g
Bologna	221	62.4	14.8	15.9	3.3	3.6		9	112	2.2	1,300	230	0	0.18	0.19	2.7	0	117	2 slices, ⅛ × 4 in.	211
Boston brown bread	219	44.5	4.8	2.1	2.6	46	0.3	185	158	2.9	280	360	140	0.13	0.17	1.9	0	105	1, ¾ in. slice	48
Brains	125	78.9	10.4	8.6	1.4	0.8	0	16	330	3.6	150	340	0	0.23	0.26	4.4	18	106	3 oz	86
Bran flakes	292	3.6	10.8	1.9	4.9	78.8	3.9	61	622	5.1	1,400	1,200	0	0.46	0.23	8.7	0	117	1 cup	40
Brazil nuts (shelled)	646	5.3	14.4	65.9	3.4	11	2.1	186	693	3.4	1	670	Tr.	0.86	0.22	3.1	0	905	1 cup	140
Bread crumbs (dry)	385	8.5	11.9	4.5	2.6	72.5	0.2	111	129	2.6			0	0.27	0.22		0	339	1 cup	88
Broccoli, raw	29	89.9	3.3	0.2	1.1	5.5	1.3	130	76	1.3	16	400	3,500	0.1	0.21	1.1	118	25	1 cup	120
Broccoli, cooked	29	89.9	3.3	0.2	1.1	5.5	1.3	130	76	1.3			3,400	0.07	0.15	0.8	74	44	1 cup	150
Broccoli, frozen	30	90.2	3.4	0.3	0.8	5.3	1.1	61	63	0.8	16	244	2,850	0.07	0.13	0.6	62	36	1 cup	120
Brussels sprouts, raw	47	84.9	4.4	0.5	1.3	8.9	1.3	34	78	1.3	11	450	400	0.08	0.16	0.7	94	47	1 cup	100
Brussels sprouts, cooked	47	84.9	4.4	0.5	1.3	8.9	1.3	34	78	1.3			400	0.04	0.12	0.5	47	60	1 cup	130
Brussels sprouts, frozen	36	88.4	3.3	0.2	0.9	7.3	1.3	31	64	1.2	11	300	550	0.1	0.12	0.6	83	36	1 cup	100
Buckwheat flour	348	12	6.4	1.2	0.9	79.5	0.5	11	88	1			0	0.08	0.04	0.4	0	342	1 cup	98
Butter	716	15.5	0.6	81	2.5	0.4	0	20	16	0	980	23	3,300	Tr.	0.01	0.1	0	100	1 tbsp	14
Buttermilk	36	90.5	3.5	0.1	0.8	5.1	0	118	93	0.1	130	140	Tr.	0.04	0.18	0.1	1	86	1 cup	244
Butterscotch	410	5	0	8.9	0.5	85.6	0	20	7	1.8			0	0	Tr.	Tr.	0	20	¾ in. sq. × ⅜ in.	5
Cabbage, raw	24	92.4	1.4	0.2	0.8	5.3	1	46	31	0.5	5	230	80	0.06	0.05	0.3	50	24	1 cup shredded	100
Cabbage, cooked	24	92.4	1.4	0.2	0.8	5.3	1	46	31	0.5			90	0.05	0.05	0.3	31	40	1 cup diced	170
Candied peel, citron	314	18	0.2	0.3	1.3	80.2	1.4	83	24	0.8	290	120						89	1 oz	28
Candied peel, ginger root	340	12	0.3	0.2	0.4	87.1	0.7											85	1 small piece	25
Candied peel, lemon, orange, grapefruit	316	17.4	0.4	0.3	1.3	80.6	2.3				50	12						32	1 small piece	10
Cantaloupe	20	94	0.6	0.2	0.6	4.6	0.6	17	16	0.4	12	230	3,420	0.05	0.04	0.5	33	37	½, 5 in. diam.	385
Caramels	415	7	2.9	11.6	1	77.5	0	126	90	2.3			170	0.02	0.14	0.1	Tr.	42	⅞ in. sq. × ½ in.	10
Cashew nuts (roasted)	578	3.6	18.5	48.2	2.7	27	1.3	46	428	5	200[c]	560[c]		0.63	0.19	2.1		810	1 cup	140
Cauliflower, raw	25	91.7	2.4	0.2	0.8	4.9	0.9	22	72	1.1	24	400	90	0.11	0.10	0.6	69	31	1¼ cups	125
Cauliflower, cooked	25	91.7	2.4	0.2	0.8	4.9	0.9	22	72	1.1			90	0.06	0.08	0.5	28	30	1 cup	120
Cauliflower, frozen	22	92.7	2.1	0.2	0.6	4.3	0.9	18	45	0.6	11	234	33	0.06	0.06	0.4	55	27	1¼ cups	125
Caviar, sturgeon	243	57	26.9	15				30	300	1.4								208	3 oz	86
Celery	18	93.7	1.3	0.2	1.1	3.7	0.7	50	40	0.5	110	300	0	0.05	0.04	0.4	7	18	1 cup diced	100
Chard leaves, raw	27	91	2.6	0.4	1.2	4.8	0.8	105	36	2.5	84	380	8,720	0.06	0.18	0.4	38	27	1½ cups	100
Chard leaves, cooked	21	91.8	1.4	0.2	2.2	4.4	0.9	105	36	2.5			3,110	0.04	0.06	0.4	17	30	1 cup	145
Cheddar cheese (processed)	370	40	23.2	29.9	4.9	2	0	673	787	0.9	1,500	80	1,300	0.02	0.41	Tr.	0	105	1 oz	28
Cherries	61	83	1.1	0.5	0.6	14.8	0.3	18	20	0.4	1	260	620	0.05	0.06	0.4	8	94	1 cup pitted	154
Chestnuts (fresh)	191	53.2	2.8	1.5	1	41.5	1.1	48	48	4.1	2	410	0	0.08	0.24	1	0	95	20	250
Chicken, fryers (raw)	112	74.5	20.5	2.7	1.1	0	0	15	188	1.8	78	320	0	0.1	0.24	5.6	0	210	1 breast	224
Chicken, roasters (raw)	200	66	20.2	12.6	1	0	0	14	200	1.5	110	250	0	0.08	0.16	8	0	227	4 oz	115
Chicken, canned	199	61.9	29.8	8	2.4	0	0	14	148	1.8			0	0.04	0.16	6.4	0	169	3 oz	86

	Proximate composition							Minerals					Vitamins[d]					Total calories[b]	Average portion	
	Calories[b]	Water, g	Protein, g	Fat, g	Ash, g	Total carbohydrates, g	Crude fiber, g	Ca, mg	P, mg	Fe, mg	Na, mg	K, mg	A, IU	B_1, mg	B_2, mg	Niacin, mg	C, mg		Measure[e]	Weight, g
Chicken liver	141	69.6	22.1	4	1.7	2.6	0	16	240	7.4	51	160	32,200	0.20	2.46	11.8	20	106	2 medium livers	75
Chicory, French endive	21	94.2	1.6	0.3	1	2.9	0.8	18	21	0.7			10,000	0.05	0.20		15	3	¼ small head	15
Chili con carne	200	66.9	10.3	14.8	2.2	5.8	0.2	38	152	1.4			150	0.02	0.12	2.2		170	⅓ cup	85
Chives	52	86	3.8	0.6	1.8	7.8	2	48	57	1.9	43	430	390	0.15	0.03		11	33	1,3 in. diam.	50
Chocolate																				
milk	503	1.1	6	33.5	1.7	55.7	0.5	216	283	4	86	420	150	0.1	0.38	0.8	0	30	¾ × 1½ × ¼ in.	6
bitter	501	2.3	5.5	52.9	3.2	29.2	2.6	98	446	4.4	4	830	60	0.05	0.24	1.1	0	30	¾ × 1½ × ¼ in.	6
plain	471	1.4	2	29.8	1.4	62.7	1.4	63	287	2.8	35	230	30	0.03	0.15	0.6	0	28	¾ × 1½ × ¼ in.	6
Chocolate creams	394	9	4	14	1	72					10	110	55				0	55	1¼ in. diam. × ¾ in.	14
Chocolate-flavored milk	74	83	3.2	2.2	0.8	10.6	0	109	91	0.1	4	33	90	0.03	0.16	0.1	1	185	1 cup	250
Chocolate syrup	209	39	1.2	1.1	0.6	56.6	0.6	15	86	1.4	60	130						40	1 tbsp	19
Clams (raw)	81	80.3	12.8	1.4	2.1	3.4	0	96	139	7	180	240	110	0.1	0.18	1.6		92	4 oz	115
Cocoa, breakfast	293	3.9	8	23.8	5	48.9	4.6	125	712	11.6	57	1,400	30	0.12	0.38	2.3	0	15	2 tsp	5
Cocoa beverage (all milk)	95	79	3.8	4.6	0.9	10.9	0.1	119	114	0.4	16		160	0.04	0.19	0.2	1	236	1 cup	250
Coconut (dry)	556	3.3	3.6	39.1	0.8	53.2	4.1	43	191	3.6		770	0	Tr.	Tr.	Tr.	0	344	1 cup shreds	62
Cod																				
raw	74	82.6	16.5	0.4	1.2	0	0	10	194	0.4	60	360	0	0.06	0.09	2.2	2	85	4 oz	115
dried	375	12.3	81.8	2.8	7	0	0	50	891	3.8	8,100	160	0	0.08	0.45	10.9	0	106	1 oz	28
Coffee (black)	4	99	0.2	0	0.2	0.7	0	4	4	0.5	0.03	16.2						9	1 cup	230
Cola beverages	46	88				12					1	52						83	6 oz	180
Corn																				
raw	92	73.9	3.7	1.2	0.7	20.5	0.8	9	120	0.5	0.3–0.4	240–370	390	0.15	0.12	1.7	12	92	1 ear, 8 in. long	100
cooked	85	75.5	2.7	0.7	0.9	20.2	0.8	5	52	0.6			390	0.11	0.1	1.4	8	85	1 ear, 5 in.	140
canned	67	80.5	2	0.5	0.9	16.1	0.2	4	51	0.5	205	200	200	0.03	0.05	0.9	5	140	1 cup	116
Corn bread	219	49.2	6.7	4.7	2.8	36.6	0.6	139	155	1.9			130	0.17	0.23	1.3	0	103	1, 2¾ in. muffin	48
Corn flakes	385	3.6	8.1	0.4	2.9	85	0.1	11	58	2.2	660		0	0.41	0.1	2.2	0	96	1 cup	25
Corn grits	51	87.1	1.2	0.1	0.6	11	0	1	10	0.3		160	40	0.04	0.03	0.4	0	122	1 cup	242
Corned beef (canned)	216	59.3	25.3	12	3.4	0		20	106	4.3	1,300	60	0	0.02	0.24	3.4	0	180	3 oz	86
Corned beef hash (canned)	141	70.4	13.7	6.1	2.6	7.2	0.2	26	146	1.3	540		Tr.	0.03	0.14	2.9	0	120	3 oz	86
Cornmeal																				
whole	362	12	9	3.4	1.1	74.5	1	6	178	1.8		200	440	0.3	0.08	1.9	0	459	1 cup	127
degermed	363	12	7.9	1.2	0.5	78.4	0.6	6	99	2.9	0.7		300	0.44	0.26	3.5	0	527	1 cup	145
Cottage cheese	95	76.5	19.5	0.5	1.5	2		96	189	0.3	290	72	20	0.02	0.31	0.1	0	27	1 oz	28
Crabs	104	77.2	16.9	2.9	1.7	1.3		45	182	0.9	1,000	110	0	0.05	0.06	2.5	0	90	3 oz	86
Cracked wheat bread	259	36	8.5	2.2	1.9	51.4	0.5	83	126	2	620	250	0	0.25	0.19	2.5	0	60	1, ½ in. slice	23
Crackers (saltines)	431	4.6	9.2	11.8	3.3	71.1	0.4	19	92	1	1,100	120		0.06	0.04	1	0	34	2, 2 in. square	8
Cranberries	48	87.4	0.4	0.7	0.2	11.3	1.4	14	11	0.6	1	65	40	0.03	0.02	0.1	12	54	1 cup	113
Cranberry sauce	198	48.1	0.1	0.3	0.1	51.4	0.4	8	7	0.3	1	17	30	0.02	0.02	0.1	2	550	1 cup	277
Cream																				
light	204	72.5	2.9	20	0.6	4	0	97	77	0.1	50	91	830	0.03	0.14	0.1	1	30	1 tbsp	15
whipping	330	59	2.3	35	0.5	3.2	0	78	61	0	40	56	1,440	0.02	0.11	0.1	1	50	1 tbsp	15
Cream cheese	371	51	9	37	1	2	0	68	97	0.2	250	74	1,450	0.01	0.22	0.1	0	106	1 oz	28
Cucumbers	12	96.1	0.7	0.1	0.4	2.7	0.5	10	21	0.3	0.9	230	0	0.03	0.04	0.2	8	6	6, ⅛ in. slices	50
Currants, red	55	84.4	1.2	0.2	0.6	13.6	4	36	33	0.9	2	160	120	0.04	0.05		36	30	½ cup	55
Custard	114	77.3	5.3	5.4	0.8	11.2	0	114	119	0.5			340	0.05	0.20	0.1	Tr.	283	1 custard cup	248

Composition of foods, showing constituents of 100 g of edible portion[a] (cont.)

	Proximate composition							Minerals					Vitamins[a]					Average portion		
	Cal-ories[b]	Water, g	Pro-tein, g	Fat, g	Ash, g	Total carbohy-drates, g	Crude fiber, g	Ca, mg	P, mg	Fe, mg	Na, mg	K, mg	A, IU	B₁, mg	B₂, mg	Nia-cin, mg	C, mg	Total cal-ories[b]	Measure[e]	Weight, g
Dandelion greens (cooked)	44	85.8	2.7	0.7	2	8.8	1.8	187	70	3.1	76	430	15,170	0.13	0.12	0.7	16	80	1 cup greens	180
Dates (dried)	284	20	2.2	0.6	1.8	75.4	2.4	72	60	2.1	1	790	60	0.09	0.1	2.2	0	505	1 cup pitted	177
Doughnuts	425	18.7	6.6	21	1	52.7	0.2	73	286	0.7			140	0.16	0.13	1.2	0	136	1	32
Duck	322	54.3	16.1	28.6	1	0		9	172	2.4				0.12	0.4	7.9	8	370	4 oz	115
Egg																				
white (raw)	50	87.8	10.8	0	0.6	0.8	0	6	17	0.2	110	100	0	0	0.26	0.1	0	15	1 white	31
white (dried)	398	3	85.9	0	4.8	6.3	0	48	135	1.6			0	0	2.05	0.7	0	223	1 cup whites	56
yolk (raw)	361	49.4	16.3	31.9	1.7	0.7	0	147	586	7.2	26		3,210	0.27	0.35	Tr.	0	61	1 yolk	17
yolk (dried)	693	3	31.2	61.2	3.3	1.3	0	282	1,123	13.8			5,540	0.5	0.66	0.1	0	666	1 cup yolks	96
whole (raw)	162	74	12.8	11.5	1	0.7	0	54	210	2.7	81	100	1,140	0.1	0.29	0.1	0	77	1 medium egg	54
whole (dried)	592	5	46.8	42	3.6	2.5	0	190	767	8.8			3,740	0.34	1.06	0.2	0	640	1 cup	108
Eggplant	24	92.7	1.1	0.2	0.5	5.5	0.9	15	37	0.4	0.9	190	30	0.04	0.05	0.6	5	60	2 slices	250
Endive	20	93.3	1.6	0.2	0.9	4	0.8	79	56	1.7	18	400	3,000	0.07	0.12	0.4	11	90	1 lb, raw	460
Farina																				
cereal	44	89.2	1.3	0.1	0.3	9.1	0	3	13	0.2	11	10	0	0.04	0.03	0.2	0	105	1 cup	238
meal	370	10.5	10.9	0.8	0.4	77.4	0.4	28	112	1.3	2	86	0	0.37	0.26	1.3	0	625	1 cup	169
Fats, vegetable (cooking)	884	0	0	100	0	0	0	0	0	0	4	0	0	0	0	0	0	1,768	1 cup	200
Fig																				
canned	113	68.5	0.8	0.3	0.4	30	0.9	35	21	0.4	1	105	50	0.03	0.03	0.4	Tr.	130	3, 2 tbsp syrup	115
dried	270	24	4	1.2	2.4	68.4	5.8	186	111	3	34	780	80	0.16	0.12	1.7	0	57	1 large, 1 × 1 in.	21
Fig bars	350	13.8	4.2	4.8	1.4	75.8	1.7	69	69	1.3			0	0.02	0.06	0.9	0	87	1 large bar	25
Flounder (raw)	68	82.7	14.9	0.5	1.3	0	0	61	195	0.8				0.06	0.05	1.7	0	78	4 oz	115
Fondant	352	8	0	0	1	91	0	0	0	0			0	0	0	0	0	28	1 in. sq. × 5/8 in.	8
Frankfurter (cooked)	248	62	14	20	2	2	0.2	6	49	1.2		220	0	0.16	0.18	2.5	0	124	1.7 × 3/4 in.	51
French bread	270	35.5	8.1	2.7	1.7	52	0	24	71	1.8	1,100		0	0.24	0.15	2.2	0	1,225	1 lb	453
Frog legs (raw)	73	81.9	16.4	0.3	1.1	0	0	18	147	1.1			0	0.14	0.25	1.2	0	82	4 oz	115
Fruit cake	354	22.9	5.2	13.8	2.2	55.9	1.2	97	126	2.8	9	160	160	0.14	0.14	1.1	0	106	2 × 2 × 1/2 in.	30
Fruit cocktail (canned)	70	80.6	0.4	0.2	0.3	18.6	0.4	9	12	0.4			160	0.01	0.01	0.4	2	180	1 cup	257
Fudge (plain)	411	5	1.7	11.3	0.7	81.3	0.3	48	67	0.3			220	0.01	0.07	0.1	Tr.	185	2 in. sq. × 5/8 in.	45
Ginger ale	35	91				9	0				8	0.6					0	63	6 oz	180
Gingerbread	327	30.4	3.9	12	2.1	51.6	0.1	114	71	2.5			100	0.04	0.08	1		180	1, 2 in. cube	55
Goose	366	49.7	15.9	33.6	0.9	0	0	9	176	2.4				0.14			13	420	4 oz	115
Gooseberries	39	88.9	0.8	0.2	0.4	9.7	1.9	22	28	0.5	0.7	87	290				33	59	1 cup	150
Graham crackers	393	5.5	8	10	2.2	74.3	0.8	20	203	1.9	710	330	0	0.30	0.12	1.5	0	55	2 medium	14
Grape																				
American	70	81.9	1.4	1.4	0.4	14.9	0.5	17	21	0.6	3	84	80	0.06	0.04	0.2	4	84	1 cup	153
European	66	81.6	0.8	0.4	0.5	16.7	0.5	17	21	0.6	4	180	80	0.06	0.04	0.2	4	102	1 cup, 40 grapes	160
Grape juice	67	81	0.4	0	0.4	18.2		10	10	0.3	1	120		0.04	0.05	0.2	Tr.	120	6 oz	180
Grapefruit																				
raw	40	88.8	0.5	0.2	0.4	10.1	0.3	22	18	0.2	0.5	200	Tr.	0.04	0.02	0.2	40	77	1 cup sections	194
canned	72	79.8	0.6	0.2	0.4	19.1	0.2	13	14	0.3			Tr.	0.03	0.02	0.2	30	181	1 cup	249
Grapefruit juice (canned)	52	85.3	0.5	0.1	0.4	13.7	0.1	8	13	0.3	0.4	150	Tr.	0.03	0.02	0.2	35	131	1 cup	251

	Proximate composition							Minerals					Vitamins[d]					Average portion		
	Calories[b]	Water, g	Protein, g	Fat, g	Ash, g	Total carbohydrates, g	Crude fiber, g	Ca, mg	P, mg	Fe, mg	Na, mg	K, mg	A, IU	B₁, mg	B₂, mg	Niacin, mg	C, mg	Total calories[b]	Measure[e]	Weight, g
Green snap beans																				
raw	35	88.9	2.4	0.2	0.8	7.7	1.4	65	44	1.1	0.9	300	630	0.08	0.11	0.5	19	26	¼ cup	75
cooked	22	92.5	1.4	0.2	1.2	4.7	0.5	36	23	0.7			660	0.05	0.09	0.4	10	27	1 cup	125
canned	18	93.5	1	0.1	1.2	4.2	0.6	27	19	1.4	410	120	410	0.03	0.04	0.3	4	27	1 cup	125
frozen	27	91.6	1.7	0.1	0.5	6.2	1.1	45	33	0.8	16	244	2,850	0.07	0.13	0.6	62	36	1 cup	120
Guava	70	80.6	1	0.6	0.7	17.1	5.5	30	29	0.7			250	0.07	0.04	1.2	302	49	1 small	80
Haddock (cooked)	158	66.9	18.7	5.5	1.9	7	0	18	182	0.6				0.04	0.09	2.6		158	1 fillet, 4 × 3 × ½ in.	100
Halibut																				
raw	126	75.4	18.6	5.2	1	0	0	13	211	0.7	56	540	440	0.07	0.06	9.2		145	4 oz	115
cooked	182	64.2	26.2	7.8	1.9	0	0	14	267	0.8				0.06	0.07	10.5		230	1 fillet, 4 × 3 × ½ in.	126
Ham																				
fresh (raw)	344	53	15.2	31	0.8	0	0	9	168	2.3		340	0	0.74	0.18	4	0	296	3 oz	86
cured (cooked)	397	39	23	33	5.4	0.4	0	10	166	2.9	1,100	345	0	0.54	0.21	4.2	0	340	3 oz	86
Hamburger	364	47	22	30	1.1	0	0	9	158	2.8	107		0	0.08	0.19	4.8	0	316	3 oz	86
Hard candy	383	1	0	0	0	99	0	0		0			0	0	0	0	0	31	3, ¾ in. diam.	8
Heart, beef (raw)	108	77.6	16.9	3.7	1.1	0.7	0	9	203	4.6	90	160	30	0.58	0.89	7.8	6	92	3 oz	86
Herring																				
raw	191	67.2	18.3	12.5	2.7	0	0	10	256	1.1			110	0.02	0.15	3.4		191	1 small	100
kippered	211	61.0	22.2	12.9	4	0	0	66	254	1.4			0	Tr.	0.28	2.9		211	1 small	100
Honey	294	20	0.3	0	0.2	79.5	0	5	16	0.9		10	0	Tr.	0.04	0.2	4	62	1 tbsp	21
Honey Dew melon	32	90.5	0.5	0	0.5	8.5	0.4	17	16	0.4	7		40	0.05	0.03	0.2	23	49	1, 2 × 7 in. wedge	150
Ice cream (plain)	207	62.1	4	12.5	0.8	20.6	0	123	99	0.1	100	90	520	0.04	0.19	0.1	1	167	1 slice	81
Kale																				
raw	40	86.6	3.9	0.6	1.7	7.2	1.2	225	62	2.2	110	410	7,540	0.10	0.26	2	115	70	1¾ cups	175
frozen	32	89.8	3.2	0.5	0.9	5.6	0.9	132	52	1.2	29	254	8,000	0.07	0.17	0.8	60	56	1¾ cups	175
Ketchup	98	69.5	2	0.4	3.6	24.5	0.4	12	18	0.8	1,300	800	1,880	0.09	0.07	2.2	11	17	1 tbsp	17
Kidney beans, red																				
raw	336	12.2	23.1	1.7	3.6	59.4	3.5	163	437	6.9			0	0.57	0.22	2.5	2	638	1 cup	190
canned or cooked	90	76.0	5.7	0.4	1.5	16.4	0.9	40	124	1.9			0	0.05	0.05	0.8	0	230	1 cup	255
Kidneys, beef (raw)	141	74.9	15	8.1	1.1	0.9	0	9	221	7.9	210	310	1,150	0.37	2.55	6.4	13	120	3 oz	86
Lamb																				
rib chop (raw)	356	51.9	14.9	32.4	0.8	0	0	9	138	2.2	98	340	0	0.13	0.18	4.3	0	409	4 oz	115
rib chop (cooked)	418	40	24	35	1.2	0	0	11	200	3			0	0.14	0.26	5.6	0	480	4 oz	115
leg roast (raw)	235	63.7	18	17.5	0.9	0	0	10	213	2.7	78	380	0	0.16	0.22	5.2	0	202	3 oz	86
leg roast (cooked)	274	56	24	19	1.1	0	0	10	257	3.1			0	0.14	0.25	5.1	0	314	3 oz	86
Lard	902	0	0	100	0	0	0	0	0	0	0.3	0.2	0	0	0	0	0	126	1 tbsp	14
Lemon	32	89.3	0.9	0.6	0.5	8.7	0.9	40	22	0.6	0.7	130	0	0.04	Tr.	0.1	50	20	1, 2 in. diam.	100
Lemon juice	24	91.4	0.4	0.2	0.3	7.7		14	11	0.1	1.1		0	0.04	Tr.	0.1	42	4	1 tbsp	15
Lentils	339	12.2	24	1.2	2.2	60.4	1.7	34	292	7.4	3	1,200	570	0.56	0.24	2.2	5	204	¼ cup	60
Lettuce, head	15	94.8	1.2	0.2	0.9	2.9	0.6	22	25	0.5	12	140	540	0.04	0.08	0.2	8	7	2 large or 4 small leaves	50

Composition of foods, showing constituents of 100 g of edible portion[a] (cont.)

	Proximate composition							Minerals					Vitamins[d]					Average portion		
	Cal-ories[b]	Water, g	Pro-tein, g	Fat, g	Ash, g	Total carbohy-drates, g	Crude fiber, g	Ca, mg	P, mg	Fe, mg	Na, mg	K, mg	A, IU	B₁, mg	B₂, mg	Nia-cin, mg	C, mg	Total cal-ories[b]	Measure[e]	Weight, g
Lima beans, green																				
raw	128	66.5	7.5	0.8	1.7	23.5	1.5	63	158	2.3	1	680	280	0.21	0.11	1.4	32	96	½ cup	75
cooked	95	74.9	5	0.4	1.4	18.3	2	29	77	1.7			290	0.14	0.09	1.1	15	152	1 cup	160
canned	71	80.9	3.8	0.3	1.5	13.5	1.3	27	73	1.7	310	210	130	0.04	0.04	0.5	8	176	1 cup	249
frozen	100	73.2	6.1	0.2	1.5	19	1.7	23	102	2.3	181	489	220	0.11	0.06	1.14	21	75	½ cup	75
Lime	37	86	0.8	0.1	0.8	12.3	0.9	40	22	0.6	1	100	0	0.04	Tr.	0.1	27	19	1, 1½ in. long	68
Lime juice (fresh)	24	91	0.4	0	0.3	8.3	0	14	11	0.1		175		0.04	Tr.	0.1	27	57	1 cup	246
Liver																				
beef (raw)	136	69.7	19.7	3.2	1.4	6	0	7	358	6.6	110	380	43,900	0.26	3.33	13.7	31	117	3 oz	86
beef (fried)	208	57.2	23.6	7.7	1.8	9.7	0	8	486	7.8			53,500	0.26	3.96	14.8	31	118	2 oz	57
calf (raw)	141	70.8	19	4.9	1.3	4	0	6	343	10.6	110	380	22,500	0.21	3.12	16.1	36	121	3 oz	86
pork (raw)	134	72.3	19.7	4.8	1.5	1.7	0	10	362	18	77	350	14,200	0.4	2.98	16.7	23	115	3 oz	86
Liverwurst	263	59	16.7	20.6	2.2	1.5		9	238	5.4	892	149	5,750	0.17	1.12	4.6	0	150	2 oz	57
Lobster																				
raw	88	79.2	16.2	1.9	2.2	0.5	0	61	184	0.6	210	180		0.13	0.06	1.9		88	½ average	100
canned	92	77.2	18.4	1.3	2.7	0.4	0	65	192	0.8				0.03	0.07	2.2		78	3 oz	86
Loganberries	62	82.9	1	0.6	0.5	15	1.4	35	19	1.2			200	0.03	0.07	0.3	24	90	1 cup	144
Macaroni (dry)	377	8.6	12.8	1.4	0.7	76.5	0.4	22	165	2.9	1	160	0	0.88	0.37	6	0	463	1 cup dry	123
Mackerel (canned)	182	66	19.3	11.1	3.2	0	0	185	274	2.1			430	0.06	0.21	5.8		155	3 oz	86
Malted milk	104	78.2	4.6	4.4	1	11.8	0	135	123	0.3			250	0.07	0.21		1	281	1 cup	270
Margarine	720	15.5	0.6	81	2.5	0.4	0	20	16	0	1,100	58	3,300	0	0	0	0	100	1 tbsp	14
Marshmallows	325	15	3	0	1	81	0		0	0	41	6		0	0	0	0	98	5, 1¼ in. diam.	30
Mayonnaise	708	16	1.5	78	1.5	3	0	19	60	1	590	25	210	0.04	0.04	0	0	92	1 tbsp	13
Milk, cow's																				
whole (fluid)	68	87	3.5	3.9	0.7	4.9	0	118	93	0.1	50	140	160	0.04	0.17	0.1	1	166	1 cup	244
nonfat (fluid)	36	90.5	3.5	0.1	0.8	5.1	0	123	97	0.1	52	150	Tr.	0.04	0.18	0.1	1	87	1 cup	246
nonfat (dry)	362	3.5	35.6	1	7.9	52	0	1,300	1,030	0.6	528	1,130	40	0.35	1.96	1.1	7	28	1 tbsp	8
evaporated	138	73.7	7	7.9	1.5	9.9	0	243	195	0.2	100	270	400	0.05	0.36	0.2	1	346	1 cup	252
Mince pie	252	43	2.5	6.9	2	45.6	0.5	16	40	2.2			10	0.07	0.04	0.4	1	340	4 in. sec. of 9 in. pie	135
Muffins	280	37.4	8	8.4	2.2	42.1	0.1	206	191	1.6			100	0.18	0.21	1.5	0	135	1, 2¾ in. muffin	48
Mushrooms																				
raw	16	91.1	2.4	0.3	1.1	4	0.9	9	115	1	5	520	0	0.10	0.44	4.9	5	8	½ cup diced	50
canned	11	93	1.4	0.2	1	3.7		7	90	0.8	400	150		0.02	0.25	2		28	1 cup	244
Mustard greens	22	92.2	2.3	0.3	1.2	4	0.8	220	38	2.9	48	450	7,180	0.06	0.18	0.7	45	31	1 cup greens	140
Noodles, egg (cooked)	67	83.8	2.2	0.6	0.6	12.8	0.1	4	35	0.5			30	0.14	0.06	1	0	107	1 cup	60
Oat cereal	396	4	14.5	7	4.3	70.2	2	160	350	4.1			0	0.82	0.19	1.9	0	100	1 cup	25
Oatmeal	63	84.8	2.3	1.2	0.7	11	0.2	9	67	0.7	55		0	0.1	0.02	0.2	0	150	1 cup	238
Oil (salad or cooking)	884	0	0	100	0	0	0	0	0	0	0.3	0.1	0	0	0	0	0	124	1 tbsp	14
Okra (cooked)	32	89.8	1.8	0.2	0.8	7.4	1	82	62	0.7	0.2	220	740	0.06	0.06	0.8	20	28	8 pods	85
Olive																				
green	132	75.2	1.5	13.5	5.8	4	1.2	87	17	1.6	2,400	55	300	Tr.				72	10 "mammoth"	65
ripe	191	71.8	1.8	21	2.8	2.6	1.5	87	17	1.6	980	23	60	Tr.	Tr.			106	10 "mammoth"	65
Onions (mature)																				
raw	45	87.5	1.4	0.2	0.6	10.3	0.1	32	44	0.5	1	130	50	0.03	0.04	0.2	9	50	1, 2½ in. diam.	110
cooked	38	89.5	1	0.2	0.6	8.7	0.8	32	44	0.5			50	0.02	0.03	0.2	6	79	1 cup	210
Orange	45	87.2	0.9	0.2	0.5	11.2	0.6	33	23	0.4	0.3	170	190	0.08	0.03	0.2	49	70	1 medium, 3 in. diam.	215

	Proximate composition							Minerals					Vitamins[d]					Total calories[b]	Average portion	
	Calories[b]	Water, g	Protein, g	Fat, g	Ash, g	Total carbohydrates, g	Crude fiber, g	Ca, mg	P, mg	Fe, mg	Na, mg	K, mg	A, IU	B1, mg	B2, mg	Niacin, mg	C, mg		Measure[e]	Weight, g
Orange juice																				
fresh	44	87.5	0.8	0.2	0.4	11	0.1	19	16	0.2	3.6	182	190	0.08	0.03	0.2	49	108	1 cup	246
canned	44	87.5	0.8	0.2	0.4	11.1	0.1	10	18	0.3	0.5	190	100	0.07	0.02	0.2	42	135	1 cup	251
Oyster stew	91	82.6	5.3	5.4	1.4	5.3	0	117	110	1.5			280	0.06	0.18	0.4		244	1 cup, 6–8 oysters	240
Oysters (raw)	84	80.5	9.8	2.1	2	5.6	0	94	143	5.6	73	110	320	0.15	0.2	1.2		200	13–19 medium, 1 cup	238
Pancakes																				
wheat	218	55.4	6.8	9.2	2	26.6	0.1	158	154	1.3			200	0.18	0.21	1.3	Tr.	60	1, 4 in. diam.	27
buckwheat	176	62.0	6.1	8.4	2.6	20.9	0.5	249	362	1.2			110	0.16	0.16	0.9	Tr.	48	1, 4 in. diam.	27
Papaya	43	88.3	0.6	0.1		10		19	13	0.3			2,400	0.05	0.13		36	73	1, 2½ × 7 in. wedge	170
Parsley	50	83.9	3.7	1	2.4	9	1.8	193	84	4.3	8	880	8,230	0.11	0.28	1.4	193	1	1 tbsp	3.5
Peach																				
raw	46	86.9	0.5	0.1	0.5	12	0.6	8	22	0.6	0.5	160	880	0.02	0.05	0.9	8	45	1 medium, 2½ × 2 in. diam.	114
canned	68	80.9	0.4	0.1	0.4	18.2	0.4	5	14	0.4	5	31	450	0.01	0.02	0.7	4	175	1 cup	258
frozen	88	76.3	0.5	0.1	0.8	22.8	0.4	4	12	0.7	3	124	133	0.01	0.04	0.7	13	99	4 oz	112
dry	265	24	3	0.6	3	69.4	3.5	44	126	6.9	12	1,100	3,250	0.01	0.2	5.4	19	424	1 cup	160
Peanut brittle	441	2	8.3	15.5	1.3	72.8	0.8	38	124	2			0	0.09	0.05	4.9	0	66	1½ × 3 in.	15
Peanut butter	576	1.7	26.1	47.8	3.4	21	2	74	393	1.9	120	820	0	0.12	0.13	16.2	0	92	1 tbsp	16
Peanuts (roasted)	559	2.6	26.9	44.2	2.7	23.6	2.4	74	393	1.9	460[c]	700[c]	0	0.3	0.13	16.2	0	805	1 cup	144
Pear																				
raw	63	82.7	0.7	0.4	0.4	15.8	1.4	13	16	0.3	2	100	20	0.02	0.04	0.1	4	95	1, 3 × 2½ in. diam.	182
canned	68	81.1	0.2	0.1	0.2	18.4	0.8	8	10	0.2	8	52	Tr.	0.01	0.02	0.1	2	80	2 halves, 2 tbsp syrup	117
Peas, green																				
raw	98	74.3	6.7	0.4	0.9	17.7	2.2	22	122	1.9	1	370	680	0.34	0.16	2.7	26	74	½ cup	75
cooked	70	81.7	4.9	0.4	0.9	12.1	2.2	22	122	1.9			720	0.25	0.14	2.3	15	111	1 cup	60
frozen	83	80.3	5.7	0.4	0.8	12.9	1.8	24	92	2.2	160	153	670	0.33	0.10	1.9	17	124	1 cup	150
Peas, dry, split	344	10	24.5	1	2.8	61.7	1.2	33	268	5.1	42	880	370	0.77	0.28	3.1	2	689	1 cup	200
Pecans	696	3	9.4	73	1.6	13	2.2	74	324	2.4	0.3	420	50	0.72	0.11	0.9	2	752	1 cup halves	108
Peppers, green	25	92.4	1.2	0.2	0.5	5.7	1.4	11	25	0.4	0.6	170	630	0.04	0.07	0.4	120	16	1 medium	76
Pilchards (canned)	200	65.2	17.7	13.5	2.9	0.7	0	381	168	4.1	760	260	30	0.01	0.3	7.4	0	171	3 oz	86
Pineapple juice (canned)	49	86.2	0.3	0.1	0.4	13	0.1	15	8	0.5	0.5	140	80	0.05	0.02	0.2	9	121	1 cup	249
Plain cake	327	26.8	6.4	8.2	1.6	57	0.1	155	137	0.4			120	0.08	0.08	0.3	0	161	1, 2¾ in. cupcake	50
Plum																				
raw	50	85.7	0.7	0.2	0.5	12.9	0.5	17	20	0.5	0.6	170	350	0.06	0.04	0.5	5	30	1, 2 in. diam.	60
canned	76	78.6	0.4	0.1	0.5	20.4	0.3	8	12	1.1	18	110	230	0.03	0.03	0.4	1	186	1 cup	256
Popcorn	386	4	12.7	5	1.6	76.7	2.2	11	281	2.7			0	0.39	0.12	2.2	0	54	1 cup popped	14
Potato chips	544	3.1	6.7	37.1	4	49.1	1.1	30	152	1.9	2,000	240	50	0.18	0.11	3.2	11	108	10 medium, 2 in.	20
Pretzels	369	8	8.8	3.2	5.5	74.5	0.3	12	71	0.7	1,700	130	0	0.01	0.04	0.7	0	18	5 small sticks	5
Prune juice	71	80	0.4	0	0.3	19.3		25	40	1.8	2	260	0	0.03	0.08	0.4	1	170	1 cup	240
Prunes	268	24	2.3	6	2.1	71	1.6	54	85	3.9	6	600	1,890	0.10	0.16	1.7	3	94	4 large	40
Puffed rice	392	3.5	5.9	0.6	2.3	87.7	0.5	21	116	1.8	0.9	100	0	0.46	0.08	5.5	0	55	1 cup	14
Puffed wheat	355	3.8	10.8	1.6	3.6	80.2	1.7	46	329	4.2	4	340	0	0.56	0.18	6.4	0	43	1 cup	12
Pumpkin																				
raw	31	90.5	1.2	0.2	0.8	7.3	1.3	21	44	0.8	0.6	480	3,400	0.05	0.08	0.6	8	37	¾ cup	120
canned	33	90.2	1	0.3	0.6	7.9	1.2	20	36	0.7	2	240	3,400	0.02	0.06	0.5		76	1 cup	228
Pumpkin pie	202	58.9	4.2	9.6	1.5	25.8	0.6	54	81	0.8			1,910	0.03	0.12	0.3	0	265	4 in. sec. of 9 in. pie	131

Composition of foods, showing constituents of 100 g of edible portion[a] (cont.)

	Proximate composition							Minerals					Vitamins[d]					Total calories[b]	Average portion	
	Calories[b]	Water, g	Protein, g	Fat, g	Ash, g	Total carbohydrates, g	Crude fiber, g	Ca, mg	P, mg	Fe, mg	Na, mg	K, mg	A, IU	B₁, mg	B₂, mg	Niacin, mg	C, mg		Measure[e]	Weight, g
Raisin bread	284	30.2	7.1	3.1	1.8	57.8	0.2	80	104	1.8			10	0.24	0.15	2.2	0	65	1, ½ in. slice	23
Raisins	268	24	2.3	0.5	2	71.2		78	129	3.3	21	720	50	0.15	0.08	0.5	Tr.	430	1 cup	160
Raspberries, red																				
raw	57	84.1	1.2	0.4	0.5	13.8	4.7	40	37	0.9	0.5	130	130	0.02	0.07	0.3	24	70	1 cup	123
frozen	98	74.3	0.7	0.2	0.2	24.7	2.1	12	17	0.6	0.7	97	80	0.02	0.07	0.6	21	84	3 oz	86
Raspberries, black	74	80.6	1.5	1.6	0.6	15.7	6.8	40	37	0.9	0.3	190	0	0.02	0.07	0.3	24	100	1 cup	134
Rhubarb (frozen)	74	80.2	0.6	0.2	0.6	19.2	0.9	99	14	0.8	6	212	83	0.02	0.06	0.2	7	202	1 cup	273
Rice																				
brown	360	12	7.5	1.7	1.1	77.7	0.6	39	303	2	9	150	0	0.32	0.05	4.6	0	748	1 cup	208
converted	362	12	7.6	0.3	0.4	79.4	0.2	24	136	0.8	4	170	0	0.20	0.03	3.8	0	677	1 cup	187
white	362	12.3	7.6	0.3	0.4	79.4	0.2	24	136	0.8	2	130	0	0.07	0.03	1.6	0	692	1 cup	191
wild	364	8.5	14.1	0.7	1.4	75.3	1	19	339	1.8	7	220	0	0.45	0.63	6.2	0	593	1 cup	163
Rice flakes	392	3.5	5.9	0.6	2.3	87.7	0.5	21	116	1.8	720	180	0	0.46	0.08	5.5	0	117	1 cup	30
Rolls																				
plain	309	28.5	9	5.5	1.9	55.1	0.2	55	96	1.8			0	0.24	0.15	2.2	0	120	1, 1/12 lb.	39
sweet	323	28.4	8.5	7.8	1.5	53.8	0.2	63	104	1.8			0	0.24	0.15	2.2	0	178	1	55
Rye bread	244	35.3	9.1	1.2	2	52.4	0.4	72	147	1.6	590	160	0	0.18	0.08	1.5	0	57	1, ½ in. slice	23
Rye flour	318	11	16.3	2.6	2.0	68.1	2.4	54	536	4.5		860	0	0.61	0.22	2.7	0	285	1 cup	80
Salad dressing, French	394	39.6	0.6	35.5	4	20.3	0.3	0	0	0			0	0	0	0	0	60	1 tbsp	15
Salmon																				
raw	223	63.4	17.4	16.5	1	0	0		289	0.9	48	410	310	0.10	0.23	7.2	9	192	3 oz	86
canned	203	64.7	19.7	13.2	2.4	0	0	154	289	0.9	540	300	230	0.03	0.14	7.3	0	120	3 oz	86
Salt pork	783	8	3.9	85	3.5	0	0	Tr.	Tr.	0.6	1,800	27		0.18	0.04	0.9	0	470	2 oz	60
Sardines (canned)	214	57.4	25.7	11	4.7	1.2	0	386	586	2.7	510	560	220	0.02	0.17	4.8	0	182	3 oz drained	86
Sauerkraut (canned)	22	91.2	1.4	0.3	2.7	4.4	0.9	36	18	0.5	630	140	40	0.03	0.06	0.1	16	32	1 cup drained	150
Sausage, pork (raw)	450	41.9	10.8	44.8	2.1	0	0	6	100	1.6	740	140	0	0.43	0.17	2.3	0	158	2, 3½ in. long	35
Scallops (raw)	78	80.3	14.8	0.1	1.4	3.4	0	26	208	1.8	150	420	0	0.04	0.1	1.4		90	4 oz	115
Shad (raw)	168	70.2	18.7	9.8	1.4	0	0		260	0.5				0.15	0.24	8.4		191	4 oz	115
Sherbet	123	68.1	1.5	0	0.4	30		50	40	0	174	218	0	0.02	0.08	Tr.	0	118	½ cup	96
Shrimp (canned)	127	66.2	26.8	1.4	5.8	0	0	115	263	3.1	140	220	60	0.01	0.03	2.2	0	110	3 oz	86
Soybean flour	264	9	42.5	6.5	4.8	37.2	2.6	244	610	13		1,700	110	0.82	0.34	2.6	0	232	1 cup	88
defatted	228	11	44.7	1.1	5.5	37.7	2.3	265	623	13	1		70	1.1	0.35	2.9	0			
Soybean sprouts	46	86.3	6.2	1.4	0.8	5.3	0.8	48	67	1			180	0.23	0.20	0.8	13	50	1 cup of raw	107
Soybeans	331	7.5	34.9	18.1	4.7	34.8	5.0	227	586	8	4	1,900	110	1.07	0.31	2.3	Tr.	695	1 cup of dry	210
Spaghetti (cooked)	149	60.6	5.1	0.6	3.5	30.2	0.2	9	65	1.1			0	0.17	0.1	1.4	0	220	1 cup	148
Spinach																				
raw	20	92.7	2.3	0.3	1.5	3.2	0.6	81	55	3	82	780	9,420	0.11	0.2	0.6	59	22	4 oz	115
cooked	26	90.8	3.1	0.6	1.9	3.6	1	124	33	2			11,780	0.08	0.2	0.6	30	46	1 cup	80
canned	20	92.3	2.3	0.4	1.8	3.0	0.7	90	33	1.6	320	260	6,790	0.02	0.1	0.3	14	45	1 cup	232
Sponge cake	291	31.8	7.9	5	0.9	54.4		28	110	1.4			520	0.05	0.15	0.2	0	117	2 in. sec. of 8 in. cake	40
Squash, summer																				
raw	16	95	0.6	0.1	0.4	3.9	0.5	15	15	0.4	0.2	150	260	0.05	0.09	0.8	17	40	1¾ cups diced	250
frozen	21	93.4	1.4	0.1	0.4	4.7	0.6	14	32	0.6	4	169	150	0.07	0.04	0.4	6	44	1 cup cooked, diced	210
Squash, winter																				
raw	38	88.6	1.5	0.3	0.8	8.8	1.4	19	28	0.6	0.3	240	4,950	0.05	0.12	0.5	8	95	1¾ cups diced	250
frozen	33	89.2	1.2	0.4	0.51	8.8	1.2	27	33	1.3	0.2	209	4,280	0.03	0.07	0.5	7	82	1¾ cups diced	250
cooked	47	85.7	1.9	0.4	1	11	1.8	24	35	0.8			6,190	0.05	0.15	0.6	7	97	1 cup mashed	205

	Proximate composition							Minerals					Vitamins[d]					Total calories[b]	Average portion	
	Calories[b]	Water, g	Protein, g	Fat, g	Ash, g	Total carbohydrates, g	Crude fiber, g	Ca, mg	P, mg	Fe, mg	Na, mg	K, mg	A, IU	B_1, mg	B_2, mg	Niacin, mg	C, mg		Measure[e]	Weight, g
Starch (pure)	362	12	0.5	0.2	0.3	87	0.1	0	0	0	4	4	0	0	0	0	0	29	1 tbsp	8
Strawberries																				
raw	37	89.9	0.8	0.5	0.5	8.3	1.4	28	27	0.8	0.8	180	60	0.03	0.07	0.3	60	54	1 cup	149
frozen	95	74.8	0.5	0.2	0.2	24.4	0.6	13	16	0.6	1.5	107	33	0.02	0.06	0.5	43	82	3 oz	86
Succotash (frozen)	97	66.3	4.5	0.4	0.8	21.4	0.9	15	90	1.2	73	279	167	0.11	0.06	1.5	7	205	¾ cup, cooked	210
Sweetbreads (cooked)	178	67.2	22.7	9.1	0	0	0	14	596	1.6	69	243	0	0.08	0.4	0	0	204	4 oz	115
Swiss cheese	355	40	26.4	26.9	5.1	1.6	0	887	867	0.9			1,390	0.01	0.4	0.1	0	101	1 oz	28
Swordfish (cooked)	178	64.8	27.4	6.8	1.7	0	0	20	251	1.1			2,300	0.05	0.06	10.3	0	223	1 steak, 3×3½ in.	125
Tangerine	44	87.3	0.8	0.3	0.7	10.9	1	33	23	0.4	2	110	420	0.07	0.03	0.2	31	35	1 medium, 2½ in. diam.	114
Tangerine juice	39	89.2	0.9	0.3	0.4	9.2		19	16	0.2	0.6	170	420	0.06	0.03	0.2	26	95	1 cup	246
Tapioca (dry)	360	12.6	0.6	0.2	0.2	86.4	0.1	12	12	1	5	19	0	0	0	0.2	0	547	1 cup	152
Tomato																				
raw	20	94.1	1	0.3	0.6	4	0.6	11	27	0.6	3	230	1,100	0.06	0.04	0.5	23	30	1 medium, 2×2½ in.	150
canned	19	94.2	1	0.2	0.7	3.9	0.4	11	27	0.6	18	130	1,050	0.06	0.03	0.7	16	46	1 cup	242
Tomato juice	21	93.5	1	0.2	1	4.3	0.2	7	15	0.4	230	230	1,050	0.05	0.03	0.8	16	50	1 cup	242
Tomato puree	36	89.2	1.8	0.5	1.3	7.2	0.4	11	37	1.1	100		1,880	0.09	0.07	1.8	28	90	1 cup	249
Tongue, beef	207	68	16.4	15	0.9	0.4	0	9	187	2.8	800	260	0	0.12	0.29	5	0	235	4 oz	115
Tuna fish (canned)	198	60	29	8.2	2.7	0	0	8	351	1.4	800	240	80	0.05	0.12	12.8	0	170	3 oz drained solids	86
Turkey	268	58.3	20.1	20.2	1	0	0	23	320	3.8	40–92	310–320	Tr.	0.09	0.14	8	0	304	4 oz	115
Turnip greens																				
raw	30	89.5	2.9	0.4	1.8	5.4	1.2	259	50	2.4	10	440	9,540	0.09	0.46	0.8	136	15	½ cup	50
cooked	30	89.5	2.9	0.4	1.8	5.4	1.2	259	50	2.4			10,600	0.06	0.41	0.7	60	43	1 cup	145
Veal cutlet	219	60	28	11	1.4	0	0	12	258	3.5			0	0.08	0.28	6.1	0	184	3 oz	86
Vienna bread	270	35.5	8.1	2.7	1.7	52	0.2	24	71	1.8			0	0.24	0.15	2.2	0	1,225	1 lb	453
Waffles	287	40	9.3	10.6	2.3	37.8	0.1	192	204	1.8			360	0.18	0.27	1.3	0	216	1, 4½×5⅝×½ in.	75
Walnuts, English	654	3.3	15	64.4	1.7	15.6	2.1	83	380	2.1	2	450	30	0.48	0.13	1.2	3	654	1 cup of halves	100
Watercress	18	93.6	1.7	0.3	1.1	3.3	0.5	195	46	2			4,720	0.08	0.16	0.8	77	5	½ cup	20
Watermelon	28	92.1	0.5	0.2	0.3	6.9	0.6	7	12	0.2	0.3	110	590	0.05	0.05	0.2	6	97	½ slice, ¾×10 in.	345
Wheat flakes	355	3.8	10.8	1.6	3.6	80.2	1.7	46	329	4.2	1,300	320	0	0.56	0.18	6.4	0	125	1 cup	35
Wheat flour																				
80% extended	365	12	12.0	1.3	0.7	74.1	0.5	24	191	1.3	1	120	0	0.26	0.07	2	0	400	1 cup stirred	110
self-rising	350	12	9.2	1	4	73.8	0.4	272	484	2.9	1,500	90	0	0.44	0.26	3.5	0	384	1 cup stirred	110
all-purpose	364	12	10.5	1	0.4	76.1	0.3	16	87	2.9	1	86	0	0.44	0.26	3.5	0	400	1 cup stirred	110
cake	364	12	7.5	0.8	0.3	79.4	0.2	17	73	0.5			0	0.03	0.03	0.7	0	364	1 cup stirred	100
Wheat germ	361	11	25.2	10	4.3	49.5	2.5	84	1,096	8.1	2	780	50	2.05	0.8	4.6	0	246	1 cup	68
Whey (dried)	344	6.2	12.5	1.2	7.7	72.4	0	679	576	0.2			50	0.49	2.5	0.8	0	125	—	—
White bread	275	34.7	8.5	3.2	1.8	51.8	0.2	79	92	1.8	640	180	0	0.24	0.15	2.2	0	63	1, 1½ in. slice	23
Whole wheat bread	240	36.6	9.3	2.6	2.5	49	1.5	96	263	2.2	930	230	0	0.3	0.13	3	0	55	1, 1½ in. slice	23
Yeast																				
baker's (compressed)	86	70.9	10.6	0.4	2.4	13	0.3	25	605	4.9	4	360	0	0.45	2.07	28.2	0	24	1 oz	28
brewer's (dry)	273	7	36.9	1.6	7.9	37.4	0.8	106	1,893	18.2	150	1,700	0	9.69	5.45	36.2	0	22	1 tbsp	8

[a] A blank in the figure columns indicates that no value for a constituent is reported in the literature, although it seems reasonable to assume that it should be present.

[b] 1 calorie = approx. 4.19 joules.

[c] When roasted and salted.

[d] Tr. = trace amount.

[e] Approximate conversions are: 1 cup = 237 milliliters; 1 tbsp = 15 milliliters; 1 tsp = 5 milliliters; 1 oz (vol.) = 30 milliliters; 1 oz (wt.) = 28 grams; 1 lb = 454 grams; 1 in. = 2.5 centimeters.

SOURCE: Table courtesy of H. J. Heinz Company; modified from the version in Benjamin T. Burton, Human Nutrition, 3d ed., McGraw-Hill, 1976.

INDEX

Index

Asterisks indicate entries which are article titles.

Linoleic acid 367–368*, 374
  essential fatty acid function 367
  minimum requirements 368
  physiological function 367–368
  sources 367
Linolenic acid 368*
  biosynthesis 368
  essential fatty acid function 368
  nutritional requirements 368
  physiological function 368
  sources 368
  soybean oil 368
Linseed oil 247, 248, 369*
  linolenic acid 368*
Linum usitatissimum 247, 369
Linuron 338
Lipase 219, 370
Lipid 369–370*
  accumulation around damaged cells 390
  blood lipids 371
  classification 369
  dietary 374
  eggs 225
  extraction 369
  functions 389
  identification 370
  occurrence 369
  separation 369–370
  sources of abnormal accumulation 389–390
  yeast sources 685
Lipid metabolism 370–374*
  adipose tissue 370–371
  essential fatty acids 374
  fat digestion and absorption 370
  fatty acid oxidation 371
  fatty acid synthesis 373
  ketone body formation 372
  lipotropic factors 372–373
  metabolic disorders 389–390
  modification of dietary lipids 374
  phospholipid synthesis 374
  role of phosphatides 374
  small intestine 217
  triglyceride synthesis 374
Lipid storage disease 390
Lipoma 389
Lipomyces 681
Lipton process (food analogs) 309
Liqueur 221
Liquid fertilizer 239
  application 241
Litchi 375
Litchi chinensis 375
Little bluestem grass 145
Little cherry disease 185
Liver 218–219
  alcoholic cirrhosis 91
Livestock: cattle production, beef 172–176*
  cattle production, dairy 176–178*
  dressing 268–269
  feeding 64
  fungus infections 66
  judging 65
  grazing 57–58

Livestock—cont.
  pest and disease control 65–66
Livestock breeding 63–64
  breeding terminology 63
  formation of new breeds 64
  systems 63–64
Livestock farming: crop and livestock farming 58
  engineering challenges 53
  Mediterranean agriculture 58
  subsistence 56
Livestock ranching 60
Long-day plants 440
Long-stalked clover 190
Loose kernel smut (sorghum) 615
Loose smut: barley 128
  oats 420
Louping ill 374*
Low-temperature long-time pasteurizer 397
Lowbush blueberry 144
LTLT see Low-temperature long-time
Lucerne 91
Lupine 374–375*
Lupus erythematosus 388–389
Lush, Jay L. 147
Lychee 375*
Lycopersicon 650
Lycopersicon esculentum 650
Lycopersicon pimpinellifolium 650
Lysine 107, 108, 375–376*

M

Macadamia nut 376*, 417
Macadamia ternifolia 376, 417
Mace 624
Machinery: agricultural see Agricultural machinery
  dairy 210–214
McQuigg, J. D. 15
Macronutrients (fertilizer) 234
Macrophomina phaseoli 200, 204
Magnesium: fertilizer 234
  role in plant growth 463
  utilization by soil microorganisms 612
Maine Anjou cattle 173
Maize 253
Maize dwarf mosaic virus 200
Marjoram 624
Malathion 349
Maleic hydrazide (responses to weather) 62
Malignant neoplasms 392
Malignant pustule 112
Malnutrition 376–378*
  alcoholism 89–90
  basic food requirements 3
  cell requirements 377
  essential metabolite deficiencies 377
  generalized 377
  improving food availability 5–9
  kwashiorkor disease 357*, 377–378

Malnutrition—cont.
  metabolic disorders 385–392*
  pellagra 435*
  rickets 544*
  scurvy 553*
  starvation 628–630*
Malt vinegar 658
Malta fever 153
Maltase 170
Malthus, T. 1, 2
Malting (barley) 129–130
Maltose 635
Malus domestica 114
Malus malus 114
Malus pumila 114
Malus sylvestris 114
Mandarin 378*
Mandioca 544
Maneb 320
Manganese: role in plant growth 464
  utilization by soil microorganisms 612
Mangifera indica 378
Mango 378*
Manihot esculenta 171, 544
Manioc 171, 544
Manufactured food 254, 290
Manure 378*
  fertilizer alternative 29
Maple sugar 635, 637
Maranta arundinacea 116, 544
Margarine 306, 378–380*
  composition 380
  manufacture 380
  production 380
Mariculture 40
Marine fisheries 245, 380–384*
  changing patterns 382
  fishery management 383–384
  harvest of the sea 380–382
  international management 384
  United States fishing industry 382–383
Market gardening 59
Market Names of Fishery Products, Plan for 39
Marmalades 301, 302
Marshmallows 296, 297
Marssonina panattoniana 366
Martin, A. J. P. 98
Mayer, G. E. 514
Mayo (wheat) 44
Mayonnaise 231
  emulsifying and homogenizing 280
  whipping 280
MCPA (herbicide) 338
MCPB (herbicide) 338
MDMV see Maize dwarf mosaic virus
Meadow fescue 244
Meat: beef grades 174
  cattle production, beef 172–176*
  grading of market animals 65
  lamb 562
  spoilage 312
Meat products 254, 302–303
  canned meats 303
  cured and pickled meats 302
  cured and smoked meats 302–303
  fat 303

Meat products—cont.
  frozen meats 303
  tenderized fresh meats 303
Mecoprop 338
Medicago arabica 203
Medicago falcata 92, 93, 94
Medicago lupulina 203
Medicago orbicularis 203
Medicago sativa 91, 93, 94, 202
Mediterranean agriculture 57–58
Melampsora lini 248, 482
Melanconium fuligineum 332
Melilotus 190
Melilotus alba 191
Melilotus indica 190
Melilotus officinalis 191
Melizitose 425
Mellorine 343
Meloidogyne 204, 478, 618
Meloidogyne arenaria 431
Meloidogyne hapla 431
Melon: cantaloupe 160*
  Honey Dew melon 341*
  muskmelon 411–412*
  Persian melon 437*
  watermelon 670*
Melon growing 384–385*
  climate and soil requirements 384
  cultural requirements 385
  harvesting 385
Menazon 349
Mendel, Gregor 147
Mentha piperita 435
Mercaptals, sugar 409
Merino sheep 559
Metabolic disorders 385–392*
  alkaptonuria 388
  amino aciduria 388
  amyloid 387–388
  carbohydrate metabolism 390–392
  diabetes mellitus 391
  effects on cell proteins 386
  formation of abnormal proteins 387
  function of lipids 389
  galactosemia 392
  glycogen storage disease 391–392
  gout 388
  hemoglobin 387
  Hurler-Pfaundler's disease 392
  hyperproteinemia 387
  hypoproteinemia 387
  kwashiorkor disease 357*
  lipid metabolism 389–390
  lipid storage disease 390
  lipids and degenerate cells 390
  lupus erythematosus 388–389
  malignant neoplasms 392
  multiple myeloma 387
  nucleic acid structure and metabolism 388–389
  obesity, hyperlipemia, lipid tumors 389
  phenylketonuria 388

Plant disease control—*cont.*
cultural practices 491
disease resistance 492–494
eradication campaigns 496
quarantines 496–497
translocation in plants 512
Plant fiber, dietary 497–498*
cell wall fibers 497
cholesterol metabolism 498
colon cancer 498
negative properties 498
other fibers 497
relation to disease 497–498
Plant foods 253–254
Plant growth 498–508*
abscisic acid 49–51*
abscission 506–507
apical dominance 504
auxin 121–124*
brassin 146
bud dormancy 504
chemical regulators 52
cytokinins 208–210*
daily thermoperiodicity 508
dominance and germination 504–507
embryonic 500
factors affecting 498–499
field measurements 223
floral initiation and development 502–503
flower biology 503
fruit development 503
germination 504–505
gibberellin 323–325*
growing season 333–334
growth correlations 499–500
growth regulators 70–71
herbicide 336–340*
influence of pesticides 577–578
minerals essential to 462–465
periodicity 505–506
reproductive 502–503
seed germination 554–556*
temperature adaptation 67–68
thermoperiodicity 507–508
tissue culture in plants 507
vegetative meristematic activity 500–502
Plant hormones 499, 508–509*
abscisic acid 49–51*
abscission 51–52*
auxin 121–124*
brassin 145–146*
chemical classification 509
commercial uses 509
cytokinins 208–210*
flowering hormone 444
growth factors 499
physiological classification 507–508
Plant physiology 509–510
abscission 51–52*
ecology, physiological (plant) 222–224*
minerals essential to 462–465
photorespiration 444–448*
Plant regulator 508–509
Plant Quarantine Act 496
Plant translocation of organic solutes 510–513*
channels of nitrogen compounds 511

Plant translocation of organic solutes—*cont.*
import and export by leaves 511
importance of conductive tissues 510–512
mass-flow theory 512
mechanism of translocation 512–513
plant disease control 512
requirements for organic nutrients 512
sugar transport in phloem 510–511
xylem sap 511
Plant virus 513–516*
dissemination by insects 489
dissemination by man 490
establishment in the host 485–486
inoculum in plants 484–485
isolation 516
morphology 515
plant disease 476–491*
replication 516
symptoms of disease 514
transmission 514–515
Plantains 125
Plantation agriculture 58–59
Planting: broadcasters 79
drills 79
planters 79
row-crop planters 79
Plasmodiophora brassicae 158, 489, 490
Plasmopara halstedii 644
Plasmopara viticola 331
Plastic packaging material 284
Plasticizing (food preparation) 279
Pliofilm (packaging plastic) 284
Plowing 77–78
moldboard plow 77–78
disk plow 78
Plum 516–517*
diseases 517
production and economic importance 517
propagation and culture 517
types and varieties 516–517
Plum pockets (fungus disease) 517
Pneumatic malting 129
Poa compressa 145
Poa pratensis 145, 202, 333
Pod blight (soybean) 618
Pod corn 197
Podosphaera leucotricha 317
Poi 214
Polished rice 542–543
Pollution, atmospheric 118–121, 140, 479
Polyester packaging material 284
Polyethylene packaging material 284
Polymnia sonchifolia 544
Polypeptide: protein 527–532*
Polyporus 195
Polypropylene packaging material 284
Polysaccharide 161, 517–518*
carbohydrate metabolism 168–170*

Polysaccharide—*cont.*
dietary fiber 497
glycogen 327–328*
gum 334–336*
yeast sources 685
Polyspora lini 248
Polystyrene packaging material 284
Popcorn 197
Poppy seed 624
Population growth: decrease in growth rate 5–6
food supply 2
per capita wealth and growth rates 2–3
Pork fat 232
Porphyrin (deficiency) 377
Port wine 676
Postemergence herbicide 336–337
Pot barley 129
Potash (fertilizer) 238–239
Potassium: fertilizer 234
role in plant growth 463
utilization by soil microorganisms 612
Potassium chloride (potash) 238–239
Potato, Irish 518–520*, 544
constituents 519
consumption 518–519
diseases 519
production 518
varieties 518
Potato, sweet 520–522*, 544
breeding 520
diseases 521–522
processing 520–521
true yam 521
types 520
Potato blight (weather factors in control) 62
Potato harvester 81
Potato leafhopper (peanut) 430
Poultry (dressing) 268–269
Poultry production 522–526*
breeding 526
broiler production 522
brooding and rearing 523
economics of 526
egg production 522–523
feeding 523
housing 524–526
incubation 523
marketing 526
poultry health 526
products 254, 303–304
Powdery mildew: barley 129
grape 331–332
pea 428
raspberries and blackberries 537
strawberry 633
Pratylenchus brachyrus 431
Precipitation (protein preparation) 529
Preemergence herbicide 336–337
Preservatives, food 256
Preserves (fruit) 301
Pressure filter 268
vertical leaf 267
Priestley, J. 448
Primary packaging 282, 286–288

Process cheese 182, 184–185
Process control (food industry) 263–266
control center 264–265
control loop 263
new equipment 265–266
new techniques 263–264
system implementation 263
Processed food 254
Procyazine 339
Profluralin 339
Proline 107, 526–527*
Prolinemia 527
Prometryn 339
Pronamide 339
Propachlor 339
Propanil 339
Propazine 339
Propham 339
Propionibacterium freudenreicheii 665
Propionibacterium shermanii 183
Proso millet 405
Protein 251, 527–532*
albumin 88–89*
amino acid conjugation 102–103
amino acids 96–109*
analysis 530
animal-feed composition 64, 110
basic food requirements 3
biosynthesis 532
casein 170–171*
daily dietary allowances 252
deficiency 377
effects of injury to cell protein 386
eggs 225
food analogs 306–309
formation of abnormal proteins 387
functions 385
gelatin 321–323*
glutelin 327*
metabolism *see* Protein metabolism
occurrence 527–528
preparation 528–530
properties 531–532
soybean 621–623
specificity 528
structure 530–531
synthesis 385
vegetable 306–309, 619–623
Protein-calorie malnutrition 357
Protein metabolism 532–534*
digestion of protein 533–534
metabolic disorders 385–388
nutritive value of proteins 533
plasma protein synthesis 534
protein digestion in intestine 533
protein in feces formation 533–534
proteins in health and disease 532–533
role in diet 532–533
small intestine 217
tissue protein synthesis 534
utilization of absorbed amino acids 534
Proteus 156